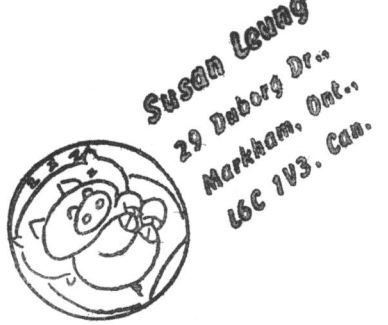

精選英漢醫學詞典

Concise Medical English-Chinese Dictionary

精選英漢醫學詞典

Concise Medical English-Chinese Dictionary

牛津大學出版社
Oxford University Press

Oxford University Press

Oxford New York
Athens Auckland Bangkok Bombay
Calcutta Cape Town Dar es Salaam Delhi
Florence Hong Kong Istanbul Karachi
Kuala Lumpur Madras Madrid Melbourne
Mexico City Nairobi Paris Singapore
Taipei Tokyo Toronto

and associated companies in

Berlin Ibadan
Oxford is a trade mark of Oxford University Press

First published 1990
This impression (Lowest digit)
3 5 7 9 10 8 6 4

English text originally published as *Concise Medical Dictionary*
by Oxford University Press in 1980. Second edition 1985.

ISBN 0 19 584912 4

Printed in Hong Kong
Published by Oxford University Press (China) Ltd.
18/F Warwick House, Taikoo Place, 979 King's Road, Quarry Bay, Hong Kong

前　　言

《精選英漢醫學詞典》根據牛津大學出版社編纂的最新英文版本編譯而成，收錄詞目達一萬多個，現今通行的重要醫學詞彙及概念在此一覽無遺。本詞典的作者爲著名醫科專家和學者，其首要對象爲醫療輔助人士，包括護士、藥劑師、物理治療師、語言治療師、社會工作者、醫院管理人員、行政人員、醫療技術員等；而對醫科學生及臨牀醫生來説，也是非常有用的案頭參考書籍。本詞典所列各條詞目除提供基本定義之外，更視乎需要加入較詳細的解説。在語言方面，本書特點是用字清楚、簡潔，絶無隱晦難懂的術語，完全符合普遍讀者的要求。因此，無論從趣味性或實用價值來看，本詞典均是家居必備的醫學參考書籍。

本詞典涉及的範圍包括解剖學、生理學、生化學、藥理學及其他主要的內、外科目；有關心理學、精神病學、社會醫學及口腔科等的較新詞彙亦包羅其中。而爲了容納這些學科的新增詞目及反映現代醫學的成果，常見於大型辭典中含糊或過時的詞目，均已刪除。這些詞目的含義，根據其綴語及接語也不難理解，且多數有關詞素在本書中已有收錄。編排方面，爲了避免詞類雜亂，派生詞（例如由各詞派生的形容詞）一律列於母詞定義之後。若干詞目並按需要附加插圖及説明。英文部分的解釋中標有「*」符號者，爲本詞典的另一獨立詞目，讀者可作進一步查閲。另有一些詞目不附解釋，而只指示讀者轉查其他詞目，這表示該詞或是與另一詞目同義，或可與另一詞目合併以作更妥善的解釋。至於一般同義詞則列於詞目後的括弧內。

A

a- (an-) *prefix denoting* absence of; lacking; not. Examples: *amastia* (absence of breasts); *amorphic* (lacking definite form); *atoxic* (not poisonous).

〔前綴〕**無，缺，不** 例如：無乳房，無定形，無毒。

ab- *prefix denoting* away from. Example: *abembryonic* (away from or opposite the embryo).

〔前綴〕**從…離** 例：胚外的，離胚的。

abarticulation *n.* **1.** the dislocation of a joint. **2.** a synovial joint (*see* diarthrosis).

①關節脫位 ②滑囊關節

abasia *n.* an inability to walk for which no physical cause can be identified. *See also* astasia.

步行不能 不能查出軀體性病因的行走能力喪失。

abdomen *n.* the part of the body cavity below the chest (*see* thorax), from which it is separated by the *diaphragm. The abdomen contains the organs of digestion – stomach, liver, intestines, etc. – and excretion – kidneys, bladder, etc.; in women it also contains the ovaries and womb. The regions of the abdomen are shown in the illustration. —**abdominal** *adj.*

腹 胸部下方的體腔。胸、腹之間以膈肌分開。腹內有消化器官胃、肝、腸等；排泄器官腎、膀胱等；婦女則有卵巢、子宮（見圖）。

abdomin- (abdomino-) *combining form denoting* the abdomen. Examples: *abdominalgia* (pain in the abdomen); *abdominothoracic* (relating to the abdomen and thorax).

〔詞幹〕**腹** 例如：腹痛，腹胸的。

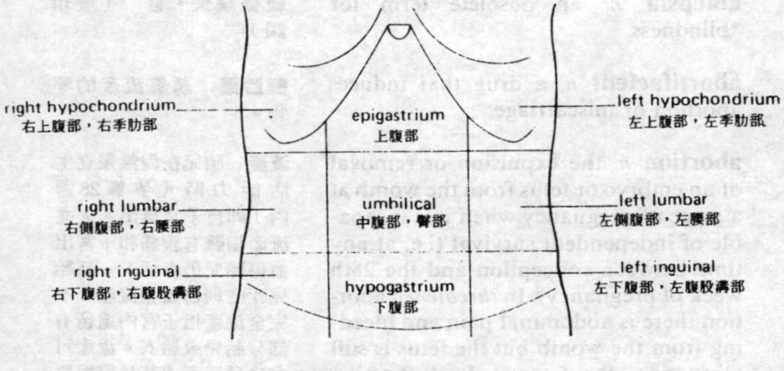

Regions of the abdomen
腹部分區圖

abdominoscopy *n. see* laparoscopy.

腹腔鏡檢法

abducens nerve the sixth *cranial nerve (VI), which supplies the lateral rectus muscle of each eyeball, responsible for turning the eye outwards.

展神經 第六對顱神經，控制兩眼外直肌，司眼球外展。

abduct *vb.* to move a limb or any other part away from the midline of the body. —**abduction** *n.*

外展 肢體或人體任何部分自人體中線向外運動。

abductor *n.* any muscle that moves one part of the body away from another or from the midline of the body.

外展肌 可使人體的一部分移離另一部分，或移離人體中線的肌肉。

aberrant *adj.* abnormal: usually applied to a blood vessel or nerve that does not follow its normal course.

異常的，迷行的 常用於描述走行異常的血管或神經。

abiotrophy *n.* degeneration or loss of function without apparent cause; for example, *retinal abiotrophy* is progressive degeneration of the retina leading to impaired vision, occurring in genetic disorders such as *retinitis pigmentosa.

生活力缺乏 無明顯原因的退化或功能缺失。例如：視網膜生活力缺失病，爲視網膜進行性退化引起，可導致視力損害，見於遺傳性疾患，如色素性視網膜炎。

ablatio *n. see* abruptio, detached retina (ablatio retinae).

剝離 如視網膜剝離。

ablation *n.* the removal of tissue, a part of the body, or an abnormal growth, usually by cutting.

部分切除術 去除人體上的部分組織或腫物，常藉切除術。

ablepharia *n.* absence of or reduction in the size of the eyelids.

無瞼 眼瞼缺失或縮小。

ablepsia *n.* an obsolete term for *blindness.

視覺缺失，盲 （廢用詞）

abortifacient *n.* a drug that induces abortion or miscarriage.

墮胎藥 誘導流產的藥物。

abortion *n.* the expulsion or removal of an embryo or fetus from the womb at a stage of pregnancy when it is incapable of independent survival (i.e. at any time between conception and the 28th week of pregnancy). In *threatened* abortion there is abdominal pain and bleeding from the womb but the fetus is still alive; once the fetus is dead abortion

流產 胎兒在尚無獨立生活能力時（孕娠28週內）即自子宮排出。先兆流產指雖有腹痛和子宮出血但胎兒仍存活。一旦胎兒死亡則爲難免流產。不完全流產指子宮內遺留有部分胎兒或胎衣。流產可有自發流產或基於醫學原

becomes *inevitable*. It is *incomplete* so long as the womb still contains some of the fetus or its membranes. Abortion may be *spontaneous* (a miscarriage) or it may be *induced* for medical or social reasons (termination of pregnancy). The *abortion rate* (the number of pregnancies lost per 1000 conceptions) is impossible to calculate precisely but is generally reckoned to be between one fifth and one third.

因以及社會原因的人工流產。流產率（每千個受孕者當中流產人數）的精確計算有困難，一般估計為$\frac{1}{5}$～$\frac{1}{3}$。

Induction or attempted induction of abortion are both criminal offences in Britain unless carried out within the terms of the Abortion Act. Two doctors have to agree that termination of pregnancy is necessary and the operation must be performed in an approved hospital or clinic. Methods in current use include vacuum *aspiration of the products of conception through a thin cannula; *dilatation and curettage: opening the womb through an abdominal incision (hysterotomy); or the use of *prostaglandins or other drugs to induce premature labour. Termination carries little risk early in pregnancy, but complications are more likely after the 13th week.

在英國除非符合流產條例中的條款，人工流產或企圖人工流產均屬犯罪行為。必須有兩個醫生同意終止妊娠，並在指定的醫院或診所進行。當前使用的方法包括：以眞空細管吸出胎塊；擴宮刮取；子宮切開術；前列腺素或其他藥物引產。早期終止孕娠危險性很小，妊娠十三週後則有可能出現併發症。

abortus *n.* a fetus, weighing less than 500 g, that is expelled from the mother's body either dead or incapable of surviving.

流產胎　母體排出重量不足500克的死胎或不能存活的胎兒。

ABO system *see* blood group.

ABO系統

abrasion *n.* **1.** a graze: a minor wound in which the surface of the skin or a mucous membrane is worn away by rubbing or scraping. **2.** the wearing of the teeth, particularly at the necks by overvigorous brushing. **3.** any rubbing or scraping action that produces surface wear.

①**擦傷**　皮膚或黏膜表面經擦或刮所致的輕傷。
②**牙齒磨損**　尤指牙齒頸部因過度刷牙的損傷。
③造成表面損傷的任何一種擦或刮的動作。

abreaction *n.* the release of strong emotion associated with a buried memory. While this can happen spontaneously, it is usually deliberately pro-

精神疏泄　深藏於記憶中的強烈情感的發泄現象。可自發出現，但通常是醫生使用心理療法、催眠

duced by a therapist using psychotherapy, hypnosis, or drugs such as amphetamines or barbiturates. The technique is used as a treatment for hysteria, anxiety state, and other neurotic conditions, especially when they are thought to be caused by *repression of memories or emotions.

術，或苯丙胺、巴比妥類藥物，有意誘導其發生。本法用於治療癔病、焦慮狀態，以及其他神經性疾患，尤其是由於記憶或情感受到壓抑所致的疾患。

abruptio (ablatio) *n.* separation. In *abruptio placentae* (*ablatio placentae*) the placenta separates from the lining of the womb before the usual time. Bleeding and pain are experienced at the point of separation, and the womb undergoes constant contraction. Severe cases involve shock. The condition is often associated with high blood pressure or *pre-eclampsia. If the neck of the womb is firm and undilated, a live fetus may be delivered by *Caesarean section.

剝離 胎盤剝離指胎盤早期與子宮內膜分離，發生剝離時有出血、疼痛，子宮持續收縮。嚴重者可有休克。本病常併發於高血壓或先兆子癇患者。如子宮頸口緊閉，保存活胎需行剖腹。

abscess *n.* a localized collection of pus anywhere in the body, surrounded and walled off by damaged and inflamed tissues. A *boil is an example of an abscess within the skin. The usual cause is local bacterial infection, often by staphylococci, that the body's defences have failed to overcome. In a *cold abscess*, sometimes due to tubercle organisms, there is swelling, but little pain or inflammation (as in acute abscesses). Antibiotics, aided by surgical incision to release pus where necessary, are the usual forms of treatment.

膿腫 人體任何部位的局部膿液聚集，四周圍以受損和發炎組織。例如：癤爲皮膚膿腫。通常由局部細菌感染所致，多爲葡萄球菌，因人體抵抗力降低而侵入。冷膿腫有時由結核菌引起，有腫脹，但疼痛或炎症較輕（與急性膿腫比較）。通常用抗生素治療，並配合以在適當部位手術切開排膿。

abscission *n.* removal of tissue by cutting.

切除 以切除方法去除組織。

Absidia *n.* a genus of fungi that sometimes cause disease in man (*see* phycomycosis).

犁頭黴屬 一屬黴菌，有時可使人致病。

absorption *n.* (in physiology) the uptake of fluids or other substances by the tissues of the body. Digested food is absorbed into the blood and lymph from the alimentary canal. Most absorption of food occurs in the small

吸收 （生理學）指人體組織吸收液體及其他物質的過程。消化道將已消化的食物吸收入血液及淋巴。食物吸收主要在小腸——即十二指腸和迴

intestine – in the jejunum and ileum – although alcohol is readily absorbed from the stomach. The small intestine is lined with minute finger-like processes (*see* villus), which greatly increase its surface area and therefore the speed at which absorption can take place. *See also* assimilation, digestion.

腸，酒精則立即被胃吸收。小腸內襯有微小指狀突起（絨毛），藉此加大吸收面積，從而迅速吸收。

abulia *n.* absence or impairment of will power. The individual still has desires but they are not put into action; initiative and energy are lacking. It is commonly a symptom of *schizophrenia.

意志缺失 無意志或意志薄弱。患者有種種願望但無行動，缺乏主動性和能量。常爲精神分裂症的症狀。

acalculia *n.* an acquired inability to make simple mathematical calculations. It is a symptom of disease in the *parietal lobe of the brain. *See* Gerstmann's syndrome.

計算不能 生後喪失做簡單數學計算的能力。爲大腦頂葉疾病的一種症狀。

acantha *n.* **1.** a spine projecting from a *vertebra. **2.** the *backbone.

①**棘** 脊椎的棘突。
②**脊柱**

acanthion *n.* the tip of the spine formed where projecting processes of the upper jaw bones (maxillae) meet at the front of the face.

前鼻棘點 兩側上頜骨的前鼻棘在臉的前面相會形成的突起尖端。

acanthosis *n.* generalized thickening of the innermost (prickle-cell) layer of the *epidermis, with abnormal multiplication and increase in the number of cells. In *acanthosis nigricans* dark warty growths occur, especially in skin folds such as the groin, armpits, and mouth. It is usually a sign of internal cancer.

棘皮症 表皮最深層的棘狀細胞層普遍增厚，伴以異常增殖和細胞數目增加。黑棘皮症出現深色疣狀物，尤以皮膚皺褶處爲最，如腹股溝、腋下和口部，這一體徵通常表示體內有癌症。

acapnia *n.* a condition in which there is an abnormally low concentration of carbon dioxide in the blood. This may be caused by breathing that is exceptionally deep in relation to the physical activity of the individual.

缺碳酸血症 血液內二氧化碳濃度過低。與個體體力活動引起的呼吸過度有關。

acariasis *n.* an infestation of mites and ticks and the symptoms, for example allergy and dermatitis, that their presence may provoke.

蟎病 受蟎和蜱侵擾並出現症狀，如變態反應和皮炎。

acaricide *n.* any chemical agent used for destroying mites and ticks.

殺蟎藥 殺滅蟎和蜱的各種化學製劑。

acarid *n.* a *mite or *tick.

蟎蜱 蟎或蜱。

Acarina *n.* the group of arthropods that includes the *mites and *ticks.

蜱蟎類 包括蟎和蜱的一類節肢動物。

Acarus (Tyroglyphus) *n.* a genus of mites. The flour mite, *A. siro* (*T. farinae*), is nonparasitic, but its presence in flour can cause a severe allergic dermatitis in flour-mill workers.

蟎屬 蟎的一屬。粉蟎係非寄生性蟎，但在麵粉中有粉蟎時可引起磨粉工人嚴重的變態反應性皮炎。

acatalasia *n.* an inborn lack of the enzyme *catalase, leading to recurrent infections of the gums (gingivitis) and mouth. It is most common in the Japanese.

缺過氧化氫酶病 先天性缺乏過氧化氫酶，可引起齒齦（齒齦炎）和口腔黏膜的反復感染。在日本最爲多見。

acceptor *n.* (in biochemistry) a substance that helps to bring about oxidation of a reduced *substrate by accepting hydrogen ions.

受體 （生物化學）通過接受氫離子以促使還原底物的氧化的一種物質。

accessory nerve (spinal accessory nerve) the eleventh *cranial nerve (XI), which arises from two roots, cranial and spinal. Fibres from the cranial root travel with the nerve for only a short distance before branching to join the vagus and then forming the recurrent laryngeal nerve, which supplies the internal laryngeal muscles. Fibres from the spinal root supply the sternomastoid and trapezius muscles, in the neck region (front and back).

副神經 第十一對腦神經。發自兩個神經根，即顱根和脊根。顱根中的副神經纖維行進很短一段距離即分支與迷走神經會合形成喉返神經，支配內部喉肌。脊根纖維在頸部（前部和後部）支配胸鎖乳突肌和斜方肌。

accommodation *n.* adjustment of the shape of the lens to change the focus of the eye. When the ciliary muscle (*see* ciliary body) is relaxed, suspensory ligaments attached to the ciliary body and holding the lens in position are stretched, which causes the lens to be flattened. The eye is then able to focus on distant objects. To focus the eye on near objects the ciliary muscles contract and the tension in the ligaments is thus lowered, allowing the lens to become rounder.

調節 調整晶體的形狀以改變眼的焦距。當睫狀肌放鬆時，附着於睫狀體上的懸韌帶（能保持晶體的位置）變緊張，致使晶體變扁。於是眼睛能對遠距離目標聚焦。眼睛對近物聚焦時，睫狀肌收縮，懸韌帶鬆弛，使晶體變圓。

accommodation reaction (convergence reaction) the constriction of the pupil that occurs when an individual focuses on a near object.

調節反應（會聚反應） 個體的兩眼對近物聚焦時瞳孔縮小。

accouchement *n.* delivery of a baby.

分娩 產出嬰兒。

acentric *n.* (in genetics) a chromosome or fragment of a chromosome that has no *centromere. Since acentrics cannot attach to the *spindle they are usually lost during cell division. They are often found in cells damaged by radiation. —**acentric** *adj.*

無着絲粒染色體 （遺傳學）不具備着絲粒的染色體或其片段。由於這種染色體無法附着紡錘體因而在細胞分裂時往往丟失。常見於受放射線損害的細胞。

acephalus *n.* a fetus without a head.

無頭畸胎 無頭胎兒。

acervulus cerebri a collection of granules of calcium-containing material that is sometimes found within the *pineal body as its calcification proceeds (normally after the 17th year): 'brain sand'.

松果體石 有時在松果體內可找到的含鈣粒狀聚集物。爲松果體鈣化的結果（通常在 17 歲後），又稱腦沙。

acetabulum (cotyloid cavity) *n.* either of the two deep sockets, one on each side of the *hip bone, into which the head of the thigh bone (femur) fits.

髖臼（髖臼腔） 髖骨兩側各一的深窩，股骨頭在其中固定。

acetanilide *n.* a drug that relieves pain and reduces fever. Since it can cause haemolytic anaemia and prolonged use may lead to *habituation, it has largely been replaced by safer analgesics.

乙醯苯胺 一種鎮痛退熱藥。自從發現本藥可致溶血性貧血並長期服用可成癮後，已很大程度爲安全的鎮痛藥所代替。

acetarsol *n.* an arsenic-containing drug administered by mouth for the treatment of amoebic dysentery, yaws, and *Vincent's angina; as vaginal tablets for vaginitis; and as a rectal *suppository for *proctitis. Possible side-effects include skin rashes (after oral administration) and local irritation (with vaginal tablets).

乙醯胂胺 一種含砷的藥物，口服可治阿米巴痢疾、雅司病、奮森氏咽峽炎；陰道片可治陰道炎；直腸栓劑可治直腸炎。可能出現的副作用有皮疹（口服後）和局部刺激（用陰道片）。

acetazolamide *n.* a *diuretic used in the treatment of glaucoma to reduce the pressure inside the eyeball. Side-effects include drowsiness and numbness and tingling of the hands and feet. Trade names: **Acetazide**, **Diamox**.

乙醯唑胺 一種利尿藥，用於治療青光眼，以降低眼球內壓。副作用有困倦、手足麻木及麻刺感。

acetoacetic acid an organic acid produced in large amounts by the liver under metabolic conditions associated with a high rate of fatty acid oxidation (for example, in starvation). The acetoacetic acid thus formed is subse-

乙醯乙酸 一種有機酸，在伴有脂肪酸高速氧化的代謝異常狀態下（例如：饑餓）由肝臟大量產生。乙醯乙酸進而轉化爲丙酮並排出體外。

quently converted to acetone and excreted. *See also* ketone.

acetohexamide *n.* a drug that reduces the level of blood sugar, used in the treatment of *diabetes mellitus. It is administered by mouth; side-effects include headache, dizziness, and nervousness. *See also* tolbutamide, chlorpropamide.

醋磺環己脲 降血糖藥，用於治療糖尿病。口服；副作用有頭痛、頭暈、神經過敏。

acetone *n.* an organic compound that is an intermediate in many bacterial fermentations and is produced by fatty acid oxidation. In certain abnormal conditions (for example, starvation) acetone and other *ketones may accumulate in the blood (*see* ketosis). Acetone is a volatile liquid that is miscible with both fats and water and therefore of great value as a solvent. It is used in chromatography and in the preparation of tissues for enzyme extraction.

丙酮 一種有機化合物，爲細菌發酵的中間產物，亦爲脂肪酸氧化的產物。在某些異常的情況下（例如：饑餓），丙酮和其他酮體可在血中蓄積（見酮病）。丙酮爲揮發性液體，可與油脂或水混合，因而爲重要溶媒。本品用於層析法，以及在提取酶時處理組織標本。

acetone body (ketone body) *see* ketone.

丙酮體（酮體）

acetonuria *n. see* ketonuria.

丙酮尿

acetylcholine *n.* the acetic acid ester of the organic base choline: the *neurotransmitter released at the synapses of parasympathetic nerves and at *neuromuscular junctions. After relaying a nerve impulse, acetylcholine is rapidly broken down by the enzyme *cholinesterase. *Atropine and curare cause muscular paralysis by blocking the action of acetylcholine at muscle membranes; *physostigmine prolongs the activity of acetylcholine by blocking cholinesterase.

乙醯膽鹼 有機膽鹼的醋酸酯：由副交感神經突觸和神經肌肉接合處釋出的神經遞質。在傳遞神經衝動後，乙醯膽鹼受膽鹼酯酶作用迅速裂解。阿托品和箭毒可阻斷乙醯膽鹼對肌細胞膜的作用致使肌肉麻痹；毒扁豆鹼可阻斷膽鹼酯酶而延長乙醯膽鹼的作用。

acetylcysteine *n.* a drug used to break down thick mucous secretions. It is administered as an aerosol, primarily for the treatment of respiratory diseases, such as bronchitis, and cystic fibrosis. Side-effects may include spasm of the bronchial muscles, nausea, vomiting, and fever.

N-乙醯半胱氨酸，痰易淨 一種能稀釋黏稠分泌物的藥物。以氣霧劑投藥，主要用於治療呼吸道疾病，如支氣管炎、肺囊性纖維變。副作用有支氣管肌肉痙攣、噁心、嘔吐、發熱。

acetylsalicylic acid *see* aspirin.

乙醯水楊酸

achalasia (cardiospasm) *n.* a condition in which the normal muscular activity of the oesophagus (gullet) is disturbed, which delays the passage of swallowed material. It may occur at any age: symptoms include difficulty in swallowing liquids and solids, slowly increasing over years; sometimes regurgitation of undigested food; and occasionally severe chest pain caused by spasm of the oesophagus. Diagnosis is by a barium X-ray examination. Treatment is by forceful stretching of the tight lower end of the oesophagus (cardia) or by surgical splitting of the muscular ring in that area (*cardiomyotomy*).

弛緩不能（賁門痙攣） 由於食道肌正常活動紊亂以致吞嚥發生困難的病症。可發生於任何年齡：症狀包括吞下液體和固體食物困難，病情逐年緩慢增重；有時發生未消化的食物返流；間或因食道痙攣引起劇烈胸痛。診斷有賴鋇餐X線檢查。治療：對食道狹窄的下端（賁門）施行擴張術，或用手術切開此處的肌肉環（賁門肌切開術）。

Achilles tendon the tendon of the muscles of the calf of the leg (the *gastrocnemius and soleus muscles), situated at the back of the ankle and attached to the calcaneus (heel bone).

跟腱 小腿後部肌肉（腓腸肌與比目魚肌）的腱。位於踝後，附着於跟骨上。

achlorhydria *n.* absence of hydrochloric acid in the stomach. Achlorhydria that persists despite large doses of histamine is associated with atrophy of the lining (mucosa) of the stomach. In this condition there is usually an absence of secretion of *intrinsic factor, which will lead to *pernicious anaemia. In some people, however, achlorhydria is not associated with any disease, produces no ill-effects, and needs no treatment.

胃酸缺乏 胃內缺乏鹽酸。頑固的胃酸缺乏（雖投與大量組胺仍不分泌胃酸）常併發於胃黏膜萎縮。在這一情況下通常造血內因子不能分泌，因而導致惡性貧血。某些人胃酸缺乏並不伴發任何疾病，無不良作用，因而無需治療。

acholia *n.* absence or deficiency of bile secretion or failure of the bile to enter the alimentary canal (for example, because of an obstructed bile duct).

無膽汁症 膽汁不分泌或不足，或不能進入消化道（如膽管阻塞）。

acholuria *n.* absence of the *bile pigments from the urine, which occurs in some forms of jaundice (*acholuric jaundice*). —**acholuric** *adj.*

無膽色素尿 尿中缺乏膽色素，發生於某些類型的黃疸。

achondroplasia *n.* an inherited disorder in which the bones of the arms and legs fail to grow to normal size due

軟骨發育不全 因軟骨和骨的缺損致使四肢不能發育為正常大小的一種先天

to a defect in both cartilage and bone. It results in a type of *dwarfism characterized by short limbs, a normal-sized head and body, and normal intelligence. —**achondroplastic** *adj.*

性疾病。可形成一型侏儒，特點爲四肢短小，但頭顱、軀體及智力正常。

achromatic *adj.* without colour.

無色的

achromatic lenses lenses specially designed for use in the eyepieces of microscopes and other scientific instruments. They give clear images, unblurred by the coloured fringes that are produced with ordinary lenses (caused by splitting of the light into different wavelengths).

消色差透鏡 專門設計用於顯微鏡和其他科學儀器的目鏡鏡片，可顯出清晰圖像，沒有一般鏡片產生的模糊的彩色邊緣（色差係因光線分解爲不同的波長所致）。

achromatopsia *n.* the inability to perceive colour. Such complete *colour blindness is very rare and is usually associated with poor *visual acuity; it is usually determined by hereditary factors.

全色盲 無感色能力。全色盲十分稀少，常伴有視敏度弱。通常由遺傳因素決定。

achylia *n.* absence of secretion. The term is usually applied to a nonsecreting stomach (*achylia gastrica*) whose lining (mucosa) is atrophied (*see* achlorhydria).

分泌液缺乏 分泌功能喪失。本詞通常用於因黏膜萎縮所致的胃液缺乏。

acidaemia *n.* a condition of abnormally high blood acidity. This may result from an increase in the concentration of acidic substances and/or a decrease in the level of alkaline substances in the blood. *See also* acidosis. *Compare* alkalaemia.

酸血症 血液酸度異常增高的狀態。可因血內酸性物質濃度增高和/或鹼性物質濃度降低所致。

acid-base balance the balance between the amount of carbonic acid and bicarbonate in the blood, which must be maintained at a constant ratio of 1:20 in order to keep the hydrogen ion concentration of the plasma at a constant value (pH 7.4). Any alteration in this ratio will disturb the acid-base balance of the blood and tissues and cause either *acidosis or *alkalosis. The lungs and the kidneys play an important role in the regulation of the acid-base balance.

酸鹼平衡 血液中的碳酸氫鹽之間的量的平衡。二者必須保持 1:20 的恒定值（pH 7.4）。恒定比例任何變動均可破壞血液和組織中的酸鹼平衡，導致酸中毒或鹼中毒。肺和腎在調節酸鹼平衡中起重要作用。

acid-etch technique a technique for bonding resin-based restorative ma-

酸蝕法 使樹脂修復體與牙齒釉質黏合的一種方

terials to the enamel of teeth. A porous surface is created by applying phosphoric acid for approximately one minute.

法。應用磷酸約一分鐘可在牙齒造成多孔的表面。

acid-fast *adj.* **1.** describing bacteria that have been stained and continue to hold the stain after treatment with an acidic solution. For example, tuberculosis bacteria are acid-fast when stained with a *carbol fuchsin preparation. **2.** describing a stain that is not removed from a specimen by washing with an acidic solution.

耐酸性 ①形容經染色後再用酸性溶液處理時仍繼續保持其顏色的細菌。如結核菌經石炭酸品紅製劑染色呈耐酸性。 ②形容標本用酸性液冲洗仍不褪色的染劑。

acidophil (acidophilic) *adj.* **1.** (in histology) describing tissues, cells, or parts of cells that stain with acid dyes (such as eosin). **2.** (in bacteriology) describing bacteria that grow well in acid media.

嗜酸性 ①在組織學中形容能被酸性染料染色（如曙紅）的組織、細胞或細胞中的某些部位。 ②在細菌學中形容在酸性培養基上生長良好的細菌。

acidosis *n.* a condition in which the acidity of body fluids and tissues is abnormally high. This arises because of a failure of the mechanisms responsible for maintaining a balance between acids and alkalis in the blood (*see* acid-base balance). In *gaseous acidosis* more than the normal amount of carbon dioxide is retained in the body, as in drowning. In *renal acidosis*, kidney failure results in excessive loss of bicarbonate or retention of phosphoric and sulphuric acids. Patients with diabetes mellitus suffer from a form of acidosis in which sodium, potassium, and *ketone bodies are lost in the urine.

酸中毒 體液和組織中酸度異常升高的狀態。這種升高是由於保持血內酸鹼平衡的機制失控引起。在呼吸性酸中毒，人體內滯留的二氧化碳遠較正常人爲高，如見於溺斃者。在腎性酸中毒，腎功能衰竭可導致碳酸氫鹽喪失過多或磷酸和硫酸留滯。糖尿病患者含併酸血症時，尿中有鉀、鈉與酮體排出。

acinus *n.* (*pl.* **acini**) **1.** a small sac or cavity surrounded by the secretory cells of a gland. Some authorities regard the term as synonymous with *alveolus, but others distinguish an acinus by the possession of a narrow passage (lumen) leading from the sac. **2.** (in the lung) the tissue supplied with air by one terminal *bronchiole. *Emphysema is classified by the part of the acinus involved (i.e. *centriacinar*, *panacinar*, or *periacinar*). —**acinous** *adj.*

①**腺泡** 腺體內由分泌細胞圍成的囊或腔。有些學者認爲本詞與 alveolus 同義，亦有人用以專指帶有腺管的腺泡。 ②**肺泡** 與細支氣管末端相通連的含氧肺組織。肺氣腫即以累及的肺泡部位分類（如中心肺泡性肺氣腫、全肺泡性肺氣腫、周圍性肺氣腫）。

aclasis *n. see* diaphysial aclasis.

骨幹性續連症

acne *n.* a skin disorder in which the sebaceous glands become inflamed. The commonest variety, *acne vulgaris*, generally starts in adolescence and is caused by overactivity of the sebaceous glands. The sebum produced by the glands cannot escape because the hair follicles become blocked by a *keratin plug and a pustule forms, with fluid leaking into the surrounding tissue. The keratin plug turns black, forming the familiar blackhead. Acne vulgaris occurs mainly on the face, chest, and back; it is usually mild, disappearing in adulthood, but can be severe and chronic, causing infected cysts and scarring of the skin. The course of this condition may be helped by regular washing, the removal of blackheads, and sometimes the use of antibiotics. There are many other varieties of acne, some being caused by contact with chemical substances (such as tar). *See also* rosacea.

痤瘡 因皮脂腺發炎而產生的皮膚病。常見的一種是尋常痤瘡（普通粉刺），通常在青春期開始，由皮脂腺分泌過剩引起。產生的皮脂由於角質栓阻塞毛囊口而不能排出，形成小膿疱，並向周圍組織滲透。角質栓色變黑，形成常見的黑頭。尋常痤瘡主要發生於面、胸、背部，通常輕微，成年後即行消失。但亦可加重並成為慢性，形成感染性囊腫並在皮上結疤。定時洗滌、去除黑頭粉刺以及適時使用抗生素有助於改善病情。痤瘡種類很多，其中有些是因接觸化學物品（如焦油）所致。

aconite *n.* the dried roots of the herbaceous plant *Aconitum napellus* (monkshood or wolfbane), containing three *analgesic substances: *aconine*, *aconitine*, and *picraconitine*. Aconite was formerly used to prepare liniments for muscular pains and a tincture for toothache, but is regarded as too toxic for use today.

烏頭 草本植物歐烏頭的乾燥根，含有三種止痛物質：烏頭原鹼、烏頭鹼和苦烏頭鹼。過去常用烏頭製備肌肉止痛搽劑和牙痛水，目前認為其毒性過大。

acoustic *adj.* of or relating to sound or the sense of hearing.

聽的，聲學的 與聲或與聽覺有關的。

acoustic holography a technique of building up a three-dimensional picture of structures within the body using *ultrasound waves. Two separate sound sources cause ultrasound waves to be transmitted through and reflected from the organs being examined. The interference patterns produced on a liquid surface are illuminated by laser light and photographed to form a *hologram*.

超聲波全息照像術 利用超聲波產生體內結構三維圖像的技術。使兩個分離的聲源產生的超聲波穿透被檢器官並自其反射回來，由此在液面產生的干擾圖像經激光照射後攝影即取得全息照片。

acoustic nerve *see* vestibulocochlear nerve.

聽神經

acquired *adj.* describing a condition or disorder contracted after birth and not attributable to hereditary causes. *Compare* congenital.

獲得性，後天性 描述出生後獲得的某種狀態或病患，並非因遺傳所致。

acquired immunodeficiency syndrome *see* AIDS.

獲得性免疫缺陷綜合徵

acrania *n.* congenital absence of the skull, either partial or complete, due to a developmental defect.

無顱畸形 先天性頭顱缺乏，分部分缺或全缺兩種，由發育缺損所致。

acriflavine *n.* a dye used as an antiseptic on skin and mucous membranes and to disinfect contaminated wounds. It may cause sensitivity of the skin to sunlight.

吖啶黃 一種染料。用於皮膚和黏膜的滅菌和受污染傷口的消毒。可使皮膚對日光過敏。

acro- *prefix denoting* **1.** extremity; tip. Example: *acrohypothermy* (abnormal coldness of the extremities (hands and feet)). **2.** height; promontory. Example: *acrophobia* (morbid dread of heights). **3.** extreme; intense. Example: *acromania* (an extreme degree of mania).

〔前綴〕 ①**肢體，尖端** 例如：手足溫度過低（四肢肢端不正常寒冷）。②**高，隆突** 例如：高處恐怖（病態懼高）。③**極端的，重度（重症）的** 例如：重躁狂（極度躁狂）。

acrocentric *n.* a chromosome in which the *centromere is situated at or very near one end. —**acrocentric** *adj.*

具近端着絲粒的 着絲粒位於或接近一端的染色體。

acrocyanosis *n.* bluish-purple discoloration of the hands and feet due to slow circulation of the blood through the small vessels in the skin.

手足發紺 皮膚小血管循環慢以致手足呈青紫色。

acrodermatitis *n.* inflammation of the skin of the feet or hands. A diffuse chronic variety produces swelling and reddening of the affected areas, followed by atrophy. The cause is unknown and there is no treatment.

肢皮炎 手或足的皮膚炎症。慢性瀰散型肢皮炎可在感染部位發生紅腫，繼之以萎縮。病因不明，無有效療法。

acrodynia *n. see* pink disease.

肢痛病

acromegaly *n.* increase in size of the hands, feet, and the face due to excessive production of *growth hormone

肢端肥大症 垂體腫瘤引起生長激素（促生長素）過度產生所致的手、足、

(somatotrophin) by a tumour of the anterior pituitary gland. The tumour can be treated with X-rays or surgically removed. *See also* gigantism.

面部增大。腫瘤可用X線治療或手術切除。

acromion *n.* an oblong process at the top of the spine of the *scapula, part of which articulates with the clavicle (collar bone) to form the *acromioclavicular joint*. —**acromial** *adj.*

肩峯 肩峯頂端的卵圓形突起，部分與鎖骨連結形成肩鎖關節。

acroparaesthesiae *n.* a tingling sensation in the hands and feet.

肢端感覺異常 手和足有麻刺感。

acrosclerosis *n.* a skin disease thought to be a type of generalized *scleroderma. It also has features of *Raynaud's disease, with the hands, face, and feet being mainly affected.

肢端硬化症 一種皮膚病。可能是全身硬皮病的一型。亦具備雷諾氏病的特點，多發於手、面、足。

acrosome *n.* the caplike structure on the front end of a spermatozoon. It breaks down just before fertilization, releasing a number of enzymes that assist penetration between the follicle cells that still surround the ovum.

頂體 精子前端的帽狀結構。在即將受精前脫落，釋出一些酶以協助精子在包圍卵子的卵泡細胞之間穿過。

acrylic resin one of a group of polymeric materials used for making denture teeth, denture bases, and formerly as a dental filling material.

乙烯樹脂 聚合體材料的一種，用以製做托牙、牙基，過去用以補牙。

ACTH (adrenocorticotrophic hormone, adrenocorticotrophin, corticotrophin) a hormone synthesized and stored in the anterior pituitary gland, large amounts of which are released in response to any form of stress. ACTH controls the secretion of *corticosteroid hormones from the adrenal gland. It is administered by injection to test adrenal function and to treat conditions such as rheumatic diseases (especially in children) and asthma.

促腎上腺皮質激素 垂體前葉合成並存貯的激素。大部分在各種應激狀態時釋出。本激素控制腎上腺皮質類甾醇的分泌。注射用可測腎上腺功能，並用以治療某些病症，諸如風濕病（尤指兒童）和哮喘。

actin *n.* a protein, found in muscle, that plays an important role in the process of contraction. *See* striated muscle.

肌纖蛋白 見於肌肉的一種蛋白，在收縮時起重要作用。

Actinobacillus *n.* a genus of Gram-negative nonmotile aerobic bacteria that are characteristically spherical or rodlike in shape but occasionally grow

放線桿菌類 一屬革蘭氏陰性無運動的需氧細菌，呈球形或柱狀並偶爾長出分支菌絲。放線桿菌能在

into branching filaments. Actinobacilli cause disease in animals. The species *A. mallei* causes *glanders, an infection of horses that can be transmitted to man.

動物中致病。鼻疽放線桿菌可致馬鼻疽，且可傳染人。

Actinomyces *n.* a genus of Gram-positive nonmotile fungus-like bacteria that cause disease in animals and man. The species *A. israeli* is the causative organism of human *actinomycosis.

放線菌屬 一屬革蘭氏陽性無運動的眞菌樣細菌，可在人畜致病。衣氏放線菌爲人類放線菌病的病原體。

actinomycin *n.* a *cytotoxic drug, produced by *Streptomyces* bacteria, that inhibits the growth of cancer cells. There are two forms, both of which are administered by injection. Actinomycin C may damage bone marrow. Actinomycin D may cause nausea, vomiting, diarrhoea, blood disorders, and bone-marrow damage.

放線菌素 一種細胞毒製劑，產生於鏈黴菌，可抑制癌細胞生長。有兩型，均注射給藥。放線菌素 C 可損害骨髓。放線菌素 D 可致噁心、嘔吐、腹瀉、血液病以及骨髓損害。

actinomycosis *n.* a noncontagious disease caused by the bacterium *Actinomyces israeli*, which most commonly affects the jaw but may also affect the lungs, brain, or intestines. The bacterium is normally present in the mouth but it may become pathogenic following an *apical abscess or extraction of a tooth. It is characterized by multiple sinuses that open onto the skin. Treatment is by drainage of pus and a prolonged course of antibiotics.

放線菌病 由衣氏放線菌所致的非接觸性傳染病，最多發於頜，亦見於肺腦或小腸。此菌正常時可存在於口腔中，僅在出現根尖膿腫或拔牙後致病。其特點爲多數竇道開口於皮膚表面。治療：引流排膿並延長抗生素療程。

actinotherapy *n.* the treatment of disorders with *infrared or *ultraviolet radiation.

放射療法 用紅外或紫外射線治療疾病的方法。

action potential the change in voltage that occurs across the membrane of a nerve or muscle cell when a *nerve impulse is triggered. It is due to the passage of charged particles across the membrane (*see* depolarization) and is an observable manifestation of the passage of an impulse.

動作電位 當發生神經衝動時在神經細胞或肌細胞膜內外發生的電壓變化。這種由於帶電粒子通過細胞膜而產生的變化是衝動通過該處的可見表現。

active transport (in biochemistry) an energy-dependent process in which certain substances (including ions, some drugs, and amino acids) are able to cross cell membranes against a concentration gradient. The process is inhi-

主動轉運 在生物化學中，指某些物質（包括離子，某些藥劑，以及氨基酸）能夠逆濃度梯度穿過細胞膜的過程。這一過程需要消耗能量，並可因細

bited by substances that interfere with cellular metabolism (e.g. high doses of digitalis).

胞代謝干擾物質（例如高劑量毛地黃）而受抑。

actomyosin *n.* a protein complex formed in muscle between actin and myosin during the process of contraction. *See* striated muscle.

肌動球蛋白 肌肉收縮時在肌動蛋白和肌球蛋白之間形成的複合體。

acupuncture *n.* a traditional Chinese system of healing in which symptoms are relieved by thin metal needles inserted into selected points beneath the skin. The needles are stimulated either by rotation or, more recently, by an electric current. Recent hypotheses suggest that the needling activates deep sensory nerves, which cause the pituitary and midbrain to release *endorphins – the brain's natural pain-killers. Acupuncture is widely used in the Far East for the relief of pain and in China itself has become an alternative to anaesthesia for some major operations. Acupuncturists in the West may be medically qualified but many are not.

針療 一種中國傳統的醫療方法。以金屬細針刺入皮膚特定的穴位以解除症狀。針的刺激可用旋轉手法產生，近年又應用電針。現時的理論認爲用針作用於深部感覺神經可使垂體和中腦釋放內啡肽——腦的天然止痛劑。針刺在遠東廣泛應用於解痛，在發源地中國則開始在某些大手術中以其替代痲醉藥。針灸醫師在西方有的取得行醫資格，多數則否。

acute *adj.* **1.** describing a disease of rapid onset, severe symptoms, and brief duration. *Compare* chronic. **2.** describing any intense symptom, such as severe pain.

急性 ①描述一種起病快、症狀嚴重、持續時間不長的疾病。 ②描述任何一種嚴重的症狀，如劇痛。

acute abdomen an emergency surgical condition caused by damage to one or more abdominal organs following injury or disease. The patient is in severe pain and often in shock. Perforation of a peptic ulcer or a severely infected appendix, or rupture of the liver or spleen following a crushing injury, all produce an acute abdomen requiring urgent treatment.

急腹症 由外傷或疾病損害一個或更多的腹部器官所致的外科緊急狀態。患者劇痛並往往休克。消化道潰瘍穿孔或嚴重闌尾感染，或因外傷後的肝、脾破裂，均出現急腹症並需緊急處理。

acute rheumatism *see* rheumatic fever.

急性風濕病

acyclovir *n.* an antiviral drug that inhibits DNA synthesis in cells infected by *herpesviruses. Administered by mouth or intravenously, it is useful in patients whose immune systems are

無環鳥苷 一種抗病毒藥，可在感染疱疹病毒的細胞內抑制 DNA 合成。口服或靜脈注射。對免疫系統紊亂的患者有效，亦

disturbed and also possibly in the treatment of genital herpes and herpes encephalitis.

用以治療生殖系統疱疹以及疱疹性腦炎。

ad- *prefix denoting* towards or near. Examples: *adaxial* (towards the main axis); *adoral* (towards or near the mouth).

〔前綴〕**向，接近** 例如：向軸的（向主軸），向口的（向口或接近口）。

adamantinoma *n.* an obsolete term for an *ameloblastoma.

釉質上皮瘤 廢詞，現用成釉〔質〕細胞瘤。

Adam's apple (laryngeal prominence) a projection, lying just under the skin, of the thyroid cartilage of the *larynx.

亞當蘋果（喉結） 喉部皮膚下甲狀軟骨的突起部位。

Adams-Stokes syndrome *see* Stokes-Adams syndrome.

亞－斯二氏綜合徵

adaptation *n.* the phenomenon in which a sense organ shows a gradually diminishing response to continuous or repetitive stimulation. The nose, for example, may become adapted to the stimulus of an odour that is continuously present so that in time it ceases to report its presence. Similarly, the adaptation of touch receptors in the skin means that the presence of clothes can be forgotten a few minutes after they have been put on.

適應 一種器官對持續或重複刺激逐漸降低反應的現象。例如：鼻子開始適應持續的臭味時就不感其臭。同理，皮膚觸覺的適應意味着穿衣後幾分鐘就感覺不到身上有衣服。

addiction *n.* a state of *dependence produced by the habitual taking of any of certain drugs. Strictly speaking, the term implies the state of physical dependence induced by such drugs as morphine, heroin, and alcohol, but it is also used for the state of psychological dependence, produced by drugs such as barbiturates. Treatment is aimed at gradual withdrawal of the drug and eventually total abstention. *See also* alcoholism, tolerance.

癮，癖 習慣攝入某種藥物而產生的一種依賴狀態。嚴格地說，本詞的含意是對嗎啡、海洛因和酒精等產生的肉體上的依賴，但亦用於對巴比妥酸鹽等藥物引起的精神上的依賴。治療：應力爭逐漸撤藥直到最後戒除。

Addison's disease a syndrome due to inadequate secretion of corticosteroid hormones by the *adrenal glands, sometimes as a result of tuberculous infection. Symptoms include weakness, loss of energy, low blood pressure, and

阿狄森氏病 因腎上腺分泌皮質甾類激素不足所致的一種綜合徵，有時是結核感染的結果。症狀包括虛弱、無力、低血壓、皮膚上有黑色素沉着。過去

dark pigmentation of the skin. Formerly fatal, the disease is now curable by replacement hormone therapy.

難免一死，當今用激素代替療法已可治癒。

adduct *vb.* to move a limb or any other part towards the midline of the body. —**adduction** *n.*

收，內收 肢體或任何部位向人體中線活動。

adductor *n.* any muscle that moves one part of the body towards another or towards the midline of the body.

收肌，內收肌 使人體的一部分向其他部位或向人體中線活動的肌肉。

aden- (adeno-) *prefix denoting* a gland or glands. Examples: *adenalgia* (pain in); *adenogenesis* (development of); *adenopathy* (disease of).

〔前綴〕**腺** 例如：腺痛，腺發生，腺病。

adenine *n.* one of the nitrogen-containing bases (*see* purine) that occurs in the nucleic acids DNA and RNA. *See also* ATP.

腺嘌呤 存在於核酸 DNA 和 RNA 中的含氮鹼類之一。

adenine arabinoside a compound with antiviral activity, particularly against *herpesviruses. It is also active against tumours but its clinical use is restricted by its toxicity.

阿拉伯糖腺嘌呤 一種有抗病毒活性的化合物。尤以對疱疹病毒有效。亦有抗腫瘤作用，但因具毒性，在臨床應用受限。

adenitis *n.* inflammation of a gland or group of glands. For example, *mesenteric adenitis* affects the lymph glands (nodes) in the membranous support of the intestines (the mesentery); *cervical adenitis* affects the lymph glands in the neck.

腺炎 單個或多個腺體發炎。例如：腸繫膜腺炎即支持小腸的膜（腸繫膜）中的淋巴腺（結）受到感染，頸腺炎即頸部淋巴腺感染。

adenocarcinoma *n.* a malignant epithelial tumour arising from the glandular structures, which are constituent parts of most organs of the body. The term is also applied to tumours showing a glandular growth pattern. These tumours may be subclassified according to the substances that they produce, for example *mucus-secreting* and *serous adenocarcinomas*, or to the microscopical arrangement of their cells into patterns, for example *papillary* and *follicular adenocarcinomas*. They may be solid or cystic (*cystadenocarcinomas*). Each organ may produce tumours showing a variety of histological types: for example, the ovary may

腺癌 自腺體組織產生的惡性上皮腫瘤。腺體組織是人體多數器官的構成部分。本詞亦用於呈腺體樣增生型的腫瘤。腺癌依據其產生的物質分類，如：黏液分泌型腺癌和漿液腺癌；或以鏡下細胞排列形狀分型，如乳突狀腺癌、濾泡狀腺癌。腺癌可爲實質性的或囊狀的（囊狀腺癌）。每一種器官產生的腫瘤可呈不同組織型；例如：卵巢既可產生黏液型囊腺癌，又可產生漿液型囊腺癌。

produce both mucinous and serous cystadenocarcinomas.

adenohypophysis *n.* the anterior lobe of the *pituitary gland.

腺性垂體 垂體前葉。

adenoidectomy *n.* surgical removal of the *adenoids, commonly combined with tonsillectomy in a child who suffers recurrent sore throats and difficulty in breathing through the nose.

增殖腺切除術 手術切除腺樣增殖體。在患有復發性咽峽炎且經鼻呼吸困難的兒童做扁桃體切除術時結合進行。

adenoids (pharyngeal tonsils) *n.* the collection of lymphatic tissue at the rear of the nose. Enlargement of the adenoids from recurrent throat infections may cause obstruction to breathing through the nose (*see* adenoidectomy).

腺樣增殖體（咽扁桃體） 鼻腔後部成團的淋巴組織。腺樣體增大是由於咽部反復感染，可阻塞鼻呼吸（見增殖腺切除術）。

adenoma *n.* a benign tumour of epithelial origin that is derived from glandular tissue or exhibits clearly defined glandular structures. Adenomas may become malignant (*see* adenocarcinoma). Some show recognizable tissue elements, such as fibrous tissue (*fibroadenomas*), while others, such as bronchial adenomas, produce active compounds giving rise to clinical syndromes (*see* argentaffinoma). Tumours in certain organs, including the pituitary gland, are often classified by their histological staining affinities, for example *eosinophil*, *basophil*, and *chromophobe adenomas*.

腺瘤 由腺組織發生的或呈現清楚腺狀結構的上皮良性腫瘤。腺瘤可轉爲惡性（見腺癌）。有些具有可以辨認的組織成分，如纖維組織（纖維腺瘤）；有些（如支氣管腺瘤）可產生活性化合物引起症狀（見嗜銀細胞瘤）。某些器官（包括垂體）的腫瘤，通常以組織染色的親合性來分類，如嗜曙紅、嗜鹼、嫌色腺瘤等。

adenosine *n.* a compound containing adenine and the sugar ribose: it occurs in ATP. *See also* nucleoside.

腺苷 一種含有腺嘌呤和核糖的化合物，出現於ATP中。

adenosine diphosphate *see* ADP.

二磷酸腺苷

adenosine monophosphate *see* AMP.

一磷酸腺苷

adenosine triphosphate *see* ATP.

三磷酸腺苷

adenosis *n.* (*pl.* **adenoses**) **1.** excessive growth or development of glands. **2.** any disease of a gland, especially of a lymph gland (node).

腺病 ①腺體過度增長或發育。 ②任何一種腺病，尤指淋巴腺（結）。

adenovirus *n.* one of a group of DNA-containing viruses causing latent infections of the upper respiratory tract that

腺病毒 一類含有DNA的病毒，可致輕微的上呼吸道感染，症狀類似感冒。

produce symptoms resembling those of the common cold.

①**黏連** 正常狀態下互相分隔的兩個面結合在一起，如關節活動面因局部炎症或受損後纖維結締組織增生而黏連（纖維組織本身亦稱黏連組織）。腹部手術後可發生腸襻間的黏連，可能阻塞消化道。一旦心包發生黏連，心動將受到限制。②**癒合** 傷口邊緣連接在一起的癒合過程。一期癒合幾乎沒有肉芽，二期癒合則創緣以肉芽連合在一起。

adhesion *n.* **1.** the union of two normally separate surfaces, such as the moving surfaces of joints, by fibrous connective tissue developing in an inflamed or damaged region. (The fibrous tissue itself is also called an adhesion.) Adhesion between loops of intestine may occur following abdominal surgery, possibly obstructing the alimentary canal. If the pericardial sac is affected by adhesion, the movements of the heart may be restricted. **2.** a healing process in which the edges of a wound fit together. In *primary adhesion* there is very little *granulation tissue; in *secondary adhesion* the two edges are joined together by granulation tissue.

adiadochokinesis *n. see* dysdiadochokinesis.

輪替運動障礙

Adie's syndrome (Holmes-Adie syndrome) an abnormality of the pupils of the eyes, often affecting only one eye. At rest the affected pupil is larger than the normal one; it reacts slowly to light and the response on convergence of the eyes is also slow. Eventually the affected pupil will constrict much more completely than its fellow. One or more tendon reflexes may be absent. The condition is almost entirely restricted to women.

艾迪氏綜合徵（霍-艾二氏綜合徵） 一種瞳孔異常，常影響單眼。休息時病側瞳孔大於正常；對光反應與會聚反應皆遲緩。偶爾受累瞳孔較另側者收縮更爲完好。一種或多種的腱反射可能消失。患者幾乎全爲婦女。

adipocere *n.* a waxlike substance, consisting mainly of fatty acids, into which the soft tissues of the body can be converted after death. This usually occurs when the body is buried in damp earth or is submerged in water. Adipocere delays post-mortem decomposition and is a spontaneous form of preservation without mummification.

屍蠟 一種主要由脂肪酸組成的蠟樣物質。死後屍體軟組織可轉變成此種物質。通常發生在葬於濕地或溺水的屍體。屍蠟可延遲屍體腐敗，是除木乃伊之外的天然的屍體保存形式。

adipose tissue fibrous *connective tissue packed with masses of fat cells. It forms a thick layer under the skin and occurs around the kidneys and in the buttocks. It serves both as an insulating

脂肪組織 充滿脂肪細胞的纖維結締組織。在皮下形成厚層，在腎臟周圍和臀部大量存在。脂肪組織既屬隔熱層又有貯藏能量

layer and an energy store; food in excess of requirements is converted into fats and stored within these cells.

的作用，食物攝入過多則轉變爲脂肪存入這種細胞內。

adiposis (liposis) *n.* the presence of abnormally large accumulations of fat in the body. The condition may arise from overeating, hormone irregularities, or a metabolic disorder. In *adiposis dolorosa*, a condition affecting women more commonly than men, painful fatty swellings are associated with defects in the nervous system. *See also* obesity.

肥胖病 人體存在大量積聚的脂肪。可因過度攝食、激素分泌紊亂或代謝失常引起。痛性肥胖病（婦女患者一般較男性爲多）常併發於神經系統疾患。

aditus *n.* an anatomical opening or passage; for example, the opening of the tympanic cavity (middle ear) to the air spaces of the mastoid process.

入口，口 解剖學上的入口或通道；例如：鼓室腔（中耳）通向乳突氣腔的開口。

adjuvant *n.* any substance used in conjunction with another to enhance its activity. Aluminium salts are used as adjuvants in the preparation of vaccines from the toxins of diphtheria and tetanus: by keeping the toxins in precipitated form, the salts increase the efficacy of the toxins as antigens.

佐劑 與其他藥物結合使用以增加其性能的任何物質。鋁鹽在製備白喉和破傷風毒素疫苗時用作佐劑；鋁鹽可使毒素保持沉澱狀，藉以增加毒素的抗原作用。

adnexa *pl. n.* adjoining parts. For example, the *uterine adnexa* are the Fallopian tubes and ovaries (which adjoin the womb).

附件 毗鄰部分。例如：子宮附件爲輸卵管和卵巢（毗鄰子宮）。

ADP (adenosine diphosphate) a compound containing adenine, ribose, and two phosphate groups. ADP occurs in cells and is involved in processes requiring the transfer of energy (*see* ATP).

二磷酸腺苷 含腺嘌呤、核糖和兩個磷酸基的化合物。存在於細胞中，參預需要能量轉移的過程。

adrenal glands (suprarenal glands) two triangular *endocrine glands, each of which covers the superior surface of a kidney. Each gland has two parts, the *medulla* and *cortex*. The medulla forms the grey core of the gland; it consists mainly of *chromaffin tissue and is stimulated by the sympathetic nervous system to produce *adrenaline and *noradrenaline. The cortex is a yellowish tissue surrounding the medulla. It is

腎上腺 兩個三角形的內分泌腺，均覆蓋在腎的上部。每個腺有兩部分：髓質和皮質。髓質形成腺的灰色的核心；主要由嗜鉻組織組成，受交感神經刺激而產生腎上腺素和去甲腎上腺素。皮質爲黃色組織，圍繞髓質。皮質是在胚胎時由中胚層衍化而來，受垂體激素刺激（主

derived embryologically from mesoderm and is stimulated by pituitary hormones (principally *ACTH) to produce three kinds of *corticosteroid hormones, which affect carbohydrate metabolism (e.g. *cortisol), electrolyte metabolism (e.g. *aldosterone), and the sex glands (oestrogens and androgens).

要是 ACTH）產生三種皮質類固醇激素，可影響碳水化合物的新陳代謝（如可的松）、電解質的新陳代謝（如醛甾醇）和性腺（雌激素和雄激素）。

adrenaline (epinephrine) *n.* an important hormone secreted by the medulla of the adrenal gland. It has the function of preparing the body for 'fright, flight, or fight' and has widespread effects on circulation, the muscles, and sugar metabolism. The action of the heart is increased, the rate and depth of breathing are increased, and the metabolic rate is raised; the force of muscular contraction improves and the onset of muscular fatigue is delayed. At the same time the blood supply to the bladder and intestines is reduced, their muscular walls relax, and the sphincters contract. *Sympathetic nerves were originally thought to act by releasing adrenaline at their endings, and were therefore called *adrenergic* nerves. In fact the main substance released is the related substance *noradrenaline, which also forms a portion of the adrenal secretion.
Adrenaline given by injection is valuable for the relief of bronchial asthma, because it relaxes constricted airways. It is also used during surgery to reduce blood loss by constricting vessels in the skin.

腎上腺素 腎上腺髓質分泌的一種重要激素。當機體處於"恐懼，追逐，逃跑，戰鬥"等狀態中時，就要靠這種激素來維持。該激素影響遍及循環、肌肉以及糖代謝：心博增快，呼吸深度與頻率增加，代謝率升高，肌肉收縮力增强並延緩疲勞。同時膀胱和腸道供血減少，其肌肉壁鬆弛，括約肌收縮。過去人們認爲交感神經的末端是釋放腎上腺素的，因而曾稱之爲腎上腺能神經。事實上釋放的主要物質是與腎上腺素近似的去甲腎上腺素。前者亦佔腎上腺分泌的一部分。腎上腺素注射可緩解呼吸道收縮，故治療支氣管哮喘有效，因其又能收縮血管，在外科手術時亦用以減少出血。

adrenergic *adj.* describing nerve fibres that release *noradrenaline as a neurotransmitter. *Compare* cholinergic.

腎上腺素能的 描述釋放神經遞質去甲腎上腺素的神經纖維。

adrenocorticotrophic hormone (adrenocorticotrophin) *see* ACTH.

促腎上腺皮質激素

adrenogenital syndrome precocious sexual development and apparent masculinization in girls, caused by overproduction of hormones by the adrenal cortex in infancy.

腎上腺性徵綜合徵 性發育早熟和女孩明顯男性化。由於嬰兒期腎上腺皮質激素過度分泌所致。

adrenolytic *adj.* inhibiting the activity of *adrenergic nerves. Adrenolytic activity is opposite to that of *adrenaline.

抗腎上腺素的　具有抑制腎上腺素能神經作用的。抗腎上腺素的作用與腎上腺的作用相反。

advancement *n.* the detachment by surgery of a muscle or tendon from its normal attachment site and its reattachment at a more advanced (anterior) point. The technique is used, for example, in the treatment of squint or in repositioning the womb.

徒前術　以手術使肌肉或腱脫離正常部位後，使與更前的位置再相接。本術用於斜視治療或子宮復位。

adventitia (tunica adventitia) *n.* **1.** the outer coat of the wall of a *vein or *artery. It consists of loose connective tissue and networks of small blood vessels, which nourish the walls. **2.** the outer covering of various other organs or parts.

外膜　①靜脉或動脉壁的外衣。由疏鬆結締組織和網狀小血管組成，起營養血管壁的作用。　②其他多種器官或結構的外被。

adventitious *adj.* **1.** occurring in a place other than the usual one. **2.** relating to the adventitia.

偶生的，外來的　①發生於非正常部位的。　②與外膜有關的。

Aëdes *n.* a genus of widely distributed mosquitoes occurring throughout the tropics and subtropics. Most species are black with distinct white or silvery-yellow markings on the legs and thorax. *Aëdes* species are not only important as vectors of *dengue, *yellow fever, *filariasis, and Group B viruses causing encephalitis but also constitute a serious biting nuisance. *A. aegypti* is the principal vector of dengue and yellow fever.

伊蚊屬　在熱帶和亞熱帶孳生且分佈廣泛的蚊屬。多數蚊種呈黑色，在腿和胸部有明顯白色或銀黃色紋記。伊蚊屬的蚊種不僅是登革熱、黃熱病、絲蟲病和乙型腦炎病毒的主要媒介，且對人叮擾嚴重。埃及伊蚊是登革熱和黃熱病的主要媒介。

aegophony *n. see* vocal resonance.

羊音

-aemia *suffix denoting* a specified condition of the blood. Example: *hyperglycaemia* (excess sugar in the blood).

〔後綴〕**血症**　血液異常狀態。例如：高血糖症（血液糖分過高）。

aer- (aero-) *prefix denoting* air or gas. Examples: *aerogastria* (gas in the stomach); *aerogenesis* (production of gas).

〔前綴〕**氣**　空氣或氣體。例如：胃積氣（胃內有氣體），產氣（產生氣體）。

aerobe *n.* any organism, especially a microbe, that requires the presence of free oxygen for life and growth. *See also* anaerobe, microaerophilic.

需氧菌　任何在生活發育中需要游離氧的生物體（尤指微生物）。

aerobic *adj.* **1.** of or relating to aerobes: requiring free oxygen for life and growth. **2.** describing a type of cellular *respiration in which foodstuffs (carbohydrates) are completely oxidized by atmospheric oxygen, with the production of maximum chemical energy from the foodstuffs.

需氧的 ①需氧菌的或與需氧菌有關的：需要游離氧生活發育。 ②描述一型細胞呼吸，其食物（碳水化合物）被大氣氧完全氧化，食物中的化學能全部產生出來。

aerodontalgia *n.* pain in the teeth due to change in atmospheric pressure during air travel or the ascent of a mountain.

航空牙痛 因航空旅行或登山時的氣壓改變引起的牙痛。

aeroneurosis *n.* a syndrome of anxiety, agitation, and insomnia found in pilots flying unpressurized aircraft and attributed to *anoxia.

飛行員神經官能症 飛行員乘無密封艙飛機飛行時因缺氧呈現的綜合徵。表現有焦慮、激動和失眠等。

aerophagy *n.* the swallowing of air. This may be done voluntarily to stimulate belching, accidentally during rapid eating or drinking, or unconsciously as a habit. Voluntary aerophagy is used to permit oesophageal speech after surgical removal of the larynx (usually for cancer).

吞氣症 吞入空氣。可隨意引起，以產生噯氣，飲食過速時可偶然發生。吞氣症有時爲一種無意識的習慣。切除喉管（通常爲治癌）的病人利用隨意性吞氣來協助食管語音的發音。

aerosol *n.* a suspension of extremely small liquid or solid particles (about 0.001 mm diameter) in the air. Drugs in aerosol form may be administered by inhalation.

氣霧劑 空氣中懸浮的氣體或固體微小粒子（直徑最大不超過0.001 mm）。藥物製成氣霧劑型可供吸入給藥。

aetiology (etiology) *n.* **1.** the study or science of the causes of disease. **2.** the cause of a specific disease.

①**病因學** 研究致病原因的科學。 ②**病因** 特定疾病的原因。

afebrile *adj.* without, or not showing any signs of, a fever.

無熱的 不發熱的或不具任何發熱徵象的。

affect *n.* (in psychiatry) a wave of emotion or the emotion associated with a particular idea. –**affective** *adj.*

情感 在精神病中指感情的波動，或伴隨某種特定觀念產生的感情。

afferent *adj.* **1.** designating nerves or neurones that convey impulses from sense organs and other receptors to the brain or spinal cord, i.e. any sensory nerve or neurone. **2.** designating blood vessels that feed a capillary network in an organ or part. **3.** designating lym-

傳入的，輸入的 ①指從感覺器官或其他感受器將衝動傳入腦或脊髓的神經或神經元。 ②指進入器官或部位的毛細血管網的血管。③指進入淋巴結的淋巴管。

phatic vessels that enter a lymph node. *Compare* efferent.

afibrinogenaemia *n.* complete absence of the coagulation factor *fibrinogen in the blood. *Compare* hypofibrinogenaemia.

無纖維蛋白原血症 血液完全缺乏凝血因子纖維蛋白原。

aflatoxin *n.* a poisonous substance produced in the spores of the fungus *Aspergillus flavus*, which infects peanuts. The toxin is known to produce cancer in certain animals and is suspected of being the cause of liver cancers in human beings living in warm and humid regions of the world, where stored nuts and cereals are contaminated by the fungus.

黃曲黴毒素 眞菌黃曲黴孢子產生的毒物，常感染花生。本毒素已知對某些動物致癌，估計其爲世界溫濕地區人類肝癌的病因。在這些地區儲存的堅果及穀物亦易被眞菌污染。

afterbirth *n.* the placenta, umbilical cord, and ruptured membranes associated with the fetus, which normally become detached from the womb and expelled within a few hours of birth.

胎盤胎膜，胞衣 與胎兒相連的胎盤、臍帶和撕破的羊膜的總稱。在正常情況下產後數小時自子宮脫落並排出。

after care long-term surveillance as an adjunct or supplement to formal medical treatment of those who are chronically sick or handicapped. After care includes the provision of special aids and the adaptation of homes to improve daily living.

醫療後監護 對慢性病或殘疾人進行長期監護。這是對正規醫療的輔助或補充措施。本措施包括提供各種專用助殘設備，並幫助患者逐漸適應日常的家庭生活。

after-image *n.* an impression of an image that is registered by the brain for a brief moment after an object is removed from in front of the eye, or after the eye is closed.

後像 映入腦內的物像在該物體消失或閉目後仍能保持短暫時刻的現象。

after-pains *pl. n.* pains in the womb during the first few days after childbirth, caused by contraction of the womb muscles as its nonpregnant dimensions are restored. After-pains can be relieved by the use of such drugs as aspirin.

產後痛 產後數日內的子宮痛，是由於子宮復舊過程中子宮肌收縮所致。產後痛可用阿司匹林等藥解除。

agalactia *n.* absence or abnormally low production of milk in a woman who has just given birth.

無乳 婦女產後無乳或泌乳過少的現象。

agammaglobulinaemia *n.* a total deficiency of the plasma protein *gamma

缺丙種球蛋白血 血漿中缺乏丙種球蛋白。

globulin. *Compare* hypogammaglobulinaemia.

agar *n.* an extract of certain seaweeds that forms a gel suitable for the solidification of liquid bacteriological *culture media. *Blood agar* is nutrient agar containing 5–10% horse blood, used for the cultivation of certain bacteria or for detecting haemolytic (blood-destroying) activity.

瓊脂 某種海草的提取物。呈凝膠狀態，用以將液體細菌培養基配製成固體培養基。血瓊脂含 5~10% 馬血，用以培養某些細菌並測定其溶血作用（破壞血液的能力）。

Age Concern (in Britain) a voluntary agency with particular interest in the problems of the aged.

老年康采恩 （英國）一個關心老齡問題的志願組織。

agenesis *n.* absence of an organ, usually due to total failure of its development in the embryo.

發育不全 某個器官缺乏。通常由於胚胎期該器官發育障礙所致。

agglutination (clumping) *n.* the sticking together, by serum antibodies called *agglutinins*, of such microscopic antigenic particles as red blood cells or bacteria so that they form visible clumps. Any substance that stimulates the body to produce an agglutinin is called an *agglutinogen*. Agglutination is a specific reaction; in the laboratory, sera containing different known agglutinins provide an invaluable means of identifying unknown bacteria. When blood of different groups is mixed, agglutination occurs because serum contains natural antibodies (*isoagglutinins*) that attack red cells of a foreign group, whether previously encountered or not. This is not the same process as occurs in *blood coagulation.

凝集 血清抗體（凝集素）使鏡下可見的顆粒狀抗原諸如血細胞或細菌等黏結爲明顯的團塊的現象。任何可刺激人體產生凝集素的物質都可稱爲凝集原。凝集爲一種特異性反應；在實驗室內備有含不同已知凝集素血清，對鑑定不明的細菌有重要意義。不同血型的血液混合會發生凝集反應。因爲血清含有天然抗原，不論它以前是否接觸過異型血液，都會破壞異型血的紅細胞。此過程與血液凝固現象迥然不同。

agglutinin *n.* an antibody that brings about the *agglutination of bacteria, blood cells, or other antigenic particles.

凝集素 一種可使細菌、血細胞或其他抗原顆粒凝集的抗體。

agglutinogen *n.* any antigen that provokes formation of an agglutinin in the serum and is therefore likely to be involved in *agglutination.

凝集原 任何可促使血清凝集素形成的抗原物質。參預凝集過程。

aglossia *n.* congenital absence of the tongue.

無舌畸形 先天性缺舌。

agnathia *n.* congenital absence of the lower jaw, either partial or complete.

無下頜畸形 先天性全部或部分下頜缺損。

agnosia *n.* a disorder of the brain whereby the patient cannot interpret sensations correctly although the sense organs and nerves conducting sensation to the brain are functioning normally. It is due to a disorder of the *association areas in the parietal lobes. In *auditory agnosia* the patient can hear but cannot interpret sounds (including speech). A patient with *tactile agnosia* (*astereognosis*) retains normal sensation in his hands but cannot recognize three-dimensional objects by touch alone. In *visual agnosia* the patient can see but cannot interpret symbols, including letters (*see* alexia).

認識不能 因腦的功能紊亂患者不能正確理解感覺到的東西。雖然此時感覺器官和把感覺傳導到腦內的神經均屬正常。本病是由於頂葉連合區的病變所致。聽覺識別不能，指病人可聽到，但不能理解聲音（包括語言）。觸覺識別不能，指病人保有正常手感，但僅以接觸不能識別物體的立體形狀。視覺識別不能，指病人可看到，但不能理解符號（包括字母）的意義。

agonal *adj.* describing or relating to the phenomena, such as cessation of breathing or change in the ECG or EEG, that are associated with the moment of death.

瀕死的 描述瀕死或與瀕死有關的現象，如呼吸停止，或死亡發生時的心電圖、腦電圖變化。

agonist (prime mover) *n.* a muscle whose active contraction causes movement of a part of the body. Contraction of an agonist is associated with relaxation of its *antagonist.

主動肌 一種在有效收縮時可致人體某一部分活動的肌肉。主動肌的收縮同時發生其抗括肌的放鬆。

agoraphobia *n.* a morbid fear of public places and/or of open spaces. *See also* phobia.

廣場恐怖，曠野恐怖 對公共場所和/或開闊地方的病態恐懼。

agranulocytosis *n.* a disorder in which there is a severe acute deficiency of certain blood cells (*neutrophils) as a result of damage to the bone marrow by toxic drugs or chemicals. It is characterized by fever, with ulceration of the mouth and throat, and rapidly leads to prostration and death. Treatment is by administration of antibiotics in large quantities. When feasible, transfusion of white blood cells may be life-saving.

粒細胞缺乏症 某種血細胞（嗜中性）的急性嚴重缺乏，爲毒藥或化學品損傷骨髓所致。特徵爲發熱，口、咽潰瘍，可迅速導致衰竭和死亡。治療可使用大劑量抗生素。如有條件，可輸入白細胞搶救。

agraphia (dysgraphia) *n.* an acquired inability to write, although the strength and coordination of the hand remain

書寫不能，失寫 後天性無書寫能力，雖然手的力量與協調作用均屬正常。

normal. It is related to the disorders of language and it is caused by disease in the *parietal lobe of the brain. *See* Gerstmann's syndrome.

本病與語言障礙有關，爲大腦頂葉病損所致。

agromania *n.* a pathologically strong impulse to live alone in open country.

野居癖　一種强烈的、病態的獨身在曠野生活的衝動。

ague *n. see* malaria.

瘧疾

AID *see* artificial insemination.

人工授精

AIDS (acquired immunodeficiency syndrome) a viral disease characterized by loss of the cell-mediated immune response due to decreased numbers of certain T-lymphocytes. After a long incubation period (up to several years), the patient suffers fever, weight loss, and enlargement of the lymph nodes, eventually succumbing to life-threatening infections (e.g. a severe pneumonia caused by the normally harmless protozoan *Pneumocystis carinii*) or cancers, particularly *Kaposi's sarcoma. The viruses, principally HIV (human immunodeficiency virus), are transmitted in blood, semen, and vaginal fluid, and in western countries AIDS is most prevalent among male homosexuals, haemophiliacs who have received transfusions of infected blood, and intravenous drug users sharing needles.

艾滋病（獲得性免疫缺陷綜合徵）　以某種T淋巴細胞減少引起細胞免疫反應喪失爲特徵的綜合徵。在長久的潛伏期後（可達3年），病人出現發熱、體重下降、淋巴結腫大等症狀，最後死於危及生命的感染（例如：通常無害的原生動物卡氏肺囊蟲引起的嚴重肺炎）、癌症（尤其是卡波濟氏肉瘤）。本病主要流行於鷄姦的男性同性戀者、血友病患者，海洛英癮者亦可感染，推測本病可經受感染的血液製品傳播。病因未肯定，一般認爲病原可能爲病毒。

AIH *see* artificial insemination.

人工授精

ainhum *n.* loss of one or more toes due to slow growth of a fibrous band around the toe that eventually causes a spontaneous amputation. The condition is found in negroes and is associated with going barefoot.

阿洪病　喪失一或多個脚趾。在趾周緩慢生長出纖維索條，最終導致自發斷趾。見於黑人，與赤脚行走有關。

air bed a bed with a mattress whose upper surface is perforated with thousands of holes, through which air is forced under pressure. The patient is thus supported, like a hovercraft, on a

氣床　墊褥上具有以千數計氣孔的床。空氣在高壓下穿透氣孔，患者就像在氣墊船上一樣，躺在一層由空氣形成的氣墊上。本

cushion of air. This type of bed is invaluable for the treatment of patients with large areas of burns.

床對大面積燒傷病人有重要作用。

air embolism an air lock that obstructs the outflow of blood from the right ventricle of the heart. Air may gain access to the circulation as a result of surgery, injury, or intravenous infusions. The patient experiences breathlessness and chest discomfort and develops acute heart failure. Tipping the patient head down, lying on the left side, may move the air lock.

氣栓 阻塞右心室血流的空氣栓塞。空氣可因手術、外傷、或靜脉輸液進入循環系統。病人感到呼吸困難、胸部不適，進而發展到急性心力衰竭。使病人頭部向下傾斜，左側臥位，可移走氣栓。

air sickness *see* travel sickness.

航空病

akinesia *n.* a loss of normal muscular tonicity or responsiveness. In *akinetic epilepsy* there is a sudden loss of muscular tonicity, making the patient fall with momentary loss of consciousness. *Akinetic mutism* is a state of complete physical unresponsiveness although the patient's eyes remain open and appear to follow movements. It is a consequence of damage to the base of the brain. —**akinetic** *adj.*

運動不能 肌肉失去緊張性或反應能力。運動不能性癲癇，指肌肉突然失去緊張性，病人跌倒，且暫時喪失知覺。運動不能性啞症，指病人身體所有的反應能力全部喪失，僅眼可張開並隨物活動。為腦基底受損的結果。

ala *n.* (*pl.* **alae**) (in anatomy) a winglike structure; for example, either of the two lateral flared portions of the external nose or the winglike part of the ilium.

翼 （解剖學）翼狀結構。例如：鼻翼，指外鼻兩側能張開的部分或髂骨翼。

alactasia *n.* absence or deficiency of the enzyme lactase, which is essential for the digestion of milk sugar (lactose). All babies have lactase in their intestines, but the enzyme disappears during childhood in about 10% of northern Europeans, 40% of Greeks and Italians, and 80% of Africans and Asians. Alactasia causes symptoms only if the diet regularly includes raw milk, when the undigested lactose causes diarrhoea and abdominal pain.

缺乳糖酶症 消化乳糖所必需的乳糖酶缺乏或不足。所有嬰兒在腸道中均有乳糖酶，但在北歐約有10%，希臘和意大利約有40%，非洲和亞洲約有80%的兒童患缺乳糖酶症。僅在那些經常飲用生乳的人中出現症狀，未消化的乳糖可致腹瀉或腹痛。

alanine *n.* *see* amino acid.

丙氨酸

alastrim *n.* a mild form of smallpox, causing only a sparse rash and low-grade fever. Medical name: **variola minor**.

乳白痘，類天花 溫和型天花，僅出現稀疏的疹子和低燒。醫學名稱：輕型天花。

Albers-Schönberg disease *see* osteopetrosis.

阿-尚二氏病，骨硬化病

albinism *n.* the inherited absence of pigmentation in the skin, hair, and eyes (*see* albino).

白化病　先天性皮膚、頭髮、眼睛缺乏色素。

albino *n.* an individual lacking the normal body pigment (melanin). Albinos have white hair and pink skin and eyes. The pink colour is produced by blood in underlying blood vessels, which are normally masked by pigment.

白化病患者　任何缺乏體內正常色素（黑色素）的人。患者出現白髮、粉紅皮膚及眼。粉紅色由皮下血管產生，這種血管在正常情況下被黑色素遮住。

albumin *n.* a protein that is soluble in water and coagulated by heat. An example is *serum albumin*, which is found in blood plasma and is important for the maintenance of plasma volume. Albumin is synthesized in the liver; the inability to synthesize it is a prominent feature of chronic liver disease (*cirrhosis).

白蛋白，清蛋白　一種可溶於水並在加熱後凝固的蛋白。例如：血清白蛋白，見於血漿，對維持血漿容量十分重要。本蛋白在肝內合成，肝病的突出特點就是喪失合成白蛋白的能力。

albuminuria (proteinuria) *n.* the presence of serum albumin, serum globulin, or other serum proteins in the urine. This may be associated with kidney or heart disease. Albuminuria is not always associated with disease: it may occur after strenuous exercise or after a long period of standing (*orthostatic albuminuria*).

蛋白尿　在尿中出現血清白蛋白、血清球蛋白或他種血清蛋白。其出現與腎、心疾患有關。本病有時與疾病無關：可發生於緊張的鍛煉或長時間的站立以後。

albumose *n.* a substance, intermediate between albumin and peptones, produced during the digestion of proteins by pepsin and other endopeptidases (*see* peptidase).

脲　蛋白質分解成腖的過程中的一種中間產物。在蛋白質被胃蛋白酶或其他肽鏈內切酶作用時產生。

alcaptonuria (alkaptonuria) *n.* congenital absence of an enzyme, homogentisic acid oxidase, that is essential for the normal breakdown of the amino acids tyrosine and phenylalanine. Accumulation of *homogentisic acid causes dark brown discoloration of the skin and eyes (*ochronosis*) and progressive damage to the joints, especially of the spine. The gene responsible for the condition is recessive, so that a child is

尿黑酸尿　先天性缺乏分解酪氨酸和苯丙氨酸等氨基酸所必須的尿黑酸氧化酶。尿黑酸積聚可使皮、眼變成棕黑色，並出現尤其父母雙方均攜帶此種缺損基因時才發病。

以脊椎關節爲明顯的進行性關節損傷。本病的致病基因是隱性的，兒童僅在

affected only if both parents are carriers of the defective gene.

alcohol *n.* any of a class of organic compounds formed when a hydroxyl group (–OH) is substituted for a hydrogen atom in a hydrocarbon. The alcohol in alcoholic drinks is *ethyl alcohol* (*ethanol*), which has the formula C_2H_5OH. It is produced by the fermentation of sugar by yeast. 'Pure' alcohol contains not less than 94.9% by volume of ethyl alcohol. It is obtained by distillation. A solution of 70% alcohol can be used as a preservative or antiseptic. When taken into the body ethyl alcohol depresses activity of the central nervous system (*see also* alcoholism). *Methyl alcohol (methanol) is extremely poisonous.

酒精 碳氫化合物中的一個氫原子被羥〔基〕置換所形成的一類有機化合物。酒精性飲料中的酒精爲乙醇，分子式爲 C_2H_5OH，爲糖類經酵母發酵產生。"純"酒精中乙醇含量不得少於按容積計的 94.9%，係經蒸餾取得。70% 酒精可用於防腐或消毒。攝入體內的乙醇可抑制中樞神經系統的活動。甲醇爲劇毒。

Alcoholics Anonymous a voluntary agency of self help that is organized and operated locally among those with alcoholic dependency and has national and international support. Members are expected to admit to their drink problems, discuss these openly and frankly at the regular meetings of the group, and also to take part in efficient family support schemes to help those members who have lapses.

嗜酒者互誡協會 一種自助的地方性的志願機構，由嗜酒者組成和管理，並得到國家和國際的支持。協會要求會員承認他們嗜酒，在定期的會議上公開地並坦率地討論問題，同時要和那些因酗酒而墮落的人的家屬在一起共同制定挽救他們的行之有效的計劃。

alcoholism *n.* the syndrome due to physical *dependence on alcohol, such that sudden deprivation may cause withdrawal symptoms – tremor, anxiety, hallucinations, and delusions (*see* delirium tremens). The risk of alcoholism for an individual and its incidence in a society depend on the amount drunk. Countries such as France, where heavy drinking is socially acceptable, have the highest incidence. Usually several years' heavy drinking is needed for addiction to develop, but the range is from one to 40 years. Alcoholism impairs intellectual function, physical skills, memory, and judgment: social skills, such as conversation, are preserved until a late stage.

醇中毒 人體因嗜酒成癮而一旦禁飲時出現的戒斷綜合徵。症狀有震顫、焦慮、幻覺以及妄想等。醇中毒對個人的危害及對社會的影響須視該人的飲酒多少而定。法國等地酗酒是合法的，因而對社會造成巨大影響。通常大量飲酒數年才能成癮，其時間自 1 至 40 年不等。醇中毒損害智力、人體技能、記憶以及判斷力；社交技能諸如談話可保留至晚期。酗酒亦可致心肌病，周圍神經炎、肝硬變、以及腸炎。本病常由精神病醫院治療，在該處首先要

Heavy consumption of alcohol also causes *cardiomyopathy, peripheral *neuritis, *cirrhosis of the liver, and enteritis. Treatment is usually given in a psychiatric hospital, where the alcoholic is first 'dried out' and then helped to understand the psychological pressures that led to his heavy drinking. Drugs such as *disulfiram (Antabuse), which cause vomiting if alcohol is taken, may help in treatment.

徹底戒酒，進而要幫助患者了解心理作用對酗酒的巨大影響。使用雙硫醒後一旦再用酒則嘔吐，因而對治療有利。

Aldomet *n. see* methyldopa.

甲基多巴

aldosterone *n.* a steroid hormone (*see* corticosteroid) that is synthesized and released by the adrenal cortex and acts on the kidney to regulate salt (potassium and sodium) and water balance. It may be given by injection as replacement therapy when the adrenal cortex secretes insufficient amounts of the hormone and also to treat shock.

醛甾酮 一種甾類激素。由腎上腺皮質合成並分泌，作用於腎臟，以調節鹽（鉀和鈉）和水的平衡。腎上腺皮質分泌本激素不足時可注射本激素作爲替代治療。並可用於治療休克。

aldosteronism *n.* overproduction of aldosterone, one of the hormones secreted by the adrenal cortex, leading to abnormalities in the amounts of sodium, potassium, and water in the body. It is one cause of raised blood pressure (hypertension).

醛甾酮增多症 腎上腺皮質的一種激素醛甾酮分泌過多，引起體內鈉、鉀、水的含量異常。爲血壓上升（高血壓）的一個因素。

Aleppo boil *see* oriental sore.

東方瘡，皮膚利什曼病

aleukaemic *adj.* describing a stage of *leukaemia in which there is no increase in the number of white cells in the blood. The stage is almost invariably followed by one in which excessive numbers of white cells are produced, as typical in leukaemia.

白細胞不增多性 形容白血病的一期，該期血內細胞不增加。本期後無例外地緊接着發生白血病典型的表現：白細胞大量增多。

alexia *n.* an acquired inability to read. It is due to disease in the left hemisphere of the brain in a right-handed person. In *agnosic alexia* (*word blindness*) the patient cannot read because he is unable to identify the letters and words, but he retains the ability to write and his speech is normal. This is a form of *agnosia. A patient with *aphasic alexia* (*visual asymbolia*) can neither

失讀症 後天性閱讀能力喪失。是慣用右手（右利）的人因左腦患病所致。識字不能性失讀症（詞盲），指因不能判定字母和單詞而不能讀字，但仍保有書寫、講話的正常能力。這是失認症的一型。患失語性失讀症（視覺性說示不能）時，既不

read nor write and often has an accompanying disorder of speech. This is a form of *aphasia. *See also* dyslexia.

能讀又不能寫並常伴以語言障礙，是失語症的一型。

alexin *n.* a former name for the serum component now called *complement.

防禦素 血清成分的舊名，現稱補體。

alexithymia *n.* a lack of psychological understanding of one's own emotions and moods. It is considered by some psychiatrists to be a way in which people develop *psychosomatic symptoms.

表達心境不能 對自身的感情和心境缺乏心理學的理解。一些精神科醫師認爲這在某些人是心身症狀的一種形式。

algesimeter *n.* a piece of equipment for determining the sensitivity of the skin to various touch stimuli, especially those causing pain.

痛覺計 一種測定皮膚對不同觸覺刺激（特別是痛覺刺激）的敏感性的儀器。

-algia *suffix denoting* pain. Example: *neuralgia* (pain in a nerve).

〔後綴〕**痛** 如神經痛。

algid *adj.* cold: usually describing the cold clammy skin associated with certain forms of malaria.

濕冷的 通常用於描述患某型瘧疾時出現的濕冷皮膚。

alienation *n.* (in psychiatry) **1.** the experience that one's thoughts are under the control of somebody else, or that other people participate in one's thinking. It is a symptom of *schizophrenia. **2.** insanity.

①**人格解體性疏離感** 感到自己的思維活動受到別人控制，或者別人的思想也參預到自己的思維活動中來的一種體驗。是精神分裂症的一種症狀。 ②**精神錯亂**。

alimentary canal the long passage through which food passes to be digested and absorbed (see illustration). It extends from the mouth to the anus and each region is specialized for a different stage in the processing of food, from mechanical breakdown in the mouth to chemical *digestion and *absorption in the stomach and small intestine and finally to faeces formation and storage in the colon and rectum.

消化道 食物所通過的並在其中被消化和吸收的較長通道（見圖）。消化道自口延伸至肛門，每一部分對所通過的食物的消化均有不同的作用，開始時在口內是機械性碎裂，繼而在胃和小腸經過化學性消化和吸收，最後形成糞便貯存在結腸和直腸。

alizarin (alizarin carmine) *n.* an orange-red dye derived from coal tar and originally isolated from the plant madder (*Rubia tinctorum*). Alizarin is insoluble in water but dissolves in

茜素 一種自煤焦油中提取的橘紅色染料。最初是自茜草屬植物分離而得。茜素不溶於水，但溶於鹼液、酒精和乙醚。用做

alkalis, alcohol, and ether. It is used as a pH indicator and as a histochemical reagent for calcium, thallium, titanium, and zirconium.

pH 指示劑及檢驗鈣、鉈、鈦和鋯的生化試劑。

alkalaemia *n.* abnormally high blood alkalinity. This may be caused by an increase in the concentration of alkaline substances and/or a decrease in that of acidic substances in the blood. *See also* alkalosis. *Compare* acidaemia.

鹼血〔症〕 血液鹼度異常升高。因血內鹼性物質濃度增加和/或酸性物質濃度減低所致。

alkaloid *n.* one of a diverse group of nitrogen-containing substances that are produced by plants and have potent effects on body function. Many alkaloids are important drugs, including *morphine, *quinine, *atropine, and *codeine.

生物鹼 植物產生的一組不同成分的含氮物質，對人體功能有巨大作用。多種生物鹼爲重要藥物，包括嗎啡、奎寧、阿托品、可卡因。

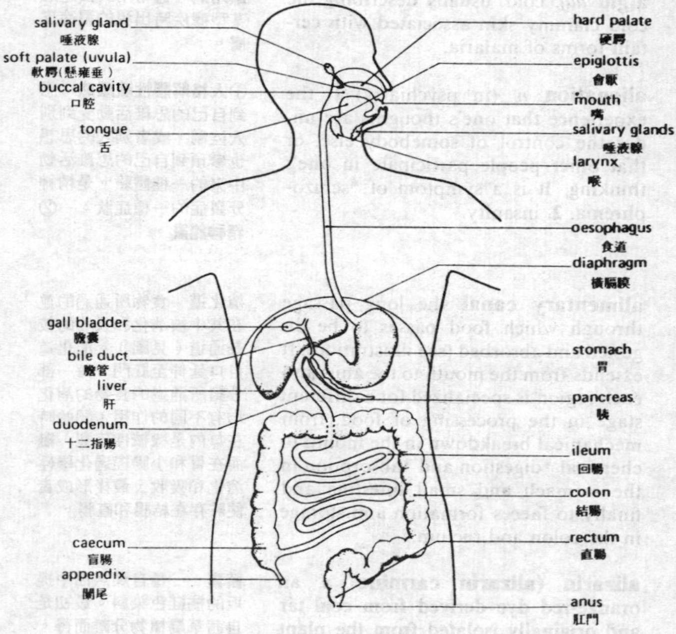

The alimentary canal
消化道

alkalosis *n.* a condition in which the alkalinity of body fluids and tissues is abnormally high. This arises because of a failure of the mechanisms that usually maintain a balance between alkalis and acids in the arterial blood (*see* acid-base balance). Alkalosis may be associated with loss of acid through vomiting or with excessive sodium bicarbonate intake. Breathing that is abnormally deep in relation to the amount of physical exercise may lead to *respiratory alkalosis.* Alkalosis may produce symptoms of muscular weakness or cramp.

鹼中毒 體液和組織內鹼度異常升高。原因爲動脈血維持酸鹼平衡的機能衰竭。亦可與嘔吐失酸或食入過多碳酸氫鈉有關。與體育鍛煉有關的異常深呼吸可導致呼吸性鹼中毒。鹼中毒可產生肌肉孱弱或痛性痙攣。

alkaptonuria *n. see* alcaptonuria.

尿黑酸尿

allantois *n.* the membranous sac that develops as an outgrowth of the embryonic hindgut. Its outer (mesodermal) layer carries blood vessels to the *placenta and so forms part of the *umbilical cord. Its cavity is small and becomes reduced further in size during fetal development (*see* urachus). —**allantoic** *adj.*

尿囊 胚胎後腸生長發育生成的膜狀囊。其外層（中胚層的）有血管通向胎盤並形成臍帶的一部分。其囊腔細小，在胚胎發育過程中進一步縮小。

allele (allelomorph) *n.* one of two or more alternative forms of a *gene, only one of which can be present in a chromosome. Two alleles of a particular gene occupy the same relative positions on a pair of *homologous chromosomes. If the two alleles are the same, the individual is *homozygous for the gene; if they are different he is *heterozygous. *See also* dominant. —**allelic** *adj.*

等位基因 基因具有的兩個或更多的交替型中的一個，但在一個染色體中僅能出現一型。在一對同源的染色體中，特殊基因的兩個等位基因各佔據同一相應的位置。如兩個等位基因相同，其個體稱爲純合子；兩個等位基因不同則其個體稱爲異合子。

allelomorph *n. see* allele.

等位基因

allergen *n.* any *antigen that causes *allergy in a hypersensitive person. Allergens are diverse and affect different tissues and organs. Pollens, fur, feathers, mould, and dust may cause hay fever; house mites have been implicated in some forms of asthma; drugs, dyes, cosmetics, and a host of other chemicals can cause rashes and dermatitis; some food allergies may cause diarrhoea or constipation or simulate

變應原 對敏感者可引起變態反應的任何抗原。變應原種類很多，且可影響不同組織和器官。花粉、皮革、羽毛、黴菌和塵土可引起乾草熱；室內蟎類與某型哮喘有關；藥物、染料、化妝品以及許多化學品可致皮疹和皮炎；有些食物變應原可致腹瀉、便秘或類似急性細菌性食

acute bacterial food poisoning. When a patient's allergen has been identified, it may be possible to attempt *desensitization to alleviate or prevent allergic attacks. —**allergenic** *adj.*

物中毒的症狀。一旦患者的變應原已確定，就有可能行脫敏療法以減少或預防變應原的侵害。

allergy *n.* a disorder in which the body becomes hypersensitive to particular antigens (called *allergens), which provoke characteristic symptoms whenever they are subsequently encountered, whether inhaled, ingested, injected, or otherwise contacted. Normally antibodies in the bloodstream and tissues react with and destroy specific antigens without further trouble. In an allergic person, however, the reaction of allergen with tissue-bound antibody (*reagin) also leads, as a side-effect, to cell damage, release of *histamine and *serotonin, inflammation, and all the symptoms of the particular allergy. Different allergies afflict different tissues and may have either local or general effects, varying from asthma and hay fever to severe dermatitis or gastroenteritis or extremely serious shock (*see* anaphylaxis). —**allergic** *adj.*

變態反應 對某種特異抗原（變應原）過敏的人在接觸到該種抗原時發生典型症狀的一種疾病。吸入、食入、注射入或經其他方式接觸抗原可發病。在正常的情況下，抗體在血流和組織中與特異性抗原起作用並將其破壞，而不致發病。在具變應體質的人，一旦變應原與組織中的抗體（反應素）起作用即可導致一些副作用，如細胞損傷、釋放組胺和血清素、炎症，以及變態反應的特異症狀。不同變應原危害不同組織，可引起局部或全身症狀，如哮喘、乾草熱以至嚴重皮炎、胃腸炎或重度休克等。

allograft *n. see* homograft.

同種移植物

alloisoleucine *n.* one of the isomers of the amino acid isoleucine.

別異亮氨酸 異亮氨酸的一種異構體。

allopathy *n.* (in homeopathic medicine) the orthodox system of medicine, in which the use of drugs is directed to producing effects in the body that will directly oppose and so alleviate the symptoms of a disease. *Compare* homeopathy.

對抗療法 （順勢療法用語）一種傳統的醫療體系。用能在體內產生與症狀直接對抗作用的藥物來使疾病症狀緩解。

allopurinol *n.* a drug used in the treatment of chronic gout. It acts by reducing the level of uric acid in tissues and blood. It is administered by mouth; side-effects include nausea, vomiting, diarrhoea, headache, fever, stomach pains, and skin rashes. Occasionally, nerve damage and enlargement of the liver may occur.

別嘌呤醇 用於治療慢性痛風的藥。其作用爲降低組織和血液內的尿酸。口服。副作用有噁心、嘔吐、腹瀉、頭痛、發熱、胃痛以及皮疹。偶爾可損傷神經或發生肝腫大。

alloxan *n.* a *pyrimidine derivative that has been used to induce diabetes in experimental animals as it destroys the cells of the pancreatic islets of Langerhans that produce insulin.

四氧嘧啶 嘧啶衍生物。因能損傷產生胰島素的胰島細胞，用以誘發實驗動物糖尿病。

allylestrenol (allyloestrenol) *n.* a synthetic female sex hormone (*see* progestogen) used in the treatment of abnormal bleeding from the womb and threatened abortion. It is administered by mouth. Trade name: **Gestanin**.

烯丙雌烯醇 用於治療不正常子宮出血及先兆流產的一種合成雌激素。口服。

almoner *n.* a former name for a *medical social worker.

救濟員 醫學社會工作人員的舊稱。

alopecia (baldness) *n.* absence of hair from areas where it normally grows. Alopecia may be hereditary (the usual progressive loss of scalp hair in men); it may be due to disease or injury, or it can occur in old age. *Alopecia areata* is a condition of unknown origin in which hair falls out in patches.

脫髮 在正常生髮區無髮。可爲遺傳性（一般爲男性進行性頭皮脫髮），可爲疾病或損傷所致，或發生於老年。斑禿指未明原因的成片脫髮。

aloxiprin *n.* a compound made from aluminium oxide and *aspirin. Its actions and uses are similar to those of aspirin, but it is said to be more stable and less liable to cause irritation and bleeding of the stomach.

氧化鋁縮乙醯水楊酸 氧化鋁與阿司匹林的化合物，作用與用途類同阿司匹林，據說較穩定，且引起胃刺激或出血的傾向較小。

alpha-fetoprotein (afp) *n.* a protein formed in the liver of the fetus and present in the *amniotic fluid in small amounts. In *anencephaly and *spina bifida the amount of afp in the fluid is greatly increased in the first six months of pregnancy, and this can be detected by *amniocentesis. As there is a 1 in 20 chance of recurrence after one child with these defects and a 1 in 10 chance or higher after two affected babies, amniocentesis early in the second trimester of the next pregnancy is advisable, with a view to termination if the afp level is abnormally high.

甲胎蛋白 胎兒肝臟形成的一種蛋白，在羊水中含有少量。胎兒如爲無腦〔畸形〕和脊柱裂，在妊娠開始的6個月內羊水甲胎蛋白明顯增加，因而可藉羊膜穿刺術檢定。如一個嬰兒出現上述畸形，則再次妊娠有1/20的機會再發；如連續兩胎罹及，則再發的機會爲1/10以上，應在下次妊娠的第三個月至第六個月內早期行羊膜穿刺術，一旦發現甲胎蛋白異常增加即終止妊娠。

alprenolol *n.* a drug used to treat arrhythmia and angina of the heart and to reduce high blood pressure (*see* beta blocker). Its actions and uses are similar

烯丙心安 一種治療心律不齊、心絞痛並降壓的藥。作用與用途類似萘心安，且較少影響呼吸功能。

to those of *propranolol, but it is less likely to affect respiratory function.

ALS **1.** *see* antilymphocytic serum. **2.** amyotrophic lateral sclerosis. *See* motor neurone disease.

①**抗淋巴細胞血清** ②**肌萎縮性〔脊髓〕側索硬化**

altitude sickness (mountain sickness) the condition that results from unaccustomed exposure to a high altitude (4500 m or more above sea level). Reduced atmospheric pressure and shortage of oxygen cause deep rapid breathing (*hyperventilation), which lowers the concentration of carbon dioxide in the blood (*see* alkalosis). Symptoms include nausea, exhaustion, and anxiety. In severe cases there may be acute shortness of breath due to fluid collecting in the lungs (pulmonary *oedema), which requires treatment by diuretics and return to a lower altitude.

高山病　不能適應高原（海拔 4500 米或其上）引起的一種疾病。低氣壓、缺氧可致深而快速的呼吸（換氣過度），以降低血液中二氧化碳的濃度。症狀有噁心、衰竭、焦慮。嚴重者可因肺水腫而致呼吸短促，需用利尿藥治療並回到海拔較低的地區去。

aluminium hydroxide a safe slow-acting antacid and *laxative. It is administered by mouth as a gel in the treatment of indigestion, gastric and duodenal ulcers, and reflux *oesophagitis.

氫氧化鋁　一種安全和作用緩慢的抗酸藥和緩瀉藥，口服。其凝膠用於治療消化不良、胃和十二指腸潰瘍，以及返流性食管炎。

alveolitis *n.* inflammation of an *alveolus or alveoli. Chronic inflammation of the walls of the lung alveoli is usually caused by inhaled inorganic dusts (*see* pneumoconiosis) or organic dusts (*see* farmer's lung). It is sometimes associated with rheumatoid arthritis or systemic sclerosis. The condition progresses slowly to the state of fibrosis, emphysema, and bronchiectasis known as *honeycomb lung*. Alveolitis can be controlled with corticosteroid therapy.

肺泡炎　肺泡的炎症。肺泡壁慢性炎症常因吸入無機塵或有機塵所致。有時與類風濕性關節炎或全身性硬化病相伴隨。本病可緩慢發展爲纖維變性、氣腫、支氣管擴張即蜂窩狀肺。治療：使用皮質類甾醇。

alveolus *n.* (*pl.* **alveoli**) **1.** (in the *lung) a blind-ended air sac of microscopic size. About 30 alveoli open out of each *alveolar duct*, which leads from a respiratory *bronchiole. The *alveolar walls*, which separate alveoli, contain capillaries. The alveoli are lined by a single layer of *pneumocytes, which thus

①**肺泡**　肺內的一種具盲端的微小的含氣囊。每一個從呼吸性細支氣管延伸而成的肺泡管中約有 30 個肺泡開口。將肺泡分隔開的肺泡壁中含有毛細血管。肺泡只有一層肺細胞，因此在空氣和血液之

form a very thin layer between air and blood so that exchange of oxygen and carbon dioxide is normally rapid and complete. Children are born with about 20 million alveoli. The adult number of about 300 million is reached around the age of eight. **2.** the part of the upper or lower jawbone that supports the roots of the teeth (*see also* mandible, maxilla). After tooth extraction it is largely absorbed. **3.** the sac of a *racemose gland (*see also* acinus). **4.** any other small cavity, depression, or sac. —**alveolar** *adj.*

間衹有極薄的一層，正常時氧氣與二氧化碳的交換迅速而完全。兒童出生時有小泡 2000 萬個，至 8 歲時可達 30000 萬個左右。 ②**齒槽**　上、下頜支持牙根的部位。拔牙後齒槽可有明顯吸收。 ③**葡萄狀腺**　④任何一種小腔、陷窩、囊腔。

alveus *n.* a cavity, groove, or canal. The *alveus hippocampi* is the bundle of nerve fibres in the brain forming a depression in which the hippocampus lies.

槽　一種腔，溝，道。海馬槽指大腦的一束纖維形成的凹陷，海馬即位於該處。

Alzheimer's disease a progressive form of *dementia occurring in middle age, for which there is no treatment. It is associated with diffuse degeneration of the brain. *Compare* Pick's disease.

阿爾茨海默氏病，早老性痴呆　一種發生於中年的進行性痴呆，尙無療法。本病發生於大腦瀰漫性變性。

amalgam *n.* any of a group of alloys containing mercury. In dentistry amalgam fillings are made by mixing a silver-tin alloy with mercury.

汞齊　一種含汞的合金。牙科汞齊塡料用銀-錫與汞的合金製成。

Amanita *n.* a genus of fungi that contains several species of poisonous toadstools, including *A. phalloides* (death cap), *A. pantherina* (panther cap), and *A. muscaria* (fly agaric). They produce toxins that cause abdominal pain, violent vomiting, and continuous diarrhoea. In the absence of treatment death occurs in approximately 50% of cases, due to severe liver damage.

捕蠅蕈屬　眞菌類的一屬，其中有數種毒菌，包括條蕈（死亡帽子），瓢蕈（黑豹帽子），捕蠅蕈（蠅蘑菇）。所產生的毒素可致腹痛，劇吐，以及持續腹瀉。如不治療半數病例因肝臟受損死亡。

amantadine *n.* an antiviral drug that probably acts by preventing the penetration of the virus into the host cell. It is used in the treatment of influenza infections and parkinsonism. Common side-effects include nervousness, loss of muscular coordination, and insomnia. Trade name: **Symmetrel**.

金剛烷胺　一種抗病毒藥，其作用可能爲防止病毒穿入宿主細胞。用於治療流感和帕金森氏病。常見副作用包括神經質、肌肉共濟失調以及失眠。

amaurosis *n.* partial or complete blindness. For example, *amaurosis fugax* is a condition in which loss of vision is transient. —**amaurotic** *adj.*

黑朦 部分盲或全盲。例如，一時性黑朦爲短暫失明的狀態。

amaurotic familial idiocy *see* Tay-Sachs disease.

家族黑朦性癡獃

ambivalence *n.* (in psychology) the condition of holding opposite feelings (such as love and hate) for the same person or object. Excessive and prevalent ambivalence was thought by Bleuler to be a feature of schizophrenia.

矛盾症 在心理學上指對同一人或物具有相反的兩種感情（如愛和恨）。Bleuler 認爲嚴重矛盾症爲精神分裂症的表現。

Amblyomma *n.* a genus of hard *ticks, several species of which are responsible for transmitting tick *typhus. The bite of this tick can also give rise to a serious and sometimes fatal paralysis.

鈍緣蜱屬 硬蜱的一屬，其中有些種確認可傳播斑疹傷寒。蜱刺咬可引起嚴重甚至致命的麻痺。

amblyopia *n.* poor sight, not due to any detectable disease of the eyeball or visual system. In practice this strict definition is not always obeyed. For example, in *toxic amblyopia*, caused by tobacco, alcohol, certain other drugs, and vitamin deficiency, there is a disorder of the *optic nerve. The commonest type is *amblyopia ex anopsia*, in which factors such as squint (*see* strabismus), cataract, and other abnormalities of the optics of the eye (*see* refraction) impair its normal use in early childhood by preventing the formation of a clear image on the retina.

弱視 非由可查及的眼球或視力系統疾病所致的視力低下。在實踐中上述嚴格定義亦可變動。例如：由於煙草、酒精、某些藥品中毒和缺乏維生素引起的弱視，就有視神經損傷。最常見的一型是廢用性弱視，本型的致病因素有斜視、白內障及眼視力的其他異常，由於這些因素阻礙視網膜的清晰成像，故在孩提時即可影響視力。

amblyoscope (orthoptoscope, synoptophore) *n.* an instrument for measuring the angle of a squint and assessing the degree to which a person uses both eyes together. It consists of two L-shaped tubes, the short arms of which are joined by a hinge so that the long arms point away from each other. The subject looks into the short end and each eye sees, via a system of mirrors and lenses, a different picture, which is placed at the other end of each tube. If a squint is present, the tubes may be adjusted so that the short arms line up with the direction of each eye.

同視鏡 測量斜視角度並評定一個人雙眼視物時斜視程度的儀器。該儀器由兩個 L 形管組成，L 的短臂靠鉸鏈相連，長臂則可彼此分開。通過一組反光鏡和透鏡自短臂端觀看置於長臂端的目標，各眼可見不同圖像。如有斜視，則可調節短臂以使之與每隻眼的視線方向一致。

ambutonium *n.* a drug with actions similar to those of *atropine. It is given by mouth to treat indigestion and peptic ulcer.

胺苯丁銨 一種作用類同阿托品的藥。口服，用於治療消化不良和消化性潰瘍。

amelia *n.* congenital total absence of the arms or legs due to a developmental defect. It is one of the fetal abnormalities induced by the drug *thalidomide taken early in pregnancy. *See also* phocomelia.

無肢〔畸形〕 發育缺陷所致的先天性臂或腿全缺。爲畸胎的一種，是因妊娠早期服用肽胺哌啶酮的結果。

ameloblast *n.* a cell that forms the enamel of a tooth and disappears before tooth eruption.

成釉細胞 一種形成牙齒釉質的細胞，在牙萌出前消失。

ameloblastoma *n.* a locally malignant tumour in the jaw. It is considered to develop from ameloblasts although it does not contain enamel. The term *adamantinoma*, formerly used for this tumour, is now no longer in use as it suggests (incorrectly) a growth that is as hard as enamel.

成釉細胞瘤 頜局部的惡性腫瘤。雖不含釉質，但人們認爲是由成釉細胞發展而來。釉質上皮瘤一詞過去即指此種腫瘤，但現不再使用，因此詞泛指任何部位的硬如釉質的腫瘤。

amelogenesis *n.* the formation of enamel by *ameloblasts, which is completed before tooth eruption. *Amelogenesis imperfecta* is a hereditary condition in which enamel formation is disturbed. The teeth have an unusual surface but are not more prone to decay.

釉質發生 由成釉細胞形成釉質的過程。在牙萌出前完成。釉質生長不全爲遺傳疾病，本病發生是因爲釉質形成受阻。牙齒表面異常，但齲變率並不高於正常者。

amenorrhoea *n.* the absence or stopping of the menstrual periods. It is normal for the periods to be absent before puberty, during pregnancy and milk secretion, and after the end of the reproductive period (*see* menopause). In *primary amenorrhoea* the menstrual periods fail to appear at puberty, often because of a congenital defect (e.g. *Turner's syndrome). In *secondary amenorrhoea* the menstrual periods stop after establishment at puberty, for a great variety of reasons including disorders of the hypothalamus (a part of the brain), deficiency of ovarian hormone, *pituitary or thyroid gland deficiency, diabetes, mental disturbance, depression, anorexia nervosa, change of

經閉 無或停經。在青春期以前、妊娠期、泌乳期和育齡結束後無或停經係屬正常。原發性經閉表現爲青春期不能行經，常因先天性缺陷所致（例如：特納氏綜合徵）。繼發性經閉係在青春期已有排經後經期中止，病因多樣，包括下丘腦（大腦的一部分）疾患、卵巢激素缺乏、垂體或甲狀腺功能缺陷、糖尿病、精神障礙、抑鬱症、神經性食慾缺乏、環境改變、子宮或卵巢切除等。

surroundings, and removal of the womb or ovaries.

amentia *n.* failure of development of the intellectual faculties. *See* subnormality.

智力缺陷 智力發育障礙。

amethocaine *n.* a potent local anaesthetic. It is applied to skin or mucous membranes for eye, ear, nose and throat surgery, but it has also been employed for *spinal anaesthesia.

丁卡因 强力局部麻醉藥。用於眼、耳、鼻、喉外科的皮膚或黏膜的麻醉，亦用於脊髓麻醉。

ametropia *n.* any abnormality of *refraction of the eye, resulting in blurring of the image formed on the retina. *See* astigmatism, hypermetropia, myopia. *Compare* emmetropia.

屈光不正 眼的任何一種折射異常，結果使視網膜成像模糊。

amiloride *n.* a *diuretic that causes the increased excretion of sodium and chloride. It may produce dizziness and weakness and its continued use may lead to an excessive concentration of potassium in the blood. Trade name: **Midamor**.

氨氯吡咪 增加鈉、氯排出的利尿藥。可產生眩暈、衰弱，長期服用可致血鉀濃度過高。

aminacrine *n.* an antiseptic with the same actions and uses as *acriflavine. Unlike acriflavine, it does not cause staining.

氨基吖啶 殺菌消毒藥，作用同吖啶黃，與吖啶黃的不同處是不致黃染。

amino acid an organic compound containing an amino group ($-NH_2$) and a carboxyl group ($-COOH$). Amino acids are fundamental constituents of all *proteins. Breakdown of proteins found in the body yields the following amino acids: alanine, arginine, asparagine, aspartic acid, cysteine, cystine, glutamic acid, glutamine, glycine, histidine, isoleucine, leucine, lysine, methionine, phenylalanine, proline, serine, threonine, tryptophan, tyrosine, and valine. Some of these amino acids can be synthesized by the body; others, the *essential amino acids, must be obtained from protein in the diet. Certain amino acids present in the body are not found in proteins; these include *citrul-

氨基酸 含有一個氨基和一個羧基的有機化合物。氨基酸是蛋白質的基本成分。人體內蛋白質分解可產生下列氨基酸：丙氨酸、精氨酸、天門冬醯胺、天門冬氨酸、半胱氨酸、胱氨酸、穀氨酸、穀醯胺、甘氨酸、組氨酸、異亮氨酸、亮氨酸、賴氨酸、蛋氨酸、苯丙氨酸、脯氨酸、絲氨酸、蘇氨酸、色氨酸、酪氨酸、纈氨酸。上述氨基酸有些可在體內合成；其他必需氨基酸則攝自食物中的蛋白質。有些氨基酸在人體存在，但在蛋白質中找不到，

line, *ornithine, *taurine, and *gamma-aminobutyric acid.

包括瓜氨酸、鳥氨酸、牛磺酸、γ-氨酪酸。

aminobenzoic acid *see* para-aminobenzoic acid.

氨基苯甲酸

aminoglutethimide *n.* a drug used in the treatment of advanced breast cancer. It inhibits synthesis of adrenal steroids (medical adrenalectomy) and the peripheral conversion of androgens to oestrogens. It is administered by mouth, usually with corticosteroid replacement therapy. Side-effects, which are largely dose-related, include drowsiness, dizziness, and a transient skin rash. Trade name: **Orimeten**.

氨基乙哌啶酮 用於治療晚期乳腺癌的藥物。可抑制腎上腺甾類的合成（藥物性腎上腺切除術），並制止外周的雄激素轉化爲雌激素。口服，通常在行皮質類甾醇代替療法時同時使用。副作用與大劑量使用有關，包括嗜眠、眩暈、以及短暫皮疹。商品名：氨基導眠能。

aminophylline *n.* a drug that relaxes smooth muscle and stimulates respiration. It is widely used to dilate the air passages in the treatment of asthma and emphysema, to dilate the coronary arteries in angina pectoris, and as a *diuretic, particularly in cases of *oedema. Administered by injection or in suppositories, it may cause nausea, vomiting, dizziness, and fast heart rate. *See also* theophylline.

氨茶鹼 一種可鬆弛平滑肌並刺激呼吸的藥。廣泛用於擴張氣管以治療哮喘和肺氣腫，用於擴張冠狀動脈以治療心絞痛，亦爲利尿劑，尤多用於水腫患者。注射或製成栓劑使用，可致噁心、嘔吐、眩暈和心率加快。

amitosis *n.* division of the nucleus of a cell by a process, not involving *mitosis, in which the nucleus is constricted into two.

無絲分裂 細胞核通過壓縮過程分裂爲二。不含有絲分裂。

amitriptyline *n.* a tricyclic *antidepressant drug that has a mild tranquillizing action. Common side-effects include drowsiness, dizziness, numbness, and tingling of limbs. Trade names: **Elatrol**, **Tryptizol**.

阿米替林 一種具有輕微安定作用的三環結構的抗抑鬱藥。常見副作用有嗜眠、暈眩、痲木及四肢有痲刺感。

amnesia *n.* total or partial loss of memory following physical injury, disease, drugs, or psychological trauma (*see* confabulation, fugue, repression). *Anterograde amnesia* is loss of memory for events following some trauma; *retrograde amnesia* is loss of memory for events preceding the trauma. Some patients experience both types.

遺忘〔症〕，記憶缺失 在身體受傷、患病、用藥或精神創傷後出現的部分或全部記憶缺失。順行性遺忘，指失去對受傷後事物的記憶，逆行性遺忘，指失去對受傷前事物的記憶。有些患者兼有兩型。

amniocentesis *n.* withdrawal of a sample of the fluid (amniotic fluid) surrounding an embryo in the womb by piercing the amniotic sac through the abdominal wall. As the amniotic fluid contains cells from the embryo (mostly shed from the skin), cell cultures enable chromosome patterns to be studied so that *prenatal diagnosis of chromosomal abnormalities (such as *Down's syndrome) can be made. Metabolic errors and other diseases, such as *spina bifida, can also be diagnosed prenatally from the biochemistry of the cells or that of the fluid (*see* alpha-fetoprotein). Although the risks of amniocentesis, in skilled hands, are extremely low, there is no point in undertaking it unless the parents agree to a termination of the pregnancy if a serious abnormality is discovered. The tests must be completed by the 16th week.
Amniocentesis can also be used in the later weeks of pregnancy to assess the severity of fetal (Rh) haemolytic disease and, by measuring lecithin compounds, the risk of the baby developing the *respiratory distress syndrome.

羊膜穿刺術 針穿腹壁進入子宮羊膜腔內抽取胎兒周圍的液體（羊水）標本。羊水含有胚胎細胞（大多自胚胎皮膚脫落），經培養即能識別染色體模式，於是可在產前診斷染色體異常。新陳代謝障礙及脊椎裂等疾病，亦可通過細胞或液體的生化檢查行產前診斷。雖然在技術熟練者行羊膜穿刺術危險性很小，但除非在夫婦雙方同意一旦發現異常即中止妊娠的情況下才能採用本法。本術務於16周以前進行。
羊膜穿刺術亦在妊娠較後的幾週內進行。目的在於估測胎兒（Rh）溶血疾病的嚴重性。通過對卵磷脂化合物的檢查亦可估測嬰兒發生呼吸窘迫綜合徵的危險性。

amniography *n.* the making of X-ray pictures (*amniograms*) of the amniotic sac, which enables the placenta and umbilical cord to be visualized.

羊膜造影術 拍攝羊膜腔X線片（羊膜片）的技術。本術可使胎盤和臍帶顯影。

amnion *n.* the membrane that forms initially over the dorsal part of the embryo but soon expands to enclose it completely within the *amniotic cavity. It expands outwards and fuses with the chorion, obliterating virtually all the intervening cavity. The double membrane (*amniochorion*) normally ruptures at birth. —**amniotic** *adj.*

羊膜 開始時覆蓋胚胎背部的膜，不久即擴展爲羊膜腔，將胚胎整個包圍在內。其外伸部分與絨毛膜融合，兩者之間的腔不復存在。該雙層膜（羊膜絨毛膜）正常時在分娩時破裂。

amnioscopy *n.* examination of the inside of the amniotic sac by means of an instrument (*amnioscope*) that is passed through the abdominal wall. This allows the developing infant

羊膜鏡檢術 用羊膜鏡通過腹壁穿刺以檢查羊膜腔內部。可直接觀察羊膜腔內胎兒發育狀態。子宮頸羊膜鏡檢術是在妊娠晚期

within the cavity to be viewed directly. *Cervical amnioscopy*, performed late in pregnancy, enables the amniotic sac to be inspected through the neck of the womb, using a different instrument. When transilluminated, its fluid volume can be appraised without puncture and any meconium observed.

使用另一種器械通過子宮頸檢查羊膜腔。使用透照法則無需穿刺和觀察胎糞即可估測羊水量。

amniotic cavity the fluid-filled cavity between the embryo and the *amnion. It forms initially within the inner cell mass of the *blastocyst and later expands over the back of the embryo, eventually enclosing it completely. *See also* amniotic fluid.

羊膜腔 胎兒與羊膜之間充滿液體的腔隙。最初由胚胎內層細胞團形成，繼而在胎兒背部延伸擴大，最後包圍整個胎兒。

amniotic fluid the fluid contained within the *amniotic cavity. It surrounds the growing fetus, protecting it from external pressure. The fluid is initially secreted from the *amnion and is later supplemented by urine from the fetal kidneys. Some of the fluid is swallowed by the fetus and absorbed through its intestine. *See also* amniocentesis.

羊水 羊膜腔內的液體。包繞生長中的胎兒，保護胎兒免遭外界壓力。本液最初由羊膜分泌，其後則由胎兒腎臟排出的尿液補充。有些羊水被胎兒吞下並被其腸道吸收。

amniotomy *n.* the artificial puncturing of the membranes surrounding the baby in the womb by means of a special instrument (*amniotome*). Labour generally follows naturally, but in some cases it must be started artificially by additional measures.

羊膜刺破術 以特製器械（羊膜穿破器）人工穿破子宮內包繞嬰兒的膜。破膜後通常自然分娩。有時需人工破膜促使胎兒娩出。

amodiaquine *n.* an antimalarial drug with effects and uses similar to those of *chloroquine. It has also been used for the treatment of lupus erythematosus, leprosy, and rheumatoid arthritis. Doses used to treat malaria have almost no side-effects, but prolonged use may cause blue-grey deposits on the cornea of the eye, fingernails, and hard palate.

氨酚喹 功效與用法類同氯喹的一種抗瘧藥。亦曾用於治療紅斑性狼瘡、麻瘋和類風濕性關節炎。治療瘧疾的用量幾無副作用，但長期使用可在眼角膜、指甲及硬顎上出現藍灰色沉積。

amoeba *n.* (*pl.* **amoebae**) any single-celled microscopic animal of jelly-like consistency and irregular and constantly changing shape. Found in water, soil and other damp environ-

阿米巴 一種呈膠凍樣稠度、體形不規則且不斷變形的單細胞動物。在水、土壤以其他潮濕環境可查見，其活動和進食依賴可

ments, they move and feed by means of flowing extensions of the body (*see* pseudopodium). Some amoebae cause disease in man (*see* Entamoeba). *See also* Protozoa. —**amoebic** *adj.*

流動擴展的身體。有些阿米巴在人體致病。

amoebiasis *n. see* dysentery.

阿米巴病

amoebocyte *n.* a cell that moves by sending out processes of its protoplasm in the same way as an amoeba.

阿米巴樣細胞 靠原生質伸出突起進行活動的細胞。其活動方式與阿米巴一樣。

amoeboma *n.* a tumour that occurs in the rectum or caecum of the large intestine and is caused by the parasite **Entamoeba histolytica*, a protozoan that invades and destroys the walls of the gut. Tumours may ulcerate and become infected with pus-forming (pyogenic) bacteria, causing severe inflammation of the bowel wall. The tumours usually harden and may even obstruct the bowel.

阿米巴瘤 因溶組織內阿米巴寄生而發生於直腸或盲腸的腫瘤。是該種原生動物侵入並損害腸壁所致。腫瘤可成爲潰瘍並被化膿菌感染，在腸壁形成嚴重炎症。腫瘤堅硬，甚至阻塞腸道。

amok *n.* a sudden outburst of furious and murderous aggression, directed indiscriminately at everybody in the vicinity. It is encountered only in certain cultures, such as that of the Malays.

殺人狂 突然爆發的狂怒和殺人行爲。患者無選擇地傷害附近的任何人。本病僅發生在某些民族或種族，如馬來人。

AMP (adenosine monophosphate) a compound containing adenine, ribose, and one phosphate group. AMP occurs in cells and is involved in processes requiring the transfer of energy (*see* ATP).

一磷酸腺苷 一種含有腺嘌呤、核糖和一個磷酸基的化合物。見於細胞內，起供能作用。

ampere *n.* the basic *SI unit of electric current. It is equal to the current flowing through a conductor of resistance 1 ohm when a potential difference of 1 volt is applied between its ends. The formal definition of the ampere is the current that when passed through two parallel conductors of infinite length and negligible cross section, placed 1 metre apart in a vacuum, produces a force of 2×10^{-7} newton per square metre between them. Symbol: A.

安培 電流的基本國際單位。指電動勢爲 1 伏特時，通過電阻爲 1 歐姆的電流。正式的定義是：在眞空中兩條相距爲 1 米的無限長的平行導線（其圓截面略而不計）之間產生每平方米 2×10^{7} 牛頓的力所需的電流强度。

amphetamine *n.* a *sympathomimetic drug that has a marked stimulant action on the central nervous system. It alleviates fatigue and produces a feeling of mental alertness and well-being. The drug has been used in the treatment of *narcolepsy, mild depressive neuroses, and obesity. It is administered by mouth; side-effects include insomnia and restlessness. *Tolerance of amphetamine develops rapidly, and prolonged use may lead to *dependence.

苯丙胺 一種對中樞神經系統具有顯著興奮作用的擬交感神經藥。可減輕疲勞，使思維敏銳和情緒愉快。用於治療發作性睡病、輕度抑鬱性神經官能症、肥胖病。口服；副作用有失眠和煩躁不安。本藥耐藥性發展迅速，長期服用可產生賴藥性。

amphiarthrosis *n.* a slightly movable joint in which the bony surfaces are separated by fibrocartilage (*see* symphysis) or hyaline cartilage (*see* synchondrosis).

微動關節 只能作輕微活動的關節。骨面之間只有纖維軟骨或透明軟骨。

amphoric breath sounds *see* breath sounds.

空甕性呼吸音

amphotericin *n.* an *antibiotic, derived from the bacterium *Streptomyces griseus*, used to treat deep-seated fungal infections; it is inactive against bacteria and viruses. It can be administered by mouth, but is usually given by intravenous injection. Common side-effects include headache, fever, muscle pains, and diarrhoea. In some cases kidney damage may occur.

兩性黴素 自灰色鏈黴菌獲取的一種抗生素。用於治療內臟的黴菌感染，對細菌、病毒無效。可口服，但通常以靜脈注射給藥。常見副作用有頭痛、發熱、肌肉痛、腹瀉。在一些病例可發生腎損傷。

ampicillin *n.* an *antibiotic used to treat a variety of infections, including those of the urinary, respiratory, biliary, and intestinal tracts. It is inactivated by *penicillinase and therefore cannot be used against organisms producing this enzyme. It is given by mouth or injection; side-effects include nausea, vomiting, and diarrhoea, and some allergic reactions may occur. Trade names: **Amcill**, **Penbritin**, **Polycillin**, **Principen**.

氨芐青黴素 一種用於治療多種感染，包括泌尿道、呼吸道、膽道、腸道感染的抗生素。青黴素酶可使其滅活，因而不能殺滅產生此酶的微生物。口服或注射用；副作用有噁心、嘔吐、腹瀉，亦可發生一些過敏反應。

ampoule (ampule) *n.* a sealed glass or plastic capsule containing one dose of a drug in the form of a sterile solution for injection.

安瓿 封口的玻璃或塑料小瓶，內含供一次注射用的溶於無菌液體的藥物。

ampulla *n.* (*pl.* **ampullae**) an enlarged or dilated ending of a tube or canal.

壺腹 管道膨大或擴張的一端。內耳半規管膨大為

The semicircular canals of the inner ear are expanded into ampullae at the point where they join the vestibule. The *ampulla of Vater* is the dilated part of the common bile duct where it is joined by the pancreatic duct.

壺腹並與前庭相滙合。法特氏壺腹為總膽管的膨大部分並在該處與胰管相滙合。

amputation *n.* the removal of a limb, part of a limb, or any other portion of the body (such as a breast). The term is customarily modified by an adjective showing the particular type of amputation. Once a common operation in surgery, it is now usually performed only in cases of severe injury to limbs or, particularly in elderly people, when circulation to a limb is inadequate and gangrene develops. In planning an amputation the surgeon takes account of the patient's work and the type of artificial part (prothesis) that will be fitted.

切斷術 切除整肢或部分肢體，或切除身體任何部分（如一側乳房）。本詞習慣用法是前加定語以表明特定型的切斷術。本術過去是常用的外科手術，現只在肢體嚴重損傷或肢體血流不暢而發生壞疽者（尤指老年人）才施行。制訂切斷術方案時外科醫生應考慮病人的工作以及裝配假肢的類型。

amygdala (amygdaloid nucleus) *n.* one of the *basal ganglia: a roughly almond-shaped mass of grey matter deep inside each cerebral hemisphere. It has extensive connections with the olfactory system and sends fibres to the hypothalamus; its functions are apparently concerned with mood, feeling, instinct, and possibly memory for recent events.

杏仁核 基底神經節之一：大腦兩半球深部處兩側各一的杏仁形的灰質團塊。與嗅覺系統有廣泛聯係，並發出纖維至下丘腦；其功能與情緒、感覺、本能明顯有關，並可能影響對近事的記憶。

amylase *n.* an enzyme that occurs in saliva and pancreatic juice and aids the digestion of starch, which it breaks down into glucose, maltose, and dextrins. Amylase will also hydrolyse *glycogen to yield glucose, maltose, and dextrins.

澱粉酶 存在於唾液和胰液中的消化澱粉的一種酶，使其分解為葡萄糖、麥芽糖和糊精。澱粉酶亦可水解糖原產生葡萄糖、麥芽糖和糊精。

amyl nitrite a drug that relaxes smooth muscle, especially that of blood vessels. Given by inhalation, amyl nitrite is used mainly in the treatment of angina pectoris. It is rapidly absorbed and acts quickly, producing a fall in arterial blood pressure. Side-effects include flushing, faintness, and headache. High doses may cause restlessness,

亞硝酸〔異〕戊酯 一種平滑肌鬆弛藥，尤適用於血管。吸入給藥，主要用於治療心絞痛。吸收及作用迅速，可降動脈壓。副作用有顏面潮紅、暈厥、頭痛。大劑量可致煩躁不安、嘔吐以及皮膚藍染。

vomiting, and blue coloration of the skin.

amylobarbitone *n.* an intermediate-acting *barbiturate, administered by mouth as a *hypnotic in the treatment of insomnia, as a preoperative sedative, and to treat for anxiety. It is also injected intravenously to produce mental relaxation before psychoanalysis. Prolonged use may lead to *dependence and overdosage has serious toxic effects (*see* barbiturism). Trade names: **Amytal, Amobarbital**.

異戊巴比妥 一種中效的巴比妥類，口服，用於失眠症的催眠、術前鎮靜、以及焦慮的治療。精神分析前靜脉注入以使精神放鬆。長期使用可產生賴藥性，過量則有嚴重毒性作用。

amyloid *n.* a *glycoprotein, resembling starch, that is deposited in the internal organs in amyloidosis.

澱粉樣蛋白 一種類似澱粉的糖蛋白，沉積在澱粉樣變性患者內部器官中。

amyloidosis *n.* infiltration of the liver, kidneys, spleen, and other tissues with amyloid, a starchlike substance. In *primary amyloidosis* the disorder arises without any apparent cause; *secondary amyloidosis* occurs as a late complication of such chronic infections as tuberculosis or leprosy and also in *Hodgkin's disease. Amyloidosis is also very common in the genetic disease familial Mediterranean fever (*see* polyserositis).

澱粉樣變性 肝、腎、脾和其他組織的澱粉樣蛋白（一種類同澱粉物質）的浸潤。原發性澱粉樣變性的起病無明顯原因，繼發性澱粉樣變性爲某些慢性疾患的後期合併症，諸如結核、麻瘋以及何傑金氏病。在遺傳性疾病家族性地中海熱亦常見澱粉樣變性。

amylopectin *n.* *see* starch.

枝鏈澱粉

amylose *n.* *see* starch.

直鏈澱粉

amyotonia congenita (floppy baby syndrome) a disorder, present at birth, in which the child's muscles are weak and floppy. A gradual spontaneous improvement occurs and the child's progress is thereafter normal. It must be distinguished from the hypotonic form of *cerebral palsy, infantile *motor neurone disease, and congenital myopathy, which are usually progressive.

先天性肌弛緩（鬆軟嬰兒綜合徵） 出生時即存在的幼兒肌肉無力且鬆軟的一種疾病。病情可逐漸自行改善，進而幼兒發育正常。需與肌弛緩型的大腦麻痺、運動神經元病、先天性肌病等相鑑別。這類疾病往往是進行性的。

amyotrophy *n.* a progressive loss of muscle bulk associated with weakness of these muscles. It is caused by disease of the nerve that activates the affected muscle. Amyotrophy is a feature of any

肌萎縮 肌肉進行性萎縮並伴發軟弱無力。係由於支配患病肌肉的神經發生病變所致。肌萎縮可見於種種慢性神經疾患，並且

chronic *neuropathy and it may be the most prominent neurological symptom of diabetes mellitus and meningovascular syphilis. A combination of amyotrophy and spasticity characterizes *motor neurone disease.

可能是糖尿病和腦膜血管梅毒的最明顯的神經系統症狀。肌萎縮併發痙攣是運動神經元病的特徵。

an- *prefix. see* a-.

〔前綴〕**無，缺，不**

anabolic *adj.* promoting tissue growth by increasing the metabolic processes involved in protein synthesis. Anabolic agents are usually synthetic male sex hormones (*see* androgen); they include *ethyloestrenol, *methandienone, nandrolone, norethandrolone, oxymesterone, and stanolone. They are used to help weight gain in underweight patients, such as the elderly and those with serious illnesses, and to strengthen the bones in osteoporosis. Some anabolic steroids cause virilization in women and liver damage.

組織代謝的 增進蛋白質合成代謝以促進組織生長的。組成代謝劑通常爲人工合成的雄激素，包括乙基雌烯醇、去氫甲睾酮、諾龍、乙諾酮、羥甲睾酮和雙氫睾酮。這些藥可爲年老或重病患者等體重不足者增長體重，或骨質疏鬆症患者增强骨質等。某些組成代謝類甾醇可致婦女男性化和損傷肝臟。

anabolism *n.* the synthesis of complex molecules, such as proteins and fats, from simpler ones by living things. *See also* anabolic, metabolism.

組成代謝 生物將較簡單分子合成爲如蛋白質和脂肪之類複雜分子的過程。

anacidity *n.* a deficiency or abnormal absence of acid in the body fluids.

酸缺乏 體液內酸不足或異常地缺乏。

anacrotism *n.* the condition in which there is an abnormal curve in the ascending line of a pulse tracing. It may be seen in cases of aortic stenosis. —**anacrotic** *adj.*

升線一波脉 在脉搏曲線升肢上有一異常凹陷的現象。可見於主動脉狹窄病例。

anaemia *n.* a reduction in the quantity of the oxygen-carrying pigment *haemoglobin in the blood. The main symptoms are excessive tiredness and fatiguability, breathlessness on exertion, pallor, and poor resistance to infection. There are many causes of anaemia. It may be due to loss of blood (*haemorrhagic anaemia*), resulting from an accident, operation, etc., or from chronic bleeding, as from an ulcer or haemorrhoids. *Iron-deficiency anaemia* results from lack of iron, which is necessary for the production of haemoglobin (*see* sideropenia). *Haemolytic anaemias* re-

貧血 血內載氧色素血紅蛋白數量低下。主要症狀爲極度怠倦和疲勞，動輒氣喘，臉色蒼白，抗感染力弱等等。貧血原因很多，可能因意外傷害、手術等而失血，或因潰瘍、痔瘡等慢性出血等等（出血性貧血）。缺鐵性貧血是因缺乏造血紅蛋白必不可少的鐵而引起。溶血性貧血則由於大量（含有血色素的）紅細胞遭到破壞。這類貧血可能因化學毒品、自體免疫、寄生蟲

sult from the increased destruction of red blood cells (which contain the pigment). This can be caused by toxic chemicals; *autoimmunity; the action of parasites, especially in *malaria; or conditions such as *thalassaemia and *sickle-cell disease, associated with abnormal forms of haemoglobin, or *spherocytosis, which is associated with abnormal red blood cells. (*See also* haemolytic disease of the newborn.) Anaemia can also be caused by the impaired production of red blood cells, as in *leukaemia (when red-cell production in the bone marrow is suppressed) or *pernicious anaemia.
Anaemias can be classified on the basis of the size of the red cells, which may be large (*macrocytic anaemias*), small (*microcytic anaemias*), or normal-sized (*normocytic anaemias*). (*See also* macrocytosis, microcytosis.) The treatment of anaemia depends on the cause. —**anaemic** *adj.*

（尤其是瘧疾）的作用引起，或爲與血紅蛋白異常有關的地中海貧血和鐮狀細胞病，或由於紅細胞造血過程遭受破壞所致，如白血病（骨髓生產紅細胞受阻）或惡性貧血。
貧血可根據紅細胞之大小分類：大的稱爲大紅細胞性貧血，小的稱爲小紅細胞性貧血，正常的稱爲正常紅細胞貧血。治療均依據原因而定。

anaerobe *n.* any organism, especially a microbe, that is able to live and grow in the absence of free oxygen. A *facultative anaerobe* is a microorganism that grows best in the presence of oxygen but is capable of some growth in its absence. An *obligate anaerobe* can grow only in the absence of free oxygen. *Compare* aerobe, microaerophilic.

厭氧菌 能在缺乏游離氧情況下存活並生長的任何微生物（特別是厭氧菌）。兼性厭氧菌最適合於在有氧情況下生長，但缺氧時也能生長。專性厭氧菌僅在缺乏游離氧情況下生長。

anaerobic *adj.* **1.** of or relating to anaerobes. **2.** describing a type of cellular respiration in which foodstuffs (usually carbohydrates) are never completely oxidized because molecular oxygen is not used. *Fermentation is an example of anaerobic respiration.

①**厭氧的** 屬於或關於厭氧菌的。②**乏氧的** 描述細胞呼吸的一種類型。此時由於缺乏分子氧，食物（通常是碳水化合物）不能完全氧化。如發酵。

anaesthesia *n.* loss of feeling or sensation in a part or all of the body. Anaesthesia of a part of the body may occur as a result of injury to or disease of a nerve; for example in leprosy. The term is usually applied, however, to the medical technique of reducing or abol-

①**感覺缺乏** 身體一部分的或全部的感覺或知覺缺失。身體部分感覺缺失可能由於一條神經受傷或患病而引起，例如麻瘋病。②**麻醉法** 本詞通常指手術時減輕或消除患者疼痛

ishing an individual's sensation of pain to enable surgery to be performed. This is effected by administering drugs (*see* anaesthetic) or by the use of other methods, such as *acupuncture or hypnosis.

General anaesthesia is total unconsciousness, usually achieved by administering a combination of injections and gases (the latter are inhaled through a mask). It is induced for such major operations as removal of the stomach or a lung. Recently, anaesthesia has been used in combination with artificial lowering of the body temperature (hypothermia) in certain complex operations, such as cardiac surgery. *Local anaesthesia* abolishes pain in a limited area of the body and is used for minor operations, particularly many dental procedures. It may be achieved by injections of substances such as lignocaine (commonly used in dentistry) close to a local nerve, which deadens the tissues supplied by that nerve. Local anaesthesia may be combined with intravenous sedation. An appropriate injection into the spinal column produces *spinal anaesthesia in the lower limbs or abdomen.

的醫療措施。可以投藥，或使用針刺、催眠等方法以取得麻醉效果。

全身麻醉指神志完全喪失，通常以注射和氣體的聯合投藥而奏效（氣體經面罩吸入）。在施行胃、肺切除等大手術時宜用本法。近來在心臟外科等複雜手術中，麻醉法已與人工降低體溫（低溫）結合使用。局部麻醉是在身體的有限範圍內消除疼痛，用於小手術，尤其用於多種牙科手術中。局部麻醉是在局部神經附近注射利多卡因（牙科常用）之類藥物，使神經所支配的組織麻木。局部麻醉可與靜脉內注射鎮靜劑結合使用。在脊髓適當部位注射麻醉藥可產生下肢或腹部麻醉。

anaesthetic 1. *n.* an agent that reduces or abolishes sensation, affecting either the whole body (*general anaesthetic*) or a particular region (*local anaesthetic*). General anaesthetics, used for surgical procedures, depress activity of the central nervous system, producing loss of consciousness. *Anaesthesia is induced by short-acting *barbiturates (such as thiopentone) and maintained by inhalation anaesthetics (such as *halothane). Local anaesthetics inhibit conduction of impulses in sensory nerves in the region where they are injected or applied; they include *cocaine and *lignocaine. **2.** *adj.* reducing or abolishing sensation.

①**麻醉藥**　可降低或消除全身（全身麻醉）或特定部位（局部麻醉）感覺的藥物。外科手術用的全身麻醉藥可抑制中樞神經活動，使神志喪失。用速效巴比妥類（如硫噴妥鈉）可引起麻醉，用吸入麻醉藥（如氟烷）可維持麻醉。局部麻醉是將麻醉藥在局部注射或外敷，以抑制該部位感覺神經上的衝動的傳導。局部麻醉藥有可卡因等。　②**麻醉的**　降低或消除感覺的。

anaesthetist *n.* a medically qualified doctor who administers an anaesthetic to induce unconsciousness in a patient before a surgical operation.

麻醉師 手術前使用麻醉劑以使患者喪失意識的有行醫資格的醫師。

anákhré *n. see* goundou.

鼻骨增殖性骨膜炎

anal *adj.* of, relating to, or affecting the anus; for example an anal *fissure or an anal *fistula.

肛門的 屬於、關於或患及肛門的。例如，肛門裂，或肛門瘻。

analeptic *n.* a drug that restores consciousness to a patient in a coma or faint; for example, *ethamivan or *nalorphine. Analeptics stimulate the central nervous system to counteract the effects of large doses of narcotic drugs, which depress the central nervous system.

復甦藥，興奮藥 恢復昏迷或暈厥患者神志的藥物。例如香草醯二乙胺，烯丙嗎啡等。復甦藥刺激中樞神經系統，解除大劑量麻醉藥對中樞神經系統起的抑制作用。

analgesia *n.* reduced sensibility to pain, without loss of consciousness and without the sense of touch necessarily being affected. The condition may arise accidentally, if nerves are diseased or damaged, or be induced deliberately by the use of pain-killing drugs (*see* analgesic). Strictly speaking, local *anaesthesia should be called *local analgesia*. *See also* relative analgesia.

痛覺缺失，止痛 痛感降低但不喪失意識。觸覺或可保留。這種情況可在神經性疾患或神經受損時發生，使用止痛藥亦可引起。嚴格來說，局部麻醉應稱爲局部止痛。

analgesic **1.** *n.* a drug that relieves pain. Mild analgesics, such as *aspirin and *paracetamol, are used for the relief of headache, toothache, and mild rheumatic pain. More potent *narcotic analgesics*, such as *morphine and *pethidine, are used only to relieve severe pain since these drugs may produce *dependence and *tolerance. Some analgesics, including aspirin, *ibuprofen, *indomethacin, and *phenylbutazone, also reduce fever and inflammation and are used in rheumatic conditions. **2.** *adj.* relieving pain.

止痛藥，鎮痛藥 解除疼痛的藥物。輕止痛藥如阿司匹林、撲熱息痛等，用於緩解頭痛、牙痛和輕症風濕痛等。較强的麻醉性止痛藥如嗎啡、哌替啶等可產生賴藥性或耐藥性，所以僅用於劇烈疼痛。某些止痛藥包括阿司匹林、布洛芬、消炎痛和保泰松等具解熱消炎作用，可用於風濕性病症。 ②**止痛的**

analogous *adj.* describing organs or parts that have similar functions in different organisms although they do not have the same evolutionary origin or development. *Compare* homologous.

同功器官 在進化起源或發育均不相同的生物體中的功能相似的器官或部位。

analysand *n.* a person undergoing *psychoanalysis.

受精神分析者　接受精神分析的人。

analysis *n.* (in psychology) any means of understanding complex mental processes or experiences. There are several systems of analysis used by different schools of psychology; for example, *psychoanalysis; *transactional analysis*, in which people's relationships are explained in psychoanalytic terms; and *functional analysis*, in which a particular kind of behaviour is thoroughly described with reference to its frequency, its antecedents, and its consequences.

分析　（精神病學）瞭解複雜的心理過程或體驗的一種手段。各家心理學派使用的分析體系有幾種。例如精神分析是以精神分析學派術語解釋人際關係的交談式分析方法，功能分析是參照其發生率、前因及後果，詳盡論述特殊行爲的分析方法。

anamnesis *n.* memory, particularly the recollection by a patient of the symptoms that he noticed at the time when his disease was first contracted.

既往症　患者對其最初發病所注意到的症狀的回憶，尤指追憶。

anankastic *adj.* describing a collection of long-standing personality traits, including stubbornness, meanness, an over-meticulous concern to be accurate in small details, a disposition to check things unnecessarily, severe feelings of insecurity about personal worth, and an excessive tendency to doubt evident facts. *See* personality disorder, obsession.

强迫性人格的　指頑固、自私、過分計較細微末節、不必要地反復檢查做過的事情、嚴重的個人不安全感、對事實疑慮重重等等一系列長期存在的性格特點。

anaphase *n.* the third stage of *mitosis and of each division of *meiosis. In mitosis and anaphase II of meiosis the chromatids separate, becoming daughter chromosomes, and move apart along the spindle fibres towards opposite ends of the cell. In anaphase I of meiosis the pairs of homologous chromosomes separate from each other. *See* disjunction.

後期　有絲分裂和各次減數分裂的第三階段。在有絲分裂和減數分裂後期II時，染色單體分裂，變爲子染色體，並沿紡錘絲移向細胞的兩端。在減數分裂後期I時，成對的同源染色體各自分開。

anaphylaxis *n.* an abnormal reaction to a particular *antigen, in which histamine is released from tissues and causes either local or widespread symptoms. An allergic attack (*see* allergy) is an example of localized anaphylaxis. Rarer, but much more serious, is *anaphylactic shock*: an extreme and gener-

過敏性，過敏症，過敏反應　對特種抗原引起的一種異常反應，該時組胺從組織內釋出，並引起局部或全身症狀。變態反應即爲局部過敏反應的一種，較少見；但更嚴重的是過敏性休克，此時組胺四處

alized allergic reaction in which widespread histamine release causes swelling (oedema), constriction of the bronchioles, heart failure, circulatory collapse, and sometimes death. —**anaphylactic** *adj.*

泛濫造成浮腫、細支氣管狹窄、心力衰竭、循環性虛脫，有時致死。

anaplasia *n.* a loss of normal cell characteristics or differentiation, which may be to such a degree that it is impossible to define the origin of the cells. Anaplasia is typical of malignant tumours.

退行發育，間變 細胞喪失正常或分化特徵的過程，以致無法辨認其來源。退行發育爲惡性腫瘤的特徵。

anasarca *n.* massive swelling of the legs, trunk, and genitalia due to retention of fluid (*oedema): found in congestive heart failure and some forms of renal failure.

全身水腫 見於充血性心力衰竭或某種腎功衰竭的人，因積液而產生下肢、軀幹和陰部等處大面積浮腫。

anastomosis *n.* **1.** (in anatomy) a communication between two blood vessels without any intervening capillary network. *See* arteriovenous anastomosis. **2.** (in surgery) an artificial connection between two tubular organs or parts, especially between two normally separate parts of the intestine. *See also* shunt.

①**吻合支** （解剖學）無毛細血管介入其間的兩血管相通。 ②**吻合術**（外科）在二管狀器官或管形部分，尤指腸的二段正常分離部分之間的人工連接。

anatomy *n.* the study of the structure of living organisms. In medicine it refers to the study of the form and gross structure of the various parts of the human body. The term *morphology* is sometimes used synonymously with anatomy but it is usually used for *comparative anatomy*: the study of differences in form between species. *See also* cytology, histology, physiology. —**anatomical** *adj.* —**anatomist** *n.*

解剖學 研究生物體結構的學科。在醫學上，指對人體各部分的形狀和肉眼可見的結構的研究。有時形態學與解剖學作同義詞用，但形態學通常指比較解剖學，即對不同種系的形態差異進行研究的學科。

anatoxin *n.* a former name for *toxoid.

類毒素 toxoid 的舊稱。

anconeus *n.* a muscle behind the elbow that assists in extending the forearm.

肘〔後〕肌 位於肘之後伸展前臂的肌肉。

Ancylostoma (Ankylostoma) *n.* a genus of small parasitic nematodes (*see* hookworm) that inhabit the small intestine and are widely distributed in Eu-

鈎〔口線〕蟲屬 寄居於小腸的一屬寄生性小線蟲。廣泛分佈於歐、美、亞、非各洲。成蟲以其切齒附

rope, America, Asia, and Africa. The worms suck blood from the gut wall, to which they are attached by means of cutting teeth. Man is the principal and optimum host for *A. duodenale*.

着小腸吮血。人類是適宜其生長的主要宿主。

ancylostomiasis *n.* an infestation of the small intestine by the parasitic hookworm *Ancylostoma duodenale. See* hookworm disease.

鈎〔口線蟲〕病　十二指腸鈎口線蟲在小腸的寄生。

andr- (andro-) *prefix denoting* man or the male sex. Example: *androphobia* (morbid fear of).

〔前綴〕　**男子，雄性**　例如：恐男症（病態的）。

androblastoma (arrhenoblastoma) *n.* a tumour of the ovary, composed of Sertoli cells, Leydig cells, or both. It can produce male or female hormones and may give rise to *masculinization; in children it may cause precocious puberty. Up to 30% of these tumours are malignant, but probably as many as 85% of all cases are cured by surgery alone.

男性細胞瘤　一種卵巢腫瘤。由塞爾托利氏細胞或/和萊迪希氏細胞組成，能產生雄激素或雌激素，導致女性男性化或兒童性早熟。約 30% 爲惡性。85% 的病例單用手術切除即可治癒。

androgen *n.* one of a group of steroid hormones, including *testosterone* and *androsterone*, that stimulate the development of male sex organs and male secondary sexual characteristics (e.g. beard growth, deepening of the voice, and muscle development). The principal source of these hormones is the testis (production being stimulated by *luteinizing hormone) but they are also secreted by the adrenal cortex and ovaries in small amounts. In women excessive production of androgens gives rise to *masculinization.
Naturally occurring and synthetic androgens are used in replacement therapy (to treat such conditions as delayed puberty in adolescent boys, *hypogonadism, and impotence due to testicular insufficiency); as *anabolic agents; and in the treatment of breast cancer. Side-effects include salt and water retention, increased bone growth, and masculinization in women. Androgens should not be used in patients with cancer of

雄激素　刺激男性性器官和第二性徵（鬍鬚生長，聲音變粗和肌肉發育等）發育發生的甾類激素，包括睾丸酮和雄甾酮。主要由睾丸產生，促黃體素刺激其生成。腎上腺皮質和卵巢也分泌小量。婦女產生雄激素過量則引起男性化。
天然或人工合成的雄激素用於替代療法，治療男性青少年青春期延遲、性腺機能不足及由睾丸機能不全引起的陽萎。雄激素並具有蛋白質同化作用，還可治療乳腺癌。副作用有水、鹽瀦留，骨質增生，婦女男性化。前列腺癌患者和孕婦禁用雄激素。

the prostate gland or in pregnant women. —**androgenic** *adj.*

androsterone *n.* a steroid hormone (*see* androgen) that is synthesized and released by the testes and is responsible for controlling male sexual development.

雄甾酮 在睾丸中合成並釋放的一種甾類激素。具有調節雄性性發育的作用。

anencephaly *n.* partial or complete absence of the bones of the rear of the skull and of the cerebral hemispheres of the brain. It occurs as a developmental defect and is not compatible with life for more than a few hours. It is often associated with other defects of the nervous system, such as *spina bifida. Tests for anencephaly can be made early in pregnancy in women from families with a history of the condition (*see* amniocentesis, alpha-fetoprotein).

無腦〔畸形〕 胎兒顱骨後部及大腦半球的全部或部分缺失。是一種先天發育異常，出生後存活不超過數小時。常與神經系統其他發育缺陷如脊柱裂並存。有無腦畸形家族史的孕婦，在妊娠早期進行檢查，可作出無腦畸形的診斷。

anergy *n.* **1.** lack of response to a specific antigen or allergen. **2.** lack of energy. —**anergic** *adj.*

①**無變應性** 對特定抗原或變應原缺乏反應能力。②**無力**

aneuploidy *n.* the condition in which the chromosome number of a cell is not an exact multiple of the normal basic (haploid) number. *See* monosomy, trisomy; *compare* euploidy. —**aneuploid** *adj., n.*

非整倍性 指細胞中染色體的數目非正常基數（單倍數）之整倍數的狀態。

aneurin *n. see* vitamin B_1.

硫胺

aneurysm *n.* a balloon-like swelling in the wall of an artery. This may be due to degenerative disease or syphilitic infection, which damages the muscular coats of the vessel, or it may be the result of congenital deficiency in the muscular wall. An *aortic aneurysm* may develop anywhere in the aorta. A *dissecting aneurysm* usually affects the first part of the aorta and results from a degenerative condition of its muscular coat. This weakness predisposes to a tear in the lining of the aorta, which allows blood to enter the wall and track along (dissect) the muscular coat. A dissecting aneurysm may rupture or it may compress the blood vessels arising

動脉瘤 動脉壁上的氣球狀膨大。由變性疾病或梅毒破壞血管壁的肌層所引起，或因血管壁肌層的先天性缺陷所致。主動脉瘤可發生於主動脉的任何部位。壁間動脉瘤通常在升主動脉發生。位於主動脉壁肌層的變性損害構成的薄弱環節，引起主動脉壁內膜破裂，血液進入動脉壁並割裂肌層。壁間動脉瘤可能破裂，或壓迫由主動脉分枝的血管，造成這些血管所供血的器官的壞死。病人感到撕裂樣的胸部劇痛，並可放射至背部

from the aorta and produce infarction (localized necrosis) in the organs they supply. The patient complains of severe chest pain that has a tearing quality and often spreads to the back or abdomen. Surgical repair may help in some cases. A *ventricular aneurysm* may develop in the wall of the left ventricle after myocardial infarction. A segment of myocardium becomes replaced by scar tissue, which expands to form an aneurysmal sac. Heart failure may result or thrombosis within the aneurysm may act as a source of embolism.
Most aneurysms within the brain are congenital: there is a risk that they may burst, causing a *subarachnoid haemorrhage. *Charcot-Bouchard aneurysms* are small aneurysms found on tiny arteries within the brain of elderly and hypertensive subjects. These aneurysms may rupture, causing cerebral haemorrhage. *See also* arteriovenous aneurysm. —**aneurysmal** *adj.*

或腹部。手術治療對某些病例有效。心室動脉瘤可於心肌梗塞後在左心室壁發生，由於一部分受損的肌肉被瘢痕組織所代替，接着擴張形成動脉瘤囊。其結果可發生心力衰竭，或因動脉瘤內血栓形成而引起其它部位的栓塞。腦動脉瘤絕大多數是先天性的，可能破裂並造成蛛網膜下腔出血。夏-布二氏動脉瘤是發生於老年人或高血壓病人腦部小動脉上的小動脉瘤，有可能破裂並致腦出血。

angi- (angio-) *prefix denoting* blood or lymph vessels. Examples: *angiectasis* (abnormal dilation of); *angiopathy* (disease of); *angiotomy* (cutting of).

〔前綴〕 **血管或淋巴管** 例如，血管或淋巴管擴張，血管或淋巴管病變，血管或淋巴管切除。

angiitis (vasculitis) *n.* a patchy inflammation of the walls of small blood vessels. It may result from a variety of conditions, including *polyarteritis nodosa, acute nephritis, and serum sickness. Symptoms include skin rashes, arthritis, purpura, and kidney failure. In some cases treatment with cortisone derivatives may be beneficial.

脉管炎（血管炎） 小血管壁的斑塊狀炎症。可發生於結節性多動脉炎、急性腎炎、血清病時。出現皮疹、關節炎、紫癜和腎功能衰竭症狀。可的松類藥物對某些病例有療效。

angina *n.* a sense of suffocation or suffocating pain. *See* angina pectoris, Ludwig's angina.

窒息感或窒息痛

angina pectoris pain in the centre of the chest, which is induced by exercise and relieved by rest and may spread to the jaws and arms. Angina pectoris occurs when the demand for blood by the heart exceeds the supply of the coronary arteries and it usually results from

心絞痛 位於前胸中間部的疼痛，可放射至下頦和雙臂。運動可激發疼痛，休息後緩解。當心臟所需之血量超過心臟冠狀動脉的供血量時可發生本病，常見於冠狀動脉粥樣硬化

coronary artery *atheroma. It may be prevented or relieved by such drugs as *glyceryl trinitrate and *propranolol. If drug treatment proves ineffective, *coronary angioplasty or *coronary bypass grafting may be required, the former being less invasive than the latter.

時。三硝酸甘油酯及心得安可預防或緩解本病。當藥物治療無效時，可取病人自身的動脈或靜脈在冠狀動脈的堵塞節段行旁路移植手術，以重建通道。

angiocardiography *n.* X-ray examination of the chambers of the heart after introducing a *radio-opaque contrast medium into the blood in the heart. The contrast medium (e.g. Cardioconray) is injected directly into the atria, ventricles, or great vessels of the heart by means of a slim sterile flexible tube (*cardiac catheter*), which is manipulated into position from an accessible point, such as a vein or artery in a limb (*see* (cardiac) catheterization). Its progress through the heart is followed by a rapid series of X-ray films or by the use of cine film (*cineangiocardiography). The X-ray is called an *angiocardiogram*. Angiocardiography is an important aid in diagnosing and planning the surgical repair of heart defects.

心血管造影術 向心臟血液中注入不透 X 線的造影劑後進行的心臟各房室 X 線檢查技術。使用無菌的纖細柔韌的管子（心導管），從易達心臟的肢體靜脈或動脈插入心房、心室或心臟大血管，並將造影劑（例如碘酞葡胺-碘酞鈉複合劑）通過導管直接注入上述部位。當造影劑通過心臟時，用快速系列 X 線照片（心血管照片）或電影軟片拍攝（心血管電影熒光照像術）全過程。心血管造影術對於心臟病的診斷和手術方案的擬定，是一種重要的輔助手段。

angiography *n.* X-ray examination of blood vessels. A dye that is opaque to X-rays is injected into the artery and a rapid series of X-ray films is taken (*see* arteriography). *Fluorescein angiography* is a common method of investigation in ophthalmology. *Fluorescein sodium is injected into a vein in the arm, from which it circulates throughout the body. Light of an appropriate wavelength is shone into the eye, causing the dye in the retinal blood vessels to fluoresce. This allows the circulation through the retinal blood vessels to be observed and photographed.

血管造影術 血管的 X 射線檢查。將 X 線不透性染料注入動脈血管中，同時拍攝快速系列 X 線片。熒光血管造影術是眼科研究工作中常用的一種方法。將熒光素鈉自上臂靜脈注入後流至全身，並將適當波長的光射入眼球，使視網膜血管中的染料發射熒光，從而得以觀察並拍攝到視網膜的血流情況。

angioid *adj.* resembling a blood vessel.

血管樣的 類似血管的。

angiokeratoma *n.* a localized collection of thin-walled blood vessels covered by a cap of warty material. It is most often seen as an isolated malformation in the genital skin of the elderly

血管角質瘤，血管擴張性疣 擴張的薄壁毛細血管羣，頂端如疣狀。最常見於老年人的外陰皮膚或兒童的手足部位，係一種局

or on the hands and feet of children. It is not malignant and its cause is unknown. Angiokeratomas may be removed surgically. Multiple angiokeratomas affecting the viscera and skin are seen as a rare inherited and fatal disease (*Fabry's disease*).

部病變，良性，產生的原因不明，可用手術切除之。累及內臟和皮膚的多發性血管角質瘤則被視爲少見的致死性遺傳性疾病（法布利氏病）。

angiology *n.* the branch of medicine concerned with the structure, function, and diseases of blood vessels.

脉管學 研究血管的構造、功能及血管疾病的醫學分支學科。

angioma (arteriovenous malformation) *n.* a knot of distended blood vessels overlying and compressing the surface of the brain. It commonly causes epilepsy and less often one of the vessels may burst, causing a *subarachnoid haemorrhage. It may be associated with a purple birthmark on the face: this is called the *Sturge-Weber syndrome*. *See also* haemangioma, lymphangioma.

血管瘤（動靜脉畸形） 覆蓋於腦部表層並壓迫腦組織的擴張血管團。常引起抽搐發作。有時血管破裂，發生蛛網膜下腔出血。也有可能合併面部紫色胎痣，稱爲斯-韋二氏綜合徵。

angioneurotic oedema an allergic condition producing transient or persistent swelling of areas of skin accompanied by itching, which may be severe. It is caused by *allergy to food substances, drugs, or other allergens or it may be precipitated by heat, cold, or emotional factors. *See also* urticaria.

血管神經性水腫 不同皮膚部位發生短暫性或持續性腫脹並有瘙癢（可能很嚴重）的一種變態反應性疾病。致病原因爲對食物、藥物或其他變應原的變態反應。本病可因冷熱刺激或精神因素而誘發。

angiospasm *n. see* Raynaud's disease.

血管痙攣

angiotensin *n.* a protein in the blood, derived from a plasma protein and released by the action of an enzyme (*renin) from the kidneys, that causes an increase in the output of *aldosterone from the adrenal cortex. Angiotensin is also capable of causing constriction of blood vessels, thus raising blood pressure.

血管緊張素 血液中的一種蛋白質。在腎臟產生的一種酶（腎素）作用下，血管緊張素由一種血漿蛋白衍化而來。它可使腎上腺皮質增加醛固酮的分泌，還可直接使血管收縮，從而升高血壓。

angle *n.* **1.** (in anatomy) a corner. For example, the *angle of the eye* is the outer or inner corner of the eye; the *angle of the mouth* is the site where the upper and lower lips join on either side. **2.** the degree of divergence of two lines or planes that meet each other; the space

角 ①解剖學中的角。例如：眼角指眼睛的外角或內角，嘴角指上唇與下唇在左右兩側的結合處。②兩條相交直線或相交平面所形成的角度，即相交直線間的空間。臂外偏角

between two such lines. The *carrying angle* is the obtuse angle formed between the forearm and the upper arm when the forearm is fully extended and the hand is supinated.

爲前臂伸直，手掌外旋時上臂與前臂之間形成的鈍角。

angstrom *n.* a unit of length equal to one ten millionth of a millimetre (10^{-10} m). It is not a recommended *SI unit but is sometimes used to express wavelengths and interatomic distances: the *nanometre (1 nm = 10 Å) is now the preferred unit. Symbol Å.

埃 表示千萬分之一毫米（10^{-10}米）的長度單位。並非公認的國際單位，但有時用以表示波長及原子之間的距離。毫微米（1毫微米＝10埃）爲目前較常使用的單位。埃的符號：Å。

anhidrotic 1. *n.* any drug that inhibits the secretion of sweat, such as *parasympatholytic drugs. **2.** *adj.* inhibiting sweating.

①止汗藥 抑制汗液分泌的藥物，例如副交感神經阻滯藥。 **②止汗的**

anhydraemia *n.* a decrease in the proportion of water, and therefore plasma, in the blood.

缺水血〔症〕 血液中水分含量降低並隨之使血漿比例下降的情況。

anhydrase *n.* an enzyme that catalyses the removal of water from a compound.

脫水酶 一種催化化合物脫水的酶。

anidrosis (anhidrosis) *n.* the abnormal absence of sweating, accompanying disease or occurring as a congenital defect.

無汗〔症〕 由疾病引起或因先天發育缺陷所致的不排汗現象。

anileridine *n.* a synthetic narcotic analgesic drug, given by mouth or by injection to relieve pain or support anaesthesia. It has the same uses, actions, and toxic effects as *morphine. Drug *dependence, with marked withdrawal symptoms, is easily produced by repeated administration. Trade name: **Leritine**.

氨苄哌替啶 一種合成的麻醉鎮痛藥。口服或注射給藥，用於止痛或輔助麻醉。其用途、作用和毒性作用均與嗎啡相同。反覆使用易產生賴藥性，並有明顯的戒斷症狀。

anima *n.* (in Jungian psychology) an *archetype that is the feminine component of a male's personality.

女性意象 （容格心理學）指在男子人格中由種族遺傳來的女性意象成分。

animus *n.* the *archetype that is the masculine component of a female's personality.

男性意象 指在女子人格中由種族遺傳來的男性意象成分。

aniridia *n.* congenital absence of the iris (of the eye).

無虹膜 先天性眼球虹膜缺失。

aniseikonia *n.* a condition in which the image of an object differs markedly in size or shape in each eye.

物象不等 兩眼所見同一物體的影象的大小或形狀明顯不一致。

anisocytosis *n.* an excessive variation in size between individual red blood cells. Anisocytosis may be noted on microscopical examination of a blood film; from this a graph of the numbers of cells of different sizes may be drawn. Anisocytosis may be a feature of almost any disease affecting the blood.

紅細胞〔大小〕不均 各個紅細胞的大小過分不均。在顯微鏡下觀察血細胞的大小過分不均。在顯微鏡下觀察血細胞塗片，可見到這種現象，並繪製出不同大小的紅細胞數目的曲線圖。在幾乎任何一種影響血液的疾病中都可觀察到這一現象。

anisomelia *n.* a difference in size or shape between the arms or the legs.

對稱肢體大小不等 兩上肢或兩下肢間的大小或形狀不一致。

anisometropia *n.* the condition in which the power of *refraction in one eye differs markedly from that in the other.

屈光參差 一側眼球的屈光能力與另一側眼球的屈光能力有明顯差異。

ankle *n.* **1.** the hinge joint between the leg and the foot. It consists of the *talus (ankle bone), which projects into a socket formed by the lower ends of the *tibia and *fibula. **2.** the whole region of the ankle joint, including the *tarsus and the lower parts of the tibia and fibula.

踝 ①下肢與足之間的屈戌關節。由距骨突入脛骨和腓骨下端的關節窩形成。 ②踝關節部位，包括跖骨及脛骨和腓骨下端。

ankylosing spondylitis *see* spondylitis.

關節強硬性脊椎炎

ankylosis *n.* fusion of the bones across a joint space, either by bony tissue (*bony ankylosis*) or by shortening of connecting fibrous tissue (*fibrous ankylosis*). Ankylosis is a complication of prolonged joint inflammation, as may occur in chronic infection (e.g. tuberculosis) or rheumatic disease (e.g. ankylosing *spondylitis).

關節強硬 關節腔內的骨質融合。可因骨性組織融合（骨性關節強硬）或纖維組織短縮（纖維性關節強硬）所致。併發於遷延的關節炎症，如慢性感染（例如結核）或風濕病（例如關節強硬性脊椎炎）時。

Ankylostoma *n. see* Ancylostoma.

鈎口線蟲屬

annulus *n.* (in anatomy) a circular opening or ring-shaped structure. —**annular** *adj.*

環 解剖學中的環形孔或環狀結構。

anodontia *n.* absence of the teeth because they have failed to develop. It is more common for only a few teeth to fail to develop (*see* hypodontia).

無牙 由於發育不全所致的缺牙。通常只有數個牙齒缺失。

anodyne *n.* any treatment or drug that soothes and eases pain.

①止痛療法 ②止痛藥

anomalopia *n. Obsolete.* defective colour vision (*see* colour blindness).

色覺異常 舊詞。指色覺缺陷。

anomaloscope *n.* an instrument for testing colour discrimination. By adjusting the controls of the instrument the subject has to produce a mixture of red and green light to match a yellow light. The matching is done on a brightly illuminated disc viewed down a telescope.

色盲檢察鏡 檢察辨色能力的一種儀器。調整儀器後，讓色盲患者通過望遠鏡注視一個照亮的圓盤，可產生與黃色呈對比的紅綠混合色覺。

anomalous pulmonary venous drainage a congenital abnormality in which the pulmonary veins enter the right atrium or vena cava instead of draining normally into the left atrium. The features are those of an atrial *septal defect.

肺靜脉血旁流 肺靜脉血流入右心房或下腔靜脉以取代正常情況下流入左心房的先天性異常現象。見於房間隔缺損時。

anomaly *n.* any deviation from the normal, especially a congenital or developmental defect.

異常 任何一種偏離正常的情況，尤指先天的或發育上的缺陷。

anomia *n.* **1.** a form of *aphasia in which the patient is unable to give the names of objects, although retaining an understanding of their use and the ability to put words together into speech. **2.** absence of respect for laws and established customs, which is a feature of *psychopathy.

①命名性失語症 失去稱呼物件名稱能力的一種失語症。病人仍然能夠理解該物件的用途，並具有組句和語言能力。 **②先天性道德感缺損** 無視法律和社會習俗的一種精神變態。

anonychia *n.* congenital absence of one or more nails.

無甲〔畸形〕 先天性一指或多指指甲缺失。

Anopheles *n.* a genus of widely distributed mosquitoes, occurring in tropical and temperate regions, with some 350 species. The malarial parasite (*see* Plasmodium) is transmitted to man solely through the bite of female *Anopheles* mosquitoes. Some species of *Anopheles* may transmit the parasites of bancroftian *filariasis.

按蚊屬 在熱帶和溫帶廣泛分佈的一個蚊屬，約分350種。瘧原蟲傳播到人的唯一途徑是通過雌性按蚊的叮咬。某些按蚊蚊種能傳播班氏絲蟲。

anorchism *n.* congenital absence of one or both testes.

無睪〔畸形〕 先天性單側或雙側無睪丸。

anorexia *n.* loss of appetite.

厭食 食慾缺乏。

anorexia nervosa a psychological illness, most common in female adolescents, in which the patients have no desire to eat; eating may, in fact, be abhorrent to them. The problem often starts with a simple desire to lose weight, which then becomes an obsession. The result is severe loss of weight and sometimes even death from starvation. The cause of the illness is complicated – problems within the family and rejection of adult sexuality are often factors involved. Patients must usually be treated by *psychotherapy.

神經性厭食 一種缺乏食慾的心理性疾病。病人對進食反感，多見於青春期女性。開始時常僅爲減肥而減少進食，逐漸形成强迫觀念。其後果常是體重嚴重下降，有時因飢餓致死。病因複雜，涉及家庭糾紛、拒絕房事等因素。對病人須施以心理治療。

anosmia *n.* a loss of the sense of smell. This is most often due to a head cold but it may be caused by a fracture through the anterior fossa of the skull or a frontal brain tumour.

嗅覺缺失 喪失嗅覺。大多由感冒引起，也可因顱骨前窩骨折或大腦前部腫瘤所致。

anovular (anovulatory) *adj.* not associated with the development and release of a female germ cell (ovum) in the ovary, as in *anovular menstruation*.

不排卵的 卵巢中無卵細胞發育和排出。例如：無排卵性月經。

anoxaemia *n.* a condition in which there is less than the normal concentration of oxygen in the blood. *See also* anoxia, hypoxaemia.

缺氧血〔症〕 血液中氧濃度低於正常的狀況。

anoxia *n.* a condition in which the tissues of the body receive inadequate amounts of oxygen. This may result from low atmospheric pressure at high altitudes; a shortage of circulating blood, red blood cells, or haemoglobin; or disordered blood flow, such as occurs in heart failure. It can also result from insufficient oxygen reaching the blood in the lungs due to poor breathing movements or because disease, such as pneumonia, is reducing the effective surface area of lung tissue. *See also* hypoxia. —**anoxic** *adj.*

缺氧症 身體組織中氧供應不足的狀況。可發生於下列情況時：高原低氣壓，循環血量不足，紅細胞或血紅蛋白減少，心力衰竭等情況下的循環障礙，由於呼吸運動減弱或肺炎使肺組織有效表面積減少所致的肺部血液含氧不足等。

ansa *n.* (in anatomy) a loop; for example, the *ansa hypoglossi* is the loop formed by the descending branch of the hypoglossal nerve.

襻 （解剖學）圈，環。例如：舌下神經襻，即舌下神經降支所形成的襻。

ansiform *adj.* (in anatomy) shaped like a loop. The term is applied to certain lobules of the cerebellum.

襻狀的 （解剖學）形狀如襻的。也用於小腦某些小葉的命名。

ant- (anti-) *prefix denoting* opposed to; counteracting; relieving. Examples: *antarthritic* (relieving arthritis); *antibacterial* (destroying or stopping the growth of bacteria).

〔前綴〕 **對抗，抵消，緩解** 例如，緩解關節疼痛的，抗菌的（殺滅細菌或抑制細菌生長）。

Antabuse *n. see* disulfiram.

安塔布司，戒酒硫

antacid *n.* a drug that neutralizes the hydrochloric acid secreted in the digestive juices of the stomach. Antacids, which include aluminium hydroxide, calcium carbonate, magnesium hydroxide, and sodium bicarbonate, are used to relieve pain and discomfort in disorders of the digestive system, including peptic ulcer.

解酸藥 中和胃液中鹽酸的藥物。氫氧化鋁、碳酸鈣、氫氧化鎂、碳酸氫鈉等均屬此類。可緩解消化性潰瘍等疾病的疼痛和不適。

antagonist *n.* **1.** a muscle whose action (contraction) opposes that of another muscle (called the *agonist* or *prime mover*). Antagonists relax to allow the agonists to effect movement. **2.** a drug or other substance with opposite action to that of another drug or natural body chemical, which it inhibits. Examples are the *antimetabolites. **—antagonism** *n.*

①**拮抗肌** 與另一肌羣（主動肌或原動肌）呈反作用的肌羣。拮抗肌鬆弛時，原動肌得以運動。
②**拮抗藥，拮抗劑** 一種可與某一藥物起相反（抑制）作用的藥物，或與體內一化學物質起相反（抑制）作用的物質。例如：抗代謝物。

antazoline *n.* a short-acting *antihistamine drug, given by mouth to relieve the symptoms of allergic reactions. It is less irritating than the other antihistamines, but it produces their characteristic side-effects, such as drowsiness, dizziness, and incoordination.

安他唑啉 一種口服的短效抗組胺藥，用於解除變態反應症狀。本藥較其他抗組胺藥的刺激性低，但具有此類藥物的典型副作用，如嗜眠、頭暈、共濟失調等。

ante- *prefix denoting* before. Examples: *antenatal* (before birth); *anteprandial* (before meals).

〔前綴〕 **前** 例如：出生前的，飯前的。

anteflexion *n.* the abnormal bending forward of an organ, especially the bending of the body of the womb towards the front.

前屈 某一器官的不正常前屈，尤指子宮體的前屈。

ante mortem before death. *Compare* post mortem.

死前 死亡之前。

antenatal diagnosis *see* prenatal diagnosis.

出生前診斷

Antepar *n. see* piperazine.

枸櫞酸哌嗪，磷酸哌嗪

antepartum *adj.* occurring before the onset of labour.

分娩前的 發生於產程開始之前的。

anterior *adj.* **1.** describing or relating to the front (ventral) portion of the body or limbs. **2.** describing the front part of any organ.

前的 ①表示身體或四肢朝前的或腹側的部分。②表示某一器官的前部。

anteversion *n.* the normal forward inclination of the womb.

前傾 子宮的正常的向前傾斜。

anthelmintic **1.** *n.* any drug or chemical agent used to destroy parasitic worms (helminths), e.g. tapeworms, roundworms, and flukes, and/or remove them from the body. Anthelmintics include *dichlorophen, *mepacrine, and *piperazine. **2.** *adj.* having the power to destroy or eliminate helminths.

①**蠕蟲藥，驅腸蟲藥** 用於殺死及/或驅除寄生於人體的蠕蟲（如絛蟲、蛔蟲、各種吸蟲等）的藥物或化學制劑。 ②**抗蠕蟲的，驅腸蟲的** 具有殺滅或驅除蠕蟲（腸蟲）能力的。

anthracosis *n.* a lung disease – a form of *pneumoconiosis – caused by coal dust. It affects mainly coal miners but also other exposed workers, such as lightermen, if the lungs' capacity to accommodate and remove the particles is exceeded.

碳末沉着病 一種由煤塵引起的肺塵埃沉着病。患此病者主要是煤礦工人，但其他人暴露於煤塵的量超過肺的容納和排除能力時，也可患此病。

anthracycline *n.* any of 500 or so antibiotics synthesized or isolated from species of *Streptomyces*. *Doxorubicin is the most important member of this group of compounds, which have wide activity against tumours.

蒽環類抗生素 由鏈黴菌屬合成或分離出的約 500 種抗生素。阿黴素是這類化合物中最重要的一種，具有較廣泛的抗腫瘤作用。

anthrax *n.* an acute infectious disease of farm animals caused by the bacterium *Bacillus anthracis*, which can be transmitted to man by contact with animal hair, hides, or excrement. In man the disease attacks either the lungs, causing pneumonia (*woolsorter's disease*), or the skin, producing severe ulceration (known as *malignant pus-*

炭疽 一種由炭疽桿菌引起並可傳染給人的急性家畜傳染病。人類通過與動物皮毛或排泄物的接觸而傳染。本病或侵犯人的肺部引起肺炎（肺炭疽），或侵犯皮膚而發生嚴重的潰瘍（皮膚炭疽）。本病如不予治療則可致死，大

tule). Untreated anthrax can be fatal but administration of large doses of penicillin or tetracycline is usually effective.

劑量青黴素或四環素有良好療效。

anthrop- (anthropo-) *prefix denoting* the human race. Examples: *anthropogenesis* (origin and development of); *anthropoid* (resembling); *anthropology* (science of).

〔前綴〕**人類** 例如：人類起源，類人的，人類學。

anthropometry *n.* the taking of measurements of the human body or its parts. Comparisons can then be made between individuals of different sexes, ages, and races to determine the difference between normal and abnormal development. —**anthropometric** *adj.*

人體測量 對人體或人體某一部分的測量。通過對不同性別、年齡、種族的一些個體的測量和比較，可得出正常與異常發育的差別值。

anthropozoonosis *n.* a disease that is transmissible from an animal to man, or vice versa, under natural conditions. Diseases that are found primarily in animals and sometimes affect man include *anthrax, *rabies, and *leptospirosis.

人類動物傳染病 在自然條件下能夠從動物傳染到人，或由人傳染給動物的疾病。這類疾病主要見於動物，有時感染人類，其中包括炭疽、狂犬病和鈎端螺旋體病。

antibiotic *n.* a substance, produced by or derived from a microorganism, that destroys or inhibits the growth of other microorganisms. Antibiotics are used to treat infections caused by organisms that are sensitive to them, usually bacteria or fungi. They may alter the normal microbial content of the body (e.g. in the intestine, lungs, bladder) by destroying one or more groups of harmless organisms, which may result in infections due to overgrowth of resistant organisms. These side-effects are most likely to occur with *broad-spectrum antibiotics* (those active against a wide variety of organisms). Resistance may also develop in the microorganisms being treated (for example, through incorrect dosage), and some antibiotics may cause allergic reactions. Antibiotics should not be used for minor infections, which will clear up unaided. *See also* cephalosporin, chloramphenicol, penicillin, streptomycin, tetracycline.

抗生素 由微生物產生或衍生的能夠破壞或抑制其他微生物生長的一類物質。用於治療對其敏感的微生物（通常爲細菌或黴菌）所致之感染。抗生素也能殺滅人體內（例如腸道、肺、膀胱內）的一羣或某幾羣無害的微生物，改變正常的菌羣分佈，結果造成有抗藥性的菌羣過分繁殖而致病。這種副作用在使用廣譜抗生素時最爲多見。應用抗生素還能使細菌產生抗藥性（例如由於用藥劑量不當所致），有些抗生素能引起變態反應。輕度感染無需進行治療便可自癒，不必使用抗生素。

antibody *n.* a special kind of blood protein that is synthesized in lymphoid tissue in response to the presence of a particular *antigen and circulates in the plasma to attack the antigen and render it harmless. The production of specific antibodies against antigens as diverse as invading bacteria, inhaled pollen grains, and foreign red blood cells is the basis of both *immunity and *allergy. Antibody formation is also responsible for tissue or organ rejection following transplantation. Chemically, antibodies are proteins of the globulin type; they are classified according to their structure and function (*see* immunoglobulin).

抗體 針對某種抗原的存在，於淋巴組織中合成並循環於血液中，起着殺傷抗原使之無害的作用的一種特殊的蛋白質。針對形形色色的抗原，如細菌侵入、花粉吸入或異體紅細胞輸入等而產生的特種抗體，成爲免疫反應和過敏反應的基礎。抗體形成也是組織或器官移植後發生排斥反應的原因。抗體的化學結構爲球蛋白型，並可按其結構和功能分類。

anticholinergic *adj.* inhibiting the action of *acetylcholine. *Parasympatholytic drugs are anticholinergic.

抗膽鹼能的 有抑制乙醯膽鹼之作用的。抗副交感神經藥即屬於此類。

anticholinesterase *n.* any substance that inhibits the action of *cholinesterase, the enzyme responsible for the breakdown of the neurotransmitter acetylcholine, and therefore allows acetylcholine to continue transmitting nerve impulses. Drugs with anticholinesterase activity include *neostigmine and *physostigmine; their uses include the diagnosis and treatment of *myasthenia gravis. *See also* parasympathomimetic.

抗膽鹼酯酶 能抑制膽鹼酯酶作用的物質。膽鹼酯酶能破壞神經遞質乙醯膽鹼，故抗膽鹼酯酶能使乙醯膽鹼繼續傳遞神經衝動。抗膽鹼酯酶藥有新斯的明、毒扁豆鹼等，用於重症肌無力等的診斷和治療。

anticoagulant *n.* an agent that prevents the clotting of blood. The natural anticoagulant *heparin directly interferes with blood clotting and is active both within the body and against a sample of blood in a test tube. Synthetic drugs, such as *dicoumarol, *phenindione, and *warfarin, are effective only within the body, since they act by affecting blood *coagulation factors. They take longer to act than heparin. Anticoagulants are used to prevent the formation of blood clots or to break up clots in blood vessels in such conditions

抗凝〔血〕藥 防止血液凝結的藥物。天然抗凝藥肝素直接阻礙血液凝結，在人體內和在試管內的血液標本中作用相同。人工合成的抗凝藥，如雙香豆素、苯茚二酮、丙酮芐羥香豆素等系通過影響血液中的凝血因子而起作用，故僅在人體內有效，且發生作用較肝素慢。在血栓形成或栓塞等疾病中使用抗凝劑可以防止血管中血塊形成或使血塊破

as thrombosis and embolism. Incorrect dosage may result in haemorrhage.

壞，但使用劑量不當則可引起出血。

anticonvulsant *n.* a drug that prevents or reduces the severity of fits (convulsions) in various types of epilepsy. The choice of anticonvulsant is dictated by the type of fit and the patient's response. Some anticonvulsants, such as *sodium valproate, are used to treat all types of epileptic fits. Others are used specifically for petit mal (e.g. *ethosuximide and *troxidone) or for focal and grand mal epilepsy (e.g. *phenytoin, *primidone, *carbamazepine). The dosage must be adjusted carefully as individuals vary in their response to these drugs and side-effects may be troublesome.

抗驚厥藥，抗癲癇藥 在各型癲癇中預防癲癇發作或減輕發作程度的藥物。根據癲癇的類型和病人對藥物的反應選擇抗癲癇藥。某些（如丙戊酸鈉）用於治療各型癲癇；某些（如乙琥胺和三甲雙酮）專治癲癇小發作；某些（如苯妥因、撲癇酮、氨甲醯苯䓬）用於治療局限性發作和大發作。由於各個病人對這些藥物的反應不一樣，故必須謹慎調整劑量，否則可引起麻煩的副作用。

antidepressant *n.* a drug that alleviates the symptoms of depression. The most widely prescribed antidepressants are a group of drugs with a basic chemical structure of three benzene rings, called *tricyclic antidepressants*, which include *amitriptyline and *imipramine. These drugs are useful in treating a variety of different depressive symptoms. Side-effects commonly include dry mouth, blurred vision, constipation, drowsiness, and difficulty in urination. The other main group of antidepressants are the *MAO inhibitors, which have more severe side-effects.

抗抑鬱藥 緩解抑鬱症狀的藥物。最常應用的一組稱作三環類抗抑鬱藥，其基本化學結構式上有三個苯環，阿米替林和丙咪嗪即屬於此類。對多種抑鬱症有效，常見副作用有口乾、視力模糊、便秘、嗜眠、排尿困難等。另一類主要的抗抑鬱藥爲單胺氧化酶抑制劑，副作用較前者嚴重。

antidiuretic hormone (ADH) *see* vasopressin.

抗利尿激素

antidote *n.* a drug that counteracts the effects of a poison. For example, *dimercaprol is an antidote to arsenic, mercury, and other heavy metals.

解毒劑 解除毒物之毒性作用的藥劑。例如，二硫基丙醇爲砷、汞和其他重金屬的解毒劑。

antidromic *adj.* describing impulses travelling 'the wrong way' in a nerve fibre. This is rare but may happen in shingles, when the irritation caused by the virus in the spinal canal initiates impulses that travel outwards in nor-

逆向的，逆行的 指神經纖維衝動的傳遞方向發生錯誤。這一現象少見，但可發生於患帶狀疱疹時。病毒對脊髓的刺激經傳入神經向外傳導，致該感覺

mally afferent nerves. The area of skin that the sensory nerves supply (usually a strip on the trunk) becomes painfully blistered. Antidromic impulses cannot pass *synapses, which work in one direction only.

神經所支配的皮區（通常在軀幹上呈帶狀）出現灼痛的水疱。逆行衝動不能通過神經突觸，突觸只能向一個方向傳遞衝動。

antiemetic *n.* a drug that prevents vomiting. Various drugs have this effect, including some *antihistamines (e.g. cyclizine, promethazine) and *anticholinergic drugs. They are used for such conditions as motion sickness and vertigo and to counteract nausea and vomiting caused by other drugs.

止吐藥 防止嘔吐的藥物。許多藥物有此功效，包括某些抗組胺藥（如賽克利嗪、異丙嗪等）及抗膽鹼藥。止吐藥用於暈動病、暈眩症及由藥物引起的噁心和嘔吐。

antigen *n.* any substance that the body regards as foreign or potentially dangerous and against which it produces an *antibody. Antigens are usually proteins, but simple substances, even metals, may become antigenic by combining with and modifying the body's own proteins. These are called *haptens.* —**antigenic** *adj.*

抗原 被人體視作異物或有潛在危險並產生抗體與之對抗的任何一種物質。抗原通常爲蛋白質。但許多單純的物質，甚至金屬，可與人體內的蛋白質相結合並使之起變化，因此也帶有抗原性，稱作"半抗原"或"不全抗原"。

antihelix (anthelix) *n.* the curved inner ridge of the *pinna of the ear.

對耳輪 耳廓的曲線形內嵴。

antihistamine *n.* a drug that inhibits some of the effects of *histamine in the body, in particular its role in allergic reactions. Examples are *chlorpheniramine, *diphenhydramine, and *mepyramine. Antihistamines are used mainly for the relief of hay fever, pruritus (itching), rhinitis, urticaria (nettle rash), and other allergic reactions. Many antihistamines, e.g. *cyclizine and *promethazine, also have strong *antiemetic activity and are used to prevent motion sickness. The most common side-effect of antihistamines is drowsiness and because of this they are sometimes used to promote sleep. Other side-effects include dizziness, blurred vision, tremors, digestive upsets, and lack of muscular coordination.

抗組胺藥 抑制組胺在人體內的某些作用，特別是變態反應作用的藥物。例如：氯苯吡胺、苯海拉明和甲氧芐二胺等。主要用於治療枯草熱、瘙癢症、鼻炎、蕁麻疹和其他變態反應性疾病。許多抗組胺藥，如賽克利嗪、異丙嗪，還具有較强的止吐作用並用於治療暈動病。抗組胺藥的常見副作用爲嗜睡，因此有時用於催眠。其他副作用有頭暈、視力模糊、震顫、腸胃不適、肌肉共濟失調。

antiketogenic *n.* an agent that prevents formation of *ketones in the body.

抗生酮藥 防止體內酮體生成的藥物。

antilymphocytic serum (ALS) an *antiserum, containing antibodies that suppress lymphocytic activity, prepared by injecting an animal with lymphocytes. ALS may be given to a patient to prevent the immune reaction that causes tissue rejection following transplantation of such organs as kidneys. Administration naturally also impairs other immunity mechanisms, making infection a serious hazard.

抗淋巴細胞血清 一種含有可抑制淋巴細胞活性的抗體的抗血清。將淋巴細胞注射到動物體內可製備出這種抗血清。本品可用於器官移植（如腎臟移植）病人，以防出現引起排異現象的免疫反應。本品也可抑制人體內其他免疫反應並造成感染。

antimetabolite *n.* a drug that interferes with the normal metabolic processes within cells by combining with the enzymes responsible for them. Some drugs used in the treatment of cancer, e.g. *fluorouracil, *methotrexate, and *mercaptopurine, are antimetabolites that prevent cell growth by interfering with enzyme reactions essential for nucleic acid synthesis. Side-effects of antimetabolites can be severe, involving blood cell disorders and digestive disturbances. *See also* cytotoxic drug.

抗代謝藥 一種可與催化細胞內代謝過程的酶結合，從而干擾細胞內正常代謝進程的藥物。某些抗腫瘤藥，如氟尿嘧啶、甲氨蝶呤、巰嘌呤均屬此類。這些藥物係通過干擾核酸合成必不可少的酶促反應而抑制癌細胞生長。抗代謝藥可能產生嚴重的副作用，如血細胞變化（下降）、胃腸道反應等。

antimitotic *n.* a drug that inhibits cell division and growth, e.g. *procarbazine. The drugs used to treat cancer are mainly antimitotics. *See also* antimetabolite, cytotoxic drug.

抗有絲分裂藥 抑制細胞分裂和生長的藥物，如甲苄肼。抗腫瘤藥中多半爲抗有絲分裂藥。

antimony potassium tartrate (tartar emetic) a toxic and irritating salt of antimony. It is administered (usually by slow intravenous injection) for the treatment of *schistosomiasis and *leishmaniasis but may produce severe side-effects, particularly vomiting; it should not be used in patients with heart, kidney, or liver disease. A salt with similar effects and uses is *antimony sodium tartrate*.

酒石酸銻鉀（吐酒石） 一種有毒並帶刺激性的銻鹽。通常以緩慢靜脉注入方式給藥。用於治療血吸蟲病和利什曼病。可產生嘔吐等劇烈副作用。患有心、腎、肝臟等疾病者不宜使用。與之有類似功效和用途的銻鹽爲酒石酸銻鈉。

antimutagen *n.* a substance that can either reduce the spontaneous production of mutations or prevent or reverse the action of a *mutagen.

抗誘變劑 能減少自發性突變或阻止、逆轉誘變劑作用的物質。

antimycotic *n.* a drug active against fungi. Antimycotics are used to treat

抗眞菌藥，抗黴菌藥 有抗眞菌（黴菌）作用的藥

fungal infections; they include *griseofulvin and *nystatin.

物。用於治療眞菌（黴菌）感染。如灰黃黴素、制黴菌素等。

antiperistalsis *n.* a wave of contraction in the alimentary canal that passes in an oral (i.e. upward or backwards) direction (*compare* peristalsis). It was formerly thought that antiperistalsis occurred in vomiting but modern physiological studies indicate that it never takes place in man.

逆蠕動 消化道的向口腔方向（朝上，或往回）行進的收縮波。過去認爲嘔吐時發生逆蠕動；現代生理學研究認爲，逆蠕動從未發生於人類。

antipruritic *n.* an agent that relieves itching (*pruritus). Examples are *calamine and *crotamiton, applied in creams or lotions, and some *antihistamine drugs, used if the itching is due to an allergy.

止癢藥 緩解瘙癢的藥物。例如：爐甘石、克羅他米通，配成霜劑或洗劑搽用。某些抗組胺藥用於變態反應時的瘙癢。

antipyretic *n.* a drug that reduces fever by lowering the body temperature. Several analgesic drugs have antipyretic activity, including *aspirin, *mefanamic acid, *paracetamol, and *phenylbutazone.

退熱藥 降低體溫以解除發熱的藥物。阿司匹林、甲滅酸、撲熱息痛、保泰松等鎮痛藥均有解熱功能。

antisepsis *n.* the elimination of bacteria, fungi, viruses, and other microorganisms that cause disease by the use of chemical or physical methods.

抗菌〔法〕 使用化學的或物理的方法消滅細菌、眞菌、病毒和其他致病微生物。

antiseptic *n.* a chemical that destroys or inhibits the growth of disease-causing bacteria and other microorganisms and is sufficiently nontoxic to be applied to the skin or mucous membranes to cleanse wounds and prevent infections or to be used internally to treat infections of the intestine and bladder. Examples are *crystal violet, *dequalinium, and *hexamine.

抗菌藥，防腐藥 一種殺滅致病細菌及其他微生物或抑制其生長而且無毒的化學物質。用於清潔皮膚或黏膜創口以防止感染，或內服以治療腸道和膀胱感染。例如：結晶紫，克菌定，烏洛托品。

antiserum *n.* (*pl.* **antisera**) a serum that contains antibodies against antigens of a particular kind; it may be injected to treat, or give temporary protection (passive *immunity) against, specific diseases. Antisera are prepared in large quantities in such animals as horses. In the laboratory, they are used to identify

抗血清 含有針對某一特定抗原之抗體的血清。注入人體後可以治療或在短期內預防（被動免疫）某種疾病。用馬等動物可大量製造出抗血清。在實驗室內用抗血清可以鑑定致病微生物。

unknown organisms responsible for infection (*see* agglutination).

antispasmodic *n.* a drug that relieves spasm of smooth muscle. *See* spasmolytic.

鎮痙藥，解痙藥 解除平滑肌痙攣的藥物。

antitoxin *n.* an antibody produced by the body to counteract a toxin formed by invading bacteria or from any other source.

抗毒素 人體針對外界入侵細菌的毒素或其他來源的毒素所產生的與之相對抗的抗體。

antitragus *n.* a small projection of cartilage above the lobe of the ear, opposite the tragus. *See* pinna.

對耳屏 耳垂上方，與耳屏相對的小的軟骨突起。

antitussive *n.* a drug, such as *dextromethorphan or *pholcodine, that suppresses coughing, possibly by reducing the activity of the cough centre in the brain and by depressing respiration. Some analgesic drugs also have antitussive activity, e.g. *codeine, diamorphine (*see* heroin), and *methadone.

鎮咳藥 通過減弱大腦咳嗽中樞活動及抑制呼吸而起到鎮咳作用的藥物。例如：右甲嗎喃（美沙芬）和嗎啉乙嗎啡（福可定）。有些麻醉藥也有鎮咳作用，例如：可待因，二乙醯嗎啡和美沙酮。

antivenene (antivenin) *n.* an *antiserum containing antibodies against specific poisons in the venom of such an animal as a snake, spider, or scorpion.

抗蛇毒素 含有對抗蛇、蜘蛛、蝎等毒液中特種毒素之抗體的抗血清。

antrectomy *n.* **1.** surgical removal of the bony walls of an *antrum. *See* antrostomy. **2.** a surgical operation in which a part of the stomach (the antrum) is removed. Most secretions of acid, pepsin, and the hormone gastrin occur in the antrum and the operation is used (usually combined with *vagotomy) in the treatment of peptic ulcers.

①**鼻竇切除術** 骨質竇壁的切除手術。 ②**胃竇切除術** 切除胃竇的外科手術。大部分胃酸、胃蛋白酶和胃泌素在胃竇分泌。消化性潰瘍患者常同時施行胃竇切除術和迷走神經切斷術。

antroscope *n.* an *endoscope that can be introduced into the stomach via the oesophagus to obtain a view of the pyloric antrum, the region of the stomach wall near the pyloric sphincter.

竇透照器 一種通過食道插入胃內的內窺鏡。通過該鏡可窺見胃幽門竇及幽門括約肌附近的胃壁。

antrostomy *n.* a surgical operation to produce a permanent or semipermanent artificial opening to an *antrum in a bone, so providing drainage for any fluid. The operation is sometimes carried out to treat infection of the *paranasal sinuses.

鼻竇造口術 於鼻竇處進行永久性或半永久性人工造孔以利引流的手術。副鼻竇炎患者有時施行這種手術。

antrum *n.* **1.** a cavity, especially a cavity in a bone. The *mastoid* (or *tympanic*) *antrum* is the space connecting the air cells of the *mastoid process with the chamber of the inner ear. **2.** the part of the *stomach adjoining the pylorus (*pyloric antrum*).

①**竇** 空腔，尤指骨內空腔。乳突竇爲連接乳突空氣腔與內耳的空間。 ②**胃幽門竇** 胃的靠近幽門的部分。

anuria *n.* failure of the kidneys to produce urine. This can occur in a variety of conditions that produce a sustained drop in blood pressure. Urgent assessment is required to differentiate lack of production of urine from an obstruction to the flow of urine from the kidneys, which can readily be relieved. Anuria is associated with increasing *uraemia and may require *haemodialysis.

無尿〔症〕 腎臟不能產生尿液。在各種造成血壓持續下降的情況下都可能發生。應及時作出診斷，並將腎臟生尿不能和由堵塞造成的腎臟中尿液排出障礙加以區別。後者能及時解除。前者則可併發尿毒症並逐漸加重，有時需作血液透析。

anus *n.* the opening at the lower end of the alimentary canal, through which the faeces are discharged. It opens out from the *anal canal*, below the rectum, and is guarded by two sphincters. The anus is closed except during defecation. —**anal** *adj.*

肛門 消化道末端的開口，糞便由此排出。自直腸下端的肛管開口，有二括約肌保護。肛門平時關閉，排便時除外。

anvil *n.* (in anatomy) *see* incus.

砧骨

anxiety *n.* generalized pervasive *fear. *Anxiety state* is a form of neurosis in which anxiety dominates the patient's life. It can be treated with psychotherapy, behaviour therapy, and tranquillizing drugs.

焦慮 充滿焦慮不安的狀態。焦慮狀態是一種神經官能症，病人爲焦慮所控制。可用心理療法、行爲療法及安定藥醫治。

aorta *n.* (*pl.* **aortae** or **aortas**) the main artery of the body, from which all others derive. It arises from the left ventricle (*ascending aorta*), arches over the top of the heart (*see* aortic arch) and descends in front of the backbone (*descending aorta*), giving off large and small branches and finally dividing to form the right and left *iliac arteries. The part of the descending aorta from the aortic arch to the diaphragm is called the *thoracic aorta*; the part below the diaphragm is the *abdominal aorta*. —**aortic** *adj.*

主動脉 身體的主動脉，所有其他動脉均由此而出。自左心室上升（升主動脉），呈弓狀跨越心臟上部（主動脉弓），沿脊柱前下降（降主動脉）。自主動脉分枝出大小不同的動脉，最後分成髂右動脉和髂左動脉。從主動脉弓至橫膈的降主動脉部分稱作胸主動脉，膈下部分稱作腹主動脉。

aortic arch that part of the aorta that extends from the ascending aorta, upward over the heart and then backward and down as far as the fourth thoracic vertebra. *Stretch receptors in its outer wall monitor blood pressure and form part of the system maintaining this at a constant level.

主動脈弓 自升主動脈向上延伸，經過心臟上方，再向後向下降至第四胸椎水平的主動脈段。其外壁中的壓力感受器具有調節血壓的作用，是維持血壓於穩定水平的生理調節系統的一個組成部分。

aortic regurgitation reflux of blood from the aorta into the left ventricle during diastole. Aortic regurgitation most commonly follows scarring of the aortic valve as a result of previous acute rheumatic fever, but it may also result from other conditions, such as syphilis or dissecting aneurysm. Mild cases are symptom-free, but patients more severely affected develop breathlessness, angina pectoris, and enlargement of the heart; all have a diastolic murmur. A badly affected valve may be replaced surgically with a prosthesis.

主動脈瓣閉鎖不全 主動脈中的血液於心臟舒張期倒流入左心室。最常發生於急性風濕熱所致之主動瓣瘢痕形成之後，也可發生於梅毒或壁間動脈瘤等情況下。輕度回流無症狀，嚴重者有氣短、心絞痛、心臟擴大等，所有病例都有心臟舒張期雜音。對嚴重損害的主動脈瓣可行瓣膜置換術。

aortic stenosis narrowing of the opening of the aortic valve due to fusion of the cusps that comprise the valve. It may result from previous rheumatic fever, or from calcification and scarring in a valve that has two cusps instead of the normal three, or it may be congenital. Aortic stenosis obstructs the flow of blood from the left ventricle to the aorta during systole. Breathlessness on effort, angina pectoris, and fainting may follow. The patient has a systolic murmur. When symptoms develop the valve should be replaced surgically with a mechanical prosthesis (such as a Starr-Edwards ball-cage valve) or with an aortic valve graft.

主動脈瓣狹窄 由於主動脈瓣瓣膜交界處融合所致之主動脈瓣口狹窄。可發生於風濕熱後，或主動脈瓣由兩個瓣葉組成（正常情況下有三個瓣葉）並產生鈣化和瘢痕形成時，或爲先天性。主動脈瓣狹窄使心臟收縮期時血液由左心室流入主動脈受阻。由此可發生勞力性氣短、心絞痛，並可因之而發生暈厥。聽診可聞心臟收縮期雜音。症狀發展嚴重時應當用機械瓣膜（例如斯塔爾-愛德華氏籠罩球瓣）或主動脈瓣移植片進行置換。

aortic valve a valve in the heart, lying between the left ventricle and the aorta. It consists of three pockets, shaped like half-moons, that prevent blood returning to the ventricle from the aorta. *See also* semilunar valve.

主動脈瓣 心臟中的一種瓣膜，位於左心室和主動脈之間。由三個半月狀瓣葉組成，可阻止血液由主動脈回流入左心室。

aortitis *n.* inflammation of the aorta, which most commonly occurs as a late complication of syphilis. Aortitis principally affects the ascending thoracic aorta and may result in the formation of an aneurysm and obstruction to the coronary blood flow. Chest pain may occur from pressure on surrounding structures or from the reduced blood supply to the heart. *Aortic regurgitation may be found. The syphilitic infection is treated with penicillin but surgical repair to the aortic aneurysm or valve may be needed.

主動脈炎 主動脈的炎症。最常併發於梅毒的後期，多發生於升主動脈。可引起主動脈瘤及使冠狀動脈的血流供應受阻。因主動脈周圍組織受壓迫或心臟供血不足可發生胸痛，還可發生主動脈血回流。梅毒感染用青黴素治療。主動脈瘤或主動脈瓣病變可能需施行外科治療。

aortography *n.* X-ray examination of the aorta, which involves the injection into it of a *radio-opaque contrast medium, after which a series of X-rays is taken (*see* angiocardiography). Aortography is undertaken to reveal the extent and site of diseases such as atheromatous obstruction or aneurysm; it is an essential aid to the planning of surgical treatment.

主動脈造影術 主動脈的X射線檢查。向主動脈內注入X線不透性物質，然後拍攝一系列X線片。主動脈造影術用於顯示病變的程度和部位，例如動脈粥樣硬化性血管阻塞或動脈瘤等，對於外科治療計劃的制訂有重要輔助作用。

aperient *n.* a mild *laxative.

輕瀉藥

apex *n.* the tip or summit of an organ; for example the heart or lung. The apex of a *tooth is the tip of the root, where there is a small hole (the *apical foramen*) through which vessels and nerves pass from the pulp to the periapical tissues. —**apical** *adj.*

尖 一個器官的尖端或頂點。例如心尖或肺尖。牙尖為牙根的尖，該部位有一小孔，牙髓中的血管和神經通過小孔到達根尖周圍組織。

apex beat the impact of the heart against the chest wall during *systole. It can be felt or heard to the left of the breastbone, in the space between the fifth and sixth ribs.

心尖搏動 心臟收縮時向胸壁的衝擊。在胸骨左側第五、六肋骨間隙可觸及或聽到。

Apgar score a method of rapidly assessing the general state of a baby immediately after birth. A maximum of 2 points is given for each of the following signs: type of breathing, heart rate, colour, muscle tone, and response to stimuli. Thus an infant scoring 10 points at 60 minutes after delivery

阿普蓋爾氏記分法 新生兒出生後快速評定其一般情況的方法。包括呼吸，心率，皮膚顏色，肌肉張力，刺激反應力等各項，每項最高值2分。於出生後60分鐘測量的總分達到10分者為最佳狀態。

would be in optimum condition. When the score is low, the test is repeated at intervals as a guide to progress.

低分者應間隔適當時間重新測試，以觀察其進展。

aphakia *n.* absence of the lens of the eye: the state of the eye after a cataract has been removed.

無晶體 眼內缺少晶體。白內障摘除後眼內即無晶體。

aphasia (dysphasia) *n.* a disorder of language affecting the generation of speech and its understanding and not simply a disorder of articulation (*see* dyslalia). It is caused by disease in the left half of the brain (the dominant hemisphere) in a right-handed person. It is commonly accompanied by difficulties in reading and writing. —**aphasic** *adj.*

失語症 一種發出語言和理解語言的能力同時發生障礙的疾病。本病並非單純的構音困難，通常伴有書寫和閱讀困難。

aphonia *n.* absence of or loss of the voice through disease of the larynx or mouth: if loss of speech is due to a defect in the brain the disorder is *aphasia.

失音症 因喉或口腔疾病引起的發音能力缺失或喪失。若語言能力障礙系腦缺陷引起，則爲失語症。

aphrenia *n.* failure of development of the intellectual faculties. *See* subnormality.

癡獃 智能發育不全。

aphrodisiac *n.* an agent that stimulates sexual excitement.

催慾藥，壯陽藥 刺激性慾興奮的藥物。

aphtha *n.* (*pl.* **aphthae**) a small ulcer, occurring singly or in groups in the mouth as white or red spots. Their cause is unknown and only palliative treatment is available. —**aphthous** *adj.*

口瘡 在口腔單發或多發的小潰瘍。呈白色或紅色小斑點狀。起因不明，僅用姑息療法治療。

apical abscess an abscess in the bone around the apex of a tooth. An acute abscess is extremely painful, causing swelling of the jaw and sometimes also the face. It invariably results from death and infection of the pulp of the tooth. Treatment is drainage and *root treatment or extraction of the tooth.

根尖膿腫 牙根尖周圍之骨內膿腫。急性膿腫十分疼痛，引起頜部有時整個面部腫脹。皆爲牙髓壞死或感染所致。治療：引流和根管療法，或拔除病牙。

apicectomy *n.* (in dentistry) surgical removal of the apex of the root of a tooth. It is carried out when *root treatment cannot be done or has failed.

根尖切除術 （牙科）牙齒根尖部之切除手術。當根管療法不能施用或用而無效時可採用此術。

aplasia *n.* total or partial failure of development of an organ or tissue. *See also* agenesis. —**aplastic** *adj.*

發育不全 全部或部分器官或組織的發育不足。

apneusis *n.* a state in which prolonged inhalation occurs. It occurs when the appropriate inhibitory influences are prevented from reaching the inspiratory centre of the brain.

長吸呼吸 吸氣延長的狀態。當適當的抑制性衝動不能達到大腦吸氣中樞時即發生此情况。

apnoea *n.* temporary cessation of breathing from any cause. Attacks of apnoea are common in newborn babies and should be taken seriously although they do not necessarily indicate serious illness. —**apnoeic** *adj.*

呼吸暫停 出於任何原因之呼吸暫時停止。呼吸暫停在新生兒中最常發生。雖然不一定表示有嚴重疾病，仍應愼重對待。

apocrine *adj.* **1.** describing sweat glands that occur only in hairy parts of the body, especially the armpit and groin. These glands develop in the hair follicles and appear after puberty has been reached. The strong odours associated with sweating result from the action of bacteria on the sweat produced by apocrine glands. *Compare* eccrine. **2.** describing a type of gland that loses part of its protoplasm when secreting. *See* secretion.

①**汗臭的** 描述在身體多毛部分，尤其是在腋窩和腹股溝等部的汗腺。此類腺體在毛囊內發育，青春期後纔開始顯現。隨汗排出的惡臭即細菌作用於汗腺分泌的汗液所致。 ②**泌離的** 描述當分泌時失去部分原漿的某型腺體。

apomorphine *n.* an *emetic that produces its effect by direct action on the vomiting centre in the brain. It is given by subcutaneous injection and acts within a few minutes. It is employed in the treatment of poisoning by noncorrosive substances that have been taken by mouth. In nonemetic (lower) dosage, apomorphine has sedative, hypnotic, and expectorant actions.

阿朴嗎啡 直接作用於大腦嘔吐中樞而產生其效果的一種催吐藥。皮下注射幾分鐘內可奏效。用於治療吞服非腐蝕性毒物中毒。在使用不引起嘔吐的低劑量時，阿朴嗎啡有鎮定、催眠和袪痰等作用。

aponeurosis *n.* a thin but strong fibrous sheet of tissue that replaces a *tendon in muscles that are flat and sheetlike and have a wide area of attachment (e.g. to bones). —**aponeurotic** *adj.*

腱膜 一片菲薄而堅實的纖維性組織。代替片狀扁平肌肉的肌肉腱，與骨廣泛附着。

apophysis *n.* **1.** a projection from a bone. **2.** a projection of any other part,

①**骨突** 骨的突出部分。②**突** 任何其他部分的突

e.g. of the brain (*apophysis cerebri*: the *pineal body).

出部，比如腦的突出部：松果體。

apophysitis *n.* inflammation of one or more of the synovial joints between the posterior arches of the vertebrae (*apophyseal joints*). This may occur in rheumatoid arthritis or ankylosing *spondylitis and causes pain. It contributes to partial dislocation (subluxation) of the vertebrae in arthritis and to rigidity of the spine (due to fusion of the joints) in ankylosing spondylitis.

骨突炎 椎骨後弓間滑膜關節（骨突關節）的炎症。它可能在類風濕關節炎或强直性脊椎炎中發生，並引起疼痛。在關節炎中促使脊柱不全脫位（半脫位）；在强直脊椎炎中促使（因關節融合）脊柱强直。

apoplexy *n. see* stroke.

卒中，中風

appendectomy *n.* the usual US term for *appendicectomy.

闌尾切除術 闌尾切除術的美式拚寫。

appendicectomy *n.* surgical removal of the vermiform appendix. *See also* appendicitis.

闌尾切除術 闌尾的手術切除。

appendicitis *n.* inflammation of the vermiform *appendix. *Acute appendicitis*, which has become common this century, usually affects young people. The chief symptom is abdominal pain, first central and later (with tenderness) in the right lower abdomen, over the appendix. Unusual positions of the appendix may cause pain in different sites, leading to difficulty in diagnosis. Vomiting and diarrhoea sometimes occur, but fever is slight. If not treated by surgical removal (appendicectomy) the condition usually progresses to cause an abscess or generalized *peritonitis. Conditions that mimic appendicitis include mesenteric *lymphadenitis, acute ileitis (*see* Crohn's disease), *pyelonephritis, and pneumonia. *Chronic appendicitis* was a popular diagnosis 20–50 years ago to explain recurrent pains in the lower abdomen. It is rare, and appendicectomy will not usually cure such pains.

闌尾炎 闌尾的炎症。急性闌尾炎爲本世紀常見病，通常見於青年。主要症狀是腹痛，先在腹中央，後在腹部右下側闌尾部位，伴有壓痛。闌尾如位置異常，則疼痛部位不同，可能使診斷困難。有時有嘔吐、腹瀉、微熱。如不用手術切除（闌尾切除術），病情往往發展造成膿腫或瀰漫性腹膜炎。與闌尾炎症狀極相似的有腸系膜淋巴結炎、急性廻腸炎（克羅恩氏病）、腎盂腎炎和肺炎等。慢性闌尾炎是二十至五十年前爲解釋下腹周期性疼痛常下的診斷，現已罕見，往往手術也不能解除此類病痛。

appendicostomy *n.* an operation in which the vermiform appendix is brought through the abdominal wall

闌尾造口術 爲腸道引流或減壓從腹壁內取出闌尾在上造口的手術。此手術

and opened in order to drain or decompress the intestine. It is now rarely performed, *ileostomy, *caecostomy, or *colostomy being preferred.

現已少用而多傾向於採用廻腸造口、盲腸造口、結腸造口等手術。

appendicular *adj.* **1.** relating to or affecting the vermiform appendix. **2.** relating to the limbs: the *appendicular skeleton* comprises the bones of the limbs.

①**闌尾的** 與闌尾有關或患及闌尾的。 ②**肢體的** 與肢體有關的。肢體骨骼包含肢體的所有的骨骼。

appendix (vermiform appendix) *n.* the short thin blind-ended tube, 7–10 cm long, that is attached to the end of the caecum (a pouch at the start of the large intestine). It has no known function in man and is liable to become infected and inflamed, especially in young adults (*see* appendicitis).

闌尾 附着在盲腸（大腸始端的囊狀物）末端而另端不通的細短盲管，約 7～10 cm 長。在人體內之功能尚不明，易受感染發炎。中青年尤爲多見。

apperception *n.* (in psychology) the process by which the qualities of an object, situation, etc., perceived by an individual are correlated with his/her preexisting knowledge.

統覺 （心理學）某人將當前所感知事物、情況等的各種特性與其已有知識相互貫聯的過程。

applicator *n.* any device used to apply medication or treatment to a particular part of the body.

①**敷料器** 在身體特定部位塗敷藥物的器械。 ②作治療用的電極或聲頭。

apposition *n.* the state of two structures, such as parts of the body, being in close contact. For example, the fingers are brought into apposition when the fist is clenched, and the eyelids when the eyes are closed.

對合 身體各部的兩種結構處於密切接觸的狀態。例如：當握拳時，五指被置於對合狀態；當閉目時，上下眼瞼處於對合狀態。

apraxia (dyspraxia) *n.* an inability to make skilled movements with accuracy. This is a disorder of the *cerebral cortex resulting in the patient's inability to organize the movements rather than clumsiness due to weakness, sensory loss, or disease of the *cerebellum. It is most often caused by disease of the *parietal lobes of the brain and sometimes by disease of the frontal lobes.

失用症 對精確的技藝性動作之無能爲力。此係患者大腦皮質性疾病造成的組織動作能力喪失，而非肌無力、感覺喪失或小腦性疾病等原因造成的笨拙。常由大腦頂葉疾病，有時也因額葉疾病引起。

aproctia *n.* congenital absence of the anus or its opening. *See* imperforate anus.

鎖肛，無肛 先天性肛門或肛門孔缺失。

aprosexia *n.* inability to fix the attention on any subject, due to poor eyesight, defective hearing, or mental weakness.

注意減退 因弱視、聽力缺陷、或精神衰弱等引起的對任何事物之注意力皆不能集中。

apyrexia *n.* the absence of fever.

無熱期

aqueduct *n.* (in anatomy) a canal containing fluid. For example, the *aqueduct of the midbrain* (*cerebral aqueduct*, *aqueduct of Sylvius*) connects the third and fourth *ventricles.

導水管 （解剖學）包涵有液體的管道。例如第三腦室與四腦室之間的中腦導水管（西爾維厄氏導水管）。

aqueous humour the watery fluid that fills the chamber of the *eye immediately behind the cornea and in front of the lens. It is continually being formed – chiefly by capillaries of the ciliary processes – and it drains away into Schlemm's canal, at the junction of the cornea and sclera.

房水 充滿在前房（緊接角膜後晶狀體前）內的水狀液體。主要由睫狀突的毛細血管不斷地產生，並排入角膜與鞏膜接合處之施累姆氏管（鞏膜靜脈竇）。

arachidonic acid *see* essential fatty acid.

花生烯酸

arachnidism *n.* poisoning from the bite of a spider. Toxins from the less venomous species of spider cause only local pain, redness, and swelling. Toxins from more venomous species, such as the black widow (*Lactrodectus mactans*), cause muscular pains, convulsions, nausea, and paralysis.

蛛毒中毒 被蜘蛛咬而引起的中毒。輕毒類蜘蛛的毒素僅能引起局部疼痛紅腫。如黑衣寡婦劇毒類蜘蛛的毒素則可引起肌肉疼痛、抽搐、噁心和癱瘓。

arachnodactyly *n.* abnormally long and slender fingers: usually associated with excessive height and congenital defects of the heart and eyes in *Marfan's syndrome.

細長指（趾），蜘蛛脚樣指（趾） 手指異常纖細修長。常伴發身材過高，心臟和眼等先天性缺陷，見於馬方氏綜合徵。

arachnoid (arachnoid mater) *n.* the middle of the three membranes covering the brain and spinal cord (*see* meninges), which has a fine, almost cobweb-like, texture. Between it and the pia mater within lies the subarachnoid space, containing cerebrospinal fluid and large blood vessels; the membrane itself has no blood supply.

蛛網膜 覆蓋腦和脊髓的三層膜當中的一層有纖細的蛛網樣構造的膜。蛛網膜與軟腦〔脊〕膜之間有蛛網膜下腔，內含有腦脊〔髓〕液及大血管，蛛網膜自身無血管供應。

arachnoid villus one of the thin-walled projections outwards of the ar-

蛛網膜絨毛 由蛛網膜向外伸入硬膜血竇內的薄壁

achnoid membrane into the blood-filled sinuses of the dura, acting as a one-way valve for the flow of cerebrospinal fluid from the subarachnoid space into the bloodstream. Large villi, known as *arachnoid granulations* (or *Pacchionian bodies*), are found in the region of the superior sagittal sinus. They may be so distended as to cause pitting of the adjacent bone.

突起物。起單向閥門作用，使腦脊液由蛛網膜下腔進入血流。在上矢狀竇區可見到稱爲蛛網膜粒（或帕基奧尼氏體）的大絨毛。此類絨毛之膨起足使近鄰骨發生凹陷。

arbor *n.* (in anatomy) a treelike structure. *Arbor vitae* is the treelike outline of white matter seen in sections of the cerebellum; it also refers to the treelike appearance of the inner folds of the neck of the womb.

樹 （解剖學）樹狀結構。〔小腦〕活樹就是小腦切片中所見到的白質的樹狀形態；也指子宮頸內皺襞的樹狀外觀。

arbovirus *n.* one of a group of RNA-containing viruses that are transmitted from animals to man by insects (i.e. arthropods; hence *ar*thropod-*bo*rne viruses) and cause diseases resulting in encephalitis or serious fever, such as dengue and yellow fever.

蟲媒病毒 由昆蟲（即節肢動物）作媒介從動物傳染給人（因而又稱節肢動物傳播病毒），造成腦炎或登革熱、黃熱病之類烈性熱病的一組含核糖核酸病毒。

arc-eye *n.* a painful condition of the eyes caused by damage to the surface of the cornea by ultraviolet light from arc welding. It usually resolves if the eyes are padded for 24 hours. It is similar to *snow blindness and the condition caused by overexposure of the eye to sun-tanning lamps.

弧光眼，電弧眼 因弧焊紫外線損及角膜表面而引起疼痛的疾病。若用敷料遮蓋二十四小時通常可復原。弧光眼與雪盲或眼睛經日光燈照射過度所引起的症狀相似。

arch- (arche-, archi-, archo-) *prefix denoting* first; beginning; primitive; ancestral. Example: *archinephron* (first-formed embryonic kidney).

〔前綴〕**第一，初，原始，舊，原** 例如：原腎（最初形成的胚胎腎）。

archenteron *n.* a cavity that forms in the very early embryo as the result of gastrulation (*see* gastrula). In man it forms a tubular cavity, the *archenteric canal*, which connects the amniotic cavity with the yolk sac. —**archenteric** *adj.*

原腸 在最早期胚胎中，由原腸胚胎形成的腔。在人體中，它形成一管狀腔（神經腸管），通過卵黃囊與羊膜腔相連接。

archetype *n.* (in Jungian psychology) an inherited idea or mode of thought supposed to be present in the *unconscious mind and to derive from the

原始意象 （容格氏心理學用語）存在於潛意識中的來自全人類的集體經驗而非個人生活經驗的通過

experience of the whole human race, not from the life experience of the individual.

遺傳而獲得的觀念或思維方式。

archipallium *n.* the *hippocampal formation of the cerebrum. The term is seldom used.

舊皮質 大腦的海馬結構。此詞已少用。

arcus *n.* (in anatomy) an arch; for example the *arcus aortae* (*aortic arch).

弓 （解剖學）弓狀物。例如：主動脉弓。

arcus senilis a greyish line in the periphery of the cornea, concentric with the edge but separated from it by a clear zone. It begins above and below but may become a continuous ring. It consists of an infiltration of fatty material and is common in the elderly. When it occurs in younger people it may indicate abnormal fat metabolism, but there is great racial variation in its incidence. It never affects vision.

老人弓，老人環 在角膜周圍的一條淺灰色的線。緊貼角膜邊緣，但有一條明亮帶與角膜分開。從上、下兩方開始發生，可能漸連成環。老人弓由脂肪性物質浸潤組成，並多見於老年人。當發生在年齡較輕人中，表明可能脂肪代謝異常，但發生率在各種族中差別很大。對視力從無影響。

areola *n.* **1.** the brownish or pink ring of tissue surrounding the nipple of the breast. **2.** the part of the iris that surrounds the pupil of the eye. **3.** a small space in a tissue. —**areolar** *adj.*

①**乳暈** 在乳頭周圍的淺棕或粉紅色的組織。 ②**暈** 圍繞瞳孔的部分虹膜。 ③**細隙，小區** 組織內的細隙或小區。

areolar tissue loose *connective tissue consisting of a meshwork of collagen, elastic tissue, and reticular fibres interspersed with numerous connective tissue cells. It binds the skin to underlying muscles and forms a link between organs while allowing a high degree of relative movement.

蜂窩組織 由膠原網絡、彈性組織和含有大量結締組織細胞的網狀纖維等組成的疏鬆的結締組織。它使皮膚附着於其下層的肌肉，並充填於器官之間，爲它們的活動留有充分餘地。

Argasidae *n. see* tick.

隱喙蜱科

argentaffin cells cells that stain readily with silver salts. Such cells occur, for example, in the crypts of Lieberkühn in the intestine.

嗜銀細胞 易被銀化合物染色的細胞。例如利貝昆氏腺（腸腺）腺管中的細胞。

argentaffinoma (carcinoid) *n.* a tumour of the *argentaffin cells in the glands of the intestine. Argentaffinomas typically occur in the tip of the appendix and are among the commonest tumours of the small intestine.

嗜銀細胞瘤（類癌瘤） 腸腺中嗜銀細胞的腫瘤。嗜銀細胞瘤多發於闌尾頂端，屬最常見的小腸腫瘤。也可能發生在直腸、消化道其他部位和支氣管

They may also occur in the rectum and other parts of the digestive tract and in the bronchial tree (*bronchial carcinoid adenoma*). Argentaffinomas sometimes produce 5-hydroxytryptamine (serotonin), prostaglandins, and other physiologically active substances, which are inactivated in the liver. If the tumour has spread to the liver excess amounts of these substances are released into the systemic circulation and the *carcinoid syndrome* results – flushing, headache, diarrhoea, asthma-like attacks, and in some cases damage to the right side of the heart.

樹內（支氣管類癌腺瘤）。嗜銀細胞瘤有時產生5-羥色胺（血清素）、前列腺素和其他種種在肝內被滅活的生理活性物質。腫瘤如果蔓延及肝，釋放大量此類物質進入體循環，就會引起顏面潮紅、頭痛、腹瀉、氣喘樣發作等類癌瘤綜合徵，在某些情況下，還使右心受害。

arginine *n.* an *amino acid that plays an important role in the formation of *urea by the liver.

精氨酸 肝臟合成尿素中起重要作用的一種氨基酸。

Argyll Robertson pupil a disorder of the eyes, common to several diseases of the central nervous system, in which the *pupillary (light) reflex is absent. Although the pupils contract normally for near vision, they fail to contract in bright light.

阿蓋爾·羅伯遜氏瞳孔 幾種中樞神經疾病共有的一種眼疾患。此時瞳孔反射缺失，近視時瞳孔雖能正常收縮，但對光反射消失。

argyria *n.* a form of silver poisoning in which the skin becomes dark bluish-grey due to the accumulation of the metal in the tissues. The mucous membranes and internal organs are also affected. Argyria is now rare, due to the decline in the use of silver compounds in medicine and industry (except the photographic industry).

銀質沉着病 銀中毒的一種類型。因組織內銀聚積使皮膚變成深藍灰色。黏膜和內臟也可受損。現除照相器材業外，醫藥和工業已拒絕用銀化合物，因而本病已屬罕見。

ariboflavinosis *n.* the group of symptoms caused by deficiency of riboflavin (vitamin B_2). These symptoms include inflammation of the tongue and lips and sores in the corners of the mouth.

核黃素缺乏病 由於缺乏核黃素（維生素 B_2）而引起症候羣。症狀有舌和唇發炎，嘴角生瘡。

Arnold-Chiari malformation a congenital disorder in which there is distortion of the base of the skull with protrusion of the lower brainstem and parts of the cerebellum through the opening for the spinal cord at the base of the skull. It is commonly associated

阿-希二氏畸形 顱底骨畸形、腦幹下部及部分小腦從枕大孔突出的一種先天性疾患。經常伴有神經管缺陷和腦積水。

with *neural tube defects and *hydrocephalus.

arousal *n.* **1.** a state of alertness and of high responsiveness to stimuli. It is produced by strong motivation, by anxiety, and by a stimulating environment. **2.** physiological activation of the *cerebral cortex by centres lower in the brain, such as the *reticular activating system, resulting in wakefulness and alertness. It is hypothesized that unduly high or low degrees of arousal lead to neuropsychiatric problems, such as *narcolepsy and *mania.

①**警覺**　對刺激有戒備和產生强烈反應的狀態。具有强烈的動機、焦慮狀態和充滿刺激的環境可產生這種心理狀態。　②**覺醒**　由網狀激活系統等低級中樞對大腦皮質產生之心理激活作用，可造成清醒和警覺狀態。人們假想：覺醒程度高低不當能導致發作性睡眠和躁狂之類的神經精神性疾患。

arrhenoblastoma *n. see* androblastoma.

男性細胞瘤(卵巢)

arrhythmia *n.* any deviation from the normal rhythm (sinus rhythm) of the heart. The natural pacemaker of the heart (the sinoatrial node), which lies in the wall of the right atrium, controls the rate and rhythm of the whole heart under the influence of the autonomic nervous system. It generates electrical impulses that spread to the atria and ventricles, via specialized conducting tissues, and cause them to contract normally. Arrhythmias result from a disturbance of the generation or conduction of these impulses and may be intermittent or continuous. They include *ectopic beats (extrasystoles), ectopic *tachycardias, *fibrillation, and *heart block (which is often associated with slow heart rates). Symptoms include palpitations, breathlessness, and chest pain. In more serious arrhythmias the *Stokes-Adams syndrome or *cardiac arrest may occur. Arrhythmias may result from most heart diseases but they also occur without apparent cause.

心律失常，心律不齊　心臟之正常節律(竇性心律)發生變化。位於右心房壁之天然心臟起搏點(竇房結)在自主神經系統影響下，控制整個心臟(搏動)速度和節律。由此處發出電衝動通過特殊的傳導組織，傳播至心房和心室，使其產生正常的收縮。心律失常即由這些衝動之發生或傳導的紊亂引起，可能是間歇的或持續的。心律失常包括異位搏動(額外收縮)、異位搏動過速、纖維性顫動和常表現爲心搏遲緩的心傳導阻滯。症狀有心悸、呼吸困難和胸痛。嚴重時可能出現斯-亞二氏綜合徵或心搏停止。心律失常大多因各種心臟病引起，但也可能無明顯原因。

arsenic *n.* a poisonous greyish metallic element producing the symptoms of nausea, vomiting, diarrhoea, cramps, convulsions, and coma when ingested in large doses. Drugs used as antidotes to arsenic poisoning include *dimerca-

砷　淺灰色有毒金屬元素(縮AS)。當攝取大劑量時，能引起噁心、嘔吐、腹瀉、痛性痙攣等症狀，還能致人昏迷。砷中毒的解毒劑是二硫基丙

prol. Arsenic was formerly readily available in the form of rat poison and in fly-papers and was the poisoner's first choice during the 19th century, its presence in a body being then difficult to detect. Today detection is relatively simple. Arsenic was formerly used in medicine, the most important arsenical drugs being *arsphenamine* (*Salvarsan*) and *neoarsphenamine*, used in the treatment of syphilis and dangerous parasitic diseases. Symbol: As.

醇。砷以往多用於滅鼠劑和捕蠅紙中；十九世紀時投毒人最愛選用，因當時它在人體中之存在是難以檢出的。如今檢驗方法相當簡單。以往砷用於醫藥，最主要的是用以治療梅毒和危害性寄生蟲病的砷凡拉明（灑爾佛散）和新砷凡拉明。

artefact *n. see* artifact.

人爲現象

arter- (arteri-, arterio-) *prefix denoting* an artery. Examples: *arteriopathy* (disease of); *arteriorrhaphy* (suture of); *arteriovenous* (relating to arteries and veins).

〔前綴〕**動脈**　例如：動脈病，動脈縫合術，動靜脈的（與動脈和靜脈有關的）。

arteriectomy *n.* surgical excision of an artery or part of an artery. This may be performed as a diagnostic procedure (for example, to take an arterial biopsy in the diagnosis of arteritis) or during reconstruction of a blocked artery when the blocked segment is replaced by a synthetic graft.

動脈切除術　一條或一段動脈的手術切除。可用作診斷（例如：動脈炎時取動脈活組織作診斷用）或用於阻塞動脈重建手術，以人造動脈置換阻塞部分。

arteriogram *n.* a tracing of the wave form of an arterial pulse. This can be made directly, by means of an arterial needle puncture and pressure recording, or indirectly, by a recorder placed on the skin over an artery. The tracing may be recorded on a paper strip or on a screen (oscilloscope). Some heart defects produce characteristic pulse wave forms.

動脈搏描記圖　動脈搏動波形圖。此可以利用動脈穿刺針和記錄裝置直接描記，或將記錄裝置放在動脈上面的皮膚上間接描記。圖像可描記在紙帶或熒光屏（示波儀）上。有些心臟疾患產生具有特徵性的搏動波圖形。

arteriography *n.* X-ray examination of an artery that has been outlined by the injection of a *radio-opaque contrast medium. The major uses of arteriography are to demonstrate the site and extent of atheroma, especially in the coronary arteries (*coronary angiography*) and leg arteries (*femoral angiography*), and to reveal the site of aneurysms within the skull or cerebral tumours

動脈造影術　注射不透X線的造影劑以顯現動脈輪廓的X-線檢查法。動脈造影術主要用以顯示冠狀動脈（冠狀血管造影術）和股動脈（股血管造影術）內粥樣化所在部位及其範圍；和顯示顱內動脈瘤或大腦腫瘤所在部位（頸動脈和椎動脈血管造

(*carotid* and *vertebral artery angiography*). 影術）。

arteriole *n.* a small branch of an *artery, leading into many smaller vessels – the *capillaries. By their constriction and dilation, under the regulation of the sympathetic nervous system, arterioles are the principal controllers of blood flow and pressure.

小動脈 與衆多微小血管-毛細血管相連接的動脈小分支。小動脈在交感神經調節下憑藉其收縮和舒張，對血流和血壓起主要控制作用。

arteriolitis *n.* inflammation of the arterioles (the smallest arteries), which may complicate severe hypertension. This produces *necrotizing arteriolitis*, which may result in kidney failure. A similar condition may affect the lung in pulmonary hypertension.

小動脈炎〔症〕 小動脈（最小動脈）的炎症。可併發於嚴重高血壓。高血壓引起的壞死性小動脈炎可導致腎功衰竭。肺動脈高血壓亦可引起肺部壞死性小動脈炎，導致呼吸衰竭。

arterioplasty *n.* surgical reconstruction of an artery; for example, in the treatment of *aneurysms.

動脈成形術 動脈重建手術，如用於治療動脈瘤。

arteriosclerosis *n.* an imprecise term used for any of several conditions affecting the arteries. The term is often used as a synonym for atherosclerosis (*see* atheroma). It may also be used for *Mönckeberg's degeneration*, in which calcium is deposited in the arteries as part of the ageing process, and *arteriolarsclerosis*, in which the walls of small arteries become thickened due to ageing or hypertension.

動脈硬化 可用於表述幾種不同動脈疾病的含糊之詞。它常用作動脈粥樣硬化的同義詞，也可用於因老化動脈上有鈣沉積的門克伯格氏變性，也可用於因老化或高血壓小動脈壁增厚的小動脈硬化。

arteriotomy *n.* an incision into, or a needle puncture of, the wall of an artery. This is most often performed as a diagnostic procedure in the course of *arteriography or cardiac *catheterization. It may also be required to remove an embolus (*see* embolectomy).

動脈切開術 切開或穿刺動脈壁的手術。是在動脈造影或心導管插入術中最常施用的一種診斷性手術。在排除栓子時，也可能需用此術。

arteriovenous anastomosis a thick-walled blood vessel that connects an arteriole directly with a venule, thus bypassing the capillaries. Arteriovenous anastomoses are commonly found in the skin of the lips, nose, ears, hands and feet; their muscular walls can

動靜脈吻合 不經毛細血管而直接聯接小動脈和靜脈的厚壁血管。動靜脈吻合常見於唇、鼻、耳、手和足等的皮膚內；其肌壁能收縮或舒張以改變對這些區域的血流供應。

constrict to reduce blood flow or dilate to allow blood through to these areas.

arteriovenous aneurysm a direct communication between an artery and vein, without an intervening capillary bed. It can occur as a congenital abnormality or it may be acquired following injury or surgery. It may affect the limbs, lungs, or viscera and may be single or multiple. If the connection is large, the short-circuiting of blood may produce heart failure. Large isolated arteriovenous aneurysms may be closed surgically.

動靜脉瘤 動脉直接與靜脉相通，其間無毛細血管床介入。可能因先天性畸形，也可能因損傷或手術引起。可發生於四肢、肺或內臟，單發或多發。如果動脉瘤很大，血流短路可能引起心力衰竭。大而單獨的動靜脉瘤可用手術閉合。

arteriovenous malformation *see* angioma.

動靜脉畸形

arteritis *n.* an inflammatory disease affecting the muscular walls of the arteries. It may be part of a *collagen disease or it may be due to an infection, such as syphilis. The affected vessels are swollen and tender and may become blocked. *Temporal* or *giant-cell arteritis* occurs in the elderly and most commonly affects the arteries of the scalp. The patient complains of severe headache, and blindness may result from thrombosis of the arteries to the eyes. Treatment with cortisone derivatives is rapidly effective.

動脉炎 動脉肌壁的炎性疾病。可能屬於膠原疾病一部分，也可能由於如梅毒之類的感染。患病血管腫脹，有觸痛，並可能阻塞。顳動脉炎（或巨細胞動脉炎）多發生於老年且最常侵犯頭皮的動脉。患者主訴劇烈頭痛。通往眼部動脉的血栓形成可能造成失明。用可的松類衍化物治療見效迅速。

artery *n.* a blood vessel carrying blood away from the heart. All arteries except the *pulmonary artery carry oxygenated blood. The walls of arteries contain smooth muscle fibres (see illustration), which contract or relax under the control of the sympathetic nervous system. *See also* aorta, arteriole.

動脉 從心臟往外運送血液的血管。除肺動脉外所有動脉皆運送含氧血液。血管壁含有平滑肌纖維（見圖），其收縮與舒張均由交感神經系統調節。

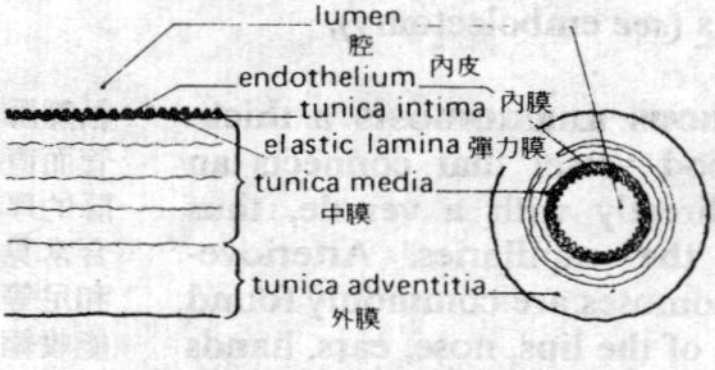

Transverse section through an artery
血管橫切面

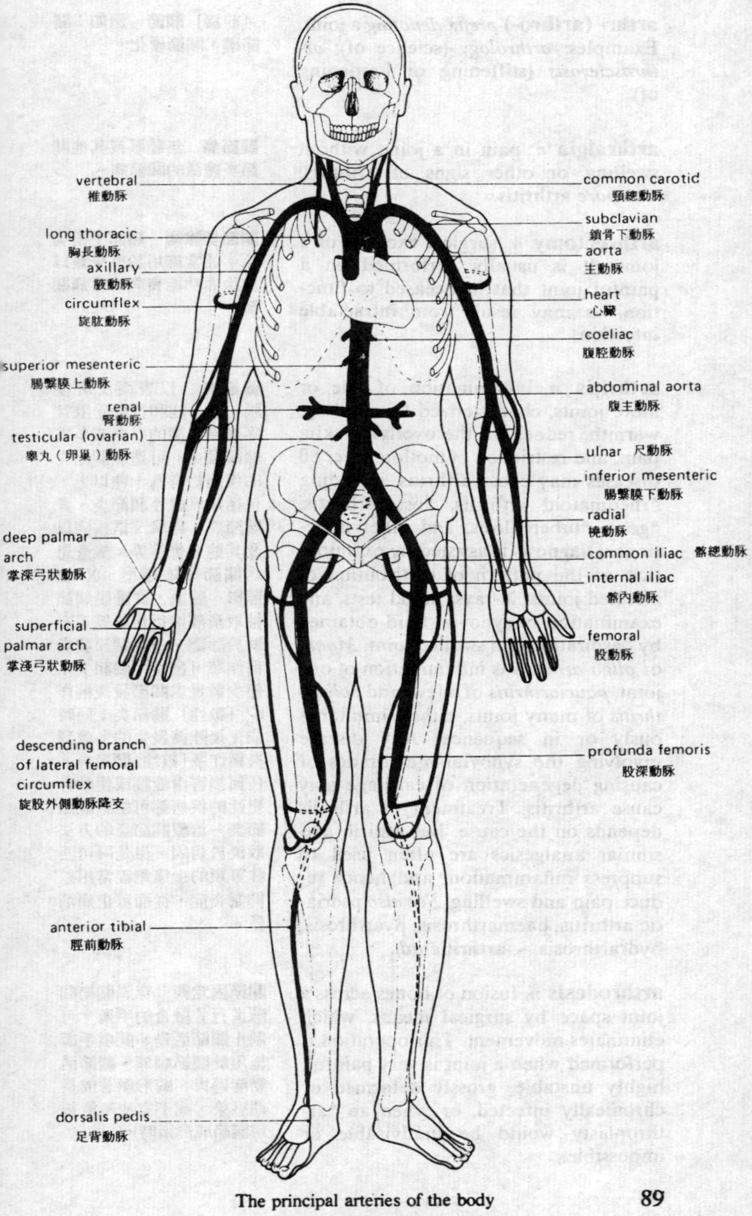
vertebral
椎動脉
long thoracic
胸長動脉
axillary
腋動脉
circumflex
旋肱動脉
superior mesenteric
腸繫膜上動脉
renal
腎動脉
testicular (ovarian)
睾丸（卵巢）動脉
deep palmar arch
掌深弓狀動脉
superficial palmar arch
掌淺弓狀動脉
descending branch of lateral femoral circumflex
旋股外側動脉降支
anterior tibial
脛前動脉
dorsalis pedis
足背動脉
common carotid
頸總動脉
subclavian
鎖骨下動脉
aorta
主動脉
heart
心臟
coeliac
腹腔動脉
abdominal aorta
腹主動脉
ulnar 尺動脉
inferior mesenteric
腸繫膜下動脉
radial
橈動脉
common iliac 髂總動脉
internal iliac
髂內動脉
femoral
股動脉
profunda femoris
股深動脉

The principal arteries of the body

人體主要動脉

arthr- (arthro-) *prefix denoting* a joint. Examples: *arthrology* (science of); *arthrosclerosis* (stiffening or hardening of).

〔前綴〕**關節**　例如：關節學，關節硬化。

arthralgia *n.* pain in a joint, without swelling or other signs of arthritis. *Compare* arthritis.

關節痛　無腫脹或其他關節炎體徵的關節痛。

arthrectomy *n.* surgical excision of a joint. It is usually performed on a painful joint that has ceased to function, as may result from intractable infection.

關節切除術　關節手術切除。通常施用於感染難以消除而功能喪失的疼痛關節。

arthritis *n.* inflammation of one or more joints, characterized by swelling, warmth, redness of the overlying skin, pain, and restriction of motion. Over 80 diseases may cause arthritis, including *rheumatoid arthritis, *osteoarthritis, *gout, *tuberculosis, and other infections. Diagnosis is assisted by examination of the pattern of distribution of affected joints, X-rays, blood tests, and examination of synovial fluid obtained by *aspiration of a swollen joint. *Mono-* or *oligo-arthritis* is inflammation of one joint, *pauciarthritis* of a few, and *polyarthritis* of many joints, either simultaneously or in sequence. Any disease involving the synovial membranes or causing degeneration of cartilage may cause arthritis. Treatment of arthritis depends on the cause, but aspirin and similar analgesics are often used to suppress inflammation, and hence reduce pain and swelling. *See also* psoriatic arthritis, haemarthrosis, pyarthrosis, hydrarthrosis. —**arthritic** *adj.*

關節炎　以表面皮膚腫脹、熱、紅和行動受限且疼痛爲特徵的一處或多處關節發炎。可造成關節炎的疾病約有八十種以上，包括類風濕性關節炎、骨關節炎、痛風、結核病以及其他感染等等。檢查患病關節分佈類型、X-線照影、驗血、從腫脹關節抽取滑液進行化驗等等有助於診斷。一處關節發炎稱作單〔發性〕關節炎；僅少數幾處關節發炎稱作少〔數性〕關節炎；同時或先後陸續發生的多處發炎稱作多〔數性〕關節炎。任何損害滑液膜或使軟骨變性的疾病都可能造成關節炎。治療關節炎的方法取決於病因，但是阿司匹林等類的止痛劑經常用以抑制炎症，從而可止痛消腫。

arthrodesis *n.* fusion of bones across a joint space by surgical means, which eliminates movement. This operation is performed when a joint is very painful, highly unstable, grossly deformed or chronically infected, or when an *arthroplasty would be inadvisable or impossible.

關節固定術　穿過關節間隙進行骨融合的手術。可制止關節活動。此項手術施用於關節劇痛、關節活動度過大、畸形顯著或長期感染，或不宜或不能施用關節成形術時。

arthrodic joint (gliding joint) a form of *diarthrosis (freely movable joint) in which the bony surfaces slide over each other without angular or rotational movement. Examples are the joints of the carpus and tarsus.

摩動關節 動關節（可自由活動的關節）中的一種：骨表面彼此互相滑動但無成角與旋轉活動的關節。例如腕關節和跗關節等。

arthrography *n.* an X-ray technique for examining joints. A *contrast medium (either air or a liquid opaque to X-rays) is injected into the joint space, allowing its outline and contents to be traced accurately.

關節照影術 檢查關節的X-線照影技術。將造影劑（不透X-射線的液體或氣體）注射入關節間隙，可精確地顯示其外形和內容。

arthropathy *n.* any disease or disorder involving a joint.

關節病 關節部位的任何疾病。

arthroplasty *n.* surgical remodelling of a diseased joint. To prevent the ends of the bones fusing after the operation, a large gap may be created between them (*gap arthroplasty*), a barrier of artificial material may be inserted (*interposition arthroplasty*), or one or both bone ends may be replaced by a *prosthesis of metal or plastic (*replacement arthroplasty*).

關節成形術 患病關節的重建手術。爲避免手術後關節骨端之間融合，可在其間形成較大間隙（間隙關節成形術），亦可插入人造材料的壁障（嵌入關節成形術），或在一骨或兩骨骨端換用金屬或塑料假骨（置換關節成形術）。

arthropod *n.* any member of a large group of animals that possess a hard external skeleton and jointed legs and other appendages. Many arthropods are of medical importance, including the *mites, *ticks, and *insects.

節肢動物 一大族具有堅硬外骨骼和節足及其他附器的動物。很多節肢動物包括蟎類、蜱類和昆蟲等在醫學上都具有重要意義。

arthroscope *n.* an instrument for insertion into the cavity of a joint in order to inspect the contents, before *biopsy or operation on the joint.

關節〔內窺〕鏡 活組織檢查或手術前，插入關節內以窺視其內容的一種器械。

arthrotomy *n.* surgical incision of a joint capsule in order to inspect the contents and drain pus (if it is present).

關節切開術 爲檢查關節內容物或在有膿時排膿而將關節囊切開的手術。

articulation *n.* (in anatomy) the point or type of contact between two bones. *See* joint.

關節 （解剖學）兩骨之間接觸的部位或方式。

articulator *n.* (in dentistry) an apparatus for relating the upper and lower models of a patient's dentition in a fixed position, usually with maximum tooth

𬌗架，咬合架 （牙科）將患者上下牙的牙列模型保持於某種固定位置的一種器械。常使上下牙儘量

contact. Some articulators can reproduce jaw movements. They are used in the construction of crowns, bridges, and dentures.

密切接觸。有些船架用於製作牙冠、牙橋和托牙。

artifact (artefact) *n.* (in microscopy) a structure seen in a tissue under a microscope that is not present in the living tissue. Artifacts, which are produced by faulty *fixation or staining of the tissue, may give a false impression that disease or abnormality is present in the tissue when it is not.

人爲現象，人工產物 在顯微鏡下組織內見到的，但在活組織中並不存在的結構。因組織固定或染色等之失誤而造成的人爲現象，可能造成某組織內有病變或異常的假象。

artificial insemination instrumental introduction of semen into the vagina in order that the woman may conceive. Insemination is timed to coincide with the day on which the woman is expected to ovulate (*see* menstrual cycle). The semen specimen may be provided by the husband (*AIH – artificial insemination husband*) in cases of *impotence or by an anonymous donor (*AID – artificial insemination donor*) in cases where the husband is sterile.

人工授精 爲求婦女受孕將精液以器械引入陰道之方法。授精時間安排應與婦女預期排卵日相符。精液可由不能行房事的配偶（人工授精丈夫）提供。配偶患不育症者，可由匿名獻精者（人工授精提供者）提供。

artificial kidney (dialyser) *see* haemodialysis.

人工腎（透析器）

artificial lung *see* respirator.

人工肺

artificial respiration an emergency procedure for maintaining a flow of air into and out of a patient's lungs when the natural breathing reflexes are absent or insufficient. This may occur after drowning, poisoning, etc., or during a surgical operation on the thorax or abdomen when muscle-relaxing drugs are administered. The simplest and most efficient method is the mouth-to-mouth technique (the '*kiss of life*'). In hospital the breathing cycle is maintained by means of a *respirator.

人工呼吸 當自然呼吸反射消失或減弱時，爲維持患者肺部空氣流通的一項救急措施。這種情況可能發生在溺水、中毒等意外事故之後，或腹部、咽喉等外科手術中服用弛緩肌肉藥物時。最簡單且最有效的方法是口對口呼吸法（救生吻）。在醫院內藉呼吸器維持患者呼吸周期。

arytenoid cartilage either of the two pyramid-shaped cartilages that lie at the back of the *larynx next to the upper edges of the cricoid cartilage.

杓狀軟骨 在喉之後鄰近環狀軟骨上緣的兩塊錐形軟骨。

asbestosis *n.* a lung disease – a form of *pneumoconiosis – caused by fibres of asbestos inhaled by those who are exposed to large amounts of the mineral. The incidence of lung cancer is high in such patients, particularly if they smoke cigarettes. *See also* mesothelioma.

石棉沉着病 接觸大量石棉礦物的人員吸入石棉纖維而引起的一種肺塵病。這種患者肺癌發病率高，吸煙者尤甚。

ascariasis *n.* a disease caused by an infestation with the parasitic worm **Ascaris lumbricoides*. Adult worms in the intestine can cause abdominal pain, vomiting, constipation, diarrhoea, appendicitis, and peritonitis; in large numbers they may cause obstruction of the intestine. The presence of the migrating larvae in the lungs can provoke pneumonia. Ascariasis occurs principally in areas of poor sanitation; it is treated with *piperazine.

蛔蟲病 因感染寄生蟲人蛔蟲而罹患的疾病。腸內成蟲能引起腹痛、嘔吐、便秘、腹瀉、闌尾炎、腹膜炎，大量蛔蟲能造成腸梗阻。肺內有移行幼蟲能激發肺炎。蛔蟲病主要發生在衛生不良地區。治療用哌嗪。

Ascaris *n.* a genus of parasitic nematode worms. *A. lumbricoides*, widely distributed throughout the world, is the largest of the human intestinal nematodes – an adult female measures up to 35 cm in length. Eggs, passed out in the stools, may be transmitted to a new host in contaminated food or drink. Larvae hatch out in the intestine and then undergo a complicated migration, via the hepatic portal vein, liver, heart, lungs, windpipe, and pharynx, before returning to the intestine where they later develop into adult worms (*see also* ascariasis).

蛔蟲屬 寄生性線蟲屬。在世界各地廣泛分佈的人蛔蟲在人類腸線蟲中最長——雌成蟲可長達 35 cm。隨糞便排出的蟲卵可在遭污染的飲食中傳播給新宿主。在腸內孵化出的幼蟲經歷一段複雜移行過程，經肝門靜脉、肝、心臟、肺、氣管和喉，然後回到腸發育爲成蟲。

ascites (hydroperitoneum) *n.* the accumulation of fluid in the peritoneal cavity, causing abdominal swelling. Causes include infections (such as tuberculosis), heart failure, *portal hypertension, *cirrhosis, and various cancers (particularly of the ovary and liver). *See also* oedema.

腹水 導致腹部膨脹的腹腔液體蓄積。病因有結核病之類的感染、心力衰竭、門靜脉高血壓、肝硬變和各種（特別是卵巢或肝的）癌。

ascorbic acid *see* vitamin C.

抗壞血酸

-ase *suffix* denoting an enzyme. Examples: *lactase*; *dehydrogenase*.

〔後綴〕**酶** 例如：乳糖酶，脫氫酶。

asepsis *n.* the complete absence of bacteria, fungi, viruses, or other microorganisms that could cause disease. Asepsis is the ideal state for the performance of surgical operations and is achieved by using *sterilization techniques. —**aseptic** *adj.*

無菌 絕無細菌、黴菌、病毒或其他致病微生物等存在的狀態。無菌是施行外科手術的理想狀態，是用滅菌技術達到的。

asparaginase *n.* an enzyme that inhibits the growth of certain tumours and is used in the treatment of acute lymphoblastic leukaemia. It may cause allergic reactions and *anaphylaxis.

天門冬醯胺酶 一種抑制某種腫瘤生長，並用以治療淋巴細胞性白血病的酶。它可能引起變態反應和過敏反應。

asparagine *n. see* amino acid.

天門冬醯胺

aspartic acid (aspartate) *see* amino acid.

天門冬氨酸

aspergillosis *n.* a rare disease in which the fungus *Aspergillus fumigatus* grows freely in pre-existing lesions in the lungs and bronchioles. Occasionally the fungus attacks the mucous membranes of the eyes, nose, or urethra or such internal organs as the lungs, liver, and kidneys.

曲黴病，曲菌病 煙曲黴菌在先有損害的肺和細支氣管中大量繁殖的一種罕見病。偶爾黴菌也侵襲眼、鼻或尿道等的黏膜，或肺、肝、腎等內臟。

Aspergillus *n.* a genus of fungi, including many common moulds, some of which cause infections of the respiratory system in man. The species *A. fumigatus* causes *aspergillosis. *A. niger* is commonly found in the external ear and can become pathogenic.

曲黴屬 包括多種常見的（其中某些致人呼吸系統感染）黴菌的黴菌屬。煙曲黴造成曲黴病，黑曲黴常見於外耳並能成爲致病黴。

aspermia *n.* strictly, a lack or failure of formation of semen. More usually, however, the term is used to mean the total absence of sperm from the semen (*see* azoospermia).

無精，精液缺乏 本詞確切含意應爲精液形成不足或精液形成不能。然而更通常指精液內毫無精子。

asphyxia *n.* suffocation: a life-threatening condition in which oxygen is prevented from reaching the tissues by obstruction of or damage to any part of the respiratory system. Drowning, choking, and breathing poisonous gas all lead to asphyxia. Unless the condition is remedied by removing the obstruction (when present) and by artifi-

窒息 呼吸系統任何一部分阻塞或受損害，阻礙氧氣到達組織而危及生命的狀況。溺水，呼吸道堵塞，和吸入有毒氣體都可導致窒息。必需解除阻塞（若有）並用人工呼吸（如需要時）進行急救，否則就可出現進行性紫

cial respiration if necessary, there is progressive *cyanosis leading to death. Brain cells cannot live for more than about four minutes without oxygen.

紺，最終導致死亡。腦細胞缺氧超過四分多鐘就不能存活。

aspiration *n.* the withdrawal of fluid from the body by means of suction using an instrument called an *aspirator*. There are various types of aspirator: some employ hollow needles for removing fluid from cysts, inflamed joint cavities, etc.; another kind is used to suck debris and water from the patient's mouth during dental treatment.

吸引術 用名爲抽吸器的工具從體內抽出液體。有不同類型抽吸器：有的用空心針管從囊腫、發炎關節腔等處抽液；另一種用在牙科治療時從患者口腔吸除殘渣和水。

aspirin (acetylsalicylic acid) *n.* a widely used drug that relieves pain and also reduces inflammation and fever. It is taken by mouth – alone or in combination with caffeine, phenacetin, or codeine – for the relief of the less severe types of pain, such as headache, toothache, neuralgias, and the pain of rheumatoid arthritis. It is also taken to reduce fever in influenza and the common cold. Aspirin may irritate the lining of the stomach, causing nausea, vomiting, pain, and bleeding. Tablets should not be held on the gum adjacent to a painful tooth as ulceration may occur. High doses cause dizziness, disturbed hearing, mental confusion, and overbreathing. *See also* analgesic.

阿司匹林（乙醯水楊酸） 一種廣泛使用的止痛、消炎和解熱的藥。爲解除如頭痛、牙痛、神經痛以及風濕類關節炎等的疼痛時，可單獨口服，或與咖啡因、非那西汀或可待因並用。在患流行性感冒和普通感冒時，亦用作解熱藥。阿司匹林可能刺激胃壁黏膜發炎造成噁心、嘔吐、疼痛、出血。藥片不得噙在貼近痛牙的牙齦上，因可能形成潰瘍。大劑量使用可造成頭暈、聽覺紊亂、精神錯亂和喘息。

assay *n.* a test or trial to determine the strength of a solution, the proportion of a compound in a mixture, the potency of a drug, or the purity of a preparation. *See also* bioassay.

測定，鑒定 爲確定溶劑的濃度、合劑中成分比、藥物性能或製劑純淨度等等而作的檢查或試驗。

assimilation *n.* the process by which food substances are taken into the cells of the body after they have been digested and absorbed.

同化〔作用〕 食物經消化和吸收後被攝入體內細胞內的過程。

association area an area of *cerebral cortex that lies away from the main areas that are concerned with the reception of sensory impulses and the start of motor impulses but is linked to them by

聯合區 處在接受感覺衝動和發出運動衝動的主區之外，但又以許多稱爲聯合纖維的神經原與這些主區相聯繫的大腦皮質區。

many neurones known as *association fibres*. The areas of association are thought to be responsible for the elaboration of the information received by the primary sensory areas and its correlation with the information fed in from memory and from other brain areas. They are thus responsible for the maintenance of many higher mental activities. *See also* body image.

據認爲聯合區負責對由初級感覺區接受的信息進行加工，並使之與由記憶和其他腦區傳送來的信息相互聯繫起來，因而負責維持多種高級神經活動。

association of ideas (in psychology) linkage of one idea to another in a regular way according to their meaning. In *free association* the linkage of ideas arising in dreams or fantasy may be used to discover the underlying motives of the individual. In *word association tests* stimulus words are produced to which the subject has to respond as quickly as possible.

聯想 （心理學）將某一概念與另一概念按其含義進行的有規律性的聯繫。在睡夢和幻想中產生的自由聯想可用來揭露某人潛在的動機。在詞聯想試驗中，受驗者必須對提問詞盡速作答。

astasia *n.* an inability to stand for which no physical cause can be found. *Astasia-abasia* is an inability to stand or walk in the absence of any recognizable physical illness. The patient's attempts are bizarre and careful examination reveals contradictory features. It is most commonly an expression of *hysteria.

起立不能 查究不出器質性病因的不能站立。立行不能，即在查找不出有任何器質性疾病下的不能站立或行走。患者意圖離奇乖僻，認眞檢查可發現有相互矛盾的現象。此爲癔病最常見的表現。

aster *n.* a star-shaped object in a cell that surrounds the *centrosome during mitosis and meiosis and is concerned with the formation of the *spindle.

星體 當細胞有絲分裂和減數分裂時，圍繞中心體出現的且與紡錘體形成有關的星狀體。

astereognosis *n. see* agnosia.

實體感缺失

asthenia *n.* weakness or loss of strength.

無力，虛弱，衰弱

asthenic *adj.* describing a personality disorder characterized by low energy, susceptibility to physical and emotional stress, and a diminished capacity for pleasure.

無力的，虛弱的 指精力衰弱，易患身心性疾患，對外界壓力的承受力減弱的人格障礙而言。

asthenopia *n. see* eyestrain.

視力疲勞

asthma *n.* a condition characterized by paroxysmal attacks of *bronchospasm, causing difficulty in breathing. *Bronchial asthma* may be precipitated by

氣喘 以陣發性支氣管痙攣造成呼吸困難爲特徵的疾病或症狀。有大批刺激因素，包括變應原（其中

exposure to one or more of a large range of stimuli, including *allergens (including some drugs, such as aspirin), exertion, emotions, and infections. The first attacks can occur at any age but are normally in early life, when – in allergic people – they may be associated with other manifestations of hypersensitivity, such as eczema and hay fever. Powerful drugs, including corticosteroids, are now available to control asthmatic attacks, which may be very serious and prolonged (*see* status asthmaticus). Avoidance of known allergens, and *desensitization to them, may help to reduce the frequency of attacks. *Cardiac asthma* occurs in left ventricular heart failure and must be distinguished from bronchial asthma, for which the treatment is different. —**asthmatic** *adj.*

包括阿司匹林之類藥物）、勞累、情緒波動和感染等等，遇到其中之一種或幾種都可促使支氣管性氣喘發作。最初發作能在任何年齡發生，但一般出現於具有濕疹、枯草熱等其他過敏性表現的幼年人。目前廣泛使用皮質類甾醇等有强效的藥物控制非常嚴重和持續的氣喘發作。對已知變應原予以廻避和施行脫敏療法或有助於減少發作。心病性氣喘因左室心力衰竭而引起，因療法不同，所以必須與支氣管性氣喘相區別。

astigmatism *n.* a defect of vision in which the image of an object is distorted, usually in either the vertical or the horizontal axis, because not all the light from it comes to a focus on the retina. Some parts of the object may be in focus but light from other parts may be focused in front of or behind the retina. This is usually due to abnormal curvature of the cornea and/or lens (*see* refraction), whose surface resembles part of the surface of an egg (rather than a sphere). The defect can be corrected by wearing *cylindrical lenses*, which produce exactly the opposite degree of distortion and thus cancel out the distortion caused by the eye itself. —**astigmatic** *adj.*

散光　來自被視物體的光線不能全部聚焦在視網膜上，因而使物像通常在垂直軸或水平軸上變形的一種視力缺陷。物體某些部分可能在視網膜上聚焦，但其他部分的光可能在視網膜前或視網膜後聚焦。通常是因角膜和/或晶狀體（其表面類似蛋形面而非球形面）的曲度反常引起。此種缺陷可配戴圓柱透鏡眼鏡予以糾正。此種眼鏡產生的變形度數恰好相反而足以抵消眼睛自身造成的變形。

astragalus *n. see* talus.

距骨

astringent *n.* a drug that causes cells to shrink by precipitating proteins from their surfaces. Astringents are used in lotions to harden and protect the skin and to reduce bleeding from minor abrasions. They are also used in mouth washes, throat lozenges, eye drops, etc., and in antiperspirants.

收斂劑　一種使細胞表面的蛋白質凝固的藥物。可導致細胞皺縮。收斂劑可用作洗劑，以强化和保護皮膚，並爲輕微擦傷止血。亦可用於漱口劑、含片、滴眼藥及止汗劑中。

astrocyte (astroglial cell) *n.* a type of cell with numerous sheet-like processes extending from its cell body, found throughout the central nervous system. It is one of the several different types of cell that make up the *glia. The cells have been ascribed the function of providing nutrients for neurones and possibly of taking part in information storage processes.

星形膠質細胞 在中樞神經系統任何部分都有的，從其自體伸出許多片狀突起的一種細胞，是組成神經膠質的幾種不同類型細胞中的一型。據認爲有給神經元提供營養的功能，或許還參與信息貯存作用。

astrocytoma *n.* a brain tumour derived from non-nervous cells (*glia), which – unlike the neurones – retain the ability to reproduce themselves by mitosis. All grades of malignancy occur, from slow-growing tumours whose histological structure resembles normal glial cells, to rapidly growing highly invasive tumours whose cell structure is poorly differentiated (*see* glioblastoma). In adults astrocytomas are usually found in the cerebral hemispheres but in children they also occur in the cerebellum.

星形細胞瘤 由一種仍保留有絲分裂能力（與神經元不同）的非神經細胞（神經膠質）生出的腦腫瘤。其惡性程度不同，從生長緩慢、其組織結構宛如正常神經膠質細胞的腫瘤，到生長迅速、侵襲性强、其組織結構分化不良的腫瘤。星形細胞瘤通常見於成人大腦半球，但在兒童小腦內亦可發生。

asymbolia *n. see* alexia.

說示不能，失示意能

asymptomatic *adj.* not showing any symptoms of disease, whether disease is present or not.

無症狀的 無論有病與否，均不見疾病之症狀的。

asynclitism *n.* the entry of the head of the baby at birth into the vagina at an oblique angle.

頭盆傾勢不均 分娩時胎兒頭以傾斜角度進入陰道。

asyndesis *n.* a disorder of thought, in which the normal *association of ideas is disrupted so that thought and speech become fragmentary. It is a symptom of schizophrenia, dementia, or confusion.

言語〔思惟〕連貫不能，失貫性言語〔思維〕 正常聯想被中斷因而語言思維支離分裂的思維性障礙。此爲精神分裂症、痴呆或精神錯亂的症狀。

asynergia *n. see* dyssynergia.

協同不能

asystole *n.* a condition in which the heart no longer beats, accompanied by the absence of complexes in the electrocardiogram. The clinical features, causes, and treatment are those of *cardiac arrest.

心搏停止 心臟停止搏動，同時心電圖複合波消失的狀況。其臨床特徵、病因和療法等均與心動停止相同。

ataraxia *n.* a state of calmness and freedom from anxiety, especially the state produced by tranquillizing drugs.

心氣和平，心神安定 一種平靜、無憂無慮狀態。尤指服用安定劑後產生的心情。

atavism *n.* the phenomenon in which an individual has a character or disease known to have occurred in a remote ancestor but not in his parents.

返祖〔現象〕，隔代遺傳 在某個人身上發生屬於遠祖而非父母的特徵或疾病的現象。

ataxia *n.* the shaky movements and unsteady gait that result from the brain's failure to regulate the body's posture and the strength and direction of limb movements. It may be due to disease of the sensory nerves or the *cerebellum. In *cerebellar ataxia* there is clumsiness of willed movements. The patient staggers when walking; he cannot pronounce words properly and has *nystagmus. *Friedreich's ataxia* is an inherited disorder appearing first in adolescence. It has the features of cerebellar ataxia, together with spasticity of the limbs. The unsteady movements of *sensory ataxia* are exaggerated when the patient closes his eyes (*see* Romberg's sign). *See also* tabes dorsalis (locomotor ataxia). —**ataxic** *adj.*

共濟失調，協調不能 因腦不能調整身體姿勢和四肢活動的力量、方向，致使步態不穩，行動搖擺。可能由感覺神經或小腦疾病引起。小腦性共濟失調中，隨意運動笨拙，患者步履蹣跚，吐字發音不準，兼有眼球震顫。弗里德賴希氏共濟失調是首先見於青春期的遺傳性疾患，具小腦性共濟失調特徵兼有四肢痙攣狀態。當感覺性共濟失調患者雙目閉合時，其行動不穩的程度更爲增强。

Atebrin *n. see* mepacrine.

阿的平

atel- (atelo-) *prefix denoting* imperfect or incomplete development. Examples: *atelencephaly* (of the brain): *atelocardia* (of the heart).

〔前綴〕**發育不全** 發育不完善或不完全的。例如：腦發育不全，心發育不全。

atelectasis *n.* failure of part of the lung to expand. This occurs when the cells lining the air sacs (alveoli) are too immature, as in premature babies, or too damaged by inhaled substances or secretions to produce the wetting agent (surfactant) with which the surface tension between the alveolar walls is overcome. The lung can usually be helped to expand by physiotherapy and supportive measures, but prolonged atelectasis becomes irreversible.

〔肺〕膨脹不全 有部分肺不能擴張。此情況發生於肺細胞過於不成熟（因嬰兒早產）；或因吸入物質或分泌液產生潤濕劑（表面活性劑）超過了肺泡壁間的表面張力而使細胞損傷過重。物理療法和輔助措施通常能有助於使肺擴展，但拖延不治，肺膨脹不全即不可恢復。

ateleiosis *n.* failure of sexual development owing to lack of *pituitary hormones. *See* infantilism, dwarfism.

性發育不全 缺乏垂體激素所致之性發育障礙。

atheroma *n.* degeneration of the walls of the arteries due to the formation in them of fatty plaques and scar tissue. This limits blood circulation and predisposes to thrombosis. It is common in adults in Western countries. A diet rich in animal fats (*see* cholesterol) and refined sugar, cigarette smoking, obesity, and inactivity are the principal causes. It may be symptomless but often causes complications from arterial obstruction in middle and late life (such as angina pectoris, heart attack, stroke, and gangrene). Treatment is by prevention, but some symptoms may be ameliorated by drug therapy (e.g. angina by glyceryl trinitrate) or by surgical bypass of the arterial obstruction.

粥樣硬化斑 動脈壁內脂肪斑塊和瘢痕組織形成而引起的動脈壁變性。動脈粥樣硬化斑限制血液循環並易引起血栓形成。在西方國家最常見於成年人。富於動物脂肪飲食和精製食糖、吸煙、肥胖以及無所事事爲主要病因。可能無症狀，但到中年和晚年因動脈阻塞往往引起心絞痛、心臟病、中風和壞疽等併發症。治療有賴於預防，但對某些症狀藥物治療可予改善（如心絞痛用硝酸甘油）或作動脈梗阻旁路手術。

atherosclerosis *n.* a disease of the arteries in which fatty plaques develop on their inner walls, with eventual obstruction of blood flow. *See* atheroma.

動脈粥樣硬化 脂肪斑〔塊〕在動脈內壁上發展，終於併發血流梗阻之動脈疾病。

athetosis *n.* a writhing involuntary movement especially affecting the hands, face, and tongue. It is usually a form of *cerebral palsy. It impairs the child's ability to speak or use his hands; intelligence is often unaffected.

手足徐動症，指痙病 主要發生在手、臉和舌部的不自主的扭曲運動。通常是大腦麻痺的一型，兒童說話或使用手的能力受到影響，通常不影響智力。

athlete's foot a fungus infection of the skin between the toes: a type of *ringworm. Medical name: **tinea pedis**.

脚氣 趾間皮膚的黴菌感染：癬的一種。醫學名稱：脚癬。

athyreosis *n.* absence of or lack of function of the thyroid gland, causing *cretinism in infancy and *myxoedema in adult life.

甲狀腺功能缺失 甲狀腺功能缺失在嬰兒期造成矮小病，成人期引起黏液〔性〕水腫。

atlas *n.* the first *cervical vertebra, by means of which the skull is articulated to the backbone.

寰椎 藉以聯接顱骨和脊柱的第一頸椎。

atony *n.* a state in which muscles are floppy, lacking their normal elasticity. —**atonic** *adj.*

張力缺乏，弛緩 肌力鬆弛，缺乏正常彈性的狀態。

atopen *n.* any substance responsible for *atopy.

異位反應原　任何引起異位反應的物質。

atopy *n.* a form of *allergy in which the hypersensitivity reaction may be distant from the region of contact with the substance (*atopen*) responsible. For example, a substance that is swallowed may give rise to a form of eczema, called *atopic dermatitis*. —**atopic** *adj.*

異位反應性　接觸刺激物（異位反應原）的部位和其所引起的過敏反應的部位可能不在一處的一種變態反應。例如：吞嚥下的某種物質可能引起稱爲異位反應性皮炎的濕疹。

ATP (adenosine triphosphate) a compound that contains adenine, ribose, and three phosphate groups and occurs in cells. The chemical bonds of the phosphate groups store energy needed by the cell, for muscle contraction; this energy is released when ATP is split into ADP or AMP. ATP is formed from ADP or AMP using energy produced by the breakdown of carbohydrates or other food substances. *See also* mitochondrion.

三磷酸腺苷　存在於細胞內的含有腺嘌呤、核糖和三個磷酸基團的化合物。磷酸基團的化學鍵貯存細胞爲肌肉收縮所需之能；三磷酸腺苷分解爲二磷酸腺苷或一磷酸腺苷時，即釋放出能。三磷酸腺苷則由一磷酸腺苷利用碳水化合物或其他食物分解所產生的能而合成。

atresia *n.* **1.** congenital absence or abnormal narrowing of a body opening. *Biliary atresia* (affecting the bile duct) causes obstructive jaundice in infancy and is lethal unless corrected surgically; *tricuspid atresia* obstructs the blood flow within the heart from the right atrium to the right ventricle. **2.** the degenerative process that affects the majority of ovarian follicles. Usually only one Graafian follicle will ovulate in each menstrual cycle. —**atretic** *adj.*

閉鎖　①身體的孔口先天性缺失或異常狹窄。膽道閉鎖於嬰兒期即引起阻塞性黃疸，若不手術矯治可致死。三尖瓣閉鎖阻塞血液由右房流往右室。　②大部分卵泡發生的退化現象。通常每次月經周期僅有一個格雷夫氏卵泡排卵。

atri- (atrio-) *prefix denoting* an atrium, especially the atrium of the heart. Example: *atrioventricular* (relating to the atria and ventricles of the heart).

〔前綴〕〔心〕房　房，尤指心房。例如：房室的（與心房和心室有關的）。

atrioventricular bundle (AV bundle, bundle of His) a bundle of modified heart muscle fibres (*Purkinje fibres*) passing from the *atrioventricular (AV) node forward to the septum between the ventricles, where it divides into right and left bundles, one for each ventricle. The fibres transmit contraction waves from the atria, via the AV node, to the ventricles.

房室束　由房室結向前通往室間隔的一束變異的心肌纖維（浦肯野氏纖維）。從室間隔再向右、左二室分爲右束和左束。房室束纖維把由心房來的收縮波經房室結傳遞到心室。

atrioventricular node a mass of modified heart muscle situated in the lower middle part of the right atrium. It receives the impulse to contract from the *sinoatrial node, via the atria, and transmits it through the *atrioventricular bundle to the ventricles.

房室結　位於右心房下中部的一團變異的心肌。房室結接受從竇房結經心房傳來的收縮衝動，並通過房室束將之傳抵心室。

atrium *n.* (*pl.* **atria**) **1.** either of the two upper chambers of the *heart. Their muscular walls are thinner than those of the ventricles; the left atrium receives oxygenated blood from the lungs via the pulmonary vein; the right atrium receives deoxygenated blood from the venae cavae. *See also* auricle. **2.** any of various anatomical chambers into which one or more cavities open. —**atrial** *adj.*

①**心房**　心臟上部兩腔之一。其肌肉壁較心室肌爲薄，左心房經由肺靜脈接受含氧的血液，右心房從腔靜脈接受脫氧的血液。②**房**　解剖學上泛指各類型的有一個或數個開口的腔室。

Atromid-S *n. see* clofibrate.

祛脂乙酯，安妥明，冠心平

atrophy *n.* the wasting away of a normally developed organ or tissue due to degeneration of cells. This may occur through undernourishment, disuse, or ageing. Forms of atrophy peculiar to women include the shrinking of the ovary at the menopause and of the *corpus luteum during the menstrual cycle. *Muscular atrophy* is associated with various diseases, such as poliomyelitis.

萎縮　由細胞變性所致正常發育之器官或組織的體積縮小。可因營養不良、廢用或老化而發生。婦女體內器官的萎縮現象，有絕經期卵巢萎縮和月經周期中的黃體萎縮。肌萎縮與脊髓灰質炎之類的疾病有關。

atropine *n.* a drug extracted from deadly nightshade (*see* belladonna) that inhibits the action of certain nerves of the autonomic nervous system (*see* parasympatholytic). Atropine relaxes smooth muscle and is used to treat biliary colic and renal colic. It also reduces secretions of the bronchial tubes, salivary glands, stomach, and intestines and is used before general *anaesthesia and to relieve peptic ulcers. It is also used to dilate the pupil of the eye. Atropine is administered by mouth, injection, or as eyedrops; common side-effects include dryness of the throat, thirst, and impaired vision.

阿托品　由顛茄中提取的能抑制自主神經系統中某種神經作用的藥物。阿托品鬆弛平滑肌，可用於治療膽絞痛和腎絞痛。本品也能減少支氣管、唾腺、胃和腸等之分泌，可作爲全身麻醉前給藥和治療消化性潰瘍，還可用於散瞳。阿托品可口服、注射或用作滴眼藥。常見副作用包括咽喉乾燥、口渴、視力障礙。

attachment *n.* (in psychology) the process of developing the first close selective relationship of a child's life, most commonly with the mother. The relationship acts to reduce anxiety in strange settings and forms a base from which children develop further relationships.

依附 （心理學）兒童時期與其最先接觸的親屬（常是母親）培養感情的過程。此種感情使兒童在陌生環境中消除焦慮不安，並形成兒童進一步發展其他感情關係的基礎。

attenuation *n.* reduction of the disease-producing ability (virulence) of a bacterium or virus by chemical treatment, heating, drying, by growing under adverse conditions, or by passing through another organism. Treated (*attenuated*) bacteria or viruses are used for many *immunizations.

減毒 用化學處理、加熱、乾燥、逆境培養、或通過其他生物傳代培養，以減低細菌或病毒致病能力（毒性）的措施。經過處理（減毒）的細菌或病毒可用作免疫接種。

attrition *n.* (in dentistry) the wearing of tooth surfaces by the action of opposing teeth. A small amount of attrition occurs with age but accelerated wear may occur in *bruxism and with certain diets.

磨損 （牙科）由相對牙齒的作用所致牙表面的損毀。輕微磨損因歲月增長而產生，但嚴重的磨損可能因夜間磨牙或某種飲食引起。

audi- (audio-) *prefix denoting* hearing or sound.

〔前綴〕①**聽** ②**聲音**

audiogram *n.* the graphic record of a test of hearing carried out on an audiometer.

聽力圖 用聽力計錄製成的聽力測驗圖像。

audiometer *n.* an apparatus for measuring hearing at different sound frequencies, so helping in the diagnosis of deafness. —**audiometry** *n.*

聽力計 測驗對不同音頻的聽力的儀器。用以對耳聾進行診斷。

auditory *adj.* relating to the ear or to the sense of hearing.

耳的，聽覺的

auditory nerve *see* vestibulocochlear nerve.

聽神經

Auerbach's plexus (myenteric plexus) a collection of nerve fibres – fine branches of the *vagus nerve – within the walls of the intestine. It supplies the muscle layers and controls the movements of *peristalsis.

奧厄巴赫氏神經叢（腸肌叢） 腸壁內的一簇神經纖維：迷走神經的細支。它支配肌層，並控制蠕動運動。

aura *n.* the forewarning of an attack. The true *epileptic aura* is felt a a breeze or coldness passing over the body. The

先兆 疾病發作的預報警告。眞性癲癇的先兆是全身寒冷。偏頭痛先兆通常

migrainous aura usually affects the patient's eyesight with brilliant flickering lights or blurring of vision. 是患者眼前金星四射或視力不清。

aural *adj.* relating to the ear. **耳的** 與耳有關的。

Aureomycin *n. see* chlortetracycline. **金黴素**

auricle *n.* **1.** a small pouch in the wall of each *atrium of the heart: the term is also used incorrectly as a synonym for *atrium*. **2.** *see* pinna. ①**心耳** 在左或右心房壁內的小囊。此詞也誤作心房的同義詞。 ②**耳廓**

auriscope (otoscope) *n.* an apparatus for examining the eardrum and the passage leading to it from the ear (external meatus). It consists of a funnel (speculum), a light, and lenses (see illustration). **耳鏡** 檢查鼓室及外耳道（由耳至鼓室之通道）之器械。由漏斗形窺器、燈、和透鏡等組成（見圖）。

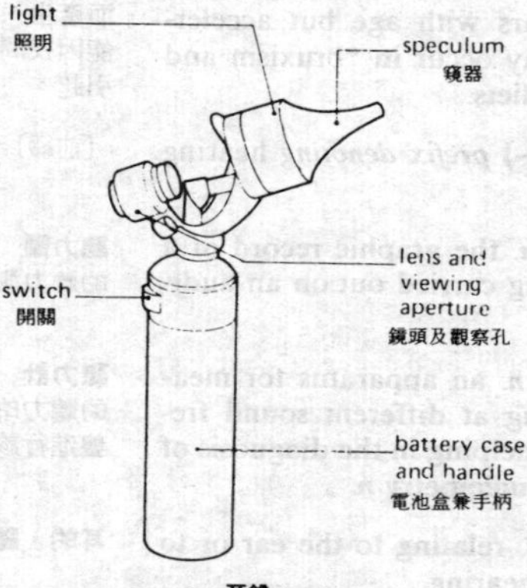

耳鏡
An auriscope

auscultation *n.* the process of listening, usually with the aid of a *stethoscope, to sounds produced by movement of gas or liquid within the body. Auscultation is an aid to diagnosis of abnormalities of the heart, lungs, intestines, and other organs according to the characteristic changes in sound pattern caused by different disease processes. —**auscultatory** *adj.* **聽診** 通常藉助聽診器聽取體內氣體或液體流動的聲音的方法。聽診是根據不同疾病所造成的特殊的聲音變化，對心、肺、腸和其他器官等的異常進行診斷的輔助手段。

auscultatory gap a silent period in the knocking sounds heard with a stethoscope over an artery, between the systolic and diastolic blood pressures, when the blood pressure is measured with a *sphygmomanometer.

聽診無音間隙 用血壓計測量血壓時，用聽診器在動脉上聽到的處於收縮壓與舒張壓之間的一段無心跳聲音的間期。

Australia antigen an antigen that has been detected by serological tests in the serum of patients suffering from serum *hepatitis. This disease is thought to be due to a virus.

澳大利亞抗原 用血清檢驗法從血清性肝炎患者的血清中查出的一種抗原。此病據認爲由病毒引起。

aut- (auto-) *prefix denoting* self. Example: *autokinesis* (voluntary movement).

〔前綴〕**自己，自體，自動，自發** 例如：自體動作（隨意運動）。

autism *n.* **1. (Kanner's syndrome, infantile autism)** a rare and severe psychiatric disorder of childhood, with an onset before the age of $2\frac{1}{2}$ years. It is marked by an inability to communicate by speech or to form abstract concepts; repetitive and limited patterns of behaviour (*see* stereotypy); and obsessive resistance to tiny changes in familiar surroundings. Autistic children are unable to form normal personal relationships but they can become emotionally attached to objects. Most (but not all) are intellectually subnormal (*see* idiot savant). Genetic factors and brain damage are probably important causes. Treatment is not specific, but lengthy specialized education is usually necessary. Behaviour problems and anxiety can be controlled with behaviour therapy and drugs (such as *phenothiazines). **2.** the condition of retreating from realistic thinking to self-centred fantasy thinking: a symptom of personality disorder and schizophrenia. **—autistic** *adj.*

孤獨癖（康納氏綜合徵，幼兒孤獨癖） 一種罕見但嚴重的發作於兩週歲半前的幼兒期精神病。特徵爲：無語言表達能力或缺乏形成抽象概念的能力，只能重復幾種有限的擧動，對日常環境中發生的細微變化亦缺乏適應能力。孤獨癖兒童不善處理人際關係，但對客觀事物却可能產生感情。大多（但非全部）智能低下。主要起因可能爲遺傳和腦損害。無特效療法，但通常需要長期的特殊教育。行爲障礙和焦慮不安等能用行爲療法和吩噻嗪之類藥物控制。 ②**自我中心主義** 逃避切合實際的想法而幻想以自我爲中心的思想狀况，係人格障礙和精神分裂症的症狀。

autoagglutination *n.* the clumping together of the body's own red blood cells by antibodies produced against them, which occurs in acquired haemolytic anaemia (an *autoimmune disease).

自體凝集〔作用〕 在後天溶血性貧血（一種自體免疫性疾病）中發生的紅細胞受到自體產生的抗體的作用而凝集成塊的現象。

autoantibody *n.* an antibody formed against one of the body's own components in an *autoimmune disease.

自體抗體 在自體免疫性疾病中產生的作用於身體自身某種組成成分的抗體。

autochthonous *adj.* **1.** remaining at the site of formation. A blood clot that has not been carried in the bloodstream from its point of origin is described as autochthonous. **2.** originating in an organ without external stimulus, like the beating of the heart.

①**原處的** 停留在形成處的。如停留在原地未被衝進血流的血塊。 ②**自發的** 起源於器官本身而非外在刺激引起的，如心搏。

autoclave **1.** *n.* a piece of equipment for sterilizing surgical instruments, dressings, etc. It consists of a chamber, similar to a domestic pressure cooker, in which the articles are placed and treated with steam at high pressure. **2.** *vb.* to sterilize in an autoclave.

①**高壓滅菌器** 對外科手術器械、敷料等進行滅菌處理的一種裝備。由一個類似家庭用高壓鍋的容器構成，物品置於其中，再用高壓蒸氣滅菌。 ②**高壓滅菌** 在高壓滅菌器內消毒。

autogenous vaccine *see* autovaccine.

自體疫苗

autograft *n.* a tissue graft taken from one part of the body and transferred to another part of the same individual. The repair of burns is often done by grafting on strips of skin taken from elsewhere on the body, usually the upper arm or thigh. Unlike *homografts, autografts are not rejected by the body's immunity defences. *See also* skin graft.

自體移植物 取自身體上的一部分，移植於同一個體上的另一部分的組織移植物。修復燒傷即從身體其他部位，經常是上肢和股部取得皮膚進行移植。與同種移植不同，自體移植物不受身體免疫反應的排斥。

autoimmune disease one of the growing number of otherwise unrelated disorders now suspected of being caused by inflammation and destruction of tissues by the body's own antibodies (*autoantibodies*). These disorders include acquired haemolytic anaemia, pernicious anaemia, rheumatic fever, rheumatoid arthritis, glomerulonephritis, and several forms of thyroid dysfunction, including Hashimoto's disease. It is not known why the body should lose the ability to distinguish between substances that are 'self' and those that are 'non-self'.

自體免疫性疾病 一組病例數日益增多的、在表面上彼此無關的、但卻被認爲是由體內自身的抗體（自體抗體）引起組織發炎與破壞的疾病。此類病包括獲得性溶血性貧血、惡性貧血、風濕熱、類風濕關節炎、腎小球性腎炎和幾種包括橋本氏病在內的甲狀腺功能障礙疾病。身體失去識別自身或非自身物質之能力的原因尙不明。

autoimmunity *n.* a disorder of the body's defence mechanisms in which antibodies (*autoantibodies*) are produced against certain components or products of its own tissues, treating them as foreign material and attacking them. *See* autoimmune disease, immunity.

自體免疫 一種身體防禦機制紊亂。此時針對自體某組成部分或其組織產物產生抗體，將自身組成部分或其組織產物視爲異物而攻擊之。

autoinoculation *n.* the accidental transfer of inoculated material from one site in the body to another. Following vaccination against smallpox, for example, satellite lesions may occur around the site of inoculation. Sometimes the conjunctiva is affected.

自體接種 接種物從身體一處向另處之意外轉移。例如，接種天花疫苗後，在接種處的四周可能發生衛星樣病損，有時還損及結膜。

autointoxication *n.* poisoning by a toxin formed within the body, in contrast to a substance swallowed or absorbed from outside.

自體中毒 並非經口或自外界吸收進入體內的而係體內形成的毒素中毒。

autolysis *n.* the destruction of tissues or cells brought about by the actions of their own enzymes. *See* lysosome.

自體溶解，自溶 由組織或細胞酶的作用而造成的自身破壞。

automatism *n.* one of the symptoms of temporal lobe *epilepsy, in which the patient performs well-organized movements. These movements may be simple and repetitive, such as hand clapping, or they may be so complex as to mimic a person's normal conscious activities.

自動症 顳葉性癲癇的一種症狀，患者完成井然有序的一系列動作。此類動作可能是簡單動作的重複，如拍掌；或者是一系列複雜的動作，就像在模倣人們平時有意識的舉動。

autonomic nervous system the part of the *nervous system responsible for the control of bodily functions that are not consciously directed, including regular beating of the heart, intestinal movements, sweating, salivation, etc. The autonomic system is subdivided into *sympathetic* and *parasympathetic nervous systems.* Sympathetic nerves lead from the middle section of the spinal cord and parasympathetic nerves from the brain and lower spinal cord. The heart, smooth muscles, and most glands receive fibres of both kinds: the interplay of sympathetic and parasympathetic reflex activity (the actions are often antagonistic) governs their working. Sympathetic nerve endings liberate

自主神經系統 神經系統中負責控制正常心搏動、腸運動、排汗、唾液分泌等等不受意識支配的身體功能活動的部分。自主神經系統分交感神經和副交感神經兩部分。交感神經從脊髓中段起始，副交感神經則起自腦和脊髓下部。心臟、平滑肌和大部分腺體均接受二者之纖維。交感和副交感反射活動（經常相反的）的相互作用調節心臟、平滑肌、腺體等的功能。交感神經末梢釋放遞質去甲腎上腺素；副交感神經末梢釋放遞質乙醯膽鹼。

*noradrenaline as a neurotransmitter; parasympathetic nerve endings release *acetylcholine.

autoploidy *n.* the normal condition in cells or individuals, in which each cell has a chromosome set consisting of *homologous pairs, which allows cell division to occur in a normal manner. —**autoploid** *adj.*, *n.*

同源性 細胞或個體的正常狀態。每一細胞皆有一套由同源偶（對）組成的染色體，使細胞分裂能在正常狀態下發生。

autopsy (necropsy, post mortem) *n.* dissection and examination of a body after death in order to determine the cause of death or the presence of disease processes.

屍體解剖（屍體剖驗，驗屍） 為明確死亡原因，或死亡過程眞象，於死後進行的身體解剖檢查。

autoradiography (radioautography) *n.* a technique for examining the distribution of a radioactive *tracer in the tissues of an experimental animal. The tracer is injected into the animal, which is killed after a certain period. Thin sections of its organs are placed in close contact with a radiation-sensitive material, such as a photographic emulsion, and observed under a microscope. Blackening of the film indicates a high concentration of radioactive material.

自體放射照相術 檢查放射性示踪劑在實驗動物組織內分佈狀況的一種技術。示踪劑注射入動物一段時間後，將動物殺死。取其器官薄片與如照相乳膠之類對放線敏感的材料密切接觸後置於顯微鏡下觀察。底片陰影處表明放射性物質濃度高。

autosome *n.* any chromosome that is not a *sex chromosome and that occurs in pairs in diploid cells. —**autosomal** *adj.*

正染色體，常染色體 在二倍體細胞內成對出現的非性染色體。

autosuggestion *n.* self-suggestion or self-conditioning that involves repeating ideas to oneself in order to change psychological or physiological states. Autosuggestion is used primarily in *autogenic training*, a technique used to help patients control their anxiety or their habits. *See* suggestion.

自我暗示 為了改變生理或心理狀態而反復進行的自我提示或自我調整的方法。自我暗示主要用於自我訓練——一種用以幫助患者控制其焦慮或習慣的技術。

autotransfusion *n.* reintroduction into a patient of blood that has been lost from the patient's circulation during surgical operation. The blood is collected by suction during the operation, filtered to remove bubbles and small blood clots, and returned into one of the patient's veins through a drip.

自體輸血 將患者手術時從循環中流失的血液再回輸入體內。當手術時，將吸取收集的血液過濾，除去氣泡及細小血塊，經點滴回輸入患者靜脈。

autotrophic (lithotrophic) *adj.* describing organisms (known as *autotrophs*) that synthesize their organic materials from carbon dioxide and nitrates or ammonium compounds, using an external source of energy. *Photoautotrophic* organisms, including green plants and some bacteria, derive their energy from sunlight; *chemoautotrophic* (*chemosynthetic*) organisms obtain energy from inorganic chemical reactions. All autotrophic bacteria are nonparasitic. *Compare* heterotrophic.

自營的（無機營養的） 指利用外界能源，從二氧化碳、氮、或銨類化合物等合成有機物質的微生物（自營生物）而言。光自營生物包括從陽光吸取能量的綠色植物和某些細菌，化學自營（化學合成）生物則從無機化學反應獲取能量。所有自營細菌都是非寄生性的。

autovaccination *n.* the use of an *autovaccine.

自體菌苗接種 使用自體菌苗進行接種。

autovaccine (autogenous vaccine) *n.* a *vaccine prepared by isolating specimens of bacteria from an infected patient, culturing them, and killing them. By injecting this vaccine back into the patient, it was hoped that the body's resistance to the infection would be stimulated. Although such vaccines were once much favoured for the treatment of boils, there is no good evidence that the dead bacteria are any more likely to stimulate immunity than the living and dead bacteria already present in the body.

自體菌苗 將染病患者體內分離出的細菌標本，經培養，滅活後製成的菌苗。人們曾經希望將菌苗回注給患者能使之產生對感染的抵抗力。此種菌苗用於治療癤腫雖曾風行一時，但無確證這種死菌較體內原有活菌和死菌更易使機體產生免疫力。

aux- (auxo-) *prefix denoting* increase; growth. Example: *auxocardia* (enlargement of the heart).

〔前綴〕**增加，生長** 例如：心擴大（心臟之增大）。

auxotroph *n.* a strain of a microorganism, derived by mutation, that requires one or more specific factors for growth not needed by the parent organism.

營養缺陷型 一種經突變而產生的，要靠某些並非其親本機體所需要的特殊因子纔能生長的微生物。

avascular *adj.* lacking blood vessels or having a poor blood supply. The term is usually used with reference to cartilage.

無血管的 缺乏血管的，或供血不良的。此詞多指軟骨而言。

aversion therapy a form of *behaviour therapy that is used to reduce the occurrence of undesirable behaviour, such as sexual deviations or drug addiction. *Conditioning is used, with repeated pairing of some unpleasant stimulus with a stimulus related to the

厭惡療法 用以矯治如性倒錯、藥癮之類惡習的一種行為療法。利用條件反射，將令人厭惡的刺激和與惡習有關的刺激反復搭配成對。例如將啤酒和電休克搭配以治療嗜酒。

undesirable behaviour. An example is pairing the taste of beer with electric shock in the treatment of alcoholism. *See also* sensitization.

avitaminosis *n.* the condition caused by lack of a vitamin. *See also* deficiency disease.

維生素缺乏〔病〕 因缺乏維生素造成的疾病。

avulsion (evulsion) *n.* **1.** the tearing or forcible separation of part of a structure. For example, a tendon may be torn from the bone to which it attaches or the skin of the scalp may be torn from the underlying tissue and bone. **2.** (in dentistry) the knocking out of a tooth by trauma. The tooth may be *reimplanted.

①**撕脫** 將結構的一部分撕開或强行分開。例如，可將腱從其所附着的骨上撕脫。 ②**牙脫落** （牙科）因外傷引起的牙脫落。此牙可再植入牙床。

axilla *n.* (*pl.* **axillae**) the armpit. —**axillary** *adj.*

腋，腋窩

axis *n.* **1.** a real or imaginary line through the centre of the body or one of its parts or a line about which the body or a part rotates. **2.** the second *cervical vertebra, which articulates with the atlas vertebra above and allows rotational movement of the head.

①**軸** 通過身體的或身體某部分中央的一根實在的或想像中的直線。或身體或身體某部分圍之旋轉的直線。 ②**樞椎** 第二頸椎。上與寰椎相聯結，頭得以轉動。

axolemma *n.* the fine cell membrane, visible only under the electron microscope, that encloses the protoplasm of an *axon.

軸膜 僅在電子顯微鏡下可見的細胞薄膜。該膜包繞軸索的原生質。

axon *n.* a nerve fibre: a single process extending from the cell body of a *neurone and carrying nerve impulses away from it. An axon may be over a metre in length in certain neurones. In large nerves the axon has a sheath (*neurilemma*) made of *myelin; this is interrupted at intervals by gaps called *nodes of Ranvier*, at which branches of the axon leave. An axon ends by dividing into several branches called *telodendria*, which make contact with other nerves or with muscle or gland membranes.

軸突 從一個神經元之細胞體伸出的，並向外輸送衝動的一根單獨的神經纖維。某些神經元的軸突可長達一米有餘。大神經中的軸突有髓磷脂形成的鞘（神經鞘），此鞘爲許多所謂郎飛氏結的缺口隔斷，由該處發出軸突分支。軸突末端分成數根稱作終樹突的支，與其他神經或與肌肉或腺體膜接觸。

axoplasm *n.* the semifluid material of which the *axon of a nerve cell is composed. It flows slowly outwards from the cell body.

軸漿，軸質　組成神經細胞軸突的半液體物質。它由細胞體徐緩流至軸突。

azapetine *n.* a short-acting drug that relieves spasm of small arteries and capillaries and improves the blood flow to the skin. Its effects and uses are similar to those of *tolazoline. Trade name: **Ilidar**.

阿嗪吡丁　緩解小動脉和毛細血管痙攣，改善皮膚血流之速效藥。藥效和用法與苄唑啉近似。

azathioprine *n.* an *immunosuppressive drug, used mainly to aid the survival of organ or tissue transplants. It has also been used in the treatment of acute and chronic leukaemias and inflammatory bowel disease (e.g. ulcerative colitis). Azathioprine may damage bone marrow, causing blood disorders. It may also cause muscle wasting and skin rashes. Trade name: **Imuran**.

硫唑嘌呤　免疫抑制劑。主要用作幫助移植器官或組織存活。也用於治療急、慢性白血病，和發炎性腸疾患（如潰瘍性結腸炎）等。硫唑嘌呤可能損害骨髓，引起血液病。也可能引起肌肉消瘦，皮膚出疹。商品名：依木蘭。

azo- (azoto-) *prefix denoting* a nitrogenous compound, such as urea. Example: *azothermia* (fever due to nitrogenous substances in the blood).

〔前綴〕**氮**　描述尿素之類含氮化合物。例如：氮血熱（血中含氮物質引起的熱病）。

azoospermia (aspermia) *n.* the complete absence of sperm from the seminal fluid. This is due either to failure of formation of sperm by the seminiferous tubules within the testes or to a blockage in the ducts that conduct sperm from the testes. A biopsy of the testis is necessary to differentiate these two causes of azoospermia; if a blockage is present it may be possible to relieve it surgically.

精子缺乏　精液中毫無精子。原因有二，一爲睾丸內細精管不能形成精子，二爲將精子輸出睾丸的導管阻塞。需行睾丸活組織檢查以辨別二者孰爲精子缺乏原因。如有阻塞，可用手術解除。

azotaemia *n.* a former name for *uraemia.

氮血症　尿毒症的舊稱。

azoturia *n.* the presence in the urine of an abnormally high concentration of nitrogen-containing compounds, especially urea.

氮尿症　尿中含氮化合物（尤其是尿素）過多。

azygos vein an unpaired vein that arises from the inferior vena cava and

奇靜脉　由下腔靜脉發出進入上腔靜脉的一條不成

drains into the superior vena cava, returning blood from the thorax and abdominal cavities.

對的靜脈。收集胸腔與腹腔的血液。

B

Babinski reflex *see* plantar reflex.

巴彬斯基反射

bacillaemia *n.* the presence of bacilli in the blood, resulting from infection.

桿菌血症 感染導致血液中存在桿菌。

bacille Calmette-Guérin *see* BCG.

卡介苗

bacilluria *n.* the presence of bacilli in the urine, resulting from a bladder or kidney infection. *See* cystitis.

桿菌尿 膀胱或腎臟感染導致尿液中含有桿菌。

bacillus *n.* (*pl.* **bacilli**) any rod-shaped bacterium. *See also* Bacillus, Lactobacillus, Streptobacillus.

桿菌，芽胞桿菌 所有桿狀細菌。

Bacillus *n.* a large genus of Gram-positive spore-bearing rodlike bacteria. They are widely distributed in soil and air (usually as spores). Most feed on dead organic material and are responsible for food spoilage. The species *B. anthracis* which is nonmotile, causes *anthrax, a disease of farm animals transmissible to man. *B. polymyxa*, commonly found in soil, is the source of the *polymyxin group of antibiotics. *B. subtilis* may cause conjunctivitis in man; it also produces the antibiotic *bacitracin.

芽胞桿菌屬，桿菌屬 革蘭氏陽性芽胞桿狀細菌屬。常以芽胞形式遍佈於土壤及空氣中。大多數以死亡有機物爲能量來源並引起食物腐敗。其中不能運動的炭疽桿菌引起牲畜炭疽並可傳染給人。多黏芽胞桿菌常存在於土壤中，是多黏菌素類抗生素的來源。枯草桿菌對人可引起結膜炎；還能產生（枯草）桿菌鈦。

bacitracin *n.* an antibiotic produced by certain strains of bacteria and effective against a number of microorganisms. It is usually applied externally, to treat infections of the skin, eyes, or nose, but can be given by mouth as an intestinal antiseptic or by injection. The principal toxic effect is on the kidneys.

（枯草）桿菌肽 一種由一定菌株產生的能有效抵禦許多微生物的抗生素。通常外用於治療皮膚、眼或鼻的感染，也可作爲腸道抗菌劑口服或注射。主要毒性反應爲腎損害。

backbone (spinal column, spine, vertebral column) *n.* a flexible bony column extending from the base of the skull to the small of the back. It encloses and protects the spinal cord, articulates with the skull, ribs, and hip girdle, and provides attachment for the muscles of the back. It is made up of individual bones (*see* vertebra) connected by discs of fibrocartilage (*see* intervertebral disc) and bound together by ligaments. The backbone of a newborn baby contains 33 vertebrae: seven cervical (neck), 12 thoracic (chest), five lumbar (lower back), five sacral (hip), and four coccygeal. In the adult the sacral and coccygeal vertebrae become fused into two single bones (sacrum and coccyx, respectively); the adult vertebral column therefore contains 26 bones (see illustration). Anatomical name: **rachis**.

脊柱 由顱骨底部向下延續至骶尾部的可彎屈的骨性支柱。它包繞並保護脊髓，與顱骨、肋骨和髖帶相關節，並爲背肌之附着點。每個脊椎骨由纖維軟骨盤（椎間盤）相連接並有韌帶附着組成整個脊柱。新生兒脊柱有 33 塊椎骨：頸椎 7，胸椎 12，腰椎 5，骶椎 5，尾椎 4。成人骶椎和尾椎分別融合爲兩塊獨立的骨頭，即骶骨和尾骨，因此成人脊柱只有 26 塊椎骨（見圖）。

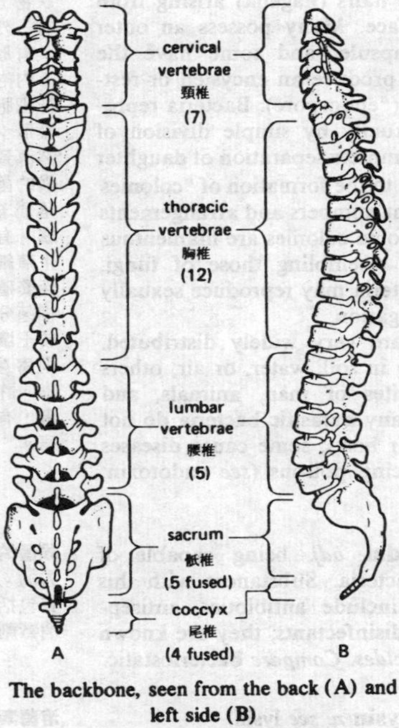

The backbone, seen from the back (A) and left side (B)
脊椎背面觀(A)和左側面觀(B)

bacteraemia *n.* the presence of bacteria in the blood: a sign of infection.

菌血症 血液中含有細菌。係感染現象之一。

bacteri- (bacterio-) *prefix denoting* bacteria. Example: *bacteriolysis* (dissolution of).

〔前綴〕**菌，細菌** 如溶菌作用。

bacteria *pl. n.* (*sing.* **bacterium**) a group of microorganisms all of which lack a distinct nuclear membrane (and hence are considered more primitive than animal and plant cells) and have a cell wall of unique composition (many antibiotics act by destroying the bacterial cell wall). Most bacteria are unicellular; the cells may be spherical (*coccus), rodlike (*bacillus), spiral (**Spirillum*), comma-shaped (**Vibrio*) or corkscrew-shaped (*spirochaete). Generally, they range in size between 0.5 and 5 μm. Motile species bear one or more fine hairs (flagella) arising from their surface. Many possess an outer slimy *capsule, and some have the ability to produce an encysted or resting form (*endospore). Bacteria reproduce asexually by simple division of cells; incomplete separation of daughter cells leads to the formation of *colonies of different numbers and arrangements of cells. Some colonies are filamentous in shape, resembling those of fungi. Some bacteria may reproduce sexually by *conjugation.

Bacteria are very widely distributed. Some live in soil, water, or air; others are parasites of man, animals, and plants. Many parasitic bacteria do not harm their hosts; some cause diseases by producing poisons (*see* endotoxin, exotoxin).

細菌 一類均缺乏明顯核膜（因而被認爲遠較動植物細胞原始），只有由單一成分組成的細胞壁的微生物（許多抗生素通過破壞細菌的細胞壁發揮作用）。大多數細菌爲單細胞；可分球狀（球菌）、桿狀（桿菌）、螺旋形（螺旋菌）、弧形（弧菌）或螺旋狀（螺旋體）。一般大小爲 0.5～5 μm。能運動的細菌有一或多個源於體表的纖細毛狀物（鞭毛）。許多細菌有一外層黏性莢膜，有些具有形成包囊或靜止狀態（內孢子）的能力。細菌經細胞簡單分裂而行無性繁殖；子細胞的不完全分裂導致細胞數量和排列各異的菌落的形成。有些菌落爲絲狀，猶如眞菌菌絲。有些細菌可經（兩個生殖細胞的）接合而行有性繁殖。

細菌分佈極廣。部分存在於土壤、水或空氣，其餘則寄生於人、動物和植物。許多寄生菌對宿主無害，有些可產生毒素而致病。

bactericidal *adj.* being capable of killing bacteria. Substances with this property include antibiotics, antiseptics, and disinfectants; they are known as *bactericides*. *Compare* bacteriostatic.

殺菌的 具有殺滅細菌能力的。具備這一特性的物質包括抗生素、防腐劑和消毒劑，統稱殺菌劑。

bacteriolysin *n. see* lysin.

溶菌素

bacteriology *n.* the science of bacteria. *See also* microbiology. —**bacteriological** *adj.* —**bacteriologist** *n.*

細菌學 研究細菌的科學。

bacteriophage (phage) *n.* a virus that attacks bacteria. In general, a phage consists of a head, tail, and tail fibres, all composed of protein molecules, and a core of DNA. The tail and tail fibres are responsible for attachment to the bacterial surface and for injection of the DNA core into the host cell. The phage grows and replicates in the bacterial cell, which is eventually destroyed with the release of new phages. Each phage acts specifically against a particular species of bacterium. This is utilized in *phage-typing*, a technique of identifying bacteria by the action of known phages on them. *See also* lysogeny.

噬菌體 侵襲細菌的一種病毒。一般來說，一個噬菌體包括頭部、尾部和尾部纖維（尾鬚），均由蛋白質分子和一個DNA核心組成。尾部及尾鬚便於噬菌體附於細菌表面和將DNA核心注入宿主細胞。它在細菌細胞內生長和複製，隨着新的噬菌體的釋放，細菌最終被消滅。一種噬菌體特異地作用於一種細菌。因而，運用噬菌體可對細菌分型，即通過已知噬菌體對細菌的作用來鑒定細菌的種類。

bacteriostatic *adj.* capable of inhibiting or retarding the growth and multiplication of bacteria. *Compare* bactericidal.

制菌的 具有抑制或延緩細菌生長和繁殖能力的。

bacterium *n. see* bacteria.

細菌

Bacteroides *n.* a genus of Gram-negative, mostly nonmotile, anaerobic rodlike bacteria. They are normally present in the alimentary and urinogenital tracts of mammals and are found in the mouth, particularly in dental plaque associated with periodontal disease. Some species cause infections (*see* Fusobacterium).

類桿菌屬 革蘭氏陰性厭氧性桿狀細菌屬，其中大部分不能運動。正常存在於哺乳動物消化道和泌尿生殖道，口腔亦可發現，尤其是在與牙周疾病有關的牙斑中。有些菌株可引起感染。

Bactrim *n. see* co-trimoxazole.

磺胺增效片 A

Baghdad boil *see* oriental sore.

巴格達瘡 東方瘡

BAL (British Anti-Lewisite) *see* dimercaprol.

二巰(基)丙醇

balanitis *n.* inflammation of the glans penis, usually associated with tightness of the foreskin (*phimosis). It is more common in childhood than in adult life. An acute attack is associated with redness and swelling of the glans.

龜頭炎 陰莖龜頭的炎症。常由包皮過緊（包莖）引起。兒童較成人多見，急性期龜頭紅腫。用抗生素治療並行包皮環切術以防復發。

Treatment is by antibiotics, and further attacks are prevented by *circumcision.

balanoposthitis *n.* inflammation of the foreskin and the surface of the underlying glans penis. It usually occurs as a consequence of *phimosis and represents a more extensive local reaction than simple *balanitis. The affected areas become red and swollen, which further narrows the opening of the foreskin and makes passing urine difficult and painful. Treatment of an acute attack is by administration of antibiotics, and further attacks are prevented by *circumcision.

龜頭包皮炎 包皮及陰莖龜頭表面的炎症。常由包皮過緊（包莖）引起，與單純龜頭炎相比，常有一些更廣泛的局部反應。炎症區域紅腫，進一步發展導致包皮開口狹窄，引起排尿困難和疼痛。急性期用抗生素治療，後行包皮環切術以防復發。

balantidiasis *n.* an infestation of the large intestine of man with the parasitic protozoan **Balantidium coli*. Man usually becomes infected by ingesting food or drink contaminated with cysts from the faeces of a pig. The parasite invades and destroys the intestinal wall, causing ulceration and *necrosis, and the patient may experience diarrhoea and dysentery. Balantidiasis is a rare cause of dysentery, mainly affecting farm workers; it is treated with various antibiotics, carbarsone, and *diiodohydroxyquinoline.

小袋蟲病 寄生性原蟲（結腸小袋蟲）引起的人體大腸感染。人常因攝入經豬糞中包囊污染的食物或飲料而感染。結腸小袋蟲入侵並破壞腸壁導致潰瘍及壞死，病人可表現爲腹瀉和痢疾。小袋蟲病引起痢疾罕見，患者多爲牧民。可用多種抗生素、卡巴胂和雙碘喹啉治療。

Balantidium *n.* a genus of one of the largest parasitic *protozoans affecting man (70 μm or more in length). The oval body is covered with threadlike cilia (for locomotion). *B. coli*, normally living in the gut of pigs as a harmless *commensal, occasionally infects man (*see* balantidiasis).

小袋蟲屬 感染人的最大的寄生性原蟲屬之一（70 μm或更長）。橢圓形軀體周圍覆以線狀纖毛（利於運動）。結腸小袋蟲通常作爲無害性共生動物棲居於豬的內臟，偶爾感染人體。

baldness *n. see* alopecia.

脫髮

ball-and-socket joint *see* enarthrosis.

球窩關節，杵臼關節

ballistocardiograph *n.* an instrument for recording the displacement of the whole body produced by the ejection of blood with each heart beat. The normal record produced by such an instrument (*ballistocardiogram*) may be altered by

心衝擊描記器 一種描記因每次心搏射出血液引起的整個身體振動的器械。由此而記錄的心衝擊描記圖可因心臟和主動脈瓣病變而改變。

disease of the heart or aortic valve (*see* aortic regurgitation, aortic stenosis).

ballottement *n.* the technique of examining a fluid-filled part of the body to detect a floating object. During pregnancy, a sharp tap with the fingers, applied to the womb through the abdominal wall or the vagina, causes the fetus to move away and then return to impart an answering tap to the examiner's hand as it floats back to its original position. This confirms that swelling of the uterus is due to a fetus rather than a tumour or other abnormality.

衝擊觸診（法） 某個浮於體內充滿液體的物體的探測方法。在孕期，經腹壁或陰道用手指向子宮施以猛烈衝擊，將胎兒推開，隨後胎兒浮回原位時檢查者能感覺到胎體對手的衝擊，藉以證實膨大的子宮是胎兒而不是腫瘤或其他異物。

balneotherapy *n.* the treatment of disease by bathing, usually in the mineral-containing waters of hot springs. The once fashionable 'water cures', taken at spas, certainly had a more psychological than physical effect. Today, specialized remedial treatment in baths, under the supervision of physiotherapists, is used to alleviate pain and improve blood circulation and limb mobility in arthritis and in nerve and muscle disorders.

浴療法 溫礦泉水洗浴是治療疾病的方法。曾一度流行的"水療"，心理作用較生理作用更大。如今，在理療師的監督管理下，專業化的輔助性浴療法運用於減輕疼痛、加速血液循環、增强關節和神經肌肉疾病患者肢體的靈活性。

bamethan *n.* a drug that relaxes smooth muscle and dilates the peripheral blood vessels. It is used in the treatment of vascular disease to relieve spasm of the arteries and improve blood flow to the tissues. Common side-effects include flushing, gooseflesh, and tingling.

巴美生 一種鬆弛平滑肌、擴張外周血管的藥物。用於治療血管疾病以解除動脈痙攣、增加組織血流量。常見副作用爲面部潮紅、起鷄皮疙瘩和刺麻感。

bandage *n.* a piece of material, in the form of a pad or strip, applied to a wound or used to bind around an injured or diseased part of the body.

綳帶 敷蓋創傷或包繞身體受傷或患病部位的塊狀或帶狀材料。

Bandl's ring *see* retraction ring.

班都氏環，子宮收縮環

Banti's syndrome a disorder in which enlargement and overactivity of the spleen occurs as a result of increased pressure within the splenic vein. The commonest cause is *cirrhosis of the liver.

班替氏綜合徵 脾靜脈壓力增高導致脾臟腫大和功能亢進的一種綜合徵。最常見的原因爲肝硬化。

barbitone (barbital) *n.* a long-acting *barbiturate, used as a hypnotic, as a sedative, for the suppression of convulsions, as an analgesic, and as an anaesthetic. Prolonged use may lead to *dependence and overdosage has serious toxic effects (*see* barbiturism). Trade name: **Veronal**.

巴比妥 一種長效巴比妥酸鹽。作爲鎮靜催眠藥用於抑制驚厥，亦用作鎮痛劑和麻醉劑。長期應用可產生賴藥性，過量使用有嚴重毒性反應。

barbitone sodium a barbiturate that has properties, uses, and side-effects similar to those of barbitone but acts more rapidly. It can be given by mouth or by injection.

巴比妥鈉 一種與巴比妥具有相同特性、用途和副作用，但顯效迅速得多的巴比妥酸鹽。可口服或注射。

barbiturate *n.* any of a group of drugs, derived from barbituric acid, that depress activity of the central nervous system. Most barbiturates, including *amylobarbitone and *pentobarbitone, are taken as sleeping pills. Very slow-acting barbiturates (such as *phenobarbitone) are used as sedatives and to control epilepsy; those with a rapid and short-lived effect (such as *thiopentone) are injected as anaesthetics. Because they produce *tolerance and psychological and physical *dependence, have serious toxic side-effects (*see* barbiturism), and can be fatal following large overdosage, barbiturates have been largely replaced in clinical use by safer drugs. The use of barbiturates with alcohol should be avoided since these drugs reinforce each other, producing serious effects.

巴比妥酸鹽 由巴比妥酸衍化而來的能抑制中樞神經系統活動的一類藥物。大多數巴比妥酸鹽包括異戊巴比妥和戊巴比妥在內，通常作爲催眠藥片劑服用。特慢效巴比妥酸鹽（如苯巴比妥）作爲鎮靜劑用於控制癲癇；快速短效類巴比妥酸鹽（如硫噴妥鈉）常作爲麻醉劑注射使用。由於易產生耐藥性及生理和心理賴藥性，有嚴重毒性副作用，且超大劑量可致死，故臨床上大部已爲較安全的藥物所取代。避免與乙醇合用，因藥理作用相互加强，產生嚴重反應。

barbiturism *n.* addiction to drugs of the barbiturate group. Signs of intoxication include confusion, slurring of speech, yawning, sleepiness, loss of memory, loss of balance, and reduction in muscular reflexes. Withdrawal of the drugs must be undertaken slowly, over 1–3 weeks, to avoid the withdrawal symptoms of tremors and convulsions, which can prove fatal.

巴比妥中毒 對巴比妥類藥物成癮。中毒症狀包括精神錯亂、語言不清、打呵欠、嗜眠、記憶喪失和肌反射減弱。必須緩慢停藥，達 1～3 週以上，以避免震顫和驚厥等致命性戒斷症狀。

baritosis *n.* a lung disease – a form of *pneumoconiosis – caused by inhaling barium dust. It gives dramatic shadows

鋇塵肺，鋇塵沉着病 吸入含鋇粉塵引起的一種肺部疾病（塵肺的一種）。

on chest X-rays but no respiratory disability.

X 線胸片有明顯陰影，但無呼吸障礙。

barium sulphate a barium salt, insoluble in water, that is opaque to X-rays and is used as a contrast medium in radiography of the stomach and intestines. *See also* enema.

硫酸鋇 不溶於水的一種鋇鹽。由於其不透 X 線，故常用作胃腸 X 線透視的造影劑。

baroreceptor (baroceptor) *n.* a collection of sensory nerve endings specialized to monitor changes in blood pressure. The main receptors lie in the *carotid sinuses and the *aortic arch; others are found in the walls of other large arteries and veins and some within the walls of the heart. Impulses from the receptors reach centres in the medulla; from here autonomic activity is directed so that the heart rate and resistance of the peripheral blood vessels can be adjusted appropriately.

壓力感受器 專門監測血壓變化的感覺神經末梢裝置。主要感受器位於頸動脈和主動脈弓；另一些位於其它一些大動脈大靜脈管壁，還有些位於心壁內。源於感受器的神經衝動傳至延髓中樞，由後者發出的自主衝動使心率和外周血管阻力得以調節在正常範圍。

barotitis *n.* discomfort in the ears due to changing air pressure during air travel.

氣壓性耳炎 空中旅行時由於空氣壓力變化引起的雙耳不適。

barotrauma *n.* damage to the middle ear or *Eustachian tube due to changes in atmospheric pressure associated with air travel.

氣壓傷 空中旅行時由於大氣壓變化引起的中耳和咽鼓管損傷。

Barr body *see* sex chromatin.

巴爾氏體

bartholinitis (vulvovaginitis) *n.* inflammation of the mucus-secreting glands alongside the vaginal opening (*Bartholin's glands). In *chronic bartholinitis* cysts may form in the glands. In *acute bartholinitis* the glands are blocked and an abscess develops.

前庭大腺炎（外陰陰道炎） 陰道開口旁黏液分泌腺（巴多林氏腺）的炎症。慢性者可形成囊腫，急性者腺管阻塞形成膿腫。

Bartholin's glands (greater vestibular glands) a pair of glands that open at the junction of the vagina and the external genitalia (vulva). Their secretions lubricate the vulva and so assist penetration by the penis during coitus. The *lesser vestibular glands*, around the vaginal opening, perform the same function.

巴多林氏腺（前庭大腺） 開口於陰道和外生殖器（外陰）連結處的一對腺體。其分泌物潤滑外陰因而利於交媾時陰莖插入陰道。前庭小腺位於陰道口周圍，功能同前庭大腺。

Bartonella *n.* a genus of parasitic rod-shaped or rounded microorganisms, usually regarded as intermediate between the bacteria and rickettsiae. They occur in the red blood cells and cells of the lymphatic system, spleen, liver, and kidneys. *B. bacilliformis* causes *bartonellosis in man.

巴爾通氏體屬 一類被認爲是介於細菌和立克次氏體之間的寄生性桿狀或球狀微生物。存在於紅細胞和淋巴系統、脾、肝和腎的細胞中。桿菌狀巴爾通氏體在人引起巴爾通氏體病。

bartonellosis *n.* an infectious disease, confined to high river valleys in Peru, Ecuador, and Columbia, caused by the parasitic microorganism **Bartonella bacilliformis*. The parasite, present in red blood cells and cells of the lymphatic system, is transmitted to man by sandflies. There are two clinical types of the disease: *Oroya fever* (*Carrion's disease*), whose symptoms include fever, anaemia, and enlargement of the liver, spleen, and lymph nodes; and *verruga peruana*, characterized by wartlike eruptions on the skin that can bleed easily and ulcerate. Oroya fever accounts for nearly all fatalities. Bartonellosis can be treated successfully with penicillin and other antibiotics and blood transfusions may be given to relieve the anaemia.

巴爾通氏體病 由寄生性微生物即桿菌狀巴爾通氏體引起的一種限發於秘魯、厄瓜多爾和哥倫比亞高原河谷的傳染病。桿菌狀巴爾通氏體存在於紅細胞和淋巴系統細胞中，由白蛉傳遞給人。該病有兩種臨床類型：奧羅亞熱（卡里翁氏病），其症狀有發熱，貧血和肝、脾、淋巴結腫大；第二類爲秘魯疣，特徵爲在皮膚上有易出血和形成潰瘍的疣狀突起物。患巴爾通氏病致死者幾乎全部是奧羅亞熱患者。青黴素或其他抗生素療效好，輸血有助於減輕貧血。

basal cell carcinoma *see* rodent ulcer.

基底細胞癌

basal ganglia several large masses of grey matter embedded deep within the white matter of the *cerebrum (see illustration). They include the *caudate* and *lenticular nuclei* (together known as the *corpus striatum*) and the *amygdaloid nucleus*. The lenticular nucleus consists of the *putamen* and *globus pallidus*. The basal ganglia have complex neural connections with both the cerebral cortex and thalamus: they are involved with the regulation of voluntary movements at a subconscious level.

基底神經節 深藏於大腦白質中的幾個大的灰質核團（見圖）。包括尾狀核和豆狀核（二者合稱紋狀體）、杏仁核。豆狀核由殼和蒼白球組成。基底神經節與大腦皮質和丘腦有複雜的神經聯系。它們參與下意識水平的隨意運動的調節。

basal metabolism the minimum amount of energy expended by the body to maintain vital processes, e.g. respiration, circulation, and digestion. It is expressed in terms of heat production per unit of body surface area

基礎代謝 維持機體生命過程如呼吸、循環和消化的最低能量消耗量。用每天每單位體表面積產熱量來表示（基礎代謝率），男性基礎代謝率平均爲每

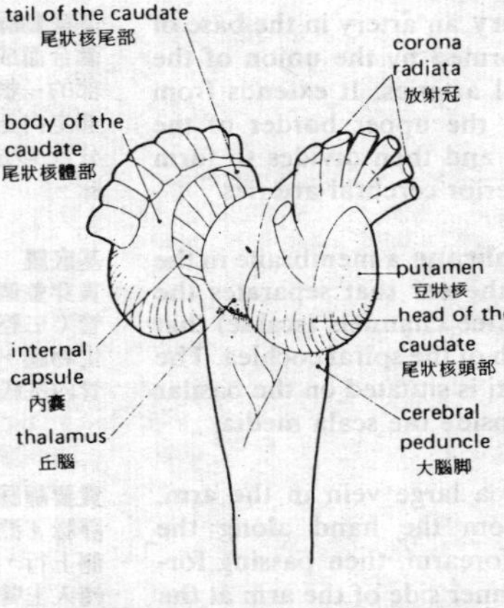

The basal ganglia and neighbouring parts
(seen from the front)

基底神經節及附近結構
（前面觀）

per day (*basal metabolic rate – BMR*), and for an average man the BMR is 1.7 Calories (7.115 kilojoules) per day. BMR may be determined by the direct method, in which the subject is placed in a respiratory chamber and the amount of heat evolved is measured, or (more normally) by the indirect method, based on the *respiratory quotient. Measurements are best taken during a period of least activity, i.e. during sleep and 12–18 hours after a meal, under controlled temperature conditions. Various factors, such as age, sex, and particularly thyroid activity, influence the value of the BMR.

天 1.7 千卡（7.115 千焦耳）。基礎代謝率可用將被測者置於呼吸室內而測量放出的熱量的直接測定法測量，或用基於呼吸商的間接測定法（更常用）測量。活動量最小時測量結果最準確，如在控制溫度情況下，進食後 12～18 小時睡眠中測量最佳。許多因素如年齡、性別，尤其是甲狀腺功能影響基礎代謝。

basement membrane the thin delicate membrane that lies at the base of an *epithelium. It is composed of mucopolysaccharide and fibres of protein.

基膜　位於上皮基底部的脆弱的薄膜。由黏多糖和蛋白纖維構成。

base pairing the linking of the two strands of a DNA molecule by means of hydrogen bonds between the bases of the nucleotides. Adenine always pairs with thymine and cytosine with guanine. *See* DNA.

鹼基對　一個 DNA 分子中的雙股多核苷酸鏈通過核苷酸內的鹼基形成的氫鍵相互聯結的形式。腺嘌呤專一與胸腺嘧啶配對，胞嘧啶和鳥嘌呤配對。

basilar artery an artery in the base of the brain, formed by the union of the two vertebral arteries. It extends from the lower to the upper border of the pons Varolii and then divides to form the two posterior cerebral arteries.

基底動脈　由兩側椎動脉滙合而成的位於大腦基底部的一根動脉。由橋腦下部走向上部邊緣，然後再分支形成兩支大腦後動脉。

basilar membrane a membrane in the *cochlea of the ear that separates the two of the three channels (scalae) that run the length of the spiral cochlea. The organ of Corti is situated on the basilar membrane, inside the scala media.

基底膜　位於耳蝸內並將貫穿整個螺旋耳蝸的耳蝸管（三腔管）一分爲二的生物膜。柯蒂氏器位於蝸管內基底膜上。

basilic vein a large vein in the arm, extending from the hand along the back of the forearm, then passing forward to the inner side of the arm at the elbow.

貴要靜脉　上臂的一條大靜脉。源於手部沿前臂背側上行，隨後向前於肘部轉入上臂內側面。

basion *n.* the midpoint of the anterior border of the large hole (foramen magnum) at the base of the *skull.

顱底點　顱骨底部枕骨大孔前緣中點。

basophil *n.* a variety of white blood cell distinguished by the presence in its cytoplasm of coarse granules that stain purple-black with *Romanowsky stains. The function of basophils is poorly understood, but they are capable of ingesting foreign particles and contain *histamine and *heparin. There are normally 0.03–0.15 × 10^9 basophils per litre of blood.

嗜鹼細胞　一種用羅曼諾夫斯基染劑染色胞漿中含有紫黑色粗大顆粒的白細胞。其功能不甚瞭解，但具有攝取外來微粒的能力，並含有組織胺和肝素。正常每升血液中含有 0.03 ~ 0.15 × 10^9。

basophilia *n.* **1.** a property of a microscopic structure whereby it shows an affinity for basic dyes. **2.** an increase in the number of certain white blood cells (*basophils) in the blood, which may occur in a variety of blood diseases.

①**嗜鹼性**　一種能對鹼性染色劑顯示親合力的顯微結構特性。　②**嗜鹼細胞增多症**　血液中嗜鹼細胞數量增加。可見於許多血液病。

basophilic *adj.* readily stainable by basic dyes: showing *basophilia.

嗜鹼（染色）的　易爲鹼性染劑着色的，顯示嗜鹼性的。

bathyaesthesia *n.* sensation experienced in the deeper parts of the body, such as the joints and muscles.

深部感覺　對軀體較深部位如關節和肌肉的感覺。

battered baby syndrome injuries inflicted on babies or young children by their parents, who are often emotionally disturbed or have themselves suffered from physical abuse in infancy or early childhood. The highest incidence of battering occurs in the first six months of life; it commonly takes the form of facial bruises, cigarette burns, bites, head injuries (often with brain damage), and fractured bones. Child abuse may be triggered by such crises as an unwanted pregnancy, unemployment, and debts; frequently, signs of older bruises, fractures, etc., are revealed when the child is brought for treatment. 60% of battered children suffer from further injury if discharged from hospital without the intensive support of a social worker and surveillance of family doctor and health visitor; a care order is often necessary to safeguard a child from further abuse.

虐待嬰兒綜合徵 父母情感障礙或他們本身在嬰幼兒期曾經受肉體虐待，遷怒於其子女，導致嬰幼兒遭受創傷。生後前6個月本病的發生率最高，常見表現有：面部青腫、煙燙傷、咬傷、頭部損傷（常合並顱腦損傷）和骨折。虐待嬰兒的行爲可由諸如非意願性懷孕、失業和欠債等危機而誘發，嬰兒在接受治療時常可見陳舊性青紫、骨折等體徵。如果沒有一些社會工作者的重點支持和家庭醫師以及保健員的監護，60% 的受害兒童在出院後將繼續遭受虐待。制訂保護兒童不再受虐待的規章制度常屬必要。

Bazin's disease a disease of young women in which tender nodules develop under the skin in the calves. The nodules may break down and ulcerate though they may clear up spontaneously. The cause is unknown but the disease may be associated with tuberculosis or, more commonly, *perniosis. Medical name: **erythema induratum**.

巴贊氏病 一種發生於年青婦女、表現爲小腿部皮下觸痛性結節的疾病。結節雖可自然痊癒，但易破裂並形成潰瘍。原因不明，可能與結核有關，但多由凍瘡引起。醫學術語：硬紅斑。

BCG (bacille Calmette-Guérin) a strain of tubercle bacillus that has lost the power to cause tuberculosis but retains its antigenic activity; it is therefore used to prepare a vaccine against the disease.

卡介苗 一種致病力喪失而抗原性尚存的結核桿菌菌株，用其製成疫苗預防結核病。

beclamide *n.* an *anticonvulsant drug used in the treatment of epilepsy. It is administered by mouth and often given together with phenobarbitone. Side-effects may include stomach upsets, dizziness, and nervousness. Trade name: **Nydrane**.

芐氯丙醯胺 一種用於癲癇治療的抗驚厥藥。口服，常與苯巴比妥合用。副作用可有胃腸不適、頭昏和神經過敏。商品名：貝克拉胺。

beclomethasone *n.* a *corticosteroid drug that reduces inflammation and is

二丙酸氯地米松 一種減輕炎症反應並外用於治療

applied externally in the treatment of various skin disorders. High dosage may cause retention of sodium and water and delayed wound healing. Trade name: **Propaderm**.

多種皮膚病的皮質類固醇藥物。大劑量可致水鈉瀦留並延緩傷口癒合。商品名：倍氯米松。

becquerel *n.* the *SI unit of activity of a radioactive source, being the activity of a radionuclide decaying at a rate of one spontaneous nuclear transition per second. It has replaced the curie. Symbol: Bq.

貝可勒爾 表示某放射源活度的國際標準單位。相當於某種放射性核素，即每秒發生一次自發原子核躍遷的速率進行衰變時的放射活度。已取代居里。符號：Bq。

bed bug a bloodsucking insect of the genus *Cimex*. *C. hemipterus* of the tropics and *C. lectularius* of temperate regions have reddish flattened bodies and vestigial wings. They live and lay their eggs in the crevices of walls and furniture and emerge at night to suck blood; although bed bugs are not known vectors of disease their bites leave a route for bacterial infection. Premises can be disinfested with *DDT.

臭蟲 臭蟲屬的一種吸血昆蟲。熱帶的熱帶臭蟲和溫帶的溫帶臭蟲有微紅色扁平軀體和發育不全的翅膀。棲息並產卵於牆壁和傢俱縫隙中，夜間出來吸血。雖然臭蟲不是已知的疾病傳播媒介，但其叮咬後的創口易致細菌感染。上述（易藏臭蟲）各處可用 DDT 消毒。

bed occupancy the number of hospital beds occupied by patients expressed as a percentage of the total beds available in the ward, specialty, hospital, area, or region. It may be recorded in relation to a defined point in time or more usefully for a period, when the calculation is based on bed-days. It is used with other indices (such as *discharge rate) to assess the demands for hospital beds in relation to diseases, specialties, or populations and hence to gauge an appropriate balance between health needs and residential (hospital) resources.

床位佔有率 指某病房、專業（科室）、醫院、地區或行政區內病人所佔床位數的百分率。可記錄時點床位佔有率或時期床位佔有率，後者更爲有用。和其它指標（如出院率）合用時可估計某疾病、某專業（科室）或人羣的醫院床位需要量，以平衡衞生保健醫療工作的供求關係。

bedsore (decubitus ulcer, pressure sore) *n.* an ulcerated area of skin caused by irritation and continuous pressure on part of the body: a hazard to be guarded against in all bedridden (especially unconscious) patients. Healing is hindered by the reduced blood supply to the area, and careful nursing

褥瘡 刺激和長期壓迫身體某部引起的皮膚潰瘍。所有臥床病人（尤其昏迷病人）都應注意預防。患病部位血流減少因而妨礙癒合，細緻的護理有助於防止局部壞疽。患者體位需經常變換，臀部、足

is necessary to prevent local gangrene. The patient's position should be changed frequently, and the buttocks, heels, elbows, and other regions at risk kept dry and clean.

跟、肘和其他患病部位應保持清潔乾燥。

bedwetting *n. see* enuresis.

遺尿

behaviourism *n.* an approach to psychology postulating that only observable behaviour need be studied, thus denying any importance to unconscious processes. Behaviourists are concerned with the laws regulating the occurrence of behaviour (*see* conditioning). —**behaviourist** *n.*

行爲主義 一種主張只需研究可觀察到的行爲的心理學派，否認潛意識過程的任何重要性。行爲主義者注重研究控制行爲發生的規律。

behaviour modification the use of the methods of behaviourist psychology (*see* behaviourism) – especially operant *conditioning – to alter people's behaviour. Behaviour modification has wider applications than *behaviour therapy, since it is also used in situations in which the client is not ill; for example, in education. *See also* chaining, prompting.

行爲矯正法 運用行爲主義心理學方法，尤其是操作行爲塑成法，以改變人的行爲。行爲矯正法較行爲療法運用廣泛。後來也用於當事人沒有疾病的情況，如教育。

behaviour therapy treatment based on the belief that psychological problems are the products of faulty learning and not the symptoms of an underlying disease. Treatment is directed at the problem or target behaviour and is designed for the particular patient, not for the particular diagnostic label that has been attached to him. *See also* aversion therapy, conditioning, desensitization.

行爲療法 基於認定心理問題是習得行爲錯誤的結果，而非某一潛在疾病的症狀這一信念制訂的治療方法。治療是針對所存在的心理問題或目標行爲表現。治療方法並非根據患者被診斷的病名，而是根據每個患者所存在的特殊情況而設計的。

bejel (endemic syphilis) *n.* a long-lasting nonvenereal form of *syphilis that occurs in the Balkans, Turkey, eastern Mediterranean countries, and the dry savannah regions of North Africa; it is particularly prevalent where standards of personal hygiene are low. The disease is spread among children and adults by direct body contact. Early skin lesions are obvious in the moist areas of the body (mouth,

非性病性梅毒（地方性梅毒） 一種病程綿長的非性病性梅毒。發生於巴爾幹半島各國、土耳其、東地中海各國和北非乾燥大草原地區。在個人衞生水平低下的地區尤爲流行。經直接身體接觸在兒童及成人中傳播。早期皮膚病損多在身體潮濕的部位（口腔、腋窩和腹股

armpits, and groin) and later there may be considerable destruction of the tissues of the skin, nasopharynx, and long bones. Wartlike eruptions in the anal and genital regions are common. Bejel, which is rarely fatal, is treated with penicillin.

溝）；後期可有明顯皮膚、鼻咽和長骨的組織破壞。肛門及生殖器部位常可見疣狀突起物。本病致死罕見，用青黴素治療。

bel *n. see* decibel.

貝爾

belladonna *n.* **1.** deadly nightshade (*Atropa belladonna*): a plant from which the drugs atropine and hyoscyamine are obtained. **2.** the poisonous alkaloid derived from deadly nightshade, from which atropine and hyoscyamine are extracted.

顛茄 ①有毒的茄屬植物（顛茄）：一種可提取阿托品和莨菪鹼的植物。②從茄屬植物中分離出並可提取阿托品和莨菪鹼的毒性生物鹼。

bell and pad a psychological method of treating bed-wetting. When the child starts to pass urine it is detected by a pad (or by sheets of metallic mesh) and this sets off a bell (or loud buzzer), which wakens the child. He then empties his bladder fully. A process of conditioning leads to his learning to be dry. It is effective in about 80% of cases.

鈴墊療法 治療遺尿的一種心理學方法。當小孩開始排尿時由一個墊子（或一個金屬網片）探知並觸響鈴（或蜂鳴器），從而喚醒小孩，然後排空膀胱。這一條件（反射）作用過程使小孩學會控制排尿。約 80% 病例有效。

Bell's palsy paralysis of the *facial nerve causing weakness of the muscles of one side of the face and an inability to close the eye. In some patients hearing may be affected so that sounds seem abnormally loud, and a loss of taste sensation may occur. The cause of this condition is unknown and recovery normally occurs spontaneously.

貝爾氏麻痺 面神經麻痺導致一側面部肌肉麻痺和閉眼不能。某些病例聽力可受累引起聽覺過敏，也可出現味覺喪失。病因不明，常自發痊癒。

belly *n.* **1.** the *abdomen or abdominal cavity. **2.** the central fleshy portion of a muscle.

①**腹** 腹部或腹腔。 ②**肌腹** 肌肉的中央肉質部。

Bence-Jones protein (Bence-Jones albumose) a protein of low molecular weight found in the urine of patients with multiple *myeloma, *lymphoma, *leukaemia, and *Hodgkin's disease.

本-周氏蛋白（本周氏朊） 存在於多發性骨髓瘤、淋巴瘤、白血病和何傑金氏病病人尿中的一種低分子量蛋白。

bendrofluazide (bendroflumethazide) *n.* a potent diuretic used in the treatment of conditions involving retention of fluid, such as congestive heart

苄氟噻嗪 一種用於治療液體瀦留狀態如充血性心力衰竭、高血壓、水腫和肥胖症的强力利尿劑。作

failure, hypertension, *oedema, and obesity. Its actions and side-effects are similar to those of *chlorothiazide.

用及副作用類似於氯噻嗪。

bends *n. see* compressed air illness.

減壓病

Benedict's test a test for the presence of sugar in urine or other liquids. A few drops of the test solution are added to *Benedict's solution*, prepared from sodium or potassium citrate, sodium carbonate, and copper sulphate. The mixture is boiled and shaken for about two minutes, then left to cool. The presence of up to 2% glucose is indicated by the formation of a reddish, yellowish, or greenish precipitate, the highest levels corresponding to the red coloration, the lowest (about 0.05%) to the green.

本尼廸特氏試驗 一種檢驗尿液或其它液體中是否存在糖的試驗。將幾滴被測溶液加入用檸檬酸鈉或檸檬酸鉀以及碳酸和硫酸銅配製的本尼廸特氏溶液中，煮沸並搖蕩約 2 分鐘，然後放冷。若葡萄糖含量達 2% 則可顯示微紅、微黃或微綠色沉澱，含糖量最高者呈紅色，最低者（約 0.05%）呈綠色。

benethamine penicillin an antibiotic effective against most Gram-positive bacteria (streptococci, staphylococci, and pneumococci). A derivative of benzylpenicillin, it can be administered by mouth but is usually given as an intramuscular injection, from which it liberates benzylpenicillin slowly. Patients hypersensitive to penicillins may suffer allergic reactions. *See also* penicillin.

苄胺青黴素 一種對大多數革蘭氏陽性菌（鏈球菌、葡萄球菌、肺炎球菌）有效的抗生素。爲苄青黴素（青黴素 G）的衍化物，可口服，但通常肌肉注射，它可緩慢釋放出青黴素 G。對青黴素類藥物過敏者禁用。

benign *adj.* **1.** describing a tumour that does not invade and destroy the tissue in which it originates or spread to distant sites in the body, i.e. a tumour that is not cancerous. **2.** describing any disorder or condition that does not produce harmful effects. *Compare* malignant.

良性的 ①形容某種不侵犯或破壞其發源組織或擴散至身體其它遠離部位的瘤，如非癌性腫瘤。 ②某些不導致有害後果的疾病或狀態。

benign intracranial hypertension (pseudotumour cerebri) a syndrome of raised pressure within the skull caused by impaired reabsorption of cerebrospinal fluid. The symptoms include headache, vomiting, double vision, and *papilloedema. It normally subsides spontaneously but treatment may be required to protect the patient's vision.

良性顱內高壓症（腦假瘤） 一種由腦脊液回流障礙引起的顱內高壓症。症狀包括頭痛、嘔吐、複視和視乳頭水腫。可自發緩解，但爲保護患者視力常需治療。

benorylate *n.* a drug, derived from *paracetamol, that relieves pain, inflammation, and fever. It is an alternative to aspirin, particularly in the treatment of rheumatoid arthritis. Side-effects may include drowsiness, noises in the ears, and skin rashes. Trade name: **Benoral**.

貝諾酯 一種由撲熱息痛衍化而來的解熱鎮痛抗炎藥。可替代阿司匹林，尤其是治療風濕性關節炎。副作用可有嗜眠、耳鳴和皮疹。商品名：撲炎痛。

benzalkonium *n.* a detergent disinfectant with the same uses and effects as *cetrimide.

新潔爾滅 用途和作用同溴棕三甲銨的去污消毒劑。

benzathine penicillin a long-acting antibiotic, given by mouth or intramuscular injection, that is slowly absorbed and effective against most Gram-positive bacteria (streptococci, staphylococci, and pneumococci). Patients hypersensitive to the penicillins suffer allergic reactions. Trade names: **Bicillin**, **Penidural**. *See also* penicillin.

苄星青黴素 一種長效、口服或肌注、吸收緩慢、對大多數革蘭氏陽性菌（鏈球菌、葡萄球菌和肺炎球菌）有效的抗生素。對青黴素類藥物過敏者禁用。商品名：長效西林。

benzethonium *n.* a detergent disinfectant with uses similar to those of *cetrimide.

苄甲乙氧胺 用途類似溴棕三甲銨的去污消毒劑。

benzhexol *n.* a drug that has actions and side-effects similar to those of *atropine. Taken by mouth, it is used mainly to reduce muscle spasm in parkinsonism. Trade names: **Artane**, **Pipanol**.

苯海索 作用和副作用類似於阿托品的一種藥物。口服，主要用於減輕帕金森氏綜合症的肌肉震顫。商品名：安坦。

benzocaine *n.* a local anaesthetic used in the form of an ointment, suppository, or aerosol to relieve painful conditions of the skin and mucous membranes. Virtually non-toxic, it can also be given by mouth to treat such conditions as lacerations of the mouth or tongue and gastric ulcers.

苯佐卡因 一種以軟膏、栓劑、噴霧劑等形式用於解除皮膚和黏膜疼痛的局部麻醉劑。無毒。亦可口服治療口腔裂傷或舌潰瘍、胃潰瘍。

benzodiazepines *n.* a group of pharmacologically active compounds used as minor *tranquillizers and hypnotics. The group includes *chlordiazepoxide, *diazepam, and *oxazepam.

苯二氮草類 一組具有弱安定藥和催眠藥療效的化合物。包括利眠寧、安定和去甲羥安定（舒寧）。

benzoic acid an antiseptic, active against fungi and bacteria, used as a preservative in foods and pharmaceuti-

安息香酸（苯甲酸） 一種能有效抵禦眞菌和細菌並用於食物和藥物製劑的

cal preparations, as well as for the treatment of fungal infections of the skin.

防腐劑。也可用於治療皮膚眞菌感染。

benzphetamine *n.* a drug with actions and side-effects similar to those of *amphetamine. It is given by mouth in the treatment of obesity. Trade name: **Didrex**.

苄甲苯丙胺　一種作用及副作用類似於苯丙胺的藥物。口服用於治療肥胖症。商品名：鹽酸苄甲苯丙胺。

benzthiazide *n.* a *diuretic used in the treatment of conditions involving fluid retention, such as congestive heart failure, *oedema, hypertension, and obesity. Trade name: **Exna**.

苄噻嗪　一種用於治療液體瀦留狀態如充血性心力衰竭、水腫、高血壓及肥胖症的利尿劑。商品名：苄硫噻嗪。

benztropine *n.* a drug similar to *atropine, but that also acts as an antihistamine, local anaesthetic, and sedative. Given by mouth it is used mainly in the treatment of parkinsonism to reduce rigidity and muscle cramps. It is well tolerated, but produces drowsiness and confusion.

苄托品（苯甲托品）　一種類似阿托品但還具有抗組胺作用、局部麻醉作用及鎮靜作用的藥物。口服，主要用於治療帕金森氏綜合症以減輕强直和肌肉痙攣。副作用小，但可產生嗜眠和精神錯亂。

benzyl benzoate an oily aromatic liquid that is applied to the body – in the form of a lotion – for the treatment of scabies. It is also useful in treating pediculosis.

苯甲酸苄酯　一種用於治療疥瘡的油性芳香性液體（以洗劑形式使用）。治療虱病亦有效。

benzylpenicillin *n. see* penicillin.

苄青黴素（青黴素 G）

beriberi *n.* a nutritional disorder due to deficiency of vitamin B_1 (thiamin). It is widespread in rice-eating communities in which the diet is based on polished rice, from which the thiamin-rich seed coat has been removed. Beriberi takes two forms: *wet beriberi*, in which there is an accumulation of tissue fluid (*oedema), and *dry beriberi*, in which there is extreme emaciation. There is nervous degeneration in both forms of the disease and death from heart failure is often the outcome.

脚氣病　缺乏維生素 B_1（硫胺）導致的一種營養性疾病。主要流行於以精製大米爲主食的國家，因富含硫胺的種衣被丟棄不用。脚氣病分兩型，即濕性脚氣病，有組織液積聚（水腫）；乾性脚氣病，有嚴重消瘦。兩種類型均有神經變性，常死於心力衰竭。

berylliosis *n.* poisoning by inhalation of beryllium or its compounds. This may be acute and sometimes fatal, but is more often chronic with the develop-

鈹中毒　吸入鈹及其化合物所致的中毒。急性中毒有時可致死，但更多見的是慢性中毒所致的全肺纖

ment of *fibrosis affecting all parts of the lungs. In Britain some workers with fluorescent light tubes were affected but this use was abolished in 1948.

維化。在英國曾有一些使用熒光燈管作業的工人中毒，但這種行業已在1948年被廢除。

beta blocker a drug that prevents stimulation of the beta-adrenergic receptors of the nerves of the sympathetic nervous system and therefore decreases the activity of the heart. Beta blockers include *oxprenolol and *propranolol, which are used to control abnormal heart rhythms, to treat angina, and to reduce high blood pressure. Blockade of beta receptors may cause constriction of air passages in the lungs and care has to be taken with the use of beta blockers in patients with any bronchial conditions. *See also* sympatholytic.

β-受體阻滯劑 一種阻止植物神經系統神經纖維的β腎上腺素能受體興奮而減弱心臟活動的藥物。包括氧烯洛爾（心得平）和普萘洛爾（心得安），用於控制異常心律、治療心絞痛和降血壓。阻斷β受體能導致肺內氣道的收縮，因而患有任何支氣管疾病的病人在使用β受體阻滯劑時都必須注意監護。

betamethasone *n.* a synthetic corticosteroid drug with effects and uses similar to those of *prednisolone. The side-effects are those of *cortisone. Trade names: **Betnelan, Betnesol, Betnovate.**

倍他米松 一種藥理作用和用途類似於强的松龍的合成皮質類固醇類藥物。副作用同可的松。

betatron *n.* a device used to accelerate a stream of electrons (*beta particles*) into a beam of radiation that can be used in *radiotherapy.

電子回旋加速器 一種將電子流（β粒子）加速，使之變爲可用於放射治療的放射束的裝置。

bethanidine *n.* a drug that lowers blood pressure. It is given by mouth and acts by blocking the sympathetic nerves that supply the blood vessels. Common side-effects include dizziness, fainting, oedema, and breathlessness. Trade names: **Bethamid, Esbatal.**

苄二甲胍 一種降壓藥。口服，通過阻斷支配血管的植物神經發揮作用。常見副作用有頭昏、暈厥、水腫和呼吸困難。商品名：硫酸苄二甲胍。

bezoar *n.* a mass of swallowed foreign material within the stomach. The material, which is usually swallowed by psychiatrically disturbed patients, accumulates and ultimately causes gastric obstruction. Its removal often requires a surgical operation. *See also* trichobezoar.

糞石 吞咽入胃的異物在胃內形成的團塊。常發生在精神病病人，吞入胃後積聚於胃中，最終導致胃阻塞，常需手術取出。

bi- *prefix* denoting two; double. Examples: *biciliate* (having two cilia); *binucleate* (having two nuclei).

二，雙 如雙纖毛的（有兩根纖毛），雙核的（有兩個核）。

biceps *n.* a muscle with two heads. The *biceps brachii* extends from the shoulder joint to the elbow (see illustration). It flexes the arm and forearm and supinates the forearm and hand. The *biceps femoris* is situated at the back of the thigh and is responsible for flexing the knee, extending the thigh, and rotating the leg outwards.

二頭肌 具有雙頭的肌肉。肱二頭肌源於肩關節止於肘部（見圖）。它使上臂和前臂屈曲並使前臂及手旋後。股二頭肌位於大腿後部，使膝關節屈曲，大腿伸直和小腿外旋。

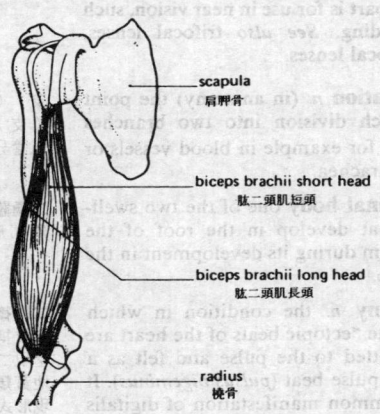

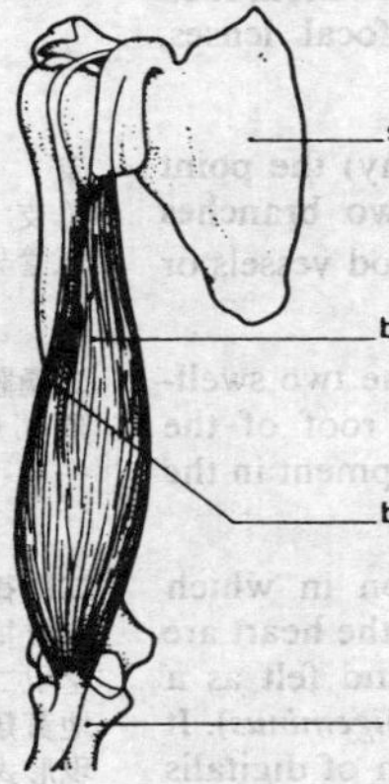

The biceps muscle of the arm

肱二頭肌

biconcave *adj.* having a hollowed surface on both sides. Biconcave lenses are used to correct short-sightedness. *Compare* biconvex.

雙凹（形）的 兩面都呈凹陷形的。雙凹透鏡用於矯正近視。

biconvex *adj.* having a surface on each side that curves outwards. Biconvex lenses are used to correct long-sightedness. *Compare* biconcave.

雙凸（形）的 兩面都呈凸出形的。雙凸透鏡用於矯正遠視。

bicornuate *adj.* having two hornlike processes or projections. The term is applied to an abnormal uterus that is divided into two separate halves at the upper end.

雙角的 具有兩個角狀突出物的。用於描述在上端分爲兩個獨立部分的異常子宮（雙角子宮）。

bicuspid 1. *adj.* having two *cusps, as in the premolar teeth and the mitral valve of the heart. **2.** *n.* (in the USA) a premolar tooth.

①**二尖的**　具有兩個尖端的。如雙尖牙和心臟二尖瓣。　②**雙尖牙**　美國用法。

bicuspid valve *see* mitral valve.

二尖瓣

bifid *adj.* split or cleft into two parts.

對裂的，兩杈的　（某物）一劈爲兩半。

bifocal lenses glasses in which the upper part of the lens is shaped to give a sharp image of distant objects and the lower part is for use in near vision, such as reading. *See also* trifocal lenses, multifocal lenses.

雙焦鏡　一種上部適於遠物清晰成像，下部適於視近物如閱讀的眼鏡。

bifurcation *n.* (in anatomy) the point at which division into two branches occurs; for example in blood vessels or in the trachea.

支　（解剖學）兩個分叉（支）的起點。如血管或氣管分叉處。

bigeminal body one of the two swellings that develop in the roof of the midbrain during its development in the embryo.

二疊體　胚胎發育時中腦頂部形成的兩個隆突之一。

bigeminy *n.* the condition in which alternate *ectopic beats of the heart are transmitted to the pulse and felt as a double pulse beat (*pulsus bigeminus*). It is a common manifestation of digitalis poisoning.

二聯律　交替出現的心臟異位搏動傳遞至脉搏使之呈現二聯脉的狀態。是洋地黃類藥物中毒的常見表現形式。

bilateral *adj.* (in anatomy) relating to or affecting both sides of the body or of a tissue or organ or both of a pair of organs (e.g. the eyes, breasts, or ovaries).

兩側的　（解剖學）涉及或影響軀體、某組織和某器官兩側的或某成對器官（如眼、乳房、卵巢）的。

bile *n.* a thick alkaline fluid that is secreted by the *liver and stored in the *gall bladder, from which it is ejected intermittently into the duodenum via the common *bile duct. Bile may be yellow, green, or brown, according to the proportions of the *bile pigments (excretory products) present; other constituents are lecithin, cholesterol, and *bile salts. The bile salts help to emulsify fats in the duodenum so that they can be more easily digested by pan-

膽汁　一種由肝臟分泌，貯存於膽囊並間斷地經膽總管排入十二指腸的碱性粘稠液體。根據膽色素（排泄產物）的含量多少可爲黃色、綠色或棕色；其它成分爲卵磷脂、固醇和膽鹽。膽鹽在十二指腸內幫助乳化脂肪，使之更易爲胰脂肪酶分解爲脂肪酸和甘油。膽鹽還與脂肪酸形成複合物，然後被轉

creatic *lipase into fatty acids and glycerol. Bile salts also form compounds with fatty acids, which can then be transported into the *lacteals. Bile also helps to stimulate *peristalsis in the duodenum.

移至乳糜管。膽鹽也可在十二指腸內幫助刺激腸蠕動。

bile acids the organic acids in bile; mostly occurring as bile salts (sodium glycocholate and sodium taurocholate). They are cholic acid, deoxycholic acid, glycocholic acid, and taurocholic acid.

膽汁酸 膽汁中的有機酸。大部分以膽鹽形式存在（甘氨膽酸鈉和牛磺膽酸鈉）。包括膽酸去氧膽酸、甘氨膽酸和牛磺膽酸。

bile duct any of the ducts that convey bile from the liver. Bile is drained from the liver cells by many small ducts that unite to form the main bile duct of the liver, the *hepatic duct*. This joins the *cystic duct*, which leads from the *gall bladder, to form the *common bile duct*, which drains into the duodenum.

膽小管 從肝臟運送出膽汁的管道。膽汁經許多微小的管道由肝細胞排出，這些微小管道集合成肝臟的主要膽管即肝管。肝管與由膽囊發出的膽囊管滙合形成膽總管，膽總管進入十二指腸。

bile pigments coloured compounds – breakdown products of the blood pigment *haemoglobin – that are excreted in *bile. The two most important bile pigments are *bilirubin*, which is orange or yellow, and its oxidized form *biliverdin*, which is green. Mixed with the intestinal contents, they give the brown colour to the faeces (*see* urobilinogen).

膽色素 隨膽汁排泄的有色化合物（血紅蛋白降解產物）。兩種最重要的膽色素是膽紅素，呈橘色或黃色；和其氧化型即膽綠素，呈綠色。膽色素和腸道內容物混合後使糞便呈棕色。

bile salts sodium glycocholate and sodium taurocholate – the alkaline salts of *bile – necessary for the emulsification of fats. After they have been absorbed from the intestine they are transported to the liver for reuse.

膽鹽 膽汁的鹼性鹽類。主要成分爲脂肪乳化必需的甘氨膽酸鈉和牛磺膽酸鈉。膽鹽經腸道吸收後被轉送至肝臟以備重新使用。

Bilharzia *n. see* Schistosoma.

血吸蟲屬

bilharziasis *n. see* schistosomiasis.

血吸蟲病

bili- *prefix denoting* bile.

〔前綴〕 **膽汁**

biliary *adj.* relating to or affecting the bile duct or bile. *See also* fistula.

膽汁的，膽管的 涉及或影響膽管或膽汁的。

biliary colic pain resulting from obstruction of the gall bladder or common bile duct, usually by a stone. The pain, which is very severe, is usually felt in

膽絞痛 膽囊或膽總管阻塞（常爲結石）引起的疼痛。疼痛異常劇烈，位於上腹中線或偏右。常於餐

the upper abdomen (in the mid-line or to the right). It often occurs about an hour after a meal (particularly if fatty), may last several hours, and is usually steady in severity (unlike other forms of *colic). Vomiting often occurs simultaneously.

後（尤以進脂肪飲食後）1小時發病，可持續數小時，疼痛程度穩定（有別於其他類型的絞痛），常伴有嘔吐。

bilious *adj.* **1.** containing bile; for example *bilious vomiting* is the vomiting of bile-containing fluid. **2.** a lay term used to describe attacks of nausea or vomiting.

膽汁（性）的 ①含膽汁的。如膽汁性嘔吐時嘔吐物爲含有膽汁的液體。②用於描述噁心和嘔吐發作（暈船）的非專業名詞。

bilirubin *n. see* bile pigments.

膽紅素

bilirubinaemia *n.* an excess of the *bile pigment bilirubin in the blood. Normally there is under 0.8 mg bilirubin per 100 ml blood; when the concentration of bilirubin is above 1–1.5 mg per 100 ml, visible *jaundice occurs.

膽紅素血症 血液中膽色素（膽紅素）超過正常範圍。正常膽紅素含量每100 mℓ血低於0.8mg，當其濃度超過1～1.5mg/100mℓ時，即可發生黃疸。

biliuria (choluria) *n.* the presence of bile in the urine: a feature of certain forms of jaundice.

膽汁尿 尿液中含有膽汁。爲某些類型黃疸的一種特徵。

biliverdin *n. see* bile pigments.

膽綠素

bimanual *adj.* using two hands to perform an activity, such as a gynaecological examination.

雙手的 用雙手進行某種活動。如婦科檢查。

binaural *adj.* relating to or involving the use of both ears.

兩耳的

binder *n.* a bandage that is wound around a part of the body, usually the abdomen, to apply pressure or to give support or protection.

綁帶 包繞身體某一部分（通常爲腹部）的一種繃帶。起加壓、支持和保護作用。

binocular *adj.* relating to or involving the use of both eyes.

雙眼的

binocular vision the ability to focus both eyes on an object at the same time, so that a person sees one image of the object he is looking at. It is not inborn, but acquired during the first few

雙眼視覺 同時將雙眼聚焦於同一物體，使被視物成爲一個影像的能力。這種能力並非先天具有的，而是在出生後頭幾個月獲

months of life. Binocular vision enables judgment of distance and perception of depth. *See also* stereoscopic vision.

得的。雙眼視覺使（人）能夠判斷距離、感覺深度。

bio- *prefix denoting* life or living organisms. Example: *biosynthesis* (formation of a compound within a living organism).

〔前綴〕 **生命，生物** 如生物合成（生物體內化合物的形成）。

bioassay *n.* estimation of the activity or potency of a drug or other substance by comparing its effects on living organisms with effects of a preparation of known strength. Bioassay is used to determine the strength of preparations of hormones or other material of biological origin when other physical or chemical methods are not available.

生物鑑定 對藥物或其他物質的活性或效力的鑑定。通過將被鑑定物和已知生物效應的標本各自對生物體的效力相比較（對照）而進行。運用於其它物理或化學方法不能鑑定的激素或其他生物源性物質的生物效應的鑑定。

biochemistry *n.* the study of the chemical processes and substances occurring in living things. **—biochemical** *adj.* **—biochemist** *n.*

生物化學 研究生物體的化學代謝過程和物質的科學。

biofeedback *n.* the giving of immediate information to a subject about his bodily processes (such as heart rate), which are usually unconscious. These processes can then be subject to operant *conditioning. This is an experimental treatment for disturbances of bodily regulation, such as hypertension.

生物反饋 把代表體內某種通常是意識不到的變化（如心率變化）的信息立即傳遞給患者的過程。這些過程可以形成操作性條件反射。此法現用於試驗治療體內調節功能紊亂，如高血壓。

biology *n.* the study of living organisms – plants, animals, and microorganisms – including their structure and working and their relationships with one another and with the inanimate world. **—biological** *adj.*

生物學 研究生物（植物、動物和微生物）的結構和活動方式、生物之間的相互關係以及生物和非生物界的相互關係的科學。

biometry *n.* the measurement of living things and the processes associated with life, including the application of mathematics, particularly statistics, to problems in biology.

生物統計 一種用數學，特別是統計學對生物及有關生命過程等生物學問題進行數據處理的方法。

bionics *n.* the science of mechanical or electronic systems that function in the same way as, or have characteristics of, living systems. *Compare* cybernetics. **—bionic** *adj.*

仿生學 研究功能和特徵與生物相同的機械和電子系統的科學。

bionomics *n. see* ecology.

個體生態學

biopsy *n.* the removal of a small piece of living tissue from an organ or part of the body for microscopic examination. Biopsy is an important means of diagnosing cancer from examination of a fragment of tumour. It is often carried out with a special hollow needle, inserted into the liver, kidney, or other organ, with relatively little discomfort to the patient.

活組織檢查 從某器官或身體某部分獲取一小塊活體組織進行顯微鏡檢查的方法。活組織檢查是用檢查腫瘤碎片診斷腫瘤的重要方法。常用一專用空針插入肝臟、腎臟或其他器官，病人可有輕微不適。

biostatistics *n.* statistical information and techniques used with special reference to studies of health and social problems. It embraces, overlaps, and is to some extent synonymous with the fields of *vital statistics* (e.g. *fertility and *mortality rates) and *demography.

生物統計學 將專門研究健康與社會問題所獲得的資料進行統計學處理的技術。它與生命統計學（如人口出生率和死亡率）和人口統計學相互交叉、重疊，並在一定程度上具有相同含意。

biotin *n.* a vitamin of the B complex that is essential for the metabolism of fat, being involved in fatty acid synthesis and *gluconeogenesis. A biotin deficiency is extremely rare in man; it can be induced by eating large quantities of raw egg white, which contains a protein – avidin – that combines with biotin, making it unavailable to the body. Rich sources of the vitamin are egg yolk and liver.

生物素，維生素 H 複合維生素B族中的一種，爲脂肪代謝包括脂肪酸合成和糖原異生所必需。生物素缺乏症在人極爲罕見，可由食入大量生蛋清引起，因爲它含有一種結合生物素的蛋白質——抗生物素蛋白（卵白素），而破壞生物素。生物素的主要來源爲蛋黃和肝臟。

bipara *n.* a woman who has been pregnant twice and has given birth to a living child at the end of each pregnancy.

產$_2$ 兩次生產並均爲活產的婦女。

biparous *adj.* giving birth to two children at the end of a pregnancy.

產雙胎的 一次懷孕分娩兩個嬰兒。

biperiden *n.* a drug with effects similar to those of atropine, used in the treatment of parkinsonism, certain forms of spasticity, and to control the muscular incoordination that may result from the use of some tranquillizers. It is given by mouth; side-effects are those of *atropine. Trade name: **Akineton**.

雙環哌丙醇 一種藥理作用類似於阿托品的藥物。用於治療帕金森氏綜合症，某些痙攣（强直）狀態和控制服用安定劑引起的肌共濟失調等，口服。副作用同阿托品。商品名：安克痙。

bipolar *adj.* (in neurology) describing a neurone (nerve cell) that has two processes extending in different directions from its cell body.

雙極的 （神經病學）指某一神經元（神經細胞）具有兩個源於胞體而向不同方向伸展的突起。

birefringence *n.* the property possessed by some naturally occurring substances (such as cell membranes) of doubly refracting a beam of light, i.e. of bending it in two different directions. —**birefringent** *adj.*

雙折射 某些自然存在物（如細胞膜）具有的使一束光折射成雙的特性，即將其轉變爲兩個不同的方向。

birth *n.* (in obstetrics) *see* labour.

分娩

birth control the use of *contraception or *sterilization (male or female) to prevent unwanted pregnancies.

節制生育 利用避孕或絕育方法（男或女）預防非意願性懷孕。

birthmark *n.* a skin blemish or mark present at birth. The cause is unknown but most birthmarks grow before the baby is born. *See* naevus.

胎記，胎痣 出生時就具有的皮膚斑記。原因不明，大多數在嬰兒出生前即長出。

birth rate *see* fertility rate.

出生率

bisacodyl *n.* a *laxative that acts on the large intestine to cause reflex movement and bowel evacuation. It is administered by mouth or in a suppository. The commonest side-effect is the development of abdominal cramps. Trade name: **Dulcolax**.

雙醋苯啶 一種作用於大腸引起反射運動和排便的輕瀉藥。口服或用栓劑。最常見副作用爲腸痙攣。

bisexual *adj.* **1.** describing an individual who is sexually attracted to both men and women. **2.** describing an individual who possesses the qualities of both sexes.

兩性的 ①指某人對男性或女性均能產生性戀。②指某人具有男女兩性的特徵。

Bismarck brown a basic aniline dye used for staining and counterstaining histological and bacterial specimens.

苯胺棕 一種用於對組織和細菌標本進行直接染色和對比染色的鹼性苯胺染料。

bistoury *n.* a narrow surgical knife, with a straight or curved blade (see illustration).

細長刀 一種刃口爲直形或彎形的狹長外科手術刀（見圖）。

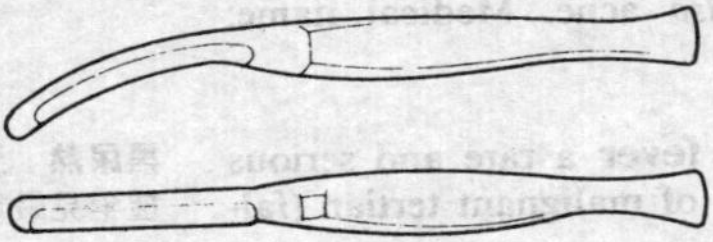

Types of bistoury
細長刀類型

bite-raiser *n.* an appliance to prevent normal closure of the teeth in the treatment of the *temporomandibular joint syndrome.

撐殆器 治療顳下頜關節綜合徵時用於阻止牙齒閉合的一種器械。

bite-wing *n.* a dental X-ray film that provides a view of the crowns of the teeth in part of both upper and lower jaws. This view is used in the diagnosis of caries and periodontal disease.

殆翼片 一種顯示部分上下牙冠的牙科 X 線片。用於診斷齲齒和牙周疾病。

bivalent *n.* (in genetics) a structure consisting of homologous chromosomes attached to each other by *chiasmata during the first division of *meiosis. —**bivalent** *adj.*

二價染色體 （遺傳學）指減數分裂初期存在的一種經交叉而相互依附的同源染色體結構。

blackdamp (chokedamp) *n.* (in mining) the poisonous gas containing carbon dioxide, carbon monoxide, or other suffocating material, sometimes found in pockets in underground workings. *Compare* firedamp.

窒息性氣體 （礦業）有時存在於地下礦穴的包含一氧化碳、二氧化碳或其它窒息性物質的毒性氣體。

Black Death *see* plague.

黑死病，鼠疫

black eye bruising of the eyelids.

黑眼（眼瞼皮下瘀血） 眼瞼的挫傷瘀血。

black fly a small widely distributed bloodsucking insect of the genus *Simulium*. Black flies are also known as buffalo gnats from their humpbacked appearance. Female flies can inflict painful bites and constitute a serious pest to man at certain times of the year. *S. damnosum* in Africa and *S. ochraceum* in Central America and Venezuela transmit the parasites causing *onchocerciasis.

黑蠅 一種微小、分佈廣泛的蚋屬吸血昆蟲。據其駝背的體形俗稱牛蚋。雌性黑蠅叮咬時疼痛，並在一年的某些時期對人構成嚴重危害。非洲憎蚋和中美洲以及委內瑞拉淡黃蚋傳播盤尾絲蟲病。

blackhead *n.* a plug formed of fatty material (sebum and keratin) in the outlet of a *sebaceous gland in the skin. Oxidation of the keratin in the blackhead is the cause of the black coloration. *See also* acne. Medical name: **comedo**.

黑頭粉刺 皮膚皮脂腺開口處脂肪物質（皮脂和角蛋白）形成的栓。其中角蛋白氧化是導致黑色的原因。醫學術語：粉刺。

blackwater fever a rare and serious complication of malignant tertian (fal-

黑尿熱 惡性間日瘧的一種罕見嚴重併發症。由於

ciparum) *malaria in which there is massive destruction of the red blood cells, leading to the presence of the blood pigment haemoglobin in the urine. The condition is probably brought on by inadequate treatment with *quinine; it is marked by fever, bloody urine, jaundice, vomiting, enlarged liver and spleen, anaemia, exhaustion, and – in fatal cases – a reduced flow of urine resulting from a blockage of the kidney tubules. Treatment involves rest, administration of alkaline fluids and intravenous glucose, and blood transfusions.

大量紅細胞破壞，導致血紅蛋白從尿中排出。可能是因不恰當地運用奎寧所致。特徵爲發熱、血尿、黃疸、嘔吐、肝脾腫大、貧血、全身衰竭（虛脫），嚴重病例可因腎小管阻塞導致尿量減少。治療包括休息、鹼化尿液和靜滴葡萄糖以及輸血。

bladder *n.* **1. (urinary bladder)** a sac-shaped organ that has a wall of smooth muscle and stores the urine produced by the kidneys. Urine passes into the bladder through the *ureters; the release of urine from the bladder is controlled by a sphincter at its junction with the *urethra. **2.** any of several other hollow organs containing fluid, such as the *gall bladder.

①**膀胱**　一個具有平滑肌壁貯存腎臟分泌的尿液的囊狀器官。尿液經輸尿管入膀胱。膀胱的排尿則由位於與尿道交界處的括約肌控制。　②**囊**　其他一些包含液體的囊狀器官如膽囊。

bladderworm *n. see* cysticercus.

囊尾蚴

-blast *suffix denoting* a formative cell. Example: *osteoblast* (formative bone cell).

〔**後綴**〕　**成…細胞**　表示形成某種細胞的前體。如成骨細胞。

blastema *n.* any zone of embryonic tissue that is still differentiating and growing into a particular organ. The term is usually applied to the tissue that develops into the kidneys and gonads.

胚基，芽基　所有尚在分化與生長爲某種特定器官的胚胎組織區（帶）。常用於描述行將分化爲腎臟和性腺的組織。

blasto- *prefix denoting* a germ cell or embryo. Example: *blastogenesis* (early development of an embryo).

〔前綴〕　**胚，芽**　表示胚細胞或胚胎。如胚源發生（某胚胎的早期發育）。

blastocoele *n.* the fluid-filled cavity that develops within the *blastocyst. The cavity increases the surface area of the embryo and thus improves its ability to absorb nutrients and oxygen.

胚泡腔　位於胚泡內的充滿液體的腔隙。此腔擴大了胚胎的表面積，因而有利於提高其吸收營養物質及氧的能力。

blastocyst *n.* an early stage of embryonic development that consists of a hollow ball of cells with a localized thickening (the *inner cell mass*) that will develop into the actual embryo; the remainder of the blastocyst is composed of *trophoblast (see illustration). At first the blastocyst is unattached, but it soon implants in the wall of the womb (uterus). *See also* implantation.

胚泡　胚胎發育的早期階段。係一個由細胞構成的中空球狀物，球內有一塊局部增厚區（泡內細胞羣），胚胎即由此區發育而成，其餘部分由滋養層（如圖）組成。最先胚泡呈游離狀，但很快即植入子宮壁。

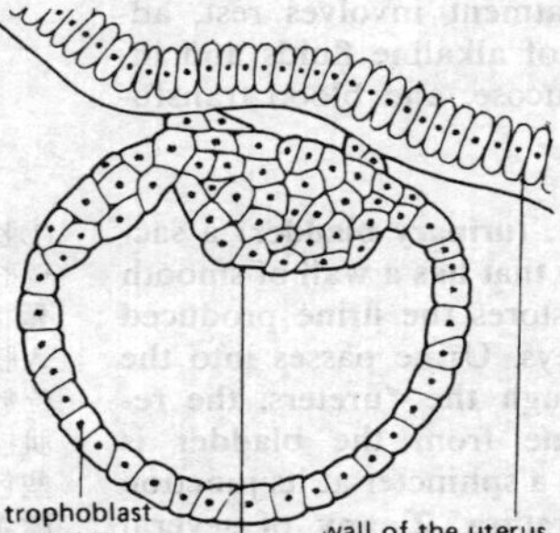

Section through a blastocyst
胚泡斷面觀

blastomere *n.* any of the cells produced by *cleavage of the zygote, comprising the earliest stages of embryonic development until the formation of the *blastocyst. Blastomeres divide repeatedly without growth and so decrease in size.

卵裂球，分裂球　合子卵裂形成的所有細胞。是胚泡形成以前胚胎發育的最早階段。卵裂球迅速分裂但不生長，故此其體積縮小。

blastomycosis *n.* any disease caused by parasitic fungi of the genus *Blastomyces*, which may affect the skin (forming wartlike ulcers and tumours on the face, neck, hands, arms, feet, and legs) or involve various internal tissues, such as the lungs, bones, liver, spleen, and lymphatics. There are two principal forms of the disease: *North American blastomycosis* (*Gilchrist's disease*), caused by *B. dermatitidis*; and *South American blastomycosis*, caused by *B. brasiliensis*. Both diseases are treated with antibiotics (such as amphotericin).

芽生菌病　由芽生菌屬寄生性眞菌引起的所有疾病。可累及皮膚（形成疣狀潰瘍和面部、頸部、手部、臂部、足部和腿部腫塊）或影響各內部組織如肺、骨、肝、脾和淋巴管。有兩種主要類型：北美芽生菌病，由皮炎類芽生菌引起；和南美芽生菌病，由巴西芽生菌引起。兩種疾病均用抗生素治療（如二性黴素）。

blastopore *n.* the opening that forms as a result of invagination of the surface layer of the early embryo (*gastrula). It is very much reduced in man, in which it gives rise to the archenteric canal (*see* archenteron).

胚孔 早期胚胎（原腸胚）表層反折（凹入）所形成的開口。在人極其微小，神經原腸管即在其內形成。

blastula *n.* an early stage of the embryonic development of many animals. The equivalent stage in mammals (including man) is the *blastocyst.

囊胚，囊胚泡 許多動物胚胎發育的早期階段。哺乳動物（包括人）的相等時期爲胚泡。

bleeding *n. see* haemorrhage

出血

blenn- (blenno-) *prefix denoting* mucus. Example: *blennorrhagia* (excessive production of).

〔前綴〕 **黏液** 如淋病有大量黏液溢出。

blennophthalmia *n. Obsolete.* *conjunctivitis in which there is a sticky yellow discharge from the eye.

眼濃溢 廢用詞。有黏性黃色分泌物的眼結膜炎。

blennorrhagia *n.* a copious discharge of mucus, particularly from the urethra. This usually accompanies *urethritis and sometimes acute *prostatitis. Treatment is directed to clearing the underlying causative organism by antibiotic administration.

淋病 有大量黏液從尿道溢出的一種疾病。常伴有尿道炎，有時伴有急性前列腺炎。治療爲使用抗生素消滅病源體。

blennorrhoea *n.* a profuse watery discharge from the urethra. This, like *blenorrhagia, is associated with either prostatitis or urethritis, and is cleared by the usual measures undertaken in the treatment of these conditions.

尿道液溢 有大量水性分泌物自尿道排出的一種疾病。和淋病一樣，與前列腺炎和尿道炎有關，並用治療這些疾病的常用方法治療。

bleomycin *n.* an antibiotic with action against cancer cells, used in the treatment of Hodgkin's disease and other lymphomas and in squamous-cell carcinoma. It is administered by injection and can cause toxic side-effects in the skin and lungs; it should not be used in patients with impaired kidney function or lung disease.

博來黴素（爭光黴素） 一種能殺傷腫瘤細胞，用於治療何傑金氏病和其它淋巴瘤以及鱗狀細胞癌的抗生素。注射給藥，對皮膚和肺有毒性副作用。腎功能損害和肺臟疾病患者禁用。

blephar- (blepharo-) *prefix denoting* the eyelid. Example: *blepharotomy* (incision into).

〔前綴〕 **眼瞼** 如眼瞼切開術。

blepharitis *n.* inflammation of the eyelids. In *squamous blepharitis*, often

瞼炎 眼瞼的炎症。鱗屑性瞼炎常與頭皮脫屑同時

associated with dandruff of the scalp, white scales accumulate among the lashes. *Chronic ulcerative blepharitis* is characterized by yellow crusts overlying ulcers of the lid margins. The lashes become matted together and tend to fall out or become distorted. *Allergic blepharitis* may occur in response to drugs or cosmetics put in the eye or on the eyelids.

發生，有白色鱗屑在睫毛中堆積。慢性潰瘍性瞼緣炎的潰瘍處有黃痂覆蓋，睫毛纏結並倒伏或屈曲。過敏性瞼炎可由於在眼部或眼瞼使用藥物或化妝品引起。

blepharon *n. see* eyelid.

眼瞼

blepharophimosis *n.* narrowing of the aperture between the eyelids. It may be congenital but can be acquired if the skin contracts at the outer corner of the eye as a result of chronic inflammation.

瞼裂狹小 雙瞼間距離狹小。可爲先天性，也可由於慢性炎症導致眼外眦部皮膚收縮而引起。

blepharoplasty (tarsoplasty) *n.* any operation to repair or reconstruct the eyelid. It involves either rearrangement of the tissues of the lid or the use of tissue from other sites (e.g. skin or mucous membrane).

瞼成形術 修復或重建眼瞼的手術。包括重新調整眼瞼組織或運用其他部位的組織（如皮膚或黏膜）修復。

blepharospasm *n.* involuntary tight contraction of the eyelids, usually in response to painful conditions of the eye.

瞼痙攣 眼瞼非隨意性緊張性收縮。常爲對眼部疼痛的反應。

blindness *n.* the inability to see. Lack of all light perception constitutes total blindness but there are degrees of visual impairment far less severe than this that may be classed as blindness for administrative or statutory purposes. For example, marked reduction in the *visual field is classified as blindness, even if objects are still seen sharply. The commonest causes of blindness are *trachoma, *onchocerciasis, and vitamin A deficiency (*see* night blindness) but there is wide geographic variation. In Great Britain the commonest causes are diabetes mellitus, myopic degeneration, and *glaucoma.

盲，視覺缺失 視覺喪失。全部光感喪失是爲全盲。除去政策中規定的具有法律意義的盲人以外，還有許多較前者爲輕的程度不等的視力缺失。例如，視野的明顯縮小也爲視覺缺失之一種，雖然患者仍能看清物體。盲的最常見原因爲沙眼、（眼）盤尾絲蟲病和維生素 A 缺乏症。但病因的地區差異很大，在英國，最常見的原因爲糖尿病、近視性變性和青光眼。

blind register (in Britain) a list of persons who are technically blind due to reduced visual acuity (inability to read a car number plate from a distance

視力缺失注册薄 對視敏度下降造成就業困難的視力缺乏（3 米遠不能看清汽車牌號）或有嚴重的視

of three metres) or who have severely restricted fields of vision (*see* blindness). Such people are entitled to special education and to financial and other social benefits. *See also* partially sighted register.

野縮小者的登記薄。他們有享受特殊教育和經濟補助及其他社會福利的權利。

blind spot the small area of the *retina of the eye where the nerve fibres from the light-sensitive cells (*see* cone, rod) lead into the optic nerve. There are no rods or cones in this area and hence it does not register light. Anatomical name: **punctum caecum**.

盲點 由光敏感細胞發出的神經纖維集合進入視神經的眼底視網膜微小區域。該區域沒有視桿細胞和視錐細胞，因而不能感光。

blind trial *see* intervention study.

盲法試驗

blinking *n.* the action of closing and opening the eyelids, which wipes the front of the eyeball and helps to spread the *tears. Reflex blinking may be caused by suddenly bringing an object near to the eye: the eyelids close involuntarily in order to protect the eye.

瞬目 開閉眼瞼的活動。能擦洗眼球前部並利於淚液擴佈，突然將某物靠近眼時可引起瞬目反射：眼瞼自行閉合以保護眼睛。

blister *n.* a swelling containing watery fluid (serum) and sometimes also blood (*blood blister*) or pus, within or just beneath the skin. Blisters commonly develop as a result of unaccustomed friction on the hands or feet or at the site of a burn. Blisters may be treated with antiseptics and dressings. An unduly painful blister may be punctured with a sterile needle so that the fluid is released.

疱 皮內或皮下的含有水樣液體（血清），有時爲血（血疱）或膿的腫物。常因手、足的異常摩擦或燒傷而引起。治療：使用抗菌藥物，敷料包紮。劇烈疼痛的水疱可用無菌空針穿刺以排除液體。

block *n.* any interruption of physiological or mental function, brought about intentionally (as part of a therapeutic procedure) or by disease. *See also* heart block, nerve block.

阻滯 人爲的（作爲治療的一部分）或由疾病引起的生理或精神功能的阻斷。

blocking *n.* (in psychiatry) **1.** a sudden halting of the flow of thought or speech. Blocking of thought, accompanied by the sensation of thoughts being removed from the mind, is a symptom of *schizophrenia. Blocking of speech may be a consequence of thought

中斷 （精神病學）①思維或語言突然中斷的現象。思維中斷伴有腦中的思想被挖空了的感覺，爲精神分裂症的一個症狀。語言中斷可是思維中斷的結果，或由機械性語言障礙

block or a result of a mechanical impediment in speech, such as *stammering. 2. failure to recall a specific event, or to explore a specific train of thought, because of its unpleasant associations.

如口吃引起。 ②由於不愉快的聯想，而不能回憶某個特定的事件，或不能按特定的思維邏輯程序進行思考。

blood *n.* a fluid tissue that circulates throughout the body, via the arteries and veins, providing a vehicle by which an immense variety of different substances are transported between the various organs and tissues. It is composed of *blood cells, which are suspended in a liquid medium, the *plasma. An average individual has approximately 70 ml of blood per kilogram body weight (about 5 litres in an average adult male).

血液 一種循環於全身的液體組織，流經動脈和靜脈，爲大量不同物質在各種不同器官和組織之間進行交換的媒介（場所）。由懸浮於液體媒介（血漿）中的血細胞組成。人體平均含量約 70mℓ/kg（成年男性平均約 5 升）。

blood bank a department within a hospital or blood transfusion centre in which blood collected from donors is stored prior to transfusion. Blood must be kept at a temperature of 4°C and may be used up to three weeks after collection.

血庫 醫院或輸血中心中貯存供血者血液以備輸血用的部門。血液必須保存在 4℃，並在採集後 3 週內用完。

blood-brain barrier the mechanism whereby the circulating blood is kept separate from the tissue fluids surrounding the brain cells. It is a semipermeable membrane allowing solutions to pass through it but excluding solid particles and large molecules.

血腦屏障 將循環血液和環繞腦細胞的組織液分隔開的機構。它是一個允許溶液通過，但固體微粒和大分子不能通過的半滲透膜。

blood cell (blood corpuscle) any of the cells that are present in the blood in health or disease. The cells may be subclassified into two major categories, namely red cells (*erythrocytes), and white cells (*leucocytes), which include granulocytes, lymphocytes, and monocytes (see illustration). Blood cells and *platelets account for approximately 40% of the total volume of the blood in health; red cells comprise the vast majority.

血細胞 正常或疾病時血液中存在的所有細胞。血細胞可分爲兩大類：紅細胞和白細胞，後者包括粒細胞、淋巴細胞和單核細胞（見圖）。血細胞和血小板正常約相當於血液總容積的 40%；紅細胞佔絕大多數。

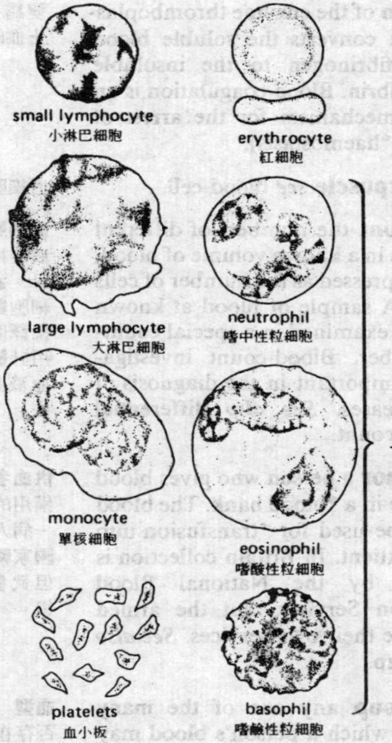

Types of blood cells
血細胞類型

blood clot a solid mass formed as the result of *blood coagulation, either within the blood vessels and heart or elsewhere (*compare* thrombus). A blood clot consists of a meshwork of the protein *fibrin in which various blood cells are trapped.

血栓 血管、心臟或其它部位內的血液凝固形成的固體組織塊。由包含各種血細胞的纖維蛋白網絡組成。

blood clotting *see* blood coagulation.

凝血

blood coagulation (blood clotting) the process whereby blood is converted from a liquid to a solid state. The process may be initiated by contact of blood with a foreign surface (*intrinsic system*) or with damaged tissue (*extrinsic system*). These systems involve the interaction of a variety of substances (*coagulation factors) and lead to the

血液凝固（凝血） 血液由液體狀態轉變爲固體狀態的過程。可由血液接觸異常表面（內源性系統）或損傷組織（外源性系統）而觸發。這些系統參與凝血因子的相互作用並導致凝血活酶的生成，後者使可溶性纖維蛋白原轉

production of the enzyme thromboplastin, which converts the soluble blood protein *fibrinogen to the insoluble protein *fibrin. Blood coagulation is an essential mechanism for the arrest of bleeding (*haemostasis).

變為不溶性纖維蛋白。為止血的原發機制。

blood corpuscle *see* blood cell.

血細胞

blood count the numbers of different blood cells in a known volume of blood, usually expressed as the number of cells per litre. A sample of blood at known dilution is examined in a special counting chamber. Blood-count investigations are important in the diagnosis of blood diseases. *See also* differential leucocyte count.

血細胞計數 計算已知血液容積內不同血細胞的數目。通常用每升血液中的細胞數來表示。將已知其稀釋度的血液標本置於專用計數室內檢查，是診斷血液疾病的重要檢查方法。

blood donor a person who gives blood for storage in a *blood bank. The blood can then be used for *transfusion into another patient. In Britain collection is organized by the National Blood Transfusion Services, but the armed forces have their own services. *See also* blood group.

供血者 獻血貯存於血庫備用的人。血液可輸給另一病人。在英國，採血由國家輸血機構組織實施，但武裝力量有其獨立機構。

blood group any one of the many types into which a person's blood may be classified, based on the presence or absence of certain inherited antigens on the surface of the red blood cells. Blood of one group contains antibodies in the serum that react against the cells of other groups.

There are more than 30 blood group systems, one of the most important of which is the *ABO system*. This system is based on the presence or absence of antigens A and B: blood of groups A and B contains antigens A and B, respectively; group AB contains both antigens and group O neither. Blood of group A contains antibodies to antigen B; group B blood contains anti-A antibodies; group AB has neither antibody and group O has both. A person whose blood contains either (or both) of these antibodies cannot receive a transfusion of blood containing the corresponding

血型 根據紅細胞表面是否存在某種遺傳性抗原而將人體血液進行分類所得的所有類型。一種血型血清中的抗體可與另一型細胞發生反應。

共有三十多種血型系統，最重要的一種為 ABO 血型系統。這個系統基於 A 抗原和 B 抗原的存在與否而劃分：A 型血和 B 型血各含有 A 抗原和 B 抗原；AB 型血含A,B 抗原，O 型血無 A,B 抗原。A 型血含抗 B 抗原的抗體；B 型血含抗 A 抗原的抗體；AB 型血無抗體；O 型血含抗 A 抗原和抗 B 抗原兩種抗體。血液中含有某類抗體的人不能接受血液中含有相應抗原的血液，如果血液中兩種抗體都有，則對

antigens. The table illustrates which blood groups can be used in transfusion for each of the four groups.

含有不同抗原的血都不能接受。下表列出四種血型的使用方法。

Donor's blood group 供血者血型	Blood group of people donor can receive blood from / 供血者可接受其血液的人的血型	Blood group of people donor can give blood to 供血者可供血給他的人的血型
A	A, O	A, AB
B	B, O	B, AB
AB	A, B, AB, O	AB
O	O	A, B, AB, O

blood plasma *see* plasma.

血漿

blood poisoning the presence of either bacterial toxins or large numbers of bacteria in the bloodstream causing serious illness. *See* pyaemia, septicaemia, toxaemia.

膿毒敗血症　存在於血流中的細菌毒素或大量細菌引起的嚴重疾病。

blood pressure the pressure of blood against the walls of the main arteries. Pressure is highest during *systole, when the ventricles are contracting (*systolic pressure*), and lowest during *diastole, when the ventricles are relaxing and refilling (*diastolic pressure*). Blood pressure is measured – in millimetres of mercury – by means of a *sphygmomanometer at the brachial artery of the arm, where the pressure is most similar to that of blood leaving the heart. The normal range varies with age, but a young adult would be expected to have a systolic pressure of around 120 mm and a diastolic pressure of 80 mm. These are recorded as 120/80.

Individual variations are common. Muscular exertion and emotional factors, such as fear, stress, and excitement, all raise systolic blood pressure (*see* hypertension). Systolic blood pressure is normally at its lowest during sleep. Severe shock may lead to an abnormally low blood pressure and possible circulatory failure (*see* hypo-

血壓　血液對大動脈管壁的側壓力。心收縮期，即心室收縮時最高（收縮壓）；心舒張期，即心室舒張和再充盈時最低（舒張壓）。血壓用 mmHg 表示，通過置於上臂肱動脈部位的血壓計測量，該部壓力與血液離開心臟時的壓力極爲近似，其正常範圍隨年齡而變化，但正常青壯年收縮壓的預期値爲 120 mmHg，舒張壓 80 mmHg 左右，簡寫爲 120/80。

個體差異常見，肌肉勞累和情緒因素如恐懼、緊張和激動均可使收縮壓增高。通常睡眠時收縮壓最低，嚴重休克可導致異常低血壓甚或循環衰竭。血壓由於交感神經系統和激素的控制得以維持於正常水平。

tension). Blood pressure is adjusted to its normal level by the *sympathetic nervous system and hormonal controls.

blood serum *see* serum.

血清

blood sugar the concentration of glucose in the blood, normally expressed in millimoles per litre. The normal range is 3.5–5.5 mmol/l. Blood-sugar estimation is an important investigation in a variety of diseases, most notably in diabetes mellitus. *See also* hyperglycaemia, hypoglycaemia.

血糖 血液中葡萄糖的濃度。常用每升中的毫摩爾數(m moℓ/ℓ)表示。正常值爲3.5～5.5 m moℓ/ℓ。血糖測定是許多疾病尤其是糖尿病的一個重要檢查項目。

blood test any test designed to discover abnormalities in a sample of a person's blood, such as the presence of alcohol, drugs, or bacteria, or to determine the *blood group.

血液檢驗 揭示人體血液標本中異常的檢驗。如檢測乙醇、藥物、細菌或確定血型。

blood transfusion *see* transfusion.

輸血

blood vessel a tube carrying blood away from or towards the heart. Blood vessels are the means by which blood circulates throughout the body. *See* artery, arteriole, vein, venule, capillary.

血管 載送血液離開或流向心臟的管道。血管是全身血液循環的通道。

blue baby an infant suffering from congenital malformation of the heart as a result of which some or all of the blue (deoxygenated) blood is pumped around the body instead of passing through the lungs to be oxygenated. The skin and lips have a purple colour. Advances in cardiac surgery have enabled remedial operations or even total correction to be performed, usually in the first few days or weeks of life. Those that cannot be corrected or improved may survive for months or years with persistent *cyanosis.

青紫嬰兒 患某類先天性心臟畸形的小兒。由於部分或全部靜脉血液（未氧合血）不通過肺臟進行氧合而直接被心臟泵至周身，皮膚和口唇呈現青紫。由於心臟外科的進展，修補甚或徹底矯正術常可在出生後幾天或幾週內施行。不能矯正或改善的患兒，紫紺持續存在，可存活數月或數年。

body *n.* **1.** an entire animal organism. **2.** the trunk of an individual, excluding the limbs. **3.** the main or largest part of an organ (such as the stomach or uterus). **4.** a solid discrete mass of tissue; e.g. the carotid body. *See also* corpus.

體 ①完整的動物機體。②除肢體以外的軀幹。③器官主要或最大的部分（如胃體或子宮體）。④獨立的實質性組織塊，如頸動脉體。

body image (body schema) the individual's concept of the disposition of his limbs and the identity of the different parts of his body. It is a function of the *association areas of the brain. *See also* Gerstmann's syndrome.

體象（軀體圖式） 一個人識別其四肢的位置和身體各部分的概念。爲大腦聯想區域的功能。

body temperature the intensity of heat of the body, as measured by a thermometer. Body temperature is accurately controlled by a small area at the base of the brain (the *hypothalamus); in normal individuals it is maintained at about 37°C (98.4°F). Heat production by the body arises as the result of vital activities (e.g. respiration, heart beat, circulation, secretion) and from the muscular effort of exercise and shivering. A rise in body temperature occurs in fever.

體溫 體熱的强度。可用溫度計測量。體溫由位於腦底部的微小區域（丘腦下部）精確控制。正常維持在 37℃（98.4℉）左右，機體的生命活動（如呼吸、心臟搏動、循環、分泌）和肌肉運動及顫抖導致產熱增加，發熱時體溫升高。

body type (somatotype) the characteristic anatomical appearance of an individual, based on the predominance of the structures derived from the three germ layers (ectoderm, mesoderm, endoderm). The three types are described as *ectomorphic, *mesomorphic, and *endomorphic.

體型 個體的特徵性解剖學表現。體型特徵取決於三個胚層（外胚層、中胚層、內胚層）演化形成的結構優勢，分別稱爲外胚層體型、中胚層體型和內胚層體型。

boil *n.* a tender inflamed area of the skin containing pus. The infection is usually caused by the bacterium *Staphylococcus aureus* entering through a hair follicle or a break in the skin, and local injury or lowered constitutional resistance may encourage the development of boils. Boils usually heal when the pus is released or with antibiotic treatment, though occasionally they may cause more widespread infection. Medical name: **furuncle**.

癤 含膿觸痛性皮膚炎症，常由經毛囊或皮膚破損入侵的金黃色葡萄球菌引起，局部損傷或機體抵抗力降低可促發癤腫。一般在膿液排出或抗生素治療後痊癒，偶見感染擴散。

bolus *n.* a soft mass of chewed food that is ready to be swallowed.

食團 咀嚼後適於吞咽的食物軟團。

bonding *n.* **1.** (in psychology) the development of a close and selective relationship, such as that of *attachment. *Mother-child bonding* is the supposed process in which physical contact between mother and child in the child's

①**依附** （心理學）選擇性親密關係的形成，如依戀。人們假想嬰兒生後數小時內，母子身體接觸可促進母親對嬰兒的愛戀和關懷。此過程稱爲母子依

first hours of life promotes the mother's loving and caring for her baby. **2.** (in dentistry) the attachment of dental restorations, sealants, and appliances to teeth. Bonding may be mechanical (*see* acid-etch technique) or chemical, by the use of adhesive *cements.

附。②**黏合**（牙科）將補牙的修復體、密封劑和各種鑲牙材料黏固在牙面上的過程。黏合可爲機械性的或化學性的，如使用黏固粉黏合。

bone *n.* the hard extremely dense connective tissue that forms the skeleton of the body. It is composed of a matrix of collagen fibres impregnated with bone salts (chiefly calcium carbonate and calcium phosphate). *Compact* (or *cortical*) *bone* forms the outer shell of bones; it consists of a hard virtually solid mass made up of bony tissue arranged in concentric layers (*Haversian systems*). *Spongy* (or *cancellous*) *bone*, found beneath compact bone, consists of a meshwork of bony bars (*trabeculae*) with many interconnecting spaces containing marrow. (See illustration.)
Individual bones may be classed as long, short, flat, or irregular. The outer layer of a bone is called the *periosteum. The *medullary cavity* is lined with *endosteum and contains the marrow. Bones not only form the skeleton but also act as stores for mineral salts and play an important part in the formation of blood cells.

骨 構成人體骨骼的堅硬的緻密結締組織。由充滿骨鹽（主要爲碳酸鈣和磷酸鈣）的膠原纖維基質組成。密質骨（骨皮質）形成骨的外殼，是呈同心圓層狀排列的骨性組織（哈佛氏系統），形成堅硬的實體層。松質骨（骨髓質）位於密質骨內部，由骨小梁網絡及存在於骨小梁之間的相互貫通的許多含有骨髓的腔隙組成（見圖）。骨可分爲長骨、短骨、扁骨和不規則骨。骨的外層稱爲骨膜，骨髓腔有骨內膜覆蓋並含有骨髓。骨不僅形成骨骼，而且還是無機鹽貯庫，在血細胞形成中也起重要作用。

bone marrow (marrow) the tissue contained within the internal cavities of the bones. At birth, these cavities are filled entirely with blood-forming *myeloid tissue* (*red marrow*) but in later life the marrow in the limb bones is replaced by fat (*yellow marrow*). Samples of bone marrow may be obtained for examination by *aspiration through a stout needle or by *trephine biopsy. *See also* haemopoiesis.

骨髓 存在於骨髓腔的組織。出生時，全部骨髓腔充滿造血骨髓組織（紅骨髓），隨後，四肢骨的骨髓逐漸被脂肪取代（黃骨髓）。用於檢查的骨髓標本可經粗針骨髓穿刺或環鑽活檢而獲得。

bony labyrinth *see* labyrinth.

骨迷路

borax *n.* a mild astringent with a weak antiseptic action, applied externally to skin and mucous membranes. Borax and boric acid are used in mouth and

硼砂 溫和並有微弱抗菌作用的收斂劑，外用於皮膚及黏膜。硼砂和硼酸可用於口腔和鼻腔沖洗、含

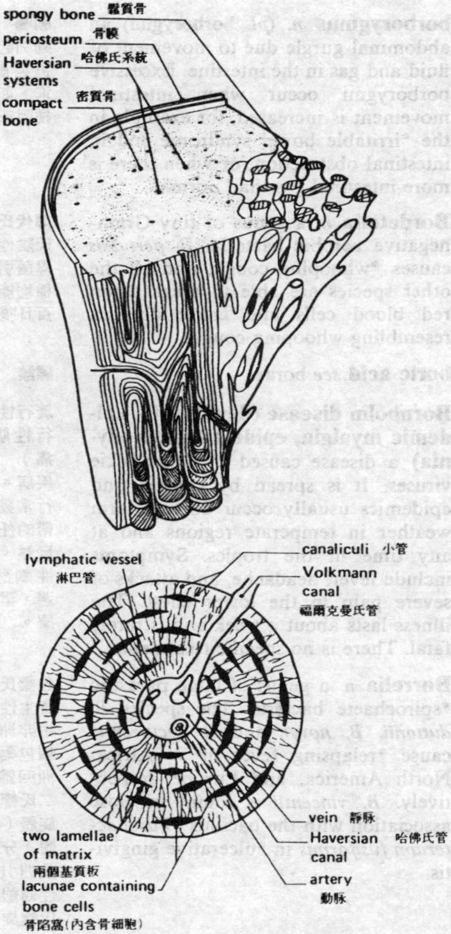

Section of the shaft of a long bone (above) with detail of a single Haversian system (below)

長骨幹(上)和一個哈佛氏系統(下)的微細構造圖

nasal washes, gargles, eye lotions and contact-lens solutions, and in dusting powder. Side-effects from external application are rare; most reported cases of poisoning are in infants.

漱、洗眼、浸泡角膜接觸鏡和撲撒患部。外用副作用罕見，報道的中毒病例多爲嬰兒。

borborygmus *n.* (*pl.* **borborygmi**) an abdominal gurgle due to movement of fluid and gas in the intestine. Excessive borborygmi occur when intestinal movement is increased, for example in the *irritable bowel syndrome and in intestinal obstruction, or when there is more intestinal gas than normal.

腸鳴 腸內液體和氣體運動引起的腹部咕嚕聲。腸道運動增强時腸鳴音亢進，如腸過敏綜合徵、腸梗阻或腸積氣時。

Bordetella *n.* a genus of tiny Gram-negative aerobic bacteria. *B. pertussis* causes *whooping cough, and all the other species are able to break down red blood cells and cause diseases resembling whooping cough.

博代氏桿菌屬 微小革蘭氏陰性需氧菌屬。百日咳桿菌引起百日咳，其它菌種均能破壞紅細胞，導致百日咳樣疾病。

boric acid *see* borax.

硼酸

Bornholm disease (devil's grip, epidemic myalgia, epidemic pleurodynia) a disease caused by *Coxsackie viruses. It is spread by contact and epidemics usually occur during warm weather in temperate regions and at any time in the tropics. Symptoms include fever, headache, and attacks of severe pain in the lower chest. The illness lasts about a week and is rarely fatal. There is no specific treatment.

流行性胸痛（鬼抓風，流行性肌痛，流行性胸膜痛） 柯薩基病毒引起的疾病。通過接觸傳染，流行常發生於溫帶熱季和熱帶的任何季節。症狀包括發熱、頭痛和下胸部陣發性劇烈疼痛。病程約一週，罕見死亡。無特效治療。

Borrelia *n.* a genus of large parasitic *spirochaete bacteria. The species *B. duttonii*, *B. novyi*, and *B. recurrentis* cause *relapsing fever in W Africa, North America, and Europe, respectively. *B. vincentii* is found in close association with the bacillus **Fusobacterium fusiformis* in *ulcerative gingivitis.

包柔氏螺旋體屬 大型的寄生性螺旋體菌屬。其中中非洲回歸熱螺旋體（達頓包柔氏螺旋體）、北美洲回歸熱螺旋體（諾-包二氏螺旋體）和回歸熱螺旋體（回歸熱包柔氏螺旋體）分別在西非、北美和歐洲引起回歸熱。在潰瘍性齒齦炎中，可發現奮森氏螺旋體與梭狀梭形桿菌同時存在。

botulism *n.* a serious form of *food poisoning from foods containing the toxin produced by the bacterium **Clostridium botulinum*. The toxin selectively affects the central nervous system; in fatal cases, death is often caused by heart and lung failure resulting from a malfunction of the cardiac and respira-

肉毒中毒 含有肉毒梭狀芽胞菌毒素的食物引起的重型食物中毒。毒素選擇性作用於中樞神經系統，危重病例常因腦部心血管及呼吸中樞功能紊亂而心肺衰竭致死。肉毒桿菌在保存不當的食物中繁殖。

tory centres of the brain. The bacterium thrives in improperly preserved foods, typically canned raw meats. The toxin, being rather unstable to heat, is invariably destroyed in cooking.

肉毒桿菌毒素對熱極不穩定，烹飪中全被破壞。

bougie *n.* a hollow or solid cylindrical instrument, usually flexible, that is inserted into tubular passages, such as the oesophagus (gullet), rectum, or urethra. Bougies are used in diagnosis and treatment, particularly by enlarging *strictures (for example, in the urethra).

探條　中空或實心的圓柱狀器械，常柔軟易屈，用以插入某些管腔如食管、直腸或尿道。用於疾病的診斷和治療，尤其是擴張狹窄（如擴張尿道狹窄）。

bowel *n. see* intestine.

腸

Bowen's disease a type of carcinoma of the squamous epidermal cells of the skin that does not spread to the basal layers.

博溫氏病　未擴散至基底層的皮膚鱗狀上皮細胞癌。

bow-legs *pl. n.* abnormal out-curving of the legs, resulting in a gap between the knees on standing. A certain degree of bowing is normal in small children, but persistence into adult life, or later development of this deformity, results from abnormal growth of the *epiphysis (as in *Still's disease) or arthritis. The condition can be corrected by *osteotomy or interposition *arthroplasty. Medical name: **genu varum**.

膝內翻　雙腿異常外曲，以致站立時雙膝不能並攏。正常小兒可有一定程度的彎曲，但骨骼異常生長（斯提爾氏病）或關節炎時，可致畸形加重或持續至成年。用截骨術或插入物關節成型術可矯正。

Bowman's capsule the cup-shaped end of a *nephron, which encloses a knot of blood capillaries (*glomerulus*). It is the site of primary filtration of the blood into the kidney tubule.

鮑曼氏囊　腎單位之杯狀末端，包繞着毛細血管球（腎小球）。原尿由此通過濾過作用進入腎小管。

brachi- (brachio-) *prefix denoting* the arm. Example: *brachialgia* (pain in).

〔前綴〕　**臂**　如臂痛。

brachial *adj.* relating to or affecting the arm.

臂的，肱的

brachial artery an artery that extends from the axillary artery, at the armpit, down the side and inner surface of the upper arm to the elbow, where it divides into the radial and ulnar arteries.

肱動脉　腋動脉在腋窩處的分枝，於上臂內側下行至肘即分為橈動脉和尺動脉。

brachialis *n.* a muscle that is situated at the front of the upper arm and contracts to flex the forearm (see illustration). It works against the triceps brachii.

肱肌 位於上臂前面的臂肌，作用爲屈肘關節（見圖）。與肱三頭肌拮抗。

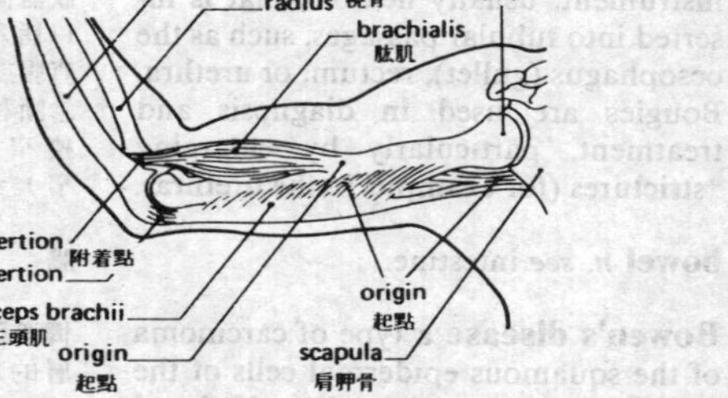

Brachialis and triceps muscles
肱肌和三頭肌

brachial plexus a network of nerves, arising from the spine at the base of the neck, from which arise the nerves supplying the arm, forearm and hand, and parts of the shoulder girdle (see illustration). *See also* radial nerve.

臂叢 源於頸部脊髓的神經叢，其分支支配上臂、前臂、手和部分肩胛帶（見圖）。

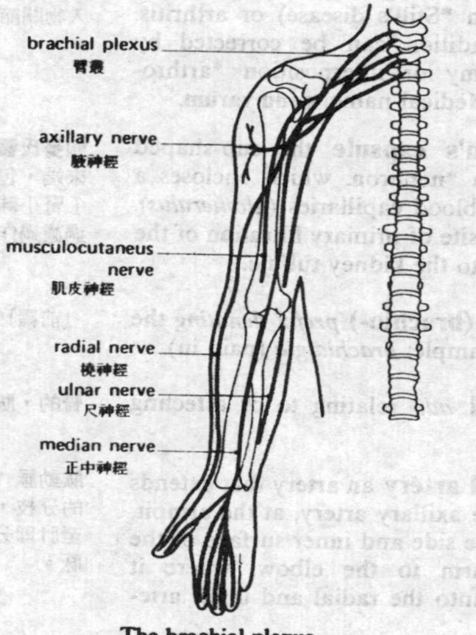

The brachial plexus
臂叢

brachiocephalic artery *see* innominate artery.

頭臂動脈

brachium *n.* (*pl.* **brachia**) the arm, especially the part of the arm between the shoulder and the elbow.

臂 臂部，尤指肩關節到肘關節間的上臂。

brachy- *prefix denoting* shortness. Example: *brachydactylia* (shortness of the fingers or toes).

〔前綴〕 **短** 如短指（趾）畸形（手指或脚趾短小）。

brachycephaly *n.* shortness of the skull, with a *cephalic index of about 80. —**brachycephalic** *adj.*

短頭（畸形） 顱骨短小，頭指數約爲 80。

brady- *prefix denoting* slowness. Example: *bradylalia* (abnormally slow speech).

〔前綴〕 **遲緩** 指緩慢或遲鈍。如語言遲鈍（言語異常緩慢）。

bradycardia *n.* slowing of the heart rate to less than 50 beats per minute. *Sinus bradycardia* is often found in healthy individuals, especially athletes, but it is also seen in some patients with reduced thyroid activity, jaundice, hypothermia, or *vasovagal attacks. Bradycardia may also result from *arrhythmias, especially complete *heart block, when the slowing is often extreme and often causes loss of consciousness.

心動過緩 心率低於 50 次/分。竇性心動過緩在健康人尤其運動員中較常見，但亦見於甲狀腺功能低下、黃疸、體溫過低或血管迷走神經性緊張的病人。心動過緩也可由心律失常，尤其是完全性傳導阻滯引起。嚴重心動過緩常導致意識喪失。

bradykinesia *n.* a symptom of *parkinsonism comprising a difficulty in initiating movements, slowness in executing movements, and an inability to make adjustments to the posture of the body.

運動遲緩 帕金森綜合徵症狀之一，包括起始運動困難、完成動作緩慢和不能調節身體姿勢。

bradykinin *n.* a naturally occurring polypeptide consisting of nine amino acids. Bradykinin is a very powerful vasodilator and causes contraction of smooth muscle; it is formed in the blood under certain conditions and is thought to play an important role as a mediator of inflammation. *See* kinin.

緩激肽 9 個氨基酸組成的天然多肽。是强力血管舒張劑，並可導致平滑肌收縮，於一定條件下在血液中形成，並認爲是一種炎症介質，在炎症中起重要作用。

braille *n.* an alphabet, developed by Louis Braille (1809–1852) in 1837, in which each letter is represented by a

布萊葉盲字 1837 年由路易斯・布萊葉發明的盲人用字。每個字母由突起

pattern of raised dots, which are read by feeling with the finger tips. It is the main method of reading used by the blind today.

的點狀模型代表，靠指尖感覺閱讀。是現代盲人閱讀的主要方法。

brain *n.* the enlarged and highly developed mass of nervous tissue that forms the upper end of the *central nervous system (see illustration). The average adult human brain weighs about 1400 g (approximately 2% of total body weight) and is continuous below with the spinal cord. It is invested by three connective tissue membranes, the *meninges, and floats in *cerebrospinal fluid within the rigid casing formed by the bones of the skull. The brain is divided into the hindbrain (rhombencephalon), consisting of the *medulla oblongata, *pons Varolii, and *cerebellum; the *midbrain (mesencephalon); and the forebrain (prosencephalon), subdivided into the *cerebrum and the *diencephalon (including the *thalamus and *hypothalamus). Anatomical name: **encephalon**.

腦 形成中樞神經系統上端的高度發達的膨大的神經組織團（見圖）。平均成人腦重約 1400g（約爲體重的 2%），向下移行爲脊髓。腦由三層結締組織膜（腦膜）覆蓋，浮於腦脊液中並由堅硬的顱骨包繞。腦分爲由延腦、橋腦和小腦組成的後腦（菱腦）、中腦以及前腦，後者又分爲大腦和間腦（包括丘腦和下丘腦）。

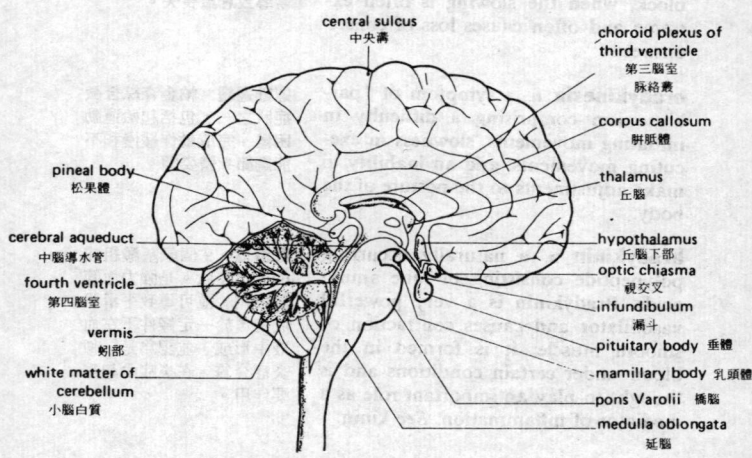

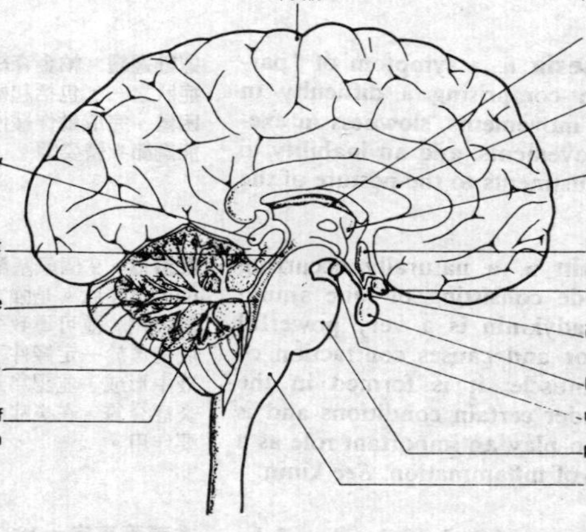

The brain (midsagittal section)
腦（矢狀面）

brain death *see* death.

腦死亡

brainstem *n.* the enlarged extension upwards within the skull of the spinal cord, consisting of the medulla oblongata, the pons, and the midbrain. The pons and medulla are together known as the *bulb*, or *bulbar area*. Attached to the midbrain are the two cerebral hemispheres. *See* brain.

腦幹 脊髓向上延伸至顱內的膨大部分，包括延腦、橋腦和中腦。橋腦和延腦稱爲球部，大腦半球附於中腦。

brain tumour *see* cerebral tumour.

腦腫瘤

branchial arch *see* pharyngeal arch.

鰓弓

branchial cleft *see* pharyngeal cleft.

鰓裂

branchial cyst a cyst that arises at the site of one of the embryonic *pharyngeal pouches due to a developmental anomaly.

鰓囊腫 胚胎期咽囊發育異常形成的囊腫。

branchial pouch *see* pharyngeal pouch.

鰓囊

breakbone fever *see* dengue.

登革熱

breast *n.* **1.** the mammary gland of a woman: one of two compound glands that produce milk. Each breast consists of glandular lobules – the milk-secreting areas – embedded in fatty tissue (see illustration). The milk passes from the

①**乳房** 女性乳腺。泌乳腺體之一。由包埋於脂肪組織中的乳腺小葉（乳汁分泌區）組成（見圖）。乳汁經乳腺小葉進入乳腺小管，漸次滙合形成 15

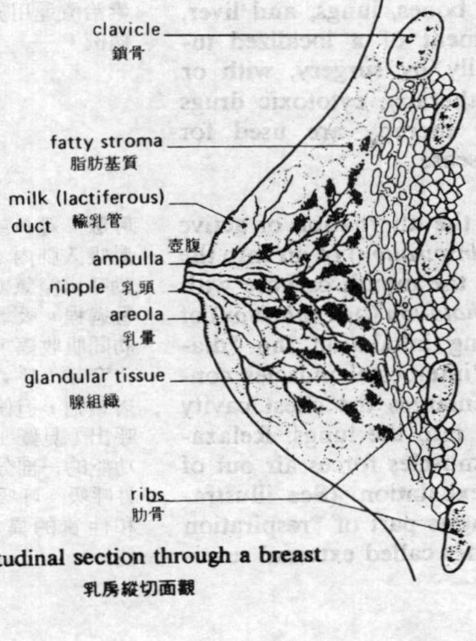

Longitudinal section through a breast
乳房縱切面觀

lobules into ducts, which join up to form 15–20 *lactiferous ducts*. Near the front of the breast the lactiferous ducts are dilated into *ampullae*, which act as reservoirs for the milk. Each lactiferous duct discharges through a separate orifice in the nipple. The dark area around the nipple is called the *areola*. *See also* lactation. Anatomical name: **mamma. 2.** the front part of the chest (thorax).

～20個輸乳管。靠近乳房前部處，輸乳管擴大成壺腹狀以貯存乳汁。每根輸乳管在乳頭各有一個開口。乳頭周圍的較暗區域稱乳暈。 ②**胸部**

breastbone *n. see* sternum.

胸骨

breast cancer a malignant tumour of the breast, usually a *carcinoma but sometimes a *sarcoma. It is rare in men but is the commonest form of cancer in women, in some cases involving both breasts. The cause is not known but it tends to run in families, and in countries such as Japan, where prolonged breast feeding is the rule, the incidence of breast cancer is very low.
The classic sign is a lump in the breast, which is often noticed after minor local injury; bleeding or discharge from the nipple may occur infrequently. Sometimes the first thing to be noticed is a lump in the armpit, which is due to spread of the cancer to the drainage lymph nodes. The tumour may also spread to the bones, lungs, and liver. Current treatment of a localized tumour is usually by surgery, with or without radiotherapy; cytotoxic drugs and hormone therapy are used for widespread disease.

乳癌 乳房的惡性腫瘤。通常為癌，但有時為肉瘤。男性罕見，但為女性最常見之腫瘤，部分病例累及雙乳。病因尚不清楚，但有家族發病傾向。在日本，由於長期哺乳的習俗，乳癌的發生率很低。典型體徵是乳房腫塊，且常在輕微局部損傷後被發現；乳頭出血或溢液較少見，有時首發表現為腋窩腫塊，為腫瘤擴散至局部引流淋巴結所致。乳癌亦可轉移至骨、肺和肝。局限性腫瘤的現代治療通常是手術，輔以或不輔以放射治療。化療和激素治療運用於廣泛轉移的病例。

breathing *n.* the alternation of active *inhalation* (or *inspiration*) of air into the lungs through the mouth or nose with the passive *exhalation* (or *expiration*) of the air. During inhalation the *diaphragm and *intercostal muscles contract, which enlarges the chest cavity and draws air into the lungs. Relaxation of these muscles forces air out of the lungs at exhalation. (See illustration.) Breathing is part of *respiration and is sometimes called external respi-

呼吸 經口或鼻將空氣主動吸入肺內（吸氣）和被動呼出空氣（呼氣）的交替過程。吸氣時，膈肌和肋間肌收縮，擴大胸腔吸入空氣；呼氣時，這些肌肉鬆弛，迫使空氣由肺中呼出（見圖）。這是呼吸功能的一部分，有時亦稱外呼吸。呼吸頻率、節律和性質的異常有許多類型。

ration. There are many types of breathing in which the rhythm, rate, or character is abnormal. *See also* apnoea, bronchospasm, Cheyne-Stokes respiration, dyspnoea, stridor.

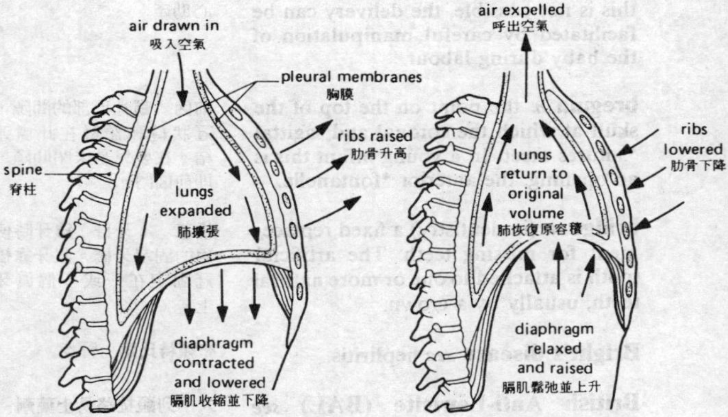

Position of the diaphragm (from the side) during breathing
呼吸時膈的位置（側面觀）

breathlessness *n. see* dyspnoea.

氣促

breath sounds the sounds heard through a stethoscope placed over the lungs during breathing. Normal breath sounds are soft and called *vesicular* – they may be increased or decreased in disease states. The sounds heard over the larger bronchi are louder and harsher. Breath sounds transmitted through consolidated lungs in pneumonia are louder and harsher; they are similar to the sounds heard normally over the larger bronchi and are termed *bronchial breath sounds*. *Crepitations and *rhonchi are sounds added to the breath sounds in abnormal states of the lung. *Amphoric* or *cavernous* sounds have a hollow quality and are heard over cavities in the lung; the amphoric quality may also be heard in voice sounds and on percussion.

呼吸音 通過置於胸部的聽診器聽到的肺部呼吸的聲音。正常呼吸音柔和，稱爲肺泡呼吸音，在疾病狀態下可增强或減弱。大支氣管部位呼吸音較響亮而粗糙。肺炎時呼吸音通過實變肺臟傳遞變得響亮而粗糙，類似於正常在大支氣管部位聽到的聲音，故名支氣管呼吸音。捻髮音和乾囉音是異常狀況時的呼吸附加音。空甕或空洞呼吸音音調呈空甕性，在肺部空洞的相應體表部位聞及，這種空甕性質亦可表現在語音和叩診中。

breech presentation the position of a baby in the womb such that it is delivered buttocks first (instead of the normal head-first position). Since this can result in a difficult birth, the baby is often turned head first before labour; if this is not possible, the delivery can be facilitated by careful manipulation of the baby during labour.

臀先露 胎兒在子宮內的位置，分娩時臀部首先娩出（而不是正常時的頭先露胎位）。可導致難產，胎兒常需在生產前糾正為頭先露，否則分娩時需細心助產。

bregma *n.* the point on the top of the skull at which the coronal and sagittal *sutures meet. In a young infant this is an opening, the anterior *fontanelle.

前囟 顱骨頂部的間隙，冠狀縫和額縫在此處連結。在嬰兒是未閉間隙，即前囟門。

bridge *n.* (in dentistry) a fixed replacement for missing teeth. The artificial tooth is attached to one or more natural teeth, usually by a crown.

橋基 （牙科）鑲牙時使用的固定牙橋。假牙靠橋冠固定在一或多個眞牙上。

Bright's disease *see* nephritis.

布賴特氏病 腎炎。

British Anti-Lewisite (BAL) *see* dimercaprol.

大不列顛抗路易士藥劑 二硫基丙醇。

British thermal unit a unit of heat equal to the quantity of heat required to raise the temperature of 1 pound of water by 1° Fahrenheit. 1 British thermal unit = 1055 joules. Abbrev.: Btu.

大不列顛熱量單位 熱量單位，相當於使 1 磅水溫度昇高華氏 1 度所需的熱量。1 大不列顛熱量單位 = 1055 焦耳。縮寫為 Btu。

Broca's area the area of cerebral motor cortex responsible for the initiation of speech. It is situated in the left frontal lobe in most (but not all) right-handed people, in the region of *Brodmann areas 44 and 45.

布羅卡氏區 支配語言的大腦運動皮質區域。在大多數（但非全部）右利人中位於左前葉，布勞德曼氏皮質區 44 和 45 區。

Brodie's abscess an abscess of bone: a form of chronic bacterial *osteomyelitis, not due to tuberculosis or syphilis. Treatment is by surgical drainage and antibiotics.

布羅廸氏膿腫（幹骺端膿腫） 骨膿腫、非結核或梅毒所致的慢性細菌性骨髓炎的一種。治療：外科引流和使用抗生素。

Brodmann areas the numbered areas (1–47) into which a map of the *cerebral cortex may conveniently be divided for descriptive purposes, based upon the arrangement of neurones seen

布勞德曼氏皮質區 根據顯微鏡下染色切片中的神經元排列情況而劃分的便於敘述的大腦皮質區域（1～47 區）。例如 4 區

in stained sections under the microscope. On the map area 4, for example, corresponds to primary motor cortex, while the primary visual cortex comes into area 17.

相當於原始運動皮質區，17 區爲原始感覺皮質區。

bromhexine *n.* an *expectorant that acts by increasing the volume and reducing the viscosity of bronchial secretions. It is used in the treatment of bronchitis and may cause nausea. Trade name: **Bisolvon**.

溴苄環己胺 祛痰劑。通過擴張支氣管和降低支氣管分泌物粘滯度而起作用。用於治療支氣管炎，能導致噁心。商品名：必嗽平。

bromides *pl. n.* salts of bromine, including potassium bromide, once widely used as sedatives because of their depressant action on the central nervous system. *See also* bromism.

溴化物 溴鹽，包括溴化鉀，由於其對中樞神經系統的鎮靜抑制作用曾廣泛作爲鎮靜劑。

bromidrosis *n.* bacterial breakdown of sweat, usually in the armpit or on the feet, which causes an unpleasant smell.

汗臭 汗液通過細菌性分解產生的異常氣味，通常發生於腋窩及足部。

bromism *n.* a group of symptoms caused by excessive intake of *bromides. Overuse for long periods leads to mental dullness, weakness, drowsiness, loss of sensation, slurred speech, and sometimes coma. A form of acne may also develop. Treatment is by immediate withdrawal.

溴中毒 攝入過多溴化物引起的一組症狀。長期過量應用溴化物會導致精神抑鬱、虛弱、嗜眠、喪失知覺、語言模糊，有時昏迷。也可產生痤瘡。治療：立即停藥。

bromodiphenhydramine *n.* an *antihistamine given by mouth to relieve the symptoms of allergic reactions, especially hay fever and rhinitis. It is also used to prevent travel sickness. Common side-effects include drowsiness, dizziness, dryness of the throat, and digestive upsets. Trade name: **Ambodryl**.

溴苯海拉明 口服抗組織胺藥。用於解除過敏反應，尤其是枯草熱和鼻炎。也可用於預防暈動病。常見副作用有嗜眠、頭昏、咽喉乾燥和消化紊亂。

brompheniramine *n.* an antihistamine that has the same uses and side-effects as *bromodiphenhydramine. Trade name: **Dimetane**.

溴苯吡胺 抗組織胺藥。作用及副作用同溴苯海拉明。

bromsulphthalein *n.* a blue dye used in tests of liver function. A small quantity of the dye is injected into the bloodstream, and its concentration in the blood is measured after 5 and then

溴磺酞鈉 檢查肝功能的藍色染料。小劑量注入血流後 5 分鐘和 45 分鐘分別測定血液中濃度，45 分鐘血液中的量大於注射

45 minutes. The presence of more than 10% of the dose in the circulation after 45 minutes indicates that the liver is not functioning normally.

量的 10% 提示肝功能異常。

bronch- (broncho-) *prefix denoting* the bronchial tree. Examples: *broncho-pulmonary* (relating to the bronchi and lungs); *bronchotomy* (incision into).

〔前綴〕 **支氣管的** 如支氣管肺（指支氣管和肺）；支氣管切開術。

bronchial tree a branching system of tubes conducting air from the trachea (windpipe) to the lungs: includes the bronchi (*see* bronchus) and their subdivisions and the *bronchioles.

支氣管樹 氣管與肺之間運送空氣的管狀分支系統。包括支氣管及分支和細支氣管。

bronchiectasis *n.* widening of the bronchi or their branches. It may be congenital or it may result from infection (especially whooping cough or measles in childhood) or from obstruction, either by an inhaled foreign body or by a growth (including cancer). Pus may form in the widened bronchus so that the patient coughs up purulent sputum, which may contain blood. Diagnosis is on the clinical symptoms and by X-ray. Treatment consists of antibiotic drugs to control the infection and physiotherapy to drain the sputum. Surgery may be used if only a few segments of the bronchi are affected.

支氣管擴張 支氣管及分支擴大。可爲先天性，或由感染所致（在兒童尤以百日咳或痲疹多見），也可由吸入異物或支氣管腫物（包括癌）造成的阻塞所致。膿液在擴張的支氣管中形成，故患者咳膿痰並可帶血。診斷靠臨床症狀和 X 線檢查。治療包括抗生素控制感染和體位排痰。手術僅限於病變局限於少數幾段支氣管者。

bronchiole *n.* a subdivision of the bronchial tree that does not contain cartilage or mucous glands in its wall. Bronchioles open from the fifth or sixth generation of bronchi and extend for up to 20 more generations before reaching the *terminal bronchioles*. Each terminal bronchiole divides into a number of *respiratory bronchioles*, from which the *alveoli open. Each terminal bronchiole conducts air to an acinus in the *lung. —**bronchiolar** *adj.*

細支氣管 管壁上無軟骨或黏液腺的支氣管樹分枝。由第 5 或第 6 級支氣管分出，後不斷分支至約第 20 級變爲終末性支氣管。每個終末性細支氣管又分爲許多呼吸性細支氣管，下爲肺泡。每一終末性細支氣管將空氣輸送至一組肺泡。

bronchiolitis *n.* inflammation of the bronchioles, due to infection by bacteria or viruses. These very small tubes easily become blocked with mucopus, which prevents air from reaching the

細支氣管炎 細菌或病毒感染引起的細支氣管炎症。細小狹窄的管道易爲黏膿阻塞，從而阻礙空氣到達肺泡。患者表現缺

alveoli of the lungs. The patient becomes short of oxygen (*see* cyanosis); in infants the breathing appears difficult and ineffectual. The condition is treated with oxygen, which is paramount, and antibiotics.

氧，嬰兒表現爲呼吸困難。最重要的治療是給氧，另用抗生素。

bronchitis *n.* inflammation of the bronchi (*see* bronchus). *Acute bronchitis* is caused by viruses or bacteria and is characterized by coughing, the production of mucopurulent sputum, and narrowing of the bronchi due to spasmodic contraction (*see* bronchospasm). In *chronic bronchitis* the patient coughs up excessive mucus secreted by enlarged bronchial mucous glands; the bronchospasm cannot be relieved by bronchodilator drugs. It is not primarily an inflammatory condition, although it is frequently complicated by acute infections. The disease is particularly prevalent in Britain in association with cigarette smoking, air pollution, and *emphysema.

支氣管炎 支氣管的炎症。急性支氣管炎由病毒或細菌引起，特點是咳嗽、咳黏液膿性痰和支氣管痙攣性收縮導致狹窄。慢性支氣管炎病人由於支氣管黏液腺增殖，咳出大量黏液，支氣管痙攣不能爲支氣管擴張劑所緩解。雖然本病常繼發於急性感染，但並非以炎症疾患爲主。在英國甚爲流行，與吸煙、空氣污染和肺氣腫有關。

bronchoconstrictor *n.* a drug that causes narrowing of the air passages by producing spasm of bronchial smooth muscle.

支氣管收縮劑 使支氣管平滑肌收縮導致氣道變狹窄的藥物。

bronchodilator *n.* an agent that causes widening of the air passages by relaxing bronchial smooth muscle. *Sympathomimetic drugs that stimulate betareceptors, e.g. *ephedrine, *isoprenaline, and *salbutamol, are potent bronchodilators and are used for relief of bronchial asthma and chronic bronchitis. These drugs are often administered as aerosols, giving rapid relief, but at high doses they may stimulate the heart.

支氣管擴張劑 使支氣管平滑肌鬆弛導致氣道擴張的藥物。刺激 β 受體的擬交感神經藥如麻黃鹼（素）、異丙基腎上腺素和羥甲叔丁腎上腺素（舒喘靈）是強力支氣管擴張劑，用於治療支氣管哮喘和慢性支氣管炎。常作噴霧劑使用，生效迅速，但大劑量可刺激心臟。

bronchography *n.* X-ray examination of the bronchial tree after it has been made visible by the injection of *radioopaque dye or the inhalation of radioopaque particles, such as tantalum. It is used particularly in the diagnosis of *bronchiectasis.

支氣管造影 注入不透 X 線的造影劑或吸入不透 X 線的微粒劑如鉭後使支氣管樹顯影進行 X 線檢查的方法。診斷支氣管擴張尤爲適宜。

bronchophony *n. see* vocal resonance.

支氣管語音

bronchopneumonia *n. see* pneumonia.

支氣管肺炎

bronchoscope *n.* an instrument used to look into the trachea and bronchi. In addition to the rigid tubular metal type, used for many years, there is now a narrower flexible *fibre-optic instrument with which previously inaccessible bronchi can be inspected. With either instrument the bronchial tree can be washed out, and samples of tissue and foreign bodies can be removed with long forceps. **—bronchoscopy** *n.*

支氣管鏡 窺視氣管及支氣管的器械。除了沿用早年的金屬硬管外，現有一種較細小易屈曲的纖維支氣管鏡，可檢查硬管達不到的支氣管。兩者均可用於冲洗支氣管樹，用長鉗經鏡可取出組織標本和異物。

bronchospasm *n.* narrowing of bronchi by muscular contraction in response to some stimulus, as in *asthma and *bronchitis. The patient can usually inhale air into the lungs, but exhalation may require visible muscular effort and is accompanied by expiratory noises that are clearly audible (*see* wheeze) or detectable with a stethoscope. The condition in which bronchospasm can be relieved by bronchodilator drugs is known as *reversible obstructive airways disease* and includes asthma; that in which bronchodilator drugs have no effect is *irreversible obstructive airways disease* and includes chronic bronchitis.

支氣管痙攣 某些刺激引起支氣管平滑肌收縮導致的支氣管狹窄。如哮喘或支氣管炎患者常可順利吸氣，但呼氣時需要所有呼吸肌運動，且伴有可淸晰聞及或用聽診器可聽到的呼氣音。能由支氣管擴張劑所緩解者，稱爲可逆性氣道阻塞性疾病，包括哮喘；支氣管擴張劑無效者，稱不可逆性氣道阻塞性疾病，包括慢性支氣管炎。

bronchospirometry *n.* a technique used to assess the efficiency of ventilation of a lung or of a segment of the lung. A catheter with an inflatable cuff is passed into the appropriate airway, through a *bronchoscope, and the volume and rate of gas exchange is estimated.

支氣管肺量測定法 測定一側肺或一個肺葉的通氣效率的方法。將一根帶有開合頭套的導管插入合適的氣道，通過支氣管鏡即可測量氣體的交換容積和速率。

bronchus *n.* (*pl.* **bronchi**) any of the air passages beyond the *trachea (windpipe) that has cartilage and mucous glands in its wall (see illustration). The trachea divides into two main bronchi,

支氣管 由氣管向下延續的管壁上含有軟骨及黏液腺的所有氣道（見圖）。氣管分爲兩支主支氣管，後者連續分支爲 5 個葉支

which divide successively into five *lobar bronchi*, 20 *segmental bronchi*, and two or three more divisions. *See also* bronchiole. —**bronchial** *adj.*

氣管，20 個段支氣管以及 2～3 級或更多分支。

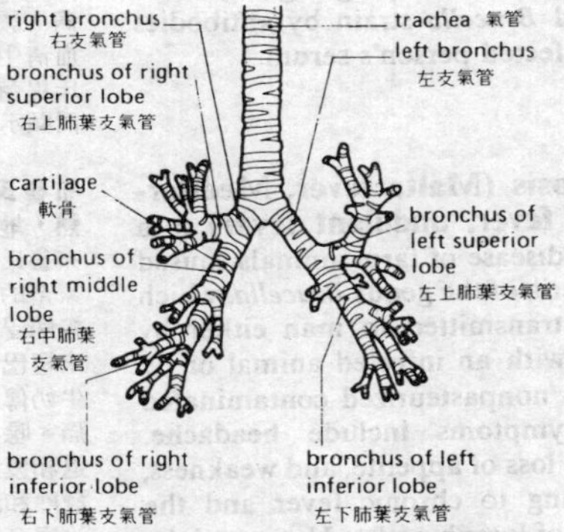

The bronchi and their principal (lobar) branches
支氣管及其主要(葉)分支

brown fat a form of fat in adipose tissue that is a rich source of energy and can be converted rapidly to heat. There is speculation that a rapid turnover of brown fat occurs to balance excessive intake of food and unnecessary production of white fat (making up the bulk of adipose tissue). Some forms of obesity may be linked to lack of – or inability to synthesize – brown fat.

棕色脂肪 脂肪的一種。是豐富的能量貯庫，能迅速轉化爲熱量。據推測棕色脂肪的迅速轉化是爲了避免由於進食過多生成不必要的白色脂肪（形成大量脂肪組織）。某些肥胖症可能與缺少或不能合成棕色脂肪有關。

Brown-Séquard syndrome the neurological condition resulting when the spinal cord has been partly cut through. In those parts of the body supplied by the damaged segment there is a flaccid weakness and loss of feeling in the skin. Below the lesion there is a spastic paralysis on the same side and a loss of pain and temperature sensation on the opposite side.

布朗-塞卡爾氏綜合徵 脊髓部分橫斷時導致的神經症狀。損傷節段所支配的區域有麻痹和皮膚感覺喪失。損傷脊髓節段以下同側痙攣性麻痹，對側痛覺和溫度覺喪失。

Brucella *n.* a genus of Gram-negative aerobic spherical or rodlike parasitic bacteria responsible for *brucellosis (undulant fever) in man and contagious

布魯氏桿菌屬 革蘭氏陰性需氧球狀或桿狀寄生菌屬，在人引起布魯氏桿菌病（波狀熱），在牛、

abortion in cattle, pigs, sheep, and goats. The principal species are *B. abortus* and *B. melitensis*. *Brucella ring test* is a diagnostic test for brucellosis involving the clumping together of a standard *Brucella* strain by antibodies in an infected person's serum.

豬、綿羊和山羊引起感染性流產。主要菌種爲流產布魯氏桿菌和馬耳他布魯氏桿菌。布魯氏桿菌環狀試驗用於診斷布魯氏桿菌病，該試驗係用受感染人血清中的抗體與標準布魯氏桿菌菌株發生凝集反應而顯示。

brucellosis (Malta fever, Mediterranean fever, undulant fever) *n.* a chronic disease of farm animals caused by bacteria of the genus *Brucella*, which can be transmitted to man either by contact with an infected animal or by drinking nonpasteurized contaminated milk. Symptoms include headache, sickness, loss of appetite, and weakness, progressing to chronic fever and the swelling of lymph nodes. Untreated the disease may last for years but prolonged administration of antibiotics and sulphonamides is effective.

布魯氏桿菌病（馬耳他熱，地中海熱，波狀熱） 布魯氏桿菌屬細菌引起的家畜的慢性疾病，能通過接觸受感染的動物或飲用未經巴士德法消毒的污染牛奶傳染給人。症狀有頭痛、噁心、嘔吐、食慾減退和疲乏無力，繼而慢性發熱和淋巴結腫大。如不治療可持續數年，但長期應用抗生素和磺胺有效。

Brufen *n. see* ibuprofen.

布洛芬

Brugia *n.* a genus of threadlike parasitic worms (*see* filaria). *B. malayi* infects man throughout southeast Asia, causing *filariasis and *elephantiasis (especially of the feet and legs). *B. pahangi*, a parasite of wild cats and domestic animals, produces an allergic condition in man, with coughing, breathing difficulty, and an increase in the number of *eosinophils in the blood. *Brugia* undergoes part of its development in mosquitoes of the genera *Anopheles* and *Mansonia*, which transmit the parasite from host to host.

馬來絲蟲屬 線狀寄生性蠕蟲屬。在全東南亞，馬來絲蟲感染人引起絲蟲病和橡皮病（尤其是腿和脚）。寄生於野貓和家畜的彭亨絲蟲在人引起過敏狀態：咳嗽、呼吸困難和血中嗜酸性粒細胞數量增加。生活史部分時間是在按蚊屬和曼蚊屬蚊蟲體內，後者將絲蟲從宿主傳給另一宿主。

bruise (contusion) *n.* an area of skin discoloration caused by the escape of blood from ruptured underlying vessels following injury. Initially red or pink, a bruise gradually becomes bluish, and then greenish yellow, as the haemoglobin in the tissues breaks down chemically and is absorbed. It may be necessary to draw off blood from very severe bruises through a needle, to aid healing.

挫傷 外傷時由於血液從破裂血管中逸出形成的局部皮膚變色。最初爲紅色或櫻紅色，由於血紅蛋白在組織中化學分解和吸收，逐漸變藍再變成黃綠色。嚴重挫傷可用空針吸出積血，以利迅速痊癒。

bruit *n. see* murmur. 雜音

Brunner's glands compound glands of the small intestine, found in the duodenum and the upper part of the jejunum. They are embedded in the submucosa and secrete mucus.
布倫內氏腺 小腸複管腺，存在於十二指腸和空腸上段，位於黏膜下層並分泌黏液。

brush border *see* microvillus. **刷狀緣**

bruxism *n.* a habit in which an individual grinds his teeth, which leads to excessive wear.
磨牙症 一種磨牙的習慣。易致牙質過多磨損。

bubo *n.* a swollen inflamed lymph node in the armpit or groin, commonly developing in venereal disease, bubonic plague, and leishmaniasis.
腹股溝淋巴結炎 腋窩和腹股溝部淋巴結腫脹發炎。通常發生於性病、腺鼠疫和利什曼氏病。

bubonic plague *see* plague. **腹股溝淋巴結鼠疫**

buccal *adj.* **1.** relating to the mouth or the hollow part of the cheek. **2.** describing the surface of a tooth adjacent to the cheek.
頰的 ①與口腔或面頰中空部位有關的部分。 ②牙與面頰之間的部位。

buccal cavity the cavity of the mouth, which contains the tongue and teeth and leads to the pharynx. Here food is tasted, chewed, and mixed with saliva, which begins the process of digestion.
口腔前庭 包括舌、牙的口腔部。由此通向咽部。食物在此品嚐、咀嚼並與唾液混合，開始消化過程。

buccal glands small glands in the mucous membrane lining the mouth. They secrete material that mixes with saliva.
頰腺 口腔黏膜內的小腺體，其分泌物和唾液混合。

buccinator *n.* a muscle of the cheek that has its origin in the maxilla and mandible (jaw bones). It is responsible for compressing the cheek and is important in mastication.
頰肌 源於上頜骨和下頜骨的頰部肌肉。功能爲收縮頰部利於咀嚼。

buclizine *n.* an *antihistamine with marked sedative properties. Given by mouth, it is used to treat mild anxiety states and tension, as well as for allergic conditions and vertigo. Side-effects include drowsiness, dizziness, dryness of the throat, and gastro-intestinal upsets. Occasionally teratogenic effects may occur. Trade names: **Softran, Vibazine.**
氯苯丁臻 具有明顯鎮痛作用的抗組織胺藥。口服，用以治療極度焦慮緊張、過敏和暈眩。副作用有嗜睡、頭昏、咽喉乾燥、胃腸不適。偶見致畸作用。商品名：安其敏。

Budd-Chiari syndrome a rare condition that follows obstruction of the
伯-齊二氏綜合徵 血栓或腫瘤阻塞肝靜脈所致的

hepatic vein by a blood clot or tumour. It is characterized by ascites and cirrhosis of the liver.

一種罕見綜合徵。其特徵爲腹水和肝硬化。

Buerger's disease an inflammatory condition affecting the arteries, especially in the legs, of young male Jews who smoke cigarettes. Intermittent *claudication (pain due to reduced blood supply) and gangrene of the limbs may develop. Coronary thrombosis may occur and venous thrombosis is common. The treatment is similar to that of *atheroma but cessation of smoking is essential to prevent progression of the disease. Medical name: **thromboangiitis obliterans**.

伯格氏病 一種發生於男性吸煙猶太青年的動脈炎性疾患。多見於下肢。可發生間歇性跛行（血流供應不足引起疼痛）和肢體壞疽，血栓性靜脈炎常見，冠狀動脈血栓形成亦可發生。治療類似於動脈粥樣硬化，戒煙可防止病情發展。醫學術語：血栓閉塞性脈管炎。

buffer *n.* a solution whose hydrogen ion concentration (pH) remains virtually unchanged by dilution or by the addition of acid or alkali. The chief buffer of the blood and extracellular body fluids is the bicarbonate (H_2CO_3/HCO_3) system. *See also* acid-base balance.

緩衝劑 稀釋或加酸加鹼後不能改變其氫離子濃度（pH）值的溶液。血液和細胞外液的主要緩沖劑爲碳酸氫鹽系統（H_2CO_3/HCO_3）。

bulb *n.* (in anatomy) any rounded structure or a rounded expansion at the end of an organ or part.

球 （解剖學）某器官或某部分末端的圓形結構或圓形擴張。

bulbar *adj.* **1.** relating to or affecting the medulla oblongata. **2.** relating to a bulb. **3.** relating to the eyeball.

①延髓的 ②球的 ③眼球的

bulbourethral glands *see* Cowper's glands.

尿道球腺

bulimia *n.* insatiable over-eating. This symptom may be psychogenic, occurring, for example, as a phase of *anorexia nervosa (*bulimia nervosa*); or it may be due to neurological causes, such as a lesion of the *hypothalamus.

食慾亢進 食慾無法滿足。可以是心因性的，如爲神經性厭食的一個階段（神經性食慾亢進），也可由神經性原因如丘腦下部損傷所致。

bulla *n.* (*pl.* **bullae**) **1.** a large blister, containing serous fluid. **2.** (in anatomy) a rounded bony prominence. **3.** a thin-walled air-filled space within the lung, arising congenitally or in *emphysema. It may cause trouble by rupturing into the pleural space (*see* pneumothorax), by adding to the air that does not contribute to gas exchange, and/or by

①大疱 含有漿液的大水疱。 **②骨疱** （解剖學）圓形骨性突出物。 **③肺大泡** 肺內充滿空氣的薄壁空隙，可爲先天性或見於肺氣腫，可破裂入胸腔，增加不能參與交換的氣體量，和/或壓迫周圍肺組織影響通氣效率。

compressing the surrounding lung and making it inefficient. —**bullous** *adj.*

bundle *n.* a group of nerve fibres situated close together and running in the same direction; e.g. the *atrioventricular bundle.

束 一組走向一致的密切聯繫在一起的神經纖維，如房室束。

bundle branch block a defect in the specialized conducting tissue of the heart (*see* arrhythmia) that is recognised as an electrocardiographic abnormality. Left or right bundle branch blocks, affecting the respective ventricles, may be seen. Occasionally both left and right bundle branch blocks occur simultaneously and the patient develops complete *heart block. The causes are similar to those of complete heart block.

束枝傳導阻滯 能爲心電圖所顯示的心臟特殊傳導組織的病變。左或右束枝傳導阻滯分別影響左室或右室，偶見左右束枝同時發生傳導阻滯導致完全性心傳導阻滯。病因類似於完全性心傳導阻滯。

bundle of His *see* atrioventricular bundle.

希氏束

bunion *n.* a swelling of the joint between the great toe and the first metatarsal bone. A *bursa often develops over the site and the great toe becomes displaced towards the others. Bunions are usually caused by ill-fitting shoes and may require surgical treatment.

蹈囊腫 蹈趾蹠趾關節的囊腫。常向周圍生長，致使蹈趾移位。通常由穿不合適的鞋引起。常需外科治療。

buphenine *n.* a drug whose main action is to dilate blood vessels, particularly those in skeletal muscles. Taken by mouth, it is used to increase the blood flow to muscle, especially in vascular disease due to spasm of the arteries. It may cause palpitations and stimulate gastric secretion. Trade names: **Arlidin, Perdilatal**.

苄丙酚胺 主要作用爲擴張血管尤其是骨骼肌血管的藥物。口服，用於增加肌肉血流量，多用於動脈痙攣性血管疾病，可致心悸和刺激胃的分泌。商品名：布福寧。

buphthalmos (hydrophthalmos) *n.* infantile or congenital glaucoma: increased pressure within the eye due to a defect in the development of the tissues through which fluid drains from the eye. Since the outer coat (sclera) of the eyeball of children is distensible, the eye enlarges as the inflow of fluid continues. It affects both eyes and may accompany congenital malformations

牛眼症（眼積水） 嬰兒或先天性青光眼：由於引流房水的組織發育缺陷導致眼內壓增高。兒童眼球鞏膜可膨脹，房水不斷產生時眼球擴大。本病常累及雙眼並可伴有身體其他部位的先天畸形。手術治療，如前房角切開術，能增加房水的吸收。在完全

in other parts of the body. Treatment is by surgical operation, e.g. *goniotomy, to improve drainage of fluid from the eye. Spontaneous arrest of buphthalmos may occur before vision is completely lost.

失明前本病可自然停止發展。

bupivacaine *n.* a potent local anaesthetic, used mainly for regional *nerve block. It is significantly longer-acting than many other local anaesthetics. It has been used in childbirth, but may cause slowing of the baby's heart, with a risk of death. Trade name: **Marcain**.

布比卡因 主要用於區域神經阻滞的强力局麻藥。作用時間長於許多其他局麻藥。已用於產婦分娩，但可引起嬰兒心跳减慢甚或死亡。商品名：麻卡因。

bur (burr) *n.* a cutting drill that fits in a dentist's handpiece. Burs are mainly used for cutting cavities in teeth.

牙鑽 牙科醫生用於牙齒鑽洞的鑽頭。

Burkitt's tumour (Burkitt's lymphoma) a malignant tumour of the lymphatic system, most commonly affecting children and largely confined to tropical Africa in a zone 15° north and south of the equator. It can arise at various sites, most commonly the facial structures, such as the jaw, and in the abdomen. Complications affecting the nervous system occur in up to 50% of cases. Viruses may possibly play a role in the origin and growth of the tumour, which has been shown to be very sensitive to *cytotoxic drug therapy.

伯基特氏腫瘤（伯基特氏淋巴瘤） 淋巴系統惡性腫瘤，大部發生於兒童及熱帶非洲赤道南北各 15° 地帶內。腫瘤可發生於任何部位，最常見的是頭面部（如頸）和腹部。約 50% 病例有神經系統併發症。病毒可能是腫瘤發生和生長的因素之一。對化療非常敏感。

burn *n.* tissue damage caused by such agents as heat, chemicals, electricity, sunlight, or nuclear radiation. A *first-degree burn* affects only the outer layer (epidermis) of the skin. In a *second-degree burn* both the epidermis and the underlying dermis are damaged. A *third-degree burn* involves damage or destruction of the skin to its full depth and damage to the tissues beneath. Burns cause swelling and blistering, due to loss of plasma from damaged blood vessels. In serious burns, affecting 15% or more of the body surface in adults (10% or more in children), this loss of plasma results in severe *shock and requires immediate transfusion of

燒傷 由熱、化學物質、電、日光或核放射引起的組織損傷。I 度燒傷僅累及皮膚表層（上皮層）。II 度燒傷累及上皮層和下面眞皮。III 度燒傷皮膚全層受損並傷及皮下組織。由於血漿從受傷血管滲出，導致腫脹和水疱。嚴重燒傷病例即成人燒傷面積達 15% 或更多（兒童 10% 或更多）時，血漿大量喪失導致嚴重休克，必須立即輸血或輸注含鹽溶液。燒傷也可致細菌感染，但可用抗生素預防。III 度燒傷需植皮。

blood or saline solution. Burns may also lead to bacterial infection, which can be prevented by administration of antibiotics. Third-degree burns may require skin grafting.

burr *n. see* bur.

（牙）鑽，圓頭銼

bursa *n.* (*pl.* **bursae**) a small sac of fibrous tissue that is lined with *synovial membrane and filled with fluid (synovia). Bursae occur where parts move over one another; they help to reduce friction. They are normally formed round joints and in places where ligaments and tendons pass over bones. However, they may be formed in other places in response to unusual pressure or friction.

黏(滑)液囊　一種內襯滑膜的充滿液體（滑液）的纖維組織囊。黏液囊位於運動部位，有助於減輕摩擦。正常時其包繞關節，位於韌帶和肌腱通過骨的地方。但它們也可在有異常壓力或摩擦的地方發生。

bursitis *n.* inflammation of a *bursa, resulting from injury, infection, or rheumatoid *synovitis. It produces pain and tenderness and sometimes restricts movement at a nearby joint; for example, at the shoulder. Treatment of bursitis not due to infection is by rest and corticosteroid injection. *See also* housemaid's knee.

滑囊炎，黏液囊炎　由於損傷、感染或風濕性滑膜炎引起的黏液囊的炎症。可引起附近關節如肩的疼痛、觸痛和運動受限。非感染性滑囊炎的治療是休息和皮質類固醇注射。

busulphan *n.* a drug that destroys cancer cells by acting on the bone marrow. It is administered by mouth, mainly in the treatment of chronic myeloid leukaemia. It may cause blood disorders producing bleeding. Trade name: **Myleran**.

二甲磺酸丁酯　一種作用於骨髓而殺死腫瘤細胞的藥物。口服，主要用於治療慢性骨髓性白血病。可引起出血。商品名：馬利蘭。

butacaine *n.* a local anaesthetic used to produce surface anaesthesia, mainly in eye, ear, nose, and throat surgery. Trade name: **Butyn**.

對氨苯酸二丁氨丙酯　一種用於表面麻醉的局部麻醉劑。主要用於五官科手術。商品名：布大卡因。

butobarbitone (butobarbital) *n.* an intermediate-acting *barbiturate, used for the treatment of insomnia and for sedation. It produces sleep within 30 minutes when given by mouth and its sedative effect lasts for about six hours. Prolonged administration may lead to *dependence and its use with alcohol should be avoided; overdosage has se-

正丁基乙基巴比妥　一種中效巴比妥酸鹽，用於治療失眠和鎮靜。口服後30分鐘內顯效，藥效持續約6小時。長期服用可發生賴藥性。避免與酒精合用。超大劑量有嚴重副作用。　商品名：正丁巴比妥。

rious effects (*see* barbiturism). Trade name: **Soneryl**.

byssinosis *n.* an industrial disease of the lungs caused by inhalation of dusts of cotton, flax, or hemp. The patient characteristically has chest tightness and *wheeze after the weekend break, which wears off during the working week. The causal agent has not been identified.

棉屑肺，棉屑沉着病 一種由於吸入棉花、亞麻、大麻微粒引起的肺部職業病。其特徵爲週末休息後有胸部緊迫感和喘鳴，但在工作日中逐漸消失。致病因子尚未確定。

C

cac- (caco-) *prefix denoting* disease or deformity. Example: *cacosmia* (unpleasant odour).

〔前綴〕 **惡，臭** 指病態或畸形。例如：惡臭幻覺或惡臭（難聞的氣味）。

cachet *n.* a flat capsule containing a drug that has an unpleasant taste. The cachet is swallowed intact by the patient.

扁囊劑 扁形膠囊。用以包裹有不良味道的藥物，患者可整粒吞嚥。

cachexia *n.* a condition of abnormally low weight, weakness, and general bodily decline associated with chronic disease. It occurs in such conditions as cancer, pulmonary tuberculosis, and malaria.

惡病質 患慢性病時出現的一種體重異常減輕、虛弱與全身狀況惡化的狀態。見於癌症、肺結核、瘧疾等。

cacosmia *n.* a disorder of the sense of smell in which scents that are inoffensive to most people are objectionable to the sufferer or in which a bad smell seems to be perpetually present. The disorder is usually due to damage to pathways within the brain rather than in the nose or olfactory nerve.

惡臭幻覺 一種嗅覺障礙。此時患者或是對正常人認爲無所謂的氣味感到難以忍受，或是經常感到有一種難聞的氣味存在。多見於顱內嗅徑損傷。鼻與嗅神經損傷引起者少見。

cadmium *n.* a silvery metallic element that can cause serious lung irritation if the fumes of the molten metal are inhaled. Long-term exposure may also cause kidney damage. Symbol: Cd.

鎘 一種與銀類似的金屬元素。吸入該金屬的蒸氣對肺可產生劇烈刺激。長期與之接觸尙可導致腎損傷。符號：Ｃｄ。

caecostomy *n.* an operation in which the caecum is brought through the

盲腸造口術 一種將盲腸外置並造瘻的手術。用於

abdominal wall and opened in order to drain or decompress the intestine, usually when the colon is obstructed or injured.

腸管減壓與引流。此術多用於結腸損傷或梗阻。

caecum *n.* a blind-ended pouch at the junction of the small and large intestines, situated below the *ileocaecal valve. The upper end is continuous with the colon and the lower end bears the vermiform appendix. *See* alimentary canal.

盲腸 小腸與大腸交接處的盲端小袋。位於回盲瓣下方。其上端與結腸相延續，下端附有闌尾。

caeruloplasmin *n.* a copper-containing protein present in blood plasma. Congenital deficiency of caeruloplasmin leads to abnormalities of the brain and liver (*see* Wilson's disease).

血漿銅藍蛋白 存在於血漿中的一種含銅蛋白質。先天缺乏此種蛋白質可引起肝腦病變。

Caesarean section a surgical operation for delivering a baby through the abdominal wall: it should not be performed before the 28th week of gestation. It is carried out when there are risks to the baby from natural childbirth; for example if it is too large to pass through the birth canal or shows signs of lack of oxygen (anoxia); in a breech presentation that cannot be turned; or if the placenta obstructs the outlet of the womb and may cause dangerous bleeding. It is also performed for the safety of the mother, for example in acute *toxaemia of pregnancy, failure to induce labour, or prolonged ineffectual labour.

剖腹產術 使嬰兒通過腹壁娩出的手術。此術於妊娠滿28週前禁止施行。當胎兒自然分娩有生命危險時方可使用。例如：胎體過大不能通過產道或有缺氧表現；無法轉位的臀先露；或胎盤阻塞宮口並有出血危險等。有時手術目的是保護母親安全，例如：急性妊娠毒血症，引產失敗，或分娩無力產程過長等。

caesium-137 *n.* an artificial radioactive isotope of the metallic element caesium. The radiation given off by caesium-137 is employed in the technique of *radiotherapy. Symbol: Cs^{137}. *See also* telecurietherapy.

銫-137 金屬元素銫的人工放射性同位素。本同位素產生的射線用於放療。符號：Cs^{137}。

caffeine *n.* an alkaloid drug, obtained from coffee and tea, that has a stimulant action, particularly on the central nervous system. It is used to promote wakefulness and increase mental activity; it also possesses diuretic properties and will help relieve certain forms of

咖啡因 自咖啡與茶葉中提取的生物鹼藥。對中樞神經系統有顯著興奮作用。用於提神醒腦，增强腦力活動。同時具有利尿作用，並能緩解某些類型的頭痛。常與阿司匹林、

headache. It is often administered with aspirin, codeine, or phenacetin as an analgesic preparation.

可待因或非那西汀做爲止痛劑合併使用。

caisson disease *see* compressed air illness.

潛水員病 （亦稱減壓病）

calamine *n.* a preparation of zinc carbonate used as a mild astringent on the skin in the form of a lotion, cream, or ointment.

爐甘石 用碳酸鋅製備的皮膚用緩和收斂劑。有洗劑、乳劑與軟膏劑等劑型。

calc- (calci-, calco-) *prefix denoting* calcium or calcium salts.

〔前綴〕 **鈣** 指鈣元素或鈣鹽。

calcaneus (heel bone) *n.* the large bone in the *tarsus of the foot that forms the projection of the heel behind the foot. It articulates with the cuboid bone in front and with the talus above.

跟骨 足的跗骨中的一塊大骨。於足後方跟部形成突起，前與骰骨成關節。

calcar *n.* a spurlike projection. The *calcar avis* is the projection in the medial wall of the lateral ventricle of the brain.

距 刺狀突起。側腦室內壁的刺狀突起稱爲禽距。

calcicosis *n.* *pneumoconiosis in marble cutters. The term is not in current use.

灰石沉着病 採石工人的塵肺病。此詞現已廢用。

calciferol *n. see* vitamin D.

骨化醇

calcification *n.* the deposition of calcium salts in tissue. This occurs as part of the normal process of bone formation (*see* ossification).

鈣化 組織中鈣鹽沉積。爲骨生成正常過程中的一部分。

calcinosis *n.* the abnormal deposition of calcium salts in the tissues. This may occur only in the fat layer beneath the skin or it may be more widespread.

鈣質沉着 組織中發生的不正常的鈣鹽沉積。可局限於皮下脂肪層，亦可廣泛發生。

calcitonin *n. see* thyrocalcitonin.

降鈣素

calcium *n.* a metallic element essential for the normal development and functioning of the body. Calcium is an important constituent of bones and teeth: the matrix of *bone, consisting principally of calcium phosphate, accounts for about 99% of the body's calcium. It is present in the blood at a concentration of about 10 mg/100 ml, being maintained at this level by hor-

鈣 對人體正常功能與發育至關重要的一種金屬元素。是骨與牙基質的重要成分，主要以磷酸鈣形式存在，約佔全身鈣量99%。血鈣濃度靠激素維持，約爲10mg/100mℓ。在許多代謝過程中鈣都佔有重要地位，如神經活動、肌肉收縮與凝血等。

mones (*see* thyrocalcitonin, parathyroid hormone). It is essential for many metabolic processes, including nerve function, muscle contraction, and blood clotting.
The normal dietary requirement of calcium is about 1 g per day: dairy products (milk and cheese) are the principal sources. Its uptake by the body is facilitated by *vitamin D; a deficiency of this vitamin may therefore result in such conditions as *rickets, *osteoporosis, and *osteomalacia. A deficiency of calcium in the blood may lead to *tetany. Excess calcium may be deposited in the body as *calculi (stones), especially in the gall bladder and kidney. Symbol: Ca.

人體對飲食中鈣的正常需要量每日約爲1g，乳製品（奶與奶酪）爲主要來源。維生素D促進其吸收，故缺乏維生素D可導致佝僂病、骨質疏鬆病與骨質軟化病等。血鈣缺乏可導致手足搐搦症。鈣量過高可在體內沉積成結石，多見於膽囊與腎臟。符號：Ca。

calculosis *n.* the presence of multiple calculi (stones) in the body. *See* calculus.

結石病 體內出現多發結石。

calculus *n.* (*pl.* **calculi**) **1.** a stone: a hard pebble-like mass formed within the body, particularly in the gall bladder (*see* gallstone) or anywhere in the urinary tract (*see* cystolithiasis, nephrolithiasis). Calculi in the urinary tract are commonly composed of calcium oxalate and are usually visible on X-ray examination. Most of these stones cause pain, whether sited in the kidney, ureter, or bladder; stones passing down a duct (such as the ureter) cause severe colicky pain. Such stones are usually removed surgically to prevent or cure urinary obstruction and infection. **2.** a calcified deposit that forms on the surfaces of teeth. *Supragingival calculus* forms above the *gingivae (gums), principally in relation to the openings of the salivary gland ducts. *Subgingival calculus* forms beneath the crest of the gingivae. Calculus hinders the cleaning of teeth.

①**結石** 體內形成的堅硬的卵石樣物質。多見於膽囊或泌尿道某處。泌尿道結石通常由草酸鈣組成，X線檢查多可發現。此類結石無論在腎臟、輸尿管或膀胱多可引起疼痛，沿管道（如輸尿管）移動時可產生劇烈絞痛，通常用外科手術摘除結石以防止梗阻與感染。
②**牙石** 牙表面形成的鈣質沉積物。齦上牙石形成於牙齦上方，多在唾液腺管開口附近。齦下牙石形成於牙齦嵴下方。牙石有礙於牙齒刷洗。

calibrator *n.* **1.** an instrument used for measuring the size of a tube or opening. **2.** an instrument used for dilating a tubular part, such as the gullet.

①**管徑測量器** ②**管道擴張器** 如食管擴張器

calliper (caliper) *n.* **1.** an instrument with two prongs or jaws, used for measuring diameters: used particularly in obstetrics for measuring the diameter of the pelvis. **2.** (also called **calliper splint**) a leg splint that consists of metal rods attached to a padded ring at the top of the leg, taking the weight of the body at the pelvis. Calliper splints can be used to exert *traction on a deformed or paralysed leg as part of orthopaedic treatment.

①**測徑器**　一種鉸形具雙翼的測徑器械。多用於產科測量盆徑。②**雙腳規形夾**　此夾用兩根金屬桿通過墊圈支托於下肢頂端，於骨盆處支持體重。在矯形治療中用於對畸形或痳痹下肢施行牽引。

callosity (callus) *n.* a hard thick area of skin occurring in parts of the body subject to pressure or friction. The soles of the feet and palms of the hands are common sites, and if much hard dead skin develops a callosity can become painful. A *corn is a type of callosity.

胼胝　身體受壓或受摩擦部位皮膚變硬與增厚。多見於手掌與足底。如胼胝中有大量死硬皮膚形成可引起疼痛。鷄眼即爲胼胝之一種。

callus *n.* **1.** a mass of blood and *granulation tissue, containing bone-forming cells, that forms around the bone ends following a fracture. Callus formation is an essential part of the process of healthy union in a fractured bone. The callus, which is visible on X-ray as a slightly opaque area, eventually becomes calcified and modelled. **2.** *see* callosity.

①**骨痂**　骨折斷端附近形成的由血液與肉芽組織組成的團塊，含有成骨細胞。骨痂形成是骨折康復癒合的重要環節，X線下可見輕度透亮區，最終鈣化成型。　②**胼胝**

calor *n.* heat: one of the classical signs of inflammation in a tissue, the other three being *rubor (redness), *dolor (pain), and *tumor (swelling). An inflamed region has a higher temperature than normal because of the distended blood vessels, which allow an increased flow of blood.

熱　組織炎症表現的典型體徵之一。其他三者爲紅、痛、腫。炎症區溫度高於正常是由於血管擴張，以獲得較多的血液供應。

calorie *n.* a unit of heat equal to the amount of heat required to raise the temperature of 1 gram of water from 14.5°C to 15.5°C (the 15° calorie). One Calorie (also known as the *kilocalorie* or *kilogram calorie*) is equal to 1000 calories; this unit is used to indicate the energy value of foods. Except in this

卡　熱量單位。使1g水的溫度自14.5C升高至15.5C所需的熱量（15°卡）。1大卡（亦稱千卡）等於1000卡。此單位用於表達食物熱量值。其他情況下多用焦耳代替卡（1卡=4.1855焦耳）。

context, the calorie has largely been replaced by the *joule (1 calorie = 4.1855 joules).

calorimeter *n.* any apparatus used to measure the heat lost or gained during various chemical and physical changes. For example, calorimeters may be used to determine the total energy values of different foods in terms of calories. —**calorimetry** *n.*

熱量計 在各種物理化學變化中用以測量熱量增減的儀器。例如：熱量計可用以測量不同食物總熱量的卡值。

calvaria *n.* the vault of the *skull.

顱蓋

calyx *n.* (*pl.* **calyces**) a cup-shaped part, especially any of the divisions of the pelvis of the *kidney. Each calyx receives urine from the urine-collecting tubes in one sector of the kidney.

盞 杯形物。尤指腎盂的分支部分。每隻腎盞自該部分的腎集合小管中收集尿液。

camphor *n.* a crystalline substance obtained from the tree *Cinnamomum camphora* that has been used to treat flatulence. It is used in the form of *camphorated oil* (camphor in cottonseed oil) in liniments as a counterirritant.

樟腦 自樟樹製得的結晶物質。曾用於治療腹脹，現以樟腦油形式（棉子油溶液）作爲擦劑外用，以對抗刺激作用。

campimetry *n.* a method of assessing the central part of the *visual field. The patient looks steadily with one eye at a target in the centre of a black screen two metres away. A small object on the end of a black rod is moved onto the screen and the patient tells the examiner when he sees it. This is repeated many times from different directions until a map is built up of the area in front of the eye in which such an object can be seen. Campimetry allows examination only of that part of the field of vision within 30° in all directions from the centre.

平面視野檢查法 檢查中央視野的方法。患者用一目凝視兩米遠處的黑色屏幕中心的目標。檢查者將另一微小的目標物置於黑色桿端向屏幕移動，直至受檢者告知已視及該物爲止。用此法自不同方向反復檢查，最終在患者眼前屏幕上繪製出一個圖形，在此圖形區域內患者可以視到該物。此法只能檢查到視野中心周圍30°範圍內的視野部分。

camptodactylia *n.* congenital inward bending of a finger, most commonly the little finger.

屈曲指 先天性指內屈。多見於小指。

canal *n.* a tubular channel or passage; e.g. the *alimentary canal and the auditory canal of the ear.

管，道 管狀通道。例如：消化管，聽道等。

canaliculus *n.* (*pl.* **canaliculi**) a small channel or canal. Canaliculi occur, for example, in compact bone, linking lacunae containing bone cells. *Bile canaliculi* are minute channels within the liver that transport bile to the bile duct.

小管 小的管道。例如：在密質骨中有骨小管把含有骨細胞的骨腔隙聯接起來。在肝臟中有膽小管把膽汁輸送至膽管。

cancellous *adj.* lattice-like: applied to the bony tissue laid down by *osteoblasts during development of bone and in the *consolidation stage of fracture repair.

網狀的 網格狀的。用以描述成骨細胞在骨發育和骨折癒合的骨化期所建立的骨組織的狀態。

cancer *n.* any *malignant tumour, including *carcinoma and *sarcoma. It arises from the abnormal and uncontrolled division of cells that then invade and destroy the surrounding tissues. Spread of cancer cells (*metastasis) may occur via the bloodstream or the lymphatic channels or across body cavities such as the pleural and peritoneal spaces, thus setting up secondary tumours at sites distant from the original tumour. Each individual primary tumour has its own pattern of local behaviour and metastasis; for example, bone metastasis is very common in breast cancer but very rare in cancer of the ovary.

There are probably many causative factors, some of which are known; for example, cigarette smoking is associated with lung cancer, radiation with some bone sarcomas and leukaemia. Some tumours, such as retinoblastoma, are inherited. Treatment of cancer depends on the type of tumour, the site of the primary tumour, and the extent of spread.

惡性腫瘤 包括癌和肉瘤在內的任何惡性腫瘤。

細胞發生無限制的異常的分裂，並侵犯、破壞周圍組織。癌瘤細胞可通過血流或淋巴道、體腔（胸腔或腹腔）擴散（轉移），因此在遠離原發瘤的部位發生續發性瘤。各種原發瘤皆有其局部特徵及轉移易發部位。如乳腺癌多發生骨轉移而卵巢癌則少見。

致病因素可能是多方面的，其中有些業已查明。如肺癌與吸煙有關，骨肉瘤及白血病與放射線照射有關。有些是遺傳性的，如成視網膜細胞瘤。治療則隨腫瘤類型、原發部位與擴散程度而有所不同。

cancrum (canker) *n.* ulceration, mainly of the lips and mouth (*cancrum oris*).

壞疽性潰瘍 主要發生於口唇部的潰瘍，如走馬疳。

candela *n.* the *SI unit of luminous intensity, equal to the intensity in a horizontal direction of a surface of 1/600,000 square metre of a black body at a temperature of 2040 kelvins and a pressure of 101,325 pascals. Symbol: cd.

坎〔德拉〕 亮度的國際單位（ＳＩ單位）。相當於黑體1/600,000平方米表面於2040開爾文的溫度與101,325帕斯卡的壓力下沿水平方向發射的亮度。符號：cd。

candicidin *n.* a fungicide, produced by the bacterium *Streptomyces griseus* and used to treat candidiasis, particularly of the vagina.

殺念珠菌素 一種由灰色鏈黴菌屬製得的殺眞菌素。用以治療念珠菌病，尤其是陰道念珠菌病。

Candida *n.* a genus of yeastlike fungi (formerly called *Monilia*) that inhabit the vagina and alimentary tract and can – under certain conditions – cause *candidiasis. The species *C. albicans*, a small oval budding fungus, is primarily responsible for candidiasis of the mouth, lungs, intestine, vagina, skin, and nails.

念珠菌屬 酵母樣眞菌的一屬。寄生於陰道與消化道，在一定條件下可致病。白色念珠菌屬——一種小的卵圓形芽生菌——是口腔、肺、腸、陰道、皮膚與指甲念珠菌病的主要病原體。

candidiasis *n.* infection with a yeastlike fungus of the genus **Candida*, usually the species *C. albicans*. The infection – formerly called *moniliasis* – is usually superficial, occurring in moist areas of the body, such as the skin folds, mouth, respiratory tract, and vagina (candidiasis of the mouth and vagina is popularly known as *thrush*). Rarely, candidiasis infection may spread throughout the body. Candidiasis of the mouth appears as white patches on the tongue or inside the cheeks. Candidiasis sometimes develops in patients receiving broad-spectrum antibiotics. It is treated with antibiotics – especially *nystatin – applied locally, inhaled, or taken by mouth.

念珠菌病 酵母樣眞菌——念珠菌屬——引起的感染。以白色念珠菌爲多見。感染通常發生在淺表、潮濕的部位，如皮膚皺褶處、口腔、呼吸道與陰道。口腔念珠菌病俗稱鵝口瘡。波及全身的病例是罕見的。患口腔念珠菌病時舌部或頰內出現白色斑點。接受廣譜抗生素治療的患者可發生本病。治療：抗生素，主要是制黴菌素，可局部外用、吸入或口服。

canine *n.* the third tooth from the midline of each jaw. There are thus four canines, two in each jaw, in both the permanent and deciduous (milk) *dentitions. It is known colloquially as the *eye tooth*.

尖牙 自中線向外數第三顆牙。上、下、左、右各具一個。俗稱犬齒。

canities *n.* loss of pigment in the hair, which causes greying or whitening. It is usually part of the ageing process, when it starts at the temples. White patches may occur as a result of *alopecia areata or *vitiligo.

灰髮症 頭髮色素脫失。頭髮變灰或變白，自顳部開始者多爲衰老過程的表現。斑狀白髮可能爲白癜瘋或斑禿所致。

canker *n. see* cancrum.

壞疽性潰瘍

cannabis *n.* a drug prepared from the Indian hemp plant (*Cannabis sativa*), also known as *pot*, *marihuana*, *hashish*, and *bhang*. Smoked or swallowed, it produces euphoria and hallucinations and affects perception and awareness, particularly of time. Cannabis has no therapeutic value and its use is illegal: there is evidence that prolonged use may cause brain damage and lead the user onto 'hard' drugs, such as heroin. *See also* dependence.

大蔴 由植物印度大蔴製得的蔴醉品。供吸入或吞入，可產生欣快感與幻覺，導致意識與知覺障礙，尤其是時間觀念的障礙。本品無治療價值，服用是非法的。已經證實長期使用可引起腦損傷，如同海洛因一樣可成癮。

cannula *n.* a hollow tube designed for insertion into a body cavity, such as the bladder, or a blood vessel. The tube contains a sharp pointed solid core (*trocar*), which facilitates its insertion and is withdrawn when the cannula is in place.

套管 用以插入膀胱、血管或體腔的中空插管。內有尖銳堅硬的管芯（套管針），以便於插入，就位後即行拔除。

cantharidin *n.* the active principle of *cantharides*, or *Spanish fly* (the dried bodies of a blister beetle, *Lytta vesicatoria*). A toxic and irritant chemical, cantharidin causes blistering of the skin and was formerly used in veterinary medicine as a counterirritant and vesicant. If swallowed it causes nausea, vomiting, and inflammation of the urinary tract, the latter giving rise to its reputation as an aphrodisiac. It is very dangerous and may cause death.

斑蝥素 斑蝥的有效成分。本品係一具有毒性與刺激性的化合物，能使皮膚起疱，獸醫曾用做抗刺激劑與起疱劑。吞入可引起噁心、嘔吐與泌尿系炎症，後者使本品獲有春藥之稱。服用本品十分危險，有死亡可能。

canthus *n.* either corner of the eye; the angle at which the upper and lower eyelids meet. —**canthal** *adj.*

眥 眼兩側的角部。上下眼瞼在此處會合。

cap *n.* a covering or a cover-like part. The *duodenal cap* is the superior part of the duodenum as seen on X-ray after a barium meal.

冠、帽、蓋 十二指腸冠即進鋇餐後X線顯示的十二指腸上部。

Capgras' syndrome (illusion of doubles) the delusion that a person closely involved with the patient has been replaced by an identical-looking impostor. It is often, but not necessarily, a form of paranoid *schizophrenia.

卡普格臘斯綜合徵（易人錯覺） 類偏執狂型精神分裂症常見的表現。患者產生一種妄想，把他非常熟悉的人，看做是他人冒充頂替的騙子。

capillary *n.* an extremely narrow blood vessel, approximately 5–20 μm in diameter. Capillaries form networks in most tissues; they are supplied with blood by arterioles and drained by venules. The vessel wall is only one cell thick, which enables exchange of oxygen, carbon dioxide, water, salts, etc., between the blood and the tissues (see illustrations).

毛細血管 極細的血管。直徑約5～20 μ m。在多數組織內形成毛細血管網。它從小動脈接受血液，然後把血液排向小靜脈。血管壁極薄，只有一層細胞，因此，血液與組織間的氧、二氧化碳、水、鹽等能在此處進行交換（見圖）。

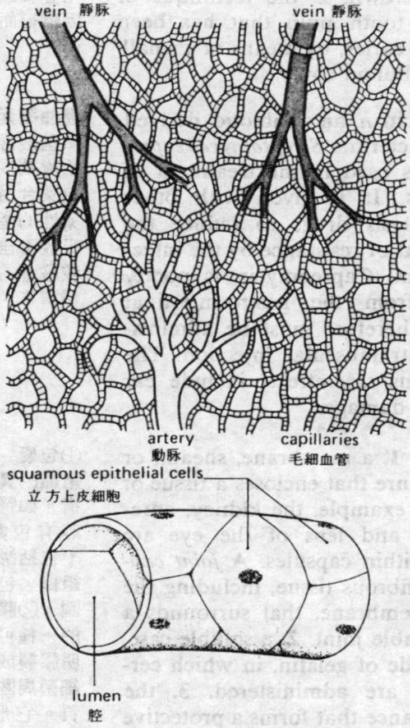

A network of capillaries (above); a single capillary (below)

毛細血管網（上）與單一毛細血管（下）

capitate *adj.* head-shaped; having a rounded extremity.

頭狀的 末端爲圓形的。

capitate bone a bone of the wrist (*see* carpus). It articulates with the scaphoid and lunate bones behind and with the third metacarpal bone in front.

頭狀骨 腕骨之一。在後方與舟骨、月骨相關節，前方與第三掌骨相關節。

capitellum *n. see* capitulum.

小頭

capitulum *n.* the small rounded end of a bone that articulates with another bone. For example, the *capitulum humeri* (or *capitellum*) is the round prominence at the elbow end of the humerus that articulates with the radius.

小頭 骨的小的圓形末端，與其它骨相關節。例如：肱骨小頭即爲肱骨肘端的圓形隆凸，與橈骨相關節。

capping *n.* (in dentistry) **1.** crowning: the technique of fitting a tooth with an *artificial crown. **2.** the technique of protecting tooth pulp that has been exposed by caries, by means of a small metal or celluloid cover.

①**造冠術** 在牙上裝配人工牙冠的技術。②**蓋髓術** 用金屬或賽璐璐覆蓋保護因齲變而暴露的牙髓的技術。

capreomycin *n.* an antibiotic, derived from the bacterium *Streptomyces capreolus*, that is used in the treatment of tuberculosis. It is given with other antituberculosis drugs to reduce the development of resistance by the infective bacteria. Capreomycin is poorly absorbed from the gastro-intestinal tract and therefore must be administered by intramuscular injection. The more serious side-effects include ear and kidney damage.

卷曲黴素 一種自卷曲鏈黴菌製得的抗生素。用以治療結核病。與其他抗結核藥合用可延緩病原菌抗藥性的產生。本品胃腸道吸收不佳，故必須肌注。較嚴重的副作用有耳與腎損害等。

capsule *n.* **1.** a membrane, sheath, or other structure that encloses a tissue or organ. For example, the kidney, adrenal gland, and lens of the eye are enclosed within capsules. A *joint capsule* is the fibrous tissue, including the synovial membrane, that surrounds a freely movable joint. **2.** a soluble case, usually made of gelatin, in which certain drugs are administered. **3.** the slimy substance that forms a protective layer around certain bacteria. It is usually made of *polysaccharide.

①**包囊** 包繞某種器官或組織的囊膜、鞘或其他結構。如腎、腎上腺、晶體等有包囊包繞。關節囊（包括滑膜）係一種纖維組織，包繞在可動關節周圍。②**膠囊** 包含有藥物的一種可溶性囊。通常由明膠製成。③**莢膜** 某些細菌周圍的一層粘液狀物質。它形成菌體的保護層，通常由多糖構成。

capsulitis *n.* inflammation of the capsule surrounding a joint.

關節囊炎

capsulotomy *n.* an incision into the capsule of the lens. In some operations for cataract the lens capsule is not removed and tends to become opaque. A tiny knife (*cystitome*) is inserted into

晶體囊切開術 一種切開晶體囊的手術。在某些白內障手術中保留的晶體囊會變混濁。可使用晶體囊刀在晶體囊中央切一小

the eye and a hole cut in the centre of the capsule, thus providing a clear path for light rays to reach the retina.

孔，讓光線通過此孔到達網膜。

caput succedaneum a temporary swelling of the soft parts of the head of a newly born infant that occurs during birth, due to compression by the muscles of the neck of the womb.

先鋒頭 新生兒娩出時頭部軟組織產生的暫時性腫脹。由於受宮頸肌肉壓迫所致。

carbachol *n.* a *parasympathomimetic drug used to relieve pressure within the eye in glaucoma. It is also used after surgical operations to restore the function of inactive bowels or bladder. Side-effects may include sweating, nausea, and faintness. Trade name: **Carcholin**.

氯化氨甲醯膽鹼 擬副交感神經藥。用於減低青光眼患者眼內壓，亦用於手術後恢復腸道與膀胱機能。

carbamazepine *n.* an *anticonvulsant drug used in the treatment of epilepsy and to relieve the pain of trigeminal neuralgia. Common side-effects include drowsiness, dizziness, and muscular incoordination; abnormalities of liver and bone marrow may occur with long-term treatment. Trade name: **Tegretol**.

氨甲醯氮䓬 抗驚厥藥。用於治療癲癇，亦可用於三叉神經痛止痛。常見副作用有嗜眠、頭昏與共濟失調等。長期使用可引起肝與骨髓損害。商品名：痛驚寧。

carbenicillin *n.* a synthetic penicillin: an antibiotic that is effective against a wide range of bacterial infections. It is poorly absorbed from the gastrointestinal tract and must be given by intramuscular injection. Allergic reactions are common side-effects. Trade name: **Pyopen**.

羧苄青黴素 一種廣譜的合成青黴素。本品胃腸道吸收不佳，必須肌注。過敏反應常見。

carbenoxolone *n.* a drug that reduces inflammation, used mainly to promote healing in the treatment of gastric ulcers or ulcers of the mouth. It is given by mouth; side-effects include the retention of salt and water (*see* oedema), weight gain, and raised blood pressure. Trade names: **Biogastrone**, **Bioral**.

生胃酮 消炎藥。主要用於促進胃潰瘍與口腔潰瘍癒合。口服。副作用有水鹽瀦留、體重增加與血壓升高等。

carbimazole *n.* a drug used to reduce the production of thyroid hormone in cases of overactivity of the gland (thyrotoxicosis). It is administered by mouth; some allergic reactions may occur and high dosage may cause enlargement of the thyroid gland,

甲亢平 甲狀腺素分泌抑制藥。用於甲狀腺機能亢進。口服。可有過敏反應。大劑量可導致甲狀腺腫大甚致堵塞氣管。

which may obstruct the windpipe. Trade names: **Bimazol**, **Neo-Mercazole**.

carbinoxamine *n.* a short-acting antihistamine, given by mouth in the treatment of allergic conditions, particularly hay fever and rhinitis, and to prevent travel sickness. Trade name: **Clistin**.

氯苯吡醇胺 短效抗組胺藥。口服。用於治療枯草熱、鼻炎等過敏性疾患及暈動病。

carbohydrate *n.* any one of a large group of compounds, including the *sugars and *starch, that contain carbon, hydrogen, and oxygen and have the general formula $C_x(H_2O)_y$. Carbohydrates are important as a source of energy: they are manufactured by plants and obtained by animals and man from the diet, being one of the three main constituents of food (*see also* fat, protein). All carbohydrates are eventually broken down in the body to the simple sugar *glucose, which can then take part in energy-producing metabolic processes. Excess carbohydrate, not immediately required by the body, is stored in the liver and muscles in the form of *glycogen. In plants carbohydrates are important structural materials (e.g. cellulose) and storage products (commonly in the form of starch). *See also* disaccharide, monosaccharide, polysaccharide.

碳水化合物 一大組含有碳、氫、氧的化合物的總稱。包括各種糖與澱粉，其共同的分子式爲 Cx（H_2O）y。它是能量的重要來源，由植物製造。動物和人類從食物中攝取。是食物的三大主要成分之一。所有的碳水化物在體內最終分解爲單糖——葡萄糖，參預供能代謝過程。沒有被機體立即利用的多餘的碳水化合物以糖原的形式貯存於肝臟與肌肉內。在植物中碳水化合物是重要的結構物質（如纖維素），也是貯存物質（通常以澱粉的形式）。

carbol fuchsin a red stain for bacteria and fungi, consisting of carbolic acid and *fuchsin dissolved in alcohol and water.

石炭酸品紅 用於細菌與眞菌染色的紅色染劑，含有石炭酸與品紅的酒精與水溶液。

carbolic acid *see* phenol.

石炭酸

carbon dioxide a colourless gas formed in the tissues during metabolism and carried in the blood to the lungs, where it is exhaled (an increase in the concentration of this gas in the blood stimulates respiration). Carbon dioxide occurs in small amounts in the atmosphere; it is used by plants in the process of *photosynthesis. It forms a solid (dry ice) at –75°C (at atmospheric

二氧化碳 無色氣體。由組織代謝產生，並由血液攜帶至肺臟呼出（血液中二氧化碳濃度增加時可刺激呼吸）。大氣中含有少量二氧化碳，植物用以進行光合作用。在 -75℃（標準大氣壓下）時形成固體（乾冰），用做冷凍劑。分子式：CO_2。

pressure) and in this form is used as a refrigerant. Formula: CO_2.

carbon monoxide a colourless almost odourless gas that is very poisonous. When breathed in it combines with haemoglobin in the red blood cells to form *carboxyhaemoglobin, which is bright red in colour. This compound is chemically stable and thus the haemoglobin can no longer combine with oxygen. Carbon monoxide is present in coal gas and motor exhaust fumes. Formula: CO.

一氧化碳 無色、幾乎無臭、有劇毒的氣體。吸入後與紅細胞內的血紅蛋白形成鮮紅色的碳氧血紅蛋白。此化合物十分穩定，因此血紅蛋白不再能與氧結合。一氧化碳存在於煤氣與汽車廢氣中。分子式：CO。

carbon tetrachloride a pungent volatile fluid used as a dry-cleaner. When inhaled or swallowed it may severely damage the heart, liver, and kidneys, causing cirrhosis and nephrosis, and it can also affect the optic nerve and other nerves. Treatment is by administration of oxygen.

四氯化碳 有刺激性的揮發性液體。用做乾洗劑。吸入或嚥入可嚴重損害心、肝、腎，導致肝硬化與腎病，亦可損害視神經或其他神經。治療：吸氧。

carboxyhaemoglobin *n.* a substance formed when carbon monoxide combines with the pigment *haemoglobin in the blood. Carboxyhaemoglobin is incapable of transporting oxygen to the tissues and this is the cause of death in carbon monoxide poisoning. Large quantities of carboxyhaemoglobin are formed in carbon monoxide poisoning, and low levels are always present in the blood of smokers and city dwellers.

碳氧血紅蛋白 一氧化碳與血紅蛋白在血液中結合的產物。碳氧血紅蛋白無輸氧至組織的能力，此即一氧化碳中毒的死因。一氧化碳中毒時有大量碳氧血紅蛋白形成。吸煙者與城市居民血中經常有少量碳氧血紅蛋白存在。

carboxylase *n.* an enzyme that catalyses the addition of carbon dioxide to a substance.

羧酶 催化某物質羧基化的酶。（羧基化即二氧化碳與有機物質的加成反應。）

carbromal *n.* a weak sedative and hypnotic, given by mouth and used in the treatment of mild insomnia. Its action lasts for a few hours but prolonged use may lead to *dependence.

二乙溴乙醯脲 弱催眠藥與鎮靜藥。口服，用於治療輕度失眠。作用持續數小時。長期服用能產生賴藥性。

carbuncle *n.* a collection of *boils with multiple drainage channels. The infection is usually caused by *Staphylococcus aureus* and normally results in an

癰 聚集在一起的癤腫。其間有許多竇道相通。多由金黃色葡萄狀球菌引起，可導致大面積死皮脫

extensive slough of skin. Treatment is with antibiotics and sometimes also by surgery.

落。治療：抗生素。有時需行手術切開。

carcin- (carcino-) *prefix denoting* cancer or carcinoma. Example: *carcinogenesis* (development of).

〔前綴〕**癌** 例如：致癌作用。

carcinogen *n.* any substance that, when exposed to living tissue, may cause the production of a *carcinoma. Such substances are known to exist in cigarette smoke and may cause lung cancer. The chemical benzidine, once used in medical laboratories, is also known to be a carcinogen. Many chemicals known to produce cancer in laboratory animals have yet to be proved to do so in man. —**carcinogenic** *adj.*

致癌物質 任何與活組織接觸後能誘發癌的物質。已知香煙中存在此種物質，可引起肺癌。在醫學化驗室中使用的聯苯胺亦屬此類物質。許多在實驗動物身上能誘發癌的化學物質對人類的致癌作用尚待證實。

carcinoid *n. see* argentaffinoma.

類癌瘤

carcino-embryonic antigen (CEA) a protein produced in the fetus but not in normal adult life. It may be produced by carcinomas, particularly of the colon, and is a rather insensitive marker of malignancy.

癌胚抗原 胎兒體內產生的一種蛋白質。正常成人體內不存在。在患癌症時，尤其是結腸癌時又可產生，但陽性率較低。

carcinoma *n.* any *cancer that arises in epithelium, the tissue that lines the skin and internal organs of the body. It may occur in any tissue containing epithelial cells. In many cases the site of origin of the tumour may be identified by the nature of the cells it contains. Organs may exhibit more than one type of carcinoma; for example, an adenocarcinoma and a squamous carcinoma may be found in the cervix (but not usually concurrently). Treatment depends on the nature of the primary tumour, different types responding to different drug combinations. —**carcinomatous** *adj.*

癌 上皮組織的惡性腫瘤。內臟與體表皆有上皮組織覆蓋，任何含有上皮細胞的組織都可能發生癌。癌瘤的原發部位多可由所含細胞的特徵來判定。同一器官亦可發生不同類型的癌，如腺癌和鱗狀癌皆可在子宮頸發生（同時併發者少見）。治療：取決於原發癌的性質。對不同類型的癌採用不同的綜合藥物療法。

carcinomatosis *n.* carcinoma that has spread widely throughout the body. Spread of the cancer cells occurs via the lymphatic channels and bloodstream

癌病 癌瘤在體內廣泛擴散。擴散方式有淋巴轉移、血行轉移與體腔移植，如通過腹腔移植。

and across body cavities, for example the peritoneal cavity.

carcinosarcoma *n.* a malignant tumour of the cervix, uterus, or vagina containing a mixture of *adenocarcinoma, sarcoma cells, and stroma. It is often bulky and polypoid, with grape-like fronds (*sarcoma botryoides*). Tissues of mesodermal origin, such as bone, cartilage, or striated muscle, may also be present.

癌肉瘤 宮頸、子宮體或陰道內的一種混合性惡性腫瘤。內含腺癌、肉瘤細胞與間質，通常巨大而呈息肉狀，並具葡萄簇樣外觀，有時含有骨、軟骨或橫紋肌等來自中胚層的組織。

cardi- (cardio-) *prefix denoting* the heart. Examples: *cardiomegaly* (enlargement of); *cardiopathy* (disease of).

〔前綴〕 **心** 例如：心臟擴大，心臟病。

cardia *n.* **1.** the opening at the upper end of the *stomach that connects with the oesophagus (gullet). **2.** the heart.

①**賁門** 胃的上口，與食道聯結處。②**心臟**

cardiac *adj.* **1.** of, relating to, or affecting the heart. **2.** of or relating to the upper part of the stomach (*see* cardia).

①**心臟的** ②**賁門的**

cardiac arrest the cessation of effective pumping action of the heart, which most commonly occurs when the muscle fibres of the ventricles start to beat rapidly without pumping any blood (ventricular *fibrillation) or when the heart stops beating completely (*asystole). There is abrupt loss of consciousness, absence of the pulse, and breathing stops. There are many causes of cardiac arrest but the most common cause is *myocardial infarction. Unless treated promptly, irreversible brain damage and death follow within minutes. Some patients may be resuscitated by massage of the heart, artificial respiration, and *defibrillation.

心搏停止 心臟的有效泵血功能喪失。多見於心室纖維震顫，此時心臟完全不能搏出血液，或心跳完全停止。患者突然意識喪失，脉搏消失，呼吸停止。病因有多種，但最多見的是心肌梗塞。如不及時治療，可發生不能恢復的腦損害，幾分鐘內即可死亡。部份患者可通過心臟按摩、人工呼吸與除顫療法得以復甦。

cardiac cycle the sequence of events between one heart beat and the next, normally occupying less than a second. The atria contract simultaneously and force blood into the relaxed ventricles. The ventricles then contract very strongly and pump blood out through the

心動週期 兩次心跳之間發生一系列變化的過程。通常歷時不到1秒。兩側心房同時收縮，把血液驅入舒張的心室，繼而心室强烈收縮，把血液驅入主動脉與肺動脉。心室收縮

aorta and pulmonary artery. During ventricular contraction, the atria relax and fill up again with blood. *See* diastole, systole.

期間，心房舒張，再度充滿血液。

cardiac muscle the specialized muscle of which the walls of the *heart are composed. It is composed of a network of branching elongated cells (fibres) whose junctions with neighbouring cells are marked by irregular transverse bands known as *intercalated discs*.

心肌 組成心壁的特殊肌肉。由長形的分支細胞（肌纖維）組成網絡，相鄰的細胞以形狀不規則的橫帶（間板）相聯結。

cardiac reflex reflex control of the heart rate. Sensory fibres in the walls of the heart are stimulated when the heart rate increases above normal. Impulses are sent to the cardiac centre in the brain, which stimulates the vagus nerve and leads to a reflex slowing of the heart rate.

心臟反射 控制心率的反射。心率高於正常時心壁內的感覺神經纖維受到刺激，把衝動傳至腦內心跳中樞，然後衝動又刺激迷走神經，反射地減緩心率。

cardinal veins two pairs of veins in the embryo that carry blood from the head (*anterior cardinal veins*) and trunk (*posterior cardinal veins*); they unite to form the *common cardinal vein*, which drains into the sinus venosus of the heart.

主靜脉 胚胎期收集頭部血液（前主靜脉）與軀幹部血液（後主靜脉）的兩對靜脉。二者滙合成總主靜脉，滙入心臟靜脉竇。

cardiology *n.* the science concerned with the study of the structure, function, and diseases of the heart. —**cardiologist** *n.*

心臟病學 研究心臟結構、功能與疾病的學科。

cardiomyopathy *n.* any chronic disorder affecting the muscle of the heart. It may be inherited but can be caused by various conditions, including virus infections, alcoholism, beriberi (vitamin B deficiency), and amyloidosis. The cause is often unknown. It may result in enlargement of the heart, *heart failure, *arrhythmias, and embolism. There is often no specific treatment but patients improve following the control of heart failure and arrhythmias.

心肌病 侵犯心肌的慢性病。本病可能是先天性的，但多由其他疾病誘發，如病毒感染、酒精中毒、腳氣病（維生素B缺乏）及澱粉樣變等。大多原因不明。本病可引起心臟擴大、心衰、心律不齊與栓塞。通常無特效療法。但心衰與心律不齊得到控制後病情可好轉。

cardiomyotomy *n. see* achalasia.

賁門肌切開術

cardiopulmonary bypass a method by which the circulation to the body is

心肺分流術 在心臟外科手術中心臟停搏時，通過

maintained while the heart is deliberately stopped during heart surgery. The function of the heart and lungs is carried out by a pump-oxygenator (*heart-lung machine) until the natural circulation is restored.

體外裝置維持循環的一種方法。在自然循環恢復前，心肺功能由泵氧合器（心肺機）代替。

cardiospasm *n. see* achalasia.

賁門痙攣

cardiotocography *n.* the automatic recording in graphic form of fetal heart rate and the amplitude, duration, and frequency of the muscular contractions of the womb during labour.

胎心與分娩力描記法 一種在分娩時自動描記宮縮頻率、幅度、持續時間與胎心的方法。

cardiotomy syndrome (postcardiotomy syndrome) a condition that may develop weeks or months after surgery to the heart and the membrane surrounding it (pericardium) and is characterized by fever and *pericarditis. Pneumonia and pleurisy may form part of the syndrome. It is thought to be an *autoimmune condition and may be recurrent. A similar syndrome (*Dressler's syndrome*) may follow myocardial infarction. It may respond to anti-inflammatory drugs, such as aspirin, indomethacin, or corticosteroids.

心切開綜合徵（心切開後綜合徵） 在心臟與心包手術後數週或數月內發生的一種以發熱與心包炎爲特徵的疾患。有一部分症狀是由胸膜炎與肺炎引起的。人們認爲這是一種自體免疫性疾病，可反復發作。心肌梗塞後可引起同樣的綜合徵（德來斯綜合徵）。阿司匹林、消炎痛與皮質固醇類藥物對之有效。

cardiovascular system (circulatory system) the heart together with two networks of blood vessels – the *systemic circulation and the *pulmonary circulation (see illustration). The cardiovascular system effects the circulation of blood around the body, which brings about transport of nutrients and oxygen to the tissues and the removal of waste products.

心血管系統（循環系統） 心臟與兩套血管網——體循環與肺循環的總稱（見圖）。血液通過心血管系統流遍全身，把營養物質與氧氣輸送到組織，並把廢物帶走。

cardioversion (countershock) *n.* a method of restoring the normal rhythm of the heart in patients with increased heart rate due to arrhythmia. A controlled direct-current shock, synchronized with the R wave of the electrocardiograph, is given through electrodes placed on the chest wall of the anaesthetized patient. The apparatus is called

心復率（抗休克） 一種使患心律不齊而心率增速的病人心率恢復正常的方法。用心復律器（改良型的除顫器）通過置於昏迷病人胸壁上的電極施以有控制的電休克刺激。刺激頻率與心電圖上的R波保持同步。

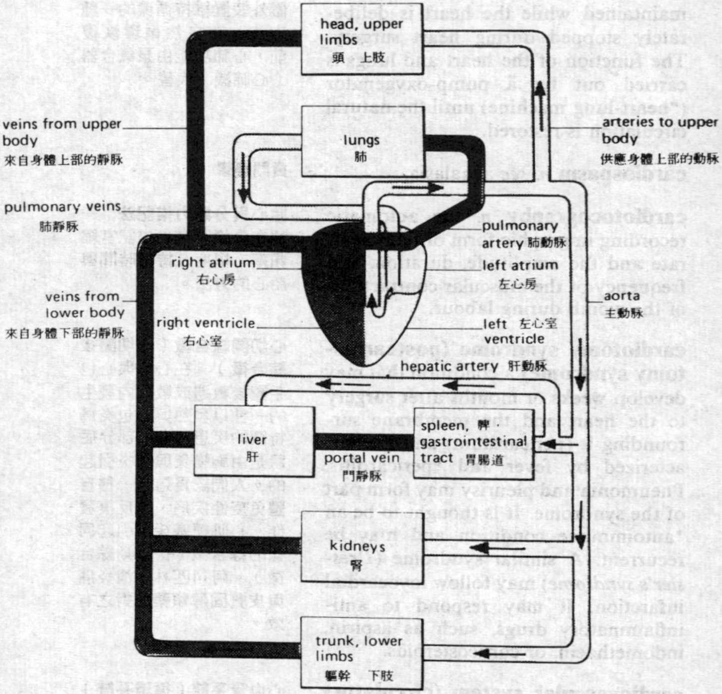

Diagram of the cardiovascular system

心血管系統

a *cardiovertor* and is a modified defibrillator (*see* defibrillation).

caries *n.* decay and crumbling of the substance of a tooth (*see* dental caries) or a bone. —**carious** *adj.*

①齲 ②骨疽

carina *n.* a keel-like structure, such as the keel-shaped cartilage at the bifurcation of the trachea into the two main bronchi.

隆凸 龍骨樣結構。例如：在氣管分成兩枝主支氣管的分叉處的龍骨樣軟骨。

cariogenic *adj.* causing caries, particularly dental caries.

生齲的

carisoprodol *n.* a drug with muscle-relaxant, analgesic, and tranquillizing

異氨甲丙二酯 一種具有鬆弛肌肉、鎮靜與止痛作

action. It is used in the treatment of spastic conditions, such as parkinsonism, and for back pain, sprains, and other injuries. It is administered by mouth; there are few side-effects, but drowsiness or dizziness may occur. Trade names: **Carisoma**, **Rela**, **Soma**.

用的藥物。用於帕金森氏病等痙攣性疾病、捩傷及其它外傷。商品名：肌安寧、異丙安寧、異丙眠爾通。

carminative *n.* a drug that relieves flatulence, used to treat gastric discomfort and colic.

驅風藥 一種消除腹脹的藥物。用以治療胃部不適與絞痛。

carneous mole a fleshy mass that develops from blood clots, membranes, or pieces of placenta left in the womb after abortion.

肉樣胎塊 流產後在子宮中留存的由胎盤碎片、羊膜與血塊混合成的肉樣塊狀物。

carotenaemia *n. see* xanthaemia.

胡蘿蔔素血症

carotene *n.* a yellow or orange plant pigment – one of the carotenoids – that occurs in three forms: alpha (α), beta (β), and gamma (γ). The most important form is β-carotene, which can be converted in the body to retinol (vitamin A). Foods containing β-carotene (milk and some vegetables) are therefore a source of the vitamin.

胡蘿蔔素 一種黃色或橘紅色的植物色素。係胡蘿蔔素類中的一種，有 α、β、γ 三種。β-胡蘿蔔素最重要，在體內可轉化爲維生素A醇。因此含此色素的食物（乳與某些植物）係人體維生素A的來源。

carotenoid *n.* any one of a group of about 100 naturally occurring yellow to red pigments found mostly in plants. The group includes the *carotenes.

胡蘿蔔素類 主要存在於植物中的一組具有自黃色至紅色間不同顏色的色素。共約百餘種，其中包括胡蘿蔔素。

carotid artery either of the two main arteries in the neck whose branches supply the head and neck. The *common carotid artery* arises on the left side directly from the aortic arch and on the right from the innominate artery. They ascend the neck on either side as far as the thyroid cartilage (Adam's apple), where they each divide into two branches, the *internal carotid*, supplying the cerebrum, forehead, nose, eye, and middle ear, and the *external carotid*, sending branches to the face, scalp, and neck.

頸動脉 向頭頸部供應血液的一對大動脉。左頸總動脉直接由主動脉發出，右頸總動脉則發自無名動脉，上升至甲狀軟骨（喉結）處各分爲兩支。頸內動脉向腦部、前額、鼻、眼、中耳供應血液，頸外動脉的分支則佈及面部、頭皮與頸部。

carotid body a small mass of tissue in the carotid sinus containing *chemoreceptors that monitor levels of oxygen, carbon dioxide, and hydrogen ions in the blood. If the oxygen level falls, the chemoreceptors send impulses to the cardiac and respiratory centres in the brain, which promote increases in heart and respiration rates.

頸動脈體 在頸動脈竇中存在的一種含有化學感受器的小體。它能感受血中氧、二氧化碳與氫離子的濃度。如含氧量減少，化學感受器就向腦內心跳中樞與呼吸中樞發放衝動，以加速心跳與呼吸。

carotid sinus a pocket in the wall of the carotid artery, at its division in the neck, containing receptors that monitor blood pressure (*see* baroreceptor). When blood pressure is raised, impulses travel from the receptors to the vasomotor centre in the brain, which initiates a reflex *vasodilatation and slowing of heart rate to lower the blood pressure to normal.

頸動脈竇 頸動脉於分支處的管壁上的小袋。袋內有壓力感受器，血壓上升時衝動自該感受器傳至腦內血管運動中樞，後者引起反射性血管擴張，減慢心率，使血壓下降至正常。

carp- (carpo-) *prefix denoting* the wrist (carpus).

〔前綴〕 **腕**

carpal 1. *adj.* relating to the wrist. **2.** *n.* any of the bones forming the carpus.

①腕的 ②腕骨

carpal tunnel the space between the carpal bones of the wrist and the connective tissue (retinaculum) over the flexor tendons. It contains the flexor tendons and the median nerve.

腕管 腕骨與屈肌腱的結締組織（支持帶）之間的空隙。其中有屈肌腱與正中神經。

carpal tunnel syndrome compression of the median nerve as it enters the palm of the hand (*see* carpal tunnel). This causes pain and numbness in the index and middle fingers and weakness of the abductor muscle of the thumb.

腕管綜合徵 正中神經在進入掌部的經路上受到壓迫產生的症候。食指與中指疼痛、麻木，拇指外展肌無力。

carphology (floccillation) *n.* plucking at the bedclothes by a delirious patient. This is often a sign of extreme exhaustion and may be the prelude to death.

捉空摸牀 譫妄患者做抓被褥狀，通常係極度衰竭的表現，或死亡前兆。

carpopedal spasm *see* spasm.

腕足痙攣

carpus *n.* the eight bones of the wrist (see illustration). The carpus articulates with the metacarpals distally and with the humerus and radius proximally.

腕骨 腕部的八塊骨頭（見圖），遠端與掌骨相關節。

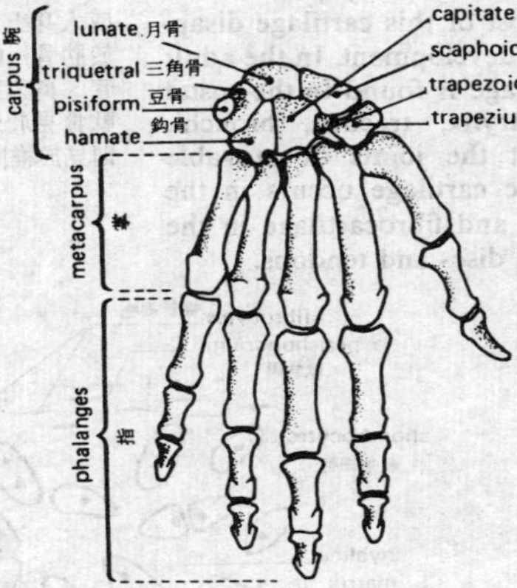

Bones of the left wrist and hand (from the front)

左腕、掌骨前面觀

carrier *n.* **1.** a person who harbours the microorganisms causing a particular disease without experiencing signs or symptoms of infection and who can transmit the disease to others. **2.** (in genetics) a person who bears a gene for an abnormal trait without showing signs of the disorder; the carrier is usually *heterozygous for the gene concerned, which is *recessive. **3.** an animal, usually an insect, that passively transmits infectious organisms from one animal to another or from an animal to man. *See also* vector.

①**病原攜帶者** 帶有某種病原微生物而無傳染病的症狀和體徵，却能把疾病傳染給他人的人。②**帶基因者** （遺傳學）帶有某種異常基因但無疾病表現的人。通常是該隱性基因的雜合子。③**媒介動物** 通常是指一種能把致病微生物從一動物機械地傳給另一動物或人的昆蟲。

cartilage *n.* a dense connective tissue composed of a matrix produced by cells called *chondroblasts*, which become embedded in the matrix as *chondrocytes*. It is a semiopaque grey or white substance, consisting chiefly of *chondroitin sulphate, that is capable of

軟骨 一種緻密結締組織。由成軟骨細胞產生的基質構成。前者變成軟骨細胞，包埋於基質內。軟骨是半透明的灰色或白色的物質，主要含有軟骨素，後者能承受巨大壓

withstanding considerable pressure. There are three types: *hyaline cartilage*, *elastic cartilage*, and *fibrocartilage* (see illustration). In the fetus and infant cartilage occurs in many parts of the body, but most of this cartilage disappears during development. In the adult hyaline cartilage is found in the costal cartilages, larynx, trachea, bronchi, nose, and at the joints of movable bones. Elastic cartilage occurs in the external ear, and fibrocartilage in the intervertebral discs and tendons.

力。共分3種：透明軟骨、彈力軟骨與纖維軟骨（見圖）。在胎兒與幼兒身上多處都有軟骨，但多數到成年期即行消失。在成人身上，透明軟骨可見於肋骨、喉、氣管、支氣管、鼻與可動關節，彈力軟骨見於外耳，纖維軟骨則見於椎間盤與肌腱。

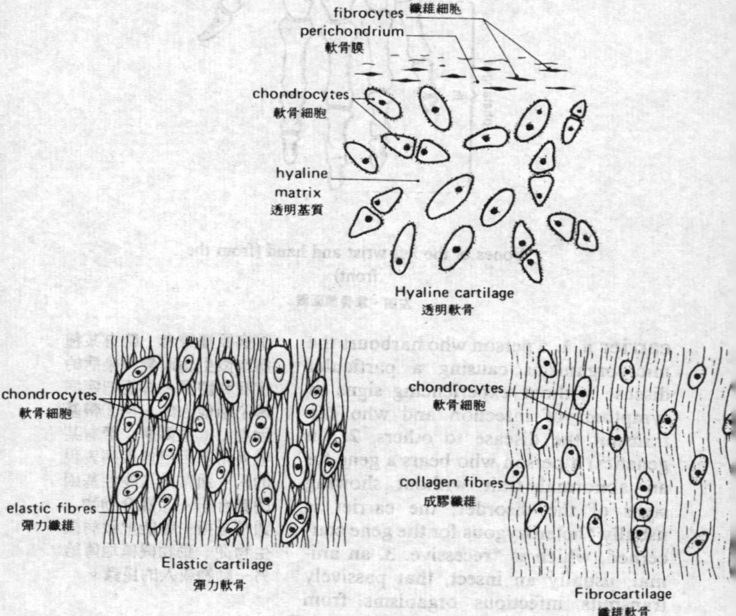

Types of cartilage
軟骨的種類

caruncle *n.* a small red fleshy swelling. The *lacrimal caruncle* is the red prominence at the inner angle of the eye. *Hymenal caruncles* occur around the mucous membrane lining the vaginal opening.

小埠 微小的紅色的肉埠。①**淚埠** 眼內角處的紅色突起。 ②**處女膜痕** 圍繞在陰道口粘膜周圍的阜狀物。

caseation *n.* the breakdown of diseased tissue into a dry cheeselike mass: a type of degeneration associated with tubercular lesions.

乾酪化 病變組織崩解成乾酪樣物質的過程。係結核病變的一種類型。

case control study comparison of a group of people who have a disease with another group free from that disease, in terms of *variables in their backgrounds (e.g. cigarette smoking in those who have died from lung cancer and in those dying from other causes). In the more precise *matched pair study* every individual with the disease is paired with a control matched on the basis of (say) age, sex, or occupation in order to place greater emphasis on a factor for which the pairs have not been matched. *Compare* cohort study, cross-sectional study.

疾病對照研究 將患某病的患者與未患該病患者的不同背景因素進行對比的研究方法。例如：將死於肺癌的吸煙者與死於其它疾病的吸煙者進行對比研究。在更精確的對照研究中，患病組與對照組中每個人的年齡、性別與職業等必須相同，以使他們之間相異的因素突出地暴露出來。

case fatality ratio the number of fatalities from a specified disease in a given period per 100 episodes of the disease arising in the same period. Unless all such deaths occur rapidly after the onset of the disease (e.g. cholera) they are likely to be the outcome of episodes that started in an earlier period (hence the term *ratio* rather than *rate*). Comparison of the annual number of admissions and fatalities in a given hospital in respect of a specific disease is known as the *hospital fatality ratio*.

病死率 某病每100名患者在特定時期內死於該病的數字。除非所有病死者在患病後短期內迅速死亡（如霍亂），則死亡數字很可能包括在此特定的時期以前即已發病的患者（因此用"比"字較用"率"字更確切一些）。醫院中每年某病的入院數與死亡數之比稱爲住院病死率。

casein *n.* a milk protein. Casein is precipitated out of milk in acid conditions or by the action of rennin: it is the principal protein of cheese. Casein is very easily prepared and is useful as a protein supplement, particularly in the treatment of malnutrition.

酪蛋白 一種牛奶蛋白。牛奶遇酸或加凝乳酶可沉澱出酪蛋白。係奶酪的主要蛋白質。製取甚易，可用做蛋白補充品，尤適用於治療營養不良。

case work *see* social services.

個案調查

cassette *n.* (in radiography) a thin light-proof box in which a piece of X-ray film is placed during the taking of an X-ray. It usually contains special screens that fluoresce under the influence of X-rays and so intensify the image that is formed on the film.

貯片盒 在X線攝影時放置X線膠片的薄壁暗盒。通常含有特殊的熒光屏，受X線照射時發出熒光，可使膠片上形成的影象更加清晰。

cast *n.* **1.** a rigid casing for a limb, made with open-woven bandage impregnated with plaster of Paris and applied while wet. A plaster cast is designed to protect a broken bone and prevent movement of the aligned bone ends until healing has progressed sufficiently. **2.** a mass of dead cellular, fatty, and other material that forms within a body cavity and takes its shape. It may then be released and appear elsewhere. For example, *granular casts appearing in the urine indicate kidney disease.

①**模型** 用浸泡着煅石膏的繃帶在未乾前纏繞在肢體上，乾固後形成的筒形石膏夾。用以保護斷骨，防止骨折斷端活動，直至充分癒合。②**管型** 死亡細胞、脂肪及其它的物質在體內某處腔隙內形成與該腔隙形狀相同的物體。該物體可排出，並在其它處所出現。例如：在尿中出現的顆粒管型提示有腎疾患。

castor oil *see* laxative.

蓖麻油

castration *n.* removal of the sex glands (the testes or the ovaries). Castration in childhood causes failure of sexual development but when done in adult life (usually as part of hormonal treatment for cancer) it produces less marked physical changes in both sexes. Castration inevitably causes sterility but it need not cause impotence or loss of sexual desire.

閹 性腺切除（睾丸或卵巢）。幼年期閹割性腺會使性活動能力喪失（通常用做對癌的激素療法的一部分）。成人期閹割後，兩性身體上發生的變化都不顯著，喪失生育能力是肯定的，但不一定會引起陽萎或性慾喪失。

cata- *prefix denoting* downward or against.

〔前綴〕 ①**向下，降** ②**對抗**

catabolism *n.* the chemical decomposition of complex substances by the body to form simpler ones, accompanied by the release of energy. The substances broken down include nutrients in food (carbohydrates, proteins, etc.) as well as the body's storage products (such as glycogen). *See also* metabolism. **—catabolic** *adj.*

分解代謝 在體內發生的由複雜的物質分解成簡單的物質並有能量釋放的化學過程。分解產物包括來自食物（糖、蛋白質等）的營養物質，也包括體內的貯存物質（如糖原）。

catalase *n.* an enzyme, present in many cells (including red blood cells and liver cells), that catalyses the breakdown of hydrogen peroxide.

過氧化氫酶 存在於許多種細胞（包括紅細胞與肝細胞）中的一種催化過氧化氫分解的酶。

catalepsy *n.* the abnormal maintenance of postures or physical attitudes, occurring in *catatonia. These may have arisen spontaneously or they may

木僵 在緊張症中出現的一種保持不變的異樣姿態。可自發出現，亦可由醫生設法誘發。對被動運

be induced by the examiner. There is no resistance to passive movements, which distinguishes it from *flexibilitas cerea.

動無抵抗，以此可與蠟樣屈曲相鑒別。

catalyst *n.* a substance that alters the rate of a chemical reaction but is itself unchanged at the end of the reaction. The catalysts of biochemical reactions are the *enzymes.

觸媒 一種能改變化學反應速度但本身在反應結束時不發生任何變化的物質。催化生化反應的觸媒稱爲酶。

catamenia *n.* *see* menstruation.

月經

cataphoresis *n.* the introduction into the tissues of positively charged ionized substances (cations) by the use of a direct electric current. *See* iontophoresis.

陽離子電泳 用直流電向組織透入帶正電荷的離子（陽離子）的方法。

cataplasia *n.* degeneration of tissues to an earlier developmental form.

組織退化 組織變化成其發育早期階段的形態的現象。

cataplexy *n.* a recurrent condition in which the patient suddenly collapses to the ground without loss of consciousness. Laughter or any strong emotion can provoke an attack. It is usually associated with *narcolepsy.

猝倒 反覆發作的並不伴有意識喪失的突然摔倒的現象。可因大笑或任何劇烈情緒波動所激發。常發生於發作性睡病。

cataract *n.* any opacity in the lens of the eye, resulting in blurred vision. The commonest type is *senile cataract*, seen frequently in the elderly, but some cataracts are congenital, while others are due to metabolic disease, such as *diabetes, *galactosaemia, and *hypocalcaemia. Cataracts may also result from direct or indirect injury to the lens and prolonged exposure of the eye to infrared rays (e.g. *glass-blowers' cataract*) or ionising radiation. Minor degrees of cataract do not necessarily impair vision seriously.
Cataract is treated by surgical removal of the affected lens (*cataract extraction*). The lens is usually removed intact (*intracapsular extraction*), but there are several techniques in which the capsule of the lens is left behind (*extracapsular extraction*).

白內障 眼內晶狀體混濁。可導致視力模糊。最常見的是老年性白內障，常見於老年人，但有些白內障是先天性的。亦可由代謝病引起，如糖尿病、半乳糖血症和低血鈣等。眼睛長期受到紅外線照射或電離輻射以及晶狀體直接與間接的外傷，亦可引起本病。輕度白內障不一定會嚴重影響視力。
治療：手術摘除病變晶狀體（晶狀體摘除術）。通常將晶狀體全部摘除（囊內摘除術），亦可保留晶狀體囊（囊外摘除術）。

catarrh *n.* the excessive secretion of thick phlegm or mucus by the mucous membrane of the nose, nasal sinuses, nasopharynx, or air passages. The term is not used in any precise or scientific sense.

卡他 自鼻腔、鼻竇、鼻咽及氣管黏膜分泌出大量黏液或痰液的現象。此術語含意不精確，科學性不强。

catatonia *n.* a syndrome of motor abnormalities associated with an abnormal mental state. The symptoms may be *excited*: *stereotypy, stilted overactivity, and purposeless violence; or *inhibited*: stupor, *catalepsy, *flexibilitas cerea, and *negativism. Commonly they are features of catatonic *schizophrenia but they are also seen in other conditions, including encephalitis and hysteria. The syndrome can often be modified by *suggestion. The symptoms usually respond transiently to intravenous *barbiturates. The major *tranquillizers are effective therapy, and *electroconvulsive therapy is sometimes used. —**catatonic** *adj.*

緊張症 精神病人出現的一種運動性異常綜合徵。興奮型的有：刻板動作，誇張的過度運動和無目的的暴力行爲。抑制型的有：木僵、蠟樣屈曲和違拗症。通常是緊張型精神分裂症的表現。亦可見於其它症患，如腦炎和癔病。本病可由暗示而緩解。靜注巴比妥類可獲暫時療效。大劑量安定藥有效。有時可用電休克療法。

catchment area the geographic area from which a hospital can expect to receive patients and on which in Britain the designated population of the hospital is based. There is no statutory requirement forcing patients to use the hospital(s) of their area, but a code of zoning practice exists for some specialties (e.g. geriatrics, mental illness). A hospital may have a smaller catchment area (e.g. a National Health Service District) for common specialties than for rarer ones, which may be shared between several districts or regions.

保健地段 在英國實行的按醫院接診患者居住範圍劃分的地區。法律上並不强制規定該地段的患者必須在該醫院看病，但規定某些專科（如老年病、精神病）的保健工作則由該地段醫院負責。各醫院負責一個較小地段內的常見病的接診工作，少見病則由幾個地段內的醫院共同負責。

catecholamines *pl. n.* a group of physiologically important substances, including *adrenaline, *noradrenaline, and *dopamine, having various different roles (mainly as *neurotransmitters) in the functioning of the sympathetic and central nervous systems. Chemically, all contain a benzene ring with adjacent hydroxyl groups (catechol) and an amine group on a side chain.

兒茶酚胺 包括腎上腺素、去甲腎上腺素、多巴胺在內的一組具有重要生理作用的物質。在交感神經與中樞神經系統內各具不同的作用（主要是遞質）。

catgut *n.* a fibrous material prepared from the tissues of animals, usually from the walls of sheep intestines, twisted into strands of different thicknesses and used to sew up wounds (*see* suture) and tie off blood vessels during surgery. The catgut gradually dissolves and is absorbed by the tissues, so that the stitches do not have to be removed later. This also minimizes the possibility of long-term irritation at the site of operation. Some catgut is treated with chromic acid for different periods during manufacture. This gives catguts of various 'lives', lasting for different lengths of time before absorption is complete.

腸線 用動物組織——通常是羊腸壁製成的纖維。將此纖維。將此纖維搓扭成不同粗細的線在手術中用以縫合傷口與結紮血管。腸線可溶解而被組織吸收，因此術後不必拆除，並可減輕對手術區組織的長期刺激。在製造時用鉻酸對腸線進行時間長短不同的處理，使之在完全吸收以前具有長短不同的"生活期"。

catharsis *n.* purging or cleansing out of the bowels by giving the patient a *laxative (cathartic) to stimulate intestinal activity.

導瀉 用輕瀉藥（導瀉藥）刺激腸管運動以清除大便的方法。

cathartic *n. see* laxative.

導瀉藥

cathepsin *n.* one of a group of enzymes found in animal tissues, particularly the spleen, that digest proteins.

組織蛋白酶 存在於動物組織（主要是脾）內的一種消化蛋白質的酶。

catheter *n.* a tube for insertion into a narrow opening so that fluids may be introduced or removed. *Urinary catheters* are passed into the bladder through the urethra to allow drainage of urine in certain disorders and to empty the bladder before abdominal operations.

導管 能插入小孔內以排出液體的管子。導尿管即在患某種疾病時用以通過尿道插入膀胱以引流尿液，或在腹腔手術前排空膀胱的小管。

catheterization *n.* the introduction of a *catheter into a hollow organ. This is most often performod as *urethral catheterization*, when a catheter is introduced into the bladder to relieve obstruction to the outflow of urine. *Cardiac catheterization* entails the introduction of special catheters into the arteries and veins of the arms or legs through which their tips are manipulated into the various chambers of the heart. Cardiac catheterization provides data on pressures and blood flow within the various chambers of the heart. It permits *angiocardiography.

導管插入術 將導管插入空腔器官的方法。最常使用的是導尿管插入術，將導管插入膀胱以解除梗阻排出尿液。心導管插入術是將一特製的導管插入上肢或下肢動脈或靜脈，使其尖端抵達各房室，以測該處的血壓。亦可通過此法行心血管造影。

cation-exchange resins complex insoluble chemical compounds that may be administered with the diet to alter the *electrolyte balance of the body in the treatment of heart, kidney, and metabolic disorders. For example, in patients on a strict low-sodium diet such resins combine with sodium in the food so that it cannot be absorbed and passes out in the faeces.

陽離子交換樹脂 一種與食物一同內服的能改變體內電解質平衡的複雜的不溶性化合物。用以治療心、腎與代謝症患。例如：嚴格進低鹽飲食的患者，用鈉鹽時併用此樹脂，可防止鈉吸收而使之隨糞便排出體外。

CAT scanner *see* computerized axial tomography.

電子計算機軸向體層掃描器

cat-scratch fever an infectious virus disease transmitted to man following injury to the skin by a cat scratch, splinter, or thorn. Mild fever and glandular swelling develop about a week after infection. In some cases serious abscess formation occurs, but generally recovery is complete.

貓抓熱 由於被貓抓傷所致的一種人類病毒性傳染病。感染後約一周有輕度發燒與淋巴結腫大，部分病例有嚴重膿腫形成，但一般均可完全康復。

cauda *n.* a tail-like structure. The *cauda equina* is a bundle of nerve roots from the lumbar, sacral, and coccygeal spinal nerves that descend nearly vertically from the spinal cord until they reach their respective openings in the vertebral column.

尾 尾樣結構。自腰、骶、尾部發出的脊髓神經集合成束稱爲馬尾。它們幾乎呈垂直下降，然後由各相應的椎間孔發出。

caudal *adj.* relating to the lower part or tail end of the body.

①尾的 ②尾側的 ③身體下部的。

caul *n.* **1.** (in obstetrics) a membrane that may cover an infant's head at birth. This membrane is part of the sac (*amnion) that encloses the fetus during pregnancy. **2.** (in anatomy) *see* omentum.

①胎頭羊膜 （產科）分娩時覆蓋胎兒頭部的一層膜。此膜係妊娠期包繞胎兒的羊膜的一部分。 **②大網膜** 解剖學術語。

causal agent a factor associated with the definitive onset of an illness (or other response, including an accident). Examples of causal agents are bacteria, trauma, and noxious agents. The relationship is more direct than in the case of a *risk factor.

致病因素 導致某種疾病（或其它情況，包括意外事故）發生的因素。例如：細菌、外傷、有毒（害）物質等。它與發病的關係比危險因素更爲直接。

causalgia *n.* an intensely unpleasant burning pain felt in a limb where there has been partial damage to the sympa-

灼痛 肢體的感覺神經與交感神經受到部分損傷時產生的一種强烈的燒灼

thetic and somatic sensory nerves. The blood supply to the limb and the growth of the skin and nails may also be abnormal.

痛。該部的血供應與皮膚和指（趾）甲的生長亦可有異常。

caustic *n.* an agent, such as silver nitrate, that causes irritation and burning and destroys tissue. Caustic agents may be used to remove dead skin, warts, etc., but care must be taken not to damage the surrounding area.

腐蝕劑 一種能刺激、燒灼並破壞組織的物質。如硝酸銀。用以去除死皮與疣等。但須注意勿傷及周圍皮膚。

caustic soda *see* sodium hydroxide.

苛性鈉

cauterize *vb.* to destroy tissues by direct application of a heated instrument (known as a *cautery*): used for the removal of small warts or other growths. —**cautery** *n.*

烙 直接使用熱的器具（烙器）破壞組織。用以去除疣與其它小的新生物。

cavernitis *n.* inflammation of the corpora cavernosa of the *penis or the corpus cavernosum of the clitoris.

海綿體炎 陰莖海綿體或陰蒂海綿體炎。

cavernous breathing *see* breath sounds.

空洞性呼吸音

cavernous sinus one of the paired cavities within the *sphenoid bone, at the base of the skull behind the eye sockets, into which blood drains from the brain, eye, nose, and upper cheek before leaving the skull through connections with the internal jugular and facial veins. Through the sinus, in its walls, pass the internal carotid artery and the abducens, oculomotor, trochlear, ophthalmic, and maxillary nerves.

海綿竇 位於顱骨底部眼眶後方的一對腔隙。它們收集來自腦、眼、鼻和頰上部的血液，於離開顱骨前，與頸內靜脉及面靜脉相滙合。

cavity *n.* **1.** (in anatomy) a hollow enclosed area; for example, the abdominal cavity or the buccal cavity (mouth). **2.** (in dentistry) **a.** the hole in a tooth caused by *caries or abrasion. **b.** the hole shaped in a tooth by a dentist to retain a filling.

①**腔** （解剖學）中空封閉的區域。如腹腔與口腔前庭。②**洞** （牙科）有兩種含義。一指齲變或磨損形成的齲洞，二指牙科醫生爲補牙而製備的備填洞。

cavity varnish (in dentistry) a solution of natural or synthetic resin in an organic solvent. It is used as a sealer for amalgam fillings or as a coating over newly inserted cement fillings.

洞襯劑 （牙科）溶於有機溶劑內的天然樹脂或合成樹脂溶液。用以封閉汞合金填料或覆蓋新充填的粘固粉。

CBW (Chemical and Biological Warfare) the use of poison gases and other chemicals, bacteria, viruses, and toxins during war.

化學生物戰 使用毒氣與其它化合物、細菌、病毒與毒劑進行的戰爭。

-cele (-coele) *suffix denoting* swelling, hernia, or tumour. Example: *gastrocele* (hernia of the stomach).

〔前綴〕 **腫物，膨出，疝** 例如：胃疝。

cell *n.* the basic unit of all living organisms, which can reproduce itself exactly (*see* mitosis). Each cell is bounded by a *cell membrane* of lipids and protein, which controls the passage of substances into and out of the cell. Cells contain *cytoplasm, in which are suspended a *nucleus and other structures (*organelles) specialized to carry out particular activities in the cell (see illustration).

細胞 能精確無誤地進行自身增殖的生物體的基本單位。每一細胞必須有一層由脂質與蛋白質組成的細胞膜，以對出入細胞的各種物質進行調節。此外，還有細胞漿，胞漿中有細胞核和執行不同功能的其他結構（細胞器）（見圖）。

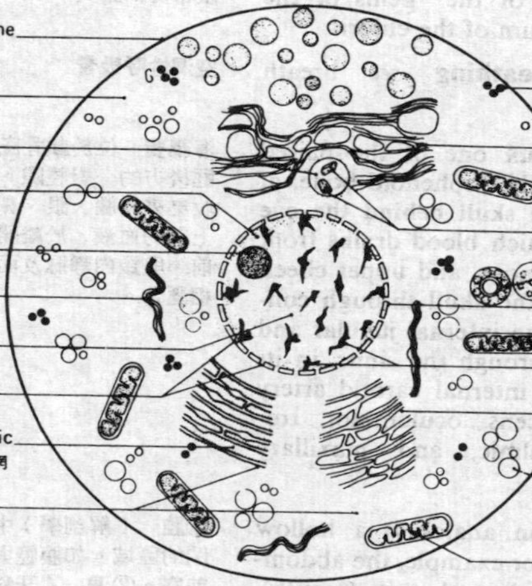

An animal cell (microscopical structure)

動物細胞（顯微鏡下結構）

Complex organisms such as man are built up of millions of cells that are specially adapted to carry out particular functions. The process of cell differentiation begins early in the development of the embryo and cells of a particular type (e.g. blood cells, liver

像人類這樣複雜的機體是由千百萬具有各種特殊功能的細胞組成的。細胞分化早在胚胎發育階段即已開始，某種特殊類型的細胞（如血細胞、肝細胞）只能產生同一類型的細胞。每個細胞含有的染色

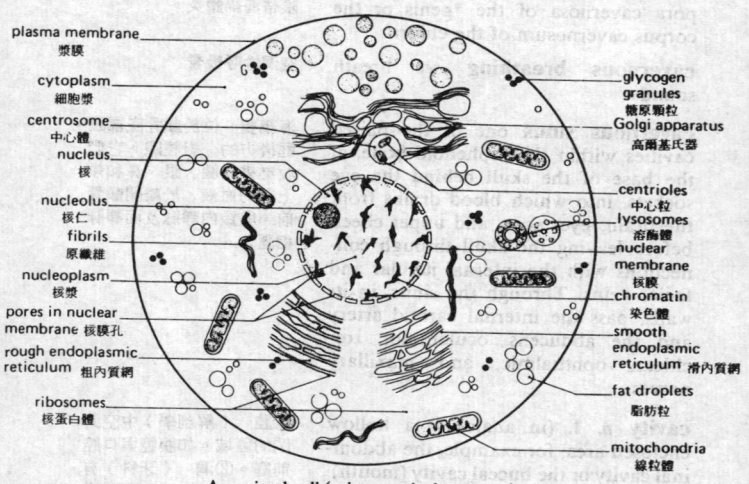

cells) always give rise to cells of the same type. Each cell has a particular number of *chromosomes in its nucleus. The sex cells (sperm and ova) always contain half the number of chromosomes of all the other cells of the body (*see* meiosis); at fertilization a sperm and ovum combine to form a cell with a complete set of chromosomes that will develop into the embryo.

體數都是一定的。性細胞（精子和卵子）的染色體只有其它體細胞的一半。受精時精子與卵子結合成具有一整套染色體的細胞，以後發育成胚胎。

cell body (perikaryon) the enlarged portion of a *neurone (nerve cell), containing the nucleus. It is concerned more with the nutrition of the cell than with propagation of nerve impulses.

胞體（核周體） 神經原（神經細胞）的膨大部份，內含有核。主要司細胞的營養功能，而與神經衝動傳導的關係不大。

cell division reproduction of cells by division first of the chromosomes (karyokinesis) and then of the cytoplasm (cytokinesis). Cell division to produce more body (somatic) cells is by *mitosis; cell division during the formation of gametes is by *meiosis.

細胞分裂 細胞通過分裂進行繁殖的過程。先是發生染色體分裂（核分裂），然後發生細胞漿分裂（胞質分裂）。體細胞通過有絲分裂進行繁殖，性細胞則通過減數分裂形成配子。

cellulitis *n.* inflammation of the connective tissue between adjacent tissues and organs. This is commonly due to bacterial infection and usually requires antibiotic treatment to prevent its spread to the bloodstream.

蜂窩纖炎 毗連的器官與組織間的結締組織的炎症。通常由細菌感染引起，須行抗生素療法，以防炎症沿血流擴散。

cellulose *n.* a carbohydrate consisting of linked glucose units. It is an important constituent of plant cell walls. Cellulose cannot be digested by man and is a component of *dietary fibre (roughage).

纖維素 以葡萄糖爲單位連結成的碳水化合物。是植物細胞壁的重要組成成分。人類不能消化纖維素，它是"食用纖維"（糙食）的成分。

Celsius temperature (centigrade temperature) temperature expressed on a scale in which the melting point of ice is assigned a temperature of 0° and the boiling point of water a temperature of 100°. For many medical purposes this scale has superseded the Fahrenheit scale (*see* Fahrenheit temperature). The formula for converting from Celsius (C) to Fahrenheit (F) is: $F = \frac{9}{5}(C + 32)$.

攝氏溫度 在刻度表上以0度爲冰點、100度爲沸點來表達的溫度。由於多種原因，醫學界多以攝氏溫度表取代華氏溫度表。換算的公式是：

華氏度＝9/5（攝氏度＋32）

cement *n.* **1.** any of a group of materials used in dentistry either as fillings or as *lutes for crowns. Glass ionomer cements are used for filling, and zinc phosphate, zinc polycarboxylate, and glass ionomer cements are used for luting. Zinc oxide–eugenol cements are widely used as temporary fillings. **2.** *see* cementum.

①**黏固粉** 牙科中用做封泥或塡料的物質。聚乙烯搪瓷黏固粉用做塡料。磷酸鋅、聚碳化鋅與聚乙烯搪瓷可用做封泥。丁香酚氧化鋅黏固粉廣泛用做可摘假牙的塡料。②**牙骨質**

cementocyte *n.* a cell found in cementum.

牙骨質細胞 牙骨質中存在的細胞。

cementoma *n.* a benign overgrowth of cementum.

牙骨質瘤 牙骨質的良性腫瘤。

cementum (cement) *n.* a thin layer of hard tissue on the surface of the root of a *tooth. It attaches the fibres of the periodontal membrane to the tooth.

牙骨質 牙根表面的一薄層硬組織。牙周膜纖維通過該層組織固定在牙齒上。

censor *n.* (in psychology) the mechanism, postulated by Freud, that suppresses or modifies desires that are inappropriate or feared. The censor is usually regarded as being located in the *superego but was also described by Freud as being in the *ego itself.

稽查 （心理學）抑制或矯正不恰當的或令人擔憂的慾望的一種心理機制，爲弗洛依德氏用語。通常認爲這種機制存在於超我，但弗洛依德氏認爲在自我中也存在。

-centesis *suffix denoting* puncture or perforation. Example: *amniocentesis* (surgical puncture of the amnion).

〔前綴〕 **穿刺術** 例如：羊膜穿刺。

centi- *prefix denoting* one hundredth or a hundred.

〔前綴〕 **百分之一**

centigrade temperature *see* Celsius temperature.

百度溫標 即攝氏溫度。

Central Manpower Committee *see* manpower committee.

中央衛生人力委員會

central nervous system (CNS) the *brain and the *spinal cord, as opposed to the cranial and spinal nerves and the *autonomic nervous system, which together form the *peripheral nervous system*. The CNS is responsible for the *integration of all nervous activities.

中樞神經系統 與組成周圍神經系統的腦神經、脊髓神經和自主神經相對應，腦與脊髓組成了中樞神經系統。中樞神經系統擔任全部神經活動的整合功能。

centre *n.* (in neurology) a collection of neurones (nerve cells) whose activities control a particular function. The *respiratory* and *cardiovascular centres*, for

中樞 （神經學）控制特定的生理功能活動的神經元（神經細胞）集團。例如：呼吸中樞與心血管運

example, are regions in the lower brainstem that control the movements of respiration and the functioning of the circulatory system, respectively.

動中樞存在於腦幹下部，各自控制着呼吸運動與循環系統的功能。

centrencephalic *adj.* (in electroencephalography) describing discharges that can be recorded synchronously from all parts of the brain. The source of this activity is in the *reticular formation of the midbrain. *Centrencephalic epilepsy* is associated with a congenital predisposition to fits.

中腦型 （腦電圖）用以描述自腦各部同時記錄下來的放電現象的某種特徵。此型放電現象來源於中腦網狀結構。中腦型癲癇的發作有遺傳因素。

centri- *prefix denoting* centre. Example: *centrilobular* (in the centre of a lobule (especially of the liver)).

〔前綴〕 **中心的，中央的** 例如：小葉中心的（尤指肝臟內的）。

centrifugal *adj.* moving away from a centre, as from the brain to the peripheral tissues.

離中的 離開中央的。例如：自腦走向末梢組織的。

centrifuge *n.* a device for separating components of different densities in a liquid, using centrifugal force. The liquid is placed in special containers that are spun at high speed around a central axis.

離心機 利用離心力對液體中不同密度的成分進行分離的器械。將液體置於特制容器內，繞中心軸高速旋轉。

centriole *n.* a small particle found in the cytoplasm of cells, near the nucleus. Centrioles are involved in the formation of the *spindle and aster during cell division. During interphase there are usually two centrioles in the *centrosome; when cell division occurs these separate and move to opposite sides of the nucleus, and the spindle is formed between them.

中心粒 存在於細胞漿中的小粒。靠近細胞核。與細胞分裂時紡錘體及星體的形成有關。於分裂間期在中心體中通常有兩顆中心粒。細胞分裂時兩者分開並移至核的兩側，其間形成紡錘體。

centripetal *adj.* moving towards a centre, as from the peripheral tissues to the brain.

向中的 由末梢走向中央的。例如：由末梢組織走向腦髓的。

centromere (kinetochore) *n.* the part of a chromosome that joins the two *chromatids to each other and becomes attached to the spindle during *mitosis and *meiosis. When chromosome division takes place the centromeres split longitudinally.

着絲粒（動原體） 聯結着兩個染色單體的染色體部分。在有絲分裂與減數分裂時附着於紡錘體。染色體分裂時着絲粒沿縱向分裂。

centrosome (centrosphere) *n.* an area of clear cytoplasm, found next to

中心體（中心球） 在未進行分裂的細胞核附近的

the nucleus in nondividing cells, that contains the *centrioles. 細胞漿的澄清區域。內含中心粒。

centrosphere *n.* **1.** an area of clear cytoplasm seen in dividing cells around the poles of the spindle. **2.** *see* centrosome. ①**中心球** 細胞分裂時在紡錘體兩極周圍的細胞漿中出現的澄清區域。②**中心體**。

centrum *n.* (*pl.* **centra**) the solid rod-shaped central portion of a *vertebra. **椎體** 椎骨中央實心的棒狀部分。

cephal- (cephalo-) *prefix denoting* the head. Example: *cephalalgia* (pain in). 〔前綴〕 **頭部** 例如：頭痛。

cephalad *adj.* towards the head. **向頭側的**

cephalexin *n.* a semisynthetic antibiotic, administered by mouth, used in the treatment of a variety of infections. *See* cephalosporin. Trade names: **Ceporex, Keflex.** **頭孢氨苄** 半合成抗生素。口服。用於各類感染。商品名：先鋒黴素IV，頭孢立新。

cephalhaematoma *n.* an egg-sized swelling on the head caused by a collection of bloody fluid between one of the skull bones (usually the *parietal bone) and its covering membrane (periosteum). It is most commonly seen in newborn infants delivered with the aid of forceps or subjected to pressures during passage through the birth canal. No treatment is necessary and the swelling disappears in a few weeks. A cephalhaematoma in an older baby or child is evidence of some recent injury to the head; occasionally an unsuspected fracture is revealed on X-ray. **頭顱血腫** 在某片顱骨（多爲頂骨）與其骨膜之間因血液集聚而出現的雞蛋大小的腫物。通常見於用產鉗助產或通過產道時受壓的新生兒。不必治療。腫物幾周內即行消失。年長兒的頭顱血腫是近期頭部外傷引起。X光下偶可意外發現骨折。

cephalic *adj.* of or relating to the head. **頭的，頭側的**

cephalic index a measure of the shape of a skull, commonly used in *craniometry: the ratio of the greatest breadth, multiplied by 100, to the greatest length of the skull. *See also* brachycephaly, dolichocephaly. **顱骨指數** 在顱骨測量術中用以表達頭顱形狀的一種指數：最大顱寬×100與最大顱長之比。

cephalic version a procedure for turning a fetus that is lying in a breech or transverse position so that its head will enter the birth passage first. It cannot be performed after labour is well advanced. **胎頭倒轉術** 臀位或橫位時旋轉兒頭使之進入產道的一種手法。在分娩進程中如爲時過晚則不能施行。

cephalin *n.* one of a group of *phospholipids that are constituents of cell membranes and are particularly abundant in the brain.

腦磷脂 磷脂類的一種。細胞膜的成分。腦內含量尤豐。

cephalocele *n. see* neural tube defects.

腦膨出

cephaloglycin *n.* a semisynthetic antibiotic, given by mouth for the treatment of urinary tract infections. The main side-effects are gastrointestinal irritation and allergy. Cross-sensitivity with the penicillins may occur and cephaloglycin should be used with caution in patients known to be sensitive to these drugs. *See* cephalosporin.

頭孢甘氨酸 一種半合成抗生素。口服。治療尿道感染。主要副作用爲消化道刺激與過敏反應。與青黴素可發生交叉過敏反應，故對青黴素過敏者用本品時需愼重。

cephalogram *n.* a special standardized X-ray picture that can be used to measure alterations in the growth of skull bones.

腦圖 用以檢查顱骨生長情況的標準化的腦X線圖像。

cephalometry *n.* the study of facial growth by examination of standardized lateral radiographs of the head. It is used mainly for diagnosis in *orthodontics.

顱測量術 用頭部標準側位X線攝影檢查頜面部發育情況的方法。主要用於口腔正畸科診斷。

cephaloridine *n.* a semisynthetic antibiotic, given by intravenous or intramuscular injection. It is used in the treatment of a variety of severe infections, including those of bones, joints, the bloodstream, and the urinary and respiratory tracts. *See* cephalosporin. Trade name: **Loridine**.

頭孢噻啶 一種半合成抗生素。靜注或肌注。用以治療各種嚴重感染，包括骨、關節、血流、泌尿道和呼吸道。商品名：頭孢黴素Ⅱ，先鋒黴素Ⅱ。

cephalosporin *n.* any one of a group of semisynthetic antibiotics, derived from the mould *Cephalosporium*, which are effective against a wide range of microorganisms and are therefore used in a variety of infections (*see* cephalexin, cephaloglycin, cephaloridine, cephalothin sodium). Cross-sensitivity with penicillin may occur and the principal side-effects are allergic reactions and irritation of the digestive tract.

頭孢菌素 自頭孢子菌屬提取的一組半合成抗生素。抗菌譜極廣，因而用於各種感染。與青黴素可產生交叉過敏反應，主要副作用爲過敏反應與消化道刺激。

cephalothin sodium a semisynthetic antibiotic, given by intramuscular or

頭孢噻吩鈉 一種半合成抗生素。肌注或靜注。用

intravenous injection in the treatment of a number of infections. *See* cephalosporin. Trade name: **Keflin**.

於多種感染。商品名：頭孢菌素 IV 鈉。

cercaria *n.* (*pl.* **cercariae**) the final larval stage of any parasitic trematode (*see* fluke). The cercariae, which have tails but otherwise resemble the adults, are released into water from the snail host in which the parasite undergoes part of its development. Several thousand cercariae may emerge from a single snail in a day.

尾蚴　各種寄生性吸蟲幼蟲發育的最後階段。尾蚴除有尾外，其他方面都與成蟲類似，在宿主螺類體內完成部分發育階段後，脫離宿主進入水中，每日每隻釘螺可產生數千隻尾蚴。

cerebellum *n.* the largest part of the hindbrain, bulging back behind the pons and the medulla oblongata and overhung by the occipital lobes of the cerebrum. Like the cerebrum, it has an outer grey cortex and a core of white matter. Three broad bands of nerve fibres – the inferior, middle, and superior cerebellar peduncles – connect it to the medulla, the pons, and the midbrain respectively. It has two hemispheres, one on each side of the central region (the *vermis*), and its surface is thrown into thin folds called *folia* (see illustration). Within lie four pairs of nuclei.
The cerebellum is essential for the maintenance of muscle tone, balance, and the synchronization of activity in

小腦　腦中的最大的部分。突出於橋腦、延腦背側，其上方為大腦枕葉遮蓋。與大腦一樣，小腦也有外層的灰質和內部的白質。有三條粗大的神經纖維束（上、中、下小腦腳）分別與中腦、橋腦、延腦相聯繫。在中央部（蚓部）兩側各有一個半球，表面形成微細的皺褶，稱為葉（見圖），內部含有四對神經核。小腦在維持肌緊張、平衡與各組肌肉的同步活動中起重要作用，使隨意運動變得協調一致，但不能引起運動，在意識、感覺及智力活動方面亦無作用。

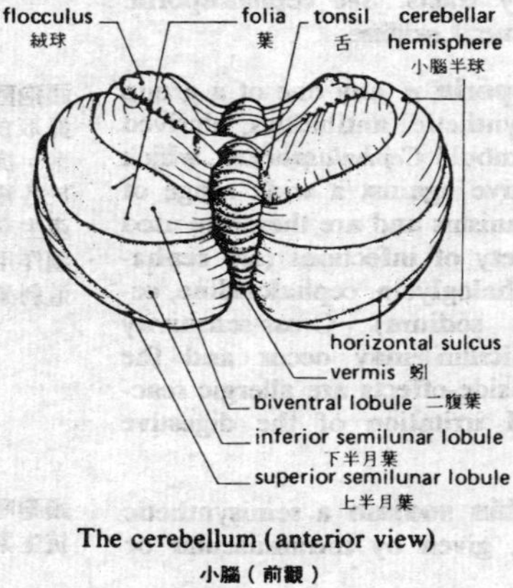

The cerebellum (anterior view)
小腦（前觀）

groups of muscles under voluntary control, converting muscular contractions into smooth coordinated movement. It does not, however, initiate movement and plays no part in the perception of conscious sensations or in intelligence. —**cerebellar** *adj.*

cerebr- (cerebri-, cerebro-) *prefix denoting* the cerebrum or brain.

〔前綴〕 **大腦，腦**

cerebral aqueduct (aqueduct of Sylvius) the narrow channel, containing cerebrospinal fluid, that connects the third and fourth *ventricles of the brain.

大腦導水管 溝通第三腦室與第四腦室的狹窄的管道。內含腦脊液。

cerebral cortex the intricately folded outer layer of the *cerebrum, making up some 40% of the brain by weight and composed of an estimated 15 thousand million neurones (*see* grey matter). This is the part of the brain most directly responsible for consciousness, with essential roles in perception, memory, thought, mental ability, and intellect, and it is responsible for initiating voluntary activity. It has connections, direct or indirect, with all parts of the body. The folding of the cortex provides a large surface area, the greater part lying in the clefts (*sulci*), which divide the upraised convolutions (*gyri*). On the basis of its microscopic appearance in section, the cortex is mapped into *Brodmann's areas; it is also divided into functional regions; including *motor cortex, *sensory cortex, and *association areas. Within, and continuous with it, lies the *white matter, through which connection is made with the rest of the nervous system.

大腦皮質 呈密集皺褶外觀的大腦外層。約佔腦重的40%，由大約150億個神經元組成。是腦部直接承擔意識功能的部位，在感覺、記憶、思維、精神活動及智力活動中起重要作用，同時又是產生隨意運動的所在。它與全身各部都有直接的或間接的聯繫。皺褶的皮質提供了廣大的表面面積，在隆起的腦廻之間的腦溝有着更爲廣大的表面。根據切片在顯微鏡下所見，皮質可按布勞德曼氏法劃分成若干區域。亦可按功能劃分爲運動區、感覺區與聯繫區等。在其內方，有白質向下延續，與神經系統其他部分相聯繫。

cerebral haemorrhage bleeding from a cerebral artery into the tissue of the brain. It is usually caused by degenerative disease of the blood vessels and high blood pressure. The extent and severity of the symptoms depend upon the site and volume of the haemorrhage; they vary from a transient weak-

腦出血 血液自腦血管流出到腦組織內的現象。通常由血管變性性病變或高血壓引起。症狀的多少與嚴重程度取決於出血的部位與出血量。有一過性衰弱或麻木感直至深度昏迷或死亡等不同表現。

ness or numbness to profound coma and death. *See also* atheroma, hypertension, stroke.

cerebral hemisphere one of the two paired halves of the *cerebrum.

大腦半球

cerebral palsy a developmental abnormality of the brain resulting in weakness and incoordination of the limbs. The brain damage may be caused by injury during birth, haemorrhage, lack of oxygen before birth, meningitis, viral infection, or faulty development. The most common disability is a *spastic paralysis (an affected child is called a *spastic*), which may slowly increase from contractures to cause fixed deformities of the limbs. Defective sensory perception, including lack of balance, is always present in some degree, and intelligence is often impaired. Posture and speech may be severely affected. Other disabilities that may occur include involuntary writhing movements (*athetosis) and epilepsy. Management of cerebral palsy is aimed at improving movement (by physiotherapy and other means), combined with prevention or surgical amelioration of fixed deformities due to muscle imbalance and the judicious use of appliances or locomotor aids. Speech therapy may also be required.

大腦性麻痹 一種能引起肢體運動障礙與共濟失調的大腦發育異常。此種腦疾患可由產傷、出血、產前缺氧、腦炎、病毒感染或發育缺陷引起。最多見的是痙攣性麻痹（此種患兒稱爲痙攣兒），攣縮的肢體可逐漸導致肢體畸形。常有一定程度的感覺障礙與平衡障礙，智能亦常受損。姿態與語言皆有嚴重異常。其他異常表現有不自主的扭曲運動（手足徐動症）與癲癇等。治療目的在於改善運動功能（用理療或其他方法），預防或用外科方法糾正肢體因肌張力失衡導致的永久性畸形，合理使用活動輔助裝置。

cerebral tumour an abnormal multiplication of brain cells. This forms a swelling that compresses or destroys the healthy brain cells and – because of the rigid nature of the skull – increases the pressure on the brain tissue. Malignant tumours grow rapidly, spreading through the otherwise normal brain tissue and causing progressive neurological disability. Benign tumours grow slowly and compress the brain tissue, sometimes causing epileptic fits.

腦腫瘤 一部分腦細胞異常增殖的現象。由此產生的腫物破壞或壓迫健康的腦細胞。顱骨是堅硬性的組織，因此腫物就增加對腦組織的壓力。惡性腫瘤生長迅速，向正常腦組織不斷擴散，引起進行性神經症狀。良性腫瘤生長緩慢，壓迫腦組織時可引起癲癇發作。

cerebration *n.* **1.** the functioning of the brain as a whole. **2.** the unconscious activities of the brain.

精神活動 ①腦的全部功能活動。 ②腦的潛意識活動。

cerebroside *n.* one of a group of compounds occurring in the *myelin sheaths of nerve fibres. They are *glycolipids, containing *sphingosine, a fatty acid, and a sugar (usually galactose or glucose).

腦苷 存在於神經纖維髓鞘中的一種化合物。係糖脂類，含有脂肪酸鞘氨醇與糖（多爲半乳糖或葡萄糖）。

cerebrospinal fever (spotted fever) a type of *meningitis caused by the bacterium *Neisseria meningitidis.* Bacteria are transmitted by coughing and sneezing: outbreaks occur most commonly in overcrowded conditions, and children are more susceptible than adults. After an incubation period of 3–5 days, symptoms appear suddenly, including severe headache, fever, stiffness of the neck muscles, and a rash of small red spots on the trunk. Occasionally the disease enters a chronic state in which deafness, blindness, and serious mental deterioration may occur. Without treatment death can occur within a week, but administration of penicillin or sulphonamide drugs is usually effective.

流行性腦膜炎（斑疹熱） 由奈瑟氏腦膜炎菌屬引起的一種腦膜炎。細菌通過咳嗽與噴嚏傳播。暴發流行多見於密集人羣。兒童較成人易感。經過3～5天潛伏期，症狀突然出現，有劇烈頭痛、發燒、項強和軀幹部細小點狀紅色皮疹，偶可轉爲慢性，出現聾、盲及重症精神變態。如不治療一週內即可死亡，但使用青黴素與磺胺類藥物每可奏效。

cerebrospinal fluid (CSF) the clear watery fluid that surrounds the brain and spinal cord. It is contained in the *subarachnoid space and circulates in the *ventricles of the brain and in the central canal of the spinal cord. The brain floats in the fluid (its weight so being reduced from about 1400 g to less than 100 g) and is cushioned by it from contact with the skull when the head is moved vigorously. The CSF is secreted by the *choroid plexuses in the ventricles, circulates through them to reach the subarachnoid space, and is eventually absorbed into the bloodstream through the *arachnoid villi. Its normal contents are glucose, salts, enzymes, and a few white cells, but no red blood cells.

腦脊液 存在於脊髓周圍的澄清水樣液體。它在蛛網膜下腔內循環於腦室與脊髓中央管之間。腦髓即懸浮於該液體內（因此腦髓的重量自1400 g 減輕至100 g 以下）。頭部劇烈運動時，腦脊液可在腦髓顱骨之間起到緩衝作用。腦脊液由腦室內的脉絡叢分泌，通過腦室循環至蛛網膜下腔，最終由蛛網膜絨毛吸收入血液。正常時含有葡萄糖、鹽、酶及少量白細胞，但無紅細胞。

cerebrovascular disease any disorder of the blood vessels of the brain and its covering membranes (men-

腦血管疾病 腦與腦膜血管的疾病。多由動脉粥樣硬化與/或高血壓引起。

inges). Most cases are due to atheroma and/or hypertension, clinical effects being caused by rupture of diseased blood vessels (*cerebral or *subarachnoid haemorrhage) or inadequacy of the blood supply to the brain (ischaemia), due to cerebral thrombosis or embolism. The term *cerebrovascular accident* is sometimes given to the clinical syndrome accompanying a sudden and severe attack, which leads to a *stroke.

病變血管破裂（腦出血或蛛網膜下出血）或由腦栓塞或腦血栓引起的腦部供血不足可產生種種臨床表現。腦血管意外一詞有時用於表達突發的、嚴重的腦卒中綜合征。

cerebrum (telencephalon) *n.* the largest and most highly developed part of the brain, composed of the two *cerebral hemispheres*, separated from each other by the *longitudinal fissure* in the midline (see illustration). Each hemisphere has

大腦（終腦） 腦的最大的、發育程度最高的部分。由自中線縱裂分開的兩側大腦半球組成（見圖）。每側半球具有灰質外層（大腦皮質），其下

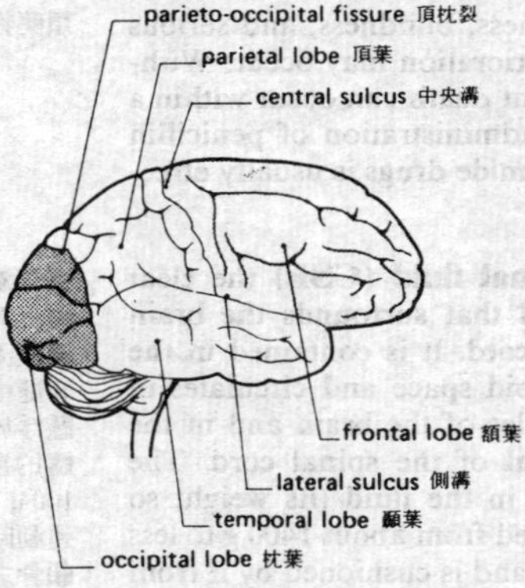

Lobes of the cerebrum (from the right side)

大腦葉（右面觀）

an outer layer of grey matter, the *cerebral cortex, below which lies white matter containing the *basal ganglia. Connecting the two hemispheres at the bottom of the longitudinal fissure is the *corpus callosum*, a massive bundle of nerve fibres. Within each hemisphere is a crescent-shaped fluid-filled cavity (lateral *ventricle), connected to the central third ventricle in the *dienceph-

爲白質，白質內含有基底神經節。在縱裂底部有由神經纖維組成的粗大的神經束（胼胝體）將兩側半球聯結起來。各半球內有新月形的、充滿液體的腔（側腦室），與間腦的第三腦室相通。大腦產生並協調身體的全部隨意運動，主宰神經系統低級部

alon. The cerebrum is responsible for the initiation and coordination of all voluntary activity in the body and for governing the functioning of lower parts of the nervous system. The cortex is the seat of all intelligent behaviour. —**cerebral** *adj.*

位的種種功能活動。大腦皮層是智力活動的部位。

cerumen (earwax) *n.* the waxy material that is secreted by the sebaceous glands in the external auditory meatus of the outer ear. Its function is to protect the delicate skin that lines the inside of the meatus.

耵聹 由外耳道皮脂腺分泌的蠟樣物質。其作用是保護外耳道表面的脆嫩的皮膚。

cervic- (cervico-) *prefix denoting* **1.** the neck. Example: *cervicodynia* (pain in). **2.** the cervix, especially of the uterus. Example: *cervicectomy* (surgical removal of).

〔前綴〕**頸** ①頭頸，如頸痛。②頸部，尤指子宮頸部，如宮頸切除術。

cervical *adj.* **1.** of or relating to the neck. **2.** of, relating to, or affecting the cervix (neck region) of an organ, especially the cervix of the womb.

①頸的 ②頸部的 某器官頸部的，尤指子宮頸部的。

cervical cancer cancer in the neck (cervix) of the womb. The growth can be detected at an early stage by periodic microscopical examination of cells released from the affected region (*see* cervical smear), and it can then be eradicated before it has been able to spread. Vaginal discharge, especially with blood, may be a symptom.

宮頸癌 子宮頸部的癌。對病變部位定期進行顯微鏡細胞學檢查（宮頸塗片）可早期發現，因此可在其擴散前早期切除。陰道分泌物增加係本病症狀。血性分泌物尤具特徵性。

cervical smear a specimen of cellular material scraped from the neck (cervix) of the womb and examined under a microscope in order to determine whether cancer is present.

宮頸塗片 塗擦宮頸所得的細胞學標本，用以鏡檢確定有否癌存在。

cervical vertebrae the seven bones making up the neck region of the *backbone. The first cervical vertebra – the *atlas* – consists basically of a ring of bone that supports the skull by articulating with the occipital condyles (*see* occipital bone). The second vertebra – the *axis* – has an upward-pointing process (the *odontoid process* or *dens*) that forms a pivot on which the atlas

頸椎 組成脊椎頸部的7塊骨頭。第一塊爲寰椎，係一環狀骨，與枕髁相關節以支撐顱骨；第二塊爲樞椎，有一向上的尖突（齒突）形成支軸，寰椎可在此軸上旋轉，頭部因之可以轉動。

can rotate, enabling the head to be turned. *See also* vertebra.

cervicitis *n.* inflammation of the neck (cervix) of the womb.

宮頸炎

cervix *n.* a necklike part, especially the *cervix uteri*, the narrow passage at the lower end of the uterus (womb), which connects with the vagina. Its cavity is normally filled with mucus, the viscosity of which changes throughout the menstrual cycle. The cervix is capable of very wide dilation during childbirth.

頸部 頸樣部分。尤指宮頸，即子宮下端與陰道相連接的狹窄通道。頸腔內通常充滿黏液，其黏稠度在月經週期中有所變化。分娩時宮頸可極度擴張。

cestode *n. see* tapeworm.

絛蟲

cetrimide *n.* a detergent disinfectant, used for cleansing skin surfaces and wounds, sterilizing surgical instruments and babies' napkins, and in shampoos. There are few adverse reactions from external application; most toxic effects are due to poisoning from ingestion. Trade name: **Cetavlon**.

溴化十六烷基三甲銨 防腐除污劑。用於清洗皮膚表面和傷口、消毒外科器械與嬰兒尿布，亦用於洗髮劑中。外用時副作用極少。誤服則有强烈毒性作用。商品名：溴棕三甲銨。

cetylpyridinium *n.* a detergent disinfectant, used for the disinfection of skin, wounds, and burns and as a mouthwash.

十六烷基吡啶 防腐除污劑。用於皮膚傷口與燒傷創面的消毒。亦可用做含漱劑。

Chagas' disease a disease caused by the protozoan parasite **Trypanosoma cruzi*. It is transmitted to man when the trypanosomes, present in the faeces of nocturnal bloodsucking *reduviid bugs, come into contact with wounds and scratches on the skin or the delicate internal tissues of the nose and mouth. The presence of the parasite in the heart muscles and central nervous system results in serious inflammation and lesions, which can prove fatal. The disease, limited to poor rural areas of South and Central America, is especially prevalent in children and young adults. There is no effective treatment. *See also* trypanosomiasis.

恰加斯氏病 由寄生性原蟲克氏錐蟲引起的疾病。病原體存在於夜間吸血的錐鼻屬蝽的大便內，通過傷口、搔抓處皮膚或口鼻等脆弱的內部組織傳入人體。存在於心臟與中樞神經系統的寄生蟲可引起致死的嚴重炎症與病損。本病僅出現於中美、南美的貧困區，主要見於兒童與青、中年。無特效療法。

chaining *n.* a technique of *behaviour modification in which a complex skill is taught by being broken down into its separate components, which are gradu-

連鎖法 一種行為矯正療法。在教授患者一種複雜的技能時，先把這種技能分解成各個單獨的成分進

ally built up into the full sequence. Usually the last component in the sequence is taught first, as it is this component that is followed by *reinforcement: this is termed *backwards chaining*.

行教授，然後才逐漸把它們建立成完整的程序。通常首先教授程序中的最後的一個成分，因爲緊跟這個成分之後就可進行强化。這種方法稱爲逆向連鎖法。

chalazion (meibomian cyst) *n.* a swollen sebaceous gland in the eyelid, caused by chronic inflammation following blockage of the gland's duct. The gland becomes converted into a jelly-like mass, producing disfigurement of the lid. It may become secondarily infected, when it will be painful and may discharge. Treatment is by application of antibiotic ointments or surgical incision and curettage of the gland.

霰粒腫（瞼板腺囊腫） 眼瞼皮脂腺由於慢性炎症引起的腫脹。係腺管阻塞的後果。腺體變成膠凍樣物質，眼瞼亦隨之變形。可因繼發感染而導致疼痛與分泌物增加。治療：抗生素類油膏外用，外科切開，腺體刮治。

chalicosis *n.* pneumoconiosis occurring in stone cutters: a variety of *silicosis. The term is not in current use.

石末肺 發生於石匠的一種肺石末沉着病。矽肺的一種。此詞現已廢用。

chancre *n.* a painless ulcer that develops on the lips, penis, urethra, or eyelid as the primary symptom of such infections as sleeping sickness and syphilis.

下疳，初瘡 發生在唇、陰莖、尿道或眼瞼上的疼痛性潰瘍。係昏睡性腦炎與梅毒等傳染病的初發症狀。

chancroid *n. see* soft sore.

軟下疳

Charcot-Leyden crystals fine colourless sharp-pointed crystals seen in the sputum of asthmatics.

夏-萊二氏晶體 哮喘患者痰液中出現的一種細小、無色、尖形的晶體。

Charcot-Marie-Tooth disease (peroneal muscular atrophy) an inherited disease of the peripheral nerves causing a gradually progressive weakness and wasting of the muscles of the legs and the lower part of the thighs. The hands and arms are eventually affected.

夏-馬-圖三氏病（腓骨肌萎縮） 一種能引起大腿下端與小腿肌肉漸進性無力與萎縮的遺傳性周圍神經疾患。最後，病變亦將蔓延至上肢與手部。

Charcot's joint a damaged, swollen, and deformed joint, often the knee, resulting from repeated minor injuries of which the patient is unaware because the nerves that normally register pain

夏科氏關節 由於反覆輕微外傷引起的關節腫脹與變形。通常發生在膝關節。因爲痛覺神經喪失功能，患者於受傷時並不感到疼痛。本病可見於梅

are not functioning. The condition may occur in syphilis, diabetes mellitus, and syringomyelia.

毒、糖尿病與脊髓空洞症。

Charnley clamps parallel metal rods driven through the ends of two bones that are to be joined to form an *arthrodesis. The rods are connected on each side of the joint by bolts bearing wing nuts; tightening of the screw arrangements forces the surfaces of the bones together. When the two bones have joined, by growth and reshaping, the clamps can be removed.

查恩氏鉗 爲固定關節而分別釘入兩骨端的一對相互平行的金屬鑽桿。鑽桿聯軸節處皆由有翼狀螺母的螺釘相連接。扭緊螺釘可使兩側骨面靠攏。當兩骨生長成形而融合時，即可拆除該鉗。

cheil- (cheilo-) *prefix denoting* the lip(s). Example: *cheiloplasty* (plastic surgery of).

〔前綴〕**唇** 例如唇成形術。

cheilitis *n.* inflammation of the lips.

唇炎

cheiloplasty *n. see* labioplasty.

唇成形術

cheiloschisis *n. see* harelip.

唇裂 兔唇

cheilosis *n.* swollen cracked bright-red lips. This is a common symptom of many nutritional disorders, including ariboflavinosis (vitamin B_2 deficiency).

唇乾裂 唇呈鮮紅色，乾裂，腫脹。許多營養不良疾患如核黃素缺乏（維生素 B_2 缺乏）的常見症狀。

cheir- (cheiro-) *prefix denoting* the hand(s). Examples: *cheiralgia* (pain in); *cheiroplasty* (plastic surgery of).

〔前綴〕**手** 例如手痛、手成形術。

cheiropompholyx *n.* a type of eczema affecting the sides and fronts of the palms and fingers, with a similar distribution on the feet. The thickness of the skin in these areas prevents the eczema vesicles from breaking and eventually the skin peels after a period of intense itching. Attacks start suddenly, often in the summer, and last up to six weeks. Secondary infection is common.

掌蹠汗疱 在手掌與足蹠掌部、側部及指間出現的一種濕疹。這些部位皮膚較厚，濕疹水疱不能破裂，故爾在劇烈搔癢之後出現脫皮現象。發病突然，通常在夏季，持續約六週。常見繼發感染。

chelating agent a chemical compound that forms complexes by binding metal ions. Some chelating agents, including *desferrioxamine and *penicillamine, are drugs used to treat metal poisoning: the metal is bound to the drug and excreted safely. Chelating

螯合劑 能把金屬離子螯合成絡合物的化合物。有些螯合劑如去鐵胺、青黴胺等用於治療金屬中毒。金屬與此類藥物結合而安全排出體外。酶的活性中心亦常爲螯合劑。

agents often form the active centres of enzymes.

cheloid *n. see* keloid.

瘢痕疙瘩

chem- (chemo-) *prefix* denoting chemical or chemistry.

〔前綴〕 **化合物，化學**

chemoreceptor *n.* a cell or group of cells that responds to the presence of specific chemical compounds by initiating an impulse in a sensory nerve. Chemoreceptors are found in the taste buds and in the mucous membranes of the nose. *See also* receptor.

化學感受器 能對某種化學物質產生反應並在感覺神經內引起衝動的一個或一組細胞。此種感受器存在於味蕾與鼻黏膜內。

chemosis *n.* swelling (oedema) of the *conjunctiva. It is usually due to inflammation but may occur if the drainage of blood and lymph from around the eye is obstructed.

球結膜水腫 通常由炎症引起。眼周圍的血液循環與淋巴循環發生障礙時亦可發生。

chemotaxis *n.* movement of a cell or organism in response to the stimulus of a gradient of chemical concentration.

趨化性 細胞或微生物受到某種化學成分的刺激而向之運動的現象。

chemotherapy *n.* the prevention or treatment of disease by the use of chemical substances. The term is sometimes restricted to the treatment of infectious diseases with antibiotics and other drugs or to the control of cancer with antimetabolites and similar drugs (in contrast to *radiotherapy).

化學療法 使用化學物質防治疾病的方法。此詞有時僅用以指對傳染病的抗生素（或其類似藥物）療法與對癌的抗代謝藥（或類似藥物）療法。

chest *n. see* thorax.

胸，胸廓

Cheyne-Stokes respiration a striking form of breathing in which there is a cyclical variation in the rate, which becomes slower until breathing stops for several seconds before speeding up to a peak and then slowing again. It occurs when the sensitivity of the respiratory centres in the brain is impaired, particularly in states of coma.

陳-施氏呼吸 呼吸速度發生明顯周期性變化的一種呼吸型。呼吸逐漸變慢，直至停止，數秒鐘後，又開始呼吸，逐漸加快，至頂峯後又開始變慢，如此周而復始。見於腦內呼吸中樞感受性受損時。多發生於昏迷狀態。

chiasma *n.* (*pl.* **chiasmata**) **1.** (in genetics) the point at which homologous chromosomes remain in contact after they have started to separate in the first division of *meiosis. Chiasmata occur from the end of prophase to anaphase

①**交叉** 在遺傳學中指同源染色體在減數分裂第一期中已開始分離但仍保持接觸的階段。自前期末延續至後期，此時遺傳物質互相交換。②**視交叉**

and represent the point at which mutual exchange of genetic material takes place (*see* crossing over). **2.** *see* optic chiasma.

chickenpox *n.* a mild highly infectious disease caused by a *herpesvirus that is transmitted by airborne droplets. After an incubation period of 11–18 days a mild fever develops, followed within 24 hours by an itchy rash of dark red pimples. The pimples spread from the trunk to the face, scalp, and limbs; they develop into blisters and then scabs, which drop off after about 12 days. The only treatment is bed rest and the application of calamine lotion to the spots to discourage scratching. Scarring is unusual. The patient is infectious from the onset of symptoms until all the spots have gone. Since an attack in childhood generally confers life-long immunity, chickenpox is rare among adults. Medical name: **varicella**.

水痘 一種由疱疹病毒通過空氣飛沫傳播引起的傳染病。病情輕，但傳染性很强。潛伏期11～18天，起病時輕度發燒，24小時內出現暗紅色瘙癢性丘疹。丘疹自軀幹部向頭部、頭皮及四周播散，繼而演變成水疱，最後結痂，約經12天全部消退。治療：卧牀，患者塗抹爐甘石洗劑止癢。極少形成疤痕。自發病起至皮疹退盡爲止皆有傳染性。兒童期患病通常產生終生免疫，因此成人期患病少見。

chiclero's ulcer a form of *leishmaniasis of the skin caused by the parasite *Leishmania tropica mexicana*. The disease, occurring in Panama, Honduras, and the Amazon, primarily affects men who visit the forests to collect chicle (gum) and takes the form of an ulcerating lesion on the ear lobe. The sore usually heals spontaneously within six months.

糖膠樹膠工人潰瘍 由墨西哥熱帶利什曼原蟲引起的一種皮膚利什曼病。本病見於巴拿馬、洪都拉斯與亞馬遜河流域，主要侵犯赴森林中採糖膠、樹膠的男性成人，表現爲耳廓處的潰瘍性病變。潰瘍通常於6個月內自行癒合。

Chief Administrative Medical Officer a physician at Area level under the NHS (Scotland) Act. *See* National Health Service.

行政區主管醫師 根據蘇格蘭全國衞生法令，某一保健地段的負責醫師。

chigger *n. see* Trombicula.

恙蟎

chigoe *n. see* Tunga.

沙蚤

Chikungunya fever a disease, occurring in Africa and Asia, caused by an *arbovirus and transmitted to man by mosquitoes of the genus *Aëdes*. The disease is similar to *dengue and symptoms include fever, headache, generalized body pain, and an irritating rash.

契昆根亞熱 一種由蟲媒病毒引起的通過伊蚊傳染人類的疾病。發生於亞洲與非洲。症狀類似登革熱，有發熱、頭痛、全身疼痛與瘙癢性皮疹。治療：止痛，退燒。

The patient is given drugs to relieve the pain and reduce the fever.

chilblain *n.* a red round itchy swelling of the skin, occurring generally on the fingers or toes in cold weather. Chilblains form part of a group of related conditions (*see* perniosis). Treatment is by keeping the limbs warm, though vasodilator drugs may help. Medical name: **pernio**.

凍瘡 通常發生於冬天的指（或趾）部的紅腫現象。呈圓形，有瘙癢感。是一組凍傷病的表現之一。治療：血管擴張藥可能奏效。主要依靠肢體保溫。

childbed *n. see* puerperium.

產褥

childbirth *n. see* labour.

分娩

child health clinic (CHC) (in Britain) a special clinic for the routine care of infants and preschool children, formerly known as a *child welfare centre*. Sometimes these clinics are staffed by doctors, *health visitors, and clinic nurses employed by District Health Authorities; the children attending them are drawn from the district around the clinic. Alternatively general practitioners may run their own CHC, say once a week, with health visitors and other staff in attendance; it is unusual for children not registered with the practice to attend such clinics. The service provides screening tests for congenital dislocation of hips, suppressed squint (*see* cover test), and impaired speech and/or hearing. The *Guthrie test may also be performed if this has not been done before the baby leaves hospital. The staff of CHCs also educate mothers (especially those having their first child) in feeding techniques and hygiene and see that children receive the recommended immunizations against infectious diseases. They also ensure that the families of handicapped children receive maximum support from health and social services and that such children achieve their maximum potential in the preschool period.

兒童保健站 英國特有的一種對幼兒與學齡前兒童提供常規保健服務工作的機構。舊稱兒童福利中心。保健站的工作人員有時是由地段衛生機構僱用的醫生、保健員以及保健護士組成，他們對居住在保健站附近兒童提供衛生保健服務。有時開業的全科醫生也可以開辦自己的兒童保健站。例如：他們可會同衛生檢查員及其它工作人員每週進行一次這種保健服務活動。絕大多數兒童都在這種保健站登記接受服務。該站對先天性髖關節脫位、隱斜視及言語與聽力障礙等疾病進行普查。如果兒童出院前未做過加斯里試驗，他們將補做這種試驗。他們還對母親（特別是初產婦）進行餵養技術與衛生方面的教育，並監督各種傳染病預防接種的施行。此外，他們還負責保證那些殘廢兒童的家庭能從社會福利機構獲得一切他們應有的補助，並使這些兒童在學齡前期能充分發展他們可能發揮的能力。

chir- (chiro-) *prefix denoting* the hand(s). *See also* cheir-.

〔前綴〕手

chiropody (podiatry) *n.* the study and care of the foot, including its normal structure, its diseases, and their treatment. —**chiropodist** *n.*

足病科　對足的正常結構、足病及其治療進行研究的專門學科。

chiropractic *n.* a system of treating diseases by manipulation, mainly of the vertebrae of the backbone. It is based on the theory that nearly all disorders can be traced to the incorrect alignment of bones, with consequent malfunctioning of nerves and muscle throughout the body.

捏脊療法　利用按摩手法以治病的一種方法。主要是按摩脊椎骨。其理論根據是：所有的疾病都是由於骨頭聯結不當，以致造成全身神經肌肉功能障礙引起的。

Chlamydia *n.* a genus of virus-like microorganisms that cause disease in man and birds. Some *Chlamydia* infections of birds can be transmitted to man (*see* ornithosis, parrot disease). *Chlamydia trachomatis* is the causative agent of the eye disease *trachoma. The organisms appear to resemble bacteria but are of similar size to viruses and all are obligate parasites.

衣原體　一種能引起人類與鳥類疾病的病毒樣微生物。某些鳥類的衣原體疾病能傳染給人類。沙眼的病原體即沙眼衣原體。衣原體形態類似細菌，而大小類似病毒，屬專性寄生物。

chloasma (melasma) *n.* the appearance of brown patches, up to several centimetres in diameter, mainly on the forehead, temples, and cheeks. It is due to a localized increase in the dark pigment *melanin and occurs sometimes in pregnancy (when the nipples also turn brown), as well as during the menopause. Women taking the contraceptive pill may also develop chloasma.

褐黃斑　主要見於前額、顳部或頰部的褐色斑。直徑可達數厘米。是局部黑色素增生的結果。可見於妊娠期與經絕期。服用避孕藥的婦女亦可出現此斑。

chlor- (chloro-) *prefix denoting* **1.** chlorine or chlorides. **2.** green.

［前綴］　**①氯，氯化物　②綠色**

chloracne *n.* an occupational acne-like skin disorder that occurs after regular contact with chlorinated hydrocarbons. These chemicals are derived from oil and tar products; 'cutting oils' used in engineering also cause the disease. The skin develops blackheads, papules, and pustules, mainly on hairy parts (such as the forearm). Warts and skin cancer may develop after many years of exposure to these chemicals.

氯痤瘡　與氯化烴類經常接觸引起的一種痤瘡樣職業皮膚病。這些化合物係石油與瀝青的衍生物。接觸機油亦可引起本病。皮膚出現黑頭粉刺、丘疹、膿疱，多見於前額髮際。長年接觸可產生疣與皮膚癌。

chloral hydrate a sedative and hypnotic drug used, mainly in children and the elderly, to induce sleep or as a daytime sedative. It is rapidly absorbed from the alimentary canal and is usually given by mouth as a syrup, although it can be administered rectally. Toxic effects are usually only seen with overdosage. Prolonged use may lead to *dependence. Trade names: **Noctec**, **Somnos**.

水合氯醛 常用於兒童與老年人的一種鎮靜催眠藥。消化道吸收迅速，常以糖漿劑口服，亦可直腸投藥。僅使用過量時才有毒性。長期服用可形成賴藥性。商品名：羅克特，索姆洛斯。

chlorambucil *n.* a drug that destroys cancer cells. It is given by mouth and used mainly in the treatment of chronic leukaemias. Prolonged large doses may cause damage to the bone marrow. Trade name: **Leukeran**.

苯丁酸氮芥 一種能破壞癌細胞的藥物。口服。通常用於治療慢性白血病。長期大量使用可損害骨髓。商品名：瘤可寧。

chloramphenicol *n.* an antibiotic, derived from the bacterium *Streptomyces venezuelae* and also produced synthetically, that is effective against a wide variety of microorganisms. However, due to its serious side-effects, especially damage to the bone marrow, it is usually reserved for serious infections (such as typhoid fever) when less toxic drugs are ineffective. Trade names: **Chloromycetin**, **Mycinol**, etc.

氯黴素 由委內瑞拉鏈霉菌培養液中分離出的一種廣譜抗生素。亦可人工合成。由於副作用嚴重，尤其是對骨髓有損害作用，本品僅用於其它毒性較輕的藥物無效時的嚴重感染（如腸傷寒）。

chlorbutol *n.* an antibacterial and antifungal agent used as a preservative in injection solutions, in eye and nose drops, in powder form for topical use in irritational skin conditions, and occasionally by mouth as a mild sedative in travel sickness.

三氯叔丁醇 一種抗細菌與抗黴菌藥。在注射液、眼藥與滴鼻藥中用做防腐劑。患皮膚病時亦可以其粉劑局部外用。患暈動病時偶可做爲輕鎮靜劑內服。

chlorcyclizine *n.* an *antihistamine drug that is slow-acting but produces long-lasting effects. Given by mouth, it is used mainly to relieve the symptoms of allergic reactions and to prevent travel sickness. Principal side-effects are drowsiness, dizziness, and dryness of the mouth and throat. Trade names: **Di-paralene**, **Histantine**.

氯二苯甲基嗪 一種作用緩慢但效果持久的抗組織胺藥。口服。主要用於解除變態反應症狀與防止暈動病。主要副作用有嗜眠、頭暈、口咽乾燥。商品名：氯環嗪。

chlordantoin *n.* an antifungal drug, used mainly for the treatment of fungus infections (candidiasis) of the vagina. It

氯海因 主要用於治療陰道黴菌（念珠菌）感染的一種抗黴菌藥。製成乳膏

is applied in the form of a cream or pessaries, and local skin reactions occasionally occur.

或栓劑使用。偶有局部皮膚反應。

chlordiazepoxide *n.* a sedative and tranquillizing drug with *muscle relaxant properties, used to relieve tension, fears and anxiety and in the treatment of alcoholism. It is administered by mouth or injection. Common side-effects are nausea, skin reactions, and muscular incoordination. Trade names: **Librium**, **Diapox**, **Elenium**. *See also* tranquillizer.

甲氯二氮䓬 鎮靜安定藥。具有肌肉鬆弛作用。用於解除緊張、恐懼、焦慮及酒精中毒。口服或注射。常見副作用為噁心、皮膚反應與肌肉共濟失調。商品名：利眠寧。

chlorhexadol *n.* a sedative and hypnotic drug with uses similar to those of *chloral hydrate. Trade name: **Medodorm**.

氯醛己醇 鎮靜安眠藥。作用與水化氯醛相同。

chlorhexidine *n.* an antiseptic used as a general disinfectant for skin and mucous membranes or as a preservative (for example, in eye drops). Chlorhexidine is used in solution, creams, gels, and lozenges and in some preparations is combined with *cetrimide. In very dilute solutions it can be used as an effective mouthwash for the control of infections of the mouth. Skin sensitivity to chlorhexidine occurs rarely. Trade name: **Hibitane**.

氯苯胍亭 皮膚、黏膜消毒藥與防腐劑（例如用於眼藥中）。本品可制成溶液、乳膏、凝膠與含片，亦可與溴棕三甲銨混合製成某種製劑。用其稀溶液漱口可控制口腔感染。皮膚過敏現象罕見。商品名：洗必太。

chlorination *n.* the addition of noninjurious traces of chlorine (often one part per million) to water supplies before human consumption to ensure that disease-causing organisms are destroyed.

加氯消毒法 以非中毒量（百萬分之一）的氯加入水源，以達到在人使用前消滅病菌的目的。

chlorine *n.* an extremely pungent gaseous element with antiseptic and bleaching properties. It is widely used to sterilize drinking water and purify swimming baths. In high concentrations it is toxic; it was used in World War I as a poison gas in the trenches. Symbol: Cl.

氯 一種具抑菌與漂白效果的、有强烈刺激性的氣體元素。廣泛用於消毒飲水與清潔游泳池水。高濃度時有毒性。第一次世界大戰時曾用做軍用毒氣。符號：Cl。

chlormadinone *n.* a synthetic sex hormone (*see* progestogen) that was formerly used in oral contraceptives as a

氯地孕酮 一種合成的性激素（孕激素類）。過去是唯一的按期口服的避孕

sequential and progestogen-only pill. Chlormadinone produces variations in the length of the menstrual cycle and abnormal bleeding; nausea, vomiting, and weight gain may also occur.

藥。本品能引起經期紊亂、不規則出血、噁心、嘔吐及體重增加。

chlormethiazole *n.* a *sedative and hypnotic drug used to treat insomnia in the elderly (when associated with confusion, agitation, and restlessness) and drug withdrawal symptoms (especially in alcoholism). It is administered by mouth or injection and the most common side-effects are tingling sensations in the nose and sneezing. Trade name: **Heminevrin**.

氯乙甲噻唑 用於老年人的一種鎮靜催眠藥。適用於有精神混亂、激動不安與戒斷症出現時（特別是戒煙）。口服或注射。常見副作用：鼻內酸感，噴嚏。商品名：氯甲噻唑。

chlormezanone *n.* a tranquillizing drug used in the treatment of mild anxiety and tension, including premenstrual tension. It is also used to relieve pain and muscle spasm. Chlormezanone is administered by mouth; the most common side-effects are drowsiness and dizziness. Trade name: **Trancopal**.

氯甲噻酮 治療輕度焦慮與緊張的安定藥。適用於經前期緊張。亦可止痛鎮痙。口服。常見副作用有嗜眠與頭昏。商品名：芬那露。

chlorocresol *n.* an antiseptic derived from phenol, used as a general disinfectant and, at low concentrations, as a preservative in injections, creams, and lotions and also in eye drops. Strong solutions applied to the skin may cause sensitivity reactions.

氯甲酚 消毒藥。苯酚的衍生物。做一般消毒劑用。低濃度用做注射劑、乳膏劑、洗劑與眼藥的防腐劑。高濃度溶液用於皮膚時可引起過敏反應。

chloroform *n.* a volatile liquid formerly widely used as a general anaesthetic. Because its use as such causes liver damage and affects heart rhythm, chloroform is now used only in low concentrations as a flavouring agent and preservative, in the treatment of flatulence, and in liniments as a *rubefacient.

氯仿 過去廣泛用做全身麻醉劑的一種揮發性液體。由於本品能引起肝損害與心率障礙，現僅以其低濃度用做矯味劑、防腐劑、驅風劑等。亦可在搽劑中用做導赤劑。

chloroma *n.* a tumour that arises in association with *myeloid leukaemia and consists essentially of a mass of leukaemic cells. A freshly cut specimen of the tumour appears green, but the colour rapidly disappears on exposure

綠色（肉）瘤 骨髓性白血病伴發的一種主要由白血病細胞組成的腫瘤。新鮮切片標本呈綠色，但暴露於空氣中顏色迅速消失。用紫外線照射可發紅

to air. It shows red fluorescence with ultraviolet light and responds to specific antileukaemic treatment.

色荧光。用特效抗白血病療法治療有效。

chlorophenothane *n.* *see* DDT.

滴滴涕

chlorophyll *n.* one of a group of green pigments, found in all green plants and some bacteria, that absorb light to provide energy for the synthesis of carbohydrates from carbon dioxide and water (photosynthesis). The two major chlorophylls, a and b, consist of a porphyrin/magnesium complex.

葉綠素 一組綠色色素中的一種色素。見於植物和某些細菌中，能吸收光線提供能量，使二氧化碳和水合成爲碳水化合物（光合作用）。兩種主要的葉綠素 a 和 b 是由卟啉/鎂絡合物組成的。

chloropsia *n.* green vision: a rare symptom of digitalis poisoning.

綠視症 視物呈綠色。洋地黃中毒的一種少見的症狀。

chloropyrilene *n.* an *antihistamine administered by mouth to treat allergies and other reactions involving release of histamine.

氯噻吡二胺 抗組織胺藥。口服。用於治療過敏及其它釋放組織胺的反應。

chloroquine *n.* a drug used principally in the treatment and prevention of malaria but also used in rheumatoid arthritis, certain liver infections and skin conditions, and lupus erythematosus. It is administered by mouth or injection; a side-effect of prolonged use in large doses is eye damage. Trade names: **Avloclor**, **Nivaquine**.

氯喹 一種主要用於防治瘧疾的藥物。亦可用於類風濕性關節炎、某類肝臟傳染病、皮膚病與紅斑性狼瘡。口服或注射。長期大劑量使用可產生眼損害。

chlorosis *n.* a severe form of *anaemia produced by gross deficiency of iron, so called because of the greenish skin pallor that it produces.

萎黃病 嚴重缺鐵引起的一種重型貧血。患者皮膚在蒼白的基礎上帶綠色調，故名。

chlorothiazide *n.* a *diuretic used to treat fluid retention (oedema) and high blood pressure (hypertension). It is administered by mouth and may cause skin sensitivity reactions, stomach pains, nausea, and reduced blood potassium levels. Trade name: **Saluric**.

氯噻嗪 治療水分瀦留（水腫）與高血壓的藥物。口服。可產生皮膚過敏反應、胃痛、噁心和低血鉀。商品名：克尿塞。

chlorotrianisene *n.* a synthetic *oestrogen administered by mouth to treat symptoms of the menopause, to suppress lactation in mothers not breast

三對甲氧苯氯乙烯 合成雌激素類藥。口服。治療經絕期症狀，退乳，並可緩解前列腺癌症狀。

feeding, and to relieve symptoms in cancer of the prostate gland. Trade name: **Tace**.

chloroxylenol *n.* an *antiseptic, derived from *phenol but less toxic and more selective in bactericidal activity, used mainly in solution as a skin disinfectant. Trade name: **Dettol**.

對氯間二甲酚　消毒藥。苯酚衍生物。毒性較輕，殺菌力較强。主要用其溶液行皮膚消毒。

chlorphenesin *n.* a compound, active against bacteria and fungi, that is applied to the skin as a cream or dusting powder to treat fungal infections, such as athlete's foot. Trade name: **Mycil**.

氯酚甘油醚　抗細菌與眞菌化合物。用其乳膏劑或粉劑治療皮膚眞菌感染，如足癬。商品名：氯酚醚。

chlorpheniramine *n.* a potent *antihistamine used to treat such allergies as hay fever, rhinitis, and urticaria. It is administered by mouth or, to relieve severe conditions, by injection. Trade name: **Piriton**.

右旋氯苯吡胺　一種高效抗組織胺藥。用於枯草熱、鼻炎與蕁麻疹等過敏性疾患。口服。重症時可注射。商品名：右撲爾敏。

chlorphenoxamine *n.* a drug with atropine-like and *antihistamine action, administered by mouth to treat muscle stiffness in parkinsonism; it does not affect tremor. Trade name: **Clorevan**.

氯苯氧胺　一種同時具有阿托品作用與抗組織胺作用的藥品。口服。治療帕金森氏病的肌肉僵硬，對震顫無效。商品名：氯甲苯海拉明。

chlorphentermine *n.* a drug used to suppress appetite in the treatment of obesity. It has a similar action to *amphetamine but is less potent. It is administered by mouth and may cause dizziness, insomnia, or drowsiness.

氯苯丁胺　食慾抑制劑。治療肥胖。與苯丙胺作用相同，但效力較低。口服。可引起頭昏、失眠、嗜眠等。

chlorproguanil *n.* a drug administered by mouth to prevent and treat malaria. Side-effects are rare, but large doses may cause stomach discomfort and vomiting.

氯丙二胍　口服抗瘧藥。副作用少。大劑量服用可引起胃不適與嘔吐。

chlorpromazine *n.* a major *tranquillizer and antipsychotic drug. It is used in the treatment of *schizophrenia and *mania; to control severe anxiety and agitation; and to control nausea and vomiting. It also enhances the effects of *analgesics and is used in terminal illness and preparation for anaesthesia. Chlorpromazine is administered by mouth or injection or as a rectal suppo-

氯丙嗪　一種重要的安定藥與抗精神病藥。用以治療精神分裂症與躁狂症，控制重度焦慮、激動、噁心、嘔吐等。亦可增强止痛藥的效果，故用於疾病臨終期或製備痲醉藥。口服或注射，亦可用直腸栓劑。常見副作用爲嗜眠與口乾。亦可引起運動障礙

sitory; common side-effects are drowsiness and dry mouth. It also causes abnormalities of movement, especially *dystonias, *dyskinesia, and *parkinsonism. Trade names: **Chloractil, Largactil**.

與張力障礙或帕金森氏病。

chlorpropamide *n.* a drug that reduces blood sugar levels and is used to treat diabetes in adults. It is administered by mouth and can cause such side-effects as skin sensitivity reactions and digestive upsets. Trade names: **Diabinese, Melitase**. *See also* sulphonylurea.

氯磺丙脲 降血糖藥。用以治療成人糖尿病。口服。副作用有皮膚過敏與消化不良。

chlorprothixene *n.* a major *tranquillizer and sedative used to treat agitation, anxiety, insomnia, delusions, and hallucinations. It is administered by mouth; common side-effects are dry mouth and drowsiness. Trade name: **Taractan**.

氯丙硫蒽 一種重要的鎮靜安定藥。用以治療激動、焦慮失眠、譫妄與幻覺。口服。常見副作用有口乾與嗜眠。商品名：泰爾登。

chlortetracycline *n.* an *antibiotic active against many bacteria and fungi. It is administered by mouth or injection or as ointment or cream (for skin and eye infections); side-effects are those of the other *tetracyclines. Trade names: **Aureomycin, Chlortetrin, Deteclo**.

氯四環素 廣譜抗生素。亦可抑制黴菌。口服或注射。亦可製成油膏或乳膏使用（治療皮膚與眼感染）。副作用與四環素同。商品名：金黴素。

chlorthalidone *n.* a *diuretic used to treat fluid retention (oedema) and high blood pressure (hypertension). It is administered by mouth and may cause skin sensitivity reactions, stomach pains, nausea, and reduced blood potassium levels. Trade name: **Hygroton**.

氯噻酮 利尿藥。用以治療水瀦留（水腫）與高血壓。口服。可引起皮膚過敏反應、胃痛、噁心與低血鉀。

choana *n.* (*pl.* **choanae**) a funnel-shaped opening, particularly either of the two openings between the nasal cavity and the pharynx.

漏斗 漏斗狀開口，尤指鼻腔與咽喉之間的兩個孔或二者之一。

chokedamp *n. see* blackdamp.

烏煙，窒息性氣體

chol- (chole-, cholo-) *prefix denoting* bile. Example: *cholemesis* (vomiting of).

[前綴] **膽汁**。例如嘔膽。

cholagogue *n.* a drug that stimulates the flow of bile from the gall bladder and bile ducts into the duodenum.

利膽藥 一種能促使膽汁自膽囊與膽管流向十二指腸的藥物。

cholangiography *n.* X-ray examination of the bile ducts, used to demonstrate the site and nature of any obstruction to the ducts or to show the presence of stones within them. A medium that is opaque to X-rays is introduced into the ducts either by injection into the bloodstream (*intravenous cholangiography*); direct injection into the liver (*percutaneous transhepatic cholangiography*); direct injection into the bile ducts at operation (*operative cholangiography*); or by injection into the duodenal opening of the ducts through a *duodenoscope (*endoscopic retrograde cholangiopancreatography*; *see* ERCP).

膽管造影術 顯示膽管梗阻部位與性質或膽石的X線檢查法。造影劑可注射入血流（靜脉膽管造影術），直接注射入肝臟（經皮肝膽管造影術），手術中直接注射入膽道（術中膽管造影術），或通過十二指腸內窺鏡注射入膽道開口部（內窺鏡逆行性膽管胰腺造影術）。

cholangiolitis *n.* inflammation of the smallest bile ducts (*cholangioles*). *See* cholangitis.

膽小管炎

cholangioma *n.* a rare tumour originating from the bile duct.

膽管瘤 在膽道發生的一種少見的腫瘤。

cholangitis *n.* inflammation of the bile ducts. It usually occurs when the ducts are obstructed, especially by stones, or after operations on the bile ducts. Symptoms include intermittent fever, usually with *rigors, and intermittent jaundice. Initial treatment is by antibiotics, but removal of the obstruction is essential for permanent cure. Liver abscess is a possible complication, and recurrent episodes of cholangitis lead to secondary biliary *cirrhosis.

膽管炎 通常於膽道梗阻，特別是膽石梗阻時引起的膽道炎症。有時發生於膽道手術後。症狀有反復的發燒，常伴有寒顫與間歇性黃疸。首先要用抗生素控制感染。根治則有賴於解除梗阻。可能併發肝膿腫。反覆發作可導致繼發性膽汁性肝硬化。

cholecalciferol *n. see* vitamin D.

膽骨化醇 即維生素D。

cholecyst- *prefix denoting* the gall bladder. Example: *cholecystotomy* (incision of).

[前綴] **膽囊** 例如：膽囊切開術。

cholecystectomy *n.* surgical removal of the gall bladder, usually for *cholecystitis or gallstones.

膽囊切除術 通常由於患膽囊炎或膽石病而將膽囊外科切除的手術。

cholecystenterostomy *n.* a surgical procedure in which the gall bladder is joined to the small intestine. It is performed in order to allow bile to pass from the liver to the intestine when the

膽囊小腸吻合手術 一種將膽囊與小腸吻合起來的手術。目的是當總膽管內的梗阻無法解除時，使膽汁由肝臟直接流入小腸。

common bile duct is obstructed by an irremovable cause.

cholecystitis *n.* inflammation of the gall bladder. *Acute cholecystitis* is due to bacterial infection, causing fever and acute pain over the gall bladder. It is usually treated by rest and antibiotics. *Chronic cholecystitis* is often associated with *gallstones and causes recurrent episodes of upper abdominal pain. Recurrent bacterial infection may be the cause, but the physical processes leading to gallstone formation may also be important. It may require treatment by *cholecystectomy. *See also* cholesterosis.

膽囊炎 膽囊的炎症。急性膽囊炎係細菌感染引起，有發熱與膽囊區疼痛。治療：卧床休息，使用抗生素。慢性膽囊炎多由膽石引起，伴有反覆發作的上腹部疼痛。反覆細菌感染可能是致病原因，但導致膽石生成的體質因素亦不可忽視。本病常須行膽囊切除術。

cholecystoduodenostomy *n.* a form of *cholecystenterostomy in which the gall bladder is joined to the duodenum.

膽囊十二指腸吻合術 膽囊小腸吻合術的一種。本術將膽囊吻合在十二指腸上。

cholecystogastrostomy *n.* a form of *cholecystenterostomy in which the gall bladder is joined to the stomach. It is rarely performed.

膽囊胃吻合術 膽囊小腸吻合術的一種。本術將膽囊與胃相吻合。很少用。

cholecystography *n.* X-ray examination of the gall bladder. A compound containing iodine and therefore opaque to X-rays is taken by mouth, absorbed by the intestine, and excreted by the liver into the bile, which is concentrated in the gall bladder. An X-ray photograph (*cholecystogram*) of the gall bladder indicates whether or not it is functioning, and gallstones may be seen as contrasting (nonopaque) areas within it. A fatty meal is usually also given, to demonstrate the ability of the gall bladder to contract.

膽囊造影術 膽囊的X線檢查法。口服一種不透X線的含碘化合物，本品在腸吸收後又經肝臟排至膽汁，在膽囊內濃縮。自膽囊X線照片中可看出膽囊功能情況，通過與造影劑的對比亦可顯示膽石。為了觀察膽囊的收縮功能，亦常給予脂肪食。

cholecystokinin-pancreozymin *n.* a hormone from the small intestine (duodenum) that causes contraction of the gall bladder and expulsion of bile into the intestine and stimulates the production of digestive enzymes by the pancreas. *See also* pancreatic juice.

縮膽囊素-促胰酶素 一種由小腸（十二指腸）生成的激素。能引起膽囊收縮，促使膽汁排入小腸，並能刺激胰腺分泌消化酶。

cholecystotomy *n.* a surgical operation in which the gall bladder is opened, usually to remove gallstones. It is performed only when *cholecystectomy would be impracticable or dangerous.

膽囊切開術 切開膽囊摘除膽石的手術。本術僅在膽囊切除術無法施行或有危險時才進行。

choledoch- (choledocho-) *prefix denoting* the common bile duct. Example: *choledochoplasty* (plastic surgery of).

[前綴] **總膽管** 例如：總膽管成形術。

choledocholithiasis *n.* stones within the common bile duct. The stones usually form in the gall bladder and pass into the bile duct, but they may develop within the duct after *cholecystectomy.

總膽管結石 總膽管內的結石。結石通常形成於膽囊然後進入膽道。它們可能在膽囊切除術後發生。

choledochotomy *n.* a surgical operation in which the common bile duct is opened, to search for or to remove stones within it. It may be performed at the same time as *cholecystectomy or if stones occur in the bile duct after cholecystectomy.

總膽管切開術 爲探查或摘除總膽管內的結石而施行切開總膽管的手術。可與膽囊切除術同時進行。在膽囊切除術後如膽道內又出現膽石時亦可施行。

cholelithiasis *n.* the formation of stones in the gall bladder (*see* gallstone).

膽石病 膽囊內膽石生成。

cholelithotomy *n.* removal of gallstones by *cholecystotomy.

膽石切除術 用膽囊切開術摘取膽石。

cholera *n.* an acute infection of the small intestine by the bacterium *Vibrio cholerae*, which causes severe vomiting and diarrhoea (known as *ricewater stools*) leading to dehydration. The disease is contracted from food or drinking water contaminated by faeces from a patient. Cholera often occurs in epidemics; outbreaks are rare in good sanitary conditions. After an incubation period of 1–5 days symptoms commence suddenly; the resulting dehydration and imbalance in the concentration of body fluids can cause death within 24 hours. Treatment involves intravenous infusion of salt solution; antibiotics only hasten recovery. The mortality rate in untreated cases is over 50%. Vaccination against cholera is effective for only 6–9 months.

霍亂 由霍亂弧菌引起的小腸急性傳染病。發生嚴重嘔吐與腹瀉（米湯樣便）而致脫水。係患者糞便污染飲水與食物而引起。常呈暴發流行，且多見於衞生不良的條件下。經1～5日潛伏期突然發病，脫水與體液分配失衡可於24小時內引起死亡。治療：含鹽溶液靜脉輸注。抗生素僅能加速恢復。未接受治療者病死率高達50％以上。霍亂疫苗接種有效期僅6～9個月。

choleresis *n.* the production of bile by the liver.

膽汁分泌

choleretic *n.* an agent that stimulates the secretion of bile by the liver thereby increasing the flow of bile.

利膽劑 促使膽汁分泌以增加膽流的物質。

cholestasis *n.* failure of normal amounts of bile to reach the intestine, resulting in obstructive *jaundice. The cause may be a mechanical block in the bile ducts, such as a stone (*extrahepatic biliary obstruction*), or liver disease, such as that caused by the drug *chlorpromazine in some hypersensitive individuals (*intrahepatic cholestasis*). The symptoms are jaundice with dark urine, pale faeces, and usually itching (pruritus).

膽汁阻塞 膽汁不能正常地抵達小腸而致黃疸。病因可能是膽道內機械性梗塞，如膽石（肝外性膽汁阻塞）；或是肝臟疾患，如高血壓患者服用藥物氯丙嗪引起（肝內性膽汁阻塞）。

cholesteatoma *n.* a mass consisting mainly of cellular debris in which cholesterol crystals may be demonstrated. Cholesteatomas occur mainly in the middle ear and, by pressure, cause destruction of surrounding structures. They may also occur in other parts of the skull and nervous system.

膽脂瘤 主要由細胞碎屑組成的腫物。其中可見膽固醇結晶。多見於中耳，由於壓迫作用，可破壞周圍組織。亦可見於其他部位，如顱部與神經系統等。

cholesterol *n.* a fatlike material (a *sterol) present in the blood and most tissues, especially nervous tissue. Cholesterol and its esters are important constituents of cell membranes and are precursors of many steroid hormones and bile salts. Western dietary intake is approximately 500–1000 mg/day. Cholesterol is synthesized in the body from acetate, mainly in the liver, and blood concentration is normally 140–300 mg/100 ml (3.6–7.8 mmol/l). Elevated blood concentration is often associated with *atheroma, of which cholesterol is a major component. Cholesterol is also a constituent of *gallstones.

膽固醇 存在於血液、大多數組織尤其是神經組織中的一種類脂物質。膽固醇及其酯類是細胞膜的重要成分，也是許多固醇類激素與膽鹽的前體。西方飲食攝入量約500～1000毫克/日。膽固醇在體內（主要在肝臟）係由乙酸鹽合成，血濃度正常爲140～300毫克/100毫升（3.6～7.8毫克分子/升）。血膽固醇升高常見於動脈粥樣化。膽固醇係構成該種病變的主要成分。膽固醇亦爲膽結石的成分。

cholesterosis *n.* a form of chronic *cholecystitis in which small crystals of cholesterol are deposited on the internal wall of the gall bladder, like the

膽固醇沉着病 慢性膽囊炎的一型。膽囊內壁有細小的膽固醇結晶沉着，似草莓種子狀，故又稱草莓

pips of a strawberry: hence its descriptive term *strawberry gall bladder*. The crystals may enlarge to become *gallstones.

樣膽囊。結晶可增大形成膽石。

cholestyramine *n.* a drug that binds with bile salts so that they are excreted. It is administered by mouth to relieve conditions due to irritant effects of bile salts – such as the itching that occurs in obstructive jaundice – and also to lower the blood levels of cholesterol and other fats. Common side-effects include constipation, diarrhoea, heartburn, and nausea. Trade names: **Cuemid, Questran**.

膽苯烯胺 一種能與膽鹽結合並促其排出的藥物。口服。用以解除膽鹽的刺激症狀，如阻塞性黃疸引起的瘙癢。亦可降底血膽固醇及其它血脂含量。常見副作用爲便秘、腹瀉、發燒、噁心。商品名：消膽胺，降膽敏。

cholic acid (cholalic acid) *see* bile acids.

膽酸

choline *n.* a basic compound important in the synthesis of phosphatidylcholine (lecithin) and other *phospholipids and of *acetylcholine. It is also involved in the transport of fat in the body. Choline is sometimes classed as a vitamin but, although it is essential for life, it can be synthesized in the body.

膽鹼 在合成乙醯膽鹼與磷脂醯膽鹼（卵磷脂）及其它磷脂類的過程中極重要的一種鹼性化合物。亦參預體內脂肪的運輸。有人認爲它是一種維生素，對生命活動至關重要，但可在體內合成。

cholinergic *adj.* describing nerve fibres that release *acetylcholine as a neurotransmitter. *Compare* adrenergic.

膽鹼能的 描述能釋放神經遞質乙醯膽鹼的神經纖維。

choline salicylate an analgesic, related to *aspirin, that is applied locally to relieve earache, mouth ulcers, and other painful conditions. Trade names: **Audax, Bonjela, Teejel**.

水楊酸膽鹼 類似阿司匹林的一種止痛藥。治療耳痛、口腔潰瘍與其他疼痛疾病。

cholinesterase *n.* an enzyme that breaks down a choline ester into its choline and acid components. The term usually refers to *acetylcholinesterase*, which breaks down the neurotransmitter *acetylcholine into choline and acetic acid. It is found in all *cholinergic nerve junctions, where it rapidly destroys the acetylcholine released during the transmission of a nerve impulse so that subsequent impulses may pass. Other cholinesterases are found in the blood and other tissues.

膽鹼酯酶 一種能將膽鹼酯分解成膽鹼與酸性部分的酶。有時即指乙醯膽鹼酯酶。該酶能將神經遞質乙醯膽鹼分解成膽鹼和乙酸。在所有膽鹼能神經接頭處都有此酶，能將傳導神經衝動時釋放的乙醯膽鹼迅速破壞，俾使下一個衝動得以通過。在血液與其他組織中亦有此酶存在。

choline theophyllinate a drug used to dilate the air passages in asthma and chronic bronchitis. It is administered by mouth and can cause digestive upsets and nausea. Trade name: **Choledyl**.

膽茶鹼 支氣管擴張藥，用於支氣管哮喘與慢性支氣管炎。口服。可引起消化不良與噁心。

choluria *n.* bile in the urine, which occurs when the level of bile in the blood is raised, especially in obstructive *jaundice. The urine becomes dark brown or orange, and bile pigments and bile salts may be detected in it.

膽汁尿 尿中出現膽汁。見於血中膽汁濃度升高時，尤其於阻塞性黃疸。尿呈暗褐色或橘黃色，可檢出膽色素與膽鹽。

chondr- (chondro-) *prefix denoting* cartilage. Example: *chondrogenesis* (formation of).

〔前綴〕 **軟骨** 例如：軟骨形成。

chondrin *n.* a material that resembles gelatin, produced when cartilage is boiled.

軟骨膠 軟骨被煮沸時出現的一種類膠狀物質。

chondriosome *n. see* mitochondrion.

線粒體

chondroblast *n.* a cell that produces the matrix of *cartilage.

成軟骨細胞 產生軟骨基質的細胞。

chondroblastoma *n.* a tumour derived from *chondroblasts, having the appearance of a mass of well-differentiated cartilage.

成軟骨細胞瘤 由成軟骨細胞產生的腫瘤。外觀呈分化良好的軟骨腫塊。

chondrocalcinosis *n.* the presence of calcium phosphate crystals in joint cartilage, as seen by X-ray in *pseudogout.

軟骨鈣化病 關節軟骨中出現磷酸鈣結晶。如假痛風之X線所見。

chondroclast *n.* a cell that is concerned with the absorption of cartilage.

破軟骨細胞 一種與軟骨吸收有關的細胞。

chondrocranium *n.* the embryonic skull, which is composed entirely of cartilage and is later replaced by bone. *See also* meninx.

軟骨顱 胚胎期的顱骨。完全由軟骨組成。以後將由骨組織所代替。

chondrocyte *n.* a *cartilage cell, found embedded in the matrix.

軟骨細胞 埋植於基質中的軟骨細胞。

chondrodysplasia (chondro-osteodystrophy, chondrodystrophy, Morquio-Brailsford disease) *n.* a hereditary disorder of cartilage formation, due to a defect in mucopolysaccharide metabolism. It results in deformities in the weight-bearing bones, which leads to dwarfism. *Osteoporosis is marked, and

軟骨發育不良 由於黏多糖代謝障礙導致軟骨形成不良的遺傳症病。由於負重骨畸形而發生侏儒病。有顯著的骨質疏鬆現象，心臟與角膜亦發生病變。診斷有賴於X線（骨骺出現典型病變）與驗尿。

the cornea and heart may also develop abnormally. The condition is diagnosed by X-rays, which show characteristic malformation of the growing ends (epiphyses) of the bones, and examination of the urine.

chondrodystrophy *n. see* chondrodysplasia.

軟骨營養障礙 即軟骨發育不良。

chondroitin sulphate a mucopolysaccharide that forms an important constituent of cartilage, bone, and other connective tissues. It is composed of glucuronic acid and N-acetyl-D-galactosamine units.

硫酸軟骨素 軟骨、骨與其結締組織中的一種重要的黏多糖。由葡萄糖醛酸與N－乙醯半乳糖胺組成。

chondroma *n.* a benign tumour of cartilage-forming cells, which may occur at the growing end of any bone but is found most commonly in the bones of the feet and hands. *See also* dyschondroplasia, enchondroma, ecchondroma.

軟骨瘤 成軟骨細胞的一種良性腫瘤。可發生於任何骨的生長端，但以手足部最多見。

chondromalacia *n.* degeneration of cartilage at a joint. *Chondromalacia patellae* is a roughening of the inner surface of the kneecap, resulting in a pain, a grating sensation, and a feeling of instability on movement.

軟骨軟化 關節軟骨變性。髕骨軟骨軟化時髕骨內面粗糙不平，引起疼痛、摩擦感和行動不穩。

chondro-osteodystrophy *n. see* chondrodysplasia.

骨軟骨營養障礙 即軟骨發育不良。

chondrosarcoma *n.* a malignant tumour of cartilage cells, occurring in a bone. Treatment is by surgical removal, which may necessitate amputation of a limb, and radiotherapy.

軟骨肉瘤 骨組織中發生的一種軟骨細胞惡性腫瘤。治療：外科切除。可能需截肢與施行放射線療法。

chord- (chordo-) *prefix denoting* **1.** a cord. Example: *chordotomy* (surgical incision of the spinal cord). **2.** the notochord.

［前綴］ **索狀物，帶狀物** ①**脊髓** 例如：脊髓切斷術。②**脊索**

chorda *n.* (*pl.* **chordae**) a cord, tendon, or nerve fibre. The *chordae tendineae* are stringlike processes in the heart that attach the margins of the mitral and tricuspid valve leaflets to projections of the wall of the ventricle (*papillary muscles*). Rupture of the chordae, through injury, endocarditis, or degen-

索 腱索、脊索或神經纖維。腱索係心臟內繩索樣的突起，它將二尖瓣的瓣葉與心室內的乳頭肌連接起來。外傷、心內膜炎或變性變化可引起腱索斷裂，而發生二尖瓣閉鎖不全。

erative changes, results in *mitral incompetence.

chordee *n.* acute angulation of the penis. In *Peyronie's disease, this is due to a localized fibrous plaque in the penis, which fails to engorge on erection. As a result, the penis angulates at this point making intercourse impossible. In a child, downward chordee is an associated deformity in *hypospadias and the more severe forms are corrected surgically.

塑形陰莖 陰莖勃起時呈現銳角彎曲。在佩羅尼氏病中陰莖內有局限性纖維組織疤痕，在勃起時影響陰莖充血，使陰莖彎曲而無法性交。兒童畸形陰莖下裂亦可使陰莖向下彎曲。嚴重者須行手術糾正。

chorditis *n.* inflammation of a vocal cord. *See* laryngitis.

聲帶炎

chordoma *n.* a tumour arising from remnants of the embryologic *notochord. The classical sites are the base of skull and the region of the sacrum.

脊索瘤 由胚胎期脊索的殘餘產生的腫瘤。多見於顱底是骶部。

chorea *n.* a jerky involuntary movement particularly affecting the shoulders, hips, and face. Each movement is sudden but the resulting posture may be prolonged for a few seconds. The symptoms are due to disease of the *basal ganglia. In *Huntington's chorea* the involuntary movements are accompanied by a progressive *dementia: there is widespread neuronal degeneration throughout the brain. It is inherited as a *dominant characteristic, appearing in half of the children of the patients with this condition. *Senile chorea* occurs sporadically in elderly people and there is no dementia. *Sydenham's chorea* affects children and is associated with rheumatic fever. It responds to mild sedatives.

舞蹈病 主要發生於肩、面、髖部的一種抽搐樣不自主運動。突然發生，但所形成的姿勢可持續數秒鐘。係基底節疾病的症狀。在杭廷頓氏舞蹈病中不自主運動伴有進行性痴呆，此時腦內有廣泛的神經元變性。本病係顯性症狀的遺傳性疾病，患者子女半數出現這種症狀。老年性舞蹈病散見於老人中，無痴呆。西登哈姆氏舞蹈病係兒童疾病，與風濕熱有關。用輕鎮靜藥有效。

chorion *n.* the embryonic membrane that totally surrounds the embryo from the time of implantation. It is formed from *trophoblast lined with mesoderm and becomes closely associated with the *allantois. The blood vessels (supplied by the allantois) are concentrated in the

絨毛膜 自胚泡在宮內植入時起即整個包被胚胎的一層胚膜。由滋養層與間胚層組成，以後與尿囊緊密相連。血管（來自尿囊）集中於絨毛膜附於宮壁的部分，形成胎盤。

region of the chorion that is attached to the wall of the womb and forms the *placenta. *See also* villus. —**chorionic** *adj.*

chorionepithelioma (choriocarcinoma) *n.* a rare form of cancer originating in the outermost of the membranes (chorion) surrounding the fetus and affecting the womb or the site of a pregnancy outside the womb, e.g. a Fallopian tube (*see* ectopic pregnancy). Chorionepithelioma, which rapidly invades and causes secondary deposits, is highly malignant; it may occur after *hydatidiform mole, pregnancy, or abortion.

絨毛膜上皮癌 一種來自包圍胎兒的最外層的膜（絨毛膜）的少見的癌。可發生於孕婦宮內或宮外，如輸卵管。生長迅速並可轉移。惡性程度極高。發生於葡萄胎、妊娠或流產後。

chorionic gonadotrophin (human chorionic gonadotrophin, HCG) a hormone, similar to the pituitary *gonadotrophins, produced by the placenta during pregnancy. Large amounts are excreted in the urine, and this is used as the basis for most *pregnancy tests. HCG maintains the secretion of *progesterone by the corpus luteum of the ovary, the secretion of pituitary gonadotrophins being blocked during pregnancy. HCG is given by injection to treat delayed puberty, undescended testes, premenstrual tension, and (with *follicle-stimulating hormone) sterility due to lack of ovulation.

絨毛膜促性腺激素 妊娠時由胎盤產生的一種與腦垂體促性腺素類似的激素。由尿大量排出，是大多數妊娠試驗的根據。在妊娠期間，垂體促性腺素分泌停止，卵巢內黃體分泌孕酮的功能則由絨毛膜促性腺激素來維持。注射給藥，用以治療青春期延遲、月經期前緊張症、不孕（與卵泡刺激素合用）。亦可用於睾丸未降（隱睾病）。

choroid *n.* the layer of the eyeball between the retina and the sclera. It contains blood vessels and a pigment that absorbs excess light and so prevents blurring of vision. *See* eye.

脉絡膜 眼球上居於視網膜鞏膜之間的一層膜。含有血管與色素，可吸收過强的光線以防止視力模糊。

choroiditis *n.* inflammation of the choroid layer of the eye. It may be inflamed together with the iris and ciliary body, but often is involved alone and in patches (*focal* or *multifocal choroiditis*). Vision becomes blurred but the eye is usually painless. *See* uveitis.

脉絡膜炎 眼脉絡膜的炎症。可能與虹膜睫狀體同時發炎，但多單獨發生。炎症呈斑狀（病竈性或多病竈性脉絡膜炎）。此時視力減退，但眼部通常無痛感。

choroid plexus a rich network of blood vessels, derived from those of the pia mater, in each of the brain's ventricles. It is responsible for the production of *cerebrospinal fluid.

脉絡叢 在各側腦室內的由軟腦膜血管形成的密集的血管網。由此處生成腦脊液。

Christmas disease a disorder that is identical in its effects to *haemophilia, but is due to a deficiency of a different blood coagulation factor, the *Christmas factor* (Factor IX).

克里斯馬斯病 臨床表現類似血友病的一種疾病。但其缺乏的是另一種不同的凝血因子——克里斯馬斯因子（第IX因子）。

chrom- (chromo-) *prefix denoting* colour or pigment.

〔前綴〕 **顏色，色素**

chromaffin *n.* tissue in the medulla of the *adrenal gland consisting of modified neural cells containing granules that are stained brown by chromates. Adrenaline and noradrenaline are released from the granules when the adrenal gland is stimulated by its sympathetic nerve supply. *See also* neurohormone.

嗜鉻組織 在腎上腺髓質中的一種由變異的神經細胞構成的組織。這種細胞內含有可被鉻染成褐色的顆粒。當腎上腺受到交感神經刺激時，即由這些顆粒釋放腎上腺與去甲腎上腺素。

-chromasia *suffix denoting* staining or pigmentation.

〔後綴〕 **色**

chromat- (chromato-) *prefix denoting* colour or pigmentation.

〔前綴〕 顏色，色素沉着

chromatid *n.* one of the two threadlike strands formed by longitudinal division of a chromosome during *mitosis and *meiosis. They remain attached at the *centromere. Chromatids can be seen between early prophase and metaphase in mitosis and between diplotene and the second metaphase of meiosis, after which they divide at the centromere to form daughter chromosomes.

染色單體 染色體在有絲分裂與減數分裂時通過縱向分裂形成的兩條細線。它們繼續附着於着絲粒。染色單體可出現於有絲分裂的前期與中期之間，及減數分裂的兩線期與第二中期之間。然後它們在着絲粒處分裂生成子染色體。

chromatin *n.* the material of a cell nucleus that stains with basic dyes and consists of DNA and protein: the substance of which the chromosomes are made. *See* euchromatin, heterochromatin.

染色質 細胞核內的一種由蛋白和脫氧核糖核酸組成並能被鹼性染料染色的物質。染色體即由此種物質組成。

chromatography *n.* any of several techniques for separating the components of a mixture by selective absorption. Two such techniques are quite

色譜法 利用選擇性吸收的原理對混合物中不同成分進行分離的技術。在分離氨基酸混合物時，在醫

widely used in medicine, for example to separate mixtures of amino acids. In one of these, *paper chromatography*, a sample of the mixture is placed at the edge of a sheet of filter paper. As the solvent soaks along the paper, the components are absorbed to different extents and thus move along the paper at different rates. In *column chromatography* the components separate out along a column of a powdered absorbent, such as silica or aluminium oxide.

學上有兩種廣泛應用的方法。一爲紙色譜法：將混合物標本置於濾紙的邊緣，以溶劑浸漬濾紙時，由於混合物中不同成分吸收的程度不同，其擴散的速度亦各異。另一爲柱色譜法：混合物置於粉狀吸收劑如氧化矽或氧化鋁中進行分離。

chromatolysis *n.* the dispersal or disintegration of the microscopic structures within the nerve cells that normally produce proteins. It is part of the cell's response to injury.

染色質溶解 神經細胞內顯微結構的分散或崩解。該結構正常時可產生蛋白質。係細胞對損傷的一種反應。

chromatophore *n.* a cell containing pigment. In man chromatophores containing *melanin are found in the skin, hair, and eyes.

色素細胞 含有色素的細胞。人類的色素細胞含有黑色素，存在於皮膚、頭髮與眼內。

chromatopsia *n.* abnormal coloured vision: a rare symptom of various conditions. Sometimes everything looks reddish to patients after removal of their cataracts; patients suffering from digitalis poisoning may see things in green or yellow. Similar disturbances of colour may be experienced by people recovering from inflammation of the optic nerve.

色視症 色視覺異常。係不同疾病中出現的一種少見的症狀。有些病人晶體摘除後視物皆呈紅色，洋地黃中毒患者視物呈綠色或黃色。有些患視神經炎的病人恢復後亦出現此類症狀。

chromoblastomycosis (chromomycosis) *n.* a chronic fungal infection of the skin usually caused by injury; for example, a wound from a wood splinter. It produces pigmented wartlike lumps – mainly on the feet and legs – that sometimes ulcerate. The disease is often found in rural communities.

着色眞菌病 通常由於外傷引起的皮膚慢性眞菌感染。例如：由木片刺傷引起。皮膚出現有色素沉着的疣狀腫塊，多見於足與腿部，有時發展成潰瘍。本病多發生於農村。

chromosome *n.* one of the threadlike structures in a cell nucleus that carry the genetic information in the form of *genes. It is composed of a long double filament of *DNA coiled into a helix together with associated proteins, with

染色體 細胞核中以基因形式攜帶遺傳信息的線樣結構。由一對長的脫氧核糖核酸細絲與相關的蛋白質盤繞成螺旋狀，基因即沿其長軸呈線狀排列，細

the genes arranged in a linear manner along its length. It stains deeply with basic dyes during cell division (*see* meiosis, mitosis). The nucleus of each human somatic cell contains 46 chromosomes, 23 being of maternal and 23 of paternal origin (see illustration). Each chromosome can duplicate an exact copy of itself between each cell division (*see* interphase) so that each new cell formed receives a full set of chromosomes. *See also* chromatid, centromere, sex chromosome. —**chromosomal** *adj.*

胞分裂時能被鹼性染料深度染色。每個人類體細胞核內有46個染色體，23個來自母體，23個來自父體（見圖）。每一個染色體在每次細胞分裂時都能複製出與自身完全同樣的產物，因此，每一個新形成的細胞都接受一整套染色體。

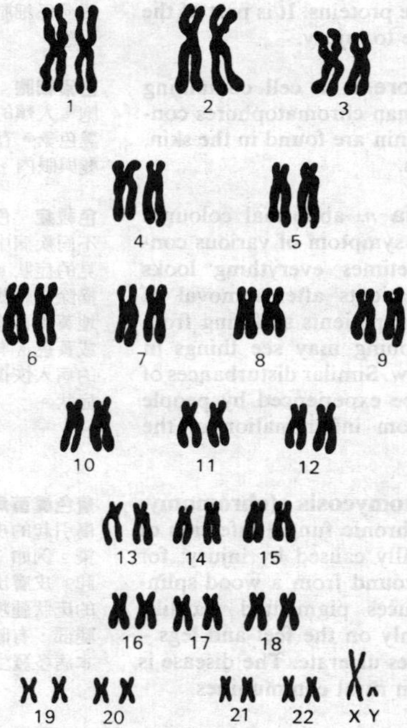

Human male chromosomes, arranged in numbered pairs according to a standard classification. The female set differs only in the sex chromosomes (XX instead of XY).

男性染色體，按標準分類法編號成對排列。女性染色體僅用××取代男性染色體即可。

chron- (chrono-) *prefix denoting* time. Example: *chronophobia* (abnormal fear of).

〔前綴〕 **時間** 例如：時間恐怖（對時間變化產生的一種異常的恐懼感）。

chronaxie *n.* a measurement of the electrical excitability of a nerve or muscle, formerly used in the detection of damage to the motor nerves. Its use has largely been superseded by *electromyography, the direct recording of electrical activity in the muscles.

時值 測量神經或肌肉電興奮性的一種數值。過去用於檢查運動神經損傷。現已多爲直接記錄肌肉電活動的肌電描記法所取代。

chronic *adj.* describing a disease of long duration involving very slow changes. Such disease is often of gradual onset. The term does not imply anything about the severity of a disease. *Compare* acute.

慢性 描述一種病程長、變化慢的疾病。這種病發病往往是逐漸的。本詞所指與疾病嚴重程度毫無關係。

Chronic Sick and Disabled Persons Act (1970) (in Britain) an Act providing for the identification and care of those suffering from a chronic or degenerative disease for which there is no cure and which can be only partially alleviated by treatment. Such patients are usually distinguished from the elderly who may also suffer from chronic diseases. It is the responsibility of local authorities to identify those with such problems and to ensure that services are available to meet their needs and that the people concerned are aware of the available services. Identification can be difficult unless doctors and health visitors notify the appropriate Social Service Departments, but there is no compulsion to make such notifications.

殘疾人法令 英國於1970年頒佈的一項有關殘疾人的法令。此法令規定，對那些無法治療或通過治療僅能獲得部分好轉的慢性病或變性性疾病患者進行鑑定並提供福利照顧。這種殘疾人尚需和患慢性病的老年人區別開來。地方當局負責對他們進行鑑定，保證提供服務以滿足他們的需求，並使有關人員了解他們可能得到何種福利照顧。如果社會福利部門沒有得到醫師和保健員的通知，這種鑑定可能發生困難。法令並未對醫務人員是否必須簽署通知書做出硬性規定。

chrys- (chryso-) *prefix denoting* gold or gold salts.

[前綴] **金，金鹽**

Chrysops *n.* a genus of bloodsucking flies, commonly called deer flies. Female flies, found in shady wooded areas, bite man during the day. Certain species in Africa may transmit the tropical disease *loiasis to man. In the USA *C. discalis* is a vector of *tularaemia.

斑虻屬 吸血蠅屬。雌蠅在蔭密林區晝間叮咬人類。非洲的某種斑虻能使人感染熱帶病——羅阿氏絲蟲病。美國的中室斑虻是傳播土拉倫斯病的媒介昆蟲。

chrysotherapy *n.* the treatment of disease by the administration of gold or its compounds. The injection of gold salts is claimed by some authorities to be extremely effective in the treatment of arthritis. However, many patients develop severe side-effects, including blood disorders, dermatitis, and upsets of liver and kidney function.

金療法 使用金或金化合物治療疾病的一種方法。某些權威學者宣稱金鹽注射治療關節炎效果卓著。但許多患者出現嚴重副作用，如血液病、皮炎、肝腎功能紊亂等。

chyle *n.* an alkaline milky liquid found within the *lacteals after a period of absorption. It consists of lymph with a suspension of minute droplets of digested fats, which have been absorbed from the small intestine. It is transported in the lymphatic system to the thoracic duct, which drains into the subclavian vein.

乳糜 食物在腸道吸收後，經一定時間，在乳糜管內出現的一種鹼性的乳樣液體。除淋巴液外，尚有自小腸吸收的消化了的脂肪微粒懸浮於其中。乳糜液通過淋巴系統運輸到胸導管，後者又進入鎖骨下靜脉。

chylomicron *n.* a microscopic particle of fat present in the blood after fat has been digested and absorbed from the small intestine.

乳糜微粒 脂肪在小腸消化吸收後在血液中出現的一種微小的脂肪顆粒。

chyluria *n.* the presence of *chyle in the urine.

乳糜尿 尿中出現乳糜。

chyme *n.* the semiliquid acid mass that is the form in which food passes from the stomach to the small intestine. It is produced by the action of *gastric juice and the churning movements of the stomach.

食糜 食物由胃進入小腸時形成的一種半液體狀酸性團塊。是由胃液及胃的攪拌作用造成的。

chymotrypsin *n.* a protein-digesting enzyme (*see* peptidase). It is secreted by the pancreas in an inactive form, *chymotrypsinogen*, that is converted into chymotrypsin in the duodenum by the action of *trypsin.

胰凝乳蛋白 一種蛋白消化酶。胰腺分泌一種無活性的胰凝乳蛋白酶原，在十二指腸內通過胰蛋白酶作用轉化成凝乳蛋白酶。

chymotrypsinogen *n. see* chymotrypsin.

胰凝乳蛋白酶原

cicatrix *n.* a scar: any mark left after the healing of a wound, where the damaged tissues fail to repair themselves completely and are replaced by connective tissue.

瘢痕 創傷癒合後遺留下的痕跡。該處損傷組織修復不全，而爲結締組織所代替。

-cide *suffix denoting* killer or killing. Examples: *bactericide* (of bacteria); *infanticide* (of children).

［後綴］ **殺死** 例如：殺菌劑，殺嬰。

ciliary body the part of the *eye that connects the choroid with the iris. It consists of three zones: the *ciliary ring*, which adjoins the choroid; the *ciliary processes*, a series of about 70 radial ridges behind the iris to which the suspensory ligament of the lens is attached; and the *ciliary muscle*, contraction of which alters the curvature of the lens (*see* accommodation).

睫狀體 眼內聯結脉絡膜與虹膜的部分。共分三帶：睫狀環，與脉絡膜相連；睫狀突，在虹膜後呈放射排列的約70根突起，與晶體懸韌帶相連；睫狀肌，收縮時可改變晶體曲率。

cilium *n.* (*pl.* **cilia**) **1.** a hairlike process, large numbers of which are found on certain epithelial cells and on certain (ciliate) protozoa. Cilia are particularly characteristic of the epithelium that lines the upper respiratory tract, where their beating serves to remove particles of dust and other foreign material. **2.** an eyelash or eyelid. —**ciliary** *adj.*

①纖毛 在某種上皮細胞和某種原蟲上大量存在的毛髮樣突起。上呼吸道的上皮細胞纖毛尤具特殊性，由於他們的抖動，灰塵顆粒與其它異物得以排出體外。**②睫**

cimetidine *n.* a drug that reduces secretion of acid in the stomach and is used to treat stomach and duodenal ulcers, inflammation of the oesophagus, and other digestive disorders. It is administered by mouth or injection and the most common side-effects are dizziness, diarrhoea, muscular pains, and rash. Trade name: **Tagamet**.

甲氰咪胍 一種抗胃酸藥。用於治療胃十二指腸潰瘍、食管炎及其它消化道疾病。口服或注射。常見副作用有頭昏、腹瀉、肌痛及皮疹。

Cimex *n. see* bed bug.

臭蟲屬

cinchocaine *n.* a local anaesthetic used in dental and other operations and to relieve pain. It is applied directly to the skin or mucous membranes or injected at the site where anaesthesia is required or into the spine. Side-effects such as yawning, restlessness, excitement, nausea, vomiting, and allergic reactions sometimes occur.

地布卡因 局部麻醉藥。用於牙科及其它手術。可在皮膚黏膜表面局部外用，或注射需麻醉部位，或注射入脊髓腔。有時可見嗜眠、不安、興奮、噁心、嘔吐及過敏反應等副作用。

cinchona *n.* the dried bark of *Cinchona* trees, formerly used in medicine to stimulate the appetite and to prevent haemorrhage and diarrhoea. Taken over prolonged periods, it may cause *cinchonism. Cinchona is the source of *quinine.

金雞納樹皮 金雞納樹的乾燥樹皮。過去入藥用於開胃、止血、止瀉。長期服用引起金雞納中毒。奎寧即取自金雞納樹皮。

cinchonism *n.* poisoning caused by an overdose of cinchona or the alkaloids quinine, quinidine, or cinchonine derived from it. The symptoms are commonly ringing noises in the ears, dizziness, blurring of vision (and sometimes complete blindness), rashes, fever, and low blood pressure. Treatment with *diuretics increases the rate of excretion of the toxic compounds from the body.

金雞納中毒 過量服用金雞納樹皮或生物鹼奎寧、奎尼丁或其衍生物辛可寧等引起的中毒。症狀通常有耳鳴、頭暈、視力模糊（有時全盲）、皮疹、發熱與低血壓。治療：投以利尿劑以促進毒物自體內排出。

cineangiocardiography *n.* a form of *angiocardiography in which the X-ray pictures are recorded on cine film. This allows the dynamic movements of the heart to be studied when the film is projected.

心血管電影照像術 將X線所見拍攝在電影膠片上的一種心血管照像術。放映電影時則可觀察研究心臟的運動。

cinefluorography *n.* the technique of taking a rapid succession of photographs of the fluorescent screen of a *fluoroscope, so that the recorded events may be later analysed.

熒光電影照像術 將熒光屏上一系列迅速變化的圖像拍攝下來的技術。在進行某項特殊的X線研究時可將迅速發生的變化拍攝在膠片上。

cineradiography *n.* the technique of taking a rapid succession of X-ray photographs, to capture on film events that occur rapidly during a particular radiographic investigation.

熒光放射照像術 將放射線檢查時發生的一系列迅速的變化拍攝到膠片上的技術。

cingulectomy *n.* surgical excision of the cingulum. The procedure is sometimes carried out as *psychosurgery for intractable mental illness.

扣帶回切除術 切除扣帶的外科手術。有時用於精神外科治療難治的精神病。

cingulum *n.* (*pl.* **cingula**) **1.** a curved bundle of nerve fibres in each cerebral hemisphere, nearly encircling its connection with the corpus callosum. *See* cerebrum. **2.** a small protuberance on the lingual surface of the crowns of incisor and canine teeth.

①**扣帶** 各側大腦半球具有的一條環形的神經纖維束。幾乎全部包繞與胼胝體的連接部分。
②**頰帶** 切牙和尖牙冠舌面的小突起。

circle of Willis a circle on the under-surface of the brain formed by linked branches of the arteries that supply the brain (see illustration). This helps to maintain the blood supply in the event of a feeding vessel being blocked. Most cerebral *aneurysms occur on or near the circle of Willis.

韋利斯環 顱底表面由向腦部供血的動脈交通支形成的動脉環（見圖）。當某一血管發生阻塞時此環可維持血供。多數顱內動脉瘤發生於此環上或在此環附近。

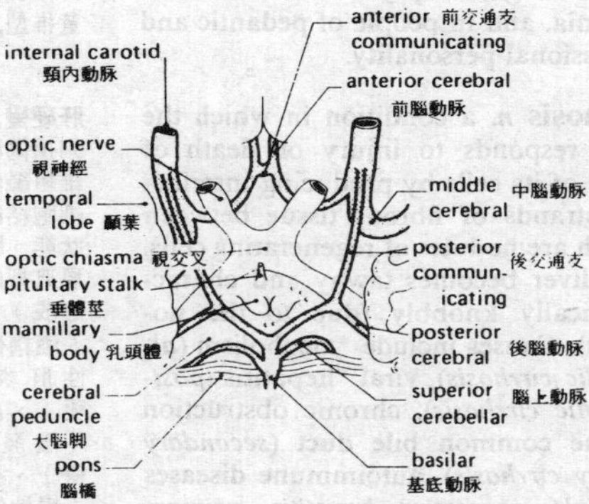

Arterial branches forming the circle of Willis (from below)
動脈交通支形成韋林斯環（下面觀）

circulatory system *see* cardiovascular system. 循環系統

circum- *prefix denoting* around; surrounding. Example: *circumanal* (around the anus). 〔前綴〕**環繞，周圍** 例如：肛周。

circumcision *n.* surgical removal of the foreskin of the penis. This operation is usually performed for religious and ethnic reasons but is sometimes required for medical conditions, mainly *phimosis and *paraphimosis. **包皮環切術** 切除陰莖包皮的外科手術。此術多由於少數民族傳統習俗與宗教信念等原因而施行。有時由於醫治疾病的目的，如包莖與箝頓包莖等。

circumduction *n.* a circular movement, such as that made by a limb. **環形運動** 例如上肢所做的環形運動。

circumflex nerve a mixed sensory and motor nerve of the upper arm. It arises from the fifth and sixth cervical segments of the spinal cord and is distributed to the deltoid muscle of the shoulder and the overlying skin. **腋神經** 上臂的一枝感覺與運動的混合神經。自第五與第六頸段發出，支配三角肌並分佈於該區皮膚上。

circumoral *adj.* situated around the mouth. **口周**

circumstantiality *n.* a disorder of thought in which thinking and speech proceed slowly and with many unnecessary trivial details. It is sometimes **瑣談症** 表現爲思維與語言緩慢並贅述許多不必要的細節的一種病症。有時見於器質性精神病、精

seen in organic *psychosis, in *schizophrenia, and in people of pedantic and obsessional personality.

神分裂症、强迫型人格與童稚型人格。

cirrhosis *n.* a condition in which the liver responds to injury or death of some of its cells by producing interlacing strands of fibrous tissue between which are nodules of regenerating cells. The liver becomes tawny and characteristically knobbly (due to the nodules). Causes include *alcoholism (*alcoholic cirrhosis*), viral *hepatitis (*postnecrotic cirrhosis*), chronic obstruction of the common bile duct (*secondary biliary cirrhosis*), autoimmune diseases (*chronic aggressive hepatitis, primary biliary cirrhosis*), and chronic heart failure (*cardiac cirrhosis*). In at least half the cases of cirrhosis no cause is found (*cryptogenic cirrhosis*). Complications include *portal hypertension, *ascites, *hepatic encephalopathy, and *hepatoma. Cirrhosis cannot be cured but its progress may be stopped if the cause can be removed. This particularly applies in alcoholism (when all alcohol must be prohibited); in hepatitis (in which corticosteroid treatment may reduce inflammation); in secondary biliary cirrhosis (in which surgery may relieve obstruction); and in cardiac failure that can be treated. —**cirrhotic** *adj.*

肝硬變 肝臟細胞由於受到損傷與死亡而產生的纖維組織索條，與再生的肝細胞結節縱橫交錯存在的狀態。肝變成黃褐色並出現典型的疙瘩（由於結節形成）。病因：酒精中毒（酒精性肝硬變）、病毒性肝炎（壞死後肝硬變）、總膽管慢性阻塞（繼發性膽汁性肝硬變）、自體免疫性疾病（慢性侵襲性肝炎、原發性膽汁性肝硬變）與慢性心力衰竭（心臟性肝硬變）。至少有半數肝硬變病因不明（病因不明性肝硬變）。合併症有門靜脈高壓、腹水、肝性腦病與肝瘤。肝硬變無法根治，但去除病因後可制止病情發展，如酒精中毒者徹底戒酒，肝炎用皮質醇類藥物可減輕炎症，繼發性膽汁肝硬變做外科手術可解除梗阻，心力衰竭者可予以相應治療。

cirs- (cirso-) *prefix denoting* a varicose vein. Example: *cirsectomy* (excision of).

［前綴］ **靜脈曲張** 如靜脈曲張切除術。

cirsoid *adj.* describing the distended knotted appearance of a varicose vein. The term is used for a type of tumour of the scalp (*cirsoid aneurysm*), which is an arteriovenous aneurysm.

曲張的 描述靜脈擴張糾纏的外觀。此詞用於描述頭皮的一種動靜脈瘤——曲張狀動靜瘤。

cisplatinum *n.* a heavy-metal compound: a *cytotoxic drug that impedes cell division by damaging DNA. Administered intravenously, it is important in the treatment of testicular and ovarian tumours. It is highly toxic; side-

順氯氨鉑 一種重金屬化合物。係細胞毒類藥物，能破壞脫氧核糖核酸以制止細胞分裂，供靜脈注射，是治療睪丸與卵巢腫瘤的重要藥物。毒性極

effects include nausea, vomiting, kidney damage, peripheral neuropathy, and hearing loss. Trade name: **Neoplatin.**

高，副作用有噁心、嘔吐、腎損害、末梢神經疾患與重聽。

cisterna *n.* (*pl:* **cisternae**) **1.** one of the enlarged spaces beneath the *arachnoid that act as reservoirs for cerebrospinal fluid. The largest (*cisterna magna*) lies beneath the cerebellum and behind the medulla oblongata. **2.** a dilatation at the lower end of the thoracic duct, into which the great lymph ducts of the lower limbs drain.

池　①蛛網膜下腔貯積腦脊液的擴大部分。最大的是小腦延髓池，位於小腦之下、延髓之後。②胸導管下端的擴大部分。來自下肢的淋巴管由此進入胸導管。

cistron *n.* the section of a DNA or RNA chain that controls the amino-acid sequence of a single polypeptide chain in protein synthesis. A cistron can be regarded as the functional equivalent of a *gene.

順反子　在蛋白質合成中控制某一多肽鏈中氨基酸排列順序的脫氧核糖核酸或核糖核酸鏈中的部分。一般認爲其功能與基因是等同的。

citric acid an organic acid found naturally in citrus fruits. Citric acid is formed in the first stage of the *Krebs cycle, the important energy-producing cycle in the body.

枸橼酸　在柑橘類果實中自然存在的一種有機酸。出現於體內重要的產能反應三羧酸循環的開始階段。

citric acid cycle *see* Krebs cycle.

枸橼酸循環　即三羧酸循環。

citrullinaemia *n.* an inborn lack of one of the enzymes concerned with the chemical breakdown of proteins to urea: in consequence both the amino acid citrulline and ammonia accumulate in the blood. Affected children fail to thrive, and show signs of mental retardation.

瓜氨酸尿症　先天缺乏一種把蛋白質分解爲尿素的酶。缺乏此酶，血內瓜氨酸與氨同時增加。患兒發育障礙，並有智力遲鈍。

citrulline *n.* an *amino acid produced by the liver as a by-product during the conversion of ammonia to *urea.

瓜氨酸　由肝臟生成的一種氨基酸。係氨轉變成尿素時的一種副產物。

clamp *n.* a surgical instrument designed to compress a structure, such as a blood vessel or a cut end of the intestine (see illustration). A variety of clamps have been designed for specific surgical procedures. Blood-vessel clamps are used to stop bleeding from the cut vessels. Intestinal clamps pre-

鉗　用以壓迫組織的外科器械。可壓迫血管或腸斷端（見圖）。爲了不同的外科手術操作目的，有不同的鉗夾。血管鉗用於血管斷端止血。腸鉗用於腸管手術時防止腸內容物溢入腹腔。腸鉗對腸壁無損。

vent the intestinal contents from leaking into the abdominal cavity during operations on the intestines and are designed not to damage the intestinal wall.

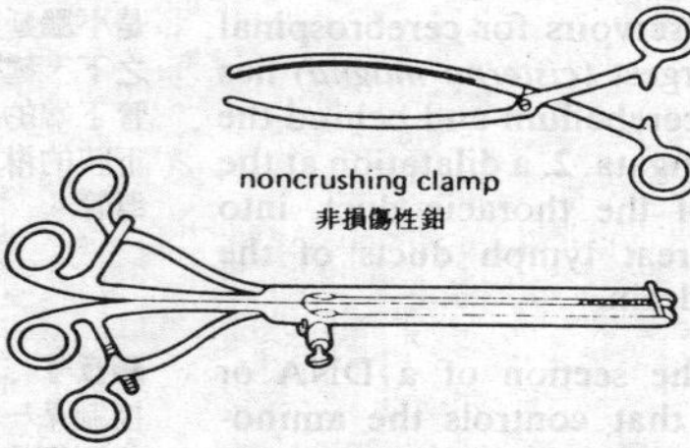

Intestinal clamps

腸鉗

clasmocyte *n. see* macrophage.

大吞噬細胞

clasp *n.* (in dentistry) the part of a *denture that keeps it in place. It is made of flexible metal.

卡環 托牙中固位的部分。常由可塑性金屬製成。

claudication *n.* limping. *Intermittent claudication* is a cramping pain, induced by exercise and relieved by rest, that is caused by an inadequate supply of blood to the affected muscles. It is most often seen in the calf and leg muscles as a result of *atheroma of the leg arteries. The leg pulses are often absent and the feet may be cold. The treatment is that of atheroma.

間歇性跛行 本病係一種痙攣性疼痛。運動時發生，休息時緩解。由患肌供血不足引起。多見於腿部或小腿。係下肢動脈粥樣硬化所致。下肢脈搏常消失，足部寒冷。治療原發病。

claustrophobia *n.* a morbid fear of enclosed places. *See also* phobia.

幽閉恐怖 被關閉獨處時的一種病態的恐懼感。

claustrum *n.* a thin vertical layer of grey matter* in each cerebral hemisphere, between the surface of the *insula and the lenticular nucleus (*see* basal ganglia).

屏狀核 存在於各側大腦半球內的垂直的薄層灰質。位於腦島與豆狀核之間。

clavicle *n.* the collar bone: a long slender curved bone, a pair of which form the front part of the shoulder girdle. Each clavicle articulates

鎖骨 一對位於肩胛帶前方的細長彎曲的骨頭。外與肩胛骨相關節，內與胸骨柄相關節。

laterally with the *scapula and medially with the manubrium of the sternum (breastbone). —**clavicular** *adj.*

clavus *n.* **1.** *see* corn. **2.** a sharp pain in the head, as if a nail were being driven in.

①**雞眼** ②**釘腦感** 腦內感到釘鑽般疼痛。

claw-foot *n.* an excessively arched foot, giving an unnaturally high instep. In most cases the cause is unknown, but the deformity may sometimes be due to an imbalance between the muscles flexing the toes and the shorter muscles that extend them; this type is found in some neuromuscular diseases, such as Friedreich's *ataxia. Surgical treatment is effective in childhood but less so in adult life. Medical name: **pes cavus**.

爪形足 極度的弓形足。腳背不自然地高高隆起。多數病例病因不明。有時係由屈趾肌與伸趾短肌力量失衡引起，此型可見於某種神經肌肉疾患，如家族性共濟失調。兒童期可行手術治癒，成人則無效。

claw-hand *n.* flexion and contraction of the fingers with extension at the joints between the fingers and the hand, giving a claw-like appearance. Any kind of damage to the nerves or muscles may lead to claw-hand; causes include injuries, *syringomyelia, and leprosy. *See also* Dupuytren's contracture.

爪形手 由於掌指關節伸直手指攣縮屈曲而出現的一種鷹爪樣外觀。神經肌肉的各種損傷都可引起。原因有外傷、脊髓室洞症、麻瘋。

clearance (renal clearance) *n.* a quantitative measure of the rate at which waste products are removed from the blood by the kidneys. It is expressed in terms of the volume of blood that could be completely cleared of a particular substance in one minute.

清除率（腎清除率） 對血液中的廢物通過腎臟排出的速度進行定量測定的一種方法。用某種物質在一分鐘內自血液完全排出所需的血液量來表示。

clearing *n.* (in microscopy) the process of removing the cloudiness from microscopical specimens after *dehydration by means of a *clearing agent*. This increases the transparency of the specimens. Xylene, cedar oil, methyl benzoate plus benzol, and methyl salicylate plus benzol are commonly used as clearing agents.

透明 製做顯微鏡標本時，脫水後用透明劑除掉其模糊現象的方法。可增加標本的透明度。常用的透明劑有二甲苯、香柏油、苯甲酸甲酯加苯、水楊酸甲酯加苯。

cleavage *n.* (in embryology) the process of repeated cell division of the fertilized egg to form a ball of cells that becomes the *blastocyst. The cells

卵裂 胚胎期受精卵不斷分裂的過程。結果形成細胞球——胚泡。這些細胞（裂球）在繼續分裂中不

(*blastomeres*) do not grow between divisions and so they decrease in size.

再生長，故其體積反而縮小。

cleft palate a fissure in the midline of the palate due to failure of the two sides to fuse in embryonic development. Only part of the palate may be affected, or the cleft may extend the full length with bilateral clefts at the front of the maxilla; it may be accompanied by a *harelip and disturbance of tooth formation. Cleft palates can be corrected by surgery.

腭裂 胚胎期兩側腭未能融合而在中線處形成的裂。腭裂可以是部分性的，亦可沿兩側腭的全長直達上頜骨前方，伴有兔唇與牙齒生長障礙。本病可用手術糾正。

cleid- (cleido-, clid-, clido-) *prefix denoting* the clavicle (collar bone). Example: *cleidocranial* (of the clavicle and cranium).

〔前綴〕 **鎖骨** 鎖骨頭顱的。

cleidocranial dysostosis a congenital defect of bone formation in which the skull bones ossify imperfectly and the collar bones (clavicles) are absent.

鎖骨顱骨發育不全 一種先天性骨發育障礙。本病有顱骨骨化不全與鎖骨缺乏。

clemizole *n.* an *antihistamine used to treat such allergies as hay fever and urticaria. It is administered by mouth or injection or applied to the skin as a cream.

氯咪唑 抗組織胺藥。用以治療枯草熱與蕁麻疹等過敏反應。口服或注射，亦可製成乳膏劑外用。

client-centred therapy (Rogerian therapy) a method of psychotherapy in which the therapist refrains from directing his client in what he should do and instead concentrates on communicating understanding and acceptance. Frequently he reflects the client's own words or feelings back to him. The aim is to enable the client to solve his own problems.

患者中心治療法 一種精神療法。醫生不指導病人去做他所應該做的事情，而只是致力於和病人交流思想以達到使之理解和接受。常常把病人說過的話或感覺反而向病人提出來。使他自己去解決自己的問題。

climacteric *n.* **1.** *see* menopause. **2.** declining sexual drive and fertility in men, usually occurring in middle age.

①絕經期 ②更年期現象 通常發生於中年的性慾與生育能力下降的現象。

clindamycin *n.* an *antibiotic used to treat serious bacterial infections. It is administered by mouth; possible side-effects are nausea, vomiting, diarrhoea, and occasional hypersensitivity reactions.

氯林可黴素 用以治療嚴重細菌感染的一種抗生素。口服。可有噁心、嘔吐、腹瀉等副作用，偶見過敏反應。

clinic *n.* **1.** an establishment or department of a hospital devoted to the treatment of particular diseases or the medical care of out-patients. **2.** a gathering of instructors, students, and patients, usually in a hospital ward, for the examination and treatment of the patients.

①**臨床科室** 醫院中治療各專科疾病和門診病人的機構或部門。②**大查房** 導師、醫學生一起在病房進行檢查和治療的活動。

clinical medicine the branch of medicine dealing with the study of patients in bed and the diagnosis and treatment of disease at the bedside, as opposed to the study of disease by *pathology or other laboratory work.

臨床醫學 醫學的一種分枝學科。與病理學和化驗室工作相反，臨床醫學是在病床邊對卧床病人進行診斷、治療、研究的學科。

clioquinol *n.* an iodine-containing antiseptic active against amoebae and other microorganisms. It is used to treat bowel infections, such as dysentery, and skin infections and is administered by mouth, as suppositories, or in ointments, creams, or lotions.

氯碘喹啉 一種含碘的抗阿米巴與抗菌藥，治療痢疾等腸道感染與皮膚感染。口服。亦可製成栓劑、油膏劑、乳膏劑或洗劑使用。

clitoris *n.* the female counterpart of the penis, which contains erectile tissue (*see* corpus cavernosum) but is unconnected with the urethra. Like the penis it becomes erect under conditions of sexual stimulation, to which it is very sensitive.

陰蒂 女性的相當於男性陰莖的部分。內有勃起組織，但與尿道不通聯。在性興奮時，可以像陰莖一樣勃起。此部位對性刺激十分敏感。

clivus *n.* (in anatomy) a surface that slopes, such as occurs in part of the sphenoid bone.

斜坡 （解剖學用語）指傾斜的表面。如蝶骨斜坡。

cloaca *n.* the most posterior part of the embryonic *hindgut. It becomes divided into the rectum and the urinogenital sinus, which receives the bladder together with the urinary and genital ducts.

泄殖腔 胚胎期後腸的最後部分。以後分成直腸和尿生殖竇，後者與膀胱及尿生殖管聯接起來。

clofibrate *n.* a drug that reduces the levels of blood lipids, including cholesterol, and is used to treat atherosclerosis and angina. It is administered by mouth; side-effects can include stomach discomfort, nausea, and diarrhoea. Trade names: **Atromid-S**, **Liprinal**.

祛脂乙酯 降血脂（包括膽固醇）藥。治療動脉粥樣硬化心絞痛。口服。副作用有胃部不適、噁心與腹瀉。商品名：安妥明。

clomipramine *n.* a drug used to treat various depressive states (*see* antidepressant). It is administered by mouth or injection; common side-effects are dry mouth and blurred vision. Trade name: **Anafranil.**

氯丙咪嗪　抗抑鬱藥。口服或注射。常見副作用有口乾與視力模糊。

clomocycline *n.* an *antibiotic used to treat infections caused by a variety of microorganisms and also used for long-term treatment of acne. It is administered by mouth and may cause digestive upsets and allergic reactions. Trade name: **Megaclor.**

羥甲金黴素　一種抗生素。用於治療多種微生物感染，亦用於長期治療痤瘡。口服。可引起消化不良與過敏反應。

clonazepam *n.* a drug with *anticonvulsant properties, used to treat epilepsy and other conditions involving seizures. It is administered by mouth or injection; drowsiness is a common side-effect. Trade name: **Rivotril.**

氯硝安定　抗驚厥藥。治療癲癇及其他伴有驚厥發作的疾病。口服或注射。常見副作用爲嗜眠。

clone 1. *n.* a group of cells (usually bacteria) descended from a single cell by asexual reproduction and therefore genetically identical to each other and to the parent cell. **2.** *vb.* to form a clone.

①**克隆**　由單一細胞通過無性繁殖產生的一組細胞羣。因此它們彼此或與親本細胞在遺傳學上相同。②做動詞用時，意爲克隆化。

clonic *adj.* of, relating to, or resembling clonus. The term is most commonly used to describe the rhythmical limb movements in convulsive epilepsy (*see* grand mal).

陣攣性的　與陣攣有關或類似陣攣的。本詞常用於描述癲癇大發作時肢體的有節律的運動。

clonidine *n.* a drug used to treat high blood pressure (hypertension) and migraine. It is administered by mouth or injection and commonly causes drowsiness and dry mouth. Trade name: **Catapres.**

氯壓定　治療高血壓與偏頭痛藥。口服或注射。常引起嗜眠和口乾。商品名：可樂寧。

clonorchiasis *n.* a condition caused by the presence of the fluke *Clonorchis sinensis* in the bile ducts. The infection, common in the Far East, is acquired through eating undercooked, salted, or pickled freshwater fish harbouring the larval stage of the parasite. Symptoms include fever, abdominal pain, diarrhoea, liver enlargement, loss of appetite, emaciation and – in advanced cases

枝睾吸蟲病　華枝睾吸蟲進入膽道引起的疾病。多見於遠東，由於進食帶有活囊蚴的鹹、腌或未煮熟的淡水魚類引起。症狀有發熱、腹痛、腹瀉、肝大、食慾減退、消瘦。晚期可有肝硬變及黃疸。治療：雖然磷酸氯喹對部分病例有效，但仍不滿意。

– cirrhosis and jaundice. Treatment is unsatisfactory although *chloroquine diphosphate has proved beneficial in some cases.

Clonorchis *n.* a genus of liver flukes, common parasites of man and other fish-eating mammals in the Far East. The adults of *C. sinensis* cause clonorchiasis. Eggs are passed out in the stools and the larvae undergo their development in two other hosts, a snail and a fish.

枝睾吸蟲屬 肝吸蟲屬。遠東食魚動物與人類身上的一種常見的寄生蟲。華枝睾吸蟲的成蟲是枝睾吸蟲病的病因。蟲卵隨糞便排出。幼蟲發育通過兩種中間宿主：螺和魚。

clonus *n.* rhythmical contraction of a muscle in response to a suddenly applied and then sustained stretch stimulus. It is most readily obtained at the ankle when the examiner bends the foot sharply upwards and then maintains an upward pressure on the sole. It is caused by an exaggeration of the stretch reflexes and is usually a sign of disease in the brain or spinal cord.

陣攣 突然牽伸某肌並持續維持伸張狀態引起的有節律的收縮。此現象極易出現於踝部。當受檢查者的足突然向上扳，並在足底持續加壓時即可出現。這是牽張反射過强引起的，通常是腦或脊髓疾患的體徵。

clopamide *n.* a *diuretic used to treat fluid retention (oedema) and high blood pressure (hypertension). It is administered by mouth and side-effects are uncommon. Trade name: **Brinaldix**.

氯哌醯胺 利尿藥。用以治療水腫與高血壓。口服。副作用少。

clorazepate potassium a tranquillizing drug used to relieve anxiety, tension, and agitation. It is administered by mouth; side-effects can include dizziness, digestive upsets, blurred vision, and, occasionally, drowsiness. Trade name: **Tranxene**.

氯氮革二鉀 安定藥。用以治療焦慮、激動、緊張。口服。副作用有頭暈、消化不良、視力模糊，偶見嗜眠。

clorexolone *n.* a *diuretic with prolonged action, used to treat fluid retention (oedema) and high blood pressure (hypertension). It is administered by mouth; common side-effects are nausea and loss of appetite, and reduced blood potassium levels may develop. Trade name: **Nefrolan**.

氯環吲酮 長效利尿藥。用以治療水腫與高血壓。口服。常見副作用有噁心、食慾減退。可能發生低血鉀。

clorindione *n.* an *anticoagulant used to prevent further blood clotting in coronary and other thromboses. It is

氯苯茚二酮 抗凝血藥。用以防止冠狀動脉與其他部位的血栓發展。口服。

administered by mouth and side-effects can include nausea, diarrhoea, hair loss, itching, and skin damage.

副作用有噁心、腹瀉、脫髮、瘙癢與皮膚病。

Clostridium *n.* a genus of mostly Gram-positive anaerobic spore-forming rodlike bacteria commonly found in soil and in the intestinal tract of man and animals. Many species cause disease in man and animals and produce extremely potent *exotoxins. *C. botulinum* grows freely in badly preserved canned foods, producing a toxin causing serious food poisoning (*botulism). *C. histolyticum*, *C. oedematiens*, and *C. septicum* all cause *gas gangrene when they infect wounds. *C. tetani* lives as a harmless *commensal in the intestine of animals and man but causes *tetanus on contamination of wounds (with manured soil). The species *C. welchii* (*C. perfringens*) – Welch's bacillus – causes blood poisoning, *food poisoning, and gas gangrene.

梭狀芽胞桿菌屬 通常存在於泥土與人類及動物腸道中的桿狀菌屬。大部分爲革蘭氏陽性，厭氧，能形成芽胞。許多種菌能引起人類與動物疾病並產生强烈的外毒素。肉毒梭狀芽胞桿菌能在保存不好的罐頭食品中迅速生長，其毒素引起嚴重的食物中毒（肉毒桿菌中毒）。溶組織梭狀芽胞桿菌、水腫梭狀芽胞桿菌及敗血梭狀芽胞桿菌感染傷口時可引起氣性壞疽。破傷風梭狀芽胞桿菌係人類與動物腸道中無害的共生菌，但污染傷口（通過糞土）可引起破傷風。魏氏梭狀芽胞桿菌可引起血液中毒、食物中毒、氣性壞疽。

clotrimazole *n.* an antiseptic used to treat all types of fungal skin infections, including ringworm and infections of the genital organs. It is applied to the infected part as cream or solution or as vaginal pessaries and occasionally causes mild burning or irritation. Trade name: **Canesten**.

克黴唑 抗眞菌藥。治療皮膚一切眞菌感染（包括癬）與生殖器官感染。可製成乳膏劑、溶液或陰道栓劑使用。偶有輕微燒灼刺激感。

clotting factors *see* coagulation factors.

凝血因子

clotting time *see* coagulation time.

凝血時間

cloxacillin sodium an antibiotic, derived from penicillin, used to treat many bacterial infections. It is administered by mouth or injection; diarrhoea sometimes occurs and hypersensitivity reactions occur in penicillin-sensitive patients. Trade name: **Orbenin**.

鄰氯青黴素鈉 從青黴素衍生出的一種抗生素。用以治療多種細菌感染。口服或注射。有時有腹瀉。在對青黴素過敏的病人亦會發生過敏反應。

clubbing *n.* thickening of the tissues at the bases of the finger and toe nails so that the normal angle between the nail and the digit is filled in. The nail

杵狀變（指趾） 指或趾基底部組織增厚以致指（趾）甲與指（趾）節間的角度消失。甲面隆起，

becomes convex in all directions and in extreme cases the digit end becomes bulbous like a club or drumstick. Clubbing is seen in pulmonary tuberculosis, bronchiectasis, empyema, infective endocarditis, cyanotic congenital heart disease, and lung cancer and as a harmless congenital abnormality.

重度者指（趾）端呈球形，類似球棒或鼓槌。本症可見於肺結核、支氣管擴張、肺氣腫、感染性心內膜炎、青紫簇先天性心臟病、肺癌。亦可爲無害的先天性畸形。

club-foot (talipes) *n.* a deformity of one or both feet in which the patient cannot stand with the sole of the foot flat on the ground. In the most common variety (*talipes equinovarus*) the foot is twisted downwards and inwards so that the patient walks on the outer edge of the upper surface of his foot. Other varieties are *talipes varus*, in which the sole of the foot is turned inwards, and *talipes valgus*, in which it is twisted outwards. The defect is present at birth and can be corrected by orthopaedic splinting in the early months of infancy. It may also occur as a complication of muscular paralysis due to poliomyelitis.

畸形足 單足或雙足畸形以致患者不能用足底在地面平穩站立。最常見的是馬蹄內翻足，足部下垂內翻，患者用足背外側邊緣部行走。其他尚有內翻足、外翻足等。先天性者可於嬰兒早期用矯形夾板糾正。本病亦可爲脊髓灰質炎所致肌肉麻痹的合併症。

clumping *n. see* agglutination.

凝集

Clutton's joint a swollen joint, usually the knee, caused by inflammation of the synovial membranes due to congenital syphilis.

克勒頓氏關節 由滑膜炎引起的關節（通常是膝關節）腫大。由先天性梅毒引起。

clyster *n.* an old-fashioned term for an *enema.

灌腸法 舊名。

CNS *see* central nervous system.

中樞神經系統

coagulant *n.* any substance capable of converting blood from a liquid to a solid state. *See* blood coagulation.

促凝劑 能夠將血液從液態轉變爲固態的任何物質。

coagulase *n.* an enzyme, formed by disease-producing varieties of certain bacteria of the genus *Staphylococcus*, that causes blood plasma to coagulate. Staphylococci that are positive when tested for coagulase production are classified as belonging to the species *Staphylococcus aureus*.

凝固酶 某些致病性葡萄球菌產生的一種能使血漿凝固的酶。在實驗中能產生此酶的都屬於金黃色葡萄球菌。

coagulation *n.* the process by which a colloidal liquid changes to a jellylike mass. *See* blood coagulation.

凝固 膠態液體轉變成膠凍樣固體的過程。

coagulation factors (clotting factors) a group of substances present in blood plasma that, under certain circumstances, undergo a series of chemical reactions leading to the conversion of blood from a liquid to a solid state (*see* blood coagulation). Although they have specific names, most coagulation factors are referred to by an agreed set of Roman numerals. Lack of any of these factors in the blood results in the inability of the blood to clot. *See also* haemophilia.

凝血因子 在一定條件下能通過一系列化學反應將血液由液態轉變成固態的存在於血漿中的一組物質。雖然各物質名目繁多，但缺少其中任何一種因子，都不能發生凝固。

coagulation time (clotting time) the time taken for blood or blood plasma to coagulate (*see* blood coagulation). When measured under controlled conditions and using appropriate techniques, coagulation times may be used to test the function of the various stages of the blood coagulation process.

凝血時間 血液或血漿凝固所需的時間。使用相應技術在控制的條件下測定凝血時間，可以檢查凝血過程不同階段的功能狀態。

coagulum *n.* a mass of coagulated matter, such as that formed when blood clots.

凝塊 因物質凝固而形成的團塊。如血凝塊。

coalesce *vb.* to grow together or unite. **—coalescence** *n.*

併合 融合或連合。

coarctation *n.* (of the aorta) a congenital narrowing of a short segment of the aorta. The most common site of coarctation is just beyond the origin of the left subclavian artery from the aorta. This results in high blood pressure (*hypertension) in the upper part of the body and arms and low blood pressure in the legs. The defect is corrected surgically.

縮窄 主動脉縮窄是發生在主動脉一小段上的先天性狹窄。最常見的縮窄部位是在左鎖骨下動脉的遠端，故可引起上肢高血壓與下肢低血壓。本病可用手術糾正。

cobalamin *n.* *see* vitamin B_{12}.

鈷胺[素]

cobalt *n.* a metallic element. The artificial radioisotope *cobalt-60*, or *radiocobalt*, is a powerful emitter of gamma radiation and is used in the radiation treatment of cancer (*see* radiotherapy, telecurietherapy). Cobalt itself forms part of the *vitamin B_{12} molecule. Symbol: Co.

鈷 金屬元素。人工放射性同位素鈷-60（放射性鈷）能發射强大的γ射線，用於治療癌（放射線療法，遠距居里療法）。鈷是維生素B_{12}的組成部分。符號：Co。

cobalt-chromium *n.* a silver-coloured nonprecious alloy of cobalt and chromium used for the metal frame of partial *dentures.

鈷鉻合金 鈷和鉻形成的一種銀色的非貴重金屬。用於製做部分托牙的骀架。

cocaine *n.* an alkaloid, derived from the leaves of the coca plant (*Erythroxylon coca*) or prepared synthetically, sometimes used as a local anaesthetic in eye, ear, nose, and throat surgery. It constricts the small blood vessels at the site of application and therefore need not be given with *adrenaline. Since it causes feelings of exhilaration and may lead to psychological *dependence, cocaine has largely been replaced by safer anaesthetics.

可卡因 自古柯屬植物葉中提取或人工合成的一種生物鹼。有時在眼、耳、鼻、喉手術中用做局部麻醉藥。本品能收縮用藥部位的小血管，故不必合用腎上腺素。因爲有致欣快感作用並能成癮，現已多被較安全的麻醉藥代替。

cocainism *n.* **1.** the habitual use of, or addiction to, *cocaine in order to experience its intoxicating effects. **2.** the mental and physical deterioration resulting from addiction to cocaine.

①**可卡因癮** 爲了享受可卡因毒性作用引起的欣快感而養成使用可卡因的習癖或對之成癮。②**可卡因中毒** 由於對可卡因成癮導致身心狀態惡化。

cocarcinogen *n.* a substance that enhances the effect of a *carcinogen.

輔致癌物質 能加强致癌物作用的物質。

coccidioidomycosis *n.* an infection caused by inhaling the spores of the fungus *Coccidioides immitis.* In the primary form there is an influenza-like illness that usually resolves within about eight weeks. In a few patients the disease becomes progressive and resembles tuberculosis. Severe or progressive infections are treated with intravenous injections of amphotericin-B. The disease is endemic only in the southwestern US, Mexico, and Venezuela.

球孢子菌病 吸入粗球孢子菌的孢子所致的感染。最初感染類似流感，通常八週內痊癒。某些患者病情進展類似結核病，嚴重病例可用二性黴素靜注。本病僅在委內瑞拉、墨西哥、美國西南部流行。

coccobacillus *n.* a rod-shaped bacterium (bacillus) that is so small that it resembles a spherical bacterium (coccus). Examples of such bacteria are **Bacteroides* and **Brucella*.

球桿菌 體積甚小以致類似球菌的桿菌。如擬桿菌與布氏桿菌。

coccus *n.* (*pl.* **cocci**) any spherical bacterium. *See also* gonococcus, menin-

球菌 所有的球狀細菌。參見淋球菌、腦膜炎雙球

gococcus, Micrococcus, pneumococcus, Staphylococcus, Streptococcus.

菌、小球菌屬、肺炎雙球菌、鏈球菌、葡萄球菌等。

coccy- (coccyg-, coccygo-) *prefix denoting* the coccyx. Example: *coccygectomy* (excision of).

[前綴] **尾** 如尾骨切除術。

coccydynia *n.* pain in the lowermost segment of the spine (coccyx) and the neighbouring area.

尾骨痛 脊柱最低的節段（尾骨）及其附近區域疼痛。

coccyx *n.* (*pl.* **coccyges** or **coccyxes**) the lowermost element of the *backbone: the vestigial human tail. It consists of four rudimentary *coccygeal vertebrae* fused to form a triangular bone that articulates with the sacrum. *See also* vertebra. —**coccygeal** *adj.*

尾骨 脊椎骨的最下部分：殘留的人尾。由4塊退化的尾椎融合成一塊三角形的骨頭，與骶椎形成關節。

cochlea *n.* the spiral organ of the *labyrinth of the ear, which is concerned with the reception and analysis of sound. As vibrations pass from the middle ear through the cochlea, different frequencies cause particular regions of the basilar membrane to vibrate: high notes cause vibration in the region

耳蝸 耳迷路中的螺旋形器官。具有接受與分析聲音的功能。當震動由中耳傳向耳蝸時，不同的頻率可引起基膜不同部位的震動。高音使靠近中耳的部位產生震動，低音使耳蝸頂部產生震動。位於中心

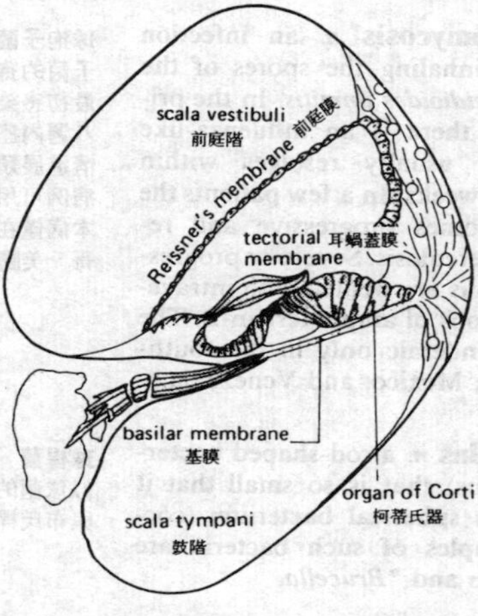

Section through a turn of the cochlea
耳蝸經螺旋切面

nearest the middle ear; low notes cause vibration in the region nearest the tip of the spiral. The *organ of Corti*, which lies within a central triangular membrane-bound canal (*scala media* or *cochlear duct*), contains sensory hair cells attached to an overlying *tectorial membrane* (see illustration). When the basilar membrane vibrates the sensory cells become distorted and send nerve impulses to the brain via the *cochlear nerve. —**cochlear** *adj.*

呈三角形的膜性管道（中階或蝸管）中的柯蒂氏器含有感覺性毛細胞，毛細胞上方覆有蓋膜（見圖）。基膜震動時感覺細胞變形並沿耳蝸神經向大腦輸送衝動。

cochlear duct (scala media) *see* cochlea.

蝸管（中階）

cochlear nerve the nerve connecting the cochlea to the brain and therefore responsible for the nerve impulses relating to hearing. It forms part of the *vestibulocochlear nerve (cranial nerve VIII).

耳蝸神經　將耳蝸與大腦聯係並將聽覺衝動傳送至大腦的神經。是前庭耳蝸神經的一部分（第Ⅷ對腦神經）。

codeine *n.* an *analgesic derived from morphine but less potent as a pain killer and sedative and less toxic. It is administered by mouth or injection to relieve pain and also to suppress coughs. Common side-effects include constipation, nausea, vomiting, dizziness, and drowsiness, but *dependence is uncommon.

可待因　由嗎啡製成的止痛藥。但止痛鎮靜作用較小，毒性較輕。口服或注射。用於止痛、鎮咳。常見副作用有便秘、噁心、嘔吐、頭暈、嗜眠，但很少成癮。

codon *n.* the unit of the *genetic code that determines the synthesis of one particular amino acid. Each codon consists of a section of the DNA molecule, and the order of the codons along the molecule determines the order of amino acids in each protein made in the cell.

密碼子　在蛋白質合成中決定某一特定氨基酸位置（順序）的遺傳密碼的單位。每一個密碼子都由一個脫氧核糖核酸片段組成，密碼子在分子內排列的順序決定細胞中合成的蛋白質中氨基酸的排列順序。

-coele *suffix denoting* **1.** a body cavity. Example: *blastocoele* (cavity of blastocyst). **2.** *see* -cele.

［後綴］①**體腔**　如囊腔。②**疝，膨出瘤，腫大**

coeli- (coelio-) *prefix denoting* the abdomen or belly. Example: *coeliectasia* (abnormal distention of).

［前綴］　**腹腔，內臟**　如腹脹（腹部異常脹大）。

coeliac *adj.* of or relating to the abdominal region. The *coeliac trunk* is a branch of the abdominal *aorta supplying the stomach, spleen, liver, and gall bladder.

腹部的 屬於或與腹部有關的。腹腔幹是腹主動脉向胃、脾、肝、膽囊供血的分支。

coeliac disease a condition in which the small intestine fails to digest and absorb food. It affects 0.1–0.2% of the population and is due to sensitivity of the intestinal lining to the protein gliadin, which is contained in *gluten in the germ of wheat and rye and causes atrophy of the digestive and absorptive cells of the intestine. Symptoms include stunted growth, distended abdomen, and pale frothy foul-smelling stools; the disease can be diagnosed by *biopsy of the jejunum and is treated successfully by a strict and lifelong gluten-free diet. Medical name: **gluten enteropathy**.

麥膠過敏性腸病 一種小腸消化吸收食物功能發生障礙的疾病。發病率0.1～0.2%。由腸黏膜對小麥與稞麥胚芽谷蛋白內含有的一種麥醇溶蛋白過敏引起。腸的消化與吸收細胞發生萎縮。症狀有生長發育障礙、腹脹、蒼白色多泡沫惡臭的大便。空腸組織活檢可診斷。治療：終身禁食含麩質食物。

coelioscopy *n.* the technique of introducing an *endoscope through an incision in the abdominal wall to examine the intestines and other organs within the abdominal cavity.

體腔鏡檢查 一種將內窺鏡通過腹壁切口插入腹腔以檢查腸管與其他腹腔臟器的技術。

coelom *n.* the cavity in an embryo between the two layers of mesoderm. It develops into the body cavity.

原始體腔 胚胎期兩層中胚層之間的腔隙。以後發育成體腔。

coenzyme *n.* a nonprotein organic compound that, in the presence of an *enzyme, plays an essential role in the reaction that is catalysed by the enzyme. Coenzymes, which frequently contain the B vitamins in their molecular structure, include *coenzyme A, *FAD, and *NAD.

輔酶 一種非蛋白質有機化合物。在酶存在的情況下，對酶所催化的反應起重要作用。在其分子結構中通常含有維生素B。其中有輔酶A、黃素腺嘌呤二核苷酸、煙醯胺腺嘌呤二核苷酸。

coenzyme A a *nucleotide containing pantothenic acid, which is an important coenzyme in the Krebs cycle and in the metabolism of fatty acids.

輔酶A 一種含有泛酸的核苷。是三羧循環與脂肪代謝中重要的輔酶。

cofactor *n.* a nonprotein substance that must be present in suitable amounts before certain *enzymes can act. Cofactors include *coenzymes and metal ions (e.g. sodium and potassium ions).

轉因子 酶起作用時必需適量存在的一種非蛋白質物質。包括輔酶與某種金屬離子（鈉離子、鉀離子等）。

Cogwheel division *see* medical committee (hospital).

嵌齒輪部門 醫學委員會中的一個部門。

cohort study (longitudinal study, prospective study) a systematic follow-up of a group of people for a defined period of time or until the occurrence of a specified event (e.g. retirement or death) in order to observe their pattern of disease and/or cause of death. On the basis of factors prevailing at the outset of the study or arising during the period of follow-up, two or more separate cohorts may be identified and compared in relation to outcome.

隊列研究(前瞻性研究) 爲了觀察疾病譜和/或致死原因，對一組對象在一定時期內或直至發生某種特殊事件爲止(如退休或死亡)進行的系統性的隨訪。根據隨訪開始時基本條件的不同以及隨訪過程中情況變化，可將研究對象分成兩組或多組，以便對結果進行鑑別與比較。

coitus (sexual intercourse, copulation) *n.* sexual contact between a man and a woman during which the erect penis enters the vagina and is moved within it by pelvic thrusts until *ejaculation occurs. *See also* orgasm. **—coital** *adj.*

性交 男女之間發生的性行爲。此時勃起的陰莖插入陰道，並由骨盆部的挺伸而運動，直至射精爲止。

coitus interruptus a contraceptive method in which the penis is removed from the vagina before ejaculation of semen (orgasm). The method is unreliable (10–20 pregnancies per 100 woman-years) and it may lead to sexual disharmony and anxiety in one or both partners.

中斷性交 一種避孕方法。於射精前即將陰莖拔出陰道。此法並不可靠(妊娠率 10~20% 人年)，而且會引起性生活不協調和單方或雙方的焦慮症。

col- (coli-, colo-) *prefix denoting* the colon. Example: *coloptosis* (prolapse of).

[前綴] **結腸** 如腸下垂。

colchicine *n.* a drug obtained from the meadow saffron (*Colchicum autumnale*), used to relieve pain in attacks of gout. It is administered by mouth; common side-effects are nausea, vomiting, diarrhoea, and stomach pains.

秋水仙鹼 自植物秋水仙屬提取的一種藥物。用於痛風發作時止痛。口服。常見副作用有噁心、嘔吐、腹瀉、胃痛。

cold (common cold) *n.* a widespread infectious virus disease causing inflammation of the mucous membranes of the nose, throat, and bronchial tubes. The disease is transmitted by coughing and sneezing. Symptoms commence 1–2 days after infection and include a

感冒 一種廣泛存在的病毒性傳染病。能引起鼻、咽喉與支氣管的炎症。由咳嗽與噴嚏傳播。感染1~2天後出現症狀：咽痛、鼻塞或流鼻涕、頭痛、咳嗽與全身無力。症

sore throat, stuffy or runny nose, headache, cough, and general malaise. The disease is mild and lasts only about a week but it can prove serious to young babies and to patients with a pre-existing respiratory complaint.

狀輕微，僅持續約一週。但在幼嬰與原有呼吸道疾病者病情可能加重。

cold sore (herpes simplex) *see* herpes.

脣疱疹（單純疱疹）

colectomy *n.* surgical removal of the colon. *Total colectomy* is removal of the whole colon, usually for extensive *colitis; *partial colectomy* is removal of a segment of the colon. *See also* hemicolectomy, proctocolectomy.

結腸切除術 對結腸行手術切除。全結腸切除術是將結腸全部切除，通常用於廣泛性結腸炎，部分結腸切除術是切除結腸的某一段。

colic *n.* severe abdominal pain, usually of fluctuating severity, with waves of pain seconds or a few minutes apart. *Infantile colic* is common among babies, due to wind in the intestine associated with feeding difficulties. *Intestinal colic* is due to partial or complete obstruction of the intestine or to constipation. Colic arising from the small intestine is felt in the upper abdomen; colic from the colon is felt in the lower abdomen. Medical names: **enteralgia**, **tormina**. *See also* biliary colic.

絞痛 每間隔數秒鐘或數分鐘發作一次的、疼痛程度呈波動性變化的嚴重的腹痛。嬰兒腹絞痛在嬰兒中常見，係餵飼困難腸內脹氣引起。腸絞痛係完全性腸梗阻、部分性腸梗阻或便秘所引起。小腸絞痛出現於上腹部，結腸絞痛出現於下腹部。

coliform bacteria a group of Gram-negative rodlike bacteria that are normally found in the gastrointestinal tract and have the ability to ferment the sugar lactose. It includes the genera *Enterobacter*, **Escherichia*, and **Klebsiella*.

大腸桿菌羣 正常時即存在於腸道的一羣革蘭氏陰性桿菌。能使乳糖發酵。包括腸桿菌屬、埃希氏桿菌屬與克雷白氏桿菌屬。

colistin *n.* an *antibiotic administered by mouth to treat gastroenteritis and other bacterial infections. Colistin is a mixture of antimicrobial substances produced by a strain of the bacterium *Bacillus polymyxa*. Trade name: **Colomycin**.

黏菌素 一種口服抗生素。用於治療胃腸炎與其它細菌感染。黏菌素是由多黏芽胞桿菌屬某一菌株產生的抗菌物質的混合物。商品名：多黏菌素E。

colitis *n.* inflammation of the colon. The usual symptoms are diarrhoea, sometimes with blood and mucus, and

結腸炎 發生在結腸的炎症。常見症狀有腹瀉，有時伴有黏液血便與下腹

lower abdominal pain. It is diagnosed by demonstrating inflammation of the colon's lining (mucosa) by *sigmoidoscopy or barium *enema X-ray. Colitis may be due to infection by **Entamoeba histolytica* (*amoebic colitis*) or by bacteria (*infective colitis*); it may also occur in *Crohn's disease (*Crohn's colitis*). *Ulcerative colitis* (*idiopathic proctocolitis*) almost always involves the rectum (*see* proctitis) as well as a varying amount of the colon, which become inflamed and ulcerated. Its cause is unknown. It varies in severity from month to month, relapses being treated by drugs, including corticosteroids and sulphasalazine (as tablets, injections, or enemas), and bed rest. Severe, continuous, or extensive colitis may be treated by surgery (*see* colectomy, proctocolectomy). Diarrhoea or pain where inflammation is absent is often due to *mucous colitis* (*see* irritable bowel syndrome).

痛。用乙狀結腸鏡觀察結腸腸黏膜或用鋇劑灌腸行X線照影可確定診斷。病因有溶組織腸阿米巴（阿米巴性結腸炎）或細菌（傳染性結腸炎）。克羅恩氏病（克羅恩氏結腸炎）、潰瘍性結腸炎（特發性直腸炎）亦可引起本病。後者幾乎經常同時侵犯直腸與一部分結腸，引起炎症與潰瘍。病因不明，病情逐月變化，通過柳氮磺胺吡啶、可地松類（口服、注射、灌腸）藥物治療與休息，仍反覆復發。嚴重持續而廣泛的結腸炎需手術治療。出現腹瀉腹痛但查無炎症存在時，多爲黏液性結腸炎。

collagen *n.* a protein that is the principal constituent of white fibrous connective tissue (as occurs in tendons). Collagen is also found in skin, bone, cartilage, and ligaments. It is relatively inelastic but has a high tensile strength.

膠原 白色纖維結締組織（如肌腱）中重要的成分——蛋白質。在皮膚、軟骨、肌腱中亦存在。彈性較小，但可伸度頗强。

collagen disease (connective-tissue disease) any one of a group of diseases that are characterized by degenerative changes in collagen – the principal component of connective tissue. Collagen diseases, which affect any part of the body in which collagen is found, include *dermatomyositis, *lupus erythematosus, and *polyarteritis nodosa.

膠原病 結締組織的重要成分膠原發生變性的一組疾病。本病可發生在體內任何存在有膠原組織的部位，包括皮肌炎、紅斑性狼瘡、結節性動脈周圍炎。

collar bone *see* clavicle.

鎖骨

collateral **1.** *adj.* accessory or secondary. **2.** *n.* a branch (e.g. of a nerve fibre) that is at right angles to the main part.

①副的，次要的 **②側方橫向分支** 如某一神經纖維的分支。

collateral circulation **1.** an alternative route provided for the blood by

①側支循環 某一主要血管發生阻塞後血液通過次

secondary vessels when a primary vessel becomes blocked. **2.** the channels of communication between the blood vessels supplying the heart. At the apex of the heart, where the coronary arteries form *anastomoses, these are very complex.

要的血管代以完成供血任務。②**心臟血管間交通支**。冠狀動脈在心尖部形成極爲複雜的動脈吻合網。

Colles' fracture fracture of the wrist, across the lower end of the *radius, usually caused by a fall on the outstretched hand. The hand and wrist below the fracture are displaced backwards. The bone is restored to its normal position under anaesthesia, and a plaster slab is applied. The fracture usually unites within six weeks. *Malunion is a common complication, resulting in deformity.

科勒斯骨折 骨折線越過撓骨下端的腕部骨折。跌倒時手臂處於外伸的姿勢容易發生。骨折遠端的手與腕部向後移位。應於麻醉下復位並上石膏夾板。骨折通常於6週內癒合。骨連接不正是常見的併發症，可產生畸形。

colliculus *n.* (*pl.* **colliculi**) a small protuberance or swelling. Two pairs of colliculi, the *superior* and *inferior colliculi*, protrude from the roof of the midbrain (*see* tectum).

丘、小阜 微小的隆起。中腦上有兩對丘，上丘與下丘。

collimation *n.* the production of a thin parallel-sided beam of radiation by means of adjustable slits placed at strategic points along the beam. A collimated beam of radiation is necessary in the technique of scintigraphy, when an organ is scanned for radioactivity (*see* scintigram).

準直 通過調節光線徑路上各點的縫隙以產生細小的平行的光束的方法。爲檢查某一器官的放射性而進行閃爍掃描時，準直光束十分必要。

collodion *n.* a syrupy solution of nitrocellulose in a mixture of alcohol and ether. When applied to the surface of the body it evaporates to leave a thin clear transparent skin, useful for the protection of minor wounds. Flexible collodion also contains camphor and castor oil, which allow the skin to stretch a little more.

火棉膠 硝化纖維素與酒精及乙醚混合的糖漿樣溶液。本品可塗沫於體表，揮發後遺留一層透明的薄膜，用以保護微小傷口。彈性火棉膠尚含有樟腦與蓖麻油，其下的皮膚可輕微伸展。

collyrium *n.* a medicated solution used to bathe the eyes.

洗眼劑 用於眼的藥性溶液。

coloboma *n.* a defect in the development of the eye causing abnormalities

缺損 能導致畸形的眼發育缺陷。嚴重程度不等。

ranging in severity from a notch in the lower part of the iris, making it pear-shaped, to defects in the lower part of the retina and choroid (the inner layers of the eyeball). Vision is usually poor in the severer cases. A coloboma of the eyelid is a congenital notch in the lid margin.

輕者僅在虹膜下部出現切跡，使之呈梨形，重者網膜與脈絡膜（眼球內房）下部完全缺乏。重症患者視力減弱。眼瞼缺損是一種先天性的瞼緣切跡樣缺損。

colon *n.* the main part of the large intestine, which consists of four sections – the *ascending*, *transverse*, *descending*, and *sigmoid colons* (see illustration). The colon has no digestive function but it absorbs large amounts of water and electrolytes from the undigested food passed on from the small intestine. At intervals strong peristaltic movements move the dehydrated contents (faeces) towards the rectum. —**colonic** *adj.*

結腸 大腸的主要部分，包括升結腸、橫結腸、降結腸和乙狀結腸（見圖）。結腸無消化功能，但能吸收來自小腸的未被消化食物中的大量水分和電解質。通過間斷性的蠕動性運動，把失去水分的腸內容物（糞便）推向直腸。

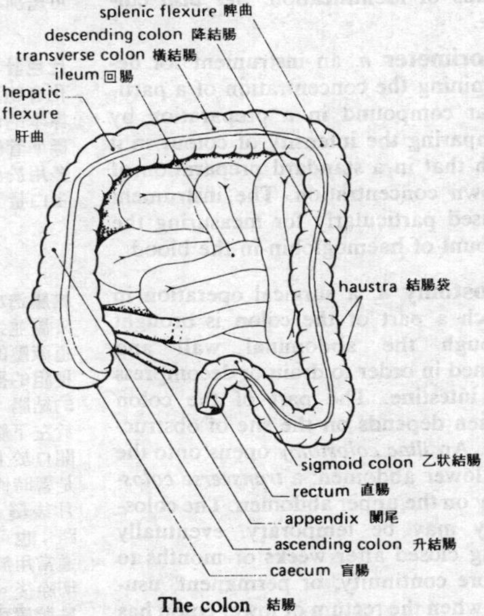

The colon 結腸

colonic irrigation washing out the contents of the large bowel by means of copious enemas, using either water, with or without soap, or other medication.

結腸灌洗術 使用大量灌腸劑將結腸內容物灌洗出來的方法。可用水（加或不加肥皂）或其他藥物。

colonoscopy *n.* a procedure for examining the interior of the entire colon and rectum using a flexible illuminated *fibreoptic instrument (*colonoscope*) introduced through the anus and guided up the colon by a combination of visual and X-ray control. It is possible to obtain specimens for microscopic examination using flexible forceps passed through the colonoscope and to remove polyps using a *diathermy snare.

結腸鏡檢查 檢查全部結腸與直腸內壁的一種方法。用一種帶有光源的彈性光學纖維器械（結腸鏡）插入肛門，在目視與X線的配合下直達結腸。可用一種彈性鉗通過結腸鏡獲取供顯微鏡檢的標本，亦可用燒灼勒除器切除息肉。

colony *n.* a discrete population or mass of microorganisms, usually bacteria, all of which are considered to have developed from a single parent cell. Bacterial colonies that grow on agar plates differ in shape, size, colour, elevation, translucency, and surface texture, depending on the species. This is used as a means of identification. *See also* culture.

菌落 由微生物（通常爲細菌）形成的單獨的羣落。其中的菌體皆來自一種親本細胞。由於菌種的不同，在瓊脂平板培養基上生長的菌落的形狀、大小、顏色、厚度、透明度、表面性狀各異。據此可鑑別不同菌種。

colorimeter *n.* an instrument for determining the concentration of a particular compound in a preparation by comparing the intensity of colour in it with that in a standard preparation of known concentration. The instrument is used particularly for measuring the amount of haemoglobin in the blood.

比色計 測定標本中某種化合物濃度的儀器。將該標本的色度與已知濃度的標準管的色度進行比較。多用於測定血液中的血紅蛋白量。

colostomy *n.* a surgical operation in which a part of the colon is brought through the abdominal wall and opened in order to drain or decompress the intestine. The part of the colon chosen depends on the site of obstruction. An *iliac colostomy* opens onto the left lower abdomen; a *transverse colostomy* on the upper abdomen. The colostomy may be temporary, eventually being closed after weeks or months to restore continuity; or permanent, usually when the rectum or lower colon has been removed. An appliance is usually worn over the colostomy opening (*stoma) to prevent soiling the clothes.

結腸造口術 將部分結腸外置並造口以引流或行腸道減壓的外科手術。根據梗阻的部位選擇不同部分的結腸。回腸造口術開口於左下腹；橫結腸造口術開口於上腹部。本術可能是暫時性的，於數週或數月後縫合以恢復腸管通路；也可能是永久性的，通常用於直腸或下段結腸切除後。開口處通常用特殊裝置覆蓋，以防糞便污染衣物。

colostrum *n.* the first secretion from the breast, occurring shortly after, or

初乳 分娩後（有時在分娩前）由孕婦乳房分泌出

sometimes before, birth. It contains serum, white blood cells, and protective antibodies.

的最初的一部分乳液。內含血漿、白細胞與保護性抗體。

colour blindness any of various conditions in which certain colours are confused with one another. True lack of colour appreciation is extremely rare (*see* monochromat), but some defect of colour discrimination is present in about 8% of Caucasian males, and 0.4% of Caucasian females. The most common type of colour blindness is *Daltonism* (*protanopia*) – red-blindness – in which the person cannot distinguish between reds and greens. Occasional cases are due to acquired disease of the retina but in the vast majority it is inherited. The defect is thought to be in the functioning of the light-sensitive cells in the retina responsible for colour perception (*see* cone). *See also* deuteranopia, trichromatic.

色盲　缺乏區別不同顏色能力的疾病。完全缺乏識別顏色能力者（全色盲）十分罕見。缺乏識別部分顏色能力者在男性白種人中約佔8%，女性白種人中約佔0.4%。最常見的類型是紅綠色盲（紅色盲），患者不能區別紅色與綠色。本病大多數是遺傳性的，偶見於網膜疾病之後。一般認爲本病係由網膜中具有色感的感光細胞（視錐細胞）功能缺陷引起。

colp- (colpo-) *prefix denoting* the vagina. Example: *colpoplasty* (plastic surgery of).

〔前綴〕**陰道**　例如：陰道成形術。

colpocele (vaginocele) *n.* **1.** a hernia protruding into the vagina. **2.** *see* colpoptosis.

①**陰道疝**　②**陰道脫垂**

colpoperineorrhaphy (colpoperineoplasty) *n.* a tissue grafting operation for repairing tears in the vagina and the area surrounding its opening (perineum).

陰道會陰縫合術（陰道會陰成形術）　修復陰道與會陰區裂傷的組織移植手術。

colpopexy *n.* the stitching of a displaced vagina to the abdominal wall. Loss of the normal position of the vagina may be caused by the action of gravity if the supporting tissues are weak.

陰道固定術　將移位的陰道縫於腹壁上的手術。陰道移位可由於支持組織虛弱、重力作用所致。

colpoptosis (colpocele) *n.* the dropping of the vagina from its normal position, which may happen under the action of gravity if the supporting tissues are weak. The condition can be corrected by *colpopexy.

陰道脫垂　陰道自其正常位置下垂。由於支持組織虛弱，重力作用所致。本病可用陰道固定術糾正。

colporrhaphy *n.* stitching of the vagina (by 'pleating') in order to reduce its laxity in cases of prolapse of the bladder (*anterior colporrhaphy*) or rectum (*posterior colporrhaphy*).

陰道縫合術 為克服陰道壁的鬆弛而將其褶疊縫合的手術。膀胱脫垂時行前陰道縫術，直腸脫垂時行後陰道縫術。

colposcope (vaginoscope) *n.* an instrument that is inserted into the vagina and permits visual examination of the neck of the womb and the upper part of the vagina in which it lies. **—colposcopy** *n.*

陰道鏡 插入陰道觀察子宮頸與陰道上部的器械。

colpotomy *n.* an incision made into the wall of the vagina.

陰道切開術 切開陰道壁的手術。

columella *n.* (in anatomy) a part resembling a small column. For example, the *columella cochleae* (*modiolus*) is the central pillar of the cochlea, around which the spiral cochlear canal winds. The *columella nasi* is the anterior part of the nasal septum.

小柱，軸 小柱狀的部分（解剖學）。例如：耳蝸軸即螺旋狀蝸管盤繞於其上的中央柱。鼻小柱係鼻中隔的前部。

column *n.* (in anatomy) any pillar-shaped structure, especially any of the tracts of grey matter found in the spinal cord.

柱 柱狀結構（解剖學）。尤指脊髓中灰質束。

coma *n.* a state of unrousable unconsciousness. Its severity is sometimes graded according to the presence or absence of withdrawal responses to painful stimuli and pupillary and corneal reflexes.

昏迷 不能喚醒的意識喪失狀態。有時可根據患者對疼痛有無退縮反應、瞳孔反射與角膜反射是否存在等來劃分昏迷的程度。

comedo *n.* (*pl.* **comedones**) *see* blackhead.

粉刺

commando operation a major operation performed to remove a malignant tumour from the head and neck. Extensive dissection, often involving the face, is followed by reconstruction to restore function and cosmetic acceptability.

頭頸部清掃術 切除頭頸部惡性腫瘤的大手術。廣泛性切除經常累及面部。為了恢復功能及美容目的，術後須行再建手術。

commensal *n.* an organism that lives in close association with another of a different species without either harming or benefiting it. For example, some microorganisms living in the gut obtain both food and a suitable habitat but

共生體 與另一不同種的生物密切共同生活並對之不產生任何利害影響的生物體。例如：某些生活在腸道中的微生物，它們在其中獲得合適的生境與食

neither harm nor benefit man. *Compare* symbiosis. —**commensalism** *n.*

物，而對人類沒有利或害的作用。

comminuted fracture a fracture in which the bone is broken into more than two pieces. A crushing force is usually responsible and there is often extensive injury to surrounding soft tissues.

粉碎性骨折 骨頭斷裂成兩塊以上的碎片的骨折。通常由擠壓傷引起，多件有廣泛軟組織損傷。

commissure *n.* **1.** a bundle of nerve fibres that crosses the midline of the central nervous system, often connecting similar structures on each side. **2.** any other tissue connecting two similar structures.

連合 ①跨越中樞神經系統中線連接兩側同樣結構的神經纖維束。②連接兩個同樣結構的任何其它組織。

communicable disease (contagious disease, infectious disease) any disease that can be transmitted from one person to another. This may occur by direct physical contact, by common handling of an object that has picked up infective microorganisms (*see* fomes), through a disease *carrier, or by spread of infected droplets coughed or exhaled into the air. The most dangerous communicable diseases are on the list of *notifiable diseases.

傳染病 能從一人傳染給他人的疾病。身體直接接觸，共同使用染菌物品，通過帶菌者或患者咳出或呼出的傳染性飛沫皆可造成傳染。最危險的傳染病見法定傳染病表。

communicans *adj.* communicating or connecting. The term is applied particularly to blood vessels or nerve fibres connecting two similar structures.

交通的 相通與相連的。此詞多用於描述血管或連接兩個同樣結構的神經纖維。

community dentistry the branch of NHS dentistry under the control of the health authorities. It is principally concerned with the treatment of children. Its staff are all salaried.

牙醫公會 國家保健局下屬的一個國民保健服務制的分支組織。主要處理兒童牙科疾病。該組織成員有工資待遇。

Community Health Council (CHC) (in Britain) a group of local residents (usually one per district) appointed to voice the views of patients in relation to the *National Health Service. Serviced by a salaried secretary, these Councils have no executive power but their views must be sought by District Health Authorities (DHA) on all matters that affect the provision of health services in

衛生議事公會 英國的一種地區性民衆團體。其職能是代表患者對國民保健服務制發表意見。在該組織任職的幹事享受工資待遇。本公會無行政職權，但地方保健局在制訂各項有關該地區的衛生條例時必需徵詢他們的意見，並聽取和研究他們的年度報

the district. The DHA must also receive and consider the annual report of each CHC within its district. Members of a CHC may pay site visits to hospitals or other health service property but not to the private premises of general practitioners. Patients who are dissatisfied with treatment may be advised by the CHC as to how to submit complaints to the DHA; indeed a letter from the secretary of the CHC showing an interest in such a complaint will usually ensure serious consideration even though the CHC lack the authority of the *health service commissioner to investigate complaints.

告。他們可視察醫院或其它醫療機構，但不能視察私人診所。患者對治療有所不滿時，亦可求助於該組織以向地方保健局提出申訴。雖然他們沒有衛生官員調查申訴的權力，但由幹事寫一封支持申訴的信常能引起當局認眞對待。

community medicine the branch of medicine concerned with assessing needs and trends in health and disease of populations as distinct from individuals. Formerly known as *social medicine*, it includes *epidemiology, public health, *preventive medicine, health care planning, and evaluation of services.

公共醫學 研究羣體健康與疾病等的發展趨勢與需求的醫學分支科學。與研究個體疾病與健康的醫學有別。舊稱社會醫學，包括流行病學、公共衞生、預防醫學、衞生工作計劃與評價等。

community nurses (in Britain) a generic term for *health visitors, *domiciliary midwives, and *home nurses. *See also* domiciliary services.

公共保健護士 英國對保健員、家庭助產士、家庭護士的統稱。

community physician (in Britain) a doctor of consultant status with special postgraduate training in community medicine. Community physicians undertake executive functions at each tier of the *National Health Service, as *Regional Medical Officer* (*RMO*) or *District Medical Officer* (*DMO*). In most appointments the DMO also acts as *Proper Officer* to the appropriate local authority, giving epidemiological and other medical advice to the *Environmental Health Officer. Other *Specialists in Community Medicine* (*SCM*) have responsibility for advising on and coordinating appropriate services (e.g. child health, social service, information and planning, and manpower).

公共保健醫師 在英國受過公共醫學研究生教育的具有經治醫師資格的醫師。他們在國民保健服務制各級機構中任職，擔任地區級或地段級主管醫師。地段級主管醫師大多兼任地方當局的專務幹事，對環境衞生官員提供流行病學與其它醫學方面的諮詢意見。公共醫學的其他專家有責任對如何協調各種衞生服務工作（例如：兒童保健，社會服務，信息與計劃，人員調動）提供意見。

community services *see* domiciliary services.

公共保健服務 爲居民提供的衛生保健服務工作。

comparative mortality figure *see* occupational mortality.

相對死亡率數字

compatibility *n.* the degree to which the body's defence systems will tolerate the presence of intruding foreign material, such as blood when transfused or a kidney when transplanted. Complete compatibility exists between identical twins: a blood transfusion between identical twins will evoke no *antibody formation in the recipient. In severe *incompatibility*, for example between completely unrelated people, there are likely to be swift immune reactions as antibodies attack and destroy any offending antigenic material. *See also* histocompatibility, immunity. —**compatible** *adj.*

相容性 機體免疫保衞系統對外來異物（如輸血或腎移植時）的耐受能力。在同卵雙胎之間存在有完全相容性。在他們之間輸血時不會產生抗體。在血型完全不配合的人們之間輸血，即存在嚴重的不容性時，由於抗體能結合並破壞輸入的抗原物質，可立即產生免疫反應。

compensation *n.* the act of making up for a functional or structural deficiency. For example, compensation for the loss of a diseased kidney is brought about by an increase in size of the remaining kidney, so restoring the urine-producing capacity.

代償 對機體中的功能或結構缺陷進行彌補的過程。例如：病腎摘除後遺留的健腎體積增大，以恢復尿液生成的能力。

complement *n.* a substance in the blood, consisting of a group of nine different fractions, that aids the body's defences when antibodies combine with invading antigens. Complement is involved with the breaking up (*lysis), *agglutination, and *opsonization of foreign cells. Following antibody-antigen reaction it may also attract scavenging cells (*phagocytes) to the area of conflict. *See also* immunity.

補體 在血液中存在的一組幫助機體內抗體抵抗外來抗原的物質。共有9種不同的成分。它們參預溶解反應、凝集反應與對外來細胞的調理素反應。在發生抗原抗體反應之後，補體還能將具有清掃功能的細胞（吞噬細胞）吸引到反應部位來。

complement fixation the binding of *complement to the complex that is formed when an antibody reacts with a specific antigen. Because complement is taken up from the serum only when such a reaction has occurred, testing for the presence of complement after mixing a suspension of a known organism

補體結合反應 抗體與特異抗原發生反應形成的複合物與補體相結合的現象。僅當抗原抗體發生反應時才自血漿中吸收補體。因此，將患者血漿與已知病原體懸液相混合後再測定補體是否存在，可

with a patient's serum can give confirmation of infection with a suspected organism. The *Wasserman reaction for diagnosis of syphilis is a complement-fixation test.

以證實該患者是否受到該病原體感染。診斷梅毒的乏色曼反應就是一種補體結合試驗。

complex *n.* (in psychoanalysis) an emotionally charged and repressed group of ideas and beliefs that is capable of influencing an individual's behaviour. The term in this sense was originally used by Jung, but it is now widely used in a looser sense to denote an unconscious motive.

情結，情綜　可以影響患者行爲的一組充滿感情的而又被壓抑着的思想和信念（精神分析用語）。容氏最初按此含意使用該術語，但現在含意已不嚴格，廣泛用於指某種潛意識的動機。

complication *n.* a disease or condition arising during the course of or as a consequence of another disease.

合併症　在某種疾病過程中併發的或續發的其他疾病。

composite resin a tooth-coloured filling material for anterior teeth. It is composed of two different materials: an inorganic filler held in an organic resin.

復合樹脂　前牙用的與牙同色的填料。由無機填料與有機樹脂兩種不同物質組成。

compress *n.* a pad of material soaked in hot or cold water and applied to an injured part of the body to relieve the pain of inflammation.

敷布　在冷水或熱水中浸泡過的織物墊。用以敷貼患部以減輕炎症引起的疼痛。

compressed air illness (caisson disease) a syndrome occurring in people working under high pressure in diving bells or at great depths with breathing apparatus. On return to normal atmospheric pressure nitrogen dissolved in the bloodstream expands to form bubbles, causing pain (the *bends*) and blocking the circulation in small blood vessels in the brain and elsewhere (*decompression sickness*). Pain, paralysis, and other features may be eliminated by returning the victim to a higher atmospheric pressure and reducing this gradually, so causing the bubbles to redissolve. Chronic compressed air illness may cause damage to the bones (*avascular necrosis*), heart, and lungs.

壓縮空氣病（潛水員病）　在高壓艙中或配戴呼吸裝置在深水作業的人們所出現的症候羣。當他們回到常壓環境中時，在血流中溶解的氮游離集聚成氣泡，引起疼痛（沉箱病），堵塞腦或其他部位小血管（減壓病）。將患者送回高壓環境中再逐漸減壓，使氣泡重新溶解，疼痛、麻痹及其他症狀即可消失。慢性壓縮空氣病可引起骨（缺血性壞死）、心、肺等損害。

compulsion *n.* an *obsession that takes the form of a motor act, such as

強迫症　一種強迫行爲。如由於怕髒而反覆盥洗。

repetitive washing based on a fear of contamination.

compulsory admission (in Britain) the entry and detention of a person within an institution (hospital or Part III Accommodation) without his consent, either because of mental illness (*see* Mental Health Act) or severe social deprivation (*see* National Assistance Act). Application by a *mental welfare officer or *social worker supported by a general practitioner and/or a suitably qualified specialist must be approved by a court of law except in emergencies relating to mental illness, in which the patient must either agree to stay as a voluntary admission or the emergency order is ratified by a court within seven days. When a patient has committed a dangerous act the court may order compulsory admission to a hospital with special security arrangements (e.g. Broadmoor). *Compare* voluntary admission.

强迫收容 對精神病患者或嚴重喪失正常社會生活能力的人，不經本人同意而在三類調節機構實行監禁和拘留（英國）。由負責精神病患者的福利的官員或社會工作者會同醫師和/或具有一定資格的有關專家提出强迫收容申請，必須由法院批准方可施行，唯精神病的緊急情況屬例外。但事後必須徵求本人同意，否則必須在7日內取得法院批准。患者有危險行爲時法院可命令醫院實行特殊保安措施。

computerized axial tomography (CAT) a development of diagnostic radiology for the examination of the soft tissues of the body. For example, within the skull it can be used to reveal the normal anatomy of the brain, the ventricles, and other structures and to distinguish pathological conditions, such as tumours, abscesses, and haematomas. The technique involves the recording of 'slices' of the body with an X-ray scanner (*CAT scanner*); these records are then integrated by computer to give a cross-sectional image. This investigation is without risk to the patient. *See also* tomography. *Compare* positron emission tomography (PET).

電子計算機軸向體層照像術 檢查體內軟組織的一種X線診斷新技術。可用以揭示顱內腦組織、腦室與其它結構的正常解剖形態並區分諸如腫瘤、膿腫和血腫等不同病理狀態。利用X線掃描儀對體內組織進行多層次掃描，掃描結果通過計算機綜合處理後，產生一種多切面交叉重合圖像。本檢查法對患者無害。

conation *n.* the group of mental activities (including drives, will, and *instincts) that leads to purposeful action.

意動 心理活動的一類（包括慾望、意念、本能）。它引起有目的的行動。

conception *n.* **1.** (in gynaecology) the start of pregnancy, when a male germ

①受孕 （產科學）妊娠的開始。指精子與卵子在

cell (sperm) fertilizes a female germ cell (ovum) in the *Fallopian tube. **2.** (in psychology) an idea or mental impression.

輸卵管中的結合。②**概念**　某種觀念或心理印象。

conceptus *n.* the products of conception: the developing infant and its enclosing membrane at all stages in the womb.

孕體　妊娠的產物。指在宮內發育各階段的胎兒與其包膜。

concha *n.* (*pl.* **conchae**) (in anatomy) any part resembling a shell. For example, the *concha auriculae* is a depression on the outer surface of the pinna (auricle), which leads to the external auditory meatus of the outer ear. *See also* nasal concha.

甲　（解剖學）介殼樣結構。如耳甲，即耳朵外面的凹陷部分。它與外耳道相通連。

concordance *n.* similarity of any physical characteristic that is found in both of a pair of twins.

一致性　雙胞胎身體上存在的相類似的特徵。

concretion *n.* a stony mass formed within such an organ as the kidney, especially the coating of an internal organ (or a foreign body, such as a urinary catheter) with calcium salts. *See also* calculus.

結石　在某臟器（如腎臟）內形成的石頭樣物質。多由鈣鹽包裹異物或某種置於內臟中的器械（如導尿管）而生成。

concussion *n.* a limited period of unconsciousness caused by injury to the head. It may last for a few seconds or a few hours. There is no recognizable structural damage to the brain, although repeated concussion eventually causes symptoms suggesting brain damage. *See also* punch drunk syndrome.

腦震蕩　由頭部外傷引起的短期意識喪失。可持續數秒鐘或數小時。腦內無可見的結構性損害，但反復發生腦震顫最終可產生腦損害症狀。

condenser *n.* (in microscopy) an arrangement of lenses beneath the stage of a microscope. It can be adjusted to provide correct focusing of light on the microscope slide.

聚光器　顯微鏡臺架下方的透鏡裝置。可調節光線使焦點聚在載物片上。

conditioned reflex a reflex in which the response occurs not to the sensory stimulus that normally causes it but to a separate stimulus, which has been learnt to be associated with it. In Pavlov's classic experiments, dogs learned to associate the sound of a bell

條件反射　對無關刺激所產生的反射。這種刺激正常時不能引起該種反射，而是在通過與正常的感覺刺激相聯繫的訓練而產生這種作用的。在巴甫洛夫的經典實驗中，教會狗把

with feeding time and would salivate at the bell's sound whether food was then presented to them or not.

進食時間和鈴聲刺激聯繫起來，以後不論給予食物與否，狗都會對鈴聲產生唾液分泌反應。

conditioning *n.* the establishment of new behaviour by modifying the stimulus/response associations. In *classical conditioning* a stimulus not normally associated with a particular response is presented together with the stimulus that evokes the response automatically. This is repeated until the first stimulus evokes the response by itself (*see* conditioned reflex). In *operant conditioning* a response is rewarded (or punished) each time it occurs, so that in time it comes to occur more (or less) frequently (*see* reinforcement).

條件反射化 改變刺激-反應之間的聯繫以建立新行爲方式的方法。經典的條件反射化是將無關刺激與能自動引起某種特殊反應的刺激相聯繫而建立起來的。兩者反復同時出現，直至無關刺激單獨就能引起反應爲止。操作性條件反射化是在每次出現反應時予以獎勵（或懲罰），最後終於使該反應能經常（或不常）出現。

condom (French letter, rubber) *n.* a sheath made of latex rubber, plastic, or silk that is fitted over the penis during sexual intercourse. Use of a condom protects both partners against the transmission of venereal diseases and, carefully used, it is a reasonably reliable contraceptive (between 2 and 10 pregnancies per 100 woman-years).

陰莖套 性交時用以套在陰莖上的護套。由乳膠、塑料或絲綢製成。使用陰莖套可保護雙方免受性病傳染，小心使用亦爲一種經濟可靠的避孕器具（妊娠率爲 2～10/100 婦女-年）。

condylarthrosis (condyloid joint) *n.* a form of *diarthrosis (freely movable joint) in which an ovoid head fits into an elliptical cavity. Examples are the knee joint and the joint between the mandible (lower jaw) and the temporal bone of the skull.

髁狀關節 由卵圓形關節頭與橢圓形關節腔形成的可動關節。例如：膝關節和顳下頜關節。

condyle *n.* a rounded protuberance that occurs at the ends of some bones, e.g. the *occipital bone, and forms an articulation with another bone.

髁 某些骨（如枕骨）末端的圓形突起。可與其他骨形成關節。

condyloma *n.* a raised wartlike growth. The commonest type, *condyloma acuminatum*, is found on the vulva, under the foreskin, or on the skin of the anal region. Condylomas are infectious and are probably transmitted during sexual contact. *Condyloma latum* is an infectious warty lesion of the secondary

濕疣 呈疣狀突起的新生物。最常見的類型尖銳濕疣見於外陰部、包皮下或肛門區的皮膚。濕疣有傳染性，可能通過性接觸傳播。扁平濕疣是二期梅毒的有傳染性疣狀病變，見於外陰或肛門周圍。

stage of syphilis, occurring around the vulva or anus.

cone *n.* one of the two types of light-sensitive cells in the *retina of the eye (*compare* rod). The human retina contains 6–7 million cones; they function best in bright light and are essential for acute vision (receiving a sharp accurate image). The area of the retina called the *fovea contains the greatest concentration of cones. Cones can also distinguish colours. It is thought that there are three types of cone, each sensitive to the wavelength of a different primary colour – red, green, or blue. Other colours are seen as combinations of these three primary colours.

視錐細胞 視網膜中兩種光感細胞之一。人類視網膜含有六七百萬個視錐細胞，它們在光亮下功能最佳，對精密視覺（感受精細準確的形像）至關重要。網膜上稱爲中央凹的部位含視錐細胞最多。視錐細胞亦能分辨顏色。一般認爲有三類視錐細胞，分別能感受紅、綠、藍三種不同原色的波長。其它顏色則是這三種原色的不同結合。

confabulation *n.* the invention of circumstantial but fictitious detail about events supposed to have occurred in the past. Usually this is to disguise an inability to remember past events. It may be a symptom of any form of loss of memory, but typically occurs in *Korsakoff's syndrome.

虛談症 對假想中的發生於過去的事件的經過與細節進行任意的虛構。往往是對喪失回憶往事能力的一種掩飾。可能是各種記憶力喪失疾病的症狀。柯薩柯夫氏綜合徵中所見者最爲典型。

confection *n.* (in pharmacy) a sweet substance that is combined with a medicinal preparation to make it suitable for administration.

糖膏〔劑〕 與藥物相混合使之適於口服的有甜味的物品。

conflict *n.* (in psychology) the state produced when a stimulus produces two opposing reactions. The basic types of conflict situation are *approach–approach*, in which the individual is drawn towards two attractive – but mutually incompatible – goals; *approach–avoidance*, where the stimulus evokes reactions both to approach and to avoid; and *avoidance–avoidance*, in which the avoidance reaction to one stimulus would bring the individual closer to an equally unpleasant stimulus. Conflict has been used to explain the development of neurotic disorders, and the resolution of conflict remains an important part of psychoanalysis. *See also* conversion.

衝突 （心理學）一種刺激引起兩種相反的反應的狀態。有三種基本類型。接近-接近衝突：患者被吸引向兩個相互矛盾的目標；接近-迴避衝突：一種刺激同時引起患者的接近反應和迴避反應；迴避-迴避反應：患者在迴避一種刺激的同時又去接近另一種同樣不愉快的刺激。衝突曾用來解釋神經症的發生。解決衝突是精神分析的一項重要課題。

confluence *n.* a point of coalescence. The *confluence of the sinuses* is the meeting point of the superior sagittal, transverse, straight, and occipital venous sinuses in the dura mater in the occipital region of the skull.

滙合 接合點。竇滙是上矢狀竇、横竇、直竇與枕骨區硬膜內的枕靜脉竇的滙合點。

congenital *adj.* describing a condition that is recognized at birth or that is believed to have been present since birth. Congenital malformations include all disorders present at birth whether they are inherited or caused by an environmental factor.

先天的 形容出生時就被認出的或肯定從出生時起就一直存在的疾病。先天性畸形包括遺傳性的和環境因素引起的出生時就存在的畸形。

congestion *n.* an accumulation of blood within an organ, which is the result of back pressure within its veins (for example congestion of the lungs and liver occurs in heart failure). Congestion may be associated with *oedema (accumulation of fluid in the tissues). It is relieved by treatment of the cause.

充血 由於靜脉回流障礙、血壓增高導致的某一器官內的血液集聚。如心力衰竭時發生的肺鬱血與肝鬱血。充血時可能伴發水腫（液體在組織中積蓄）。可通過病因治療獲得緩解。

Congo red a dark-red or reddish-brown pigment that becomes blue in acidic conditions. It is used as a histological *stain. *Amyloidosis is indicated if over 60% of the dye disappears from the blood within one hour of injection.

剛果紅 一種暗紅色或紅棕色的色素。遇酸即變成藍色。用做組織染色的染劑。如注射後一小時即有60% 以上的剛果紅自血液中消失，提示有澱粉樣變。

coniine *n.* an extremely poisonous alkaloid, found in hemlock (*Conium maculatum*), that paralyses the nerves, mainly the motor nerves. Coniine has been included in drug preparations for the treatment of asthma and whooping cough.

歐毒芹鹼 一種劇毒生物鹼。獲自傘形科的一種有毒植物。對神經（主要是運動神經）有痲痹作用。在某些治療支氣管哮喘與百日咳的成藥中含有本生物鹼。

conization *n.* surgical removal of a cone of tissue. The technique is commonly used in excising a portion of the cervix (neck) of the womb.

錐形切除術 對組織行錐形切除的外科手術。多用於子宮頸部分切除。

conjugate (conjugate diameter, true conjugate) *n.* the distance between the front and rear of the pelvis measured from the most prominent part of the sacrum to the back of the

骨盆直徑 自骶骨最突出部至耻骨聯合後測得的骨盆前後徑。因盆骨直徑無法於生前測出，只好自對角徑（耻骨聯合下緣至骶

pubic symphysis. Since the true conjugate cannot normally be measured during life it is estimated by subtracting 1.3–1.9 cm from the *diagonal conjugate*, the distance between the lower edge of the symphysis and the sacrum (usually about 12.7 cm). If the true conjugate is less than about 10.2 cm, delivery of an infant through the natural passages may be difficult or impossible, and *Caesarean section may have to be performed.

骨，一般約 12.7 cm）減去 1.3 ～ 1.9 cm 大致估計。如果直徑小於 10.2 cm，胎兒由自然產道分娩就有困難或不可能，應考慮行剖腹產。

conjugation *n.* the union of two microorganisms in which genetic material (DNA) passes from one organism to the other. In some bacteria a minute projection on the donor 'male' cell (a *pilus*) forms a bridge with the recipient 'female' cell through which the DNA is transferred. Conjugation is comparable to sexual reproduction in higher organisms.

接合　在兩個微生物之間形成的能傳遞遺傳物質（脫氧核糖核酸）的連合。有些細菌"雄性"供體細胞上的微小突起（菌毛）與"雌性"受體細胞搭橋。脫氧核糖核酸通過此橋進行傳遞。接合有點類似高等生物體的有性生殖。

conjunctiva *n.* the delicate mucous membrane that covers the front of the eye and lines the inside of the eyelids. The conjunctiva lining the eyelids contains many blood vessels but that over the eyeball contains few and is transparent. —**conjunctival** *adj.*

結膜　覆蓋於眼球前部與眼瞼內部的一層脆弱的黏膜。瞼結膜有豐富的血管。球結膜的血管甚少，因而是透明的。

conjunctivitis (pink eye) *n.* inflammation of the conjunctiva, which becomes red and swollen and produces a watery or pus-containing discharge. It causes discomfort rather than pain and does not usually affect vision. Conjunctivitis is caused by infection (in which case it usually spreads rapidly to the other eye), allergy, or physical or chemical irritation. The patient usually recovers with no after-effects in one to three weeks; bacterial infections respond to antibiotic eye drops. *See also* trachoma, ophthalmia neonatorum.

結膜炎　結膜的炎症。結膜紅腫，並有水樣與膿性分泌物。僅有不適感，而無疼痛，通常不影響視力。病因有感染（此時炎症迅速由一眼傳染至他眼）、變態反應、物理或化學刺激等。患者通常在 1 至 3 週內痊癒，無後遺症。抗生素類眼藥對細菌感染者有效。

connective tissue the tissue that supports, binds, or separates more specialized tissues and organs or functions as

結締組織　支持、聯接或分隔其它分化程度較高的組織或器官的一種組織。

a packing tissue of the body. It consists of an amorphous *ground substance* of mucopolysaccharides in which may be embedded white (collagenous), yellow (elastic), and reticular fibres, fat cells, *fibroblasts, *mast cells, and *macrophages (see illustration). Variations in chemical composition of the ground substance and in the proportions and quantities of cells and fibres give rise to tissues of widely differing characteristics, including bone, cartilage, tendons, and ligaments as well as *adipose, *areolar, and *elastic tissues.

在機體中具有固定和充填作用。由黏多糖類無定形基質與嵌於其中的白色膠原纖維、黃色彈力纖維、網狀纖維、脂肪細胞、成纖維細胞、肥大細胞與巨噬細胞組成（見圖）。由於基質中化學成分的不同，以及各種細胞與纖維的比例與數量的不同，結締組織可有多種不同的種類，諸如骨、軟骨、肌腱、韌帶以及脂肪組織、疏鬆結締組織與彈力組織等。

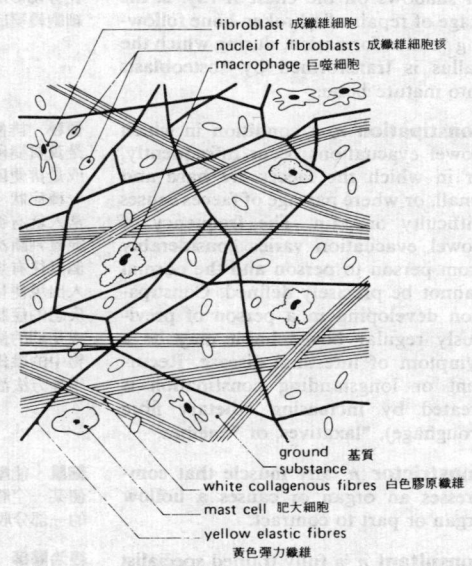

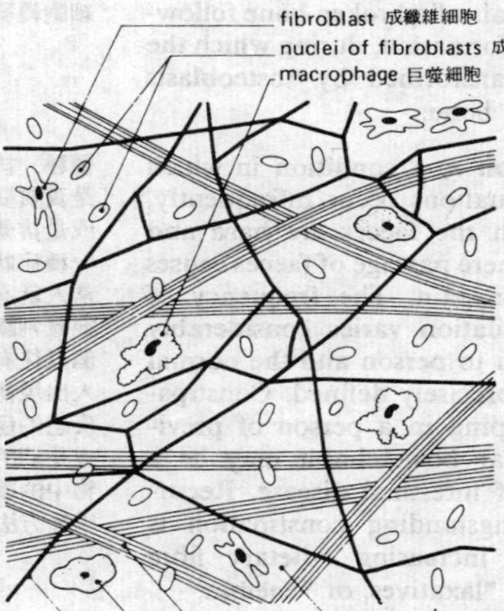

Loose (areolar) connective tissue
疏鬆結締組織

connective-tissue disease *see* collagen disease.

結締組織病　即膠原疾病。

consanguinity *n.* relationship by blood; the sharing of a common ancestor within a few generations.

血親　血緣關係。在近幾代內有共同的祖先。

conservative treatment treatment aimed at preventing a condition from becoming worse, in the expectation that either natural healing will occur or progress of the disease will be so slow that no drastic treatment will be justified. *Compare* radical treatment.

保守療法 旨在防止疾病惡化，等待疾病自然好轉的一種治療方法。在病程緩慢、不宜投予烈性藥時亦使用之。

consolidation *n.* **1.** the state of the lung in which the alveoli (air sacs) are filled with fluid produced by inflamed tissue, as in *pneumonia. It is diagnosed from its dullness to *percussion, bronchial breathing (*see* breath sounds) in the patient, and from the distribution of shadows on the chest X-ray. **2.** the stage of repair of a broken bone following *callus formation, during which the callus is transformed by *osteoblasts into mature bone.

實變 肺泡被炎性分泌物充滿（如肺炎時）的狀態。可由叩診出現濁音、聽診出現支氣管性呼吸音及X線胸透出現陰影做出診斷。②**骨化** 骨折修復過程的一個階段。發生在骨痂形成後。此時成骨細胞轉變成成熟骨細胞。

constipation *n.* a condition in which bowel evacuations occur infrequently, or in which the faeces are hard and small, or where passage of faeces causes difficulty or pain. The frequency of bowel evacuation varies considerably from person to person and the normal cannot be precisely defined. Constipation developing in a person of previously regular bowel habit may be a symptom of intestinal disease. Recurrent or longstanding constipation is treated by increasing *dietary fibre (roughage), *laxatives, or *enemas.

便秘 排便次數減少，或是糞質變硬、糞量減少，或是排便困難並有疼痛的一種症狀。排便次數在正常人就有很大差異，因此很難判斷次數多少。在一個以往有規律排便習慣的人出現便秘，可能是腸道疾患的症狀。反復發生的或長期的便秘可以增加食物中的纖維、緩瀉劑或灌腸等方法治療。

constrictor *n.* any muscle that compresses an organ or causes a hollow organ or part to contract.

縮肌 能壓迫某一器官或使某一空腔器官或該器官的一部分收縮的肌肉。

consultant *n.* a fully trained specialist in a branch of medicine who accepts total responsibility for patient care. In Britain consultants are usually responsible for the care of patients in hospital wards but they are allowed to opt for some sessions in private practice in addition to any National Health Service commitments. After registration, doctors continuing in hospital service are appointed successively *senior house*

經治醫師 具備某一專科完備的知識並對患者全面負責的專家。在英國經治醫師一般是負責治療住院患者，但除去履行國民保健服務制規定的職責外，還可以利用部分時間開業。在取得經治醫師資格後，仍在醫院任職者可逐級晋升爲主治醫師、副主任醫師及主任醫師（責任

officer, *registrar*, and *senior registrar* (all full-time training grades with increasing responsibilities). While in the training grades specialist examinations are taken and consultant appointment is based on a combination of qualifications by examination and practical experience in post. *See also* doctor.

遞增的各級專業職稱）。晋升時都要通過考試。經治醫師資格的取得，一方面要通過考試，另一方面還要根據實際的臨床經驗。

consumption *n.* any disease causing wasting of tissues, especially (formerly) pulmonary tuberculosis. —**consumptive** *adj.*

癆病 引起組織消耗的疾病。過去多指肺結核。

contact *n.* transmission of an infectious disease by touching or handling an infected person or animal (*direct contact*) or by *indirect contact* with airborne droplets, faeces, etc., containing the infective microorganism.

接觸傳染 傳染病傳播的一種方式。通過接觸或處理病人或病獸（直接接觸）或含有病原體的飛沫或糞便等（間接接觸）而感染。

contact lenses glass or plastic lenses worn directly against the eye, separated from it only by a film of tear fluid. *Corneal microlenses* cover only the cornea, while *haptic lenses* cover some of the surrounding sclera as well. Contact lenses are used mainly in place of glasses to correct long and short sightedness and other errors of refraction, but they may be used in a protective capacity in some types of corneal disease.

隱形眼鏡 直接戴在眼睛上的玻璃或塑料鏡片。與眼睛只有一薄層淚液相隔。角膜鏡片只覆蓋角膜，眼白鏡片還覆蓋周圍的鞏膜。隱形眼鏡主要用於糾正近視、遠視與其他屈光不正。有時亦用以保護某些角膜疾病。

contact therapy a form of *radiotherapy in which a radioactive substance is brought into close contact with the part of the body being heated. Needles or capsules of the isotope may be implanted in or around a tumour so that the radiation they emit will destroy it. *Compare* telecurietherapy.

接觸放射線療法 放射線療法的一種。此時放射性物質與機體受照射的部位密切接觸。將製成針狀或膠囊狀的同位素植入腫瘤中或腫瘤周圍以便射線直接破壞腫瘤。

contagious disease originally, a disease transmitted only by direct physical contact: now usually taken to mean any *communicable disease.

接觸性傳染病 過去指通過身體直接接觸傳染的疾病。現泛指所有的流行病。

contra- *prefix denoting* against or opposite. Example: *contraversion* (turning away from).

〔前綴〕 **反，抗，逆，對** 如：反轉。

contraception *n.* the prevention of unwanted pregnancy. Fertilization may be prevented by mechanical methods, including *coitus interruptus, the *condom, or the *diaphragm; by fitting the woman with an intrauterine contraceptive device (*IUD); by *sterilization; or by altering the woman's hormonal balance by regular doses of an *oral contraceptive (the Pill) or by long-acting injections of a hormonal drug (a *progestogen). Couples whose religious beliefs forbid the use of mechanical or hormonal contraceptives may use the *rhythm method, in which intercourse is limited to those days in the menstrual cycle when conception is least likely.

避孕 不願生育時避免受精的措施。可使用體外射精法，配戴陰莖套、子宮帽，放置宮內避孕器，行絕育手術，口服避孕藥（按期服用規定劑量藥物以破壞婦女內分泌平衡）及注射長效內分泌製劑（孕酮）等。由於宗教信仰而不能使用以上方法者可在安全期內性交，即在月經周期中懷孕可能最小的日期內性交。

contraction *n.* the shortening of a muscle in response to a motor nerve impulse. This generates tension in the muscle, usually causing movement.

收縮 運動神經的刺激引起的肌肉短縮。此時肌肉緊張，通常都會引起運動。

contracture *n.* *fibrosis of muscle tissue producing shrinkage and shortening of the muscle without generating any strength. It is usually a consequence of pain in or disuse of a muscle or limb. *See also* Dupuytren's contracture.

攣縮 能引起肌肉短縮的肌組織纖維性變。此時不能產生任何力量，通常係肌肉疼痛或廢用性萎縮的結果。

contraindication *n.* any factor in a patient's condition that makes it unwise to pursue a certain line of treatment. For example, an attack of pneumonia in a patient would be a strong contraindication against the use of a general anaesthetic.

禁忌症 禁用某種治療方法的疾病因素。例如：全身麻醉就是肺炎的絕對禁忌症。

contralateral *adj.* on or affecting the opposite side of the body: applied particularly to paralysis (or other symptoms) occurring on the opposite side of the body from the brain lesion that caused them.

對側的 發生於身體另一側的，或影響到身體另一側的。多用於描述腦病變時發生於身體另一側的麻痹（或其它症狀）。

contrast medium any substance that is used to improve the visibility of structures during radiography. Barium, given orally or as an enema to show up the alimentary tract on X-ray, is an

造影劑 在 X 線透視檢查中爲了使體內結構清晰地顯露出來所用的一種物質。口服鋇劑或用鋇劑灌腸以在 X 線下顯露消化

example of a contrast medium. Air is occasionally useful as a contrast medium; it may be used to displace the cerebrospinal fluid during X-ray examination of the ventricles of the brain. *See also* radio-opaque.

道即爲一例。空氣亦有時用做造影劑。在用 X 線檢查腦室時可用以取代腦脊液的位置。

contrecoup *n.* injury of a part resulting from a blow on its opposite side. This may happen, for example, if a blow on the back of the head causes the front of the brain to be pushed against the inner surface of the skull.

對衝傷 一側受到打擊時引起的另一側的損傷。例如：腦後部受到打擊時，腦前部會與顱腔內壁碰撞而發生損傷。

contusion *n. see* bruise.

挫傷

conus arteriosus the front upper portion of the right ventricle adjoining the pulmonary arteries.

動脉圓錐 右心室與肺動脉相連接的前上部分。

conus medullaris the conical end of the spinal cord, at the level of the lower end of the first lumbar vertebra.

脊髓圓錐 脊髓的圓錐形末端。位於第一腰椎下緣水平。

convergence *n.* (in neurology) the formation of nerve tracts by fibres coming together into one pathway from different regions of the brain.

集合束 （神經學）來自腦髓不同部位的神經纖維集合成一條通路的神經束。

conversion *n.* (in psychiatry) the expression of *conflict as physical symptoms. Psychiatrists believe that the repressed instinctual drive is manifested as motor or sensory loss, such as paralysis, rather than as speech or action. This is thought to be one of the ways in which *hysteria is produced.

變形發泄-轉換 （心理學）內心衝突以軀體症狀顯示出來的現象。精神病醫生認爲被壓抑的本能衝動表現於語言與行動者較少見，而表現爲運動痲痹與感覺喪失者較多見。一般認爲係癔病原因之一。

convolution *n.* a folding or twisting, such as one of the many that cause the fissures, sulci, and gyri of the surface of the *cerebrum.

廻 一種卷曲或褶疊的結構。例如：大腦表面的溝廻。

convulsion *n.* an involuntary contraction of the muscles producing contortion of the body and limbs. Rhythmic convulsions of the limbs are part of *grand mal epilepsy. *Febrile convulsions* are provoked by fever in otherwise healthy infants and young children. An afebrile *infantile convulsion* is likely to be due to birth injury or a developmental defect of the brain.

驚厥 引起軀幹和肢體扭曲的不自主的肌肉收縮。陣發性肢體驚厥見於癲癇大發作。

Cooley's anaemia *see* thalassaemia. **庫利氏貧血** 地中海貧血。

Coomb's test a means of detecting antibodies on the surface of red blood cells that can precipitate simple proteins (globulins) in the blood serum. The test is used in the diagnosis of haemolytic *anaemia (resulting from the destruction of red blood cells). **庫姆斯試驗** 檢查紅細胞表面抗原的一種方法。此時血漿中的簡單蛋白質（球蛋白）沉澱於細胞表面上。本試驗用於診斷溶血性貧血（由紅細胞破壞引起的貧血）。

copr- (copro-) *prefix denoting* faeces. Example: *coprophobia* (abnormal fear of). 〔前綴〕 **糞** 如糞便恐怖（對糞便產生的一種異常的畏懼感）。

coprolalia *n.* the repetitive speaking of obscene words. It can be involuntary, as part of the *Gilles de la Tourette syndrome. **穢褻語言** 反復使用猥褻字眼說話。可能是不自主的，見於多發性抽搐穢語綜合徵。

coprolith *n.* a mass of hard faeces within the colon or rectum, due to chronic constipation. It may become calcified. **糞石** 由慢性便秘引起的結腸或直腸中堅硬的糞塊。可能發生鈣化。

coproporphyrin *n.* a *porphyrin compound that is formed during the synthesis of protoporphyrin IX, a precursor of *haem. Coproporphyrin is excreted in the faeces during the process of red blood cell formation. **糞卟啉** 在原卟啉 IX 合成過程中生成的卟啉化合物。係血紅素的前體。在生成紅細胞的過程中由糞便排出。

copulation *n. see* coitus. **交媾** 性交

cor *n.* the heart. **心臟**

coracoid process a beaklike process that curves upwards and forwards from the top of the *scapula, over the shoulder joint. **喙突** 由肩胛骨上部向前上方彎曲的鳥嘴樣突起。位於肩關節上方。

cord *n.* any long flexible structure, which may be solid or tubular. Examples include the spermatic cord, spinal cord, umbilical cord, and vocal cord. **索，帶** 空心的或是實心的柔軟的長條。如精索、脊索、臍帶、聲帶等。

cordectomy *n.* surgical removal of a vocal cord. **聲帶切除術** 以外科手術切除聲帶。

cordotomy *n.* a surgical procedure for the relief of severe and persistent pain in the pelvis or lower limbs. The nerve fibres transmitting the sensation of pain **脊髓前側柱切斷術** 爲解除盆腔與下肢嚴重而持久的疼痛而進行的外科手術。痛覺在脊髓內通過特

to consciousness pass up the spinal cord in special tracts (the *spinothalamic tracts*). In cordotomy the spinothalamic tracts are severed in the cervical (neck) region.

殊的傳導束（脊髓丘腦束）向上傳導到感覺區。本手術是在頸段將脊髓丘腦束切斷。

Cordylobia *n. see* tumbu fly.

瘤蠅屬

core-and-cluster *n.* a form of housing for handicapped or subnormal people. Institutional organizations are replaced by small self-contained living units associated with a central facility providing more intensive resources.

分居式收養院 收容殘疾人或缺乏正常社會生活能力的人的一種機構。在此被收養者並非集中居住在一起，而是分散居住在獨立的生活小區裏。大型服務項目則由院方另設機構集中統一供應。

corectopia *n.* displacement of the pupil towards one side from its normal position in the centre of the iris. When present from birth, the displacement is usually inwards towards the nose. Scarring of the iris from inflammation may also draw the pupil out of position.

瞳孔異位 瞳孔自虹膜中央的正常位置向一側移位。先天性者通常向鼻側移位。虹膜炎症後的瘢痕亦可引起瞳孔移位。

corium *n. see* dermis.

眞皮

corn *n.* an area of hard thickened skin on or between the toes: a type of *callosity produced by ill-fitting shoes. The horny skin layers form an inverted pyramid that presses down into the deeper skin layers, causing pain. A corn may be treated by soaking in hot water or applying softening agents. Medical name: **clavus**.

鷄眼 足趾間或底部的皮膚變硬增厚部分。係胼胝的一種，由穿不合適的鞋引起。皮膚角質層形成逆向生長的錐體，壓迫皮膚深層，產生疼痛。治療：用熱水浸泡，使用軟化劑。

cornea *n.* the transparent circular part of the front of the eyeball. It refracts the light entering the eye onto the lens, which then focuses it onto the retina. The cornea contains no blood vessels and it is extremely sensitive to pain. —**corneal** *adj.*

角膜 眼球前部的圓形透明部分。它能將進入眼內的光線折射到晶體上，最後聚焦在網膜上。角膜上無血管，對痛覺極爲敏感。

corneal graft *see* keratoplasty.

角膜移植

cornification *n. see* keratinization.

角化

cornu *n.* (*pl.* **cornua**) (in anatomy) a horn-shaped structure, such as the

角 角狀結構。如舌骨與甲狀軟骨的角狀突起。

horn-shaped processes of the hyoid bone and thyroid cartilage. *See also* horn.

corona *n.* a crown or crownlike structure. The *corona capitis* is the crown of the head.

冠　冠與冠狀結構。頭頂即頭的冠部。

coronal *adj.* relating to the crown of the head or of a tooth. The *coronal plane* divides the body into dorsal and ventral parts (see illustration).

冠的　用以描述頭頂部的或牙冠部的結構。冠狀面指將身體分成前後兩部分的切面（見圖）。

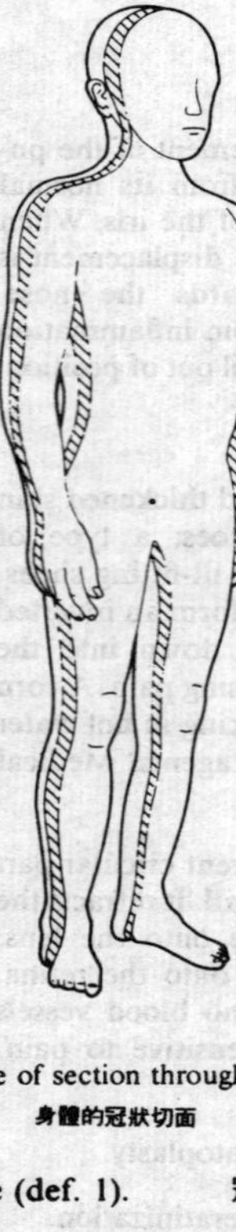

Coronal plane of section through the body

身體的冠狀切面

coronal suture *see* suture (def. 1).

冠狀縫

corona radiata 1. a series of radiating fibres between the cerebral cortex and the internal capsule of the brain. **2.** a

放射冠　①大腦皮質與內囊之間呈放射狀排列的神經纖維。　②新排出的卵

layer of follicle cells that surrounds a freshly ovulated ovum. The cells are elongated radially to the ovum when seen in section.

子周圍的一層呈放射狀排列的柱狀卵泡細胞。

coronary arteries the arteries supplying blood to the heart. The *right* and *left coronary arteries* arise from the aorta, just above the aortic valve, and form branches that encircle the heart.

冠狀動脉　向心臟供血的動脉。左右冠狀動脉起自主動脉略高於主動脉瓣處，形成分支包繞整個心臟。

coronary thrombosis the formation of a blood clot (thrombus) in the coronary artery, which obstructs the flow of blood to the heart. This is usually due to *atheroma and results in the death (infarction) of part of the heart muscle. For symptoms and treatment *see* myocardial infarction.

冠脉血栓形成　冠狀動脉內血凝塊形成的過程。可阻斷心臟的血流。通常由粥樣硬化引起，可引起心肌壞死。症狀與治療參見心肌梗死。

coroner *n.* the official who presides at an *inquest. He must be either a medical practitioner or a lawyer of at least five years standing.

驗屍官　主持驗屍的官員。該官員必須是有五年以上工作經驗的醫師或律師。

coronoid process 1. a process on the upper end of the *ulna. It forms part of the notch that articulates with the humerus. **2.** the process on the ramus of the *mandible to which the temporalis muscle is attached.

①**尺骨喙突**　尺骨上端的突起。是肘關節的一部分。　②**下頜骨冠突**　下頜支上的突起，顳肌即附着於該處。

cor pulmonale enlargement of the right ventricle of the heart that results from diseases of the lungs or the pulmonary arteries. Such diseases include those affecting the structure of the lungs (e.g. emphysema) or their function (e.g. obesity) except when these changes result from congenital heart disease or diseases primarily affecting the left side of the heart.

肺性心臟病　肺疾患或肺動脉疾患引起的右心室擴大。本病包括肺結構異常（肺氣腫）及肺功能障礙（肥胖）引起者，但不包括先天性心臟病及原發性左心病。

corpus *n.* (*pl.* **corpora**) any mass of tissue that can be distinguished from its surroundings.

體　有別於外圍的組織結構。

corpus albicans the residual body of scar tissue that remains in the ovary at the point where a *corpus luteum has regressed after its secretory activity has ceased.

白體　卵巢中的黃體分泌活動停止後退化形成的殘餘瘢痕組織。

corpus callosum the broad band of nervous tissue that connects the two cerebral hemispheres, containing an estimated 300 million fibres. *See* cerebrum.

胼胝體 連接兩側大腦半球的闊帶狀神經組織。其中約含3億條神經纖維。

corpus cavernosum either of a pair of cylindrical blood sinuses that form the erectile tissue of the *penis and clitoris. In the penis a third sinus, the corpus spongiosum, encloses the urethra and extends into the glans. All these sinuses have a spongelike structure that allows them to expand when filled with blood.

海綿體 陰莖與陰蒂中的一對有勃起作用的圓柱形血竇組織。在陰莖中還有一條尿道海綿體，包繞尿道並直達龜頭。這些血竇皆具有海綿樣結構，充血時即膨脹。

corpuscle *n.* any small particle, cell, or mass of tissue.

小體 微小的顆粒，細胞或組織團塊。

corpus luteum the glandular tissue in the ovary that forms at the site of a ruptured *Graafian follicle after ovulation. It secretes the hormone *progesterone, which prepares the womb for implantation. If implantation fails the corpus luteum becomes inactive and degenerates. If an embryo becomes implanted the corpus luteum continues to secrete progesterone until the fourth month of pregnancy, by which time the placenta has taken over this function.

黃體 排卵後在卵巢的破裂的格雷夫氏卵泡處形成的腺體組織。分泌孕酮以備子宮受精着床。如果沒有受精，黃體發生變性，停止活動。如果胚胎形成，黃體便繼續分泌孕酮，直至妊娠第四個月，以後其功能由胎盤代替。

corpus spongiosum the blood sinus that surrounds the urethra of the male. Together with the corpora cavernosa, it forms the erectile tissue of the *penis. It is expanded at the base of the penis to form the urethral bulb and at the tip to form the glans penis.

尿道海綿體 男性尿道周圍的血竇組織。與陰莖海綿體共同形成陰莖的勃起組織。在其兩端的膨大部形成尿道球和陰莖頭。

corpus striatum the part of the *basal ganglia in the cerebral hemispheres of the brain consisting of the caudate nucleus and the lentiform nucleus.

紋狀體 大腦半球基底神經節的一部分。含有尾狀核和豆狀核。

correlation *n.* (in statistics) the extent to which one of a pair of characteristics affects the other in a series of individuals. Such pairs of observations can be plotted as a series of points on a graph. If all the points on the resulting *scatter diagram* are in a straight line (which is neither horizontal nor vertical), the

相關 （統計學用語）在一組個體中，一對特徵因素的某一個對另一個的影響程度。這種成對的觀測值可以繪製成點圖。如果各點的連線係一直線（既非水平線，亦非垂直線），相關系數為零，則

correlation coefficient of 0 indicates no dependence of the one characteristic on the other of a straight line type. The *regression coefficient* is the average extent to which a unit increase of one characteristic influences the increase/decrease of the other. Where several factors appear to correlate with the onset of disease the relative importance of each may be calculated by the statistical technique known as *multivariate analysis*.

表示兩個特徵因素並無線性依賴關係。回歸系數則表示某一特徵因素的數量增加時影響另一特徵因素（使之增加或減少）的平均程度。當幾種因素看來都與某種疾病有關時，通過多變量分析的統計學技術，即可算出各種因素的重要程度來。

cortex *n.* (*pl.* **cortices**) the outer part of an organ, situated immediately beneath its capsule or outer membrane; for example, the *adrenal cortex* (*see* adrenal glands), *renal cortex* (*see* kidney), or *cerebral cortex. —**cortical** *adj.*

皮質 直接位於包膜或外膜下的某器官的外表部分。如腎上腺皮質、腎皮質或大腦皮質。

corticosteroid (corticoid) *n.* any steroid hormone synthesized by the adrenal cortex. There are two main groups of corticosteroids. The *glucocorticoids* (e.g. *hydrocortisone (cortisol), *cortisone, and corticosterone) are essential for the utilization of carbohydrate, fat, and protein by the body and for a normal response to stress. Naturally occurring and synthetic glucocorticoids have very powerful anti-inflammatory effects and are used to treat conditions involving inflammation. The *mineralocorticoids* (e.g. *aldosterone) are necessary for the regulation of salt and water balance.

皮質類固醇 由腎上腺皮質合成的固醇類激素。有兩大類。糖類皮質激素（氫化可的松、可的松、皮質酮）對體內糖、脂肪、蛋白質的代謝十分重要，並與應激反應有關。天然的與人工合成的糖類激素有强大的消炎作用，可用於治療炎性疾病。鹽類激素（醛固酮）與水鹽代謝密切相關。

corticosterone *n.* a steroid hormone (*see* corticosteroid) synthesized and released in small amounts by the adrenal cortex.

皮質酮 由腎上腺皮質合成與分泌的固醇類激素。爲量甚小。

corticotrophin *n. see* ACTH.

促腎上腺皮質激素

cortisol *n. see* hydrocortisone.

可的索

cortisone *n.* a naturally occurring *corticosteroid that is used mainly to treat deficiency of corticosteroid hormones in *Addison's disease and following surgical removal of the adrenal glands. It is administered by mouth or injection and may cause serious side-effects such as stomach ulcers and

可的松 天然存在的皮質類固醇。主要用於阿狄森氏病的皮質類固醇缺乏與腎上腺摘除術後。口服或注射。可有嚴重副作用，如胃潰瘍與出血，神經與內分泌紊亂，肌肉、骨骼、眼的損害等。

bleeding, nervous and hormone disturbances, muscle and bone damage, and eye changes.

cor triloculare a rare congenital condition in which there are three instead of four chambers of the heart due to the presence of a single common ventricle. *Cyanosis (blueness) is common. Most patients die in infancy.

三腔心 一種少見的先天性心臟病。本病只有一個共同的心室，故不具有正常心臟的四腔而只有三個腔。常有紫紺。多於嬰兒期死亡。

Corynebacterium *n.* a genus of Gram-positive, mostly aerobic, nonmotile rodlike bacteria that frequently bear club-shaped swellings. Many species cause disease in man, domestic animals, birds, and plants; some are found in dairy products. The species *C. diphtheriae* (*Klebs-Loeffler bacillus*) is the causative organism of *diphtheria, producing a powerful *exotoxin that is harmful to heart and nerve tissue. It occurs in one of three forms: *gravis*, *intermedius*, and *mitis*.

棒狀桿菌屬 一組革蘭氏陽性、多數爲需氧性、無活動能力的桿狀細菌。一端常膨大呈棒狀。其中多數係人類、家畜、鳥類與植物的致病菌。痢疾的致病菌痢疾桿菌（克呂二氏桿菌）能產生强烈的外毒素，導致心臟與神經組織損害，可引起重型、普通型或輕型痢疾。

coryza (cold in the head) *n.* a catarrhal inflammation of the mucous membrane in the nose due to either a *cold or *hay fever. *See also* catarrh.

鼻卡他 由感冒或枯草熱引起的鼻黏膜卡他性炎症。

cost- (costo-) *prefix denoting* the rib(s). Example: *costectomy* (excision of).

〔前綴〕 **肋** 如肋骨切除術。

costal *adj.* of or relating to the ribs.

肋的

costal cartilage a cartilage that connects a *rib to the breastbone (*sternum). The first seven ribs (true ribs) are directly connected to the sternum by individual costal cartilages. The next three ribs are indirectly connected to the sternum by three costal cartilages, each of which is connected to the one immediately above it.

肋軟骨 肋骨與胸骨連結部的軟骨。上七根肋骨（眞肋）以各自的肋軟骨直接與胸骨相連，下三根肋骨的軟骨只與上一根肋骨相連。

costalgia *n.* pain localized to the ribs. This term is now rarely used.

肋痛 局限於肋骨區的疼痛。此詞現已罕用。

costive *adj.* constipated.

便秘的

costochondritis *n. see* Tietze's syndrome.

肋軟骨炎 痛性非化膿性肋軟骨腫大。

cot death the death of a baby, usually occurring overnight while it is in its cot, from an unidentifiable cause. Some 20% of infant deaths in the UK occur in this way. The causes may include virus infections or allergic reactions, but evidence is growing that cot deaths are less likely in breast-fed babies and more likely in households with very low income levels.

嬰兒猝死症 在襁褓中的嬰兒由不明原因引起的突然死亡。在英國約 20% 的嬰兒死於本病。病因可能是病毒感染或變態反應。但日益增加的證據表明，本病很少發生於母乳餵養的嬰兒，而多見於經濟收入極低的家庭。

co-trimoxazole *n.* an antibacterial drug consisting of *sulphamethoxazole and *trimethoprim. Since both these drugs are well absorbed and rapidly excreted – and each potentiates the action of the other – co-trimoxazole is taken by mouth and is particularly useful for treating urinary-tract infections (such as cystitis). Side-effects are those of the *sulphonamides. Trade names: **Bactrim**, **Septrin**.

增效磺胺甲基異噁唑 含甲氧苄氨嘧啶和磺胺甲基異噁唑的抗菌藥。二者吸收良好，排泄迅速，並能相互增强效果。口服。多用於泌尿道感染（如膀胱炎）。副作用同磺胺類藥物。商品名：複方新諾明。

cotyledon *n.* any of the major convex subdivisions of the mature *placenta. Each cotyledon contains a major branch of the umbilical blood vessels, which branch further into the numerous villi that make up the surface of the cotyledon.

胎盤葉 成熟胎盤由淺溝分成的微凸的小區。每個胎盤葉都有臍血管的大分支，它們再繼續分支分佈到構成胎盤葉表面的大量絨毛上。

cotyloid cavity *see* acetabulum.

髂臼

couching *n.* an operation for cataract in which the lens is pushed out of the pupil downwards and backwards into the jelly-like vitreous humour by a small knife inserted through the edge of the cornea. It was widely employed in ancient Hindu civilizations and has been practised ever since. Its sole advantage is speed of performance, but modern developments in surgery and anaesthesia leave little place for it today. The complication rate is very high.

內障摘除術 一種摘除內障的手術。用一小刀沿角膜邊緣插入，將晶體自瞳孔向下或向後撥入膠凍樣玻璃體液中。古印度廣泛使用此術，並沿襲至今。唯一優點是手術迅速。現代外科與麻醉的發展，已使本手術失去實用價值。此手術合併症極多。

coughing *n.* a form of violent exhalation by which irritant particles in the airways can be expelled. Stimulation of

咳嗽 能將呼吸道中刺激物質咳出的猛烈的呼氣動作。咳嗽反射的刺激引起

the cough reflexes results in the glottis being kept closed until a high expiratory pressure has built up, which is then suddenly released. Medical name: **tussis**.

聲門緊閉，在產生强大的呼氣壓後又突然開放。

coulomb *n.* the *SI unit of electric charge, equal to the quantity of electricity transferred by 1 ampere in 1 second. Symbol: C.

庫倫 電量的標準國際單位。即每秒鐘通過一安培電流的電量。符號：C。

counselling *n.* a method of approaching psychological difficulties in adjustment that aims to help the client work out his own problems. The counsellor listens sympathetically, attempting to identify with the client, tries to clarify current problems, and sometimes gives advice. It involves less emphasis on insight and interpretation than does psychotherapy or psychoanalytic therapy. *See also* client-centred therapy.

諮詢 一種解除適應性心理障礙的方法。和心理療法不同的是，本法並不着重於深入分析患者的內心世界，而是滿懷同情地聽取患者的陳述，爭取和患者打成一片，努力澄清現存的問題，有時也提出若干勸告，以幫助患者自已解決問題。

counterextension *n.* an orthopaedic procedure consisting of *traction on one part of a limb, while the remainder of the limb is held steady: used particularly in the treatment of a fractured femur (thigh bone).

對抗牽伸術 在肢體其餘部分固定的情況下，對某一部分施行牽引的矯形外科手法。主要用於股骨骨折。

counterirritant *n.* an agent, such as methyl salicylate, that causes irritation when applied to the skin and is used in order to relieve more deep-seated pain or discomfort. —**counterirritation** *n.*

抗刺激劑 一種塗搽於皮膚上能產生刺激作用的物質。如水楊酸甲酯。用以減輕深部的疼痛與不適。

countertraction *n.* the use of a balancing opposing force during *traction, when a strong continuous pull is applied to a limb so that broken bones can be kept in alignment during healing. To arrange that traction on a limb by weights and pulleys does not pull the patient out of bed, countertraction is often produced by applying tension to metal pins temporarily inserted into the opposite end of the bone.

對抗牽引 對肢體施加能保持平衡的相反作用力的强力持續牽引，以使骨折端能對位癒合。使用重物與滑輪進行肢體牽引時，要確保患者不致從牀上跌下來。通常在臨時打入骨折對端的金屬釘上加重，以產生對抗牽引力。

couvade *n.* **1.** a custom in some tribes whereby a father takes to his bed during or after the birth of his child. **2.** a

①**父代母育** 一種原始部落的風俗。母親生育時或生育後，父親亦臥牀不

symptom of abdominal pain experienced by a man in relation to his wife's giving birth. It may be due to hysteria, anxiety, or sympathy.

起。②夫代妻痛 一種由焦慮、癔病或同情引起的症狀。妻子分娩時丈夫感到腹痛。

cover-slip *n.* an extremely thin square or circle of glass used to protect the upper surface of a preparation on a microscope slide.

蓋玻片 方形或圓形的極薄的玻璃片。用以保護顯微鏡載物片上的標本。

cover test a test used to detect suppressed *strabismus (squint) in children. The child is asked to look fixedly at an object with one eye while the other is kept open but covered by the hand of the observer. The hand is then withdrawn: if the eye that had been covered is seen to move towards the nose to adjust to the focus of the uncovered eye the child is assumed to have a divergent squint; movement of the eye away from the nose implies a convergent squint.

覆蓋試驗 檢查兒童隱斜視的一種方法。令兒童用一目注視某物，另一目同時睜開，但被檢查者用手遮住。然後取開此手。如果被遮目爲了調節到與注視目相等的焦距而向鼻側移動，可能有外隱斜視；如果向顳側移動則可能有內隱斜視。

Cowper's glands (bulbourethral glands) a pair of small glands that open into the urethra at the base of the penis. Their secretion contributes to the seminal fluid, but less than that of the prostate gland or seminal vesicles.

庫珀氏腺（尿道球腺） 在陰莖底部開口於尿道的一對小的腺體。該腺的分泌物是精液的組成部分，但較前列腺與精囊的分泌物爲少。

cowpox *n.* a virus infection of cows' udders, transmitted to man by direct contact, causing very mild symptoms similar to *smallpox. An attack confers immunity to smallpox. Medical name: **vaccinia**.

牛痘 牛乳腺的一種病毒感染。通過直接接觸傳染至人。症狀類似天花，但十分輕微。患病後能對天花產生免疫。

cox- (coxo-) *prefix denoting* the hip. Example: *coxalgia* (pain in).

〔前綴〕 **髖** 如髖關節。

coxa *n.* (*pl.* **coxae**) **1.** the hip bone. **2.** the hip joint.

①髖 ①髖關節

Coxiella *n.* a genus of rickettsia-like microorganisms that cause disease in animals and man. They are smaller than *rickettsiae, are transmitted by air-borne droplets rather than by insects, and they produce diseases characterized by inflammation of the lungs, without a rash (*compare* typhus). The species *C. burnettii* causes *Q fever.

柯克斯體屬 能引起人、獸患病的一組立克次體樣微生物。比立克次體小，多通過空氣飛沫傳染，少數通過媒介昆蟲。伯納特柯克斯體能引起昆士蘭熱。

Coxsackie virus one of a group of RNA-containing viruses that are able to multiply in the gastrointestinal tract (*see* enterovirus). About 30 different types exist. *Type A Coxsackie viruses* generally cause less severe and less well-defined diseases, although some cause meningitis and severe throat infections (*see* herpangina). *Type B Coxsackie viruses* cause inflammation or degeneration of brain, skeletal muscle, or heart tissue (*see* Bornholm disease).

柯薩奇病毒屬 脫氧核糖核酸病毒羣中的一組。可在胃腸道繁殖，約有 30 種不同類型。甲型柯薩奇病毒有些可引起腦膜炎和嚴重喉頭感染，但大多引起症狀輕微、界限不清的疾病。乙型柯薩奇病毒引起腦、骨骼肌與心肌組織的炎症或變性。

crab louse *see* Phthirus.

陰蝨

cradle *n.* a framework of metal strips or other material that forms a cage over an injured part of the body of a patient lying in bed, to protect it from the pressure of the bedclothes.

支架 用金屬條或其他物質製成的籠罩。置於臥牀病人身體患部，以避免受到被褥壓蓋。

cramp *n.* prolonged painful contraction of a muscle. It is sometimes caused by an imbalance of the salts in the body, but is more often a result of fatigue, imperfect posture, or stress. Spasm in the muscles making it impossible to perform a specific task but allowing the use of these muscles for any other movement is called *occupational cramp*. It most often affects the hand muscles for writing (*writer's cramp*).

痛性痙攣 肌肉持續的疼痛性收縮。有時由體內鹽類失衡引起，但多發生於疲勞、姿勢不當或受到壓迫時。發生痛性痙攣時，肌肉如果不能完成某種特殊任務但能進行其他活動稱爲職業性痙攣。最多見的是書寫痙攣。

crani- (cranio-) *prefix denoting* the skull. Example: *cranioplasty* (plastic surgery of).

〔前綴〕 **顱** 如顱成形術。

cranial nerves the 12 pairs of nerves that arise directly from the brain and leave the skull through separate apertures; they are conventionally given Roman numbers, as follows: I *olfactory; II *optic; III *oculomotor; IV *trochlear; V *trigeminal; VI *abducens; VII *facial; VIII *vestibulocochlear; IX *glossopharyngeal; X *vagus; XI *accessory; XII *hypoglossal. *Compare* spinal nerves.

腦神經 通過顱骨的不同孔隙由腦直接發出的 12 對神經。習慣上用羅馬數字命名：Ⅰ嗅，Ⅱ視，Ⅲ動眼，Ⅳ滑車，Ⅴ三叉，Ⅵ外展，Ⅶ面，Ⅷ前庭耳蝸，Ⅸ舌咽，Ⅹ迷走，Ⅺ副，Ⅻ舌下。

cranioclasm (cranioclasis, cranioclasty) *n.* the crushing of the head of the fetus in the womb by means of a special

碎顱術 用特殊器械（碎顱鉗）將子宮內胎頭壓碎的手術。用於難產。

instrument (*cranioclast*). This may be done in difficult childbirth.

craniopagus (dicephalus) *n.* *Siamese twins united by their heads.

顱部聯胎 頭部聯結在一起的連體雙胎。

craniopharyngioma *n.* a brain tumour derived from remnants of *Rathke's pouch*, an embryologic structure from which the pituitary gland is partly formed. The patient may show raised intracranial pressure and *diabetes insipidus due to reduced secretion of the hormone *vasopressin. An X-ray of the skull typically shows calcification within the tumour and loss of the normal skull structure around the pituitary gland.

顱咽管瘤 由胚胎結構臘特克氏囊的殘餘組織生長成的腦腫瘤。腦垂體腺部分由此囊構成。患者顱內壓升高，並由於後葉加壓素分泌減少出現尿崩症。顱骨 X 線典型所見為瘤體內發生鈣化，垂體腺周圍顱骨正常結構受到破壞。

craniostenosis *n.* premature closing of the *sutures between the cranial bones during development, resulting in deformities of the skull.

顱狹小 顱縫早期癒合引起的顱畸形。

craniotomy *n.* **1.** surgical removal of a portion of the skull, performed to expose the brain and *meninges for inspection or biopsy or to relieve excessive intracranial pressure (as in a subdural *haematoma). **2.** surgical perforation of the skull of a dead fetus during difficult labour, so that delivery may continue.
For both operations the instrument used is called a *craniotome*.

①**顱骨切開術** 切除部分顱骨以暴露腦與軟腦膜的手術。用以觀察病變，取活體組織，或減低顱內壓（如在硬膜下血腫時）。②**穿顱術** 難產時將死胎頭顱穿破的手術。使胎兒便於娩出。以上兩種手術的器械都稱為開顱器。

cranium *n.* the part of the skeleton that encloses the brain. It consists of eight bones connected together by immovable joints (*see* skull). —**cranial** *adj.*

顱 包含腦髓的骨腔。由八塊以不動關節連結在一起的骨頭組成。

creatinase (creatine kinase) *n.* an enzyme involved in the metabolic breakdown of creatine to creatinine.

肌酸酶 催化肌酸分解成肌酸酐的代謝過程的酶。

creatine *n.* a product of protein metabolism found in muscle. Its phosphate, *creatine phosphate* (*phosphocreatine, phosphagen*), acts as a store of high-energy phosphate in muscle and serves to maintain adequate amounts of *ATP

肌酸 肌肉中蛋白質代謝的產物。其磷酸化合物磷酸肌酸是肌肉中的高能磷酸酯庫，能保持足量的三磷酸腺苷（肌肉收縮的能量來源）。

(the source of energy for muscular contraction).

creatinine *n.* a substance derived from creatine and creatine phosphate in muscle. Creatinine is excreted in the urine.

肌酸酐 肌肉中肌酸與磷酸肌酸的代謝產物。由尿排出。

creatinuria *n.* an excess of the nitrogenous compound creatine in the urine.

肌酸尿 尿中出現大量的含氮化合物——肌酸。

creatorrhoea *n.* the passage of excessive nitrogen in the faeces due to failure of digestion or absorption in the small intestine. It is found particularly in pancreatic failure. *See* cystic fibrosis, pancreatitis.

肉質泄瀉 由於小腸消化吸收不良而在糞便中排出大量氮質。多見於胰腺功能障礙。

Credé's method 1. a technique for expelling the placenta from the womb. Downward pressure is applied to the womb through the abdominal wall in the direction of the birth canal. **2.** the application of 1% silver nitrate solution to the eyes of a newborn baby whose mother has gonorrhoea. The treatment aims to prevent the development of *ophthalmia neonatorum in the infant.

①**腹外用手壓出胎盤法** 用手在腹壁向下朝產道的方向加壓排出胎盤。 ②**新生兒硝酸銀滴眼法** 對淋病患者所生兒用 1% 硝酸銀溶液點眼以預防新生兒眼炎。

creeping eruption (larva migrans) a skin disease caused either by larvae of certain nematode worms (e.g. *Ancylostoma braziliense*) normally parasitic in dogs and cats or by the maggots of certain flies (*see* Hypoderma, Gasterophilus). The larvae burrow within the skin tissues, their movements marked by long thin red lines that cause the patient intense irritation. The nematode infections are treated with diethylcarbamazine or thiabendazole; maggots can be surgically removed.

匐形疹（遊走性幼蟲病）由某種正常時寄生於狗、貓的線蟲（巴西鈎口線蟲）的幼蟲或某種蠅類的蛆引起的皮膚病。幼蟲在皮膚組織內掘溝，外表呈現一條長細的紅線，劇烈刺癢。線蟲感染用乙胺嗪或噻苯咪唑治療。蛆則用外科切除。

crenation *n.* an abnormal appearance of red blood cells seen under a microscope, in which the normally smooth cell margins appear crinkly or irregular. Crenation may be a feature of certain blood disorders, but most commonly occurs as a result of prolonged storage of a blood specimen prior to preparation of a blood film.

皺縮紅細胞 顯微鏡下紅細胞的一種異常的外觀。此時平滑的邊緣變成不規則的鋸齒狀。可能是某種血液病的表現，但常由於血標本製做血片前保存過久所致。

crepitation (rale) *n.* a soft fine crackling sound heard in the lungs through the stethoscope. Crepitations are made either by air passages and alveoli (air sacs) opening up during inspiration or by air bubbling through fluid. They are not normally heard in healthy lungs but their interpretation is somewhat controversial.

捻髮音（囉音） 用聽診器在肺部聽到的一種輕微細小的破裂音。細支氣管或肺泡於吸氣時開放，或是氣泡通過液體時都會產生此音。在正常健肺不出現此音，但對其產生原因的解釋尚不一致。

crepitus *n.* **1.** a crackling sound or grating feeling produced by bone rubbing on bone or roughened cartilage, detected on movement of an arthritic joint. Crepitus in the kneejoint is a common sign of *chondromalacia patellae in the young and *osteoarthritis in the elderly. **2.** a similar sound heard with a stethoscope over an inflamed lung when the patient breathes in.

①**骨摩擦音（感）** 骨與骨摩擦或與粗糙的軟骨摩擦產生的咿軋音或摩擦感。出現於發炎的關節活動時。年輕人患軟骨軟化或老年人患骨關節炎時於膝關節常出現骨摩擦音。②**捻髮音** 用聽診器在肺炎患者肺部吸氣時聽到的囉音。

cresol *n.* a strong antiseptic effective against many microorganisms and used mostly in soap solutions as a general disinfectant. It is sometimes used in low concentrations as a preservative in injections. Cresol solutions irritate the skin and if taken by mouth are corrosive and cause pain, nausea, and vomiting.

煤酚 一種常用的對多種微生物皆有殺菌效果的消毒劑。多用其肥皂溶液。有時用其低濃度做爲注射液的防腐劑。對皮膚有刺激作用，口服則因腐蝕作用引起疼痛、噁心、嘔吐。

crest *n.* a ridge or linear protuberance, particularly on a bone. Examples include the crest of fibula and the iliac crest (of the ilium).

嵴 線形隆起或脊狀結構。尤指骨上的，如腓骨嵴與髂嵴。

cretinism *n.* a syndrome of *dwarfism, mental retardation, and coarseness of the skin and facial features due to lack of thyroid hormone from birth (congenital *hypothyroidism).

克汀病 表現爲身材矮小、智力低下、皮膚粗糙和特殊容貌的一種綜合徵。係先天缺乏甲狀腺激素所致。

cribriform plate *see* ethmoid bone.

篩板

cricoid cartilage the cartilage, shaped like a signet ring, that forms part of the anterior and lateral walls and most of the posterior wall of the *larynx.

環狀軟骨 形狀類似圖章戒指的軟骨。形成喉的前壁和側壁的一部分，後壁的大部分。

crisis *n.* **1.** the turning point of a disease, after which the patient either improves or deteriorates. Since the ad-

①**極期** 疾病發生好轉或惡化的轉折點。由於抗生素的使用，傳染病已很少

vent of antibiotics, infections seldom reach the point of crisis. **2.** the occurrence of sudden severe pain in certain diseases. *See also* Dietl's crisis.

發展到極期。 ②**危象** 某種疾病過程中劇烈的疼痛。如游走腎危象。

crista *n.* (*pl.* **cristae**) **1.** the sensory structure within the ampulla of a *semicircular canal within the inner ear (see illustration). The cristae respond to changes in the rate of movement of the head, being activated by pressure from the fluid in the semicircular canals. **2.** one of the infoldings of the inner membrane of a *mitochondrion. **3.** any anatomical structure resembling a crest.

壺腹嵴 內耳半規管壺腹內的感覺末梢器（見圖）。能接受半規管淋巴液壓力的刺激，對頭部運動速度的變化發生反應。 ②**線粒體嵴** 線粒體內膜向內折疊的部分。 ③任何類似嵴狀的解剖結構。

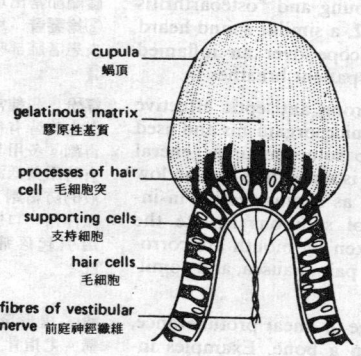

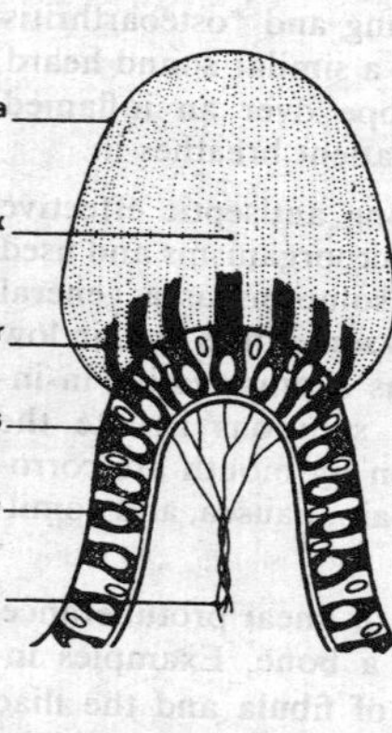

A crista in the ampulla of a semicircular canal
內耳半規管的壺腹嵴

Crohn's disease a condition in which segments of the alimentary tract become inflamed, thickened, and ulcerated. It usually affects the terminal part of the ileum; its acute form (*acute ileitis*) may mimic *appendicitis. Chronic disease often causes partial obstruction of the intestine, leading to pain, diarrhoea, and *malabsorption. *Fistulae around the anus, between adjacent loops of intestine, or from intestine to skin, bladder, etc., are characteristic complications. The cause is unknown. Treatment includes rest, corticosteroids, immunosuppressive drugs, antibiotics, or

克羅恩氏病 一種在消化道按節段分佈出現炎症、增厚與潰瘍的疾病。多侵犯回腸末端，急性型（急性回腸炎）頗似闌尾炎。慢性型常引起部分腸梗阻，發生腹痛、腹瀉與吸收不良。肛周、鄰近腸襻之間或由腸管到皮膚形成瘻管係本病典型的併發症。病因不明。治療：休息，投予皮質醇類、免疫抑制劑、抗生素。部分病例行患部手術切除。本病又名局限性腸炎、局限性回腸炎。

(in some cases) surgical removal of the affected part of the intestine. Alternative names: **regional enteritis, regional ileitis.**

cromolyn sodium a drug used to prevent and treat asthma and allergic bronchitis. It is administered by inhalation and may cause throat irritation. Trade name: **Intal**.

色甘酸鈉 治療支氣管哮喘與變態反應性支氣管炎藥。供吸入用。可引起喉頭刺激。

crossbite *n.* a condition in which some or all of the lower teeth close outside the upper teeth when the mandible is as far back as it will go.

反𬌗 下頜儘力內收時下牙仍全部或部分突出於上牙之外。

crossing over (in genetics) the exchange of sections of chromatids between pairs of homologous chromosomes, which results in the recombination of genetic material. It occurs during *meiosis at a *chiasma.

交換 遺傳學用語。在成對的同源染色體之間部分染色單體進行交換的現象。可產生遺傳物質重組，發生於減數分裂染色體交叉時。

cross-over trial *see* intervention study.

防治研究實驗

cross-sectional study the collection and analysis of information relating to persons in a population or group at a defined point in time, with particular reference to their individual characteristics and exposure to factors thought likely to predispose to disease.

橫面調查 在一特定的時間對某一組人羣的流行病學資料進行收集並分析調查。着重了解他們的個體特徵及與可疑致病因素的接觸情況。

crotamiton *n.* a drug that destroys mites and is used to treat scabies and similar skin infections and also to relieve itching. It is applied to the skin as a lotion or ointment and sometimes causes reddening and hypersensitivity reactions. Trade name: **Eurax**.

克羅他米通 殺蟎藥。用以治療疥瘡與類似的皮膚感染。亦可用於止癢。製成洗劑或軟膏劑外用。有時導致皮膚發紅或過敏。商品名：優樂散。

croup *n.* inflammation and obstruction of the larynx in young children (usually aged between six months and two years). In the past diphtheria was the most common cause, but now croup generally results from a viral infection of the respiratory tract (*see* **laryngotracheobronchitis**). The symptoms are those of *laryngitis, accompanied by signs of obstruction – harsh difficult

格魯布 幼兒（通常6個月至兩歲之間）喉部的炎症與梗阻。過去以白喉最為多見，現多由呼吸道一種病毒感染引起。出現喉炎症狀，伴有喉梗阻徵——喘鳴性呼吸困難，脈速，青紫。增加室內空氣濕度與使用輕鎮靜劑只能緩解表面症狀，反而使

breathing (*see* stridor), a rising pulse rate, restlessness, and *cyanosis. Treatment by humidification and mild sedation usually reverses the alarming symptoms. In severe cases the obstruction may require treatment by *tracheostomy or nasotracheal *intubation. *See also* epiglottitis.

人放鬆警惕。嚴重梗阻病例可能需行氣管切開或經鼻行氣管插管。

crown *n.* **1.** the part of a tooth normally visible in the mouth and usually covered by enamel. **2.** a dental *restoration that covers most or all of the natural crown. It may be made of porcelain, gold, a combination of these, or less commonly other materials. Most crowns are like thimbles and are custom made to fit over a trimmed-down tooth. A *post crown* is used to restore a tooth when insufficient of the natural crown remains. A post is inserted into the root and the missing centre of the tooth is built up; over it is fitted a thimble-like crown to restore the natural shape of the tooth. *Root treatment is required before such a crown can be made.

冠 ①正常時口腔內牙齒的可見部分。通常由釉質覆蓋。 ②覆蓋全部或部分牙冠的牙科修復體。有瓷製的，金製的，或瓷金合製的，其他材料少見。多數係罩冠，要根據修整好了的牙齒預先定製，以便嵌戴。自然牙冠殘缺時則使用樁冠。冠樁釘入牙根以維持重心，外面再加用罩冠以恢復牙齒自然外形。造冠術前需做根管治療。

crowning *n.* **1.** the stage of labour when the upper part of the infant's head is tightly encircled by the margins of the vaginal opening. Only the top of the head is visible at this stage. **2.** the fitting of an artificial *crown to a tooth.

①**着冠** 分娩的一個階段。此時陰道口緊緊包住胎頭上部，只有胎頭頂顯露在外。 ②**造冠術**

crude rate the total number of events (e.g. cases of lung cancer) expressed as a percentage (or rate per 1000, etc.) of the whole population. When factors such as age structure or sex of populations may seriously affect their rates (as in *mortality or *morbidity rates) it is more meaningful to compare age/sex specific rates using one or more age groups of a designated sex (e.g. lung cancer in males aged 55–64 years). More complex calculations, which take account of the age bias of a population as a whole, can produce *standardized rates* or – as currently used for deciding resource allocation in the British Na-

總發生率 按百分比或千分比表示的全體人口中出現某一事例（如肺癌）總數。如總人口中性別和年齡結構因素對該數字影響很大（如死亡率和發病率），則在一個或幾個指定性別的年齡組中求出按年齡和性別的特殊比率，其意義就更大（例如：55～64 歲的男性中肺癌發病率和死亡率）。更加複雜的計算法還要考慮總人口中年齡結構的差異，以求出標準化率或標準化死亡率。英國國民保健服

tional Health Service – *standardized mortality ratios* (SMR). In these the ratios of subgroups are expressed as percentages of that for a designated or standard population (e.g. England and Wales), particularly applied to the age bracket 15–64 years.
務制當局在決定財政撥款時即使用標準化死亡率。此時各分組的比率是以指定的或標準的人口中的百分比來表示的（如英格蘭和威爾士）。這種方法尤適用於 15～64 歲年齡組。

crural *adj.* **1.** relating to the thigh or leg. **2.** relating to the crura cerebri (*see* crus).
①脚的　②大腦脚的

crus *n.* (*pl.* **crura**) an elongated process or part of a structure. The *crus cerebri* is one of two symmetrical nerve tracts situated between the medulla oblongata and the cerebral hemispheres.
脚　突起呈長條形的結構。大腦脚即在大腦半球與延腦之間的一對相互對稱的神經束。

cry- (cryo-) *prefix denoting* cold.
〔前綴〕　**冷**

cryaesthesia *n.* **1.** exceptional sensitivity to low temperature. **2.** a sensation of coldness.
①冷覺過敏　②冷覺

cryoglobulin *n.* an abnormal protein – an *immunoglobulin (*see* paraprotein) – that may be present in the blood in certain diseases. Cryoglobulins become insoluble at low temperatures, leading to obstruction of small blood vessels in the fingers and toes in cold weather and producing a characteristic rash. The presence of cryoglobulins (*cryoglobulinaemia*) may be a feature of a variety of diseases, including *macroglobulinaemia, systemic *lupus erythematosus and certain infections.
冷沉球蛋白　患某種疾病時血中出現的一種異常的免疫球蛋白。遇低溫便產生沉澱。天氣寒冷時能引起指趾小血管阻塞而出現典型的皮疹。冷沉蛋白血症可出現於多種疾病，如巨球蛋白血症、系統性紅斑狼瘡與某些感染。

cryoprecipitate *n.* a precipitate produced by freezing and thawing under controlled conditions. An example of a cryoprecipitate is the residue obtained from fresh frozen blood plasma that has been thawed at 4°C. This residue is extremely rich in a clotting factor, Factor VIII (antihaemophilic factor), and is used in the control of bleeding in *haemophilia.
冷沉澱物　在人工控制的條件下進行冷凍與解凍後沉澱下來的物質。如冷凍新鮮血漿於 4℃ 解凍時產生的沉澱物。某種凝血因子（Ⅷ因子，抗血友病因子）含此物頗多，可用於血友病出血的治療。

cryoprobe *n. see* cryosurgery.
冷刀

cryostat *n.* **1.** a chamber in which frozen tissue is sectioned with a *microtome. **2.** a device for maintaining a specific low temperature.

①冷凍切片機 ②低溫控制器

cryosurgery *n.* the use of extreme cold in a localized part of the body to freeze and destroy unwanted tissues. Cryosurgery is usually undertaken with an instrument called a *cryoprobe*, which has a fine tip cooled by allowing carbon dioxide or nitrous oxide gas to expand within it. Cryosurgery is commonly used for the removal of cataracts and the destruction of certain bone tumours.

冷凍手術 使身體局部高度冷却以冷凍和破壞該處組織的方法。通常使用一種稱爲冷刀的器械，其微細的尖端因其中含有的二氧化碳或氧化亞氮膨脹而致冷。本術常用於摘除內障及破壞某些骨腫瘤。

cryotherapy *n.* the use of cold in the treatment of disorders. *See* cryosurgery, hypothermia (def. 2). *Compare* thermotherapy.

冷凍療法 利用寒冷治療疾病的方法。

crypt *n.* a small sac, follicle, or cavity; for example, the crypts of Lieberkuhn (*see* Lieberkuhn's glands), which are intestinal glands.

①隱窩 ②濾泡 ③腺體 如利貝昆氏腺（腸腺）。

crypt- (crypto-) *prefix denoting* concealed. Example: *cryptogenic* (of unknown origin).

〔前綴〕 **隱** 隱蔽的。如隱原性的，原因不明的。

cryptococcosis (torulosis) *n.* a rare disease occurring in the USA, caused by the fungus *Cryptococcus neoformans.* The fungus attacks the lungs, causing tumour-like lesions (*torulomas*), but it may also spread to the brain, causing meningitis. Treatment with *amphotericin B may be effective.

隱球菌病 發生於美國的一種由新型隱球菌引起的少見病。眞菌侵犯肺部，引起腫瘤樣病變，亦可擴散至腦引起腦膜炎。二性黴素 B 可能有療效。

Cryptococcus *n.* a genus of unicellular yeastlike fungi that cause disease in man. They are found in soil (particularly when enriched with pigeon droppings), and they are common in pigeon roosts and nests. The species *C. neoformans* causes *cryptococcosis.

隱球菌屬 一種能引起人類疾病的單細胞酵母樣眞菌屬。存在於土壤中。尤多見於含有大量鴿糞的土壤，如鴿棚與鴿巢內。新型隱球菌可引起隱球菌病。

cryptomenorrhoea *n.* absence of blood flow when the internal symptoms of menstruation are present. The condi-

隱發月經 月經周期的內部變化存在而無月經流出的現象。由陰道入口處處

tion may arise because the hymen at the entrance to the vagina lacks an opening or because of some other obstruction.

女膜閉鎖或其他原因的阻塞引起。

cryptophthalmos *n.* apparent absence of the eyes due to the skin having grown over the eyeballs during embryonic development.

隱眼畸形 由於胚胎期皮膚生長過度遮蓋眼球，引起眼球完全被掩蔽。

cryptorchidism (cryptorchism) *n.* the condition in which the testes fail to descend into the scrotum and are retained within the abdomen or inguinal canal. The operation of *orchidopexy is necessary to bring the testes into the scrotum before puberty to allow subsequent normal development; it is thought that the higher temperature in the abdomen interferes with sperm production. **—cryptorchid** *adj., n.*

隱睾病 睾丸未能降入陰囊而停留於腹腔或腹股溝內。於青春期前需行睾丸固定術將睾丸置入陰囊以保證進一步正常發育。一般認爲腹腔內的高溫會影響精子生長成熟。

crystal violet (gentian violet) an antiseptic dye used to treat some skin infections due to bacteria and fungi and also some worm infestations. Crystal violet is administered by mouth, as pessaries, or as ointments, paints, and solutions; side-effects are uncommon but can include nausea, vomiting, and diarrhoea. The dye is also used to stain tissues and microorganisms for microscopical study.

結晶紫（龍膽紫）一種有抗菌防腐作用的染料。用以治療皮膚細菌與眞菌感染，亦可治療某些蠕蟲感染。口服。亦可製成栓劑、軟膏劑、塗劑與溶液。副作用少見。有噁心、嘔吐與腹瀉等。亦用於顯微鏡下組織標本與微生物標本染色。

CSF *see* cerebrospinal fluid.

腦脊髓液

CS gas a powerful incapacitating gas used in warfare and riot control. The sufferer experiences a burning sensation in the eyes, difficulty in breathing, tightness of the chest, nausea, vomiting, and streaming from the eyes and nose. In confined spaces the gas can prove fatal.

CS 毒氣 用於戰爭或防暴的一種烈性毒氣。接觸者眼內有燒灼感，呼吸困難，胸悶，噁心，嘔吐，眼淚鼻涕不止。在通氣不良環境中可致死。

cubital *adj.* relating to the elbow or forearm; for example the *cubital fossa* is the depression at the front of the elbow.

肘的 肘部的或前臂的。如肘窩即肘前部的凹陷處。

cuboid bone the outer bone of the *tarsus, which articulates with the fourth and fifth metatarsal bones in front and with the calcaneus (heel bone) behind.

骰骨 最外側的一塊跗骨。前與第四、第五蹠骨成關節，後與跟骨成關節。

cuirass *n. see* respirator.

護胸甲

culdoscope *n.* a tubular instrument with lenses and a light source, used for direct observation of the womb, ovaries, and Fallopian tubes (*culdoscopy*). The instrument is passed through the wall of the vagina behind to the neck of the womb. *See also* endoscope.

後穹窿鏡 直接檢查子宮、卵巢與輸卵管用的管狀器械。裝有透鏡和光源。本鏡通過子宮頸後部穿過陰道壁。

Culex *n.* a genus of mosquitoes, worldwide in distribution, of which there are some 600 species. Certain species are important as vectors of filariasis (*see also* Wuchereria) and viral encephalitis.

庫蚊屬 全球廣泛存在的蚊屬。約有600種。有幾種是絲蟲病與病毒性腦炎的傳播媒介，具有臨牀重要性。

culicide *n.* an agent that destroys mosquitoes or gnats.

殺蚊劑 殺滅蚊蚋的藥劑。

culmen *n.* an area of the upper surface of the *cerebellum, anterior to the declive and posterior to the central lobule and separated from them by deep fissures.

山頂 小腦頂部表面部分。位於小腦山坡前，中央小葉後，與兩者有深溝相隔。

culture 1. *n.* a population of microorganisms, usually bacteria, grown in a solid or liquid laboratory medium (*culture medium*), which is usually *agar, broth, or *gelatin. A *pure culture* consists of a single bacterial species. A *stab culture* is a bacterial culture growing in a plug of solid medium within a bottle (or tube); the medium is inoculated by 'stabbing' with a bacteria-coated straight wire. A *stock culture* is a permanent bacterial culture, from which subcultures are made. *See also* tissue culture. **2.** *vb.* to grow bacteria or other microorganisms in cultures.

①**培養物** 在固體或液體培養基中生長的微生物（通常是細菌）種羣。培養基多用瓊脂、肉湯或明膠製做。純培養物只含有一種細菌。針刺培養物是用染菌的直金屬絲刺入瓶（或試管）內的固體培養基中進行接種生長。存儲培養物是一種恒久細菌培養物，用以進行次代培養。 ②**培養** 使細菌或其他微生物在培養基內生長。

cumulative action the toxic effects of a drug produced by repeated administration of small doses at intervals that are not long enough for it to be either broken down or excreted by the body.

蓄積作用 重復用藥所產生的毒性作用。用藥後在藥物尚未分解或排出體外又重復用藥，雖然量小亦會產生毒性作用。

cumulus oophoricus a cluster of follicle cells that surround a freshly ovulated ovum. By increasing the effective size of the ovum they may assist its

卵丘 發育初期的卵細胞周圍的卵泡細胞羣。能使卵細胞有效體積增加，使之易於進入輸卵管，受精

entrance into the end of the Fallopian tube. They are dispersed at fertilization by the contents of the *acrosome.

時為精子頂體所含的酶溶解。

cuneiform bones three bones in the *tarsus – the *lateral* (external), *intermediate* (middle), and *medial* (internal) cuneiform bones – that articulate respectively with the first, second, and third metatarsal bones in front. All three bones articulate with the navicular bone behind.

楔骨 跗部的三塊骨頭。有外側楔骨、中間楔骨、內側楔骨，前與第一、第二、第三蹠骨成關節，後與舟狀骨成關節。

cuneus *n.* a wedge-shaped area of *cerebral cortex that forms the inner surface of the occipital lobe.

楔葉 大腦皮層中形成枕葉內表面的楔形部分。

Cuniculus *n.* a genus of large forest-dwelling rodents, the pacas or spotted cavies, found in South and Central America. In Brazil these animals are a natural reservoir of the parasite *Leishmania braziliensis*, which causes espundia (*see* leishmaniasis).

隧鼠屬 生活於森林中的大型嚙齒動物之一屬。如花斑豚鼠，見於中南美洲。在巴西係巴西利什曼原蟲的自然保蟲宿主，能引起鼻咽黏膜利什曼病。

cupola *n.* **1.** the small dome at the end of the cochlea. **2.** any of several dome-shaped anatomical structures.

頂 ①耳蝸末端的小圓頂。 ②任何穹窿狀的解剖結構。

cupping *n.* the former practice of applying a heated cup to the skin and allowing it to cool, which causes swelling of the tissues beneath and an increase in the flow of blood in the area. This was thought to draw out harmful excess blood from diseased organs nearby and so promote healing. In *wet cupping* the skin was previously cut, so that blood would actually flow into the cup and could be removed.

杯吸術 過去使用的一種治療方法。於杯中加熱置於皮膚上，冷却後即引起下面的皮膚組織腫脹充血。一般認為能吸出鄰近病變器官中過多的有害的血液，促進痊癒。濕杯吸術是事先將皮膚切開，血液確能流入杯內以去除之。

cupula *n.* a small dome-shaped structure consisting of sensory hairs embedded in gelatinous material, forming part of a *crista in the ampullae of the semicircular canals of the ear.

蝸頂 內耳壺腹嵴上的小圓頂樣結構。內含浸埋於膠樣物質中的感覺毛。

curare *n.* an extract from the bark of South American trees (*Strychnos* and *Chondodendron* species) that relaxes and paralyses voluntary muscle. Used for centuries as an arrow poison by South American Indians, curare was

箭毒鹼 自南美馬錢屬與剛多防已類樹皮獲取的浸出物。具有鬆弛與麻痹隨意肌的作用。數世紀來南美洲印第安人用做箭毒。在醫療上曾用以控制破傷

formerly employed to control the muscle spasms of tetanus and, more recently, as a muscle relaxant in surgical operations. It has now been replaced in surgery by *tubocurarine.

風時肌肉痙攣，後又在手術中用做肌鬆藥。但現已被筒箭毒所代替。

curettage (curettement) *n.* the scraping of the internal surface of an organ or body cavity by means of a spoon-shaped instrument (*curette*). Curettage is usually performed to remove diseased tissue or to obtain a specimen for diagnostic purposes. *See also* dilatation and curettage.

刮除術 用一種勺形器械（刮匙）刮擦器官或體內某個腔隙內表面的手術。多用於去除病變組織或取診斷標本。

curette *n.* a spoon-shaped instrument for scraping tissue from a cavity (*see* curettage).

刮匙 自腔隙內刮除組織用的匙形器械。

curie *n.* a former unit for expressing the activity of a radioactive substance. It has been replaced by the *becquerel. Symbol: Ci.

居里 過去使用的放射性物質的放射性單位。現已被貝可取代。符號：Ci。

Curschmann's spirals elongated *casts of the smaller bronchi, which are coughed up in bronchial asthma. They unroll to a length of 2 cm or more and have a central core ensheathed in mucus and cell debris.

庫施曼螺旋 支氣管哮喘時咳出的細支氣管管型。舖開總長約 2 cm 或更長些，核心部爲黏液與細胞碎片所包繞。

Cushing's syndrome the condition resulting from excess amounts of *corticosteroid hormones in the body. Symptoms include weight gain, reddening of the face and neck, excess growth of body and facial hair, raised blood pressure, loss of mineral from the bones (osteoporosis), raised blood glucose levels, and sometimes mental disturbances. The syndrome may be due to overstimulation of the adrenal glands by excessive amounts of the hormone ACTH, secreted either by a tumour of the pituitary gland (*Cushing's disease*) or by a malignant tumour in the lung or elsewhere. Other causes include a benign or malignant tumour of the adrenal gland(s) resulting in excess activity of the gland and prolonged therapy with high doses of corticosteroid drugs (such as prednisone).

庫興氏綜合徵 體內皮質醇類激素過多引起的疾病。症狀有體重增加，頸面部潮紅，體毛與鬍鬚過多，血壓升高，骨內礦物質脫失（骨質疏鬆病），血糖增多，有時有精神障礙。本病可能係大量的促皮質素對腎上腺刺激過强所致。腦垂體腺腫瘤（庫興氏病）或肺部等其他部位的腫瘤都會分泌大量的促皮質素。其他病因尚有腎上腺本身的可引起腺體活動增强的良性或惡性腫瘤，以及長期使用大劑量皮質醇類藥物（如潑尼松）治療等。

cusp *n.* **1.** any of the cone-shaped prominences on teeth, especially the molars and premolars. **2.** a pocket or fold of the membrane (endocardium) lining the heart or of the layer of the wall of a vein, several of which form a *valve. When the blood flows backwards the cusps fill up and become distended, so closing the valve.

牙尖 牙齒（尤指磨牙與前磨牙）上的圓錐形突起。 ②**瓣尖** 心內膜或靜脉壁內層形成的折疊物或小袋。集合構成瓣口。血液逆流充滿並擴張瓣尖，使瓣口關閉。

cutaneous *adj.* relating to the skin.

皮膚的

cuticle *n.* **1.** the *epidermis of the skin. **2.** a layer of solid or semisolid material that is secreted by and covers an *epithelium. **3.** a layer of cells, such as the outer layer of cells in a hair.

①**表皮** 皮膚的外表層。②**護膜** 由某種上皮細胞分泌出的固體層或半固體層。覆蓋於該細胞之上。③**角質層** 一層細胞。如毛髮細胞的外層。

cutis *n. see* skin.

皮膚

cyan- (cyano-) *prefix denoting* blue.

〔前綴〕 **青紫色，藍色**

cyanide *n.* any of the notoriously poisonous salts of hydrocyanic acid. Cyanides combine with and render inactive the enzymes of the tissues responsible for cellular respiration, and therefore they kill extremely quickly; unconsciousness is followed by convulsions and death. Hydrogen cyanide vapour is fatal in less than a minute when inhaled. Sodium or potassium cyanide taken by mouth may also kill within minutes. Prompt treatment with amyl nitrite and sodium thiosulphate or cobalt EDTA may save life. Cyanides give off a smell of bitter almonds.

氰化物 衆所周知的有毒的氫氰酸鹽類。氰化物與組織內的細胞呼吸酶相結合，抑制了酶的活性，因而迅速引起死亡。患者意識喪失，繼而驚厥、死亡。吸入氫氰酸蒸氣一分鐘內即死亡。口服氰化鉀或氰化鈉於幾分鐘內亦可致死。用亞硝酸異戊酯與硫代硫酸鈉或依地酸鈷及時治療或可挽救生命。氰化物具有苦杏仁氣味。

cyanocobalamin *n. see* vitamin B_{12}.

鈷氰胺 即維生素 B_{12}。

cyanopsia *n.* a condition in which everything looks bluish.

藍視症 視物皆呈藍色的一種病症。

cyanosis *n.* a bluish discoloration of the skin and mucous membranes resulting from an inadequate amount of oxygen in the blood. Cyanosis is associated with heart failure, lung diseases, the breathing of oxygen-deficient at-

紫紺 由於血氧供應不足而使皮膚、黏膜變藍的症狀。發生於心力衰竭、肺疾患、吸入含氧不足的空氣與窒息時，亦見於患先天性心臟病的青紫嬰兒。

mospheres, and asphyxia. Cyanosis is also seen in *blue babies, because of congenital heart defects. —**cyanotic** *adj.*

cybernetics *n.* the science of communication processes and automatic control systems in both machines and living things: a study linking the working of the brain and nervous system with the functioning of computers and automated feedback devices. *See also* bionics.

控制論 研究機械與生物體內信息傳遞過程與自動控制系統的科學。這門科學把腦及神經系統的活動與計算機及自動反饋裝置的功能聯繫起來。

cycl- (cyclo-) *prefix denoting* **1.** cycle or cyclic. **2.** the ciliary body. Example: *cyclectomy* (excision of).

〔前綴〕 ①**環** 圓形的。 ②**睫狀體** 如睫狀體切除術。

cyclamate *n.* either of two compounds, sodium or calcium cyclamate, that are thirty times as sweet as sugar and, unlike saccharin, stable to heat. Cyclamates were used as sweetening agents in the food industry until 1969, when their use was banned because they were suspected of causing cancer.

環己氨磺酸鹽 比糖甜 30 倍的兩種化合物：環己氨磺酸鈉或環己氨磺酸鈣。本品耐熱，這點與糖精不同。在 1969 年以前食品工業用做甜味劑，後因疑有致癌作用而禁用。

cyclandelate *n.* a *vasodilator drug used to improve circulation in cerebrovascular disease and other conditions in which blood flow is reduced. It is administered by mouth; side-effects are rare but high doses sometimes cause nausea, digestive upsets, and flushing. Trade name: **Cyclospasmol**.

環扁桃酯 血管擴張藥。用以改善腦血管疾病與其它供血不足性疾病的血液循環。口服。副作用少見。大劑量有時引起噁心、消化不良、顏面潮紅。商品名：安脉生。

cyclitis *n.* inflammation of the *ciliary body of the eye (*see* uveitis).

睫狀體炎

cyclizine *n.* a drug with *antihistamine properties, used to prevent and relieve nausea and vomiting in travel sickness, vertigo, disorders of the inner ear, and postoperative sickness. It is administered by mouth; common side-effects are drowsiness and dizziness. Trade names: **Marzine, Valoid**.

苯甲嗪 抗組胺藥。可防治噁心嘔吐。用於暈動病、暈眩、內耳疾患與術後嘔吐等。口服。常見副作用有嗜眠與頭昏。商品名：賽克利嗪。

cyclobarbitone *n.* a *barbiturate drug used as a hypnotic and sedative in cases of insomnia and anxiety. It is administered by mouth and prolonged use can

環巴比妥 巴比妥類催眠鎮靜藥。用於治療失眠與焦慮。口服。長期使用可產生賴藥性。

cause *dependence. Trade name: **Phanodorm**.

cyclodialysis *n.* an operation for *glaucoma in which part of the *ciliary body is separated from its attachment to the sclera, producing a cleft between the two. The aqueous humour comes into contact with the exposed surface of the ciliary body and some of it is absorbed from this surface. The pressure within the eye will be reduced if this absorption adds significantly to the drainage of fluid from the eye.

睫狀體分離術 治療青光眼的手術。將睫狀體部分與鞏膜分離，在二者之間留一裂隙，使房水得以與暴露出來的睫狀體表面相接觸，部分房水則可由此處吸收。如果引流效果顯著，可減低眼壓。

cyclomethycaine *n.* a local anaesthetic applied to the skin in solution to relieve discomfort in cuts, abrasions, and minor skin irritations. It sometimes causes skin sensitivity reactions.

環甲卡因 局麻藥。製成溶液供皮膚外用。可用於割傷、擦傷與輕癢。本藥有時可引起皮膚過敏反應。

cyclopentamine *n.* a drug that constricts small blood vessels and raises blood pressure (*see* sympathomimetic). It is administered by injection to maintain blood pressure during surgery and is also used in nasal decongestants. Large doses sometimes cause giddiness, headache, nausea, and vomiting.

環戊丙甲胺 血管收縮藥。能升高血壓，注射劑用於手術中維持血壓。亦用以滴鼻以減輕鼻黏膜充血。大劑量有時引起頭暈、頭痛、噁心與嘔吐。

cyclopenthiazide *n.* a *diuretic used to treat fluid retention (oedema), high blood pressure (hypertension), and heart failure. It is administered by mouth and may cause skin sensitivity reactions, nausea, constipation, diarrhoea, and reduced blood potassium levels. Trade name: **Navidrex**.

環戊氯噻嗪 利尿藥。用以治療水腫、高血壓、心力衰竭。口服。可引起皮膚過敏反應、噁心、嘔吐、便秘、腹瀉與低血鉀。

cyclopentolate *n.* a drug, similar to *atropine, that is used in eye drops to paralyse the ciliary muscles and dilate the pupil for eye examinations and to treat some types of eye inflammation. Trade names: **Mydrilate**, **Cyclopentolate Hydrochloride Minims**.

環戊醇胺酯 散瞳藥。作用與阿托品類似，點眼時可麻痹睫狀肌。用於檢查眼底與治療某些眼部炎症。商品名：環戊通。

cyclophoria *n.* a type of squint (*see* strabismus) in which the eye, when covered, tends to rotate slightly clockwise or anticlockwise.

旋轉隱斜視 斜視的一種類型。眼球被遮蓋時輕度沿順行鐘或逆時鐘方向轉動。

cyclophosphamide *n.* a drug used to treat some cancers, often in combination with other *cytotoxic drugs. It also has *immunosuppressive properties and is used in prolonging the survival of tissue transplants and in other conditions requiring reduced immune response. Cyclophosphamide is administered by mouth or by injection; common side-effects are nausea, vomiting, and – particularly at high doses – hair loss. Trade name: **Endoxana**.

環磷醯胺 抗腫瘤藥。常與其他細胞毒類藥物併用。本品同時有免疫抑制作用，可用於延長移植組織的壽命及其他需要減輕免疫反應的疾病。口服或注射。常見副作用有噁心、嘔吐，大劑量可引起脫髮。商品名：安道生。

cycloplegia *n.* paralysis of the ciliary muscle of the eye (*see* ciliary body). This causes inability to alter the focus of the eye and is usually accompanied by paralysis of the muscles of the pupil, resulting in fixed dilation of the pupil (*mydriasis*). It is induced by the use of atropine or similar drugs in order to rest the muscle in cases of inflammation of the iris and ciliary body. It may also occur after injuries to the eye.

睫狀肌麻痺 眼內睫狀肌發生麻痺的現象。此時眼調節焦距的能力喪失。常伴有瞳孔肌麻痺，使瞳孔固定於擴張狀態。患虹膜睫狀體炎時爲了使瞳孔肌休息，可用阿托品類藥物引起。睫狀肌麻痺亦可由眼外傷引起。

cyclopropane *n.* a general *anaesthetic, administered by inhalation for all types of surgical operation. It can cause postoperative nausea, vomiting, and headache.

環丙烷 全身麻醉藥。在各種手術中供吸入用。手術後可有噁心、嘔吐與頭痛。

cycloserine *n.* an *antibiotic, active against a wide range of bacteria, used as supporting treatment in tuberculosis and in some infections of the urinary tract. It is administered by mouth; side-effects, which can be severe, include dizziness, drowsiness, convulsions, and mental confusion.

環絲氨酸 廣譜抗生素。治療結核病的輔助藥品。亦用於治療某些泌尿道感染。口服。副作用有時很嚴重，包括頭暈、嗜眠、驚厥與精神錯亂等。

cyclosporin A a drug that suppresses the immune system and is administered to prevent and treat rejection of a transplanted organ or bone marrow.

環孢菌素 A 免疫抑制藥。用於防治移植器官與骨髓引起的排異反應。

cyclothymia *n.* the occurrence of marked swings of mood from cheerfulness to misery. These fluctuations are not as great as those of *manic-depressive psychosis. They usually represent a

循環情感性氣質 情緒在快樂與憂愁之間發生明顯的交替性變化。這種波動不像燥狂抑鬱性精神病那樣明顯，通常僅是變態人

personality disorder, for which *psychotherapy is sometimes helpful.

格的一種表現，進行心理治療有時奏效。

cyclotron *n.* a machine in which charged particles following a spiral path within a magnetic field are accelerated by an alternating electric field. It produces electromagnetic radiation, which has been used in the treatment of certain cancers.

迴旋加速器 通過交替改變電場的方法使帶電粒子在磁場中沿螺旋路線加速前進的裝置。這種加速器可產生電磁輻射，用以治療某些癌症。

cyesis *n. see* pregnancy.

妊娠

cyn- (cyno-) *prefix denoting* a dog or dogs. Example: *cynophobia* (morbid fear of).

〔前綴〕 **犬** 如犬恐怖（對狗發生的一種病態的恐懼）。

cyproheptadine *n.* a potent *antihistamine administered by mouth to treat allergies and itching skin conditions; it is also used to stimulate the appetite. Drowsiness is a common side-effect. Trade name: **Periactin**.

賽庚啶 高效抗組胺藥。口服。用以治療變態反應與皮膚瘙癢性疾患。亦用以刺激食慾。常見副作用有嗜眠。

cyproterone *n.* a steroid drug that inhibits the effects of male sex hormones (androgens) and is used to treat various sexual disorders in men. It is administered by mouth and common side-effects include tiredness, loss of strength, inhibition of sperm formation, infertility, and breast enlargement (gynaecomastia).

去乙醯環丙氯地孕酮 一種具有抑制雄激素效果的固醇類藥。用以治療各種男子性功能障礙。口服。常見副作用有怠倦、無力、精子發育障礙、男子不育與乳房增大（男子女性型乳房）。

cyrtometer *n.* a device for measuring the shape of the chest and its movements during breathing.

胸圍計 一種測量胸圍形狀及其呼吸時運動的器械。

cyst *n.* **1.** an abnormal sac or closed cavity lined with *epithelium and filled with liquid or semisolid matter. There are many varieties of cysts occurring in different parts of the body. *Retention cysts* arise when the outlet of a glandular duct is blocked, as in *sebaceous cysts. Some cysts are congenital, due to abnormal embryonic development; for example, *dermoid cysts. Others are tumours containing cells that secrete mucus or other substances, and another type of cyst is formed by parasites in the body (*see* hydatid cyst). Cysts may

①**囊腫** 襯以上皮組織並充滿液體或半液狀物質的囊袋或封閉的腔隙。在體內不同部分會發生許多種不同的囊腫。瀦留囊腫發生於腺管出口阻塞時，如皮脂囊腫。有些囊腫是先天性的，由胚胎期發育異常引起，如皮樣囊腫。有些囊腫是腫瘤內含有分泌粘液或其他物質的細胞所致，有些是體內寄生蟲產生的包囊。口腔內亦會出現囊腫，如牙尖處的牙囊

occur in the jaws: a *dental cyst* occurs at the apex of a tooth, a *dentigerous cyst* occurs around the crown of an unerupted tooth, and an *eruption cyst* forms over an erupting tooth. *See also* ovarian cyst. **2.** a dormant stage produced during the life cycle of certain protozoan parasites of the alimentary canal, including **Giardia* and **Entamoeba*. Cysts, passed out in the faeces, have tough outer coats that protect the parasites from unfavourable conditions. The parasites emerge from their cysts when they are eaten by a new host. **3.** a structure formed by and surrounding the larvae of certain parasitic worms.

腫，未萌出牙的牙冠周圍的含牙囊腫，萌生牙上方的萌牙囊腫。 ②**包囊期** 消化道內某些寄生原蟲（如賈第蟲屬與阿米巴屬）生活周期中的休眠階段。由糞便排出的包囊有一層堅韌的外殼，以保護寄生蟲能在不利的環境中生存。被新的宿主食入後，寄生蟲又自包囊中脫出。 ③**包囊** 在某些寄生蟲周圍形成的包膜。

cyst- (cysto-) *prefix denoting* **1.** a bladder, especially the urinary bladder. Example: *cystoplasty* (plastic surgery of). **2.** a cyst.

〔前綴〕 ①**膀胱** 如膀胱成形術。 ②**囊**

cystadenoma *n.* an *adenoma showing a cystic structure.

囊腺瘤 具有囊樣結構的腺瘤。

cystalgia *n.* pain in the urinary bladder. This is common in *cystitis and when there are stones in the bladder and is occasionally present in bladder cancer. Treatment is directed to the underlying cause.

膀胱痛 產生於膀胱部位的疼痛。常見於膀胱炎與膀胱結石。偶見於膀胱癌。治療：針對病因。

cystectomy *n.* surgical removal of the urinary bladder. This is necessary in the treatment of certain bladder conditions, notably cancer. The ureters draining the urine from the kidneys are reimplanted into the colon (*see* ureterosigmoidostomy) or into an isolated segment of intestine (usually the ileus), which is brought to the skin surface as a spout (*see* ileal conduit).

膀胱切除術 對膀胱行外科切除的手術。在某些膀胱疾患，特別是膀胱癌時必須施行。輸尿管可移植於結腸上，或移植於切除的一段小腸（多爲回腸）上，再由皮膚表面開口排出尿液。

cysteine *n.* a sulphur-containing *amino acid that is an important constituent of many enzymes. The disulphide (S–S) links between adjacent cysteine molecules in polypeptide chains contribute to the three-dimensional molecular structure of proteins.

半胱氨酸 一種含硫氨基酸。係多種酶的重要組成成分。多肽鏈中兩個相鄰半胱氨酸分子間的二硫鍵構成了蛋白質的立體分子結構。

cystic *adj.* **1.** of, relating to, or characterized by cysts. **2.** of or relating to the gall bladder or urinary bladder.

①囊的，包囊的 ②膽囊的 ③膀胱的

cystic duct *see* bile duct.

膽囊管

cysticercosis *n.* a disease caused by the presence of tapeworm larvae (*see* cysticercus) of the species **Taenia solеum* in any of the body tissues. Man becomes infected on ingesting tapeworm eggs in contaminated food or drink. The presence of cysticerci in the muscles causes pain and weakness; in the brain the symptoms are more serious, including mental deterioration, paralysis, giddiness, epileptic attacks, and convulsions, which may be fatal. There is no specific treatment for this cosmopolitan disease although surgical removal of cysticerci may be necessary to relieve pressure on the brain.

囊尾蚴病 有鈎絛蟲的幼蟲存在於人體組織中所引起的疾病。人類因食入被蟲卵汚染的飲食而感染。肌肉內的囊尾蚴引起疼痛與無力，腦內者則引起較嚴重的症狀，有智力衰退、痲痹、癲癇和驚厥，可致死。雖然爲了減低顱內壓可能必須將囊尾蚴切除，但對此世界性疾病尚無特效療法。

cysticercus (bladderworm) *n.* a larval stage of some *tapeworms in which the scolex and neck are invaginated into a large fluid-filled cyst. The cysts develop in the muscles or brain of the host following ingestion of tapeworm eggs. *See* cysticercosis.

囊尾蚴 某類絛蟲的幼蟲期。幼蟲的頭節與頸節反折入一個大的充滿液體的包囊內。宿主食入蟲卵後包囊在肌肉或腦內生長。

cystic fibrosis (fibrocystic disease of the pancreas, mucoviscidosis) a hereditary disease affecting the exocrine glands (including mucus-secreting glands, sweat glands, and others). The abnormality results in the production of thick mucus, which obstructs the intestinal glands (causing meconium *ileus in newborn babies), pancreas (causing deficiency of pancreatic enzymes), and bronchi (causing *bronchiectasis). Respiratory infections, which may be severe, are a common complication. The sweat contains excessive amounts of sodium and chloride, which is an aid to diagnosis. Treatment consists of minimizing the effect of the disease by administration of pancreatic enzymes and bronchial physiotherapy and by preventing and combating secondary infection.

囊腫性纖維變性（胰纖維性囊腫病，胰管黏稠物阻塞症） 外分泌腺（包括黏液腺、汗腺及其它）產生病變的一種遺傳性疾病。本病產生黏稠的液體，阻塞腸腺引起新生兒胎糞性腸梗塞，阻塞胰腺引起胰酶缺乏症，阻塞支氣管引起支氣管擴張。呼吸道感染是常見的併發症，可能十分嚴重。汗腺內含有大量氯化鈉，此點有助於診斷。治療僅限於對症：口服胰酶，支氣管理療，防治繼發感染。

cystine *n. see* amino acid.

胱氨酸

cystinosis *n.* an inborn defect in the absorption and metabolism of amino acids, leading to abnormal accumulation of the amino acid cystine in the blood, kidneys, and lymphatic system. Excess excretion of cystine in the urine (*cystinuria*) leads to the formation of cystine stones in the kidneys. *See also* Fanconi syndrome.

胱氨酸病 由於氨基酸吸收與代謝障礙引起血、腎與淋巴系統中胱氨酸大量積聚的先天性疾病。尿中胱氨酸過多（胱氨酸尿）可於腎中產生胱氨酸結石。

cystinuria *n. see* cystinosis.

胱氨酸尿

cystitis *n.* inflammation of the urinary bladder, often caused by infection (most commonly by the bacterium *Escherichia coli*). It is usually accompanied by the desire to pass urine frequently, with a degree of burning. More severe attacks are often associated with the painful passage of blood in the urine, accompanied by a cramplike pain in the lower abdomen persisting after the bladder has been emptied. An acute attack is treated by antibiotic administration and a copious fluid intake.

膀胱炎 主要由埃舍利希氏桿菌感染引起的膀胱炎症。常有尿頻，排尿時有一定程度的燒灼感。嚴重時有痛性血尿，膀胱排空後下腹部仍有持續性絞痛。急性發作期用抗生素治療，並大量飲水。

cystitome *n.* a small knife with a tiny curved or hooked blade, used to cut the lens capsule in the type of operation for cataract in which the capsule is left behind (*extracapsular cataract extraction*). *See also* capsulotomy.

晶狀體囊刀 帶有微小彎曲或鈎形刀口的微型手術刀。在晶狀體囊外切除術（保留晶狀體囊）中用以切開晶狀體囊。

cystocele *n.* prolapse of the base of the bladder in women. It is usually due to weakness of the pelvic floor after childbirth and causes bulging of the anterior wall of the vagina on straining. When accompanied by stress incontinence of urine, surgical repair (anterior *colporrhaphy) is indicated.

膀胱突出 女性膀胱基底部脫垂。通常由於產後骨盆底鬆弛導致陰道前壁於用力時向前膨出。如有嚴重尿失禁可行手術修復。

cystography *n.* X-ray examination of the urinary bladder after the injection of a contrast medium. The X-ray photographs or films thus obtained are known as *cystograms*. Cystography is most commonly performed to detect reflux of urine from the bladder to the

膀胱造影術 於注射造影劑後對膀胱進行X線檢查的方法。用此法拍下的照片稱爲膀胱X線照片。多用於檢查尿液自膀胱向輸尿管返流的病變（主要是兒童）。如果是

ureters, usually in children (*see* vesicoureteric reflux). If films are taken during voiding then the ureters can also be observed (*see* urethrography).

在膀胱排空時拍片則輸尿管亦可顯影。

cystolithiasis *n.* the presence of stones (calculi) in the urinary bladder. The stones are either formed in the bladder, due to obstruction, urinary retention, and infection (*primary calculi*), or pass to the bladder after being formed in the kidneys (*secondary calculi*). They cause pain, the passage of bloody urine, and interruption of the urinary stream and should be removed surgically. *See* calculus.

膀胱結石病 膀胱內出現結石。由於梗阻、尿潴留、感染，結石可能在膀胱內形成（原發性結石），也可能在腎內形成然後排入膀胱（繼發性結石），可引起疼痛、血尿與排尿障礙，應行手術摘除。

cystometer *n.* an apparatus for measuring pressure within the bladder. Modern investigations also include measurement of urine flow, and the resultant bladder pressure/flow study (*urodynamic investigation*) provides useful information regarding bladder function.

膀胱內壓測量器 一種用於測量膀胱內壓力的器械。現代技術尚包括尿流量測定。膀胱內壓力/流量研究（尿流動力學）結果能提供有關膀胱功能的重要資料。

cystopexy (vesicofixation) *n.* a surgical operation to fix the urinary bladder (or a portion of it) in a different position. It may be performed as part of the repair or correction of a prolapsed bladder.

膀胱固定術 將膀胱（或其一部分）固定在另一部位上的手術。本術亦是脫垂膀胱修復術的一部分。

cystosarcoma phylloides a malignant tumour of the connective tissue of the breast: it accounts for approximately 1% of all breast cancers. Such tumours may show a wide variation in cell structure. The best treatment for a localized tumour is simple *mastectomy.

葉狀囊性肉瘤 乳房的惡性結締組織腫瘤。約佔乳腺全部惡性腫瘤的1%。有多種不同的細胞結構。對局限性腫瘤的首選療法是單做乳房切除術。

cystoscopy *n.* examination of the bladder by means of an instrument (*cystoscope*) inserted via the urethra. The cystoscope consists of a metal sheath surrounding a telescope and light-conducting bundles. Irrigating fluid is conducted via the sheath into the bladder and additional channels are available for the catheters to be inserted into the ureters, diathermy electrodes

膀胱鏡檢查 用膀胱鏡插入尿道檢查膀胱的方法。膀胱鏡由望遠鏡與光導纖維束構成，外罩一層金屬套管。灌洗液自金屬套管中注入，其他通道用以向尿道中插入導管，去除息肉用的透熱電極和取腫瘤或其他新生物用的活體組織鉗等。

for removing polyps, etc., or biopsy forceps for taking specimens of tumours or other growths.

cystostomy *n.* the operation of creating an artificial opening between the bladder and the anterior abdominal wall. This provides a temporary or permanent drainage route for urine.

膀胱造口術 在前腹壁與膀胱之間做人工造口的手術。可對尿液行長期或暫時引流。

cystotomy *n.* surgical incision into the urinary bladder, usually by cutting through the abdominal wall above the pubic symphysis (*suprapubic cystotomy*). This is necessary for such operations as removing stones or tumours from the bladder and for gaining access to the prostate gland in the operation of transvesical *prostatectomy.

膀胱切開術 切開膀胱的手術。常用的術式是在恥骨聯合上方的腹壁切開。在摘除膀胱腫瘤與結石時，以及在經膀胱前列腺切除術中，爲了達到前列腺，均必需施行此手術。

cyt- (cyto-) *prefix denoting* **1.** cell(s). **2.** cytoplasm.

〔前綴〕 **①細胞 ②細胞質**

cytarabine *n.* a *cytotoxic drug used to suppress the symptoms of some types of leukaemia. It is administered by injection and can damage the bone marrow, leading to various blood cell disorders. Other side-effects are nausea, vomiting, mouth ulcers, and diarrhoea. Trade name: **Cytosar**.

阿糖胞苷 可減輕某些類型的白血病症狀的細胞毒藥。注射用。可損害骨髓，引起各種血細胞病變。其他副作用有噁心、嘔吐、口腔潰瘍與腹瀉。

-cyte *suffix denoting* a cell. Examples: *chondrocyte* (cartilage cell); *osteocyte* (bone cell).

〔後綴〕 **細胞** 如軟骨細胞，骨細胞。

cytidine *n.* a compound containing cytosine and the sugar ribose. *See also* nucleoside.

胞嘧啶核苷 胞嘧啶與核糖組成的化合物。

cytochemistry *n.* the study of chemical compounds and their activities in living cells.

細胞化學 研究活細胞的化學組成及其活動的學科。

cytochrome *n.* a compound consisting of a protein linked to *haem. Cytochromes act as electron transfer agents in biological oxidation-reduction reactions, particularly those associated with the mitochondria in cellular respiration. *See* electron transport chain.

細胞色素 含有血色素蛋白質的一種化合物。細胞色素是生物氧化還原反應中的電子傳遞體，與細胞呼吸中的線粒體關係尤爲密切。

cytogenetics *n.* a science that links the study of inheritance (genetics) with that of cells (cytology); it is concerned mainly with the study of the *chromosomes, especially their origin, structure, and functions.

細胞遺傳學 一門把細胞學與遺傳學結合起來的科學。主要研究染色體及其來源、結構及功能等。

cytokinesis *n.* division of the cytoplasm of a cell, which occurs at the end of cell division, after division of the nucleus, to form two daughter cells. *Compare* karyokinesis.

胞質分裂 在細胞分裂末期，細胞核分裂以後發生的細胞質分裂的現象。由此分成兩個子細胞。

cytology *n.* the study of the structure and function of cells. The examination of cells under a microscope is used in the diagnosis of various diseases, e.g. cancer (*see* cervical smear). *See also* biopsy. **—cytological** *adj.*

細胞學 研究細胞的構造與功能的科學。顯微鏡下細胞學檢查用於診斷多種疾病，如癌。

cytolysis *n.* the breakdown of cells, particularly by destruction of their outer membranes.

細胞溶解 細胞的分解。特別是由於破壞了細胞的外膜引起的分解。

cytomegalovirus (CMV) *n.* a member of the herpes group of viruses (*see* herpesvirus). It commonly occurs in man and normally produces symptoms milder than the common cold. However, in individuals whose immune systems are disturbed (e.g. by cancer) it can cause more severe effects, and it has been found to be the cause of congenital handicap in infants born to women who have contracted the virus during pregnancy.

巨細胞病毒 疱疹病毒屬中的一種。常侵犯人類，但引起的症狀比感冒還輕。在免疫力低下的患者（如癌症）則可能出現嚴重症狀。現已發現婦女妊娠期感染本病毒者會分娩出先天畸形的胎兒。

cytometer *n.* an instrument for determining the number of cells in a given quantity of fluid, such as blood, cerebrospinal fluid, or urine. *See* haemocytometer.

血細胞計數器 計算在一定量的液體（如血、腦脊液、尿）中細胞數的儀器。

cytomorphosis *n.* the changes undergone by a cell in the course of its life cycle.

細胞變形 細胞在其生活周期的過程中所發生的形態變化。

cytopenia *n.* a deficiency of one or more of the various types of blood cells. *See* eosinopenia, erythropenia, lymphopenia, neutropenia, pancytopenia, thrombocytopenia.

血細胞減少症 一種或多種血細胞減少。

cytophotometry *n.* the study of chemical compounds in living cells by means of a *cytophotometer*, an instrument that measures light intensity through stained areas of cytoplasm.

細胞光度測定法 一種使用細胞光度計測定活細胞中化學成分的方法。這種儀器可測定細胞漿染色區域的透光度。

cytoplasm *n.* the jelly-like substance that surrounds the nucleus of a cell. *See also* ectoplasm, endoplasm, protoplasm. **—cytoplasmic** *adj.*

細胞漿 細胞核周圍的膠凍樣物質。

cytoplasmic inheritance the inheritance of characters controlled by factors present in the cell cytoplasm rather than by genes on the chromosomes in the cell nucleus. Cytoplasmic inheritance is known to occur in lower animals and in plants but has not so far been found in man.

細胞質遺傳 由細胞質的因素而非細胞核染色體上的基因所控制的某種特徵的遺傳。僅見於低等動物與植物，至今仍未在人類中發現。

cytosine *n.* one of the nitrogen-containing bases (*see* pyrimidine) that occurs in the nucleic acid DNA.

胞嘧啶 存在於脫氧核糖核酸中的一種含氮鹼基。

cytosome *n.* the part of a cell that is outside the nucleus.

細胞質體 細胞核以外的部分。

cytotoxic drug a drug that damages or destroys cells and is used to treat various types of cancer, with or without the use of *radiotherapy. Examples are *cyclophosphamide, *cytarabine, and *mustine; they offer successful treatment in some conditions and help reduce symptoms and prolong life in others. Cytotoxic drugs destroy cancer cells by inhibiting cell division (i.e. they are *antimitotic*) but they also affect normal cells, particularly in bone marrow, skin, stomach lining, and fetal tissue, and dosage must be carefully controlled. *See also* antimetabolite.

細胞毒類藥 一種對細胞有損傷與破壞作用的藥物。用以治療各類癌症。可與放射療法合併使用，亦可單獨使用。如環磷醯胺、阿糖胞苷、氮芥等。它們對某些癌症療效顯著，對其它亦能減輕症狀或延長壽命。細胞毒類藥物是通過抑制細胞分裂（抗有絲分裂）而產生抗癌作用的，因此對正常細胞，尤其是骨髓、皮膚、胃黏膜與胎兒組織亦有影響。劑量需小心控制。

cytotrophoblast *n.* the part of a *trophoblast that retains its cellular structure and does not invade the maternal tissues. It forms the outer surface of the *chorion.

細胞滋養層 滋養層中仍保持本身細胞結構的部分。它不侵入母體組織，而構成絨毛膜的外表面。

D

dacry- (dacryo-) *prefix denoting* **1.** tears. **2.** the lacrimal apparatus.
〔前綴〕 ①淚液 ②淚器

dacryoadenitis *n.* inflammation of the tear-producing gland (*see* lacrimal apparatus). It usually occurs only in people who are in generally poor health.
淚腺炎 產生淚液的腺體的炎症。通常僅見於健康不良者。

dacryocystitis *n.* inflammation of the lacrimal sac (in which tears collect), usually occurring when the duct draining the tears into the nose is blocked (*see* lacrimal apparatus).
淚囊炎 淚囊（收集淚液的裝置）的炎症。通常發生於引流淚液入鼻腔的導管阻塞時。

dacryocystorhinostomy *n.* an operation to relieve blockage of the nasolacrimal duct (which drains tears into the nose), in which a communication is made between the lacrimal sac and the nose by removing the intervening bone. *See* dacryocystitis, lacrimal apparatus.
淚囊鼻腔造口術 一種通過切除中間的骨塊，使淚囊與鼻腔溝通，從而解除鼻淚管（引流淚液入鼻腔的導管）阻塞的手術。

dacryops *n. Obsolete.* a watering eye.
淚眼

dactyl- *prefix denoting* the digits (fingers or toes). Examples: *dactylomegaly* (abnormal size of); *dactylospasm* (painful contraction of).
〔前綴〕 **指，趾** 例如：指、趾巨大（指、趾大小異常），指趾痙攣（指、趾疼痛性收縮）。

dactylitis *n.* inflammation of a finger or toe caused by bone infection (as in tuberculous *osteomyelitis) or rheumatic disease.
指（趾）炎 由骨感染（如結核性骨髓炎）或風濕病引起的指或趾的炎症。

dactylology *n.* the representation of speech by finger movements: deaf and dumb language.
手語 藉手指的動作表達語言，聾啞人語言。

Daltonism (protanopia) *n.* red-blindness: a defect in colour vision in which a person cannot distinguish between reds and greens. The term has been used to refer to *colour blindness in general.
色盲（紅色盲） 一種色覺缺陷。患者不能區別紅色與綠色。本詞過去一直用以泛指色盲。

damp *n.* (in mining) any gas encountered underground other than air. *See* blackdamp, firedamp.
礦內毒氣 地下（礦內）遇到的空氣以外的任何氣體。

D and C *see* dilatation and curettage.

擴張術和刮除術（D 和 C）

dandruff (scurf) *n.* a common condition in which the scalp is covered with small flakes of dead skin. The flakes, which come away when the hair is brushed or combed, represent an increase in the normal loss of the outermost skin layer. Some types of dandruff are accompanied by inflammation of the scalp to give a type of seborrhoeic dermatitis (*see* eczema). If too little sebum is produced the hair becomes dry and brittle, with the formation of white skin flakes; too much sebum gives greasy hair and yellow flakes. Treatment is by regular washing with a detergent shampoo. Medical name: **pityriasis capitis.**

頭皮屑　頭皮上覆蓋着的死亡的皮膚鱗片。此係常見現象。梳頭時有頭皮屑掉落，表示皮膚最外層的正常耗損有所增加。某些類型的頭皮脫屑同時伴有頭皮炎症，係脂溢性皮炎的表現。如果皮脂產生過少，頭髮變得乾而脆，同時形成白色皮屑；皮脂過多，則頭髮油潤並有黃色皮屑。治療：定時用洗髮精洗頭。

dangerous drugs *see* Misuse of Drugs Act (1971).

危險藥物

danthron *n.* a *laxative administered by mouth; it sometimes colours the urine pink or red.

二羥蒽醌　口服緩瀉劑。有時可使尿染成粉紅色或紅色。

dapsone *n.* a drug (*see* sulphone) used to treat leprosy and some types of dermatitis. It is administered by mouth or injection; the commonest side-effects are allergic skin reactions.

氨苯砜　治療麻瘋和某些類型皮炎的藥物。口服或注射。最常見的副作用爲皮膚變應性反應。

dark adaptation the changes that take place in the retina and pupil of the eye enabling vision in very dim light. Dark adaptation involves activation of the *rods – the cells of the retina that function best in dim light – and the reflex enlargement of the pupil (*see* pupillary reflex). *Compare* light adaptation.

暗適應　眼睛的視網膜和瞳孔在極弱光下爲了視物所發生的變化。暗視應包括視桿細胞（一種在弱光下發揮最佳功能的視網膜細胞）的激活以及瞳孔的反射性開大。

day blindness comparatively good vision in poor light but poor vision in good illumination. The condition is usually congenital and associated with poor *visual acuity and defective colour vision. Acquired cases occur when the *cones (light-sensitive cells) at the

晝盲　在弱光下視力尚好而在良好照明下視力反而差的現像。此症通常爲先天性，伴有視敏度差和色覺缺陷。患病時如果視網膜後部的視錐細胞（一種對光敏感的細胞）遭到選

back of the retina are selectively destroyed by disease. Medical name: **hemeralopia**. *Compare* night blindness.

擇性破壞，則可發生獲得性晝盲。

day hospital a hospital in which patients spend a substantial part of the day under medical supervision but do not stay overnight. Day hospitals are mainly used for the treatment of elderly patients and those with mental disorders.

晝間醫院 一種患者白天大部分時間在院接受醫護觀察而晚間不過夜的醫院。晝間醫院主要爲老年患者和精神病患者服務。

DDT (chlorophenothane, dicophane) *n.* a powerful insecticide that has been in wide use for many years against lice, fleas, flies, bed bugs, cockroaches, and other disease-carrying and destructive insects. It is a relatively stable compound that is stored in animal fats, and the quantities now present in the environment – in the form of stores accumulated in animal tissues – raise the question of possible harmful effects on the body. Acute poisoning, from swallowing more than 20 g, produces nervous irritability, muscle twitching, convulsions, and coma, but only a few fatalities have been reported.

二二三（滴滴涕，氯苯乙烷） 强有力的殺蟲劑，曾多年廣泛用於殺滅蝨子、跳蚤、蒼蠅、臭蟲、蟑螂及其他傳播疾病和有害的昆蟲。爲相對穩定的化合物，可在動物脂肪內蓄積。現時由於在環境中（以在動物組織中蓄積的形式）大量存在，從而產生了可能對人體有害的問題。吞入二二三20g 以上引起急性中毒，出現神經興奮性過高、肌肉顫搐、驚厥以及昏迷，但報告死亡者不多。

de- *prefix denoting* **1.** removal or loss. Examples: *demineralization* (of minerals from bones or teeth); *devascularization* (of blood supply). **2.** reversal.

〔前綴〕 ①**脫，去** 除去或丟失。例如脫礦質作用（骨或牙失去礦物質），血供阻斷（失去血液供應）。 ②**逆轉，反向**

deafness *n.* partial or total loss of hearing in one or both ears. *Conductive deafness* is due to a defect in the conduction of sound from the external ear to the internal ear, most commonly an infection affecting the small bones in the middle ear (*otitis media) but also caused by an abnormal condition of the inner ear (*see* otosclerosis) that affects the conduction of sound. *Perceptive deafness* is due to a lesion of the *cochlea in the inner ear, the auditory nerve, or the auditory centres in the brain. It may be present from birth (for example if the mother was affected with

聾 一耳或雙耳完全或部分喪失聽力。由於聲音從外耳向內耳傳導障礙所致的聾稱爲傳導性聾，其最常見的原因爲感染波及中耳聽小骨（中耳炎），也可以是內耳病變影響聲音傳導。由於內耳的耳蝸、聽神經或腦內的聽中樞的損害所致的聾稱爲感音性聾，此種聾可以與生俱來（如母親在妊娠期患過風疹）；成人發生的原因爲損傷、疾病（梅尼爾氏病）或長時間受强烈噪聲

German measles during pregnancy). In adults it may be brought on by injury, disease (e.g. *Ménière's disease), or prolonged exposure to loud noises; progressive perceptive deafness (*presbyacusis*) is common with advancing age. The type of deafness can be diagnosed by various hearing tests (*see* Rinne's test, Weber's test), and the treatment depends on the cause. *See also* hearing aid.

影響。進行性感音性聾常發生於老年期（老年性聾）。聾的類型可用各種聽力試驗予以診斷。根據致聾原因採取相應治療措施。

deamination *n.* a process, occurring in the liver, that occurs during the metabolism of amino acids. The amino group ($-NH_2$) is removed from an amino acid and converted to ammonia, which is ultimately converted to *urea and excreted.

脫氨基作用 在肝內氨基酸代謝中發生的過程。氨基酸上的氨基（$-NH_2$）被移除而變爲氨，後者最終變爲尿素而被排出。

death *n.* absence of vital functions. Medically, death used to be defined as permanent cessation of the heart beat. More recently emphasis has switched to *brain death*, defined as permanent functional death of the centres in the brainstem that control the breathing, pupillary, and other vital reflexes. Usually two independent medical opinions are required before brain death is agreed, but organs such as kidneys may then legally be removed for transplantation surgery before the heart has stopped.

死亡 生命機能的喪失。醫學上，死亡過去定義爲心跳永久停止。晚近轉而强調所謂腦死亡。其定義爲腦幹內控制呼吸、瞳孔及其它生命重要反射中樞的永久性機能喪失。通常需要兩分獨立進行的醫學鑑定才能確定爲腦死亡；此時即使心跳尚未停止，取下腎臟之類的器官用於移植外科，在法律上是許可的。

death certificate a medical certificate stating the cause of a person's death, usually also stating the deceased's marital status, occupation, and age. A doctor's diagnosis of the main cause of death, and any contributory causes of death, and his signature are registered in Great Britain at Somerset House. Death certificates are required by law in the majority of countries throughout the world.

死亡證書 記述個體死亡原因，通常還包括死者婚姻狀況、職業和年齡的醫學證書。在英國，醫生對死亡的主要原因以及與死亡有關的任何原因所作的診斷及其簽名，須在薩默塞特院登記備案。全世界多數國家法律對死亡證書有所規定。

debridement *n.* the process of cleaning an open wound by removal of foreign material and dead tissue, so that healing may occur without hindrance.

清創術 清除開放性傷口內的異物和壞死組織的過程。目的是使傷口順利癒合。

debrisoquine *n.* a potent drug used to treat high blood pressure (hypertension). It is administered by mouth; common side-effects are nausea, headache, sweating, and general malaise. Trade name: **Declinax**.

異喹胍 用於高血壓的强效藥物。口服。常見副作用爲噁心、頭痛、出汗、全身不適。

dec- (deca-) *prefix denoting* ten.

〔前綴〕 **十，癸**

Decadron *n. see* dexamethasone.

地塞米松

decalcification *n.* loss or removal of calcium salts from a bone or tooth.

脫鈣 骨或牙內鈣鹽的丟失或移除。

decapitation *n.* removal of the head, usually the head of a dead fetus to enable delivery to take place. This procedure is very rare nowadays, being undertaken only in dire circumstances when the fetal head is too large to pass through the birth canal, the mother's life is endangered, and Caesarean section impossible.

斷頭術 將頭截除。通常是截除死胎頭使分娩得以進行。現今已絕少採用，僅在胎頭過大難以通過產道，危及產婦生命，而又不能施行剖腹產的情況下，方用斷頭術。

decapsulation *n.* the surgical removal of a *capsule from an organ; for example, the stripping of the membrane that envelops the kidney.

被膜剝除術 用外科手術去除器官的被膜。例如腎包膜剝除術。

decay *n.* (in bacteriology) the decomposition of organic matter due to microbial action.

腐敗 由於細菌作用而發生的有機物分解（細菌學）。

decerebration *n.* the removal of the higher centres of the brain or cutting across the brain below the cerebrum so that cerebral functions are eliminated. This procedure is carried out on experimental animals, but certain injuries to the brain in man may cause the same severe neurological signs as occur in an animal that has been decerebrated.

去大腦 切除大腦高級中樞或在大腦以下將腦橫切，以消除大腦的機能。此手術一般在實驗動物上進行，但人類有些大腦損傷時也會發生類似去大腦動物的嚴重神經病學體徵。

deci- *prefix denoting* a tenth.

〔前綴〕 **十分之一**

decibel (db) *n.* one tenth of a bel: a unit for comparing levels of power (especially sound) on a logarithmic scale. A power source of intensity *P* has a power level of 10 $\log_{10} P/P_0$ decibels, where P_0 is the intensity of a reference source. The decibel is much more widely used than the bel. Silence is 0 db; a whisper has an intensity of 20 db,

分貝 十分之一貝爾：用對數值表示功率（特別是聲功率）水平的單位。強度的功率源 P 等於 $10 \log_{10} P / P_0$ 分貝的功率水平，P_0 爲參照系的强度。分貝較貝爾使用廣泛得多。寂靜爲0分貝，耳語的强度爲20分貝，正

normal speech 50 db, heavy traffic 80 db, and a jet aircraft 120 db. 常說話爲50分貝，交通繁忙時的强度爲80分貝，噴氣式飛機則達到120分貝。

decidua *n.* the modified mucous membrane that lines the wall of the uterus (womb) during pregnancy and is shed with the afterbirth at parturition (*see* endometrium). There are three regions: the *decidua capsularis*, a thin layer that covers the embryo; the *decidua basalis*, where the embryo is attached; and the *decidua parietalis*, which is not in contact with the embryo. —**decidual** *adj.*

蛻膜 妊娠期鋪襯在子宮內壁上的發生了變化的黏膜。此膜分娩時隨胎盤胎膜一起脫落。蛻膜分三部分：覆蓋胚胎的一層菲薄的包蛻膜；胚胎附着處的基蛻膜；與胚胎不相接觸的壁蛻膜。

deciduoma *n.* a mass of tissue within the womb derived from remnants of *decidua. *See also* chorionepithelioma (malignant deciduoma).

蛻膜瘤 子宮內殘留的蛻膜組織塊。

deciduous teeth the primary teeth, which are shed just before eruption of their permanent successors. In the absence of permanent successors they can remain functional for many years. *See* dentition.

乳牙 初生牙。在恒牙臨萌出前脫落。在恒牙闕如的情況下，乳牙可維持功能多年。

decigravida *n.* a woman who has been pregnant ten times.

孕$_{10}$ 妊娠十次的婦女。

decipara *n.* a woman who has been pregnant at least ten times and has given birth to a child capable of survival after each of ten pregnancies.

產$_{10}$ 妊娠至少十次且十次均爲活產的婦女。

declive *n.* an area of the upper surface of the *cerebellum, posterior to the culmen and anterior to the folium of the middle lobe.

山坡 小腦上部表面、山頂之後中央小葉之前的區域。

decomposition *n.* the gradual disintegration of dead organic matter, usually foodstuffs or tissues, by the chemical action of bacteria and/or fungi.

腐敗分解 死亡的有機體（通常爲食物或組織）藉細菌和/或眞菌的化學作用而發生的逐漸分解過程。

decompression *n.* **1.** the reduction of pressure on an organ or part of the body by surgical intervention. Surgical decompression can be effected at many sites: the pressure of tissues on a nerve

減壓 ①用外科手段減輕對器官或身體局部的壓力。外科減壓可在許多部位發揮作用：切開組織可減除對神經的壓迫；切開

may be relieved by incision; raised pressure in the fluid of the brain can be lowered by cutting into the *dura mater; and cardiac compression – the abnormal presence of blood or fluid round the heart – can be cured by cutting the sac (pericardium) enclosing the heart. **2.** the gradual reduction of atmospheric pressure for deep-sea divers, who work at artificially high pressures. *See* compressed air illness.

硬腦脊膜可使過高的腦脊液壓力下降；切開包裹心臟的心包可以消除心臟壓迫（心包腔內積存血液或液體的異常狀態）。②對在人工高壓下工作的深水潛水員實施逐漸減低大氣壓力的過程。

decompression sickness *see* compressed air illness.

減壓病

decongestant *n.* an agent that reduces or relieves nasal congestion. Most nasal decongestants are *sympathomimetic drugs, applied either locally, in the form of nasal sprays or drops, or taken by mouth.

減充血劑 減輕或消除鼻黏膜充血的藥物。多爲擬交感藥物。局部滴入或噴霧，也有口服的。

decortication *n.* **1.** the removal of the outside layer (cortex) from an organ or structure, such as the kidney. **2.** an operation for removing the blood clot and scar tissue that forms after bleeding into the chest cavity (haemothorax).

①去皮質 去除器官（如腎臟）或結構的外層（皮質）。 **②胸膜外纖維層剝離術** 將胸膜腔出血（血胸）後形成的血塊和瘢痕組織剝除的手術。

decubitus *n.* the recumbent position.

臥位 躺臥的體位。

decubitus ulcer *see* bedsore.

褥瘡性潰瘍

decussation *n.* a point at which two or more structures of the body cross to the opposite side. The term is used particularly for the point at which nerve fibres cross over in the central nervous system.

交叉 身體兩種或多種結構向對側跨越交叉的部位。本詞主要指中樞神經系統內神經纖維向對側跨越的部位。

deer fly *see* Chrysops.

斑虻

defence mechanism the means whereby an undesirable impulse can be avoided or controlled (*see* censor). Many defence mechanisms have been described, including *repression, *projection, and *reaction formation. They may be partly responsible for such problems as tics, stammering, and phobias.

心理防禦機制 避免或控制不需要的衝動的心理手段。已有許多機制得到描述，其中有：壓抑機制、投射（推諉）機制、反應構成機制等。它們可能是產生抽搐、口吃、恐怖症等的部分原因。

deferent *adj.* **1.** carrying away from or down from. **2.** relating to the vas deferens.

①輸出的 ②輸精管的

defervescence *n.* the disappearance of a fever, a process that may occur rapidly or take several days, depending upon the cause and treatment given.

退熱 發熱消退。由於病因或治療方法的不同，可以突然退熱，也可以在幾天內逐漸退熱。

defibrillation *n.* administration of a controlled electric shock to restore normal heart rhythm in cases of cardiac arrest due to ventricular *fibrillation. The apparatus (*defibrillator*) administers the shock either through electrodes placed on the chest wall over the heart or directly to the heart after the chest has been opened surgically.

除纖顫 對心室纖顫導致心臟停搏的病例給予可控電震，使之恢復心臟正常節律。使用的儀器稱爲除顫器，電震通過置於胸壁上心臟部位的電極而給予患者，在外科開胸情況下也可直接刺激心臟。

defibrination *n.* the removal of *fibrin, one of the plasma proteins that causes coagulation, from a sample of blood. It is normally done by whisking the blood with a bundle of fine wires, to which the strands of fibrin that form in the blood adhere.

去纖維蛋白法 從血液樣品中除去纖維蛋白（一種可以引起凝血的血漿蛋白）的方法。一般是用一束細金屬絲在血中攪動，血中形成的纖維蛋白便纏繞在絲上。

deficiency *n.* (in genetics) *see* deletion.

缺乏，不足

deficiency disease any disease caused by the lack of an essential nutrient in the diet. Such nutrients include *vitamins, *essential amino acids, and *essential fatty acids.

缺乏性疾病 由於飲食中缺乏某種基本營養素而發生的疾病。這類營養素包括維生素、必需氨基酸、必需脂肪酸等。

deflorescence *n.* a disappearance of a rash in those diseases in which a rash is a characteristic part of the illness.

退疹 指出疹性疾病中皮疹的消退。

degeneration *n.* the deterioration and loss of specialized function of the cells of a tissue or organ. The changes may be caused by a defective blood supply or by disease. Degeneration may involve the deposition of calcium salts, fat (*see* fatty degeneration), or fibrous tissue in the affected organ or tissue. *See also* infiltration.

變性，退行性變 組織或器官細胞的特殊功能的衰退或喪失。血液供應不足以及患疾病時均可發生這類病變。受累器官或組織中出現鈣鹽沉着、脂肪堆積以及纖維組織，均屬於變性範疇。

deglutition *n.* *see* swallowing.

吞嚥

dehiscence *n.* a splitting open, as of a surgical wound.

裂開 如外科傷口裂開。

dehydration *n.* **1.** loss or deficiency of water in body tissues. The condition may result from inadequate water intake and/or from excessive removal of water from the body; for example, by sweating, vomiting, or diarrhoea. Symptoms include great thirst, nausea, and exhaustion. The condition is treated by drinking plenty of water; severe cases require intravenous administration of water and salts (which have been lost with the water). **2.** the removal of water from tissue during its preparation for microscopical study, by placing it successively in stronger solutions of ethyl alcohol. Dehydration follows *fixation and precedes *clearing.

失水，脫水 ①身體組織中水分喪失或不足。其原因可爲入水量不足，和/或出水量過大（如出汗、嘔吐、腹瀉）。症狀有：煩渴、噁心、衰竭。治療措施是大量飲水。嚴重病例需靜脉給水和鹽（因鹽隨同水一起喪失）。②製備顯微鏡研究用標本時，將組織塊依次浸入濃度遞增的一系列乙醇液中，以除去組織中水分的步驟。脫水前須做固定和脫水後須採用透明措施。

dehydrogenase *n. see* oxidoreductase.

脫氫酶

déjà vu a vivid psychic experience in which immediately contemporary events seem to be a repetition of previous happenings. It is a symptom of temporal lobe *epilepsy. *See also* jamais vu.

似曾相識症 一種生動的心理體驗。表現爲對當時見到的事物覺得像是以前遇到過的事物的重現。爲顳葉癲癇的症狀之一。

deletion (deficiency) *n.* (in genetics) a type of chromosome mutation in which a part of the chromosome, and therefore the genes carried on that part, is lost.

缺失 遺傳學用語。染色體突變的一種類型。表現爲染色體的一部分（即載有基因的部分）的丟失。

Delhi boil *see* oriental sore.

德里瘡 東方瘡

delirium *n.* an acute disorder of the mental processes accompanying organic brain disease. It may be manifested by illusions, disorientation, hallucinations, or extreme excitement and occurs in metabolic disorders, intoxication, deficiency diseases, and infections.

譫妄，妄想 大腦器質性疾病時發生的一種急性精神活動障礙。表現爲錯覺、定向障礙、幻覺或極度興奮。可見於代謝性疾病、中毒、缺乏性疾病及傳染病時。

delirium tremens a psychosis caused by *alcoholism, usually seen as a withdrawal syndrome in chronic alcoholics. Typically it is precipitated by a head injury or an acute infection causing abstinence from alcohol. Features include anxiety, tremor, sweating, and vivid and terrifying visual and sensory

震顫性譫妄 由酒精中毒引起的精神病。常作爲慢性酒精中毒患者的戒斷綜合徵而出現。一般患者先有因頭部損傷或急性感染以致戒酒的病史。症狀有：焦慮、震顫、出汗、出現動物或昆蟲的逼眞嚇

hallucinations, often of animals and insects. Severe cases may end fatally.

人的視幻覺或感覺性幻覺。嚴重者可致死。

deltoid *n.* a thick triangular muscle that covers the shoulder joint (see illustration). It is responsible for raising the arm away from the side of the body.

三角肌 覆蓋肩部的三角形厚肌（見圖）。其功能是側舉上臂。

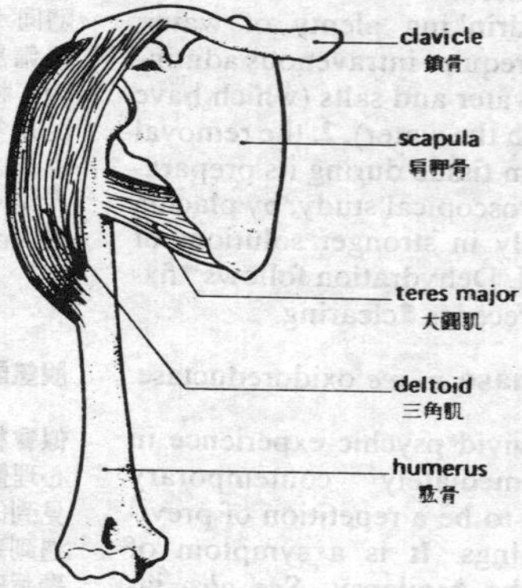

The deltoid muscle
三角肌

delusion *n.* an irrationally held belief that cannot be altered by rational argument. In mental illness it is often a false belief that the individual is persecuted by others, is very powerful, is controlled by others, or is a victim of physical disease (*see* paranoia). It may be a symptom of schizophrenia, *manic-depressive psychosis, or an organic psychosis.

妄想 用理性論證無法改變的不合理的執着的信念。在精神病中通常表現爲一種錯誤的信念，如受迫害妄想，誇大妄想，受控妄想，或者軀體疾病妄想。

dementia *n.* a chronic or persistent disorder of the mental processes due to organic brain disease. It is marked by memory disorders, changes in personality, deterioration in personal care, impaired reasoning ability, and disorientation. *Presenile dementia* occurs in young or middle-aged people. The term is sometimes reserved for Alzheimer's disease and Pick's disease, but it is important to distinguish these condi-

痴呆 由於大腦器質性疾病而發生的一種慢性頑固性精神活動障礙。其特點爲記憶障礙、性格改變、缺乏自理能力、推理能力障礙、定向障礙。青年或中年可發生早老性痴呆。本詞有時專用於阿爾茨海默氏病和皮克氏病，故須與那些可以治療的大腦疾病的痴呆相區別。

tions from those brain diseases for which curative treatment may be available.

demethylchlortetracycline *n.* an antibiotic that is active against a wide range of bacteria and is used to treat various infections. It is administered by mouth; common side-effects are nausea, diarrhoea, and symptoms resulting from the growth of organisms not sensitive to the drug. Trade name: **Ledermycin**.

去甲氯四環素　用於治療各種細菌感染的廣譜抗生素。口服。常見副作用爲噁心、腹瀉以及對本藥不敏感的細菌生長而引起的症狀。

demi- *prefix denoting* half.

〔前綴〕　半

Demodex *n.* a genus of harmless parasitic mites, the follicle mites, found in the hair follicles and associated sebaceous glands of the face. They resemble tiny worms, about 0.4 mm in length, and their presence may give rise to dermatitis.

脂蟎屬　一屬無害的寄生蟎——毛囊脂蟎。寄生於面部毛囊及其皮脂腺內。長約0.4mm，形似細小蠕蟲。可引起皮炎。

demography *n.* the study of the populations of the world, their racial make-up, movements, birth rates, death rates, and other factors affecting the quality of life within them. *See also* biostatistics.

人口學　研究世界人口、種族組成、人口轉移、出生率、死亡率以及各種影響生活水平和人口質量的因素的科學。

demulcent *n.* a soothing agent that protects the mucous membranes and relieves irritation. Demulcents form a protective film and are used in mouth washes, gargles, etc., to soothe irritation or inflammation in the mouth.

緩和藥　保護黏膜、緩和刺激的藥物。能生成一層保護膜，用於含漱、清漱咽部等，以緩和口腔刺激或炎症。

demyelination *n.* a disease process selectively damaging the *myelin sheaths in the central or peripheral nervous system. This in turn affects the function of the nerve fibres, which the myelin normally supports. Demyelination may be the primary disorder, as in *multiple sclerosis, or it may occur after head injury or strokes.

髓鞘脫失　選擇性損害中樞和周圍神經系統的髓鞘的病理過程。髓鞘脫失後，正常由髓鞘支持的神經纖維的功能遭受損害。可爲原發性病變，如見於多發性硬化症；也可發生於頭部損傷或腦卒中後。

denaturation *n.* the changes in the physical and physiological properties of a protein that are brought about by heat, X-rays, or chemicals. These

變性　蛋白質經受熱、X射線或化學物理作用而發生的物理和生理特性的改變。屬於此類的有失去活

changes include loss of activity (in the case of enzymes) and loss (or alteration) of antigenicity (in the case of *antigens).

性（酶）、失去或改變抗原性（抗原）等。

dendrite *n.* one of the shorter branching processes of the cell body of a *neurone, which makes contact with other neurones at synapses and carries nerve impulses from them into the cell body.

樹突 神經元體的較短的分支狀突起。與其他神經元在突觸部位發生接觸，並從突觸處將衝動傳入神經元體內。

dendritic ulcer a branching ulcer of the surface of the cornea caused by herpes simplex virus. A similar appearance may be produced by a healing corneal abrasion. Dendritic ulcers tend to recur because the virus lies dormant in the tissues; years may elapse between attacks.

樹枝狀潰瘍 單純疱疹病毒引起的角膜表面的分支狀潰瘍。角膜擦傷癒合時可產生相似的表現。由於病毒蟄伏於組織內，本病有復發傾向，兩次發作之間可有數年間隔。

denervation *n.* interruption of the nerve supply to the muscles and skin. The muscle is paralysed and its normal tone (elasticity) is lost. The muscle fibres shrink and are replaced by fat. A denervated area of skin loses all forms of sensation and its subsequent ability to heal and renew its tissues is impaired.

去神經支配 中斷神經對於肌肉和皮膚的支配。肌肉癱瘓，失去正常時的張力（彈性）。肌纖維變細而爲脂肪所代替。失去神經支配的皮膚則喪失全部感覺，其癒合和組織重建能力也受損害。

dengue (breakbone fever) *n.* a viral disease transmitted to man principally by the mosquito **Aëdes aegypti*. Symptoms, which last for a few days, include severe pains in the joints and muscles, headache, sore throat, fever, running of the eyes, and an irritating rash. These symptoms recur in a usually milder form after an interval of two or three days. Death rarely occurs, but the patient is left debilitated and requires considerable convalescence. Dengue occurs throughout the tropics and subtropics. Patients are given aspirin and codeine to relieve the pain and calamine lotion is helpful in easing the irritating rash.

登革熱（斷骨熱） 一種主要由埃及伊蚊傳給人的病毒性疾病。症狀持續幾天，包括：關節和肌肉劇烈疼痛、頭痛、咽喉炎、發熱、流淚、瘙癢性皮疹。這些症狀經2～3天的間隔而再次出現，但通常表現較輕，很少死亡。患者虛弱，需認眞調理。登革熱分佈於熱帶和亞熱帶地區。治療：用阿司匹林和可待因鎮痛，爐甘石洗劑可減輕皮疹癢感。

dens *n.* a tooth or tooth-shaped structure.

牙，齒 牙齒或齒狀結構。

dens invaginatus literally, an infolded tooth: a specific type of tooth malformation that mainly affects upper lateral incisors to varying degrees.

牙內陷 按字面意義即可知為陷入的牙。一種主要發生於上側切牙的輕重不等的特殊類型牙畸形。

dent- (denti-, dento-) *prefix denoting* the teeth. Example: *dentoalveolar* (relating to the teeth and associated jaw).

〔前綴〕 **牙** 例如：牙槽的（牙和與之相連的頜骨的）。

dental auxiliary any of several assistants to a dentist. A *dental hygienist* performs scaling and instruction in oral hygiene under the supervision of the dentist. A *dental surgery assistant* helps the dentist at the chairside by preparing materials, passing instruments, and aspirating the mouth. A *dental technician* constructs dentures, crowns, and orthodontic appliances in the laboratory for the dentist. A *dental therapist* performs treatment on children under the direction of a dentist in the community dental services and in hospitals.

牙科輔助人員 牙科醫生助手的統稱。例如，牙科保健員在牙科醫生監督下執行牙潔治和牙科保健的指導任務。牙外科助手則在牙科椅旁協助醫生準備材料、傳遞器械和握持吸引器。牙科技士在實驗室內為醫生製備托牙、牙冠及正畸用具。牙科治療員則在社區牙科防治站或醫院內在牙科醫生指導下對兒童進行治療。

dental caries decay and crumbling of the substance of a tooth. Dental caries is caused by the metabolism of the bacteria in *plaque attached to the surface of the tooth. Acid formed by bacterial breakdown of sugar in the diet gradually etches and decomposes the enamel of the tooth. If left unrepaired it spreads in and progressively destroys the tooth completely, first exposing the deeper dentine, causing toothache, and eventually opening the pulp to allow ingress of infection into the bone and abscess formation (*see* apical abscess). Frequent intake of sugar is a major cause, and the disease is more common in young people and has a predilection for specific sites. Repair consists of removing the decayed part of the tooth using a *drill and replacing it with a *filling. The resistance of enamel to dental caries can be increased by the application of *fluoride salts to the tooth surface from toothpastes or mouth rinses. *Fluoridation of water also makes teeth resistant to caries during the period of tooth development.

齲 牙質的腐朽和破碎。由附着於牙表面的牙斑中的細菌的代謝所致。食物中的糖經細菌分解而產生酸，後者逐漸侵蝕並使牙表面的釉質解體。若不予修補，齲向深部發展，將牙徹底破壞，先是暴露深部的牙本質引起牙痛，進而使髓腔開放，以致細菌侵入骨內，形成膿腫。經常吃糖是致齲的主要原因，因而青年人患齲最多，並且有易發部位。修補齲牙是用牙鑽去除牙齲壞的部分和置入塡料。使用含氟鹽的牙膏或漱口液，可增强牙釉質的抗齲能力。水中加氟也可增强發育期牙的抗齲能力。

dental committee (local) *see* medical committee (local).

牙科委員會（地方）

dental floss fine thread, usually of nylon, used to clean some surfaces of teeth.

牙線 用以清潔部分牙面的細線，通常爲尼龍製成。

dental nerve either of two nerves that supply the teeth. The *inferior dental nerve* supplies the lower teeth and for most of its length exists as a single large bundle; thus anaesthesia of it has a widespread effect (*see* inferior dental block). The *superior dental nerve*, which supplies the upper teeth, breaks into separate branches at some distance from the teeth and it is possible to anaesthetize these individually with less widespread effect for the patient.

牙神經 兩條支配牙的神經。下牙神經支配下列牙，幾乎全長爲一粗大的單束，因此麻醉此神經可獲得大範圍的麻醉效果。上牙神經支配上列牙，它在到達牙之前的一定距離陸續分爲數支，因此可單個地麻醉以取得較局限的麻醉效果。

dental unit a major piece of dental equipment to which are attached the dental drills, aspirator, and compressed air syringes.

牙科治療椅 牙科設備。裝配有牙鑽、吸引器及壓力氣槍等主要部件。

dentate *adj.* serrated; having toothlike projections.

齒狀的 具有齒狀突起的。

dentifrice *n.* a paste or powder for cleaning the teeth. Toothpastes contain a fine abrasive; an essential ingredient is suitable flavouring to make their use pleasant. Most toothpastes contain *fluoride salts, which help to prevent dental caries.

牙粉（膏） 清潔牙齒的粉或膏。牙膏中含有纖細的磨料，基本成分中還有適宜的香料以使人們樂於使用。多數牙膏中含有氟鹽，有防齲之功。

dentine *n.* a hard tissue that forms the bulk of a tooth. The dentine of the crown is covered by enamel and that of the root by cementum. The dentine is permeated by fine tubules, which close to the centre of the tooth contain cellular processes from the pulp. Exposed dentine is sensitive to touch, heat, and cold.

牙本質 構成牙主體的堅硬組織。牙冠部的牙本質表面被覆釉質，牙根部的牙本質則包有牙骨質。牙本質中有許多微細的小管穿透，小管在近牙中心的部位與來自牙髓的細胞突相接。暴露的牙本質對觸、熱、冷敏感。

dentinogenesis *n.* the formation of *dentine by *odontoblasts. Although dentine continues to be formed throughout life, very little is formed later than a few years after tooth

牙本質生成 由成牙質細胞形成牙本質的過程。牙本質在一生中不斷生成，但在牙萌出幾年後生成極爲緩慢。所謂牙本質生成

eruption. *Dentinogenesis imperfecta* is a hereditary condition in which dentine formation is disturbed, resulting in loss of overlying enamel.

不全是一種遺傳性病變，表現為牙本質生成障礙，並缺乏釉質覆蓋。

dentist *n.* a member of the dental profession, who in the UK must be registered with the General Dental Council unless he holds a medical qualification.

牙科醫生 牙科專業人員。在英國，牙科醫生必須在全國牙科協會註冊，否則應持有醫生證書。

dentistry *n.* the study, management, and treatment of diseases and conditions affecting the mouth, jaws, teeth, and their supporting tissues. *See* endodontics, orthodontics, periodontics, preventive dentistry.

牙科學 對口、頜、牙及其支持組織疾病進行研究、處理和治療的學科。

dentition *n.* the arrangement of teeth in the mouth. The *deciduous dentition* comprises the teeth of young children. It consists of 20 teeth, made up of incisors, canines, and molars only. The lower incisor erupts first at about 6 months of age, and all the deciduous

牙列 牙在口腔內的排列。幼兒牙組成乳牙列，共20顆牙，包括切牙、尖牙及磨牙。下切牙於6個月時最先萌出，一般2-3歲乳牙全部出齊。下切牙約於6歲時最先脫落。從6

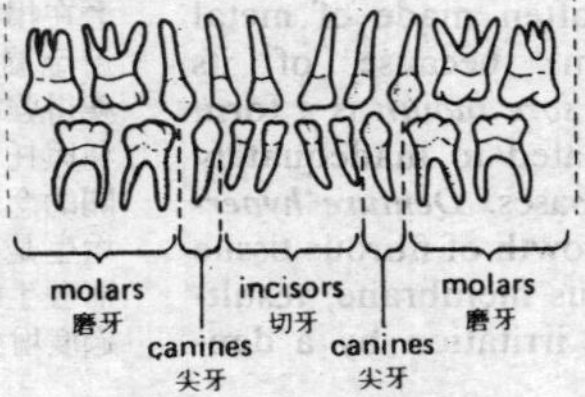

Deciduous dentition
乳牙列

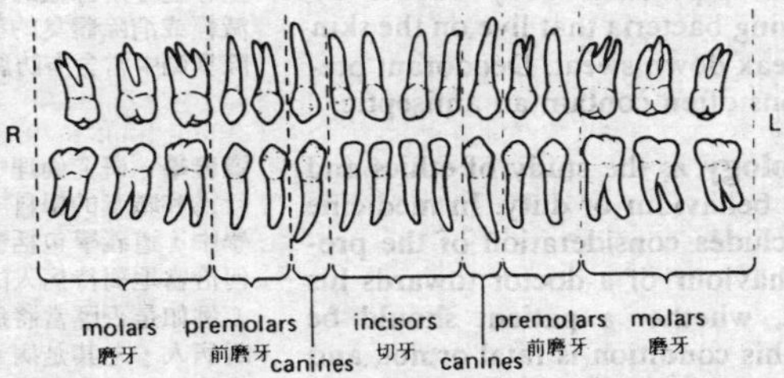

Permanent dentition
恒牙列

teeth have usually erupted by the age of 2–3. The lower incisors are shed first at about 6 years of age, and from this time until about 12 years old both deciduous and permanent teeth are present; i.e. there is a *mixed dentition*. The *permanent dentition* consists of up to 32 teeth, made up of incisors, canines, premolars, and molars. The first tooth to erupt is the first molar (at the age of 6) and most have appeared by the age of 14 years, although the third molars may not erupt until the age of 18–21 years. See illustrations.

歲至12歲左右乳牙與恒牙共存，即所謂混合牙列。恒牙列由32顆牙組成，包括切牙、尖牙、前磨牙和磨牙。最先萌出的是第一磨牙（6歲），至14歲大部分萌出，然而第三磨牙可到18～21歲才萌出（見圖）。

denture (prosthesis) *n.* a removable replacement for one or more teeth carried on some type of plate or frame. A *complete denture* replaces all the teeth in one jaw. It is usually made entirely of acrylic resin. A *partial denture* replaces some teeth because others still remain. It is designed to restore function with the least potential damage to the remaining teeth. The framework of the denture base is often made of metal (*cobalt-chromium) because of its strength. *Denture sore mouth* is a form of candidiasis related to inadequately cleaned denture bases. *Denture hyperplasia* is an overgrowth of fibrous tissue covered by mucous membrane, resulting from chronic irritation by a denture.

托牙（假牙） 裝在一定形狀的托版或支架上、可以取下的一個或多個牙的替代物。全口托牙是取代單頜的全副牙齒。通常全用丙烯酸樹脂製成。部分托牙只取代缺失的牙齒，因爲其他牙仍存留。部分托牙的設計旨在恢復功能而盡可能減小對存留牙的潛在損害。基托的支架常用金屬（鈷-鎳）製成以獲得强度。托牙口瘡是一種與托牙製備得不平整有關的念珠菌感染。托牙性增生是由於托牙慢性刺激而發生的黏膜下纖維組織過度增生。

deodorant *n.* an agent that reduces or removes unpleasant body odours by destroying bacteria that live on the skin and break down sweat. Deodorant preparations often contain an antiseptic.

除臭劑 殺滅在皮膚表面生存並分解汗液的細菌以減輕或消除體臭的藥物。除臭劑中常含有防腐劑。

deontology *n.* the study of ethics and correct behaviour or duty. In medicine this includes consideration of the proper behaviour of a doctor towards his patient, whether a patient should be told if his condition is fatal or not, and similar problems for which there may be *Hippocratic oath.

道義學 研究倫理、正確行爲和職責的學科。在醫學中，道義學包括醫生如何恰當地對待病人的問題（例如是否應當將病情告訴病人，尤其是病人患絕症時），以及可能涉及希波克拉底誓言的類似問題。

deoxycholic acid *see* bile acids.

脫氧膽酸

deoxycorticosterone *n.* a hormone, synthesized and released by the adrenal cortex, that regulates salt and water balance. *See also* corticosteroid.

脫氧皮脂酮 腎上腺皮質合成並釋放的激素，調節水、鹽平衡。

deoxyribonuclease *n.* an enzyme, located in the *lysosomes of cells, that splits DNA at specific places in the molecule.

脫氧核糖核酸酶 存在於細胞溶酶體內的一種酶。在分子內的特定部位裂解DNA。

deoxyribonucleic acid *see* DNA.

脫氧核糖核酸

Department of Health and Social Security a department of central government that supports the Secretary of State for Health and Social Services in meeting his obligations, which include the *National Health Service and the prevention and control of infectious diseases. Information is collated, priorities assessed, and resources allocated to Regional and District Health Authorities. Similar assessments and allocations are made to local authorities for *social services. The department is staffed by civil servants, including medical and nursing personnel and those from other health professions. Equivalent departments support the ministers responsible for similar services in Scotland, Wales, and Northern Ireland.

衞生與社會保障部 中央政府的一個部門。其職能是支持國家衞生與社會服務事業大臣履行職責，即：開展全國性的衞生保健和傳染病的防治工作，審核情報資料，評審重點項目，確定對地區級和地段級保健局的撥欵。有關地方社會服務部門的上列工作內容亦由該部負責。該部人員編制由醫、護及其它衞生專業的公職人員組成。在蘇格蘭、威爾士和北愛爾蘭，則有同樣的部門協助該部部長進行工作。

dependence (drug dependence) *n.* the physical and/or psychological effects produced by the habitual taking of certain drugs, characterized by a compulsion to continue taking the drug. In *physical dependence* withdrawal of the drug causes specific symptoms (*withdrawal symptoms*), such as sweating, vomiting, or tremors, that are reversed by further doses. Substances that may induce physical dependence include alcohol and the 'hard' drugs morphine, heroin, and cocaine. Dependence on 'hard' drugs carries a high mortality, partly because overdosage may be fatal and partly because their casual injection intravenously may lead to infec-

賴藥性 指由習慣性攝入某些藥物所致的、不得不持續攝入該藥物的軀體的和/或心理的效應。軀體性賴藥性的表現是：撤去藥物可引起一些特殊的症狀（戒斷症狀），諸如出汗、嘔吐、震顫等，給藥後又可消失。能引起軀體性賴藥性的物質有酒精和“硬性”藥，如嗎啡、海洛因和可卡因。對“硬性”藥產生賴藥性有很高的死亡率，部分是由於藥物過量可致死，部分是由於不嚴密消毒的靜脈內注射可以引起肝炎之類感染。治

tions such as *hepatitis. Treatment is difficult and requires specialist skills. Much more common is *psychological dependence*, in which repeated use of a drug induces reliance on it for a state of well-being and contentment, but there are no physical withdrawal symptoms if use of the drug is stopped. Substances that may induce psychological dependence include nicotine in tobacco, cannabis, and many 'soft' drugs, such as barbiturates and amphetamines.

療困難，且需要專門技術。較爲多見的是心理性賴藥性：反復攝入某種造成依賴性的藥物才能維持良好和滿足狀態，但停藥後不出現戒斷症狀。能引起心理性依賴性的物質有煙草中的煙鹼、大麻以及“軟性”藥如巴比妥類和苯丙胺類。

depersonalization *n.* a state in which a person feels himself becoming unreal or strangely altered, or feels that his mind is becoming separated from his body. Minor degrees of this feeling are common in normal people under stress. Severe feelings of depersonalization occur in anxiety neurosis, in states of *dissociation, in depression and schizophrenia, and in epilepsy (particularly temporal-lobe epilepsy). *See also* derealization.

人格解體 一種感覺自己變得不是眞實存在或發生了奇怪變化，或者感覺自己的思維與軀體相分離的狀態。正常人在應急狀態中常可產生輕度的這類感覺。嚴重的人格解體感覺發生於焦慮性神經症、分裂狀態、抑鬱症、精神分裂症及癲癇（特別是顳葉癲癇）。

depilatory *n.* an agent applied to the skin to remove hair.

脫毛劑 使皮膚脫毛的藥物。

depolarization *n.* the sudden surge of charged particles across the membrane of a nerve or muscle cell that accompanies a physicochemical change in the membrane and cancels out, or reverses, its resting potential to produce an *action potential. The passage of a *nerve impulse is a rapid wave of depolarization along the membrane of a nerve fibre.

除極化 荷電粒子突然大量透過神經細胞或肌細胞的膜，隨着出現膜的物理化學變化，使靜息電位消除或逆轉，從而產生動作電位的過程。一個神經衝動的通行即是一個沿着一條神經纖維的膜行進的快速的除極波。

depressant *n.* an agent that reduces the normal activity of any body system or function. Drugs such as general *anaesthetics, *barbiturates, and opiates are depressants of the central nervous system and respiration. *Cytotoxic drugs, such as azathioprine, are depressants of the levels of white blood cells.

抑制劑 使任何身體系統或功能的正常活動降低的藥物。如全身麻醉藥、巴比妥類、阿片之類藥物爲中樞神經系統和呼吸的抑制劑，細胞毒藥物（如硫唑嘌呤）爲白細胞抑制劑。

depression *n.* a mental state characterized by excessive sadness. Activity can

抑鬱症 以過分憂鬱爲特徵的精神狀態。活動可以

be agitated and restless or slow and retarded. Behaviour is governed by pessimistic or despairing beliefs, and sleep, appetite, and concentration are disturbed. There are several causes. *Manic-depressive psychosis causes severe depressions, in which there may be delusions of being worthless, ill, wicked, or impoverished and hallucinations of accusing voices. Loss and frustration also cause depression, which may be prolonged and disproportionate in depressive *neurosis. Treatment is with *antidepressant drugs and/or *psychotherapy. Severe cases may need *electroconvulsive therapy. *See also* endogenous, reactive.

表現爲焦慮不安，也可以表現爲緩慢、遲鈍。行爲受悲觀或絕望的信念所支配，睡眠、食慾和注意力集中均發生障礙。原因多種多樣。躁狂-抑鬱性精神病可表現嚴重的抑鬱，患者可有認爲無生存價值、生病、邪惡、無可救藥等妄想以及譴責聲音幻覺。失敗和挫折也可引起抑鬱症，這種抑鬱症可以持久不癒，在抑鬱性神經症可表現爲不均衡型。治療可用抗抑鬱藥和/或心理療法。嚴重者需用電休克療法。

depressor *n.* **1.** a muscle that causes lowering of part of the body. The *depressor labii inferioris* is a muscle that draws down and everts the lower lip. **2.** a nerve that lowers blood pressure.

①**降肌** 使身體一部下降的肌肉，如下唇方肌將下唇下拉並外翻。 ②**減壓神經** 降低血壓的神經。

dequalinium *n.* an antiseptic, active against some bacteria and fungi, used as lozenges or paint to treat mouth and throat infections.

克菌定 治療某些細菌和眞菌有效的抗菌劑。常製成錠劑或搽劑，用以治療口腔和咽喉感染。

deradenitis *n.* inflammation of the lymph nodes in the neck.

頸淋巴結炎 頸部淋巴結的炎症。

derealization *n.* a feeling of unreality in which the environment is experienced as unreal and as flat, dull, or strange. The experience is unwelcome and often frightening. It occurs in association with *depersonalization or with the conditions that cause depersonalization.

現實感喪失 一種虛幻的感覺。環境被體驗爲不是切實存在的，而是單調、暗淡或者奇形怪狀的東西。患者不喜歡這種體驗，常爲之恐懼。多與人格解體或與引起人格解體的疾病併存。

dereism *n.* undirected fantasy thinking that fails to respect the realities of life. When this becomes markedly dominant it may be a feature of *schizoid personality or of *schizophrenia.

空想癖 不切生活實際的、無定向的幻想思維。如發展嚴重，可能成爲精神分裂樣人格或精神分裂症的一種表現。

derm- (derma-, dermo-, dermat(o)-) *prefix denoting* the skin.

〔前綴〕 **皮膚**

-derm *suffix denoting* **1.** the skin. **2.** a germ layer.

〔後綴〕 ①**皮膚** ②**胚層**

Dermacentor *n.* a genus of hard *ticks, worldwide in distribution, the adults of which are parasites of man and other mammals. The wood tick, *D. andersoni*, transmits Rocky Mountain spotted fever to man in the western USA and the dog tick, *D. variabilis*, is the vector of the milder form of this disease in the east.

革蜱屬 一屬全世界廣泛分佈的硬蜱。成蟲爲人和其他哺乳動物的寄生蟲。安氏革蜱是美國西部傳播落基山斑疹傷寒給人的媒介，變異革蜱則是美國東部該病溫和型的媒介。

dermal *adj.* relating to or affecting the skin, especially the *dermis.

皮的 皮膚（尤其是眞皮）的，影響皮膚的。

Dermanyssus *n.* a genus of widespread parasitic mites. The red poultry mite, *D. gallinae*, is a common parasite of wild birds in temperate regions but can also infest poultry. It occasionally attacks and takes a blood meal from man, causing itching and mild dermatitis.

皮刺螨屬 一屬廣泛分佈的寄生螨。雞皮刺螨是溫帶地區野生鳥類最常見的寄生蟲，也可侵襲家禽。偶爾吸人血而引起瘙癢和輕度皮炎。

dermatitis *n.* inflammation of the skin caused by an outside agent: a condition with many causes. The skin is red and itchy and small blisters may develop. In most cases the condition is associated with certain typical changes in the skin that are described as *eczema (*eczematous dermatitis*). Eczematous dermatitis may result from direct irritation of the skin by a substance (such as a chemical) or it may be an allergic reaction to a particular substance that has been in contact with the skin, injected, or taken by mouth. In cases associated with a different reaction the disorder is described as *noneczematous dermatitis*. Industrial substances are a common cause of noneczematous dermatitis, which is sometimes called *occupational dermatitis*. Other types of dermatitis can be caused by soaps or detergents (for example, in nappies) or by sunlight. Treatment of dermatitis depends upon the cause.

皮炎 由外界因子引起的皮膚炎症。原因多種多樣。皮膚發紅、瘙癢，並起小水疱。大多數皮炎同時還有某些典型的皮膚改變，即所謂濕疹（濕疹性皮炎）。後者可由某些物質（如化學劑）直接刺激皮膚引起，也可以是針對某種曾經與皮膚接觸過，或注射、口服過的特定物質而發生的變應性反應。如果合併發生的皮膚反應不是濕疹，則稱爲非濕疹性皮炎。引起非濕性皮炎的常見原因是工業物質，故有時又稱爲職業性皮炎。肥皂和洗滌劑（如含於尿布內的）或日光暴晒可引起另外類型的皮炎。皮炎的治療隨原因而定。

Dermatobia *n.* a genus of nonbloodsucking flies inhabiting lowland woods and forests of South and Central

皮蠅屬 一屬棲居於中美洲和南美洲低地樹林和森林中的非吸血蠅。人皮蠅

America. The parasitic maggots of *D. hominis* can cause a serious disease of the skin in man (*see* myiasis). The maggots burrow into the skin, after emerging from eggs transported by bloodsucking insects (e.g. mosquitoes), and produce painful boil-like swellings. Treatment involves surgical removal of the maggots.

的寄生蛆可引起一種嚴重的人體皮膚病（蠅蛆病）。吸血昆蟲（如蚊）將蠅卵傳給人，卵孵化爲蛆，鑽入皮內，引起疼痛的癤腫樣腫脹。治療：手術切除蠅蛆。

dermatofibrosarcoma protuberans a tumour probably derived from *histiocytes that may occur in any part of the body. It is locally invasive but does not *metastasize. It often recurs locally despite excision.

隆凸性皮膚纖維肉瘤 一種發生於身體任何部位、可能起源於組織細胞的腫瘤。具有局部侵襲性，但不轉移。切除後常局部復發。

dermatoglyphics *n.* the study of the patterns of finger, palm, toe, and sole prints. These patterns are formed by skin ridges, the distribution of which is unique to each individual. As well as being of value in criminology, dermatoglyphics is of interest to anthropologists and to doctors studying genetic disorders. *See also* fingerprint.

皮紋學 研究指、趾、手掌、脚底和脚跟皮紋型式的學科。皮紋型式係由皮嵴形成，人各有其獨特的皮紋分佈。皮紋學不僅在犯罪學中有價值，且爲人類學家和研究遺傳病的醫生所感興趣。

dermatology *n.* the medical specialty concerned with the diagnosis and treatment of skin disorders. —**dermatological** *adj.* —**dermatologist** *n.*

皮膚病學 有關皮膚疾病診斷和治療的醫學專業。

dermatome *n.* **1.** a surgical instrument used for cutting thin slices of skin in some skin grafting operations. **2.** that part of the segmented mesoderm in the early embryo that forms the deeper layers of the skin (dermis) and associated tissues. *See* somite.

①**植皮刀** 某些皮膚移植手術時切取皮膚薄片用的外科器械。 ②**生皮節** 早期胚內形成皮膚（眞皮）深層及附屬組織中胚層體節部分。

dermatomyositis *n.* an inflammatory disorder of the skin and underlying tissues, including the muscles (where breakdown of the muscle fibres occurs). The condition is one of the *collagen diseases. A bluish-red skin eruption occurs on the face, scalp, neck, shoulders, and hands and is later accompanied by severe swelling. Dermatomyositis is often associated with internal cancer.

皮肌炎 一種皮膚及下層組織（包括肌肉——在該處發生肌纖維斷裂）的炎症性疾病。本病爲膠原性疾病的一種。表現爲顏面、頭皮、頸、肩、手部出現紫紅色皮疹，隨後併發嚴重腫脹。本病常與內臟癌症同時存在。

Dermatophagoides *n.* a genus of *mites that have been detected in samples of dust taken from houses in various parts of Europe. The mites may occasionally infest the skin of the scalp and cause dermatitis.

表皮蟎屬 一種分佈於歐洲許多地區、從室塵中檢出的蟎。有時可侵襲頭皮引起皮炎。

dermatophyte *n.* any microscopic fungus that grows on the skin and mucous membranes. There are three main genera: **Microsporum*, **Epidermophyton*, and **Trichophyton*. These do not invade the deeper tissues of the body.

皮眞菌 祇能在顯微鏡下見到的皮膚眞菌和黏膜眞菌。主要有三屬：小孢子菌屬、表皮癬菌屬、髮癬菌屬。這些眞菌均不侵犯身體深部組織。

dermatophytosis *n.* any fungus infection of the skin; more specifically, an infection caused by the parasitic fungus **Epidermophyton*.

皮眞菌病 皮膚眞菌感染。較特殊的是由表皮癬菌屬寄生眞菌引起的感染。

dermatoplasty *n.* replacement of damaged or destroyed skin by surgery. *See* plastic surgery, skin graft.

植皮術 置換受損或破潰皮膚的外科手術。

dermatosis *n.* any disease of skin, particularly one without inflammation.

皮膚病 皮膚疾病，尤指非炎症性疾病。

dermis (corium) *n.* the true *skin: the thick layer of living tissue that lies beneath the epidermis. It consists mainly of loose connective tissue within which are blood capillaries, lymph vessels, sensory nerve endings, sweat glands and their ducts, hair follicles, sebaceous glands, and smooth muscle fibres. —**dermal** *adj.*

眞皮 位於表皮下方的厚層活組織。主要由含毛細血管、淋巴管、感覺神經末梢、汗腺及其導管、毛囊、皮脂腺及平滑肌纖維的疏鬆結締組織所組成。

dermographia *n.* a local allergic reaction caused by pressure on the skin. People with such highly sensitive skin can 'write' on it with a finger or blunt instrument, the pressure producing lasting weals.

皮膚劃紋現象 一種按壓皮膚引起的局部變應性反應。有這種高度皮膚敏感的人，可用手指或鈍器在皮膚上寫出"字"來，其壓力引起持續一段時間的劃痕。

dermoid 1. *adj.* resembling the skin. **2.** *n. see* dermoid cyst.

①**皮樣的** ②**皮樣囊腫**

dermoid cyst (dermoid) a cyst containing hair, hair follicles, and *sebaceous glands, usually found at sites marking the fusion of developing sections of the body in the embryo. Sometimes a dermoid cyst may develop after an

皮樣囊腫 含有毛髮、毛囊和皮脂腺的囊腫。通常見於胚胎期體節發育融合的部位。有時外傷後可發生皮樣囊腫。治療：外科手術摘除。

injury. Treatment is by surgical removal.

Descemet's membrane the elastic membrane that lines the inner surface of the cornea of the eye, next to the aqueous humour.

後彈性層 舖襯在眼角膜內表面的彈性膜。與房水接觸。

desensitization *n.* **1.** (*or* **hyposensitization**) a method for reducing the effects of a known allergen by injecting, over a period, gradually increasing doses of the allergen, until resistance is built up. *See* allergy. **2.** a technique used in the *behaviour therapy of phobic states. The thing that is feared is very gradually introduced to the patient, first in imagination and then in reality. At the same time the patient is taught relaxation to inhibit the development of anxiety (*see* relaxation therapy). In this way he is able to cope with progressively closer approximations to the feared object or situation.

脫敏 ①使已知變應原的作用減弱的方法。方法爲每隔一定時間注射一次變應原，逐漸增量直至建立對變應原的耐受性。②用於治療恐怖症的一種行爲療法技術。先向患者解釋他懼怕的事物，然後慢慢過渡到讓患者直接接觸這個事物，同時教會患者放鬆自己以壓制焦慮的產生。患者因而得以逐漸接近所懼怕的事物或情景。

deserpidine *n.* a drug that reduces blood pressure and is used to treat essential hypertension (*see* sympatholytic). It is administered by mouth; side-effects include stuffiness of the nose, diarrhoea, nausea, headache, lethargy, and depression. Trade name: **Harmonyl**.

去甲氧利血平 治療特發性高血壓的降壓藥。口服。副作用爲鼻塞、腹瀉、噁心、頭痛、嗜眠及抑鬱。

desferrioxamine *n.* a drug that combines with iron in body tissues and fluids and is used to treat iron poisoning (including that resulting from prolonged or constant blood transfusion, as for thalassaemia), diseases involving iron storage in parts of the body (*see* haemochromatosis), and for the diagnosis of such diseases. It is administered by mouth, injection, or as eye drops; reactions and pain sometimes occur on injection. Trade name: **Desferal**.

去鐵銨 能與身體組織和體液內的鐵結合的藥物。用於鐵中毒（由於長時間或經常輸血所致，如治療地中海貧血時）和體內鐵蓄積的疾病（血色病）的治療和診斷。口服、注射或滴眼。注射有時可引起疼痛和全身不良反應。

desipramine *n.* a tricyclic *antidepressant drug administered by mouth or injection; common side-effects are dry mouth, blurred vision, insomnia, and

去甲丙咪嗪 三環結構的抗抑鬱藥。口服或注射。常見副作用爲口乾、視物模糊、失眠、步態不穩。

unsteadiness in walking. Trade name: **Pertofran**.

desmosome *n.* an area of contact between two adjacent cells, occurring particularly in epithelia. The cell membranes at a desmosome are thickened and fine fibres (*tonofibrils*) extend from the desmosome into the cytoplasm.

橋粒 兩個相鄰細胞（主要是上皮）間的接觸區。橋粒處細胞膜增厚，並有細纖維（張力原纖維）自橋粒發出進入細胞漿內。

desquamation *n.* the process in which the outer layer of the *epidermis of the skin is removed by scaling.

脫屑 皮膚外皮表層剝落的過程。

detached retina separation of the retina from the layer of the eyeball (choroid) to which it is attached. It commonly occurs when one or more holes in the retina allow fluid from the vitreous cavity of the eyeball to accumulate between the retina and choroid, which are only delicately attached. Sometimes the detachment is secondary to inflammation or tumour of the choroid or disorder of the vitreous humour. Vision is lost in the affected part of the retina. The condition can be treated surgically by creating patches of scar tissue between the retina and the choroid (by application of extreme heat or cold; *see* photocoagulation), which, combined with *plombage, stick it back into place.

視網膜脫落 眼內視網膜從所附着的脈絡膜上脫落。通常是視網膜上出現一個或幾個孔洞，眼球玻璃體腔內的液體經裂孔進入視網膜和脈絡膜之間（因兩者貼附不緊）並蓄積，遂導致視網膜脫落。有時脫落繼發於脈絡膜炎症、腫瘤或玻璃體病變。脫落的視網膜部分失去視力。可外科手術治療：用高溫或冷凍使視網膜和脈絡膜之間形成瘢痕黏連，亦可配合使用異物塡充。

detergent *n.* a synthetic cleansing agent that removes all impurities from a surface by reacting with grease and suspended particles, including bacteria and other microorganisms. Some detergents, e.g. *cetrimide, are used solely for cleansing; others may be used as *antiseptics and *disinfectants.

去垢劑 合成的清潔劑。可與含細菌及其他微生物的油脂和混懸粒子發生反應而將物體表面的污垢清除。有的去垢劑（如溴化十六烷基三甲銨）只用於清潔，有的則可用作抗菌劑和消毒劑。

detoxication (detoxification) *n.* the process whereby toxic substances are removed or toxic effects neutralized. It is one of the functions of the liver.

解毒 除去有毒物質或中和其毒性影響的過程。爲肝臟的功能之一。

detrition *n.* the process of wearing away solid bodies (e.g. bones) by friction or use.

磨耗 固體物（如骨）由於摩擦或使用而磨損的過程。

Dettol *n. see* chloroxylenol. **氯二甲酚**

detumescence *n.* **1.** the reverse of erection, whereby the erect penis or clitoris becomes flaccid after orgasm. **2.** subsidence of a swelling. ①**勃起消退** 性慾高潮過後陰莖或陰蒂變軟。 ②**消腫**。

deut- (deuto-, deuter(o)-) *prefix denoting* two, second, or secondary. 〔前綴〕 **二，第二，繼發**

deuteranopia *n.* a defect in colour vision in which reds, yellows, and greens are confused. It is thought that the mechanisms for perceiving red light and green light are in some way combined in people with this defect. *Compare* protanopia, tritanopia. *See also* colour blindness. **綠色盲** 紅、黃、綠色相混淆的色覺缺陷。一般認爲此種缺陷的患者，其分辨紅色光的機制與分辨綠色光的機制以某種方式結合在一起。

deutoplasm *n. see* yolk. **副漿**

deviance *n.* variation from normal behaviour beyond the limits acceptable to the majority of the conforming peer group; particularly (though not exclusively) applied to sexual habits (*see also* perversion). **乖僻** 行爲超出大多數相同階層人群可以接受的範圍。本詞主要（雖不是唯一）用於性習慣。

deviation *n.* (in ophthalmology) any abnormal position of one or both eyes. For example, if the eyes are both looking to one side when the head is facing forwards, they are said to be *deviated* to that side. Such deviations of both eyes may occur in brain disease. Deviations of one eye come into the category of squint (*see* strabismus). **偏斜** （眼科學）一眼或雙眼位置異常。例如，當面向前方時，如果雙眼都向一側注視，就稱爲向該側偏斜，見於腦疾患。一眼偏斜屬於斜視範疇。

Devic's disease *see* neuromyelitis optica. **視神經脳脊髓炎**

devitalization *n.* (in dentistry) removal of the pulp of a tooth. *See* root treatment. **殺髓** 牙科學用語。去除牙髓。

dexamethasone *n.* a *corticosteroid drug used principally to treat severe allergies, skin and eye diseases, rheumatic and other inflammatory conditions, and hormone and blood disorders. It is administered by mouth or injection; side-effects include sodium **地塞米松** 皮質類固醇類藥物。主要用於治療重症變應性疾病、皮膚病、眼病、風濕病及其他炎性疾病，以及內分泌病、血液病。口服或注射。副作用有水鹽瀦留、肌無力、抽

and fluid retention, muscle weakness, convulsions, vertigo, headache, and hormonal disturbances (including menstrual irregularities). Trade names: **Decadron, Oradexon**.

搐、暈眩、頭痛及內分泌失調（如月經失調）。

dexamphetamine *n.* a drug with actions and effects similar to those of *amphetamine. Trade names: **Dexamed, Dexedrine.**

右旋苯丙胺 作用和副作用均與苯丙胺相類似的藥物。

dextr- (dextro-) *prefix denoting* **1.** the right side. Example: *dextroposition* (displacement to the right). **2.** (in chemistry) dextrorotation.

〔前綴〕 ①**右** 例如：右移位。 ②**右旋**（化學）

dextran *n.* a carbohydrate, consisting of branched chains of glucose units, that is a storage product of bacteria and yeasts. Preparations of dextran solution are used in transfusions, to increase the volume of plasma.

葡聚糖，右旋糖酐 由枝鏈葡萄糖組成的碳水化合物。爲細菌和酵母的貯藏產物。右旋糖酐溶液製劑用於輸液以擴增血漿容積。

dextrin *n.* a carbohydrate formed as an intermediate product in the digestion of starch by the enzyme amylase. Dextrin is used in the preparation of pharmaceutical products (as an *excipient) and surgical dressings.

糊精 一種碳水化合物。爲澱粉酶消化澱粉過程的中間產物。用於製藥（作爲賦形劑）和外科敷料。

dextrocardia *n.* a congenital defect in which the position of the heart is a mirror image of its normal position, with the apex of the ventricles pointing to the right. It may be associated with other congenital defects and is often combined with *situs invertus*, in which the appendix and liver lie on the left side of the abdomen and the stomach lies on the right side. Isolated dextrocardia produces no adverse effects.

右位心 一種表現爲心臟位置與正常相反的先天性缺陷。心室尖部朝向右側。可與其它先天性缺陷同時存在，例如常與內臟轉位共存，其時闌尾和肝臟位於左腹部而胃居右位。單純右位心不產生有害影響。

dextromethorphan *n.* a drug used in lozenges, syrups, and linctuses to suppress coughs (*see* antitussive). It sometimes causes drowsiness, dizziness, and digestive upsets.

美沙芬 鎮咳藥。做成糖錠、糖漿和舔膏劑應用。有時可引起嗜眠、頭暈和消化紊亂。

dextromoramide *n.* an *analgesic used to relieve moderate or severe pain. It is given by mouth, injection, or as suppositories and sometimes causes

嗎散痛 鎮痛藥。用以解除中度或重度疼痛。口服、注射，或做成栓劑。有時可引起頭暈、血壓下

dizziness, reduced blood pressure, nausea, vomiting, and sleepiness. Dextromoramide is similar to *morphine and can cause morphine-type dependence. Trade name: **Palfium**.

降、噁心、嘔吐和瞌睡。與嗎啡一樣，可引起嗎啡型賴藥性。

dextropropoxyphene *n.* an *analgesic used to relieve mild or moderate pain. It is administered by mouth, often in combination with other analgesics, and sometimes causes dizziness, drowsiness, nausea, and vomiting.

右旋丙氧酚　止痛藥。用以解除輕度或中度疼痛。口服。常與其他止痛藥共用。有時可引起頭暈、嗜眠、噁心、嘔吐。

dextrose *n. see* glucose.

右旋糖

dextrothyroxine *n.* a *thyroid hormone used to reduce blood cholesterol levels in patients with normally working thyroid glands and also to treat hypothyroidism. It is administered by mouth and side-effects commonly involve chest pains due to angina.

右旋甲狀腺素　甲狀腺激素製劑。用以治療甲狀腺機能減退。對於甲狀腺機能正常的患者可降低血膽固醇水平。口服。常見副作用爲胸痛（由於心絞痛）。

dhobie itch a skin disease – a type of allergic *dermatitis – caused by clothes laundry-marked with ink used in India by native laundrymen (or women).

朶比癬　一種變應性皮炎型的皮膚病。見於印度。係由於當地洗衣婦用印度墨標記洗滌物所致。

di- *prefix denoting* two or double.

〔前綴〕　**二，雙**

dia- *prefix denoting* **1.** through. **2.** throughout or completely. **3.** apart.

〔前綴〕　**①通過　②貫穿，完全　③分開**

diabetes *n.* any disorder of metabolism causing excessive thirst and the production of large volumes of urine. Used alone, the term most commonly refers to *diabetes mellitus. *See also* diabetes insipidus, haemochromatosis (bronze diabetes). —**diabetic** *adj.*, *n.*

多尿症　以煩渴和多尿爲特徵的代謝疾病。單獨使用時多指糖尿病。

diabetes insipidus a rare metabolic disorder in which the patient produces large quantities of dilute urine and is constantly thirsty. It is due to deficiency of the pituitary hormone *vasopressin, which regulates reabsorption of water in the kidneys, and is treated by administration of the hormone.

尿崩症　一種少見的代謝病。患者排出大量低比重尿並持續口渴。係由於缺乏垂體後葉激素——加壓素（控制腎臟中水的重吸收）所致。治療：給與該種激素。

diabetes mellitus a disorder of carbohydrate metabolism in which sugars in the body are not oxidized to produce energy due to lack of the pancreatic

糖尿病　糖代謝疾病。由於缺乏胰腺激素——胰島素，體內的糖不能氧化產生能量。糖的蓄積導致糖

hormone *insulin. The accumulation of sugar leads to its appearance in the blood (*hyperglycaemia*), then in the urine; symptoms include thirst, loss of weight, and the excessive production of urine. The use of fats as an alternative source of energy leads to disturbances of the *acid-base balance, the accumulation of ketones in the bloodstream (*ketosis), and eventually to convulsions preceding *diabetic coma*. There appears to be an inherited tendency to diabetes; the disorder may be triggered by various factors, including physical stress. Diabetes that starts in childhood or adolescence is usually more severe than that beginning in middle or old age. Treatment is based on a carefully controlled diet, with adequate carbohydrate for the body's needs, together with injections of insulin or drugs (such as *tolbutamide) that are taken by mouth to lower blood-glucose levels. Lack of balance in the diet or in the amount of insulin taken leads to *hypoglycaemia. Long-term complications of diabetes include thickening of the arteries, which can affect the eyes (diabetic *retinopathy).

在血中出現（高血糖症）和隨後在尿中出現。症狀包括：口渴、體重減輕、大量排尿。由於轉而利用脂肪作爲能量來源，導致酸鹼平衡紊亂，血中酮體蓄積（酮症），最終發生抽搐以至糖尿病性昏迷。糖尿病似有遺傳傾向，可由各種因素（如體力緊張）誘發。始發於兒童和青年期的糖尿病，常較中老年糖尿病爲重。治療原則爲小心控制飲食，根據身體需要給於適量碳水化合物，同時注射胰島素或口服降血糖藥（如甲磺丁脲）。飲食失控或胰島素用量不當可引起低血糖症。糖尿病的遠期併發症有動脈變粗，後者可影響視力（糖尿病性視網膜病）。

diaclasia *n.* a fracture made deliberately by a surgeon to correct a deformity in a bone, which has usually resulted from a badly set or untreated fracture.

折骨術 外科醫生故意將骨折斷以矯正通常由於接骨不良或骨折未治所致的骨畸形。

diaclast *n.* a surgical instrument used for the destruction of the skull of a fetus. This rare procedure enables a dead fetus to be delivered through the birth canal.

穿顱器 用以破碎胎兒顱骨的外科器械。這種不常用的操作可使死胎通過產道而被娩出。

diagnosis *n.* the process of determining the nature of a disorder by considering the patient's *signs and *symptoms, medical background, and – when necessary – results of laboratory tests and X-ray examinations. *See also* differential diagnosis, prenatal diagnosis. *Compare* prognosis. —**diagnostic** *adj.*

診斷 通過對患者的症狀、體徵、醫學背景以及必要時包括化驗室和 X 綫檢查結果的分析而確定疾病本質的過程。

diakinesis *n.* the final stage in the first prophase of *meiosis, in which homologous chromosomes, between which crossing over has occurred, are ready to separate.

終變期 減數分裂前期第一時相的最後階段。其時已經發生交換的兩條同源染色體正準備分開。

dialyser *n.* a piece of apparatus for separating components of a liquid mixture by *dialysis, especially an artificial kidney (*see* haemodialysis).

透析器 藉透析作用將液體混合物中的組分分離的裝置。主要指人工腎。

dialysis *n.* a method of separating particles of different dimensions in a liquid mixture, using a thin semipermeable membrane whose pores are too small to allow the passage of large particles, such as proteins, but large enough to permit the passage of dissolved crystalline material. A solution of the mixture is separated from distilled water by the membrane; the solutes pass through the membrane into the water while the proteins, etc., are retained. The principle of dialysis is used in the artificial kidney (*see* haemodialysis).

透析 一種用薄半透膜將液體混合物中不同大小的粒子分離的方法。半透膜上的小孔只容許溶解的晶體物質通過，而蛋白質之類的大粒子則不能通過。用半透膜將混合物溶液與蒸餾水隔開，溶質通過膜進入水中，蛋白質等則被留下。人工腎即是應用透析的原理。

diamorphine *n. see* heroin.

海洛英

diamthazole *n.* a drug with antifungal activity used to treat skin infections such as athlete's foot and some types of ringworm. It is applied to the infected part as ointment, dusting powder, or tincture and sometimes causes irritation and hypersensitivity reactions.

雙胺噻唑 抗眞菌藥。用於治療脚癬和一些皮膚癬病感染。製成軟膏、撒粉或酊劑使用。有時可引起皮膚刺激和過敏反應。

diapedesis *n.* migration of cells through the walls of blood capillaries into the tissue spaces. Diapedesis is an important part of the reaction of tissues to injury (*see* inflammation).

血細胞滲出 細胞穿過毛細血管壁進入組織間隙的過程。爲損傷後組織反應的重要組成部分。

diaphoresis *n.* the process of sweating, especially excessive sweating. *See* sweat.

出汗 分泌汗液，尤其是大量分泌汗的過程。

diaphoretic (sudorific) *n.* a drug that causes an increase in sweating, such as *pilocarpine, which stimulates the sweat glands directly. *Antipyretic drugs also have diaphoretic activity,

發汗劑 引起出汗增加的藥物。如匹羅卡品直接刺激汗腺分泌。解熱藥也有發汗作用。在發熱時發汗有助於退熱。

which helps reduce the body temperature in fevers.

diaphragm *n.* **1.** (in anatomy) a thin musculomembranous dome-shaped muscle that separates the thoracic and abdominal cavities. The diaphragm is attached to the lower ribs at each side and to the breastbone and the backbone at the front and back. It bulges upwards against the heart and the lungs, arching over the stomach, liver, and spleen. There are openings in the diaphragm through which the oesophagus, blood vessels, and nerves pass. The diaphragm plays an important rôle in *breathing. It contracts with each inspiration, becoming flattened downwards and increasing the volume of the thoracic cavity. With each expiration it relaxes and is restored to its dome shape. **2.** a hemispherical rubber cap fitted inside the vagina over the neck of the womb as a contraceptive. When combined with the use of a chemical spermicide the diaphragm provides reliable contraception with a failure rate as low as 2–10 pregnancies per 100 woman-years.

①**膈肌** 爲分隔胸腔和腹腔的圓穹狀肌膜型薄肌。膈肌兩側附着於下位肋骨，前方和後方附着於胸骨和脊椎。向上方膨隆，抵着心和兩肺；圓穹下面包蓋胃、肝和脾。膈面有幾個裂孔，其間有食管、血管和神經通過。膈肌在呼吸中起重要作用。吸氣時，膈肌緊張，下降變爲扁平形，以增加胸腔容量。呼氣時，膈肌鬆弛，恢復圓穹形態。 ②**子宮帽** 橡膠製半球帽形避孕器具。放置於陰道內蓋着子宮頸部。子宮帽與殺精子化學藥物同用，其避孕失敗率低至 2～10 次妊娠/100婦女-年。

diaphysial aclasis a hereditary abnormality of cartilage and bone growth, resulting in many cartilaginous outgrowths (exostoses) from the long bones. Bone growth may also be retarded, causing stunting and deformity.

骨幹性續連症 一種遺傳性軟骨和骨生長異常。表現爲長骨上長出許多軟骨贅（外生軟骨疣）。骨生長也可停滯，以至發育不良和畸形。

diaphysis *n.* the shaft (central part) of a long bone. *Compare* epiphysis.

骨幹 長骨的中段部分。

diaphysitis *n.* inflammation of the diaphysis (shaft) of a bone, through infection or rheumatic disease. It may result in impaired growth of the bone and consequent deformity.

骨幹炎 感染或風濕病所致的骨幹炎症。可影響骨的生長而致骨畸形。

diarrhoea *n.* frequent bowel evacuation or the passage of abnormally soft or liquid faeces. It may be caused by intestinal infections, other forms of intestinal inflammation (such as *colitis

腹瀉 排便次數增多或排出異常的軟便或水樣便。原因可爲腸感染或其他類型的腸道炎症（如結腸炎、節段性回腸炎），吸

or *Crohn's disease), *malabsorption, anxiety, and the *irritable bowel syndrome. Severe or prolonged diarrhoea may lead to excess losses of fluid, salts, and nutrients in the faeces.

收障礙、焦慮症以及腸刺激綜合徵。嚴重腹瀉或長期腹瀉可導致水鹽和營養物質過度喪失。

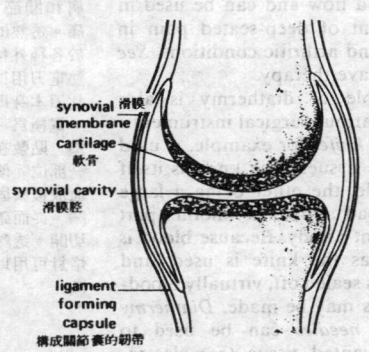

diarthrosis (synovial joint) *n.* a freely movable joint. The ends of the adjoining bones are covered with a thin cartilaginous sheet, and the bones are linked by a ligament (*capsule*) lined with *synovial membrane, which secretes synovial fluid (see illustration). Such joints are classified according to the type of connection between the bones and the type of movement allowed. *See* arthrodic joint, condylarthrosis, enarthrosis, ginglymus, saddle joint, trochoid joint.

動關節（滑囊關節） 可自由活動的關節。或關節的骨末端覆有一薄層軟骨，並藉韌帶（關節囊）而連接，囊內面襯有滑膜，分泌滑液。這類關節根據骨連接的類型及運動的型式而分類。

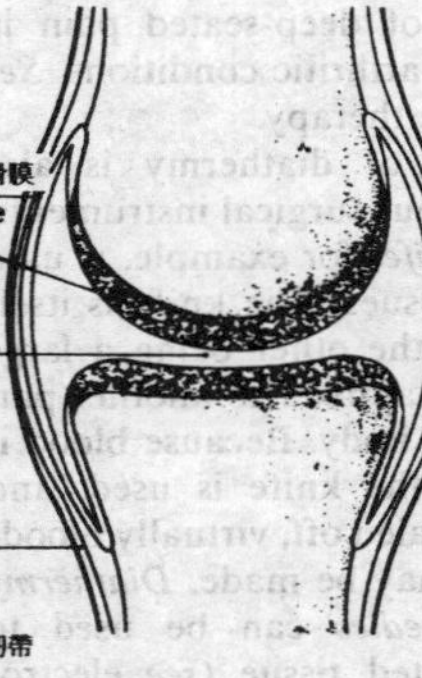

A synovial joint

動關節

diaschisis *n.* a temporary loss of reflex activity in the brainstem or spinal cord following destruction of the cerebral cortex. As time passes this state of suppressed reflex activity is replaced by one of unduly exaggerated reflexes and spasticity of the limbs.

神經機能聯系不能 大腦皮質破壞後發生的腦幹或脊髓反射性活動暫時喪失。經過一段時間，這種反射活動抑制狀態被反射性異常亢奮和肢體强直狀態所取代。

diastase *n.* an enzyme that hydrolyses starch in barley grain to produce maltose during the malting process. It has been used to aid the digestion of starch in some digestive disorders.

澱粉酶 製麥芽過程中將大麥粒中的澱粉水解爲麥芽糖的酶。在某些消化紊亂時用以幫助消化澱粉。

diastole *n.* the period between two contractions of the heart, when the muscle of the heart relaxes and allows the chambers to fill with blood. The term usually refers to *ventricular diastole*, which lasts about 0.5 seconds in a normal heart rate of about 70/minute. During exertion this period shortens, so allowing the heart rate to increase. *See also* blood pressure, systole. —**diastolic** *adj.*

舒張期 心臟兩次收縮之間的時期。此時心肌鬆弛，心腔爲血液所充盈。本詞一般指心室舒張期，在每分鐘70次的正常心律時約持續0.5秒。用力時舒張期縮短，使心率增加。

diastolic pressure *see* blood pressure.

舒張壓

diathermy *n.* the production of heat in a part of the body by means of a high-frequency electric current passed between two electrodes placed on the patient's skin. The heat generated increases blood flow and can be used in the treatment of deep-seated pain in rheumatic and arthritic conditions. *See also* microwave therapy.
The principle of diathermy is also utilized in various surgical instruments: a *diathermy knife*, for example, is used to coagulate tissues. The knife is itself one electrode, the other being a large moistened pad applied to another part of the patient's body. Because blood is coagulated as the knife is used, and small vessels sealed off, virtually bloodless incisions may be made. *Diathermy snares* and *needles* can be used to destroy unwanted tissue (*see* electrocautery).

透熱療法 在患者皮膚上放置兩個電極，通以高頻電流而在身體某部分產熱的治療方法。產生的熱使血流增加，用以治療風濕病和關節炎時的深部疼痛。透熱的原理還被應用於各種外科器械：例如透熱電刀用以使組織凝固。此刀本身即爲一電極，另一電極爲一大的浸濕的襯墊，貼敷在患者身體的另一部位。使用此刀，由於血液被凝固，小血管被封閉，從而確實地做到無血切開。透熱圈套器和透熱烙針可用以破壞無用的組織。

diathesis *n.* a higher than average tendency to acquire certain diseases, such as allergies, rheumatic diseases, or gout. Such diseases may run in families, but they are not inherited.

素質 比一般人易患某些疾病（變態反應性疾病、風濕病、痛風）的傾向。這類疾病可累及一些家庭成員，但不遺傳。

diazepam *n.* a *tranquillizer with *muscle-relaxant and *anticonvulsant properties, used to relieve anxiety and tension and in the treatment of epilepsy and muscular rheumatism. It is administered by mouth or injection; common side-effects are drowsiness and lethargy. Trade name: **Valium**.

安定 具有鬆弛肌肉和抗抽搐特性的安定藥。用於解除焦慮症和緊張症，治療癲癇和肌肉風濕。口服或注射。常見副作用爲困倦和嗜眠。

diazoxide *n.* a drug used to lower blood pressure in patients with hypertension and also used to treat conditions in which the levels of blood sugar are low (including *insulinoma). It is usually administered (by mouth or (for hypertension) injection) with a diuretic as it causes salt and water retention.

氯甲苯噻嗪 用於高血壓患者降血壓和治療血糖過低（如胰島素瘤）的藥物。口服或注射（降血壓）。因能引起水鹽豬留，須與利尿藥同用。

dibenzepin *n.* an *antidepressant drug administered by mouth. Common side-effects include dry mouth, blurred vision, constipation, sweating, drowsiness, and reduced blood pressure. Trade name: **Noveril**.

二苯氮䓬 口服抗抑鬱藥。常見副作用爲口乾、視物模糊、便秘、出汗、困倦和血壓下降。

dicephalus *n. see* craniopagus.

雙頭畸胎

dichloralphenazone *n.* a *sedative used to relieve pain, fever, and restlessness, mainly in children and elderly patients. It is administered by mouth and sometimes causes skin reactions, nausea, vomiting, and headache. It can also cause *dependence of the barbiturate-alcohol type. Trade names: **Paedo-Sed**, **Welldorm**.

二氯醛安替比林 鎮靜藥。具有鎮痛、解熱、消除不安的作用。主要用於兒童和老人。口服。有時可引起皮膚反應、噁心、嘔吐和頭痛。還可導致巴比妥、酒精型賴藥性。

dichlorophen *n.* an *anthelmintic drug used to treat human tapeworm infestation. It is administered by mouth and commonly causes abdominal pain and discomfort, diarrhoea, nausea, and vomiting. Trade name: **Anthiphen**.

雙氯酚 驅腸蟲藥。用於治療人體絛蟲感染。口服。常見副作用爲腹痛、腹部不適、腹瀉、噁心、嘔吐。

dichlorphenamide *n.* a *diuretic used to reduce pressure within the eye in the treatment of glaucoma. It is administered by mouth; side-effects include drowsiness, dizziness, digestive upsets, and skin rashes. Trade names: **Daranide**, **Oratrol**.

二氯苯二磺胺 利尿藥。用於降低眼壓，治療青光眼。口服。副作用爲困倦、頭暈、消化紊亂、皮疹。

dichromatic *adj.* describing the state of colour vision of those who can appreciate only two of the three primary colours. People with such vision match any given colour by a mixture of the two they can distinguish. *Compare* trichromatic.

二色視的 只能接受三原色中兩種原色的色覺異常。二色視者只能用他們能夠分辨的二原色來混合配色。

Dick test a test for susceptibility to *scarlet fever. If a small quantity of toxin from the bacteria responsible (haemolytic streptococci) is injected under the skin of a person not immune to the disease, a positive reaction results, causing local reddening of the skin.

狄克氏試驗 檢查猩紅熱易感性的試驗。將小量溶血性鏈球菌毒素注入對猩紅熱無免疫力的人的皮下，產生陽性反應——局部皮膚發紅。

dicophane *n. see* DDT.

二二三，滴滴涕

dicoumarol *n.* an *anticoagulant drug used in the treatment of coronary and venous thrombosis. It is administered by mouth and may cause nausea, vomiting, and diarrhoea. Dicoumarol has now largely been replaced in clinical use by *phenindione or *warfarin because it is slow acting, has unpredictable effects, and may produce bleeding from overdosage.

雙香豆素 抗凝血藥。用於治療冠狀動脈和靜脈血栓形成。口服。可引起噁心、嘔吐和腹瀉。由於起效慢，並可引起意外效應，過量可致出血，因而在目前臨床上已基本為苯茚二酮和華法令所代替。

dicrotism *n.* a condition in which the pulse is felt as a double beat for each contraction of the heart. It may be seen in typhoid fever. —**dicrotic** *adj.*

二波脉 在一次心臟收縮中能觸到兩次脉搏的現象。可見於腸傷寒。

dictyoma *n.* a tumour of the epithelium lining the *ciliary body of the eye. It may be benign or malignant.

視網膜胚瘤 眼睫狀體部的視網膜上皮的腫瘤。可為良性或惡性。

dicyclomine *n.* a drug that reduces spasms of smooth muscle and is used to relieve peptic ulcer, infantile colic, colitis, and related conditions. It is administered by mouth; side-effects include dry mouth, thirst, and dizziness. Trade name: **Merbentyl**.

雙環胺 減輕平滑肌痙攣的藥物。用於治療消化性潰瘍、嬰兒腹絞痛、結腸炎及有關疾病。口服。副作用為口乾、口渴、頭暈。

didym- (didymo-) *prefix denoting* the testis.

〔前綴〕 **睾丸**

dieldrin *n.* an insecticide that attacks the central nervous system of insects and has proved useful in the control of various beetles flies, and larvae that attack crops. Because of its toxic effects, there has been considerable anxiety over its widespread use in situations where food may be contaminated.

狄厄爾丁 殺蟲劑。作用於昆蟲中樞神經系統，用以殺滅各種甲蟲、蠅和危害穀物的昆蟲幼蟲。因有毒性，人們對其廣泛應用可能污染食物而焦慮不安。

diencephalon *n.* an anatomical division of the forebrain, consisting of the

間腦 前腦的一部分。由上丘腦、丘腦（背側丘

epithalamus, thalamus (dorsal thalamus), hypothalamus, and ventral thalamus (subthalamus). *See* brain.

腦）、下丘腦和丘腦底部（腹側丘腦）組成。

dienoestrol *n.* a synthetic female sex hormone (*see* oestrogen) administered by mouth to treat symptoms of the menopause, to suppress lactation, and to relieve symptoms in cancer of the breast or prostate. It is also applied as a cream to relieve itching or inflammation of the vagina and in acne. Trade name: **Hormofemin**.

己二烯雌酚 合成的雌性激素。口服。用於治療絕經期和斷乳症狀，亦用於減輕乳腺癌、前列腺癌症狀。製成乳膏劑還可減輕陰道搔癢或炎症及痤瘡。

diet *n.* the mixture of foods that a person eats. A *balanced diet* contains adequate quantities of all the *nutrients.

飲食 人吃的混合食物。所謂平衡的飲食含有適量的全部營養素。

dietary fibre (roughage) the part of food that cannot be digested and absorbed to produce energy. Dietary fibre falls into four groups: *cellulose*, *hemicelluloses*, *lignins*, and *pectins*. Highly refined foods, such as sucrose, contain no dietary fibre. Foods with a high fibre content include wholemeal cereals and flour, root vegetables, nuts, and fruit. Dietary fibre is considered by some to be helpful in the prevention of many of the diseases of Western civilization, such as *diverticulosis, constipation, appendicitis, obesity, and diabetes mellitus. Communities consuming high-fibre diets very rarely have any of these diseases.

食物纖維（粗糙食物） 食物中不能消化、吸收和產生能量的部分。食物纖維有四類：纖維素、半纖維素、木質素和果膠。高度精製的食物（如蔗糖）不含食物纖維。含纖維成分多的食物有：沒有去麩的粗面粉、根類蔬菜、果仁、水果。有人認爲，食物纖維有助於預防許多由西方文明帶來的疾病，諸如腸憩室病、便秘、闌尾炎、肥胖症、糖尿病等。在攝入食物纖維量大的地區，上述疾病相當少見。

dietetics *n.* the application of the principles of *nutrition to the selection of food and the feeding of individuals and groups.

飲食學 根據營養原理選擇食物爲個體或人群配食的科學。

diethylcarbamazine *n.* an anthelmintic drug that destroys filariae and is therefore used in the treatment of filariasis, loiasis, and onchocerciasis. It is administered as tablets. Side-effects may include headache, malaise, joint pains, nausea, and vomiting.

海羣生 驅腸蟲藥。有殺絲蟲作用，用於治療絲蟲病、羅阿絲蟲病和盤尾絲蟲病。製成片劑口服。副作用爲頭痛、不適、關節痛、噁心、嘔吐。

diethylpropion *n.* a drug, similar to *amphetamine, that suppresses the

二乙胺苯丙酮 一種與苯丙胺類似的藥物。具有抑

appetite and is used in the treatment of obesity. It is administered by mouth and may cause dry mouth, insomnia, depression, headache, constipation, and allergic rashes. Dependence of the amphetamine type can occur. Trade names: **Apesate, Tenuate**.

制食慾的作用，用於治療肥胖症。口服。副作用爲口乾、失眠、抑鬱、頭痛、便秘、變應性皮疹。可產生苯丙胺型賴藥性。

diethylstilboestrol *n.* a synthetic female sex hormone (*see* oestrogen) used to treat symptoms of the menopause, menstrual disorders, inflammation of the female genital organs, and cancer of the breast and prostate. It is administered by mouth or injection or as creams and pessaries; side-effects include loss of appetite, abdominal pain, and diarrhoea.

乙烯雌酚 合成的雌性激素。用於治療絕經期症狀、月經失調、女性生殖器炎症、乳腺癌和前列腺癌。

Dietl's crisis acute obstruction of a kidney causing severe pain in the loins. The obstruction usually occurs at the junction of the renal pelvis and the ureter, causing the kidney to become distended with accumulated urine (*see* hydronephrosis). Sometimes the pelvis drains spontaneously, with relief of pain, but acute decompression of the kidney may be required with surgical relief of the obstruction (*pyeloplasty).

狄特爾氏危象 引起腰部劇痛的一側急性腎梗阻。梗阻常發生於腎盂和輸尿管的接合部，腎盂因尿瀦留而擴張（腎積水）。有時梗阻可自行解除，疼痛隨之消失；但要達到腎臟迅速減壓，可能需要外科手術（腎盂成形術）解除梗阻。

differential diagnosis *diagnosis of a condition whose signs and/or symptoms are shared by various other conditions. For example, abdominal pain may be due to any of a large number of different disorders, which must be ruled out in arriving at a correct diagnosis.

鑑別診斷 對具有與其它疾病類似的症狀和/或體徵的疾病作出診斷。例如，許多不同的疾病都可有腹痛，爲達到正確診斷，必須將其他疾病予以排除。

differential leucocyte count (differential blood count) a determination of the proportions of the different kinds of white cells (leucocytes) present in a sample of blood. Usually 100 white cells are counted and classified under the microscope, so that the results can readily be expressed as percentages of the total number of leucocytes and the absolute numbers per litre of blood. The information often aids diagnosis of disease.

白細胞分類計數（血細胞分類計數） 確定血液標本中各種白細胞的比例。通常在顯微鏡下計數100個白細胞並進行分類，其結果可便捷地表示各型白細胞在總數中所佔的百分數以及每升血液中的白細胞絕對數。此項資料常有助於疾病診斷。

differentiation *n.* the process in embryonic development during which unspecialized cells or tissues become specialized for particular functions.

分化 胚胎發育中未分化的細胞或組織特化而具有特定功能的過程。

digestion *n.* the process in which ingested food is broken down in the alimentary canal into a form that can be absorbed and assimilated by the tissues of the body. Digestion includes mechanical processes, such as chewing, churning, and grinding food, as well as the chemical action of digestive enzymes and other substances (bile, acid, etc.). Chemical digestion begins in the mouth with the action of *saliva on food, but most of it takes place in the stomach and small intestine, where the food is subjected to *gastric juice, *pancreatic juice, and *succus entericus.

消化 攝入的食物在消化道內分解爲可被身體組織吸收和同化的物質的過程。消化包括咀嚼、攪拌、磨碎的機械加工和消化酶及其他物質（膽汁、胃酸等）的化學作用。化學消化始於口腔（唾液對食物的作用），主要在胃和小腸內進行，食物在胃和小腸內受到胃液、胰液和腸液的作用。

digitalis *n.* an extract from the dried leaves of foxgloves (*Digitalis* species), which contains various substances, including *digitoxin and *digoxin, that stimulate heart muscle. Used to treat heart failure, it is administered by mouth or, in emergency, by injection. High doses can cause nausea, vomiting, loss of appetite, diarrhoea, abdominal pain, and abnormal heart activity. *See also* digitalization.

洋地黃 乾毛地黃葉的提取物。含有洋地黃毒甙和地高辛等具有刺激心肌作用的成分。用於治療心力衰竭。口服，緊急時可注射。大劑量可引起噁心、嘔吐、食慾不振、腹瀉、腹痛和心律不齊。

digitalization *n.* the administration of the drug digitalis or one of its purified derivatives to a patient with heart failure until the optimum level has been reached in the heart tissues. At this stage the control of heart failure should be adequate and there should be few side-effects. The process of digitalization may take several days.

洋地黃化 給心力衰竭患者服用洋地黃或其純衍化物，使心肌組織內的藥物達到最適濃度。此時心力衰竭得到最佳控制而副作用又最小。有時須幾天才能達到洋地黃化。

digitoxin *n.* a drug that increases heart muscle contraction and is used in heart failure. It is slow-acting but the effects are prolonged. Digitoxin is administered by mouth or injection; side-effects are those of *digitalis.

洋地黃毒甙 使心肌收縮增强的藥物。用於治療心力衰竭。生效緩慢但作用能維持較長時間。口服或注射。副作用同洋地黃。

digoxin *n.* a drug that increases heart muscle contraction and is used in heart failure. It is rapidly effective and the effects are short-lived. Digoxin is administered by mouth or injection; side-effects are those of *digitalis.

地高辛 使心肌收縮力增强的藥物。用於治療心力衰竭。生效迅速但作用維持短暫。口服或注射。副作用同洋地黃。

dihydrallazine *n.* a drug used to lower blood pressure in moderate hypertension. It is administered by mouth, often in combination with reserpine or other hypotensive agents, since side-effects (fast heart rate, headache, loss of appetite, nausea, and vomiting) may be severe.

雙肼酞嗪 用於治療中度高血壓的降血壓藥。口服。常與利血平或其他降血壓藥聯合應用，以減輕其可能的嚴重副作用，如心率加快、頭痛、食慾不振、噁心、嘔吐。

dihydrocodeine *n.* a drug used to relieve pain and suppress coughs (*see* analgesic, antitussive). It is administered by mouth or injection and sometimes causes nausea, dizziness, and constipation. Dependence of the *morphine type can also occur, but this is rare.

雙氫可待因 鎮痛鎮咳藥。口服或注射。有時可引起噁心、頭暈、便秘。還可產生嗎啡型賴藥性，但較少見。

dihydroergotamine *n.* a derivative of *ergotamine used to prevent and relieve migraine attacks. It is administered by mouth or injection; side-effects are rare but nausea sometimes occurs.

雙氫麥角胺 一種麥角胺衍化物。用於預防和解除偏頭痛發作。口服或注射。副作用少，偶可有噁心。

diiodohydroxyquinoline *n.* an antiseptic used to treat bowel infections and dysentery. It is administered by mouth or as pessaries and occasionally causes irritation of the digestive system, headache, itching, and boils. Trade name: **Diodoquin**.

雙碘喹啉 抗感染藥。用於治療腸道感染和痢疾。口服或做成栓劑。偶可引起消化道刺激、頭痛、瘙癢和癤腫。

diiodotyrosine *n.* an iodine-containing substance produced in the thyroid gland from which the *thyroid hormones are derived.

二碘酪氨酸 甲狀腺產生的含碘物質，由之生成甲狀腺激素。

dilaceration *n.* a condition affecting some teeth after traumatic injury, in which the root and crown are at an abnormal angle to each other. It usually necessitates removal of the tooth.

彎曲牙 創傷所致的牙疾病，牙根與牙冠之間呈現異常的角度。一般需拔除患牙。

dilatation *n.* the enlargement or expansion of a hollow organ (such as a blood vessel) or cavity.

擴張 中空器官（如血管）或腔室的增大或擴張。

dilatation and curettage (D and C) an operation in which the neck of the womb is expanded, using an instrument called a *dilator, and the lining of the womb is peeled off with a curette (*see* curettage). It is performed for a variety of reasons, including the removal of any remaining material left after a miscarriage, remova! of cysts or tumours, and examination of the womb lining in the diagnosis of gynaecological disorders.

擴張刮除術 用擴張器擴張子宮頸管和用刮匙刮除子宮內膜的手術。用於流產後除去宮內殘留物、囊腫和腫瘤摘除，以及檢查子宮內膜作婦科疾病診斷用。

dilator *n.* **1.** an instrument used to enlarge a body opening or cavity. For example, the male urethra may become narrowed by disease and it can sometimes be restored to its original size by inserting a dilator. Dilators are also used to enlarge the canal in the neck of the womb in the procedure of *dilatation and curettage. **2.** a drug, applied either locally or systemically, that causes expansion of a structure, such as the pupil of the eye or a blood vessel. *See also* vasodilator. **3.** a muscle that, by its action, opens an aperture or orifice in the body.

①**擴張器** 用以擴張器官開口部或腔室。例如，男性尿道因病狹窄時，有時可插入擴張器使之恢復原來大小。在擴張刮除術中用擴張器擴張子宮頸管。②**擴張藥** 供局部或全身使用的可使眼瞳孔或血管之類結構擴大的藥物。③**開大肌** 使體內器官的開口部開大的肌肉。

diloxanide *n.* an antiseptic used to treat bowel infections. It is administered by mouth and occasionally causes vomiting, flatulence, itching, and skin rash.

安特醯胺 治療腸道感染的抗菌藥。口服。偶可引起嘔吐、氣脹、瘙癢和皮疹。

dimenhydrinate *n.* an *antihistamine used to prevent and treat travel sickness, nausea and vomiting due to other causes, vertigo, and inner ear disturbances. It is administered by mouth or injection and commonly causes drowsiness, dizziness, digestive upsets, dry mouth, and headache. Trade name: **Dramamine**.

乘暈寧 抗組胺藥。用於預防和治療暈車和其他原因所致的噁心、嘔吐、眩暈及內耳疾病。口服或注射。常見副作用爲困倦、頭暈、消化道不適、口乾、頭痛。

dimercaprol *n.* a drug that combines with metals in the body and is used to treat poisoning by antimony, arsenic, bismuth, gold, mercury, and thallium and in Wilson's disease. It is administered by injection and commonly

二巰基丙醇 一種能在體內與金屬結合的藥物。用於治療銻、砷、鉍、金、汞、鉈中毒及威爾遜氏病。注射。常見副作用爲噁心、嘔吐、流淚。

causes nausea, vomiting, and watering of the eyes. Trade name: **British Anti-Lewisite (BAL)**.

dimethisterone *n.* a synthetic female sex hormone (*see* progestogen) used to treat amenorrhoea and disorders of the lining of the womb and formerly used in sequential *oral contraceptives. It is administered by mouth; side-effects are abdominal pains, breast turgidity, nausea, and vertigo.

二甲炔睾酮 合成的雌性激素。用於治療閉經和子宮內膜異常。過去用作連續口服避孕藥。口服。副作用爲腹痛、乳房脹大、噁心、眩暈。

dimethothiazine *n.* an *antihistamine used to treat allergies such as hay fever. It is administered by mouth; side-effects include drowsiness, dry mouth, nausea, stomach pain, vertigo, diarrhoea, and mild headache. Trade name: **Banistyl**.

二甲噻嗪 用於治療枯草熱等變應性疾病的抗組胺藥。口服。副作用爲嗜眠、口乾、噁心、胃痛、眩暈、腹瀉、輕度頭痛。

dimethyl sulphoxide (DMSO) a chemical used in an ointment to treat skin inflammations or in combination with other topically applied drugs to improve their absorption. It may cause skin irritation.

二甲亞碸 一種化合物。可制成軟膏，用以治療皮膚炎症，或與其他外用藥聯合使用，以促進吸收。可引起皮膚刺激。

dimetria (uterus duplex, uterus didelphys) *n.* the condition of having a double womb.

雙子宮 長有一對子宮的畸形。

dioctyl sodium sulphosuccinate a softening agent that is given by mouth or in suppositories, often together with a laxative, to relieve constipation. It is also used in solution to soften ear wax.

磺琥辛酯鈉 軟化劑。口服或做成栓劑，常與輕瀉藥同用以解除便秘。也可製成溶液，軟化耳垢。

diodone *n.* an iodine-containing compound that is *radio-opaque and therefore useful in radiographic examination of parts of the body. Injected into the bloodstream, it is concentrated by the kidneys as it is excreted and forms a useful medium for showing up the urinary tract and any abnormalities that may be present (*see* pyelography).

碘吡啦啥 一種含碘造影劑。用於放射線檢查。注入血液後，在腎內集中。自腎內排出時，能使尿路和尿路中存在的各種異常顯影。

dioptre *n.* the unit of measurement of the power of *refraction of a lens. One dioptre is the power of a lens that brings parallel light rays to a focus at a point

屈光度 測量透鏡屈光能力的單位。一個屈光度是指透鏡使通過它的平行光綫在透鏡後 1 m 處聚焦的

one metre from the lens, after passing through it. A stronger lens brings light rays to a focus at a point closer to it than a weaker lens and is a higher number of dioptres in power.

能力。屈光力强的透鏡的光線聚焦點較屈光力弱的透鏡爲近，其屈光度數也較大。

dipeptidase *n.* an enzyme, found in digestive juices, that splits certain products of protein digestion (dipeptides) into their constituent amino acids. The latter are then absorbed by the body.

二肽酶　消化液内的一種酶。能使蛋白質消化產物（二肽）分解爲氨基酸。氨基酸遂被身體吸收。

dipeptide *n.* a compound consisting of two amino acids joined together by a peptide bond (e.g. glycylalanine, a combination of the amino acids glycine and alanine). *See* dipeptidase.

二肽　兩個氨基酸藉肽鍵結合成的化合物。例如甘氨酸和丙氨酸結合組成甘氨醯丙氨酸。

diphenhydramine *n.* an *antihistamine used to treat allergic conditions, such as hay fever and rhinitis, and in cough mixtures. It is administered by mouth or injection; side-effects include drowsiness, dry mouth, dizziness, and nausea. Trade name: **Benadryl**.

鹽酸苯海拉明　抗組胺藥。用於治療枯草熱、鼻炎等變應性疾病，也可作爲止咳合劑的成分。口服或注射。副作用爲嗜眠、口乾、頭暈、噁心。

diphenoxylate *n.* a drug used, often in combination with *atropine, to treat diarrhoea. It is also used after *colostomy or ileostomy to reduce the frequency and fluidity of the stools. It is administered by mouth; side-effects can include nausea, drowsiness, dizziness, skin reactions, and restlessness.

氰苯哌酯　常與阿托品同用的止瀉藥。在結腸造口術或回腸造口術後常用以減少排便次數和使大便變乾。口服。副作用有嗜眠、頭暈、皮膚反應和不安。

diphtheria *n.* an acute highly contagious infection, caused by the bacterium *Corynebacterium diphtheriae*, generally affecting the throat but occasionally other mucous membranes and the skin. The disease is spread by direct contact with a patient or carrier or by contaminated milk. After an incubation period of 2–6 days a sore throat, weakness, and mild fever develop. Later, a soft grey membrane forms across the throat, constricting the air passages and causing difficulty in breathing and swallowing; a *tracheostomy may be necessary. Bacteria multiply at the site of infection and release a toxin into the bloodstream, which damages heart and

白喉　由白喉棒狀桿菌引起的急性接觸性傳染病。傳染性極高。通常侵犯咽喉，偶爾侵犯其它黏膜和皮膚。疾病通常是與患者或帶菌者直接接觸引起，亦可通過污染的乳汁傳播。經過2～6天的潛伏期後，出現咽喉痛、虛弱、輕度發熱。稍後，咽喉出現灰色軟膜，阻礙空氣通過，引起呼吸和吞嚥困難，以致需行氣管切開術。細菌在感染部位繁殖，並向血內釋放毒素，對心臟和神經造成危害。可在4天内因心力衰竭或

nerves. Death from heart failure or general collapse can follow within four days but prompt administration of antitoxin and penicillin arrests the disease; complete recovery requires prolonged bed rest. An effective immunization programme has now made diphtheria rare in most Western countries (*see also* Schick test).

全身虛脫而死亡。及時應用抗毒素和青黴素可控制疾病，經長時間臥床可完全恢復。由於推行有效的計劃免疫，白喉在多數西方國家已屬罕見。

diphtheroid *adj.* resembling diphtheria (especially the membrane formed in diphtheria) or the bacteria that cause it.

類白喉的 與白喉（主要指白喉時形成的假膜）或白喉桿菌類似的。

diphyllobothriasis *n.* an infestation of the intestine with the broad tapeworm, **Diphyllobothrium latum*, which sometimes causes nausea, malnutrition, diarrhoea, and anaemia resulting from impaired absorption of vitamin B_{12} through the gut. The infestation, common in Baltic countries, is contracted following ingestion of uncooked fish infected with the larval stage of the tapeworm. The tapeworm can be expelled from the gut with the anthelmintic *mepacrine.

裂頭絛蟲病 由闊節裂頭絛蟲引起的腸道感染。可有噁心、營養不良、腹瀉和貧血（由於腸內維生素B_{12}吸收障礙）等表現。在波羅的海沿岸國家多見。係由於生食受裂頭絛蟲幼蟲感染的魚肉所致。可用驅腸蟲藥阿的平驅蟲。

Diphyllobothrium *n.* a genus of large tapeworms that can grow to a length of 3–10 m. The adult of *D. latum*, the broad (or fish) tapeworm, infects fish-eating mammals including man, in whom it may cause serious anaemia (*see* diphyllobothriasis). The parasite has two intermediate hosts: a freshwater crustacean and a fish (*see also* plerocercoid).

裂頭絛蟲屬 一屬可生長達3～10m長的巨大絛蟲。闊節裂頭絛蟲成蟲感染食魚的哺乳動物，包括人類，引起嚴重貧血。有兩個中間宿主：淡水甲殼類和魚類。

dipipanone *n.* a potent *analgesic drug used to relieve severe pain. It is administered by mouth or injection and may cause nausea, vomiting, dizziness, and drowsiness.

二苯哌己酮 强效鎮痛藥。用以解除劇痛。口服或注射。可引起噁心、嘔吐、頭暈和嗜眠。

dipl- (diplo-) *prefix denoting* double.

〔前綴〕 **雙倍**

diplacusis *n.* perception of a single sound as double owing to a defect of the *cochlea in the inner ear.

複聽 內耳耳蝸缺陷所致將單聲感知爲雙聲的現象。

diplegia *n.* paralysis involving both sides of the body and affecting the legs more severely than the arms. *Cerebral diplegia* is a form of *cerebral palsy in which there is widespread damage, in both cerebral hemispheres, of the brain cells that control the movements of the limbs. —**diplegic** *adj.*

兩側癱　身體兩側癱瘓。腿重於臂。大腦性兩側癱是指大腦兩半球控制肢體運動的腦細胞遭受廣泛損害所致的一種大腦性痲痹。

diplococcus *n.* any of a group of nonmotile parasitic spherical bacteria that occur in pairs. The group includes the *pneumococcus.

雙球菌　成對存在、沒有運動能力的寄生性球形細菌，例如肺炎雙球菌。

diploë *n.* the lattice-like tissue that lies between the inner and outer layers of the *skull.

板障　顱骨內板、外板之間的網格狀組織。

diploid *adj.* describing cells, nuclei, or organisms in which each chromosome except the Y sex chromosome is represented twice. *Compare* haploid, triploid. —**diploid** *n.*

二倍體的　指除 Y 性染色體外每條染色體均成雙存在的細胞、細胞核或機體。

diplopia *n.* double vision: the simultaneous awareness of two images of the one object. It is usually due to a disturbance in the coordinated movements of the muscles that move the eyeball, and covering one eye will abolish it. A very slight degree of doubling, which does not disappear when one eye is covered, may be experienced by introspective people. This is *uniocular diplopia*, and only in the rarest cases is there any abnormality of the eye.

複視　看一個物體時同時產生兩個物像。通常由於眼球運動肌的協調運動失調所致。遮蓋一眼可消除複視。有內省心理傾向的人可體驗到一種即使遮蓋一眼也無法消除的極輕微的複視。這種現象稱爲單眼複視。只有極少數病例具有眼的異常。

diplotene *n.* the fourth stage in the first prophase of *meiosis, in which *crossing over occurs between the paired chromatids of homologous chromosomes, which then begin to separate.

雙線期　減數分裂前期中的第四階段。同源染色體的成對染色單體發生交換，然後開始分離。

diprophylline *n.* a drug that relaxes bronchial muscle and stimulates heart muscle. It is used to relieve symptoms in asthma and bronchitis and to treat congestive heart failure. It is adminis-

二羥丙茶鹼　鬆弛支氣管壁肌、興奮心肌藥物。用於支氣管炎時解除哮喘症狀和治療心力衰竭。口服、注射或製成栓劑使

tered by mouth, injection, or in suppositories and may cause nausea and vomiting, headache, palpitations, and dizziness, especially following injection. *See also* bronchodilator. Trade names: **Neutraphylline**, **Silbephylline**.

用。注射後可引起噁心、嘔吐、頭痛、心悸、頭暈。

diprosopus *n.* a fetal monster with a single trunk and normal limbs but with some degree of duplication of the face.

雙面畸胎　一種不能存活的畸胎。有軀幹和正常的四肢，但面部不同程度地分裂爲二。

dipsomania *n.* morbid and insatiable craving for alcohol, occurring in paroxysms. Only a small proportion of alcoholics show this symptom. *See* alcoholism.

間發性酒狂　以發作形式出現的對酒精的病態的不可控制的渴望。嗜酒者僅少數顯示此種症狀。

Diptera *n.* a large group of insects, including *mosquitoes, gnats, midges, house flies and *tsetse flies, that possess a single pair of wings. The mouthparts of many species, e.g. mosquitoes and tsetse flies, are specialized for sucking blood; these forms are important in the transmission of disease (*see* vector). *See also* fly.

雙翅目　一大目昆蟲，包括只有一對翅膀的蚊、蚋、蠓、家蠅和彩彩蠅。其中許多種（如蚊、彩彩蠅）的口器特化而能吸血，因而在傳播疾病上具有重要作用。

Dipylidium *n.* a genus of tapeworms. *D. caninum*, a common parasite of the small intestine of dogs and cats, occasionally infects man but usually produces no obvious symptoms. Fleas are the intermediate hosts, and children in close contact with pets become infected on ingesting fleas harbouring the parasite.

複孔絛蟲屬　絛蟲中的一屬。犬複孔絛蟲是狗、猫的常見小腸寄生蟲，偶也侵襲人，但通常不產生明顯症狀。蚤爲中間宿主。當兒童與狗、猫密切接觸時，可能將帶寄生蟲的蚤吞入而被感染。

dipyridamole *n.* a drug that dilates the blood vessels of the heart. It is used to treat reduced heart activity and is given by mouth or injection. It may cause headache, stomach upsets, and dizziness.

潘生丁　擴張心臟血管藥。用於治療心臟功能低下。口服或注射。可引起頭痛、胃部不適和頭暈。

director *n.* an instrument used to guide the extent and direction of a surgical incision.

探針　外科切開時用以引導方向和測量深度的器械。

dis- *prefix denoting* separation.

〔前綴〕　**分離**

disability *n. see* handicap.

殘疾

Disabled Living Foundation (in Britain) a voluntary agency interested in all aspects of the care of those with *handicaps and in improving their quality of life. It is particularly concerned with aids to daily living, which can be inspected by clients, doctors, and others at a permanent exhibition at the headquarters of the Foundation.

殘疾人生活基金會 英國的從事對殘疾人全面照顧和改善他們生活的志願機構。該機構特別關心殘疾人的日常生活，並由委託人、醫生及基金會總部常設機構的其他人員予以督導。

disabled person *see* Employment Service Division.

殘疾人

disaccharide *n.* a carbohydrate consisting of two linked *monosaccharide units. The most common disaccharides are *maltose, *lactose, and *sucrose.

二糖 由兩個單糖單位連結而成的碳水化合物。

disarticulation *n.* separation of two bones at a joint. This may be the result of an injury or it may be done by the surgeon at operation in the course of amputation; for example of a limb, finger, or toe.

關節離斷 在關節部位將兩骨分離。可爲外傷的結果，亦可由外科醫生在截斷術（如截斷肢體、指、趾）中施行。

disc *n.* (in anatomy) a rounded flattened structure, such as an *intervertebral disc or the *optic disc.

盤 解剖學用語。扁圓形結構。例如椎間盤、視神經盤。

discharge rate the number of cases of a specified disease discharged from hospitals related to the population of the *catchment area: usually expressed regionally per 10,000.

出院率 某種疾病出院例數與聚居地區人口之比。通常以每10000人口表示。

discission *n.* an operation for cataract in which the front of the lens capsule is cut extensively by a fine knife or needle inserted through the edge of the cornea. Subsequently the lens is absorbed naturally into the surrounding fluid of the eye. It is usually necessary to perform *capsulotomy later.

內障刺開術 一種內障手術。用一小刀在晶狀體囊前面切一大口或用細針自角膜緣插入眼內，隨後晶狀體在房水內自然吸收。但以後仍常須作晶狀體囊摘除術。

disease *n.* a disorder with a specific cause and recognizable signs and symptoms; any bodily abnormality or failure to function properly, except that resulting directly from physical injury (the latter, however, may open the way for disease).

疾病 由特殊原因引起並具有可識別的症狀和體徵的異常狀態。包括一切軀體畸形與器官功能障礙。但直接物理損傷所致的障礙不包括在內（而後者却可爲疾病開闢道路）。

disimpaction *n.* the process of separating the broken ends of a bone when

嵌插分離 將骨折時在强力作用下嵌插在一起的骨

they have been forcibly driven together during a fracture. *Traction may be required to keep the bone ends separate but in good alignment.

折端分離的過程。可用牽引方法使斷端在正確的對位綫上保持分離。

disinfectant *n.* an agent that destroys or removes bacteria and other microorganisms and is used to cleanse surgical instruments and other objects. Examples are *cresol, *hexachlorophane, and *phenol. Dilute solutions of some disinfectants may be used as *antiseptics or as preservatives in solutions of eye drops or injections.

消毒劑 殺滅或除去細菌及其他微生物的藥劑。用於清潔手術器械及其他物品。例如煤酚、雙三氯酚和苯酚。某些消毒劑的稀釋液可用作抗菌劑、滴眼液或注射液中的防腐劑。

disinfection *n.* the process of eliminating infective microorganisms from contaminated instruments, clothing, or surroundings by using physical means or chemicals (*disinfectants).

消毒 用物理方法或化學劑（消毒劑）消滅被污染的器械、衣被或環境中的致病微生物的過程。

disinfestation *n.* the destruction of insect pests and other animal parasites. This generally involves the use of insecticides applied either topically, as in delousing, or as a spray for eliminating an infestation of fleas or bed bugs in the home.

殺滅病媒法 殺滅致病昆蟲及其他動物寄生蟲。通常是使用殺蟲劑。局部用以滅蝨，室內噴灑用以消滅跳蚤和臭蟲。

disintegrative psychosis *see* Heller's syndrome.

分裂性精神病

disjunction *n.* the separation of pairs of homologous chromosomes during meiosis or of the chromatids of a chromosome during *anaphase of mitosis or meiosis. *Compare* nondisjunction.

分離 減數分裂時同源染色體對的分離過程。或指有絲分裂或減數分裂後期一條染色體的染色單體的分離過程。

dislocation (luxation) *n.* displacement from their normal position of bones meeting at a joint. Dislocation of the shoulder is common in sports injuries, and congenital abnormalities may lead to repeated dislocations of the hip. The bones are restored to their normal positions by manipulation, which may require local or general anaesthesia (*see* reduction). *Compare* subluxation.

脫位 骨在關節部位離開正常位置。肩關節脫位常見於運動損傷，髖關節反復脫位則可爲先天性畸形所致。脫位的骨可藉手法恢復正常位置。但有時須在局部麻醉或全身麻醉下進行。

dismemberment *n.* the amputation of a leg, arm, or part of a limb.

截斷術 截斷腿、臂或肢體的一部分。

disoma *n.* a double-bodied fetal monster with a single head.

雙軀幹畸胎 一頭雙身畸胎。

disopyramide *n.* a *parasympatholytic drug used to treat various heart conditions involving abnormal heart rates. It is administered by mouth; side-effects such as dry mouth, blurred vision, difficulty in urination, and digestive upsets may occur. Trade names: **Norpace**, **Rythmodan**.

雙異丙吡胺 擬副交感藥。用以治療心律紊亂等各種心臟病症。口服。副作用為口乾、視物模糊、排尿困難，還可有消化道不適。

disorientation *n.* the state produced by loss of awareness of space, time, or personality. It can be the result of drugs, anxiety, or organic disease (such as dementia or *Korsakoff's syndrome).

定向力障礙 對空間、時間或人物喪失感知能力的狀態。可由藥物、焦慮症或器質性疾病（如痴呆或柯爾薩可夫氏綜合徵）引起。

dispensary *n.* a place where medicines are made up by a pharmacist according to the doctor's prescription and dispensed to patients. A dispensary is often part of an out-patient department in a hospital.

藥房 藥劑師按醫生處方為患者配製藥劑的場所。通常為醫院門診部的一部分。

displacement *n.* (in psychology) the substitution of one type of behaviour for another, usually the substitution of a relatively harmless activity for a harmful one; for example, kicking the cat instead of one's boss.

替代 心理學用語。用一種行為類型替代另一種類型。通常以較無害的行動替代有害的行動。例如，用踢貓來代替踢老板的行動。

dissection *n.* the cutting apart and separation of the body tissues along the natural divisions of the organs and different tissues in the course of an operation. Dissection of corpses is carried out for the study of anatomy.

解剖 沿着器官或不同組織間的自然分界將身體組織予以切開或分離的手術。學習解剖學要進行屍體解剖。

disseminated *adj.* widely distributed in an organ (or organs) or in the whole body. The term may refer to disease organisms or to pathological changes.

播散的 廣泛分佈於一個或多個器官以至全身的。本詞可用於描述患病機體或病理學改變。

disseminated sclerosis *see* multiple sclerosis.

播散性硬化

dissociation *n.* (in psychiatry) the process whereby thoughts and ideas can be split off from consciousness and may function independently, thus (for example) allowing conflicting opinions

分裂 精神病學用語。觀點、念頭離開意識而獨立活動。例如在同一時刻對同一客體可持有互相矛盾的觀點。分裂可為癔症性

to be held at the same time about the same object. Dissociation may be the main factor in cases of hysterical *fugue and multiple personalities.

神游和多重人格的主要因素。

distal *adj.* **1.** (in anatomy) situated away from the origin or point of attachment or from the median line of the body. For example, the term is applied to a part of a limb that is furthest from the body; to a blood vessel that is far from the heart; and to a nerve fibre that is far from the central nervous system. *Compare* proximal. **2.** (in dentistry) describing the surface of a tooth away from the midline of the jaw.

①**遠側的** （解剖學）指位於附着部（或點）遠側的或身體中線遠側的。例如，距軀幹較遠的肢體部分，遠離心臟的血管，遠離中樞神經系統的神經纖維。 ②**遠中的** （牙科學）指頜中線遠側的牙面。

distichiasis *n.* a very rare condition in which there is an extra row of eyelashes behind the normal ones. They may rub on the cornea.

雙行睫 正常眼睫毛後面又長出一排睫毛的現象。極罕見。可以造成角膜擦傷。

District Health Authority *see* National Health Service.

地段保健

District Management Team *see* National Health Service.

地段管理班子

District Medical Committee *see* medical committee.

地段醫學委員會

District Medical Officer (DMO) *see* community physician.

地段主管醫師

district nurse *see* home nurse.

地段護士

District Planning Team a multidisciplinary group of doctors, nurses, and others established in a health district to identify gaps in the services and to suggest how they can be improved. Outside agencies (e.g. *social services) are included when appropriate. Some teams are permanent (e.g. those dealing with the elderly and mentally sick); others are established on an *ad hoc* basis.

地段保健工作組 由保健地段內醫生、護士等人員組成的多科性工作組。任務爲查證醫療服務工作中的疏漏並提出改進建議。條件許可時應設置外勤機構（如社會服務）。有的工作組爲常設的（如從事老年和精神病業務的），其他則是爲特定任務而建立的。

disulfiram *n.* a drug used in the treatment of chronic alcoholism. It acts as a deterrent by producing unpleasant effects when taken with alcohol, including flushing, breathing difficulties,

雙硫醒 治療慢性酒精中毒藥物。與酒精同服，可引起顏面潮紅、呼吸困難、頭痛、心悸、噁心、嘔吐等不良反應，因而起

headache, palpitations, nausea, and vomiting. It is administered by mouth; common side-effects are fatigue, nausea, and constipation. Trade name: **Antabuse**.

威攝物的作用。口服。副作用爲疲乏、噁心和便秘。

dithiazanine *n.* an *anthelmintic drug used to treat certain worm infestations. It is administered by mouth and stains the stools bluish-green. Other side-effects include nausea, vomiting, diarrhoea, fluid retention, and fever.

噻唑青胺 驅腸蟲藥。用於治療某些蠕蟲感染。口服。可使大便染成藍綠色。其它副作用有噁心、嘔吐、腹瀉、水豬留、發熱。

dithranol *n.* a drug applied to the skin as an ointment or paste to treat ringworm infections, psoriasis, and other skin conditions. It may irritate the skin on application.

1,8,9-蒽三酚 皮膚外用藥。用其糊劑與軟膏劑治療眞菌感染、銀屑病及其他皮膚病。可引起皮膚刺激。

diuresis *n.* increased secretion of urine by the kidneys. This normally follows the drinking of more fluid than the body requires, but it can be stimulated by the administration of a *diuretic.

利尿 腎臟泌尿增加。正常飲入水量超過身體需要時便發生利尿。也可用利尿藥引起利尿。

diuretic *n.* a drug that increases the volume of urine produced by promoting the excretion of salts and water from the kidney. Examples are the *thiazide diuretics* (e.g. *chlorothiazide and *chlorthalidone), *frusemide, *spironolactone, and *triamterene. Diuretics are used to reduce the oedema due to salt and water retention in disorders of the heart, kidneys, liver, or lungs. Some mild diuretics, including *acetazolamide, are used to reduce the pressure within the eyeball in glaucoma. Diuretics are also used – in conjunction with other drugs – in the treatment of high blood pressure. Treatment with thiazide diuretics often results in potassium deficiency; this is corrected by simultaneous administration of potassium salts.

利尿藥 通過促進腎臟排鹽和水而增加尿量的藥物。代表藥物有噻嗪類（如氯噻嗪、氯噻酮）、速尿、安體舒通和氨苯喋啶。用以減輕心、腎、肝、肺疾病時水、鹽豬留所致的水腫。有些輕利尿藥（如乙醯唑胺）用於青光眼時降低眼內壓，還可與其他藥物聯合應用治療高血壓。使用噻嗪類利尿藥常引起鉀不足，因而需要同時給鉀鹽以矯正。

divagation *n.* rambling discursive thought and speech. It is not specific to any one psychiatric condition.

語無倫次 思維和言語凌亂無序。這種現象並非任何一種精神疾病所特有。

divaricator *n.* a scissor-like surgical instrument used to divide portions of

分離器 手術中用以分離組織的剪刀樣器械。

tissue into two separate parts during an operation.

diverticular disease a condition in which there are diverticula (*see* diverticulum) in the colon associated with lower abdominal pain and disturbed bowel habit. The pain is due to spasm of the muscles of the intestine and not to inflammation of the diverticula (*compare* diverticulitis).

憩室病 結腸憩室併有下腹痛和大便習慣紊亂的病症。疼痛起於腸肌痙攣而非憩室炎症。

diverticulitis *n.* inflammation of a *diverticulum, most commonly of one or more colonic diverticula. This type of diverticulitis is caused by infection and causes lower abdominal pain with diarrhoea or constipation; it may lead to abscess formation, which often requires surgical drainage. A Meckel's diverticulum sometimes becomes inflamed due to infection, causing symptoms similar to *appendicitis. Diverticula elsewhere in the alimentary tract are not subject to diverticulitis. *Compare* diverticular disease.

憩室炎 結腸憩室（常爲一個或多個）的炎症。係由細菌感染所致，可引起下腹痛、腹瀉或便秘。炎症進展形成膿腫時需外科引流。美克爾氏憩室炎有時可產生類似闌尾炎的症狀。消化道其他部位的憩室不發炎。

diverticulosis *n.* a condition in which diverticula exist in a segment of the intestine without evidence of inflammation (*compare* diverticulitis).

腸憩室病 腸管某節段存在多個無炎性憩室。

diverticulum *n.* (*pl.* **diverticula**) a sac or pouch formed at weak points in the walls of the alimentary tract. They may be caused by increased pressure from within (*pulsion diverticula*) or by pulling from without (*traction diverticula*). A *pharyngeal diverticulum* occurs in the pharynx and may cause difficulty in swallowing. *Oesophageal diverticula* occur in the middle or lower oesophagus (gullet); they may be associated with muscular disorders of the oesophagus but rarely cause symptoms. *Gastric diverticula* affect the stomach (usually the upper part) and cause no symptoms. *Duodenal diverticula* occur on the concave surface of the duodenal loop; they may be associated with *dyspepsia

憩室 在消化道管壁薄弱部分形成的囊或袋。可由於內壓增加或外部牽拉而發生，前者稱推壓性憩室，後者稱牽引性憩室。咽部發生的咽憩室可引起吞嚥困難。食管中部或下部發生的食管憩室可併發於食管肌的病變，但少有症狀。胃憩室多見於胃上部，亦無症狀。十二指腸憩室發生於十二指腸曲的凹面，可合併消化不良，但通常少有症狀。空腸憩室常爲多發性，當細菌在內繁殖時可引起腹部不適和吸收障礙。美克爾氏憩室爲先天性異常，發生於廻

but usually cause few symptoms. *Jejunal diverticula* affect the small intestine, are often multiple, and may give rise to abdominal discomfort and *malabsorption due to growth of bacteria within them. *Meckel's diverticulum* occurs in the ileum, about 35 cm from its termination, as a congenital abnormality. It may become inflamed, mimicking *appendicitis; if it contains embryonic remnants of stomach mucosa it may form a *peptic ulcer, causing pain, bleeding, or perforation. *Colonic diverticula*, affecting the colon (particularly the lowest portion), become commoner with increasing age and often cause no symptoms. However they are sometimes associated with abdominal pain or altered bowel habit (*see* diverticular disease) or they may become inflamed (*see* diverticulitis).

腸距末端約35cm處，發炎時很像闌尾炎。如該憩室內含有胃黏膜胚胎殘留物，會產生消化性潰瘍而有疼痛、出血以至穿孔。結腸（特別是下段）憩室隨年齡增長而增多，但常無症狀，有時可伴發腹痛和大便習慣改變，也可發炎。

division *n.* the separation of an organ or tissue into parts by surgery.

分割 手術中將器官或組織切割成幾塊。

divulsor *n.* a surgical instrument used to dilate forcibly any canal or cavity, usually the urethra.

擴張器 施加壓力使管道、腔室（常爲尿道）擴張的外科器械。

dizygotic twins *see* twins.

二卵雙胎

DNA (deoxyribonucleic acid) the genetic material of nearly all living organisms, which controls heredity and is located in the cell nucleus (*see* chromosome, gene). DNA is a *nucleic acid composed of two strands made up of units called *nucleotides (see illustration). The two strands are wound around each other into a double helix and linked together by hydrogen bonds between the bases of the nucleotides (*see* base pairing). The genetic information of the DNA is contained in the sequence of bases along the molecule (*see* genetic code); changes in the DNA cause *mutations. The DNA molecule

脫氧核糖核酸（DNA） 爲幾乎一切活機體所含有、位於細胞核內、控制遺傳性的遺傳物質。是由兩條核苷酸鏈構成的核酸（見圖）。兩條鏈相互纏繞呈雙螺旋結構，藉核苷酸鹼基之間的氫鍵連結在一起。DNA的遺傳信息包含在分子的鹼基順序中。DNA的改變引起突變。DNA分子通過複製過程準確無誤地生產出自已的複本，當細胞分裂時將遺傳信息傳遞給子代細胞。

can make exact copies of itself by the process of *replication, thereby passing on the genetic information to the daughter cells when the cell divides.

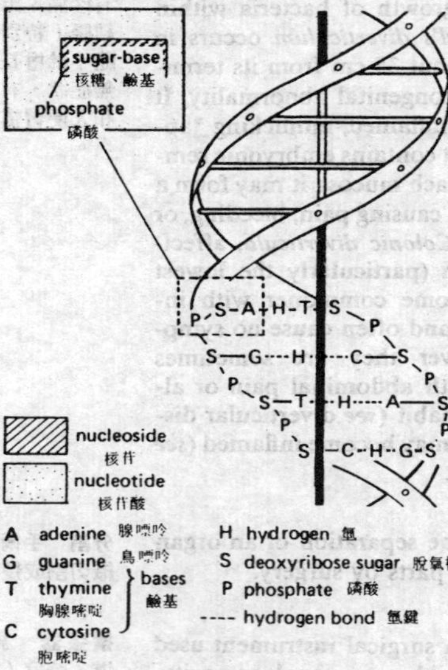

Structure of part of a DNA molecule

DNA 分子的部分結構

Doctor *n.* **1.** the title given to a recipient of a higher university degree than a Master's degree. The degree *Medicinae Doctor* (MD) is awarded by some British universities as a research degree. In the US the degree is awarded on qualification. **2.** a courtesy title given to a qualified medical practitioner, i.e. one who has been registered by the General Medical Council (GMC). Most doctors in the UK obtain bachelors' degrees in medicine and surgery (MB, BS) or the diplomas of the conjoint boards of the Royal College of Physicians and the Royal College of Surgeons (LRCP, MRCS): these degrees or diplomas and one year's hospital experience are required by the

①**博士** 高於碩士的大學學位的稱號。醫學博士（MD）學位在英國某些大學是作為一種研究成果的等級而授予的。在美國學位則是一種資格獎勵。②**醫師** 對獲得行醫資格者的（即在全國醫學委員會註册的）尊稱。在英國大多數醫師須獲得內科和外科學士學位，或持有皇家內科醫師學會和皇家外科醫師學會聯合理事會的文憑。而且要在醫院實習一年，方可在全國醫學委員會註册為醫生。正常情況下，註册前必須在指定的醫院的普通科中擔任過兩

GMC before they will register a person as a doctor. Normally it is compulsory to hold two full-time *preregistration appointments* in general subjects at hospitals recognized for this purpose. The doctor has the title *house physician* (or *surgeon*), *resident*, or *intern* and is debarred from independent practice. Surgeons in the UK do not use the title Doctor and are referred to, as a mark of distinction, as Mr. In the US qualified dentists and pharmacists also use the courtesy title Doctor. *See also* consultant.

個科的專職職務。僅具有內科病房或外科病房醫生、低年住院醫生、實習醫生稱號的醫生，不能獨立行醫。在英國外科醫生不用 Doctor 稱呼，而用 Mr. 以資區別。在美國獲得資格的牙科醫生和藥劑師也稱爲 Doctor。

dolich- (dolicho-) *prefix denoting* long. Example: *dolichocolon* (abnormally long colon).

〔前綴〕 **長的** 例如長結腸（結腸過長）。

dolichocephaly *n.* the condition of having a relatively long skull, with a *cephalic index of 75 or less. —**dolichocephalic** *adj.*

長頭 頭圍指數小於75的頭顱偏長的狀態。

dolor *n.* pain: one of the classical signs of inflammation in a tissue, the other three being *calor (heat), *rubor (redness), and *tumor (swelling). The pain in inflammation is thought to be due to the release of chemicals from damaged cells.

痛 組織發炎的典型現象之一。炎症的其他三項體徵爲熱、紅和腫。人們認爲，炎症疼痛係受損細胞釋放某些化學物質的結果。

dolorimetry *n.* the measurement of pain. *See* algesimeter.

測痛法 測量疼痛程度的方法。

domiciliary midwife (in Britain) a State Registered Nurse with special training in midwifery (both hospital and domiciliary practice). She must be registered with the Central Midwives' Board in order to practise; this requires regular refresher courses to supplement the basic qualification of *State Certified Midwife* (*SCM*). Planned home deliveries are comparatively rare, the work of domiciliary midwives is mainly concerned with antenatal and postnatal care, especially in those discharged 48 hours or less after delivery, and in some cases conducting deliveries in community hospitals.

家庭助產士 在英國受過助產專業訓練（醫院和家庭接生）的國家註册的護士。家庭助產士須在助產士全國理事會註册方可從業。助產士定期學習知識更新課程，以此作爲對國家合格助產士基本資格的補充措施。家庭助產士進行有計劃的家庭接生的機會不多，主要是做產前和產後（特別是產後48小時內）護理。她們有時是在產院內接生。

domiciliary services (in Britain) health and social services that are available in the home and are distinguished from hospital-based services. They include the services of such personnel as community nurses employed by Area Health Authorities (*see* home nurse, domiciliary midwife, health visitor) and social workers, home helps, and bath attendants employed by social service departments of local authorities. Also included are services such as meals on wheels, loan equipment for home care, and ambulatory aids. The term *community services* is also applied to these services, but strictly speaking, hospitals and other residential institutes should be included under the latter heading.

家庭服務 在英國家庭裏能得到的保健和社會服務，這種服務與醫院服務不同。工作人員包括行政區僱用的公共保健護士，當地社會服務部門僱用的工作人員、家庭服務員、助浴員。服務內容還包括車送飯食、租賃家庭護理用具以及流動服務等。所謂公共保健服務一詞也可用於上述服務，但嚴格論之，應包括醫院及其他收容患者的機構。

dominant *adj.* (in genetics) describing a gene (or its corresponding characteristic) whose effect is shown in the individual whether its *allele is the same or different. If the allele is different it is described as *recessive* and its effect is masked. —**dominant** *n.*

顯性的 遺傳學用語。指基因（或者相應特徵）的影響在等位基因相同或不同的個體中顯示出來。如果等位基因不相同，則稱爲隱性的，其影響被遮蔽。

domiphen *n.* an *antiseptic administered in the form of lozenges to treat bacterial and fungal infections of the mouth and throat. It is also used in solution for cleansing wounds and burns, for treating fungal infections of the skin, and for general disinfection of skin and mucous membranes.

杜米芬 抗菌藥。做成糖錠劑，用以治療口腔和咽喉的細菌性和眞菌性感染。其溶液可用於清潔創口和燒傷，治療皮膚眞菌感染以及一般的皮膚、黏膜消毒。

donor *n.* a person who makes his own tissues or organs available for use by someone else. For example, a donor may provide blood for transfusion (*see* blood donor) or a kidney for transplantation.

供者 提供自身器官或組織爲他人使用的人。例如，供者可提供血液用於輸血或提供腎臟用於移植。

dopa *n.* dihydroxyphenylalanine: a physiologically important compound that forms an intermediate stage in the synthesis of catecholamines (dopamine, adrenaline, and noradrenaline) from the essential amino acid tyrosine. It also plays a role itself in the functioning of

多巴 二羥苯丙氨酸。具有重要生理作用的化合物，係自必需氨基酸酪氨酸合成兒茶酚胺（多巴胺、腎上腺素、去甲腎上腺素）過程中的中間產物。還在大腦某些部分的

certain parts of the brain. The form *L-dopa* is administered for the treatment of *parkinsonism, a disease in which there is a deficiency of dopamine in the brain.

機能中發揮作用。左旋多巴用於治療大腦帕金森氏病——大腦內多巴胺缺陷的疾病。

dopamine *n.* a *catecholamine derived from dopa that is an intermediate in the synthesis of noradrenaline. It is found in high concentrations in the adrenal medulla and is also in the brain, in the caudate nucleus (*see* basal ganglia), where it may function as a *neurotransmitter.

多巴胺 多巴（去甲腎上腺素合成過程中的中間產物）的一種兒茶酚胺衍化物。以很高濃度存在於腎上腺髓質，並存在於大腦尾狀核，具有神經遞質的功能。

dopamine hypothesis the theory that schizophrenia is caused in part by abnormalities in the metabolism of *dopamine and can be treated in part by drugs (such as *chlorpromazine) that antagonize its action as a neurotransmitter.

多巴胺假說 本學說認爲，精神分裂症的發生，部分原因是由於多巴胺代謝異常，因而可用對抗其神經遞質作用的藥物（如氯丙嗪）作爲治療的一部分。

dors- (dorsi-, dorso-) *prefix denoting* **1.** the back. Example: *dorsalgia* (pain in). **2.** dorsal.

〔前綴〕 ①**背** 例如背痛。 ②**背側的**

dorsal *adj.* relating to or situated at or close to the back of the body or to the posterior part of an organ.

背側的 位於或鄰近身體背部（或器官後部）的。

dorsiflexion *n.* backward flexion of the foot or hand or their digits; i.e. bending towards the upper surface.

背屈 手、腳或指、趾向背側屈曲，亦即彎向上表面。

dorsoventral *adj.* (in anatomy) extending from the back (dorsal) surface to the front (ventral) surface.

背腹側的 解剖學用語。指從後（背）側表面向前（腹）側表面延伸。

dorsum *n.* **1.** the back. **2.** the upper or posterior surface of a part of the body; for example, of the hand. *See also* dorsal.

①**背** ②背面身體某部分的上或後表面。例如手背。

dose *n.* a carefully measured quantity of a drug that is prescribed by a doctor to be given to a patient at any one time. The *median effective dose* (*ED_{50}*) is the dose of a drug that produces desired effects in 50% of individuals tested. *See also* LD_{50}.

劑量 醫生給患者開出的處方中經仔細稱量過的一次藥物量。半數有效量（ED_{50}）是指使50%受試者產生預期效果的藥物劑量。

dosimeter *n.* a device to record the amount of radiation received by work-

放射量計 記錄接觸X射綫或其它輻射的工作人員

ers with X-rays or other radiation, usually consisting of a small piece of photographic film in a holder attached to the clothing. At regular intervals the film is examined to discover the amount of radiation it (and therefore the wearer) have received.

接受輻射量的儀器。通常由一個內裝感光膠片的可掛在衣服上的小盒組成。每隔一定時間檢查膠片，以確定其（即佩帶者）輻射接受量。

dosimetry *n.* the calculation of appropriate doses for given conditions, usually the calculation of correct amounts of radiation for the treatment of cancer in different parts of the body. *See* radiotherapy.

劑量測定 計算特定條件下的適合劑量的方法。通常是計算治療身體不同部位腫瘤所需的正確輻射量。

double-bind *n.* a disordered pattern of family relationships in which one family member gives contradictory instructions to another (as when a mother asks her child verbally for affection but simultaneously, by her gestures, indicates that the child should remain distant). The result is that any action the child makes will be wrong, and furthermore he cannot escape from the situation. This has been supposed, but not proved, to be a factor in causing schizophrenia.

矛盾性牽制 一種異常型式的家庭關係。表現爲一個家庭成員對另一成員發出矛盾的指示。例如母親口說要孩子表示親近，但同時却用手勢指示孩子保持距離，其結果是，孩子的任何行動都是錯的，而且他還不能逃避這種狀況。人們曾推測這是引起精神分裂症的一個因素，但未能證實。

double-blind trial *see* intervention study.

雙盲試驗

double vision *see* diplopia.

複視

douche *n.* a forceful jet of water used for cleaning any part of the body, most commonly the vagina. A vaginal douche is extremely unreliable as a method of contraception.

冲洗 以加壓噴頭噴水清潔身體某部分（最常爲陰道）。將陰道冲洗作爲避孕措施是極不可靠的。

Down's syndrome a form of mental subnormality due to a chromosome defect (there are three no. 21 chromosomes instead of the usual two). The main physical features are a slightly oblique slant to the eyes, as in the Mongolian races (hence the former name of this condition – *mongolism*); a round head; flat nasal bridge; fissured tongue; abnormalities of the palms, including single transverse creases and characteristic dermal ridges; small

先天愚型綜合徵 一種由於染色體缺陷（21號染色體有3條，而正常時爲2條）而發生的智力低下。主要體檢所見爲：兩眼輕度斜視，圓形顱，扁鼻樑，舌面有溝紋，手掌有單一貫通紋（通關掌）和特徵性皮嵴，耳朵小圓或多結節，身材矮小。許多上述特徵在出生時即已存在，因而早期即可診斷；

round or knotty ears; and short stature. Many of these features are present at birth, enabling an early diagnosis; the condition can also be diagnosed prenatally, by *amniocentesis. The ultimate mental attainment is about that of a five-year-old child, i.e. an IQ of 50–60. Rare partial forms of Down's syndrome occur with a slightly higher IQ (*see* mosaicism). Medical name: **trisomy 21**.

還可用羊膜腔穿刺在出生前作出診斷。智力最高可達5歲兒童水平，即智商僅爲50～60。醫學名稱：21-三體。

doxepin *n.* a drug used to relieve depression, especially when associated with anxiety (*see* antidepressant, tranquillizer). It is administered by mouth; side-effects can include drowsiness, dry mouth, blurred vision, and digestive upsets. Trade name: **Sinequan.**

多慮平 消除抑鬱症（尤其在合併焦慮症時）的藥物。口服。副作用爲嗜眠、口乾、視物模糊、消化道不適。

doxorubicin *n.* an *anthracycline antibiotic isolated from *Streptomyces peucetius caesius* and used mainly in the treatment of leukaemia and various other forms of cancer. Doxorubicin acts by interfering with the production of DNA and RNA (*see also* antimetabolite). It is administered by injection or infusion; side-effects include bone marrow depression, baldness, gastrointestinal disturbances, and heart damage. Trade name: **Adriamycin**.

亞德利亞黴素 由波賽青灰鏈黴菌分離得到的蒽環類抗生素。主要用於治療白血病和各種癌瘤。其作用爲干擾 DNA 和 RNA 合成。注射或輸注。副作用爲骨髓抑制、脫髮、胃腸道紊亂及心臟損害。

doxycycline *n.* an *antibiotic used to treat infections caused by a wide range of bacteria and other microorganisms. It is administered by mouth and side-effects are those of the other *tetracyclines. Trade name: **Vibramycin**.

强力霉素 用於治療細菌和其它微生物感染的廣譜抗生素。口服。副作用同四環素類。

DPT vaccine a combined *vaccine against diphtheria, whooping-cough, and tetanus organisms, prepared from their *toxoids and other antigens.

白百破疫苗 抗白喉、百日咳和破傷風病原體的三聯疫苗。係用上述微生物的類毒素和其他抗原製備。

drachm *n.* **1.** a unit of weight used in pharmacy. 1 drachm = 3.883 g (60 grains). **2.** a unit of volume used in pharmacy. 1 fluid drachm = 3.696 ml (1/8 fluid ounce).

打蘭 ①藥用重量單位。1打蘭＝3.883克（60格令）。②藥用容量單位。1液量打蘭＝3.696毫升（⅛液量盎斯）。

dracontiasis *n.* a tropical disease caused by the parasitic nematode *Dracunculus medinensis* (*see* guinea worm) in the tissues beneath the skin. The disease is transmitted to man via contaminated drinking water. The initial symptoms, which appear a year after infection, result from the migration of the worm to the skin surface and include itching, giddiness, difficulty in breathing, vomiting, and diarrhoea. Later a large blister forms on the skin, usually on the legs or arms, which eventually bursts and may ulcerate and become infected. Dracontiasis is common in India and West Africa but also occurs in Arabia, Iran, East Africa, and Afghanistan. Treatment involves killing the adult worms with injections of phenolthiazine.

麥地那龍線蟲病 由於麥地那龍線蟲寄生於皮下淺組織所致的熱帶病。通過飲用污染水而感染。於感染後一年出現初始症狀，係因線蟲向皮膚表面移行而引起，包括瘙癢、頭暈、呼吸困難、嘔吐和腹瀉。以後皮膚（常爲腿、臂）上出現大疱，破裂後形成潰瘍並可發生感染。本病多見於印度和西非，在阿拉伯、伊朗、東非和阿富汗亦有發生。治療：注射酚噻嗪以殺滅成蟲。

Dracunculus *n. see* guinea worm.

龍線蟲屬

dragee *n.* a *pill that has been coated with sugar.

糖衣丸 外包糖衣的藥丸。

drain 1. *n.* a device, usually a tube or wick, used to draw fluid from an internal body cavity to the surface. A drain is sometimes inserted during an operation to ensure that any fluid formed immediately passes to the surface, so preventing an accumulation that may become infected or cause pressure in the operation site. **2.** *vb. see* drainage.

①引流物 用以將體內腔隙內液體引向體表的器具。通常爲一條管子或紗布條。手術中有時插入引流物以確保生成的液體迅即被引出體外，從而避免蓄積造成感染或壓迫手術部位。 **②引流**

drainage *n.* the drawing off of fluid from a cavity in the body, usually fluid that has accumulated abnormally. For example, serous fluid may be drained from a swollen joint, pus removed from an internal abscess, or urine from an overdistended bladder. *See also* drain.

引流 從體內腔隙內引出液體（通常爲異常蓄積的液體）。例如，從腫脹的關節腔內可引流出漿液性液體，從深處膿腫內引出膿液，從脹滿的膀胱內引流尿液。

drastic *n.* any agent causing a major change in a body system or function, e.g. strong laxatives.

峻烈藥 任何使機體系統或功能發生顯著改變的藥劑。例如峻瀉劑。

draw-sheet *n.* a sheet placed beneath a patient in bed that, when one portion has been soiled or become uncomfortably wrinkled, may be pulled under the

墊單 鋪在床上與患者身體相貼的單子。當其一部分沾污或起褶使患者不適時，可從患者身下抽出，

patient so that another portion may be used. The bed does not have to be remade, and the patient does not have to leave bed.

而其它部分仍可使用。不須重新舖床，患者也不須離床。

drepanocyte (sickle cell) *n. see* sickle-cell disease.

鐮刀狀細胞

drepanocytosis *n. see* sickle-cell disease.

鐮刀狀細胞增多症

dressing *n.* material applied to a wound or diseased part of the body, with or without medication, to give protection and assist healing.

敷料 貼敷於創口或身體患病部位的物質。含或不含藥物。用以保護局部，促進恢復。

drill *n.* (in dentistry) a rotary instrument used to remove tooth substance, particularly in the treatment of caries. It consists of a handpiece that takes variously shaped *burs. Most drilling is done with an air-driven turbine handpiece, but some is performed with a much slower mechanically driven handpiece. Drills usually have a water-spray coolant.

牙鑽 一種轉動的牙科器械，用以除去牙質，主要用於治療齲病。由可裝各種形狀的鑽頭的握柄構成。最常用的是氣動渦輪牙鑽，但有時也用轉速較低的機械驅動牙鑽操作。牙鑽通常帶有噴水冷却裝置。

drip (intravenous drip) *n.* apparatus for the continuous injection (*transfusion) of blood, plasma, saline, glucose solution, or other fluid into a vein. The fluid flows under gravity from a suspended bottle through a tube ending in a hollow needle inserted into the patient's vein. The rate of flow can be adjusted according to the rate of drips seen in a transparent section of the tube, which also serves as a trap for bubbles.

輸注器（靜脉輸注器） 供連續靜脉內輸注血液、血漿、鹽水葡萄糖溶液或其它液體的裝置。液體在重力作用下從懸瓶通過管子經末端的中空針頭流入患者靜脉內。液流速度可根據觀察玻璃滴管內的液滴速度予以調節。滴管還可用以排除氣泡。

drom- (dromo-) *prefix denoting* movement or speed.

〔前綴〕 **運動，速度**

dromomania *n.* a pathologically strong impulse to travel, which is said to be present in some vagabonds.

漂泊癖 病態的想要旅行的强烈衝動。據認爲存在於某些流浪者中。

dropsy *n. see* oedema.

水腫

Drosophila *n.* a genus of very small flies, commonly called fruit flies, that breed in decaying fruit and vegetables. *D. melanogaster* has been extensively used in genetic research as it has only

果蠅屬 一屬很小的蠅。因在腐爛水果和蔬菜中繁殖而得名。果蠅曾廣泛用於遺傳學研究，因其只有4對染色體，並且其唾液

four pairs of chromosomes and those in its salivary glands are easily recognizable. Adult *D. repleta* sometimes feed on faecal matter and may transmit disease organisms.

腺的染色體易於辨認。果蠅成蟲有時食取糞便渣滓，因而可以傳播病原體。

drostanolone *n.* a synthetic male sex hormone (*see* androgen) used in the treatment of breast cancer, often in conjunction with other drug treatment or surgery. It is administered by injection and with prolonged use may cause such side-effects as growth of hair and deepening of the voice. Trade name: **Masteril**.

甲雄烷酮 合成的雄性激素。用於治療乳腺癌，常與其它藥物或手術聯合應用。注射。長期應用可發生體毛生長和嗓音低沉等副作用。

drug *n.* any substance that affects the structure or functioning of a living organism. Drugs are widely used for the prevention, diagnosis, and treatment of disease and for the relief of symptoms. The term *medicine* is sometimes preferred for therapeutic drugs in order to distinguish them from narcotics and other addictive drugs that are used illegally.

藥物 任何能影響活機體結構和功能的物質。藥物廣泛用於疾病的預防、診斷和治療以及解除症狀。藥物一詞有時主要指治療用藥物，區別於麻醉藥和其他非法應用的成癮性藥。

drug dependence *see* dependence.

賴藥性

dry socket a painful condition in which the normal healing of a tooth socket has been disturbed. Instead of being filled with a blood clot the socket is empty. The cause is not clear; treatment is palliative and the condition resolves in 10–14 days.

乾槽症 一種疼痛性牙病。牙槽的正常修復過程遭受破壞。牙槽內除血凝塊外沒有其他物質。原因不明。採取姑息治療，症狀經10～14日可解除。

Duchenne dystrophy *see* muscular dystrophy.

杜興氏肌營養不良症

duct *n.* a tubelike structure or channel, especially one for carrying glandular secretions.

管，導管 管樣結構或管道。主要指輸送腺體分泌物的管道。

ductless gland *see* endocrine gland.

無管腺

ductule *n.* a small duct or channel.

小管 小導管或小管道。

ductus *n.* a duct. The *ductus deferens* is the *vas deferens.

管，導管 例如輸精管。

ductus arteriosus a blood vessel in the fetus connecting the pulmonary artery directly to the ascending aorta,

動脉導管 胚胎期直接連通肺動脉和升主動脉，使血液繞過肺循環的血管。

so bypassing the pulmonary circulation. It normally closes after birth. Failure of the ductus to close (*patent ductus arteriosus*) produces a continuous *murmur, and the consequences are similar to those of a *septal defect. It may close spontaneously in childhood but often requires surgical closure.

正常在出生後關閉。動脉導管未閉（動脉導管開放）產生持續的雜音，其後果與房室間隔缺損相同。在兒童期有時可自然關閉，但多數須作外科手術。

dumbness *n. see* mutism.

啞

Dumdum fever *see* kala-azar.

黑熱病

dumping syndrome a group of symptoms that sometimes occur after stomach operations, particularly *gastrectomy. After a meal, especially one rich in carbohydrate, the patient feels faint and weak and may sweat and become pale. The attack lasts 30 minutes to two hours and is caused by rapid stomach emptying, leading to falls in blood sugar and the drawing of fluid from the blood into the intestine. Avoidance of carbohydrate meals may relieve the syndrome but further surgery is sometimes required.

傾倒綜合徵 胃手術（主要是胃切除）後有時發生的一組症狀。飯後（特別是進食碳水化合物豐富的食物）患者感覺虛弱無力，出汗，臉色蒼白。發作持續約30分鐘至2小時。原因爲胃內容排空過快，引起血糖降低和血中的水分被吸收到小腸內。廻避進食碳水化合物可解除此症，但有時須作外科手術。

duo- *prefix denoting* two.

〔前綴〕 **兩，二**

duoden- (duodeno-) *prefix denoting* the duodenum. Example: *duodenectomy* (excision of).

〔前綴〕 **十二指腸** 例如十二指腸切除術。

duodenal ulcer an ulcer in the duodenum, caused by the action of acid and pepsin on the duodenal lining (mucosa) of a susceptible individual. It is usually associated with an increased output of stomach acid and affects people with blood group O more commonly than others. Symptoms include pain in the upper abdomen, especially when the stomach is empty, which often disappears completely for weeks or months; vomiting may occur. Complications include bleeding, *perforation, and obstruction due to scarring. Symptoms are relieved by antacid med-

十二指腸潰瘍 十二指腸內的潰瘍。有體質性致病的傾向。係由胃酸和胃蛋白酶作用於十二指腸黏膜所致。通常同時有胃酸分泌過多。較多侵犯O型血型者。症狀有上腹痛（尤具是胃內空虛時），疼痛常可完全消失數周至數月。可有嘔吐。併發症有出血、穿孔，當有瘢痕收縮時可發生梗阻。給予制酸藥降低胃酸可使症狀緩解，有時須作手術以求根治。

icines or reduction of stomach acid; surgery is sometimes required for a permanent cure (*see* gastrectomy, vagotomy).

duodenoscope *n.* a *fibrescope for examining the interior of the duodenum. An end-viewing instrument is used for most examinations, but a side-viewing instrument is used for *ERCP.

十二指腸鏡 用於檢查十二指腸內腔的纖維窺鏡。多數檢查使用前視式窺鏡。

duodenostomy *n.* an operation in which the duodenum is brought through the abdominal wall and opened, usually in order to introduce food. *See also* gastroduodenostomy.

十二指腸造口術 引導十二指腸穿過腹壁向外開放以便灌注食物的手術。

duodenum *n.* the first of the three parts of the small *intestine. It extends from the pylorus of the stomach to the jejunum. The duodenum receives bile from the gall bladder (via the common bile duct) and pancreatic juice from the pancreas. Its wall contains various glands (including *Brunner's glands*) that secrete *succus entericus. —**duodenal** *adj.*

十二指腸 小腸三部分的第一部分。上接胃幽門，向下延伸到空腸。十二指腸接受來自膽囊（經過膽總管）的膽汁和來自胰腺的胰液。腸壁內含有分泌腸液的各種腺體（如勃倫納氏腺）。

Dupuytren's contracture forward curvature of one or more fingers (usually the third and/or fourth) due to fixation of the flexor tendon of the affected finger to the skin of the palm. The condition is treated by surgical *division of the fibrous bands joining tendon and skin.

杜普伊特倫氏攣縮 一指或多指（通常爲第三和/或第四指）由於其屈肌腱與手掌癒着而發生向前彎曲。治療：手術分離連接肌腱與皮膚的纖維索。

dura (dura mater, pachymeninx) *n.* the thickest and outermost of the three *meninges surrounding the brain and spinal cord. It consists of two closely adherent layers, the outer of which is identical with the periosteum of the skull. The inner dura extends downwards between the cerebral hemispheres to form the *falx cerebri* and forwards between the cerebrum and cerebellum to form the *tentorium*. A thin film of fluid (not cerebrospinal fluid) separates the inner dura from the arachnoid.

硬（腦脊）膜 包繞腦和脊髓的三層腦（脊）膜中最外面和最厚的一層。由相互緊密黏着的兩層組成。外層就是顱骨的骨膜。內層在大腦兩半球之間下延形成大腦鐮，在大腦和小腦之間向前延伸形成小腦幕。硬膜內層與蛛網膜之間有一薄層液體（不是腦脊液）相隔。

dural *adj.* of, relating to, or affecting the *dura.

硬（腦脊）膜的

dwarfism *n.* abnormally short stature from any cause. The most common type of dwarf is the *achondroplastic dwarf* (*see* achondroplasia). *Pituitary dwarfs* have a deficiency of *growth hormone due to a defect in the pituitary gland; they are well proportioned and show no mental retardation, but may be sexually underdeveloped. *Primordial dwarfs* have a genetic defect in their response to growth hormone. Dwarfism is also associated with thyroid deficiency (*see* cretinism), in which both physical and mental development is retarded; chronic diseases such as rickets; renal failure; and intestinal malabsorption.

侏儒 各種原因所致的身材異常矮小。最常見的類型是軟骨發育不全性侏儒。垂體性侏儒係垂體後葉缺陷以致生長激素分泌不足所致，這種侏儒身體各部勻稱，無智力發育停滯，但性發育不良。先天性侏儒其管理生長激素的基因有缺陷。侏儒還可與下述疾病併存：甲狀腺機能低下，此時智力和體格發育均停滯；佝僂病，腎功能衰竭和腸吸收障礙等慢性疾病。

dydrogesterone *n.* a synthetic female sex hormone (*see* progestogen) used to treat menstrual abnormalities (such as dysmenorrhoea) and infertility and to prevent miscarriage. It is administered by mouth and may cause mild nausea and breakthrough bleeding. Trade name: **Duphaston**.

6-去氫逆孕酮 合成的雌性激素。用於治療月經失調（如痛經）、不育症以及預防流產。口服。可引起輕度噁心和突發性出血。

dynamometer *n.* a device for recording the force of a muscular contraction. A small hand-held dynamometer may be used to record the strength of a patient's grip. A special optical dynamometer measures the action of the muscles controlling the shape of the lens of the eye.

肌力計 記錄肌肉收縮力量的儀器。一種小型手握式肌力計可測定患者的握力。另一種光學肌力計則可測量調節眼晶狀體形狀的肌肉的活動。

dyne *n.* a unit of force equal to the force required to impart to a mass of 1 gram an acceleration of 1 centimetre per second per second. 1 dyne = 10^{-5} newton.

達因 力的單位。等於1克質量獲得1釐米/秒^{2}的加速度所需的力。1達因＝10^{-5}牛頓。

-dynia *suffix denoting* pain. Example: *proctodynia* (in the rectum).

〔後綴〕 **痛** 例如肛部（直腸內）痛。

dys- *prefix denoting* difficult, abnormal, or impaired. Examples: *dysbasia* (difficulty in walking); *dysgeusia* (impairment of taste).

〔前綴〕 **困難，異常，障礙** 例如步行困難，味覺障礙。

dysaesthesiae *pl. n.* the abnormal and sometimes unpleasant sensations felt by a patient with partial damage to a peripheral nerve when his skin is touched. *Compare* paraesthesiae.

感覺異常 周圍神經部分受損的患者當皮膚觸及物體時產生的異常（有時是不舒服的）感覺。

dysarthria *n.* a speech disorder in which the pronunciation is unclear although the linguistic content and meaning are normal.

發育障礙 一種言語障礙，表現爲發音不清，然而語言內容和詞義是正常的。

dysbarism *n.* any clinical syndrome due to a difference between the atmospheric pressure outside the body and the pressure of air or gas within a body cavity (such as the paranasal sinuses or the middle ear). *See* compressed air illness.

氣壓病 一切由於外界大氣壓和體內腔室（如鼻旁竇或中耳）氣壓的差異而產生的臨床綜合徵。

dysbulia *n.* any disturbance of the will or of the mental processes that lead to purposeful action.

意志障礙 一切屬於意志和導致有目的的行動的心理過程的障礙。

dyschezia *n.* a form of constipation resulting from a long period of voluntary suppression of the urge to defecate. The rectum becomes distended with faeces and bowel movements are difficult or painful.

大便困難 由於長期有意識壓抑便意而造成的便秘類型。直腸爲糞便所膨脹，排便動作困難或有疼痛。

dyschondroplasia *n.* a condition due to faulty ossification of cartilage, resulting in development of many benign cartilaginous tumours (*see* chondroma). The bones involved may become stunted and deformed.

軟骨發育不良 由於軟骨鈣化異常以致發生多發性良性軟骨腫瘤的疾病。受累骨可生長受阻並變形。

dyscrasia *n.* an abnormal state of the body or part of the body, especially one due to abnormal development or metabolism. In classical medicine the term was used for the imbalance of the four *humours, which was believed to be the basic cause of all diseases.

體液失調 主要由於發育或代謝障礙所致的身體（或部分）異常狀態。在古典醫學中用以指人體內四種體液不平衡，當時認爲這種失衡是一切疾病的根源。

dysdiadochokinesis (adiadochokinesis) *n.* clumsiness in performing rapidly alternating movements. It is often recognized by asking the patient to tap with his fingers on the back of his other hand. It is a sign of disease of the cerebellum.

輪替運動障礙 快速變換動作不靈活。通常醫生讓患者用手指輕敲另一手背來判斷。爲小腦疾病的症狀。

dysentery *n.* an infection of the intestinal tract causing severe diarrhoea with blood and mucus. *Amoebic dysentery* (*amoebiasis*) is caused by the protozoan *Entamoeba histolytica* and results in ulceration of the intestines and occasionally in the formation of abscesses in the liver (*see* hepatitis), lungs, testes, or brain. The parasite is spread by food or water contaminated by infected faeces. Symptoms appear days or even years after infection and include diarrhoea, indigestion, loss of weight, and anaemia. Prolonged treatment with drugs, including emetine and tetracyclines, is usually effective in treating the condition. Amoebic dysentery is mainly confined to tropical and subtropical countries.

Bacillary dysentery is caused by bacteria of the genus *Shigella* and is spread by contact with a patient or carrier or through food or water contaminated by their faeces. Epidemics are common in overcrowded insanitary conditions. Symptoms, which develop 1–6 days after infection, include diarrhoea, nausea, cramp, and fever and they persist for about a week. An attack may vary from mild diarrhoea to an acute infection causing serious dehydration and bleeding from the gut. In most cases, provided fluid losses are replaced, recovery occurs within 7–10 days; antibiotics may be given to eliminate the bacteria. *Compare* cholera.

痢疾 引起嚴重腹瀉（便中帶血或黏液）的腸道感染。阿米巴痢疾由腸溶組織內阿米巴引起，其時腸內有潰瘍形成，有時可發生肝、肺、睾丸或腦膿腫。寄生蟲通過血液或被感染的糞便污染的食物或水傳播。感染後少則幾天多則幾年出現症狀：腹瀉、消化不良，體重減輕、貧血。長期藥物（吐根素和四環素）治療常能奏效。本病主要見於熱帶和亞熱帶國家。

細菌性痢疾由志賀氏桿菌屬細菌引起，係通過患者或帶菌者、或被其糞便污染的食物或水而傳播。常在居民密集、衞生條件差的地區造成流行。感染後1～6天發病。症狀爲腹瀉、噁心、腹絞痛、發熱，持續約一周。發作可多樣化：從輕型腹瀉到導致嚴重脫水和腸出血的急性感染。多數場合，只要丟失的水分得到補充，可在7～10天內恢復健康；可給予抗生菌以殺滅細菌。

dysgenesis *n.* faulty development; *gonadal dysgenesis* is failure of the ovaries or testes to develop (*see* Turner's syndrome).

發育不全 發育缺陷。卵巢或睾丸發育不全稱爲生殖發育障礙。

dysgerminoma (germinoma, gonocytoma) *n.* a malignant tumour of the ovary, thought to arise from primitive germ cells; it is homologous to the *seminoma of the testis. About 15% of such tumours affect both ovaries; outside the ovary they have been recorded in the anterior mediastinum and near the pineal gland. Dysgerminomas may

無性細胞瘤（生殖母細胞瘤） 卵巢惡性腫瘤。據認爲來自原始生殖細胞。該瘤與精原細胞瘤同源。約15%侵犯兩側卵巢。除卵巢外，尙有於前縱隔和松果體附近發生該瘤的報告。嬰兒至老年均可發生，平均發病年齡爲20歲

occur from infancy to old age, but the average age of patients is about 20 years. They are very sensitive to *radiotherapy. Dysgerminomas are also known as *large cell carcinomas* or *alveolar sarcomas of the ovary*.

左右。對放射治療極爲敏感。又稱卵巢大細胞性癌病或蜂窩狀肉瘤。

dysgraphia *n. see* agraphia.

書寫困難

dysidrosis (dyshidrosis) *n.* any abnormality of sweating or the sweat glands other than excessive sweating (*hyperhidrosis*), diminished sweating (*hypohidrosis*), or absence of sweating (*anidrosis*); for example, changes in the colour or smell of sweat.

出汗異常 不屬於出汗過多、過少和無汗的所有其它出汗異常。例如汗色和汗味的改變。

dyskinesia *n.* a group of involuntary movements that appear to be a fragmentation of the normal smoothly controlled limb and facial movements. They include *chorea, *dystonia, and those involuntary movements occurring as side-effects to the use of L-dopa and the phenothiazines.

運動障礙 一類不隨意運動。正常肢體和顏面平穩、精細的運動這時變得支離散亂。這類障礙包括舞蹈症、張力障礙以及使用左旋多巴和酚噻嗪而出現的不隨意運動副作用。

dyslalia *n.* a speech disorder in which the patient uses a vocabulary or range of sounds that is peculiar to him. It is a feature of the defective speech acquired by children who have been aphasic from birth (*see* aphasia).

出語障礙 一種言語障礙。患者用特有的詞滙或怪聲調說話。這是生後即患失語症兒童學到的有缺陷言語的表現。

dyslexia *n.* a developmental disorder selectively affecting a child's ability to learn to read and write. It is an uncommon condition, affecting boys more often than girls, and creates serious educational problems. It is sometimes called *specific dyslexia* or *developmental dyslexia* to distinguish it from acquired difficulties with reading and writing. *Compare* alexia. —**dyslexic** *adj.*

誦讀困難 選擇性影響兒童學習讀寫能力的發育障礙。不常見，男孩多於女孩，造成嚴重教育問題。有時稱爲特異性誦讀困難或發育性誦讀困難，以區別於後天性讀寫困難。

dyslogia *n.* disturbed and incoherent speech. This may be due to *dementia, *aphasia, *subnormality, or mental illness.

難語症 說話支離破碎、不連貫。見於痴呆、失語症、智力低下或精神疾病。

dysmenorrhoea *n.* painful or difficult menstruation. The most common type is *primary* (*essential*) *dysmenorrhoea*,

痛經 月經疼痛或困難。最常見類型爲原發性痛經，始於月經初潮，無明

which begins with the first period and has no apparent cause. In *secondary dysmenorrhoea* painful menstruation is experienced at some stage following the establishment of normal periods, for reasons including inflammation of the womb lining, the presence of tumours in the muscles of the womb, blockage of the blood flow, and mental disturbance.

顯原因。繼發性痛經是在正常月經周期建立後的某階段發生的月經痛。原因爲子宮內膜炎症、子宮肌瘤、月經受阻及精神障礙等。

dysmnesic syndrome a disorder of memory in which new information is not learned but old material is well remembered. *See* Korsakoff's syndrome.

記憶障礙綜合徵 對往事記憶淸楚而對新鮮信息記不住的記憶障礙。

dysmorphophobia *n.* a fixed distressing belief that one's body is deformed and repulsive, or an excessive fear that it might be so.

畸形恐怖 頑固地相信自已身體有令人厭惡的畸形並爲之苦惱不堪。或者過分懼怕自已會發生畸形。

dyspareunia *n.* painful or difficult sexual intercourse experienced by a woman. Psychological or physical factors may be responsible (*see* vaginismus).

性交困難 婦女體驗的性交痛或性交困難。可能有心理的或軀體的因素。

dyspepsia (indigestion) *n.* disordered digestion: usually applied to pain or discomfort in the lower chest or abdomen after eating and sometimes accompanied by nausea or vomiting. **—dyspeptic** *adj.*

消化不良 一種消化障礙。表現爲飯後下胸部或腹部疼痛或不適，有時可伴有噁心、嘔吐。

dysphagia *n.* a condition in which the action of swallowing is either difficult to perform, painful (*see* odynophagia), or in which swallowed material seems to be held up in its passage to the stomach. It is caused by painful conditions of the mouth and throat, obstruction of the pharynx or oesophagus by diseases of the wall or pressure from outside, or by abnormalities of muscular activity of the pharynx or oesophagus.

吞嚥困難 吞嚥動作困難或引起疼痛，或者感覺吞嚥的東西像是滯留在通向胃的中途。引起吞嚥困難的原因有口腔和咽喉的疼痛性病症、咽或食管阻塞（管壁病變或外來壓迫所致，或由於咽或食管肌緊張性異常）。

dysphasia *n. see* aphasia.

言語困難

dysphemia *n. see* stammering.

口吃

dysphonia *n.* difficulty in speaking due to a disorder of the larynx, vocal cords, tongue, or mouth. *Compare* dysarthria, aphasia.

發音困難 喉、聲帶、舌或口腔疾病所致的言語困難。

dysplasia (alloplasia, heteroplasia) *n.* abnormal development of skin, bone, or other tissues. *See also* fibrous dysplasia.

發育不良 皮膚、骨或其他組織發育異常。

dyspnoea *n.* laboured or difficult breathing. (The term is often used for a sign of laboured breathing apparent to the doctor, *breathlessness* being used for the subjective feeling of laboured breathing.) Dyspnoea can be due to obstruction to the flow of air into and out of the lungs (as in bronchitis and asthma), various diseases affecting the tissue of the lung (including pneumoconiosis, emphysema, tuberculosis, and cancer), and heart disease.

呼吸困難 須費力的呼吸或困難的呼吸。（本詞常用以描述醫生見到的呼吸體徵；所謂氣短則指費力呼吸時的主觀感覺)。呼吸困難可發生於進出肺的氣流受阻（支氣管炎或哮喘時）、各種侵犯肺組織的疾病（塵肺、肺氣腫、肺結核、癌）及心臟病等時。

dyspraxia *n. see* apraxia.

運用障礙 運用功能不全。

dyssynergia (asynergia) *n.* clumsily uncoordinated movements found in patients with disease of the cerebellum. They include *dysmetria* (the application of inappropriate force for a movement), intention *tremor, *dysdiadochokinesis, and a staggering wide-based gait.

協同失調（協同不能） 見於小腦疾病患者的精神運動不協調。其中包括辨距障礙（做一個動作時用力不當）、意向震顫、輪替運動障礙以及兩腿分開的蹣跚步態。

dystocia *n.* difficult birth, caused by abnormalities in the fetus or the mother. The most common causes of *fetal dystocia* are excessive size or *malpresentation of the baby. *Maternal dystocia* may result if the pelvis is abnormally small, the womb muscles fail to contract, or the neck of the womb fails to expand. If the cause of dystocia cannot be eliminated, it may be necessary to deliver the baby by Caesarean section or to operate in such a way that it can be removed with the minimum possible risk to the mother.

難產 胎兒或母親異常所致的分娩困難。最常見的胎兒性難產的原因是胎兒過大或胎位不正。母親性難產則可起於骨盆過小、子宮收縮無力或子宮頸開張不全。難產原因除不去，便須行剖腹術或採用對母親危險性最小的手術娩出胎兒。

dystonia *n.* a postural disorder caused by disease of the *basal ganglia in the

張力障礙 大腦基底神經節病變引起的姿態障礙。

brain. There is spasm in the muscles of the shoulders, neck, and trunk. The arm is often held in a rotated position and the head is drawn back and to one side.

表現爲肩、頸、軀幹肌肉痙攣。上臂常保持一種轉動姿勢，頭被拉向一側後方。

dystrophia myotonica a type of *muscular dystrophy in which the muscle weakness and wasting is accompanied by an unnatural prolongation of the muscular contraction after any voluntary effort (*see* myotonia). The muscles of the face, temples, and neck are especially wasted. Baldness, endocrine malfunction, and cataracts also occur. The disease can affect both sexes (it is inherited as an autosomal dominant character) and appears in early middle age.

肌强直性營養不良 一種肌營養不良類型。表現爲肌肉軟弱消瘦，每當有意識用力時便發生不自然的肌肉收縮時間過長。顏面、兩顳和頸部肌肉消瘦尤爲明顯。可伴發脫髮、內分泌障礙和白內障。男女均可罹病（爲常染色體顯性遺傳），發生於中年早期。

dystrophy (dystrophia) *n.* a disorder of an organ or tissue, usually muscle, due to impaired nourishment of the affected part. The term is applied to several unrelated conditions; for example, *muscular dystrophy and *dystrophia adiposogenitalis* (*see* Fröhlich's syndrome).

營養不良 器官或組織（常爲肌肉）在有害影響下發生營養障礙而致的病變。本詞用於一些相互沒有關聯的病症，如肌營養不良和肥胖性生殖營養不良。

dysuria *n.* difficult or painful urination. This is usually associated with urgency and frequency of urination if due to *cystitis or *urethritis. The pain is burning in nature and is relieved by curing the underlying cause. A high fluid intake usually helps.

排尿困難 排尿困難或疼痛。在膀胱炎或尿道炎情况下常與尿急、尿頻同時存在。疼痛爲燒灼性質，除去原因後即可解除。大量進水常有幫助。

E

ear *n.* the sense organ concerned with hearing and balance (see illustration). Sound waves, transmitted from the outside into the external auditory meatus, cause the eardrum (tympanic membrane) to vibrate. The small bones

耳 具有聽覺和平衡功能的感覺器官（見圖）。聲波從外界傳入外耳道，引起鼓膜振動。中耳小骨（聽骨）——錘骨，砧骨、鐙骨——將聲波的振

(ossicles) of the middle ear – the malleus, incus, and stapes – transmit the sound vibrations to the fenestra ovalis, which leads to the inner ear (*see* labyrinth). Inside the *cochlea the sound vibrations are converted into nerve impulses. Vibrations emerging from the cochlea could cause pressure to build up inside the ear, but this is released through the *Eustachian tube. The *semicircular canals, *saccule, and *utricle – also in the inner ear – are all concerned with balance.

動傳入前庭窗，再由前庭窗傳入內耳（見迷路）。在耳蝸裏，聲波振動被轉化成神經衝動。耳蝸裏的振動將在耳中產生逐漸增大的壓力，但在通過咽鼓管時被減小。內耳中的半規管、球囊、橢圓囊都與平衡有關。

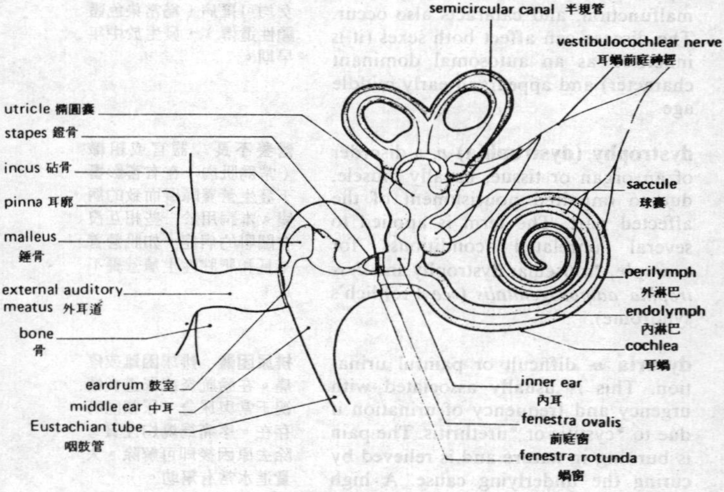

Structure of the ear

耳的結構

earache *n. see* otitis, otalgia. 耳痛

eardrum *n. see* tympanic membrane. 鼓膜

earwax *n. see* cerumen. 耳垢

eburnation *n.* the wearing down of the cartilage at the articulating surface of a bone, exposing the underlying bone. This is an end result of *osteoarthritis.

骨質緻密化　附着於骨端關節面的軟骨磨損變薄。是骨關節炎的最終結果。

ec- *prefix denoting* out of or outside. 〔前綴〕外，在……之外

ecbolic *n.* an agent, such as *oxytocin, that induces childbirth by stimulating contractions of the womb.

催產劑 刺激子宮收縮，促使胎兒娩出的一種藥物。如（後葉）催產素。

ecchondroma *n.* (*pl.* **ecchondromata**) a benign cartilaginous tumour (*see* chondroma) that protrudes beyond the margins of a bone. *Compare* enchondroma.

外生軟骨瘤 一種高出骨緣的良性軟骨瘤。

ecchymosis *n.* a bruise: an initially bluish-black mark on the skin, resulting from the release of blood into the tissues either through injury or through the spontaneous leaking of blood from the vessels (as in some blood diseases).

瘀斑 一種挫傷。皮膚上最初出現的是黑藍色斑迹。因血液從受損傷部位或（在某些血液病時）自然地從血管內滲入組織所引起。

eccrine *adj.* **1.** describing sweat glands that are distributed all over the body. Their ducts open directly onto the surface of the skin and they are densest on the soles of the feet and the palms of the hands. *Compare* apocrine. **2.** *see* merocrine.

①**外分泌的** 指分佈於全身的汗腺。汗腺導管直接開口於皮膚表面。脚底和手掌是汗腺最密集的部位。 ②**部分分泌的**

eccyesis *n. see* ectopic pregnancy.

異位妊娠

ecdemic *adj.* not occurring normally in the population of a country: applied sometimes to unusual diseases brought in from abroad by immigrants or travellers. *Compare* endemic.

外來的 不是正常地發生在某一國家人口之內的；有時指移民或旅遊者從國外帶進的不常見的疾病。

ecdysis *n.* the act of shedding skin; *desquamation.

蛻皮 皮膚脫落，脫皮。

ECG *n. see* electrocardiogram.

心電圖

echinococciasis (echinococcosis) *n. see* hydatid disease.

棘球蚴病

Echinococcus *n.* a genus of small parasitic tapeworms that reach a maximum length of only 8 mm. Adults are found in the intestines of dogs, wolves, or jackals. If the eggs are swallowed by man, who can act as a secondary host, the resulting larvae penetrate the intestine and settle in the lungs, liver, or brain to form large cysts, usually 5–10 cm in diameter (*see* hydatid disease). Two species causing this condition are *E. granulosus* and *E. multilocularis*.

棘球屬 小型寄生絛蟲屬。最長的只有8mm。在狗、狼或豹的腸道內可發現其成蟲。如蟲卵被人食入，則人可做為第二宿主，長成的幼蟲可穿腸壁進入肺、肝或腦，形成大囊腫，其直徑通常爲5～10cm。細粒棘球絛蟲和多房棘球絛蟲是產生這種病情的兩個種。

echoacousia *n.* a false sensation of echoing after normally heard sound.

回聲感覺 正常聲音後聽到的一種回聲的錯覺。

echocardiography *n.* the use of *ultrasound waves to investigate and display the action of the heart as it beats.

超聲心動描記法 在心臟跳動時，用超聲波來研究並展示出心臟活動情況的方法。

echoencephalography *n.* investigation of structures within the skull by detecting the echoes of ultrasonic pulses. The chief value of the method is in detecting those disorders causing a displacement of the midline structures of the brain.

腦超聲波檢查法 通過檢查超聲脉衝的回波來研究顱內結構的方法。其主要價值在於能查出引起大腦中線結構移位的疾病。

echography *n.* the technique of using *ultrasound waves to map out and study the internal structure of the body. Ultrasound waves are reflected to different degrees by different structures within the body. The visual recording of these reflected waves is called an *echogram*. *See also* ultrasonics.

超聲波描記術 用超聲波描記並研究體內結構的技術。超聲波可被體內不同結構不同程度地反射回來，這些反射的描記記錄叫回波圖。

echokinesis *n. see* echopraxia.

模仿運動

echolalia *n.* pathological repetition of the words spoken by another person. It may be a symptom of language disorders, *autism, *catatonia, or *Gilles de la Tourette syndrome.

模仿語言 病理性的重複他人說過的話。可能是語言障礙、孤獨癖、緊張症或圖雷特氏病的症狀。

echopraxia (echokinesis) *n.* pathological imitation of the actions of another person. It may be a symptom of *catatonia or of *latah.

模仿行動 病理性的模仿他人的行動。可能是緊張症或拉塔病的症狀。

echotomography *n. see* ultrasonotomography.

超聲斷層描記法

echovirus *n.* one of a group of about 30 RNA-containing viruses, originally isolated from the human intestinal tract, that were found to produce pathological changes in cells grown in culture, although they were not clearly associated with any specific disease. These viruses – which were accordingly termed *e*nteric *c*ytopathic *h*uman *o*rphan viruses – are now thought to be

埃可病毒 約含有30個RNA的一組病毒。在人體腸道內被首先分離，能使培養基中的細胞發生病理變化，但是否與某些特異性疾病有關還不清楚。現在，這些曾被叫做“人腸道孤兒病毒”的病毒被認爲是非特異性腦膜炎、多種胃腸道和呼吸道感染

the cause of nonspecific meningitis, many gastrointestinal and respiratory tract infections, and of many illnesses producing symptoms of the common cold. *Compare* reovirus.

及其他一些有感冒症狀的疾病的病因。

eclabium *n.* the turning outward of a lip.

脣外翻

eclampsia *n.* a rare and serious condition, affecting women either at the end of pregnancy or shortly after childbirth, in which the whole body is affected by convulsions and the patient eventually passes into a coma. Blood pressure is high, the urine contains proteins, and the ankles and other parts swell because of the accumulation of water in the tissues (oedema). Eclampsia is a threat to the life of both baby and mother. It represents an advanced stage of *toxaemia of pregnancy and can be prevented by regular antenatal examinations.

子癇 一種發生在妊娠晚期或胎兒娩出後不久的婦女身上的嚴重疾病。不常見，發病期間患者全身驚厥，最後進入昏迷狀態。患者血壓增高，有蛋白尿，由於液體在組織內聚積，踝部及其他部位水腫。子癇對胎兒及母親有生命危險。它是妊娠毒血症發展的嚴重階段。定期對孕婦進行檢查可預防此病。

ecology (bionomics) *n.* the study of the relationships between man, plants and animals, and the environment, including the way in which human activities may affect other animal populations and alter natural surroundings. —**ecological** *adj.* —**ecologist** *n.*

生態學 關於人類、植物、動物以及環境之間相互關係的一門科學。也包括研究能影響動物群及改變自然環境的人類活動的方式。

ecraseur *n.* a surgical device, resembling a *snare, that is used to sever the base of a tumour during its surgical removal.

絞勒器 外科器械，類似勒除器。用於外科切除腫瘤時除去其根底。

ecstasy *n.* a sense of extreme well-being and bliss. The word applies particularly to *trance states dominated by religious thinking. While not necessarily pathological, it can be caused by epilepsy (especially of the temporal lobe) or by schizophrenia.

入迷 一種極度幸福和喜悅的感覺。特指因被宗教思想所支配而產生的迷惘狀態。雖不一定是病理現象，但可因癲癇（特別是顳葉病變引起的）或精神分裂症而引起。

ECT *see* electroconvulsive therapy.

電驚厥療法

ect- (ecto-) *prefix denoting* outer or external.

〔前綴〕 **外，外部，外面**

ectasia (ectasis) *n.* the dilatation of a tube, duct, or hollow organ.

擴張 管、道或空心臟器膨脹。

ecthyma *n.* a skin disease – an ulcerative type of *impetigo – in which the infection spreads down to the lower layer of the skin (dermis). Ecthyma heals more slowly than ordinary impetigo and causes scarring.

深膿疱 一種皮膚病——潰瘍型膿疱病。感染向皮下層（眞皮）擴散。比一般膿疱癒合慢，且留有疤痕。

ectoderm *n.* the outer of the three *germ layers of the early embryo. It gives rise to the nervous system and sense organs, the teeth and lining of the mouth, and the *epidermis and its associated structures (hair, nails, etc.). —**ectodermal** *adj.*

外胚層 胚胎早期三胚層中的外層。神經系統、感覺器官、牙齒、口腔黏膜、表皮層及附屬結構（毛髮、指甲等）由此層發生。

ectomorphic *adj.* describing a *body type that is relatively thin, with a large skin surface in comparison to weight. —**ectomorph** *n.* —**ectomorphy** *n.*

外胚層體型的 指身材很瘦而皮膚面積與體重相比又很大的一種體型。

-ectomy *suffix denoting* surgical removal of a segment or all of an organ or part. Examples: *appendicectomy* (of the appendix); *prostatectomy* (of the prostate gland).

〔後綴〕 **切除術** 指某器官或部位部分或全部的外科切除。如：闌尾切除術，前列腺切除術。

ectoparasite *n.* a parasite that lives on the outer surface of its host. Some ectoparasites, such as bed bugs, maintain only periodic contact with their hosts, whereas others, such as the crab louse, have a permanent association. *Compare* endoparasite.

外寄生物 生活在宿主外表的寄生物。有些寄生物，如臭蟲，只是定期的與宿主接觸。而其他的，如陰蝨，却長期與宿主接觸。

ectopia *n.* **1.** the misplacement, due either to a congenital defect or injury, of a bodily part. **2.** the occurrence of something in an unnatural location (*see* ectopic beat, ectopic pregnancy). —**ectopic** *adj.*

異位 ①身體某部位因先天性缺陷或損傷而產生的錯位。 ②某事物發生在不正常的部位（如異位搏動，異位妊娠）。

ectopic beat (extrasystole) a heart beat due to an impulse generated somewhere in the heart outside the sinoatrial node. Ectopic beats are generally premature in timing; they are classified as *supraventricular* if they originate in the atria and *ventricular* if they arise from a focus in the ventricles. They may be produced by any heart disease, by nicotine from smoking, or by caffeine from excessive tea or coffee consump-

異位搏動（期外收縮） 心臟竇房結以外的部位發出的衝動所引起的心臟跳動。通常是期前收縮。異位搏動分兩種：室上性，衝動來自心房；室性，衝動來自心室。可由各種心臟病、煙草中的尼古丁引起，或因飲入大量茶、咖啡因所引起。此情況也可見於正常人。作爲患者，

tion; they are common in normal individuals. The patient may be unaware of their presence or may feel that his heart has 'missed a beat'. Ectopic beats may be suppressed by drugs such as quinidine, propranolol, and lignocaine; avoidance of smoking and reduction in excessive tea or coffee intake may help. *See* arrhythmia.

他可能意識不到異位搏動的存在，或可能感到他的心臟"漏搏"。異位搏動可被奎尼丁、心得安及利多卡因制止。不吸煙、少飲濃茶和咖啡也有助於緩解。

ectopic pregnancy (extrauterine pregnancy) the development of a fetus at a site other than in the womb. This may happen if the fertilized egg cell remains in the ovary or in the tube leading from near the ovary to the womb (the Fallopian tube) or if it lodges in the free abdominal cavity. The most common type of ectopic pregnancy is a *tubal* (or *oviducal*) *pregnancy*, which occurs in Fallopian tubes that become blocked or inflamed. The growth of the fetus may cause the tube to burst and bleed. In most cases the fetus dies within three months of conception and is absorbed into the woman's body. However, development sometimes continues to a stage at which a live baby can be delivered by Caesarean section. Medical name: **eccyesis.**

異位妊娠（宮外孕） 胎兒在子宮以外的部位發育。可因受精卵滯留在卵巢或輸卵管或腹腔裏而發生。常見的類型是輸卵管妊娠，可引起輸卵管堵塞或炎症。生長的胎兒可使輸卵管破裂和出血。多數情況下，胎兒在妊娠三個月之內即死亡，並被母體吸收。但有時，胎兒可繼續生長發育，這時就要通過剖腹產手術將活嬰取出。

ectoplasm *n.* the outer layer of cytoplasm in cells, which is denser than the inner cytoplasm (*endoplasm) and concerned with activities such as cell movement. **—ectoplasmic** *adj.*

外〔胞〕質（漿） 細胞的胞質的外層，比細胞內質稠密，並與活動（如細胞運動）有關。

ectro- *prefix denoting* congenital absence.

〔前綴〕 **先天性缺失。**

ectrodactyly *n.* congenital absence of all or part of one or more fingers.

缺指 先天性（部分或全部）缺少一個或多個手指。

ectromelia *n.* congenital absence or gross shortening (aplasia) of the long bones of one or more limbs. *See also* amelia, hemimelia, phocomelia.

缺肢 先天性單肢或多肢缺失或發育不全。

ectropion *n.* turning out of the eyelid, away from the eyeball. The commonest

瞼外翻 眼瞼離開眼球向外翻轉。常見的類型是老

type is *senile ectropion*, in which the lower eyelid droops because of loss of the elasticity of its tissues in old age. If the muscle that closes the eye (orbicularis oculi) is paralysed the lower lid also droops. Ectropion may also occur if the lining membrane (conjunctiva) of the lid is very thickened or if scarring causes contraction of the skin.

年性瞼外翻，因老年時結締組織的彈性消失而下眼瞼下垂。如眼輪匝肌麻痺，下眼瞼也會下垂。如瞼結膜很厚，或有疤痕而引起皮膚收縮，也會發生瞼外翻。

eczema *n.* a superficial inflammation of the skin, mainly affecting the *epidermis. Eczema causes itching, with a red rash often accompanied by small blisters that weep and become crusted. Subsequent scaling, thickening, or discoloration of the skin may occur. The disorder has several forms, with two major divisions: *eczematous dermatitis*, which results from external factors (*see* dermatitis); and *endogenous* (or *constitutional*) *eczema*, occurring without any obvious external cause. Classification of endogenous eczema is based on its appearance and site. The five types are *atopic*, commonly found in childhood and sometimes associated with a family history of allergy; *discoid*, characterized by small well-defined areas of eczema; *pompholyx, found on the hands and feet; *seborrhoeic*, in which scaly plaques occur in areas of the greatest sebum production (the scalp, face, etc.); and *varicose*, which develops on the legs in association with poor circulation. Treatment of eczema depends on the cause but usually includes the use of locally applied corticosteroids. —**eczematous** *adj.*

濕疹 皮膚淺表性炎症。主要發生在表皮。可引起瘙癢、紅疹，還常伴有液體流出，並有結痂。結痂部位的皮膚增厚、褪色，此種疾病有多種形式，但主要分兩種：濕疹性皮炎（由外界因素引起）與內源性濕疹，後者無明顯外因而發病。本病還可根據其表現和發生部位而繼續分類。其五種類型爲：①特應型：常見於兒童，有時，與家族過敏史有關。②盤型：範圍小，界限清楚爲特點。③汗疱型：見於手和脚。④皮脂溢型：在大量產生皮脂的部位（頭皮，臉部等），有鱗屑產生。⑤靜脉曲張型：發生於下肢，與血液循環不佳有關。濕疹的治療依病因不同而不同，但通常包括皮質類固醇的局部使用。

edentulous *adj.* lacking teeth: usually applied to people who have lost their teeth.

無牙的 沒牙的，通常指失去牙齒的人。

edrophonium *n.* a drug that stimulates skeletal muscles (*see* parasympathomimetic). It is administered by injection in a test for diagnosis of *myasthenia gravis. Side-effects can include nausea

氯化騰喜龍 一種刺激骨骼肌的藥物。注射給藥，用於診斷重症肌無力。副作用有噁心、嘔吐、流涎增多、腹瀉及胃痛。

and vomiting, increased saliva flow, diarrhoea, and stomach pains. Trade name: **Tensilon**.

EDTA (ethylenediamine tetra-acetic acid) a compound used as a *chelating agent in the treatment of poisoning with several different metals, such as lead and strontium. It is normally administered in the form of its calcium sodium salt, called *calcium sodium edetate*.

乙二胺四乙酸 一種化合物。作爲一種螯合劑用於治療某些金屬中毒。如鉛、鍶中毒。

EEG (electroencephalogram) *see* electroencephalography.

腦電圖

effector *n.* any structure or agent that brings about activity in a muscle or gland, such as a motor nerve that causes muscular contraction or glandular secretion. The term is also used for the muscle or gland itself.

效應器 能夠引起肌肉或腺體活動的任何結構或物質。如能夠引起肌肉收縮或腺體分泌的運動神經。此術語也用於肌肉或腺體本身。

efferent *adj.* **1.** designating nerves or neurones that convey impulses from the brain or spinal cord to muscles, glands, and other effectors; i.e. any motor nerve or neurone. **2.** designating vessels or ducts that drain fluid (such as lymph) from an organ or part. *Compare* afferent.

輸出的 ①指將大腦或脊髓發出的衝動轉送到肌肉、腺體或其他效應器上的神經或神經元，如所有的運動神經或神經元。②指將某器官或某部位的液體（如淋巴液）引流的脉管或管道。

effleurage *n.* a form of *massage in which the hands are passed continuously and rhythmically over a patient's skin in one direction only, with the aim of increasing blood flow in that direction and aiding the dispersal of any swelling due to *oedema.

輕撫法 一種按摩的方式。將手放在患者某部位的表面，向同一方向有規律的按壓，以增加那一部位的血運，並促進水腫的消散。

effort syndrome a condition of marked anxiety about the condition of one's heart and circulatory system. This is accompanied by a heightened consciousness of heartbeat and respiration, which in turn is worsened by the anxiety it induces. Treatment is commonly with reassurance and *tranquillizers; psychotherapy is only occasionally necessary.

奮力綜合症 對自己心臟及循環系統狀況過分擔憂的一種病症，伴有對心跳和呼吸的高度意識感。由此引起的擔憂可加重此病情。通常的治療方法是消除疑慮及服用鎮靜藥。只有在必要時進行心理療法。

effusion *n.* **1.** the escape of pus, serum, blood, lymph, or other fluid into a body cavity as a result of inflammation or the presence of excess blood or tissue fluid in an organ or tissue. **2.** fluid that has escaped into a body cavity.

①**滲漏** 某一器官或組織因炎症或血液、組織液過多而向體腔裏滲出膿汁、血清、血液、淋巴液及其它液體。②**滲漏液** 溢到體腔裏的液體。

egg cell *see* ovum.

卵細胞

ego *n.* (in psychoanalysis) the part of the mind that develops from a person's experience of the outside world and is most in touch with external realities. In Freudian terms the ego is said to reconcile the demands of the *id (the instinctive unconscious mind), the *superego (moral conscience), and reality.

自我（精神分析學）意識的一部分。來自某人對外界的體驗。與外在的現實密切相關。弗洛伊德學說認爲，自我能使伊德（本能的潛意識），超我（道德上的良心）及現實的需要之間協調一致。

eidetic *adj. see* imagery.

遺覺的

eikonometer *n.* an instrument for measuring the size of images on the retina of the eye.

影象計 測量眼中視網膜成象大小的儀器。

Eisenmenger reaction a condition in which *pulmonary hypertension is associated with a *septal defect, so that blood flows from the right to the left side of the heart or from the pulmonary artery to the aorta. This allows blue blood, poor in oxygen, to bypass the lungs and enter the general circulation. This reduces the oxygen content of the arterial blood in the aorta and its branches, resulting in a patient with a dusky blue appearance (*cyanosis) and an increased number of red blood cells (*polycythaemia). There is no curative treatment at this stage, but the patient may be helped by the control of heart failure and polycythaemia. The condition may be prevented by appropriate treatment of the septal defect before irreversible pulmonary hypertension develops.

艾森門格反應 因心室間隔缺損而產生肺高壓，使血液從心臟右側流向左側或從肺動脈流向主動脈的一種病症。這樣，低氧血就不通過肺部而直接進入體循環，使進入主動脈及其分支裏的動脈血氧含量下降。患者出現紫紺面容，紅細胞數增加。處於這一時期，是沒有治癒方法的。但可通過控制心衰及紅細胞增多使患者病情緩解。在不可逆性肺高壓到來之前，適當治療室間隔缺損可預防此病。

ejaculation *n.* the discharge of semen from the erect penis at the moment of sexual climax (orgasm) in the male. The constituents of semen are not released simultaneously, but in the following sequence: the secretion of *Cowper's glands followed by that of

射精 男性在性高潮期精液從勃起的陰莖射出的過程。精液的成分不是同時釋放出來，而是按下列順序進行的：庫珀氏腺分泌液、前列腺液和精子，最後是精囊分泌液。

the *prostate gland and the spermatozoa and finally the secretion of the *seminal vesicles. *See also* premature ejaculation.

elastic cartilage a type of *cartilage in which elastic fibres are distributed in the matrix. It is yellowish in colour and is found in the external ear.

彈性軟骨 軟骨的一種。其彈性纖維分佈在基質。微帶黃色，見於外耳。

elastic tissue strong extensible flexible *connective tissue rich in yellow *elastic fibres*. These are long, thin, and branching and are composed primarily of an albumin-like protein, *elastin*. Elastic tissue is found in the dermis of the skin, in arterial walls, and in the walls of the alveoli of the lungs.

彈性組織 彈性極强的結締組織。富於黃色彈性纖維，細長且有分支，主要由類似白蛋白的彈性硬蛋白構成。見於皮膚表皮、動脉壁及肺泡壁。

elastin *n.* protein forming the major constituent of *elastic tissue fibres.

彈性硬蛋白 構成彈性組織纖維主要成分的蛋白質。

elastosis *n.* degeneration of the yellow fibres in connective tissues and skin (*see* elastic tissue).

彈性組織變性 結締組織和皮膚中的黃色纖維變性。

elation (exaltation) *n.* a state of cheerful excitement and enthusiasm. Marked elation of mood is a characteristic of *mania or *hypomania.

得意〔洋洋〕 興高采烈並充滿熱情的狀態。明顯得意的情緒是躁狂或輕躁狂的特徵。

electroanaesthesia *n.* local or general anaesthesia (usually the latter) brought about by passing an electric current through the tissues.

電麻醉 電流通過組織而引起的局部和全身麻醉（通常是後者）。

electrocardiogram (ECG) *n.* a recording of the electrical activity of the heart on a moving paper strip (see illustration). The ECG tracing is recorded by means of an apparatus called an *electrocardiograph* (*see* electrocardiography). It aids in the diagnosis of heart disease, which may produce characteristic changes in the ECG.

心電圖 在移動的紙條上記錄下來的心臟電活動曲線（見圖）。心電圖的描繪是由心動描記器進行的。有助於診斷心臟病，後者可能在心電圖上產生特殊的改變。

electrocardiography *n.* a technique for recording the electrical activity of the heart. Electrodes connected to the recording apparatus (*electrocardiograph*) are placed on the skin of the four limbs and chest wall; the record itself is

心電描記法 記錄心臟活動的一種技術。將連接記錄儀的電極與四肢和胸壁皮膚相接觸，所做出的記錄叫心電圖。在常用的標量法中，可記錄12個導

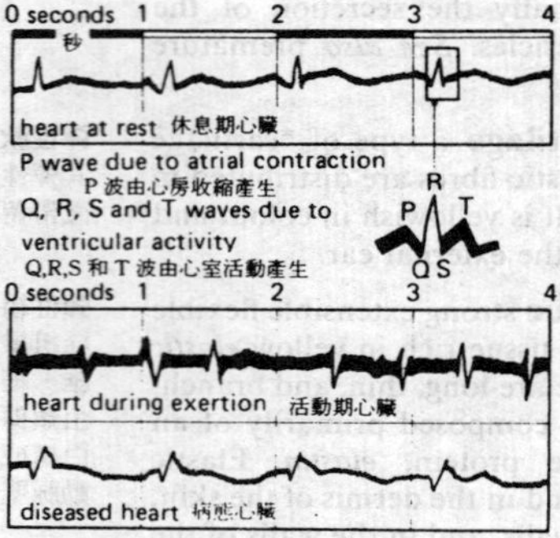

Typical electrocardiograms

典型的心電圖

called an *electrocardiogram (ECG). In conventional *scalar electrocardiography* 12 leads (*see* lead[2]) are recorded, but more may be employed in special circumstances (for example, an oesophageal lead, from an electrode within the gullet, may be used in the analysis of arrhythmias).

Vectorcardiography is less commonly used in Britain, but may be employed to obtain a three-dimensional impression of electrical activity of the heart.

聯。在特殊情況下，會使用更多的導聯（如在分析心律不齊時，可以從插入食管內的電極引出食管導聯）。

向量心電描記法在英國已很少使用，但可用來獲得心臟電活動的立體概念。

electrocardiophonography *n.* a technique for recording heart sounds and murmurs simultaneously with the ECG, which is used as a reference tracing. The sound is picked up by a microphone placed over the heart. The tracing is a *phonocardiogram*. It provides a permanent record of heart sounds and murmurs and is useful in their analysis.

心音電描記法　與心電圖同時進行的記錄心音及其雜音的一種技術。以心電圖作爲參考標記。心音由放在心臟部位胸壁上的擴音器所接收。錄下的曲線就是心音圖。它提供了心音及其雜音的永久性記錄，在其分析中很有用。

electrocautery (galvanocautery) *n.* the destruction of diseased or unwanted tissue by means of a needle or snare that is electrically heated (*see* diathermy). Warts, polyps, and other growths can be burned away by this

電烙術　用電熱針或電熱勒除器將疾病組織或不需要的組織破壞掉。疣、息肉及其他生長物可用這種方法燒除。此時，電流是不通過健康組織的。

method; the electricity does not pass through the tissues themselves.

electrocoagulation *n.* the coagulation of tissues by means of a high-frequency electric current concentrated at one point as it passes through them. Electrocoagulation, using a *diathermy knife, permits bloodless incisions to be made during operation.

電凝法 當高頻電流通過組織時，使其集中在某一點上，以此方法使該組織凝固。在手術中，根據電凝法，用透熱刀可做無血切開。

electroconvulsive therapy (ECT) a treatment for severe depression and occasionally for schizophrenia and mania. A convulsion is produced by passing an electric current through the brain. The convulsion is modified by giving a *muscle relaxant drug and an *anaesthetic, so that in fact only a few muscle twitches are produced. The means by which ECT acts is not yet known. The procedure can also produce confusion, loss of memory, and headache, which almost always pass off within a few hours. These side-effects are reduced by unilateral treatment, in which the current is passed only through the nondominant hemisphere of the brain.

電驚厥療法 對嚴重抑鬱症，偶爾對精神分裂症及躁狂症的治療方法。驚厥是電流通過大腦時引起的，可用肌肉鬆弛劑予以控制。因此，事實上只是少數肌肉發生抽搐。此療法的原理還不很清楚。電驚厥過程也能導致精神錯亂、失去記憶及頭痛。但幾小時之後，幾乎全部消失。單側治療，即電流只通過大腦的非優勢半球，會減少這些副作用。

electrodesiccation *n. see* fulguration.

電乾燥法

electroencephalogram (EEG) *n. see* electroencephalography.

腦電圖

electroencephalography *n.* the technique for recording the electrical activity from different parts of the brain and converting it into a tracing called an *electroencephalogram* (*EEG*). The machine that records this activity is known as an *encephalograph*. The pattern of the EEG reflects the state of the patient's brain and his level of consciousness in a characteristic manner. Electroencephalography is used to detect and locate structural disease, such as tumours, in the brain; it is also used in the diagnosis and management of epilepsy.

腦電描記法 從大腦不同部位記錄腦電活動並將此描繪成圖（即腦電圖）的技術。記錄這種活動的器械叫腦電圖〔描記〕儀。腦電圖可反映出患者的大腦狀態及其清醒程度的特徵。此法用來探查和確定器質性症病，如腦內腫瘤，亦可用來診斷和處理癲癇。

electrokymography *n.* the technique of recording the movements of an

電記波照像術 通過熒光屏及光電記錄系統記錄器

organ, especially the heart, by means of a *fluoroscope and a photoelectric recording system.

官（特別是心臟）運動的技術。

electrolyte *n.* a solution that produces ions (an ion is an atom or group of atoms that conduct electricity); for example, sodium chloride solution consists of free sodium and free chloride ions. In medical usage electrolyte usually means the ion itself; thus the term *serum electrolyte level* means the concentration of separate ions (sodium, potassium, chloride, bicarbonate, etc.) in the circulating blood. Concentrations of various electrolyte levels can be altered by many diseases, in which electrolytes are lost from the body (as in vomiting or diarrhoea) or are not excreted and accumulate (as in renal failure). When electrolyte concentrations are severely diminished they can be corrected by administering the appropriate substance by mouth or by intravenous drip. When excess of an electrolyte exists it may be removed by *dialysis or by special resins in the intestine, taken by mouth or by enema.

電解質 產生離子的溶液（離子是一種能導電的原子或原子團）。如：氯化鈉溶液是由自由鈉離子及自由氯離子組成的。在醫學上，電解質通常指離子本身。因此，所謂血清電解質濃度是指在循環血液中各種離子的濃度（鈉、鉀、氯、碳酸氫鹽等）。各種電解質濃度可因各種疾病而改變，使電解質從體內丟失（如嘔吐和腹瀉時）或不能排出而聚積在體內（如腎衰時）。當電解質濃度嚴重下降時，可通過口服或靜脈點滴適當物質而糾正。當電解質過多時，可通過透析或特殊樹脂而排除。後者可口服或灌腸。

electromyography *n.* continuous recording of the electrical activity of a muscle by means of electrodes inserted into the muscle fibres. The tracing is displayed on an oscilloscope. The technique is used for diagnosing various nerve and muscle disorders and assessing progress in recovery from some forms of paralysis.

肌電描記法 將電極放入肌纖維內，連續記錄肌肉電活動的方法。可在示波器中顯示出描記圖。此技術用於各種神經及肌肉疾病的診斷及估計某些麻痹症的恢復程度。

electronarcosis *n.* the induction of sleep by passing weak electrical currents through the brain. It is seldom used in Western psychiatry.

電麻醉 微弱電流通過大腦所產生的睡眠。在西方精神病學中很少使用。

electron microscope a microscope that uses a beam of electrons as a radiation source for viewing the specimen. The resolving power (ability to register fine detail) is a thousand times greater than that of an ordinary light microscope. The specimen must be examined in a vacuum, which necessi-

電子顯微鏡 用電子束做放射源來觀察標本的顯微鏡。其放大倍數是一般光學顯微鏡的一千倍。標本必須放在用特殊技術製成的眞空設備裏檢查。電子通常集中打在熒光屏上（爲直接觀察）或照像底

tates special techniques for preparing it, and the electrons are usually focused onto a fluorescent screen (for direct viewing) or onto a photographic plate (for a photograph, or *electron micrograph*). A *transmission electron microscope* is used to examine thin sections at high magnification. A *scanning electron microscope* reveals the surfaces of objects at various magnifications; its great depth of focus is advantageous.

板上（爲拍照片，即電子顯微照像）。透射電子顯微鏡用於檢查超薄切片。掃描電子顯微鏡可顯示不同放大倍數的物體表面。深焦距是其優點。

electron transport chain a series of enzymes and proteins in living cells through which electrons are transferred, via a series of oxidation-reduction reactions. This ultimately leads to the conversion of chemical energy into a readily usable and storable form. The most important electron transport chain is the *respiratory chain*, present in mitochondria and functioning in cellular respiration.

電子轉移鏈 在活細胞內，能通過一系列氧化還原反應將電子轉移的一組酶和蛋白質。最終是將化學能量轉化成使用和貯存形式的能量。最重要的電子轉移鏈，存在於線粒體內，在細胞呼吸中發揮作用。

electrooculography *n.* an electrical method of recording eye movements. Tiny electrodes are attached to the skin at the inner and outer corners of the eye, and as the eye moves an alteration in the potential between these electrodes is recorded. The size of this potential at rest also gives an indication of the health of the retina.

眼電描記法 記錄眼運動的電學方法。將微小電極與眼的內、外角相接觸，當眼移動時，電極之間的電勢變化就被記錄下來。眼休息時的電勢大小也能提示視網膜的健康狀態。

electrophoresis *n.* the technique of separating electrically charged particles, particularly proteins, in a solution by passing an electric current through the solution. The rate of movement of the different components depends upon their charge, so that they gradually separate into bands. Electrophoresis is widely used in the investigation of body chemicals, such as the analysis of the different proteins in blood serum.

電泳 電流通過溶液時，使其中帶電粒子，特別是蛋白質分離的技術。不同成分的移動速度依其電荷大小而不同。因此，它們會逐漸分離成不同的帶。電泳廣泛用於體內化學研究，如血清中不同蛋白質的分析。

electroretinography *n.* a method of recording changes in the electrical potential of the retina when it is stimulated by light. One electrode is placed on the eye in a contact lens and the

視網膜電描記法 當光線刺激視網膜時，記錄其電勢變化的方法。將裝有一電極的隱形眼鏡放在眼睛表面，另一電極放在頭後

other is usually attached to the back of the head. In retinal disease the pattern of electrical change is altered. The technique is useful in diagnosing retinal diseases when such things as cataract make it difficult to see the retina or when the disease produces little visible change in the retina.

部，在視網膜疾病時，電描記圖發生改變。此方法在診斷視網膜疾病時很有用。如白內障一類疾病使視網膜很難看清時，或視網膜發生不易看到的病變時。

electrotherapy *n.* the passage of electric currents through the body's tissues to stimulate the functioning of nerves and the muscles that they supply. The technique is used to bring about improvement in the muscles of patients with various forms of paralysis due to nerve disease or muscle disorder. *See also* faradism, galvanism.

電療法 將電流通過體內各組織，以刺激神經和肌肉發揮其應有的作用。此方法用於因神經或肌肉疾病而發生各種麻痹的患者，可使肌肉功能得到改善。

electuary *n.* a pharmaceutical preparation in which the drug is made up into a paste with syrup or honey.

藥糖劑 一種藥物製劑。在這種製劑中，藥物與糖漿和蜜一起被製成糊劑。

elephantiasis *n.* gross enlargement of the skin and underlying connective tissues caused by obstruction of the lymph vessels, which prevents drainage of lymph from the surrounding tissues. Inflammation and thickening of the walls of the vessels and their eventual blocking is commonly caused by the parasitic filarial worms *Wuchereria bancrofti* and *Brugia malayi*. The parts most commonly affected are the legs but the scrotum, breasts, and vulva may also be involved. Elastic bandaging is applied to the affected parts and the limbs are elevated and rested. Larval forms in the blood are killed with diethylcarbamazine. *See also* filariasis.

象皮病 因淋巴管堵塞，並因此使其周圍組織淋巴液的引流障礙而引起的皮膚及皮下結締組織明顯腫大。淋巴管壁炎症、增厚及最終導致的淋巴管阻塞通常是由絲蟲：班氏吳策絲蟲和馬來絲蟲引起。最常見的發病部位在腿部，但也見於陰囊、乳房及女性外陰。將患部纏上彈性綳帶，抬高並休息肢體可得到緩解。血液中的幼蟲可用乙胺嗪殺死。

elevator *n.* **1.** an instrument that is used to raise a depressed broken bone, for example in the skull or cheek. A specialized *periosteal elevator* is used in orthopaedics to strip the fibrous tissue (periosteum) covering bone. **2.** a lever-like instrument used to ease a tooth out of its socket during extraction.

①**起子** 用來托起凹陷性骨折骨（如顱骨、顴骨骨折）的工具。特製的骨膜起子用於骨科，以剝下包繞骨的纖維組織（骨膜）。 ②**牙梃** 桿狀工具。在拔牙時，用於將牙挺出齒槽。

elimination *n.* (in physiology) the entire process of excretion of metabolic waste products from the blood by the kidneys and urinary tract.

排泄 （生理學）血液中代謝廢物從體內通過腎臟及泌尿道排出的全過程。

elixir *n.* a preparation containing alcohol (ethanol) or glycerine, which is used as the vehicle for bitter or nauseous drugs.

酏劑 含有酒精或甘油的製劑。用作苦味的、令人噁心的藥物的賦形劑。

elliptocytosis *n.* the presence of significant numbers of abnormal elliptical red cells (*elliptocytes*) in the blood. Elliptocytosis may occur as a hereditary disorder or be a feature of certain blood diseases, such as *myelofibrosis or iron-deficiency *anaemia.

橢圓形紅細胞症 在血液中存在着相當數量的非正常的橢圓形紅細胞。可做為遺傳病出現，或是某些血液病的特徵，如骨髓纖維變性或缺鐵性貧血。

elutriation *n.* the separation of a fine powder from a coarser powder by mixing them with water and decanting the upper layer while it still contains the finer particles. The heavier coarse particles sink to the bottom more rapidly.

淘析法 在粗粉末中分離出細粉末。方法是將粗、細粉末用水混合，當表面層含有細顆粒時，將其傾析。較重的粗大顆粒則很快沉入底部。

em- *prefix. see* en-.

〔前綴〕 **在，……之內**

emaciation *n.* wasting of the body, caused by such conditions as malnutrition, tuberculosis, cancer, or parasitic worms.

消瘦 身體耗損。由某些原因如營養不良、結核、癌或寄生蟲引起。

emaculation *n.* the removal of spots, freckles, or similar marks from the skin, usually by surgery.

除斑術 用手術的方法將皮膚上的斑點、雀斑、或類似的斑迹除去。

emasculation *n.* strictly, surgical removal of the penis. The term is often used to mean loss of male physical and emotional characteristics, either as a result of removal of the testes (castration) or of emotional stress.

陰莖切除術 嚴格地講，指除去陰莖的手術。但本詞常用來指因除去睪丸（睪丸切除術）或感情受到刺激而喪失男性的生理特點。

embalming *n.* the preservation of a dead body by the introduction of chemical compounds that delay putrefaction. The ancient Egyptians raised the process to a fine art in the production of their mummies. Today embalming is employed mainly so that a body can be transported long distances and funeral rites can be conducted

屍體防腐 用延緩腐爛的化學藥物保存屍體。古埃及人在保護他們的木乃伊方面已將這一技術提到很高水平。今天因主要使用了屍體防腐，屍體方能長距離運送，葬禮才不至於匆忙進行。在美國，屍體防腐是常見的衛生措施。

without undue haste. In the USA embalming is a routine hygienic measure.

embedding *n.* (in microscopy) the fixing of a specimen within a mass of firm material in order to facilitate the cutting of thin sections for microscopical study. The embedding medium, e.g. paraffin wax for light microscopy or Araldite for electron microscopy, helps to keep the specimen intact.

包埋 顯微鏡學用語。將標本放入堅固的物質裏固定，使其利於做成用於顯微鏡研究的切片。包埋物質，如用於光學顯微鏡的石蠟，用於電子顯微鏡的環氧樹脂，有助於保護標本完整無損。

embolectomy *n.* surgical removal of an *embolus in order to relieve arterial obstruction. The embolus may be removed by cutting directly into the affected artery (*arteriotomy*). In some instances it is removed by a balloon *catheter, which is manipulated beyond the embolus from a small arteriotomy in an accessible artery. The catheter is then withdrawn carrying the embolus with it. In some cases of pulmonary embolism, embolectomy may be life saving. It may also prevent gangrene, with loss of a limb, in cases of a limb artery embolus.

栓子切除術 手術切除栓子，以除去動脈栓塞。可直接切開受阻動脈去除栓子（動脈切開術）。在某些情況下，還可以用氣囊導管去除栓子。將導管從易達到栓子部位的動脈的小切口中插入，越過栓子後進行操作，然後將帶着栓子的導管抽出。在一些肺動脈栓塞的病例中，栓子切除術能挽救生命。在肢體動脈栓塞時，此手術也可預防能導致截肢的壞死。

embolism *n.* the condition in which an embolus becomes lodged in an artery and obstructs its blood flow. The most common form of embolism is *pulmonary embolism, in which a blood clot is carried in the circulation to lodge in the pulmonary artery. An embolus in any other artery constitutes a *systemic embolism*. In this case a common source of the embolus is a blood clot within the heart in mitral valve disease or following *myocardial infarction. The clinical features depend upon the site at which an embolus lodges (for example, a stroke may result from a cerebral embolism and gangrene from a limb embolism).
Treatment is by *anticoagulant therapy with heparin and warfarin. Major embolism is treated by *embolectomy or *streptokinase to remove or dissolve the embolus. *See also* air embolism.

栓塞 栓子停留在動脈裏，阻礙血液循環。最常見的是肺動脈栓塞，即循環中的血塊停留在肺動脈裏。任何動脈裏的栓子都可構成體循環栓塞。在這種病例中，常見的栓子來源是二尖瓣疾病時或心肌梗塞後心臟裏的血塊。臨床特點因栓子停留的部位而不同（如腦卒中由腦栓塞引起，壞疽由肢體動脈栓塞引起）。
治療以抗凝療法爲主，使用肝素和苄丙酮香豆素。大型栓塞應行栓子切除術治療，或用鏈激酶溶解栓子。

embolus *n.* (*pl.* **emboli**) material, such as a blood clot, fat, air, amniotic fluid, or a foreign body, that is carried by the blood from one point in the circulation to lodge at another point (*see* embolism).

栓子 在循環中，由血液從一點帶到另一點並停留下來的物質，如血塊、脂肪、空氣、羊水或異物。

embrasure *n.* the space formed between adjacent teeth.

楔狀隙 相隣牙齒之間的縫隙。

embrocation *n.* a lotion that is rubbed onto the body for the treatment of sprains and strains.

擦劑 爲治療扭傷和勞損而用來摩擦身體的洗劑。

embryo *n.* an animal at an early stage of development, before birth. In man the term refers to the products of conception within the womb in the first eight weeks of development, during which time all the main organs are formed (see illustration). *Compare* fetus. —**embryonic** *adj.*

胚胎 出生之前發育早期的動物。在人類，指在子宮內生長的前八週懷孕產物。在此期間，所有的主要器官均已形成。（見圖）

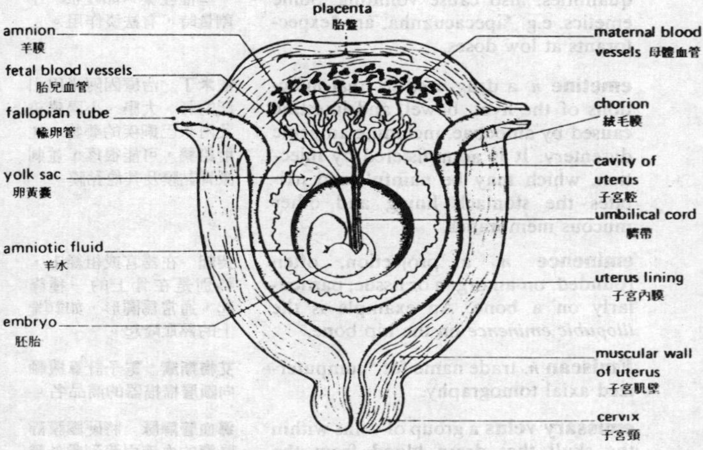

A developing embryo
胚胎的發育

embryology *n.* the study of growth and development of the embryo and fetus from fertilization of the ovum until birth. —**embryological** *adj.*

胚胎學 研究從卵子受精到胎兒出生這一時期胚胎及胎兒生長發育的科學。

embryonic disc the early embryo before the formation of *somites. It is a

胚盤 體節形成前的早期胚胎。扁平盤狀組織，背

flat disc of tissue bounded dorsally by the amniotic cavity and ventrally by the yolk sac. The formation of the *primitive streak and *archenteron in the embryonic disc determines the orientation of the embryo, which then becomes progressively elongated.

側與羊膜腔相接，腹側與卵黃囊相連。胚盤中的原條和原腸的形成決定了胚胎的定向，並使其逐漸延長。

embryotomy *n.* the cutting up of a fetus during difficult birth by means of an instrument called an *embryotome*, in order to aid delivery and reduce the danger to the mother.

碎胎術 難產時，用碎胎刀將胎兒切碎，以幫助生產和減少母體的危險。

emesis *n. see* vomiting.

嘔吐

emetic *n.* an agent that causes vomiting. Strong emetics, such as *apomorphine, are used to induce vomiting following drug overdose. Substances such as common salt, which irritate the stomach nerves if taken in sufficient quantities, also cause vomiting. Some emetics, e.g. *ipecacuanha, are *expectorants at low doses.

催吐藥 能引起嘔吐的一種藥物。强催吐藥，如阿樸嗎啡，在服藥過量時用於誘發嘔吐。某些物質，如食鹽，若食用過多，也能刺激胃神經引起嘔吐。一些催吐藥，如吐根，小劑量時，有祛痰作用。

emetine *n.* a drug used to treat infections of the liver, bowel, and intestine caused by amoebae, including amoebic dysentery. It is administered by injection, which may be painful, and irritates the stomach lining and other mucous membranes.

依米丁 治療因阿米巴引起的肝、大腸、小腸感染及阿米巴痢疾的藥物。注射給藥，可能很疼，並刺激胃黏膜及其他黏膜。

eminence *n.* a projection, often rounded, on an organ or tissue, particularly on a bone. An example is the *iliopubic eminence* on the hip bone.

突起 在器官或組織上，特別是在骨上的一種隆起，通常爲圓形，如髖骨上的髂恥隆起。

Emiscan *n.* trade name for *computerized axial tomography.

艾梅斯康 電子計算機軸向斷層掃描器的商品名。

emissary veins a group of veins within the skull that drain blood from the venous sinuses of the dura mater to veins outside the skull.

導血管靜脉 將硬腦膜靜脉竇的血液引流到顱外靜脉的一組顱內靜脉。

emission *n.* the flow of semen from the erect penis, usually occurring while the subject is asleep (*nocturnal emission*).

遺精 精液從勃起的陰莖中流出，通常發生在睡眠期間（夜間遺精）。

emmenagogue *n.* an agent that stimulates menstruation.

通經藥 刺激月經來潮的藥物。

emmetropia *n.* the state of refraction of the normal eye, in which parallel light rays are brought to a focus on the retina with the accommodation relaxed. Objects further than six metres from the eye are seen clearly without any effort to focus. *Compare* ametropia, hypermetropia, myopia.

正視眼 具有正常屈光能力的眼。即不用調節平行光線即可在視網膜上聚焦。當視物移到距眼 6 米以外時，不用調整焦距，就可以清楚地看到。

emollient *n.* an agent that soothes and softens the skin. Emollients are fats and oils, such as lanolin and liquid paraffin; they are used chiefly in skin preparations as a base for more active drugs, such as antibiotics.

潤滑劑 使皮膚光滑和柔軟的藥物。係脂肪和油脂類物質，如羊毛脂和液體石蠟。在皮膚製劑中，它們主要用做較爲速效的藥物，如抗生素的基質。

emotion *n.* a state of arousal that can be experienced as pleasant or unpleasant. Emotions can have three components: *subjective*, *physiological*, and *behavioural*. For example, fear can involve an unpleasant subjective experience, an increase in physiological measures such as heart rate, sweating, etc., and a tendency to flee from the fear-provoking situation.

情緒 能夠引起快樂或難過的心理狀態。情緒有三個組成部分：主觀上的、生理上的、行爲上的。如恐懼包括不愉快的主觀感受；生理上的反應加速，如心動過速、出汗等；及從引起恐懼的環境中逃走的傾向。

empathy *n.* the ability to understand the thoughts and emotions of another person. In a psychotherapist empathy is often considered to be one of the necessary qualities enabling successful treatment.

神入 理解他人想法和感情的能力。對進行心理治療的醫生來說，神入被認爲是能進行成功治療的必備特點之一。

emphysema *n.* air in the tissues. In *pulmonary emphysema* the air sacs (*alveoli) of the lungs are enlarged and damaged, which reduces the surface area for the exchange of oxygen and carbon dioxide. Severe emphysema causes breathlessness, which is made worse by infections. There is no specific treatment, and the patient may become dependent on oxygen. The mechanism by which emphysema develops is not understood, although it is known to be particularly common in men in Britain and is associated with chronic bronchitis, smoking, and advancing age.
In *surgical emphysema* air may escape into the tissues of the chest and neck

氣腫 組織中有氣體存在。在肺氣腫病中，肺泡腫大並被破壞，減少了氧氣和二氧化碳交換的面積。嚴重的肺氣腫可引起呼吸困難，並可因感染而加重。此病無特殊療法，患者要依靠吸氧生活。肺氣腫在英國是人人皆知和極爲常見的疾病，並與慢性氣管炎、吸烟、年齡的增長有關，但其發病機理尚未搞清。
在外科性氣腫中，氣體可能從肺和食管的裂縫中漏到胸部和頸部組織中去。在外科手術中，氣體有時

from leaks in the lungs or oesophagus; occasionally air escapes into other tissues during surgery, and bacteria may form gas in soft tissues. The presence of gas or air gives the affected tissues a characteristic crackling feeling to the touch, and it may be visible on X-rays. It is easily absorbed once the leak or production is stopped.

也會漏到其他組織中去，而且細菌也會在組織中產生氣體。因爲存在氣體，在觸摸患部組織時，有捻髮感。X線透視可見到氣體。當漏氣被阻止，或產氣停止時，氣體很容易被吸收。

empirical *adj.* describing a system of treatment based on experience or observation, rather than of logic or reason.

經驗主義的 指根據經驗或觀察而不是邏輯和推理的治療體系。

Employment Service Division (ESD) (in Britain) an integral part of the *Manpower Services Commission* (*MSC*) established in 1974 to take over responsibility from the Department of Employment for running public employment services. Along with the *Training Services Division* (*TSD*), it has special responsibility to employ and if necessary train (or retrain) those who are handicapped from any cause. Its *Disablement Resettlement Service* relies on specially trained Officers (*DRO*) who see that those with handicaps find satisfactory employment situations. Recommendations made by DRO include that of registration as *disabled people*, which helps in obtaining and retaining employment. Other ways of assisting include referral to one of 26 *Employment Rehabilitation Centres* for assessment of potential and/or reacclimatization to a working environment for those who have been absent from work through ill-health over a long period. Special training courses may be arranged for handicapped people as part of the *Training Opportunities Scheme* (*TOPS*) of the TSD. These courses, covering a wide range of skilled and semiskilled occupations and lasting about six months, may be held at colleges, *special skill centres*, or at the premises of potential employers. For the blind there are special *Blind Persons Resettlement Officers* (*BPRO*), though

雇用服務處 （在英國）於1974年建立的“人力服務委員會”的一個組成部分。該委員會接管了“雇用部”的任務，負責管理公共雇傭服務機構，與“培訓服務處”一起有特殊的雇傭責任。必要時，培訓因任何原因而殘廢的人。它的“殘廢人重新就業服務機構”主要依賴於受過專門訓練的官員，由他們來尋找殘廢人認爲滿意的工作環境。“殘廢人重新就業服務機構”頒發殘廢人登記證，有助於殘廢人得到並保留工作。另一方法是將因病長期脫離工作的人分配到26個“康復就業中心”之一，以估價其重新工作的能力和/或對工作環境的適應能力。特殊訓練班是爲殘廢人安排的，這是“培訓服務處”就業培訓大綱的一部分。這些培訓班培訓的職業項目較廣，有純技術性的和半技術性的，爲期六個月，可在學院、特殊技術中心或在雇主的單位裏舉辦。對盲人來說，還有專門的盲人重新就業辦公室，儘管全盲並不是注册的先決條件。

total blindness is not a prerequisite for registration.

empyema (pyothorax) *n.* pus in the *pleural cavity, usually secondary to infection in the lung or in the space below the diaphragm. It is a life-threatening condition, which can usually only be relieved by surgical drainage of the pus.

膿胸 胸腔積膿。常繼發於肺或膈下腔隙的感染。這是一種有生命危險的疾病。一般只有通過外科引流濃汁而緩解。

emulsion *n.* a preparation in which fine droplets of one liquid (such as oil) are dispersed in another liquid (such as water). In pharmacy medicines are prepared in the form of emulsions to disguise the taste of an oil, which is dispersed in a flavoured liquid.

乳劑 一種液體的微小顆粒（如油）分散在另一液體（如水）之中的製劑。在製藥業中，爲除去油味，藥物被製成乳劑形式。油液被分散到有香味的液體之中。

en- (em-) *prefix denoting* in; inside.

〔前 綴〕 在……之內

enamel *n.* the extremely hard outer covering of the crown of a *tooth. It is formed before tooth eruption by *ameloblasts.

釉質 牙冠的外層。極硬。在牙齒生長之前，由成釉細胞形成。

enanthema *n.* an eruption occurring on a mucus-secreting surface, such as the inside of the mouth or vagina.

黏膜疹 發生在黏膜表面的疹子，如在口腔或陰道的內表面上。

enarthrosis *n.* a ball-and-socket joint: a type of *diarthrosis (freely movable joint), e.g. the shoulder joint and the hip joint. Such a joint always involves a long bone, which is thus allowed to move in all planes.

杵臼關節 一種球囊關節。可動關節（自由移動的關節）的一種。如肩關節和髖關節。這種關節總是與長骨有關，使長骨在各種平面都能活動。

encapsulated *adj.* (of an organ, tumour, etc.) enclosed in a capsule.

包囊內的 被包囊包裹的（器官，腫瘤等）。

encephal- (encephalo-) *prefix denoting* the brain.

〔前綴〕 **腦**

encephalin (enkephalin) *n.* either of two peptides occurring naturally in the brain and having effects resembling those of morphine or other opiates. *See also* endorphin.

腦啡肽 自然產生於腦內兩種肽的任何一種。有類似嗎啡或鴉片的作用。

encephalitis *n.* inflammation of the brain. It may be caused by a viral or bacterial infection or it may be part of an allergic response to a systemic viral

腦炎 大腦炎症。可由病毒和細菌感染引起，也可是對全身病毒疾病或對接種的過敏反應的一部分。

illness or vaccination (*see* encephalomyelitis). *Viral encephalitis* is endemic in some parts of the world; it may also occur epidemically or sporadically. One form – *encephalitis lethargica* – reached epidemic proportions shortly after World War I and was marked by headache and drowsiness, progressing to coma (hence its popular name – *sleepy sickness*). Occasional cases still occur as a complication of mumps. It can cause postencephalitic *parkinsonism. Another type of encephalitis that occurs sporadically is due to herpes simplex.

病毒性腦炎是世界上一些地區的地方病，可呈流行性或散在性發病。有一種腦炎——嗜眠性腦炎——在第一次世界大戰後很快成爲流行病，並以頭痛、嗜眠及迅速進入昏迷狀態爲特點（因此，俗名又叫嗜眠病）。偶見的病例是流行性腮腺炎的併發症。它還可引起腦炎後帕金森氏綜合徵。另一種散發性腦炎由單純疱疹引起。

encephalocele *n. see* neural tube defects.

腦突出

encephalography *n.* any of various techniques for recording the structure of the brain or the activity of the brain cells. Examples are *echoencephalography, *electroencephalography, and *pneumoencephalography.

腦描記術 能記錄腦結構或腦細胞活動的各種技術。如腦超聲檢查術、腦電描記術和氣腦造影術。

encephaloid *adj.* having the appearance of brain tissue: applied to certain tumours, for example *encephaloid carcinoma of the breast*.

髓樣的 具有腦髓組織外觀的，用於描述某些腫瘤。如乳房髓樣癌。

encephalomyelitis *n.* an acute inflammatory disease affecting the brain and spinal cord. It is sometimes part of an overwhelming virus infection but *acute disseminated encephalomyelitis* is a form of delayed tissue hypersensitivity provoked by a mild infection or vaccination 7–10 days earlier. Survival through the acute phase of the illness is often followed by a remarkably complete recovery.

腦脊髓炎 腦和脊髓的急性炎症。有時是嚴重全身病毒感染的一部分。但急性瀰散性腦脊髓炎是由輕度感染或在接種後的7-10天內發生的遲發性組織過敏反應引起的。能夠渡過此病急性期的患者會很快康復。

encephalomyelopathy *n.* any condition in which there is widespread disease of the brain and spinal cord. *Necrotizing encephalomyelopathy of childhood* is a progressive illness with extensive destruction of nerve cells throughout the central nervous system. It is thought to be caused by a disorder of metabolism.

腦脊髓病 廣泛分佈於腦和脊髓的疾病的總稱。兒童壞死性腦脊髓病是一種急進性疾病，中樞神經系統的神經細胞遭到廣泛破壞。此病被認爲是代謝失常引起的。

encephalon *n. see* brain.

腦

encephalopathy *n.* any of various diseases that affect the functioning of the brain. *See* hepatic encephalopathy, Wernicke's encephalopathy.

腦病 任何損害腦功能的疾病。

enchondroma *n.* (*pl.* **enchondromata**) a benign cartilaginous tumour (*see* chondroma) occurring in the growing zone (metaphysis) of a bone and not protruding beyond its margins. Such tumours are often solitary; when multiple the condition is known as *enchondromatosis*. *Compare* ecchondroma.

內生軟骨瘤 生長在骨的生長帶（骨髓），但不超出其邊緣的一種良性軟骨瘤。這種瘤經常是單發的。當有多個這種瘤發生時，就叫做多發性內生軟骨瘤。

encopresis *n.* incontinence of faeces. The term is used for faecal soiling associated with psychiatric disturbance.

大便失禁 排便失控。此術語用來指與精神紊亂的有關的排便失禁。

encounter group a form of group psychotherapy. The emphasis is on encouraging close relationships between group members and on the expression of feelings. To this end, physical contact and confrontations between group members are arranged by the group leader. The stress of the experience can be damaging to maladjusted people.

"交朋友"小組 心理療法小組的一種形式。重點是促進小組成員密切相處和交流感情。爲達到這個目的，小組負責人根據他們能否和睦相處而給他們分組。痛苦的體驗對安排不當的小組成員來說是有害的。

encysted *adj.* enclosed in a cyst.

包囊內的 被囊包裹着的。

end- (endo-) *prefix denoting* within or inner. Example: *endonasal* (within the nose).

〔前綴〕 **在……之內，內部** 如鼻內的。

endarterectomy *n.* a surgical 're-bore' of an artery that has become obstructed by *atheroma with or without a blood clot (thrombus); the former operation is known as *thromboendarterectomy*. The inner part of the wall is removed together with any clot that is present. This restores patency and arterial blood flow to the tissues beyond the obstruction. The technique is most often applied to obstruction of the carotid arteries or of the arteries that supply the legs.

動脉內膜切除術 將帶有或不帶有血塊（栓子）的被粥樣斑塊堵塞的動脉打通。前一種手術叫做血栓動脉內膜切除術，是將動脉壁內膜與存在的血塊一起除去。這可使動脉恢復通暢，使動脉血液流到曾發生動脉阻塞的組織中去。這種手術常用於頸動脉阻塞或供應腿部血液的動脉堵塞。

endarteritis *n.* chronic inflammation of the inner (intimal) portion of the wall of an artery, which most often results from late syphilis. Thickening of the wall produces progressive arterial obstruction and symptoms from inadequate blood supply to the affected part (*ischaemia). The arteries to the brain are often involved, giving rise to meningovascular syphilis. Endarteritis of the aorta may obstruct the mouths of the coronary arteries, supplying the heart. Endarteritis of the arteries to the wall of the aorta (the vasa vasorum) contributes to *aneurysm formation. The syphilitic infection may be eradicated with penicillin.

動脈內膜炎 動脈壁內膜的慢性炎症，通常因晚期梅毒引起。動脈壁的增厚可逐漸引起動脈堵塞，並因此引起受損部位供血不足（缺血）而出現症狀。腦動脈經常受損，引起腦膜血管梅毒。主動脈內膜炎可堵塞營養心臟的冠狀動脈口。營養主動脈壁的動脈（血管滋養管）內膜炎可形成動脈瘤。青黴素可治癒梅毒性感染。

end artery the terminal branch of an artery, which does not communicate with other branches. The tissue it supplies is therefore probably completely dependent on it for its blood supply.

終末動脈 動脈的最終分支。不與其它動脈分支相交通。因此，它營養的組織要完全依靠它的血運。

endemic *adj.* occurring frequently in a particular region or population: applied to diseases that are generally or constantly found among people in a particular area. *Compare* ecdemic, epidemic, pandemic.

地方性的 在特定的區域或人羣中頻繁地發生的。指在特定的地區經常或不斷地在人羣中發生的疾病。

endemic syphilis *see* bejel.

非性病性梅毒

endocarditis *n.* inflammation of the lining of the heart cavity (endocardium) and valves. It is most often due to rheumatic fever or results from bacterial infection (*bacterial endocarditis*). Temporary or permanent damage to the heart valves may result. The main features are fever, changing heart murmurs, heart failure, and embolism. Treatment consists of rest and *antibiotics; surgery may be required to repair damaged heart valves.

心內膜炎 心臟內膜或瓣膜的炎症。主要因風濕熱或細菌性感染（細菌性心內膜炎）引起。可造成心瓣膜暫時或永久性的破壞。主要特點是發熱、多變的心臟雜音，心衰及栓塞。治療包括休息，用抗菌素；外科可修復損害的心瓣膜。

endocardium *n.* a delicate membrane, formed of flat endothelial cells, that lines the heart and is continuous with the lining of arteries and veins. At the openings of the heart cavities it is folded back on itself to form the cusps

心內膜 由扁平細胞組成的，內襯心臟的薄膜。與動、靜脈內膜相連。在心臟開口處，心內膜反折形成了心瓣膜尖部。其表面光滑，因而不妨礙血流。

of the valves. It presents a smooth slippery surface, which does not impede blood flow. —**endocardial** *adj.*

endocervicitis *n.* inflammation of the membrane lining the neck of the womb, usually resulting from infection. Surface cells (epithelium) may die, resulting in a new growth of healthy epithelium over the affected area. The condition is accompanied by a white or yellow discharge.

子宮頸內膜炎 子宮頸內膜炎症。通常由感染引起。表皮細胞（上皮細胞）可能死亡，受損部位又有新的健康上皮生長，並伴有黃或白色分泌物。

endocervix *n.* the mucous membrane (*endometrium) lining the neck (cervix) of the womb.

子宮頸內膜 覆蓋子宮頸的黏膜。

endochondral *adj.* within the material of a cartilage.

軟骨內的 在軟骨的內部。

endocrine gland (ductless gland) a gland that manufactures one or more *hormones and secretes them directly into the bloodstream (and not through a duct to the exterior). Endocrine glands include the pituitary, thyroid, parathyroid, and adrenal glands, the ovary and testis, the placenta, and part of the pancreas.

內分泌腺（無導管分泌腺） 分泌一種或多種激素並直接將其分泌入血（不是通過導管分泌到外部）的腺體。包括腦垂體、甲狀腺、甲狀旁腺及腎上腺、卵巢、睪丸、胎盤和部分胰腺。

endocrinology *n.* the study of the *endocrine glands and the substances they secrete (*hormones). —**endocrinologist** *n.*

內分泌學 研究內分泌腺及其分泌物（激素）的學科。

endoderm *n.* the inner of the three *germ layers of the early embryo, which gives rise to the lining of most of the alimentary canal and its associated glands, the liver, gall bladder, and pancreas. It also forms the lining of the bronchi and alveoli of the lung and most of the urinary tract.

內胚層 胚胎早期三胚層的內層。負責生長絕大部分消化道內膜及其附屬腺體、肝臟、膽囊及胰腺。也負責形成支氣管、肺泡及大部分泌尿道的內膜。

endodontics *n.* the study and treatment of diseases of the pulps of teeth and their sequelae. A major part of treatment is *root treatment.

牙髓病學 研究和治療牙髓病及其後遺症的科學。主要的治療手段是根管治療。

endogenous *adj.* arising within or derived from the body. For example, *endogenous depression* arises from

內生的 從體內產生的。如內生性抑鬱症就產生於體內的因素。

causes inside the body (*see* depression). *Compare* exogenous.

endolymph *n.* the fluid that fills the membranous *labyrinth of the ear.

內淋巴液 流入耳膜迷路的液體。

endolymphatic duct a blind-ended duct that leads from the sacculus and joins a duct from the utriculus of the membranous *labyrinth of the ear.

內淋巴管 從球囊發出，又與耳膜迷路橢圓囊發出的管道滙合的一側爲盲端的管道。

endometriosis *n.* the presence of membranous material of the kind lining the womb (*see* endometrium) at other sites within the cavity of the pelvis. In *direct* (*internal* or *primary*) *endometriosis*, the endometrium may penetrate the muscular wall of the womb, the ovaries, or the abdominal wall. The fragments of abnormally located tissue pass through the same periodic changes as the womb lining. Since there is no outlet for the bleeding that occurs from them, the patient suffers severe pain for several days each month. This symptom is not experienced during pregnancy or breast-feeding or after the menopause.

子宮內膜異位 子宮內膜樣物質存在於盆腔內其它部位。在直接性（子宮內或原發性）子宮內膜異位症中，子宮內膜可侵入子宮肌壁、卵巢或腹壁。這種異位組織碎片同子宮內膜一樣，隨同月經周期變化而脫落。因沒有排出的通口，患者每月都要經歷幾天嚴重的疼痛。這種症狀在孕期、哺乳期及絕經期消失。

endometritis *n.* inflammation of the membrane lining the womb (*endometrium). The condition, sometimes restricted to the neck of the womb, is a reaction to bacterial attack upon the membrane, possibly following physical damage. Ulcers may form and the membrane may be cast off. There may also be excessive menstrual bleeding and pain in the lower regions of the back and abdomen. *Decidual endometritis* occurs during pregnancy; *puerperal endometritis* is an acute form developing immediately after childbirth.

子宮內膜炎 子宮內膜炎症。有時，炎症僅限於子宮頸，是子宮內膜受損後細菌感染的結果，可產生潰瘍及黏膜脫落。也可出現月經過多及腰、下腹部疼痛。蛻膜性子宮內膜炎發生於妊娠期間。產後子宮內膜炎是分娩後迅速發生的急性病。

endometrium *n.* the mucous membrane lining the uterus (womb), which becomes progressively thicker and more glandular and has an increased blood supply in the latter part of the menstrual cycle. This prepares the en-

子宮內膜 內襯子宮的黏膜。在月經周期的後階段逐漸增厚，腺體增多，並得到更多的血液供給。這是爲胚胎的種植做準備。如果沒有妊娠，大部分子

dometrium for implantation of the embryo, but if this does not occur much of the endometrium breaks down and is lost in menstruation. If pregnancy is established the endometrium becomes the *decidua, which is shed after birth.

宮內膜將破裂並在月經期時排出體外。一旦妊娠，內膜將變成蛻膜，並在胎兒娩出後脫落。

endomorphic *adj.* describing a *body type that is relatively fat, with highly developed viscera and weak muscular and skeletal development. —**endomorph** *n.* —**endomorphy** *n.*

內胚層體形的 形容體態臃腫、內臟高度發達，而肌肉、骨骼發育較差的體型。

endomyocarditis *n.* an acute or chronic inflammatory disorder of the muscle and lining membrane of the heart. When the membrane surrounding the heart (pericardium) is also involved the condition is termed *pancarditis*. The principal causes are rheumatic fever and virus infections. There is enlargement of the heart, murmurs, embolism, and frequently arrhythmias. The treatment is that of the cause and complications. *See also* endocarditis.
A chronic condition, *endomyocardial fibrosis*, is seen in African negroes: the cause is unknown.

心肌內膜炎 心內膜和心肌的慢性或急性炎症。當心外膜（心包）也受累時，叫做全心炎。主要病因是風濕熱和病毒感染。症狀有心臟擴大、心臟雜音、栓塞及頻發的心律不齊。治療以病因和併發症爲主。一種慢性的心內膜肌纖維變性，見於非洲黑人，原因不明。

endomysium *n.* the fine connective tissue sheath that surrounds a single *muscle fibre.

肌內膜 包繞單個肌纖維的極薄的結締組織鞘。

endoneurium *n.* the layer of fibrous tissue that separates individual fibres within a *nerve.

神經內膜 在一根神經內，分隔單個纖維的纖維組織層。

endoparasite *n.* a parasite that lives inside its host, for example in the liver, lungs, gut, or other tissues of the body. *Compare* ectoparasite.

內寄生物 在宿主體內，如在肝臟、肺、腸道或其它組織內生存的寄生物。

endopeptidase *n.* a digestive enzyme (e.g. *pepsin) that splits a whole protein into small peptide fractions by splitting the linkages between peptides in the interior of the molecule. *Compare* exopeptidase. *See also* peptidase.

肽鏈內斷酶 一種消化酶（如胃蛋白酶）。通過分解分子內兩肽之間的鍵而使整個蛋白分解成若干個肽。

endophthalmitis *n.* inflammation confined to the posterior chamber of the

眼內炎 局限在眼後房的炎症。如在晶體後部。

eye, i.e. the part behind the lens. *Compare* panophthalmitis.

endoplasm *n.* the inner cytoplasm of cells, which is less dense than the *ectoplasm and contains most of the cell's structures. —**endoplasmic** *adj.*

內質 細胞內胞質，不如細胞外質稠密。具有細胞內絕大部分結構。

endoplasmic reticulum (ER) a system of membranes present in the cytoplasm of cells. ER is described as *rough* when it has *ribosomes attached to its surface and *smooth* when ribosomes are absent. It is the site of manufacture of proteins and lipids and is concerned with the transport of these products within the cell (*see also* Golgi apparatus).

內質網 細胞內胞質裏的膜系統。當其表面附有核糖體時，稱粗面內質網，反之爲滑面內質網。內質網是產生蛋白質和脂類的部位，並參與它們在細胞內的轉移。

end organ a specialized structure at the end of a peripheral nerve, acting as a receptor for a particular sensation. Taste buds, in the tongue, are end organs subserving the sense of taste.

末梢裝置 周圍神經末梢處的一種特殊結構。有接受特殊感覺的感受器作用。舌上的味蕾就是感受味覺的末梢裝置。

endorphin *n.* one of a group of chemical compounds, similar to the *encephalins, that occur naturally in the brain and have pain-relieving properties similar to those of the opiates. The endorphins are derived from a substance found in the pituitary gland called *beta-lipotropin*; they are thought to be concerned with controlling the activity of the endocrine glands.

內啡肽 與腦啡肽類似的一組化合物。產生於腦內，有類似麻醉劑的鎮痛特性。內啡肽來自腦垂體腺中一種叫做 β-趨脂素物質，並被認爲與控制內分泌腺活動有關。

endoscope *n.* any instrument used to obtain a view of the interior of the body. Examples of endoscopes include the *auriscope, used for examining the inside of the ear, and the *gastroscope, for examining the inside of the stomach. Essentially, most endoscopes consist of a tube with a light at the end and an optical system for transmitting an image to the examiner's eye. *See also* fibrescope. —**endoscopic** *adj.* —**endoscopy** *n.*

內窺鏡 用於觀察體內結構的儀器。例如耳鏡：檢查耳內結構；胃鏡：檢查胃內結構。絕大部分內窺鏡的基本結構都是由尾部帶光源的管子和將映像轉送到檢驗者眼內的光學系統組成。

endoscopic retrograde cholangiopancreatography *see* ERCP.

內窺鏡膽道胰腺逆行攝影

endospore *n.* the resting stage of certain bacteria, particularly species of the genera *Bacillus* and *Clostridium*. In adverse conditions the nucleus and cytoplasm within the normal vegetative stage of the bacterium can become enclosed within a tough protective coat, allowing the cell to survive. On return of favourable conditions the spore changes back to the vegetative form.

內孢子 某種細菌的靜止期。特別是桿菌和梭狀芽胞菌屬。在不利情況下，細菌內正常生長期的胞核和胞質可被堅硬的保護層包裹起來，使細胞免遭於害。回到有利時機時，孢子又恢復到生長期的形態。

endosteum *n.* the membrane that lines the marrow cavity of a bone.

骨內膜 覆蓋骨髓腔的膜。

endothelioma *n.* any tumour arising from or resembling endothelium. It may arise from the linings of blood or lymph vessels (*haemangioendothelioma* and *lymphangioendothelioma* respectively); from the linings of the pleural or peritoneal cavities (*see* mesothelioma); or from the meninges (*see* meningioma).

內皮瘤 起源於內皮或類似內皮的腫瘤。也可起源於血管或淋巴管內皮（血管內皮瘤及淋巴管內皮瘤）或胸膜、腹膜或腦膜。

endothelium *n.* the single layer of cells that lines the heart, blood vessels, and lymphatic vessels. It is derived from embryonic mesoderm. *Compare* epithelium.

內皮 內襯心臟、血管及淋巴管的單層細胞層。來源於胚胎的中胚層。

endothermic *adj.* describing a chemical reaction associated with the absorption of heat. *Compare* exothermic.

吸熱的 指吸收熱量的化學反應。

endotoxin *n.* a poison generally harmful to all body tissues, contained within a bacterium and released only when the bacterial cell is broken down or dies and disintegrates. *Compare* exotoxin.

內毒素 存在於細菌體內通常對人體所有組織都有害的毒物。只有在菌細胞被破壞、死亡及分解時才釋放出來。

end-plate *n.* the area of muscle cell membrane immediately beneath the motor nerve ending at a *neuromuscular junction. Special receptors in this area trigger muscular contraction when the nerve ending releases its *neurotransmitter.

終板 在神經肌結合處，直接位於運動神經末稍下的肌細胞膜的區域。當神經末稍釋放神經遞質時，該區域的特殊感受器就促使肌肉收縮。

enema *n.* (*pl.* **enemata** or **enemas**) a quantity of fluid infused into the rectum through a tube passed into the anus. An *evacuant enema* (soap or olive oil) is used to remove faeces. A *barium*

灌腸法 將一定量的液體通過從肛門進入的管子注入直腸。清洗灌腸（用肥皂或橄欖油）用於清除糞便。硫酸鋇能對X線顯

enema using barium sulphate, which is opaque to X-rays, is given to demonstrate the colon by X-ray. A *therapeutic enema* is used to insert drugs into the rectum, usually corticosteroids in the treatment of *proctocolitis.

影，所以鋇灌腸用於使結腸在X線下顯影。治療性灌腸用於把藥灌入直腸，皮質類固醇灌腸常用來治療直腸結腸炎。

enervation *n.* **1.** weakness; loss of strength. **2.** the surgical removal of a nerve.

①虛弱無力 ②神經切除

engram *n.* the supposed physical basis of an individual memory.

興奮痕迹 個體記憶的假設的生理基礎。

enkephalin *n. see* encephalin.

腦啡肽

enophthalmos *n.* a condition in which the eye is abnormally sunken into the socket. It may follow fractures of the floor of the orbit that allow the eye to sink downwards and backwards.

眼球陷沒 眼睛不正常地陷入眼眶中。眶底骨折時，眼睛可向後下方凹陷。

ensiform cartilage *see* xiphoid process.

劍突軟骨

Entamoeba *n.* a genus of widely distributed amoebae, of which some species are parasites of the digestive tract of man. *E. histolytica* invades and destroys the tissues of the intestinal wall, causing *dysentery and ulceration of the gut wall, and the parasite may spread to the liver, where it produces an abscess (*see* amoeboma). *E. coli* is a harmless intestinal parasite; *E. gingivalis*, found within the spaces between the teeth, is associated with periodontal disease and gingivitis.

內阿米巴屬 廣泛分佈的阿米巴原蟲屬。其中一些種類是人類消化道的寄生蟲。溶組織內阿米巴侵入並破壞腸壁組織，引起痢疾和腸壁潰瘍。此寄生蟲還可竄到肝臟，產生膿腫。結腸內阿米巴對腸道無害。齦內阿米巴見於兩齒之間的縫隙，與牙周病及齒齦炎有關。

enter- (entero-) *prefix denoting* the intestine. Example: *enterolith* (calculus in).

〔前綴〕**腸** 如腸結石。

enteral *adj.* of or relating to the intestinal tract.

腸的

enteralgia *n. see* colic.

腸痛

enterectomy *n.* surgical removal of part of the intestine.

腸切除術 部分腸切除手術。

enteric *adj.* relating to or affecting the intestine.

腸的 指腸或侵犯腸的。

enteric-coated *adj.* describing tablets that are coated with a substance that enables them to pass through the stomach to the intestine unchanged. Enteric-coated tablets contain drugs that are destroyed by the acid contents of the stomach.

包有腸溶衣的 指被一層物質包裹的藥片。有些藥物能被胃酸所破壞，被糖衣包裹後可使藥片通過胃進入腸道前不發生變化。

enteric fever *see* paratyphoid fever, typhoid fever.

腸熱病

enteritis *n.* inflammation of the small intestine, usually causing diarrhoea. *Infective enteritis* is caused by viruses or bacteria; *radiation enteritis* is caused by X-rays or radioactive isotopes. *See also* Crohn's disease (regional enteritis), gastroenteritis.

腸炎 小腸炎症。通常引起腹瀉。感染性腸炎由病毒和細菌引起。放射性腸炎由X線或放射性同位素引起。

enterobiasis (oxyuriasis) *n.* a disease, common in children throughout the world, caused by the parasitic nematode *Enterobius vermicularis* (*see* pinworm) in the large intestine. The worms do not cause any serious lesions of the gut wall although, rarely, they may provoke appendicitis. The emergence of the female from the anus at night irritates and inflames the surrounding skin, causing the patient to scratch and thereby contaminate fingers and nails with infective eggs. The eggs may reinfect the same child or be spread to other children. Worms may occasionally enter the vulva and cause a discharge from the vagina. Enterobiasis responds well to treatment with *piperazine compounds.

蟯蟲病 世界常見的一種兒童疾病。由寄生在大腸裏的蟯蟲引起。儘管此寄生蟲不會給腸壁造成嚴重的病變，但也可偶爾引起闌尾炎。夜間，雌蟯蟲從肛門爬出，刺激周圍皮膚並引起炎症，促使患者去抓搔，因此，患者手指及指甲被傳染性蟲卵汚染。蟲卵又可重新感染同一兒童或傳播到另一兒童。蟯蟲偶可進入陰道刺激陰道分泌。哌嗪治療蟯蟲病效果良好。

Enterobius (Oxyuris) *n. see* pinworm.

蟯蟲屬

enterocele *n.* a hernia of part of the intestine.

腸疝 部分腸道疝。

enterocentesis *n.* a surgical procedure in which a hollow needle is pushed through the wall of the stomach or intestines to release an abnormal accumulation of gas or fluid.

腸穿刺 一種外科手術。將空心針通過胃壁或腸壁刺入其內，釋放出不正常的積氣和積液。

enterocolitis *n.* inflammation of the colon and small intestine. *See also* colitis, enteritis.

小腸結腸炎 結腸和小腸炎症。

enterogastrone *n.* a hormone from the small intestine (duodenum) that inhibits the secretion of gastric juice by the stomach. It is released when the stomach contents pass into the small intestine.

腸抑胃素 小腸（十二指腸）分泌的激素。能抑制胃液的分泌。當胃內容物進入小腸時，此激素才被分泌出來。

enterogenous *adj.* borne by or carried in the intestine.

腸生的 由腸道生長的或被帶到腸內的。

enterokinase *n.* the former name for *enteropeptidase.

腸激酶 腸肽酶的舊稱。

enterolith *n.* a stone within the intestine. It usually builds up around a gallstone or a swallowed fruit stone.

腸石 腸道內的石頭。是圍繞着膽石或被吞入的果核產生的。

enteromegaly *n. Rare.* enlargement (usually increased diameter) of the intestine.

巨腸 少見。腸增大（通常是直徑增大）。

enteropathy *n.* disease of the small intestine. *See also* coeliac disease (gluten-induced enteropathy).

腸病 小腸疾病。

enteropeptidase *n.* an enzyme secreted by the glands of the small intestine that acts on trypsinogen to produce *trypsin. It is part of the *succus entericus.

腸肽酶 小腸腺分泌的一種酶。作用於胰蛋白酶原，以產生胰蛋白酶。腸肽酶是腸液中的一部分。

enteropexy *n.* a surgical operation in which part of the intestine is fixed to the abdominal wall. This was formerly performed for visceroptosis (a condition in which the abdominal organs were thought to have descended to a lower than normal position), but it is no longer carried out.

腸固定術 將部分腸管固定在腹壁上的一種外科手術。以前，此手術用來治療內臟下垂（腹腔臟器離開正常的位置而下傾）。現已不做此手術。

enteroptosis *n.* a condition in which loops of intestine (especially transverse *colon) are in a low anatomical position. At one time this was thought to cause various abdominal symptoms, and operations were devised to correct it. It is now known that no symptoms result from simple anatomical variations of this sort.

腸下垂 腸襻（特別是橫結腸）低於其固有解剖位置。曾有一時期，此情況被認爲是腹部各種症狀的原因。並設計手術予以糾正。現在已知這種單純的解剖位置變化是不會引起任何症狀的。

enterorrhaphy *n.* the surgical procedure of stitching an intestine that has either perforated or been divided during an operation.

腸縫合術 因腸穿孔或手術時腸斷離而將其縫合的一種外科手術。

enterospasm *n.* powerful contraction of the intestine, usually accompanied by pain.

腸痙攣 腸道强烈的收縮。通常伴有疼痛。

enterostomy *n.* an operation in which the small intestine is brought through the abdominal wall and opened (*see* duodenostomy, jejunostomy, ileostomy) or is joined to the stomach (*gastroenterostomy*) or to another loop of small intestine (*enteroenterostomy*).

腸造口術 將小腸經腹壁拉出並造口或將其與胃或其它腸襻相連接的手術。

enterotomy *n.* surgical incision into the intestine.

腸切開術 切開腸道的手術。

enterotoxin *n.* a poisonous substance that has a particularly marked effect upon the gastrointestinal tract, causing vomiting, diarrhoea, and abdominal pain.

腸毒素 對胃腸道有明顯作用的有毒物質。可引起嘔吐、腹瀉和腹痛。

enterovirus *n.* any virus that enters the body through the gastrointestinal tract, multiplies there, and then (generally) invades the central nervous system. Enteroviruses include *Coxsackie viruses, *echoviruses, *polioviruses, and *rhinoviruses.

腸病毒 通過胃腸道進入體內，並在腸內繁殖，然後侵犯中樞神經系統的任何病毒。包括柯薩奇病毒、埃可病毒、脊髓灰質炎病毒及鼻病毒。

enterozoon *n.* any animal species inhabiting or infecting the gut of another. *See also* endoparasite.

腸寄生物 任何寄生於他種動物腸道中的動物種類。

entoptic phenomena visual sensations caused by changes within the eye itself, rather than by the normal light stimulation process. The commonest are tiny floating spots that most people can see occasionally, especially when gazing at a brightly illuminated background (such as a blue sky).

眼內現象 因眼內本身的變化，而不是正常光線的刺激所引起的視覺。最常見的眼內變化是大多數人都能偶爾見到的小懸浮點，特別是在凝視光芒耀眼的背景（如藍天）時。

entropion *n.* inturning of the eyelid towards the eyeball. The lashes may rub against the eye and cause irritation (*see* trichiasis). The commonest type is *spastic entropion* of the lower eyelid,

瞼內翻 眼瞼向內翻向眼球。睫毛可由此磨擦眼睛，引起炎症。最常見的炎症類型是下眼瞼痙攣性內翻，因眼輪匝肌痙攣引

due to spasm of the muscle that closes the eye (orbicularis oculi). Entropion may also be caused by scarring of the lining membrane (conjunctiva) of the lid.

起。內翻也可因結膜疤痕引起。

enucleation *n.* a surgical operation in which an organ, tumour, or cyst is completely removed. In ophthalmology it is an operation in which the eyeball is removed but the other structures in the socket (e.g. eye muscles) are left in place. Commonly a plastic ball is buried in the socket to provide a firm base on which to fit an artificial eye.

剜出術 將器官、腫瘤或囊腫全部除去的手術。在眼科學中，是指將眼球除去但保留眼眶內其它結構（如眼肌）的手術。通常將一個塑料球作爲堅硬的基底埋入眼眶，再在其上嵌入人工眼。

enuresis *n.* the involuntary passing of urine, especially bedwetting at night (*nocturnal enuresis*). This can be caused by underlying disorders of the urinary tract but is usually functional in nature. The condition settles spontaneously as the child grows older, but it may persist into teenage – and rarely adult – life. The condition can be treated successfully by fluid restriction, various drugs, or use of a nocturnal alarm (*see* bell and pad). *See also* incontinence. —**enuretic** *adj.*

遺尿 無意識地排尿。特別是發生在夜間（夜遺尿）。可由潛在的泌尿道疾病引起，但通常是功能性的。隨着兒童的年齡增長，此病可逐漸停止，但也可持續到青少年。個別人還可持續到成年，直到終生。限制飲水，使用藥物，或在夜間使用鬧鐘以提醒排尿都可成功地治療此病。

environment *n.* any or all aspects of the surroundings of an organism, both internal and external, which influence its growth, development, and behaviour.

環境 生物體周圍的各個方面。包括內、外環境。能影響生物體的生長，發育和其行爲。

Environmental Health Officer (EHO) a person, employed by local authorities, with special training in such aspects of environmental health and pollution as housing, sanitation, food, clean air, and water supplies (formerly known as a *Public Health Inspector*). Though not a registered medical practitioner, the EHO is responsible for the organization of the environmental health department. If medical (epidemiological) advice is required, the appropriate *community physician (Proper Officer) acts in an advisory or consultant capacity.

環境衞生官員 當地政府雇用的在住房衞生、環境衞生、食品衞生、空氣凈化和供水衞生等方面受過專門訓練的人員（以前稱爲公共衞生檢查員）。儘管他們不是註册的醫生，但他們要負責環境衞生部門的組織工作。如果需要醫學（流行病學）諮詢，公共保健醫師將擔任顧問。

enzyme *n.* a protein that, in small amounts, speeds up the rate of a biological reaction without itself being used up in the reaction (i.e. it acts as a catalyst). An enzyme acts by binding with the substance involved in the reaction (the *substrate*) and converting it into another substance (the *product* of the reaction). An enzyme is relatively specific in the type of reaction it catalyses; hence there are many different enzymes for the various biochemical reactions. Each enzyme requires certain conditions for optimum activity, particularly correct temperature and pH, the presence of *coenzymes, and the absence of specific inhibitors. Enzymes are unstable and are easily inactivated by heat or certain chemicals. They are produced within living cells and may act either within the cell (as in cellular respiration) or outside it (as in digestion). The names of enzymes usually end in *-ase*; enzymes are named according to the substrate upon which they act (as in *lactase*), or the type of reaction they catalyse (as in *hydrolase*).
Enzymes are essential for the normal functioning and development of the body. Failure in the production or activity of a single enzyme may result in metabolic disorders; such disorders are often inherited and some have serious effects. —**enzymatic** *adj.*

酶 一種只需要少量就可以加速生化反應而其本身並不參加該反應（如起催化劑作用）的蛋白質。酶是通過與反應中的物質（底物）結合，又將該物質轉變成另一物質（反應的產物）而發揮作用的。酶對其催化反應的種類是有特異性的。因此，有很多不同的酶參與各種生化反應。爲達到其最佳活性，每種酶都需一定的條件，特別是適宜的溫度和pH值及輔酶的存在和無特異性抑制劑參與。酶是不穩定的，很容易受到熱及某些化學物質影響而失活。它們在活細胞內產生，並可在細胞內和細胞外起作用（前者如細胞呼吸，後者如消化）。酶的名稱通常以-ase結尾，並根據其作用的物質或催化的反應命名（前者如乳糖酶，後者如水解酶）。
酶對身體的正常功能和發育是必要的。一種酶的產生或活性受阻可引起代謝性疾病。這種病通常是遺傳的，有些病還可導致嚴重的後果。

eonism *n.* the adoption of female manners and dress by a man. *See* transsexualism, transvestitism.

易裝癖 男性採用女性的姿態和穿着。

eosin *n.* a red acidic dye, produced by the reaction of bromine and fluorescein, used to stain biological specimens for microscopical examination. Eosin may be used in conjunction with a contrasting blue alkaline dye taken up by different parts of the same specimen.

伊紅 紅色酸性染料，是溴和熒光素反應的產物。用來對生物標本進行染色以進行顯微鏡下檢查。伊紅可與能被同一標本不同部位所吸收的對比鹼性藍染料聯合使用。

eosinopenia *n.* a decrease in the number of eosinophils in the blood.

嗜酸性細胞減少 血液中嗜酸性紅細胞數量下降。

eosinophil *n.* a variety of white blood cell distinguished by the presence in its cytoplasm of coarse granules that stain orange-red with *Romanowsky stains. The function of the eosinophil is poorly understood, but it is capable of ingesting foreign particles, is present in large numbers in lining or covering surfaces within the body, and is involved in allergic responses. There are normally 0.04–0.4 × 10^9 eosinophils per litre of blood.

嗜酸性細胞 血液中能用羅曼諾夫斯基氏染色法將胞質內粗顆粒染成橘紅色的各種白細胞。此細胞的功能不清楚，但能消化外來顆粒，並大量存在於體內臟器的內表或外表，還與過敏反應有關。正常情況下，每升血液中有0.04-0.4×10^9個嗜酸性細胞。

eosinophilia *n.* an increase in the number of eosinophils in the blood. Eosinophilia occurs in a variety of diseases, including allergies, parasitic infestations, and certain forms of leukaemia.

嗜酸性細胞增多 血液中嗜酸細胞數量增多。可發生於各種疾病，包括過敏、寄生蟲侵襲及某些類型的白血病。

eparterial *adj.* situated on or above an artery.

動脈上的 位於動脈上，或動脈以上的。

ependyma *n.* the extremely thin membrane, composed of cells of the *glia (*ependymal cells*), that lines the ventricles of the brain and the choroid plexuses. It is responsible for helping to form cerebrospinal fluid. —**ependymal** *adj.*

室管膜 由神經膠質細胞組成的極薄的膜。內襯腦室和脉絡叢，由此產生腦脊液。

ependymoma *n.* a cerebral tumour derived from the glial (non-nervous) cells lining the cavities of the ventricles of the brain (*see* ependyma). It may obstruct the flow of cerebrospinal fluid, causing a *hydrocephalus.

室管膜瘤 生長於腦室腔內膜膠質細胞（非神經細胞的）的腦腫瘤。可堵塞腦脊液的流動，引起腦積水。

ephebiatrics *n.* the branch of medicine concerned with the common disorders of children and adolescents. *Compare* paediatrics.

青年病學 研究兒童和青少年常見病的醫學分支。

ephedrine *n.* a drug that causes constriction of blood vessels and widening of the bronchial passages (*see* sympathomimetic). It is used mainly in the treatment of asthma and other allergic conditions and chronic bronchitis. It is administered by mouth or by inhalation and may cause nausea and vomiting, insomnia, headache, and nervousness.

麻黃鹼 能使血管收縮、支氣管擴張的藥物。主要治療哮喘，某些過敏性疾病及慢性支氣管炎。口服或吸入。能引起噁心、嘔吐、失眠、頭痛及神經過敏。

epi- *prefix denoting* above or upon.

〔前綴〕 **上，在……之上**

epiblepharon *n.* an abnormal fold of skin, present from birth, stretching across the eye just above the lashes of the upper eyelid or in front of them in the lower lid. It may cause the lower lashes to turn upwards or inwards against the eye. It usually disappears within the first year of life.

瞼贅皮 出生時就存在的不正常的皮膚皺褶。佔據上眼瞼睫毛上部的整個眼部或下眼瞼睫毛的前部。可使下睫毛上翻或內翻而磨擦眼睛。

epicanthus (epicanthic fold) *n.* a vertical fold of skin from the upper eyelid that covers the inner corner of the eye. It is normal in Mongolian races and occurs abnormally in certain congenital conditions, e.g. *Down's syndrome. —**epicanthal, epicanthic** *adj.*

內眥贅皮 從上眼瞼下垂、覆蓋內眼角的垂直皮膚皺褶。在蒙古人種是正常現象，也可發生於某種先天性疾患，如伸舌樣痴呆。

epicardia *n.* the part of the *oesophagus, about 2 cm long, that extends from the level of the diaphragm to the stomach.

食管腹部 從橫膈到胃這部分食管，約2cm長。

epicardium *n.* the outermost layer of the heart wall, enveloping the myocardium. It is a serous membrane that forms the inner layer of the serous *pericardium. —**epicardial** *adj.*

心外膜 包裹心肌的心壁最外層。是一層漿膜，構成了心包漿膜層的內層。

epicondyle *n.* the protuberance above a *condyle at the end of an articulating bone.

上髁 骨關節端髁上部的突起。

epicranium *n.* the structures that cover the cranium, i.e. all layers of the scalp.

頭被 覆蓋頭顱的結構。如頭皮的各層。

epicranius *n.* the muscle of the scalp. The *frontal* portion, at the forehead, is responsible for raising the eyebrows and wrinkling the forehead; the *occipital* portion, at the base of the skull, draws the scalp backwards.

顱頂肌 頭皮中的肌肉。額部的額肌負責提眉和皺額。顱底枕部肌肉能向後牽拉頭皮。

epicritic *adj.* describing or relating to sensory nerve fibres responsible for the fine degrees of sensation, as of temperature and touch. *Compare* protopathic.

細覺的 指負責接收細微感覺如溫度、觸摸的感覺神經纖維。

epidemic *n.* a sudden outbreak of infectious disease that spreads rapidly through the population, affecting a large proportion of people. The commonest epidemics today are of influ-

流行病 突然爆發、迅速在人羣中傳播、危害大批人的傳染病。當今，最常見的流行病是流行性感冒。

enza. *Compare* endemic, pandemic. —**epidemic** *adj.*

epidemiology *n.* the study of epidemic disease, with a view to finding means of control and future prevention. This not only applies to the study of such classical epidemics as plague, smallpox, and cholera but also includes all forms of disease that relate to the environment and ways of life. It thus includes the study of the links between smoking and cancer, and diet and coronary disease, as well as *communicable diseases.

流行病學 研究控制和預防流行病的措施的科學。不僅只研究典型的流行病，如鼠疫、天花、霍亂，也研究與環境和生活方式有關的所有類型的疾病。因此，流行病學也包括研究吸煙與癌症、飲食與冠心病的關係。

epidermis *n.* the outer layer of the *skin, which is divided into four layers (see illustration). The innermost *Malpighian* or *germinative layer* (*stratum germinativum*) consists of continuously dividing cells. The other three layers are continually renewed as cells from the germinative layer are gradually pushed outwards and become progressively impregnated with keratin (*see* keratinization). The outermost layer (*stratum corneum*) consists of dead cells whose cytoplasm has been entirely replaced by keratin. It is thickest on the soles of the feet and palms of the hands. —**epidermal** *adj.*

表皮 皮膚的最外層。可分爲四層（見圖）。最內層是馬爾皮基層或生發層，由不斷分裂的細胞組成。其它三層因生發層的細胞逐漸向上推擠而不斷更新並不斷產生角蛋白。最外層由死亡細胞組成，其胞質已完全被角蛋白取代。在脚跟和手掌部位，它是最厚的。

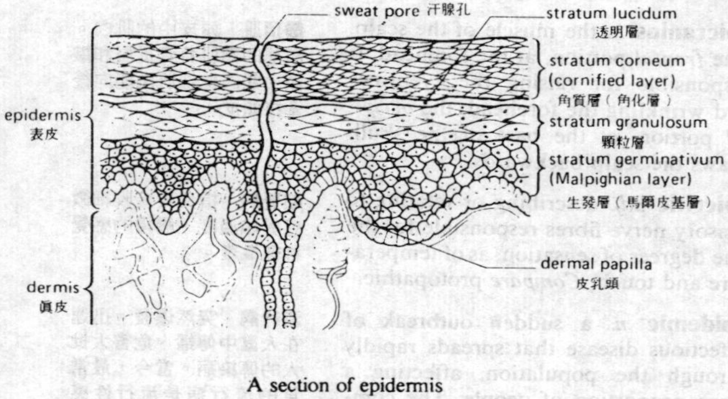

A section of epidermis
眞皮切面

epidermoid *adj.* having the appearance of epidermis (the outer layer of the skin): used to describe certain tumours of tissues other than the skin.

表皮樣的 具有表皮外觀的。用來形容某些組織而不是皮膚上的腫瘤。

epidermolysis *n.* loosening of the outer layer of the skin (epidermis), with the development of large blisters, occurring either spontaneously or after injury.

表皮鬆解 皮膚外層（表皮）疏鬆，有大疱。或是自發的，或是在損傷後產生。

Epidermophyton *n.* a genus of fungi that grow on the skin and produce the skin infections *athlete's foot and *dhobie itch.

表皮癬菌屬 生長在皮膚上的眞菌屬。可引起皮膚感染性脚癬及朵比癬。

epidiascope *n.* an apparatus for projecting a greatly magnified image of an object, such as a specimen on a microscope slide, on to a screen.

實物幻燈機 能將物體（如顯微鏡載物片上的標本）高度放大到屏幕上的投影裝置。

epididymis *n.* (*pl.* **epididymides**) a highly convoluted tube, about seven metres long, that connects the *testis to the vas deferens. The spermatozoa are moved passively along the tube over a period of several days, during which time they mature and become capable of fertilization. They are concentrated and stored in the lower part of the epididymis until ejaculation. —**epididymal** *adj.*

附睾 連接睾丸和輸精管的高度卷曲的管道。約7米長。精子沿管道被動移動需幾天的時間，在這期間精子成熟並有能力授精。精子在附睾下部濃縮並貯存，直到射精。

epididymitis *n.* inflammation of the epididymis. The usual cause is infection spreading down the vas deferens from the bladder or urethra, resulting in pain, swelling, and redness of the affected half of the scrotum. The inflammation may spread to the testicle (*epididymo-orchitis*). Treatment is by administration of antibiotics and analgesics.

附睾炎 附睾炎症。常見的原因是來自膀胱或尿道通過輸精管蔓延的感染。患側陰囊疼痛及紅腫。炎症還可擴延到睾丸。用抗生素及鎮痛藥治療。

epidural (extradural) *adj.* on or over the dura mater (the outermost of the three membranes covering the brain and spinal cord). The *epidural space* is the space between the dura mater of the spinal cord and the vertebral canal. *See also* spinal anaesthesia.

硬膜外的 在硬腦脊膜（覆蓋腦及脊髓的三層膜中的最外層）以外的。硬膜外腔是硬脊膜和椎管之間的間隙。

epigastrium *n.* the upper central region of the *abdomen. —**epigastric** *adj.*

上腹部的 腹部的中上部位。

epigastrocele *n.* a *hernia through the upper central abdominal wall.

上腹疝　中上腹壁疝。

epiglottis *n.* a thin leaf-shaped flap of cartilage, covered with mucous membrane, situated immediately behind the root of the tongue. It covers the entrance to the *larynx during swallowing.

會厭　由黏膜覆蓋的葉狀軟骨薄瓣。直接位於舌根後部。在吞咽時，蓋住喉部入口處。

epiglottitis *n.* inflammation of the mucous membrane of the epiglottis. Swelling and inflammation of the tissues at the laryngeal entrance obstructs the air flow to the lungs, causing a dangerous form of *croup.

會厭炎　會厭黏膜炎症。因喉部入口處的組織水腫、發炎，堵塞了通入肺部的氣流，可引起有生命危險的哮吼。

epilation *n.* the removal of a hair by its roots. This can be done mechanically (by pulling the hairs individually or using wax to strip an area of hair) or by electrolysis, which removes the hair permanently.

脫毛法　從根部除去毛髮。可機械性拔除（一根根地拔掉或用蠟除去某一部位的毛髮），或通過電解法除去。後者可永久除毛。

epilepsy *n.* any one of a group of disorders of brain function characterized by recurrent attacks that have a sudden onset. *Idiopathic epilepsy* is not associated with structural damage to the brain. It includes *grand mal and *petit mal, which can be controlled by the use of different *anticonvulsant drugs.
Focal (or *symptomatic*) *epilepsy* is a symptom of structural disease of the brain, and the nature of the fit depends upon the location of the disease in the brain. In *Jacksonian epilepsy* the epileptic discharge spreads over the cerebral cortex, with the resulting manifestations spreading throughout the body. In a Jacksonian motor fit the convulsive movements might spread from the thumb to the hand, arm, and face (this spread of symptoms is called the *march*). *Temporal lobe* (or *psychomotor*) *epilepsy* is caused by disease in the cortex of the temporal lobe or the adjacent parietal lobe of the brain. Its symptoms include *hallucinations of smell, taste, sight, and hearing, parox-

癲癇　一組具有腦功能失常的疾病。其特點爲反復突然性發作。特發性癲癇與腦結構受損無關。它包括大發作和小發作。可被不同種類的抗驚厥藥控制。

病竈性（症狀性）癲癇是腦結構疾病的症狀。其發作特點因疾病在腦中的位置而不同。在傑克遜氏癲癇中，癲癇性放電在大腦皮層中傳播，引起全身性發作。在傑克遜氏運動性發作中，抽搐從姆指傳到手、肩、臉（這種傳播方式稱爲進行型）。顳葉癲癇（精神運動型癲癇）是由大腦顳葉或隣近的頂葉皮質層疾病引起的。其症狀包括嗅幻覺、味幻覺、視幻覺及聽幻覺，還時常出現記憶障礙和自動症。在整個發作期間，患者始終意識不清。發作後，患者不能回憶起這一過程。

ysmal disorders of memory, and *automatism. Throughout an attack the patient is in a state of clouded awareness and afterwards he may have no recollection of the event (*see also* déja vu, jamais vu). —**epileptic** *adj.*, *n.*

epileptogenic *adj.* having the capacity to provoke epileptic fits.
引起癲癇的 具有引起癲癇發作能力的。

epiloia *n. see* tuberous sclerosis.
結節性腦硬化

epimenorrhagia *n. see* menorrhagia.
月經過多

epimenorrhoea *n.* menstruation at shorter intervals than is normal.
月經過頻 月經間期縮短。

epimysium *n.* the fibrous elastic tissue that surrounds a *muscle.
肌外膜 包繞肌肉的彈性纖維組織。

epinephrine *n. see* adrenaline.
腎上腺素

epineural *adj.* derived from or situated on the neural arch of a vertebra.
神經弓上的 源於或位於椎骨神經弓上的。

epineurium *n.* the outer sheath of connective tissue that encloses the bundles (fascicles) of fibres that make up a *nerve.
神經外膜 包繞組成神經的纖維束的結締組織外鞘。

epiphenomenon *n.* an unusual symptom or event that may occur simultaneously with a disease but is not necessarily directly related to it. *Compare* complication.
副現象 不正常的症狀或事態。可與疾病同時發生，但不一定與其有直接的關係。

epiphora *n.* watering of the eye, in which tears flow onto the cheek. It is due to some abnormality of the tear drainage system (*see* lacrimal apparatus).
淚溢 眼睛流淚，且流到頰部。因淚液引流系統不正常引起。

epiphysis *n.* **1.** the end of a long bone, which is initially separated by cartilage from the shaft (diaphysis) of the bone and develops separately. It eventually fuses with the diaphysis to form a complete bone. **2.** *see* pineal body.
①**骺** 長骨末端。最初由軟骨將其與骨幹分開，獨自生長發育。最後與骨幹融合，形成一整骨。②**松果體**

epiphysitis *n.* inflammation of the end (epiphysis) of a long bone. It may result in retardation of growth and deformity of the affected bone.
骺炎 長骨末端（骺）炎症。可使受損骨生長遲緩及變形。

epiplo- *prefix denoting* the omentum. Example: *epiplocele* (hernia containing omentum).

〔前綴〕 **網膜** 如網膜疝（含有網膜的疝）。

epiploon *n. see* omentum.

網膜

episio- *prefix denoting* the vulva. Example: *episioplasty* (plastic surgery of).

〔前綴〕 **外陰** 如外陰成形術（整形術）。

episiorrhaphy *n.* stitching together the margins of a tear in the tissues around the vaginal opening.

外陰縫合術 將陰道口周圍撕裂的組織邊緣縫合。

episiotomy *n.* an incision into the tissues surrounding the opening of the vagina (perineum) during a difficult birth, at the stage when the infant's head has partly emerged through the opening of the birth passage. The aim is to enlarge the opening in a controlled manner so as to make delivery easier and to avoid extensive tearing of adjacent tissues.

外陰切開術 將陰道口周圍組織切開。用於在胎頭部分露出產道的難產時。目的在於有限度地擴大產道口，使胎兒易於娩出及避免陰道附近組織進一步撕裂。

epispadias *n.* a congenital abnormality in which the opening of the *urethra is on the dorsal (upper) surface of the penis. Surgical correction is carried out in infancy.

尿道上裂 尿道口開在陰莖背表面（上部）的一種先天性異常。可在嬰兒時進行外科矯正。

epispastic *n. see* vesicant.

發疱藥

epistasis *n.* a type of gene action in which one gene suppresses the action of another (nonallelic) gene. The term is sometimes used for any interaction between nonallelic genes. **—epistatic** *adj.*

上位遺傳 基因作用的一種。即一種基因阻止另一基因的作用。此術語有時也用於指兩個非等位基因之間的相互作用。

epistaxis *n. see* nosebleed.

鼻出血

epithalamus *n.* part of the forebrain, consisting of a narrow band of nerve tissue in the roof of the third ventricle (including the region where the choroid plexus is attached) and the *pineal body. *See also* brain.

丘腦上部 前腦的一部分。由第三腦室頂部（包括有脉絡叢的部位）中的神經組織窄索及松果體組成。

epithalaxia *n.* loss of layers of epithelial cells from the skin or the lining of the intestine.

上皮脫屑 皮膚或腸內膜上皮細胞層脫落。

epithelioma *n.* a tumour of *epithelium, the covering of internal and exter-

上皮瘤 身體內、外表面的上皮腫瘤。上皮瘤過去

nal surfaces of the body: a former term for *carcinoma, but now also used to describe benign tumours.

指上皮癌，現也用來指良性瘤。

epithelium *n.* the tissue that covers the external surface of the body and lines hollow structures (except blood and lymphatic vessels). It is derived from embryonic ectoderm and endoderm. Epithelial cells may be flat and scalelike (*squamous*), *cuboidal*, or *columnar*. The latter may bear cilia or brush borders or secrete mucus or other substances (*see* goblet cell). The cells rest on a common *basement membrane*, which separates epithelium from underlying *connective tissue. Epithelium may be either *simple*, consisting of a single layer of cells; *stratified*, consisting of several layers; or *pseudostratified*, in which the cells appear to be arranged in layers but in fact share a common basement membrane (see illustration). *See also* endothelium, mesothelium. —**epithelial** *adj.*

上皮　覆蓋身體外表及內襯空腔結構（除血管和淋巴管）的組織。來自胚胎的內、外胚層。上皮細胞可呈扁平、鱗狀、立方或柱狀形。後者還長有纖毛，或呈刷狀緣，或分泌黏液或其它物質。細胞下面是一層基底膜，將上皮細胞與其下的結締組織分開。上皮細胞可以是單層，即由一層細胞組成；也可是複層：含有幾層細胞；或是假複層：從細胞的排列上看像多層，但事實上，這些細胞共有同一層基底膜（見圖）。

epitrichium (periderm) *n.* the most superficial layer of the skin, one cell in thickness, that is only present early in embryonic development. It protects the underlying *epidermis until it is fully formed.

皮上層　皮膚的最表層。有一層細胞厚。只存在於胚胎發育期。它保護下面表皮直至表皮完全形成。

epituberculosis *n.* enlargement of a lymph node in the thorax due to tuberculosis infection, causing the gland to press upon and occlude a bronchiole, which may result in the collapse of a lung segment (*see* atelectasis).

特異型原發性肺結核　胸淋巴結因結核感染而腫大，並由此壓迫、阻塞支氣管，使肺段萎縮。

eponychium *n. see* nail.

甲上皮

eponym *n.* a disease, structure, or species named after a particular person, usually the person who first discovered or described it. Eponyms are widespread in medicine, but they are being replaced as more descriptive terms become necessary. Thus the eponyms islets of Langerhans, aqueduct of Sylvius, and Hashimoto's disease are more

冠名名詞　用某人名字命名的一種疾病、結構或物種。通常此人是第一個發現或描述這種疾病、結構或物種的人。冠名名詞廣泛見於醫學，但現已正被取代，因更多的描述性術語是必要的。因此，屬冠名名詞的朗格罕氏島、西

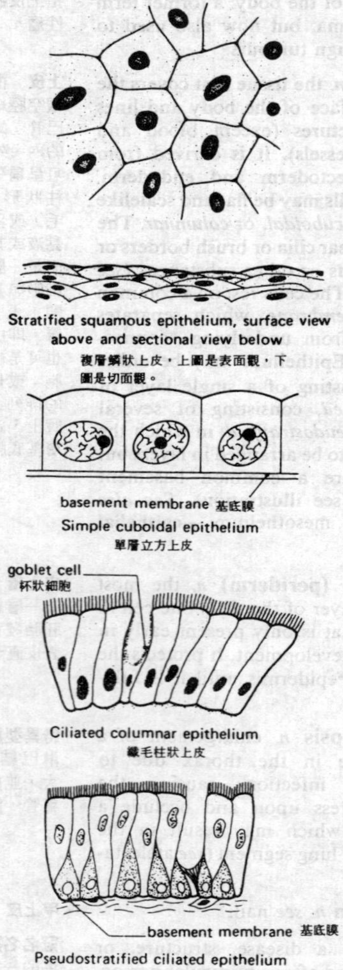

Types of epithelium

上皮的種類

likely to be designated in text books as pancreatic islands, cerebral aqueduct, and autoimmune thyroiditis, respectively. —**eponymous** *adj.*

爾維厄斯氏導水管、橋本氏病很可能在教科書中被命名爲胰島、大腦導水管，自體免疫性甲狀腺炎。

epoophoron *n. see* paroophoron.
卵巢冠

Epstein-Barr virus the virus thought to be the causative agent of *glandular fever.
愛潑斯坦-巴爾病毒 被認爲是引起腺性熱的病毒。

epulis *n.* a swelling on the gum. Most such swellings are due to fibrous hyperplasia.
齦瘤 齒齦腫大。大多數的這種腫大是由纖維增生引起。

equi- *prefix denoting* equality.
〔前綴〕 相等。

equinia *n. see* glanders.
馬鼻疽

Erb's palsy a partial paralysis of the arm caused by injury to a baby's *brachial plexus during birth. This may happen if – during a difficult delivery – excess traction applied to the head damages the fifth cervical root of the spinal cord. The muscles of the shoulder and the flexors of the elbow are paralysed and the arm hangs at the side internally rotated at the shoulder.
歐勃氏麻痹 在嬰兒出生時，損傷其臂叢引起的上肢部分麻痹。過度牽拉頭部（如在難產時）時損傷頸髓第五頸神經根可導致此病。肩部肌肉及肘部屈肌麻痹，而且上肢在肩部內旋。

ERCP (endoscopic retrograde cholangiopancreatography) a technique in which a catheter is passed through a *duodenoscope into the *ampulla of Vater of the common bile duct and injected with a radio-opaque medium to outline the pancreatic duct and bile ducts radiologically. It is now widely used in the diagnosis of obstructive jaundice and pancreatic disease. *See also* papillotomy.
內窺鏡膽管胰腺逆行造影 將導管通過十二指腸鏡進入總膽管的法特氏壺腹部，注入造影劑，使胰導管、膽管顯影。現已廣泛用於診斷阻塞性黃疸和胰腺病。

erectile *adj.* capable of causing erection or becoming erect. The penis is composed largely of erectile tissue.
能勃起的 有勃起能力的。陰莖主要是由能勃起的組織組成的。

erection *n.* the sexually active state of the penis, which becomes enlarged and rigid (due to the erectile tissue being swollen with blood) and capable of penetrating the vagina. The term is also applied to the clitoris in a state of sexual arousal.
勃起 陰莖的性興奮狀態。陰莖變得粗大、堅硬（因勃起組織充血腫大），有能力進入陰道。此術語也用來指興奮期的陰蒂。

erepsin *n.* a mixture of protein-digesting enzymes (*see* peptidase) secreted by the intestinal glands. It is part of the *succus entericus.
腸肽酶 腸腺分泌的蛋白消化酶的混合物。是腸液的一部分。

erethism *n.* **1.** a state of abnormal mental excitement or irritation. **2.** rapid response to a stimulus.

①**病態興奮** 不正常的精神興奮和煩躁狀態。
②**興奮增强** 對刺激的迅速反應。

erg *n.* a unit of work or energy equal to the work done when the point of application of a force of 1 dyne is displaced through a distance of 1 centimetre in the direction of the force. 1 erg = 10^{-7} joule.

爾格 功或能量單位。即用1達因的力使某物沿力的方向移動1 cm所做的功。1爾格＝10^{7}焦耳

erg- (ergo-) *prefix denoting* work or activity.

〔前綴〕 **功能，活動能力**

ergocalciferol *n. see* vitamin D.

麥角骨化醇

ergograph *n.* an apparatus for recording the work performed by the muscles of the body when undergoing activity. Ergographs are useful for assessment of the capabilities of athletes undergoing training.

測力器 在身體活動時，測量肌肉活動的儀器。對估價進行訓練的運動員的能力很有用。

ergometrine *n.* a drug that stimulates contractions of the womb. It is administered by injection to assist labour and to control bleeding following delivery.

麥角新鹼 刺激子宮收縮的藥物。注射給藥，以助產及控制產後出血。

ergonomics *n.* the study of man in relation to his work and working surroundings. This broad science involves the application of psychological as well as physiological principles to the design of buildings, machinery, vehicles, packaging, implements, and anything else with which man comes into contact.

人體功率學 研究人與其工作及其工作環境的科學。這一內容廣泛的科學包括運用心理學及生理學原理對建築物、機器、車輛、包裝、日用工具及其它人類所接觸的東西進行設計。

ergosterol *n.* a plant sterol that, when irradiated with ultraviolet light, is converted to ergocalciferol (vitamin D_2). *See* vitamin D.

麥角固醇 一種植物固醇。當受到紫外線照射時，可轉化成麥角骨化醇（維生素D_2）。

ergot *n.* a fungus (*Claviceps purpurea*) that grows on rye. It produces several important alkaloids, chemically related to LSD, including *ergotamine and *ergometrine, which are used in medicine in the treatment of migraine and in childbirth. Eating bread made with rye infected with the fungus has led to sporadic outbreaks of *ergotism over the centuries.

麥角 生長在黑麥上的一種眞菌。能產生出一些重要的在化學結構上屬麥角副酸二乙醯胺的生物鹼，包括麥角胺和麥角新鹼。在醫學上，它們用在偏頭痛及分娩時。過去，食用有眞菌感染的黑麥面包曾引起散發性麥角中毒，並持續了幾世紀。

ergotamine *n.* a drug that causes constriction of blood vessels and is used to relieve migraine. It is administered by mouth, injection, inhalation, or in suppositories. Common side-effects are nausea and vomiting, and ergotism may develop as a result of high doses. Trade names: **Femergin**, **Lingraine**.

麥角胺 引起血管收縮，並用來治療偏頭痛的藥物。可口服、注射、吸入或以栓劑形式給藥。常見的副作用是噁心、嘔吐。大劑量時，可引起麥角中毒。

ergotism *n.* poisoning caused by eating rye infected with the fungus *ergot. The chief symptom is gangrene of the fingers and toes, with diarrhoea and vomiting, nausea, and headache. In the Middle Ages the disease was known as *St. Anthony's fire*, because of the inflamed appearance of the tissues afflicted with gangrene and the belief that a pilgrimage to St. Anthony's tomb would result in cure.

麥角中毒 食入麥角眞菌感染的黑麥麵包而引起的中毒。主要症狀是手指、脚趾壞死，伴有腹瀉、嘔吐、噁心及頭痛。在中世紀時，此病被叫做聖安東尼火。這是因爲壞死組織呈火焰樣外觀，而且人們還認爲朝拜聖安東尼墓就可治癒此病。

erogenous *adj.* describing certain parts of the body, the physical stimulation of which leads to sexual arousal.

性慾發生的 指身體某些部位因生理性刺激而引起性興奮。

erosion *n.* **1.** an eating away of surface tissue by physical or chemical processes, including those associated with inflammation. A *cervical erosion* is an abnormal area of epithelium that may develop at the neck of the womb due to tissue damage caused at childbirth or by attempts at abortion. **2.** (in dentistry) loss of surface tooth substance, usually caused by repeated application of acid, as may occur with excessive intake of citrus fruits.

①**糜爛** 因物理和化學過程，包括炎症引起的組織表面缺損。宮頸糜爛就是在分娩或人工流產時組織損傷而引起的宮頸上皮異常。②**侵蝕** （牙科學）牙表面物質缺損。通常因反復的酸刺激引起。如大量食入柑橘類水果時。

erot- (eroto-) *prefix denoting* sexual desire or love. Example: *erotophobia* (morbid dread of).

〔前綴〕 **性慾，性愛** 如性慾恐懼。

erotomania *n.* a delusion that the individual is loved by some person, often a person of importance. Sometimes, but not always, this progresses to schizophrenia.

色情狂 某人幻想被另一人，通常是重要人物所愛。有時，這種情況可逐漸發展成精神分裂症。

eructation *n.* belching: the sudden raising of gas from the stomach.

噯氣 氣體突然從胃裏竄出。

eruption *n.* **1.** any lesion that appears at the surface of the skin and is

①**疹** 出現在皮膚表面的一種病變。特點爲紅色突

characterized by its prominence and redness. A *bullous eruption* is an eruption of blisters. **2.** (in dentistry) the emergence of a growing tooth from the gum into the mouth.

起。大疱疹是一種水疱疹。②萌出 （牙科學）在口腔內牙齒從齒齦處長出。

erysipelas *n.* an infection of the skin and underlying tissues with the bacterium *Streptococcus pyogenes*. The affected areas, usually the face and scalp, become inflamed and swollen, with the development of raised patches that may be several inches across. The patient is ill, with a high temperature. Attacks may recur in certain individuals, possibly because of a defect in their lymphatic systems. Treatment is with antibiotics.

丹毒 由丹毒鏈球菌引起的皮膚及皮下組織感染。感染部位通常是臉及頭皮。表現爲炎性水腫，伴有直徑幾英寸長的斑片狀隆起。患者發病時有高燒，個別患者其病情可反復發作。可能是因淋巴組織有缺陷所致。治療：使用抗生素。

erysipeloid (erythema serpens) *n.* an infection of the skin and underlying tissues with **Erysipelothrix rhusiopathiae*, developing usually in people handling fish, poultry, or meat. Infection enters through scratches or cuts on the hands, and is normally confined to a finger or hand, which becomes reddened; sometimes systemic illness develops. Treatment is with antibiotics.

類丹毒 豬紅斑丹毒絲菌引起的皮膚及皮下組織感染。當手被刮破或有切口時，就可因此發生感染並出現紅腫。正常情況下，感染只限於手指或手；有時，可引起全身疾病。治療：使用抗生素。

Erysipelothrix *n.* a genus of Gram-positive non-motile rod-shaped bacteria with a tendency to form filaments. They are parasites of mammals, birds, and fish. *E. rhusiopathiae* is a widely distributed species causing the disease *erysipelas in swine, which is transmissible to man.

丹毒絲菌屬 一種革蘭染色陰性、非活動性、能形成絲的桿菌屬。寄生在哺乳動物、鳥類及魚類身上。豬紅斑丹毒絲菌是廣泛分佈的菌種，能引起豬丹毒。而病豬又是人的傳染源。

erythema *n.* abnormal flushing of the skin caused by dilation of the blood capillaries. Erythema may be produced by various conditions – it is often a sign of inflammation and infection. For example, *erythema nodosum* is a disease of sudden onset, characterized by fever, joint pains, and an eruption of painful swellings on the legs. In *erythema multiforme*, a disease caused by toxins in the blood, the eruption consists of circular

紅斑 因毛細血管擴張而引起的皮膚不正常的發紅。可由各種原因產生。通常是炎症和感染的體徵。如：結節性紅斑，它是一種急性病，特點爲發熱、關節痛及腿上出現疼痛的腫脹。多形性紅斑是血液中的毒素引起的一種疾病，皮疹是由圓形或不規則形紅斑塊組成，通常發生於上肢及手的背面；

or irregular red patches, commonly occurring on the backs of the arms and hands and sometimes accompanied by systemic disease.

有時，還伴有全身性疾病。

erythr- (erythro-) *prefix denoting* **1.** redness. Example: *erythuria* (excretion of red urine). **2.** erythrocytes.

〔前綴〕 ①紅色 如紅尿症（排紅色尿）。 ②紅細胞

erythraemia *n. see* polycythaemia vera.

紅細胞增多症

erythrasma *n.* a chronic skin infection due to the bacterium *Corynebacterium minutissimum*, occurring in such areas as the armpits, groin, and toes, where skin surfaces are in contact.

紅癬 微小棒狀桿菌引起的慢性皮膚感染。發生在皮膚表面相互密切接觸的部位，如腋窩、腹股溝及脚趾間。

erythritol *n.* a drug that has a mild prolonged action in reducing blood pressure by dilating blood vessels (*see* vasodilator) and is used to treat hypertension and angina. It is administered by mouth and high doses may cause flushing, headache, fainting, and increased heart rate.

赤蘚醇 一種作用溫和、持久的降壓藥。是通過擴張血管而起作用的。用於治療高血壓和心絞痛。口服。大劑量時可引起面紅、頭痛、暈眩及心動過速。

erythroblast *n.* any of a series of nucleated cells (*see* normoblast, proerythroblast) that pass through a succession of stages of maturation to form red blood cells (*erythrocytes). Erythroblasts are normally present in the blood-forming tissue of the bone marrow, but they may appear in the circulation in a variety of diseases, (*see* erythroblastosis). *See also* erythropoiesis.

成紅細胞 經過成熟期各階段而最終形成紅細胞的一系列有核細胞中的任何一種。在正常情況下，成紅細胞存在於骨髓造血組織中。但在某些疾病時可出現在血液循環中。

erythroblastosis *n.* the presence in the blood of the nucleated precursors of the red blood cells (*erythroblasts). This may occur when there is an increase in the rate of red cell production, as in haemorrhagic or haemolytic *anaemia, or in infiltrations of the bone marrow by tumours, etc.

成紅細胞增多症 血中存在着紅細胞的前身細胞。可發生於紅細胞生成速度過快時。如在出血性和溶血性貧血時，或在骨髓受到腫瘤侵襲時。

erythroblastosis foetalis a severe but rare haemolytic *anaemia affecting newborn infants due to destruction of the infant's red blood cells by factors present in the mother's serum. It is

新生兒成紅細胞增多症 新生兒溶血性貧血。因母體血清中因素使胎兒紅細胞受到破壞而引起，很嚴重，但少見。通常因母體

usually caused by incompatibility of the rhesus blood groups between mother and infant (*see* rhesus factor).
與胎兒的血液中獼因子不配合引起。

erythrocyanosis *n.* mottled purplish discoloration on the legs and thighs, usually of adolescent girls or fat boys before puberty. The disorder sometimes occurs in older women. The condition is worse in cold weather and there is no satisfactory treatment.
紺紅皮病 在小腿和大腿上出現紫色斑紋。通常見於青春期前的少女、肥胖男孩。有時，也見於老年婦女。寒冷氣候時病情加重。尚無滿意療法。

erythrocyte (red blood cell) *n.* a *blood cell containing the pigment *haemoglobin, the principal function of which is the transport of oxygen. A mature erythrocyte has no nucleus and its shape is that of a biconcave disc, approximately 7 μm in diameter. There are normally about 5×10^{12} erythrocytes per litre of blood. *See also* erythropoiesis.
紅細胞 一種含有血紅蛋白的血細胞。主要功能是輸送氧。成熟紅細胞無核、呈雙凹形。直徑約7 μm。正常情況下，每升血液中約有 5×10^{12} 個紅細胞。

erythrocyte sedimentation rate *see* ESR.
紅細胞沉降率

erythrocytic *adj.* describing those stages in the life cycle of the malarial parasite (*see* Plasmodium) that develop inside the red blood cells (*see* trophozoite). *Compare* exoerythrocytic.
紅細胞內的 指瘧原蟲在紅細胞內生長發育的生活周期的各個階段。

erythroderma (exfoliative dermatitis) *n.* abnormal reddening, flaking, and thickening of the skin, typically affecting a wide area of the body. Commoner after the age of 50, erythroderma affects men three times as often as women and it frequently develops from a preceding skin disease, such as psoriasis.
紅皮病 皮膚不正常的紅腫，片狀脱屑及增厚。此病能侵犯身體的大面積。常見於50歲以上的患者。男性發病率是女性的三倍。多繼發於原有的皮膚病，如銀屑病。

erythroedema *n. see* pink disease.
紅皮水腫病

erythrogenesis *n. see* erythropoiesis.
紅細胞發生

erythromelalgia *n.* painful paroxysmal dilation of the blood vessels of the skin, usually affecting the feet and extremities.
紅斑性肢痛 皮膚血管陣發性擴張，疼痛。常侵犯脚及肢體。

erythromycin *n.* an *antibiotic used to treat infections caused by a wide range
紅黴素 治療細菌及其它微生物感染的廣譜抗生

of bacteria and other microorganisms. It is administered by mouth or injection. Side-effects are rare and mild, though nausea, vomiting, and diarrhoea occur occasionally. Trade names: **Erycen**, **Erythromia**, **Erythropea**, **Ilotycin**.

素。可口服也可注射。副作用少且輕。偶見噁心、嘔吐及腹瀉。

erythron *n.* that part of the blood-forming system of the body that is directed towards the production of red blood cells. The erythron is not a single organ but is dispersed throughout the blood-forming tissue of the *bone marrow. *See also* erythropoiesis.

紅細胞系 身體造血系統中，可直接產生紅細胞的那一部分。它不是單獨的器官，而是遍佈於骨髓的造血組織之中。

erythropenia *n.* a reduction in the number of red blood cells (*erythrocytes) in the blood. This usually, but not invariably, occurs in *anaemia.

紅細胞減少 血液中紅細胞數量下降。常見於貧血，但也有例外。

erythropoiesis (erythrogenesis) *n.* the process of red blood cell (*erythrocyte) production, which normally occurs in the blood-forming tissue of the *bone marrow. The ultimate precursor of the red cell is the *haemopoietic stem cell, but the earliest precursor that can be identified microscopically is the *proerythroblast. This divides and passes through a series of stages of maturation termed respectively early, intermediate, and late *normoblasts, the latter finally losing its nucleus to become a mature red cell. *See also* haemopoiesis.

紅細胞生成 紅細胞產生的過程。正常情況下，產生於骨髓的造血組織中。最早紅細胞的前身是造血幹細胞。但在顯微鏡下可識別的最早前身是原成紅細胞。它不斷分裂，並分別經過早幼、中幼、晚幼紅細胞這一系列的成熟期，最後脫核成爲成熟紅細胞。

erythropoietin *n.* a hormone secreted by certain cells in the kidney in response to a reduction in the amount of oxygen reaching the tissues. Erythropoietin increases the rate of red cell production (*erythropoiesis) and is the mechanism by which the rate of erythropoiesis is controlled.

紅細胞生成素 腎臟中某些細胞因組織內氧含量下降而分泌出來的一種激素。它能加快並控制紅細胞的生成速度。

erythropsia *n.* red vision: a rare symptom sometimes experienced after removal of a cataract and also in snow blindness.

紅視症 紅視：一種少見的症狀。有時出現在白內障手術以後，也出現在雪盲時。

eschar *n.* a scab or slough, as produced by the action of heat or a corrosive substance on living tissue.

焦痂 因熱或腐蝕物作用於活組織而產生的痂和腐肉。

escharotic *n.* a *caustic agent that produces a dry scab, or slough, when applied to the skin.

苛性藥 當作用於皮膚時，產生乾痂和腐肉的腐蝕劑。

Escherichia *n.* a genus of Gram-negative, generally motile, rodlike bacteria that have the ability to ferment carbohydrates, usually with production of gas, and are found in the intestines of man and many animals. *E. coli* – a lactose-fermenting species – is usually not harmful but under certain conditions can cause infection of the urinogenital tract and diarrhoea in children. It is also widely used in laboratory experiments for bacteriological and genetic studies.

埃希氏桿菌屬 一種革蘭氏陰性，有活動性的桿狀菌屬。能使碳水化合物發酵，並產氣，見於人類及多種動物的腸道。大腸桿菌是能發酵乳糖的菌種，通常無害。但在某些情況下可引起泌尿道感染及兒童腹瀉。大腸桿菌還被廣泛用於實驗室內細菌及遺傳學研究。

eserine *n. see* physostigmine.

毒扁豆鹼

esophoria *n.* a tendency to squint in which the eye, when covered, tends to turn inwards towards the nose. *See also* heterophoria.

內隱斜視 當閉眼時，眼睛向鼻側內移的一種斜視現象。

esotropia *n.* convergent *strabismus: a type of squint.

內斜視 會聚性斜視。斜視的一種。

espundia (mucocutaneous leishmaniasis) *n.* a disease of the skin and mucous membranes caused by the parasitic protozoan *Leishmania braziliensis* (*see* leishmaniasis). Occurring in South and Central America, espundia takes the form of ulcerating lesions on the arms and legs; the infection may also spread to the mucous membranes of the nose and mouth, causing serious destruction of the tissues.

皮膚黏膜利什曼病 由巴西利什曼原蟲引起的一種皮膚和黏膜疾病。發生於南美和中美。此病可使上肢和下肢發生潰瘍性病變。病變還可波及到鼻、口腔黏膜，使組織受到嚴重的破壞。

ESR (erythrocyte sedimentation rate) the rate at which red blood cells (erythrocytes) settle out of suspension in blood plasma, measured under standardized conditions. The ESR increases if the level of certain proteins in the plasma rises, as in rheumatic diseases, chronic infections, and malignant disease, and thus provides a simple but

紅細胞沉降率 在標準條件下測得的紅細胞在血漿懸液中沉降的速度。如果血漿中某些蛋白質增加，則沉降率增快，如在風濕病、慢性感染及惡性病時。因此在檢查惡性病時，它可做爲簡單而又有價值的普查試驗。

valuable screening test for the latter condition.

essence *n.* a solution consisting of an essential oil dissolved in alcohol.

香精劑 由酒精和溶解在其內的揮發性油組成的溶液。

essential *adj.* describing a disorder that is not apparently attributable to an outside cause; for example, essential *hypertension.

原發的 指沒有明顯外因的疾病。如原發性高血壓。

essential amino acid an *amino acid that is essential for normal growth and development but cannot be synthesized by the body. Essential amino acids are normally obtained from protein-rich foods in the diet, such as liver, eggs, and dairy products. There are eight essential amino acids: tryptophan, lysine, phenylalanine, threonine, valine, methionine, leucine, and isoleucine.

必需氨基酸 正常生長發育所必要的，而體內又不能合成的氨基酸。正常情況下，可從含蛋白質豐富的食物中攝取。如肝、蛋及乳製品。有八種必需氨基酸：色氨酸、賴氨酸、苯丙氨酸、蘇氨酸、纈氨酸、蛋氨酸、亮氨酸及異亮氨酸。

essential fatty acid one of a group of unsaturated fatty acids that are essencial for growth but cannot be synthesized by the body. The essential fatty acids are *linoleic*, *linolenic*, and *arachidonic acids*; of these, only linoleic acid need be included in the diet as the other two can be synthesized from it in the body. Large amounts of linoleic acid occur in maize (corn) oil and soya bean oil; smaller amounts in pork fat.

必需脂肪酸 體內不能合成而又是生長必需的一組非飽和脂肪酸。它們是：亞油酸、亞麻酸和花生四烯酸。其中，只有亞油酸需要加在食物中攝取。其它兩種可從進入體內的亞油酸合成。大量的亞油酸來於玉米油和豆油，少量來於豬肉脂肪。

essential oil a volatile oil derived from an aromatic plant. Essential oils are used in various pharmaceutical preparations.

揮發油 來自芳香植物的易揮發的油。用於各種藥物製劑。

esterase *n.* an enzyme that catalyses the hydrolysis of esters into their constituent acids and alcohols. For example, fatty-acid esters are broken down to form fatty acids plus alcohol.

酯酶 一種催化脂類水解，使其生成相應的酸和乙醇的酶。如脂肪酸酯可被分解成脂肪酸和乙醇。

ethacrynic acid a *diuretic used to treat fluid retention (oedema), such as that associated with heart failure and kidney and liver disorders. It is administered by mouth or injection. Com-

利尿酸 利尿藥。用於治療液體豬留（水腫），如因心衰及腎、肝疾病引起的水腫。口服或注射，常見的副作用是食慾不振，

mon side-effects are loss of appetite, difficulty in swallowing, nausea, vomiting, and diarrhoea. Trade name: **Edecrin**.

吞咽困難、噁心、嘔吐及腹瀉。

ethambutol *n.* a drug used in the treatment of tuberculosis, in conjunction with other drugs. It is administered by mouth and occasionally causes visual disturbances, which cease when the drug is withdrawn. Allergic rashes and digestive upsets may also occur. Trade name: **Myambutol**.

乙胺丁醇　與其他藥物合用的抗結核藥。口服。偶可引起視力障礙，但停藥後消失。也可引起過敏疹及消化不良。

ethamivan *n.* an *analeptic drug that stimulates breathing and is used to treat reduced or abnormal breathing, particularly in newborn babies and in cases of drug overdosage. It is administered by mouth or injection; high doses may cause restlessness, sneezing, and gasping. Trade name: **Clairvan**.

香草醯二乙胺　刺激呼吸的興奮劑。用於呼吸減弱或呼吸不正常，特別是用於新生兒及用藥過量的患者。口服或注射。大劑量可引起煩燥不安、打噴嚏及嘔吐。

ethanol (ethyl alcohol) *n. see* alcohol.

乙醇

ethchlorvynol *n.* a drug used to treat insomnia (*see* hypnotic). It is administered by mouth; side-effects include temporary giddiness, muscle incoordination, nausea, and vomiting. Trade name: **Serenesil**.

乙氯戊烯炔醇　治療失眠的藥物。口服。副作用有短暫性頭暈、肌肉活動不協調、噁心和嘔吐。

ethebenecid *n.* a *uricosuric drug used to treat gout and other conditions involving high blood levels of uric acid. It is administered by mouth and may cause skin rashes, digestive discomfort, and sedation.

二乙胺磺苯酸　促尿酸排泄藥。用於治療痛風及其他血液尿酸過高的疾病。口服。可引起皮疹、消化不良及淡漠少動。

ether *n.* a volatile liquid formerly used as an anaesthetic administered by inhalation, though now largely replaced by safer and more efficient drugs. It also has laxative action when administered by mouth. Ether irritates the respiratory tract and affects the circulation.

醚　一種揮發性液體。以前用作吸入性麻醉劑，現主要被更安全更有效的藥物所代替。口服時，還有鬆弛作用。醚能刺激消化道並損害循環系統。

ethical committee (in Britain) a group of consultants and other experts set up (especially in a hospital) to monitor investigations, concerned with teaching or research, that involve the use of human subjects. It is responsible

醫德委員會　（在英國）由顧問和專家組成的團體（特別是在醫院裏），以監督把人用於教學和科研的情況。該委員會負責讓患者充分了解科研項日的

for ensuring that patients are adequately informed of the procedures involved in a research project (including the use of dummy or placebo treatments as controls), that the tests and/or therapies are safe, and that no-one is pressurized into participating.

所有過程（包括使用對照用的安慰劑），保證實驗和治療是安全的，而且保證沒有人是被迫參加上述活動的。

ethinamate *n.* a mild *sedative used to treat insomnia. It is administered by mouth and may cause digestive discomfort.

炔己蟻胺 一種治療失眠的溫和鎮靜劑。口服。可引起消化不良。

ethinyloestradiol *n.* a synthetic female sex hormone (*see* oestrogen) administered by mouth to treat symptoms of the menopause and menstrual disorders, to suppress lactation in mothers not breast-feeding, and to treat cancer of the prostate gland. It is also used, in combination with a progestogen, in *oral contraceptives. Trade name: **Lynoral**.

炔雌醇 一種合成的雌性激素。口服，治療閉經和月經失調，抑制停止哺乳母親泌乳，還治療前列腺癌。與孕酮一起，可做爲口服避孕藥。

ethionamide *n.* a drug used to treat tuberculosis, usually in conjunction with other drugs. It is administered by mouth or in suppositories. Loss of appetite, nausea, and vomiting are common side-effects. Trade name: **Trescatyl**.

乙硫異煙胺 抗結核藥。常與其它藥合用。口服或以栓劑形式給藥。常見的副作用是食慾不振、噁心及嘔吐。

ethisterone *n.* a synthetic female sex hormone (*see* progestogen) used, often in combination with an *oestrogen, to treat menstrual disorders, particularly amenorrhoea. It was formerly used in hormone pregnancy tests. It is administered by mouth.

羥脫水孕酮 一種合成的雌激素。常與雌激素聯合使用，治療月經不調，特別是閉經。以前用於激素檢孕試驗。口服。

ethmoid bone a bone in the floor of the cranium that contributes to the nasal cavity and orbits. The part of the ethmoid forming the roof of the nasal cavity – the *cribriform plate* – is pierced with many small holes through which the olfactory nerves pass. *See also* nasal concha, skull.

篩骨 一塊構成鼻腔和眼眶的顱底的一部分的骨頭。在形成鼻腔頂部——篩骨板的部分有很多小孔，嗅神經就從中穿過。

ethnology *n.* the study of the different races of mankind and their variations: a branch of anthropology that deals

人種學 研究人類不同種族及他們不同之處的科學。是人類學的分支。人

mainly with cultural and social differences between groups and the problems, medical and otherwise, that arise from their particular ways of life. —**ethnic** *adj.*

種學主要研究不同種族之間文化及社會的區別，及因他們的特殊生活方式而出現的醫療和其他方面的問題。

ethoglucid *n.* a drug that prevents the growth of tumours and is used to treat various cancers. It is administered by injection; side-effects commonly include nausea and vomiting. Trade name: **Epodyl**.

環氧甘醚 防止腫瘤生長並治療各種癌症的藥物。注射給藥。常見的副作用有噁心、嘔吐。

ethopropazine *n.* a drug that has effects similar to those of *atropine and is used to treat parkinsonism. It is administered by mouth and may cause lethargy and drowsiness in the early stages of treatment. Trade name: **Lysivane**.

二乙異丙嗪 有類似阿托品作用的藥物。用於治療帕金森氏綜合症。口服。用藥早期，可出現嗜眠、怠睡。

ethosuximide *n.* an *anticonvulsant drug used to treat petit mal epileptic fits. It is administered by mouth; side-effects such as drowsiness, depression, and digestive disturbances may occur but are usually temporary. Trade names: **Emeside, Zarontin**.

乙琥胺 抗驚厥藥。用於治療癲癇小發作。口服。副作用有倦睡、抑鬱及消化道紊亂，但通常只是暫時性的。

ethotoin *n.* an *anticonvulsant drug used, usually in conjunction with other anticonvulsants, to treat grand mal epileptic fits. It is administered by mouth; side-effects can include digestive and visual disturbances and drowsiness. Trade name: **Peganone**.

乙基苯妥英 抗驚厥藥。常與其它抗驚厥藥聯合治療癲癇大發作。口服。副作用有消化道和視覺紊亂及怠睡。

ethyl biscoumacetate an *anticoagulant drug used to prevent blood clotting. It is administered by mouth and may cause nausea and vomiting, hair loss, and skin rash. Trade name: **Tromexan**.

新雙香豆素 預防血液凝固的抗凝藥。口服。可引起噁心、嘔吐、脫髮及皮疹。

ethylene *n.* an inflammable gas sometimes used as an anaesthetic administered by inhalation. There are usually no toxic effects, but nausea and vomiting commonly occur after its use.

乙烯 易燃性氣體。有時用作吸入性麻醉劑。通常無毒性作用。使用後常發生噁心、嘔吐。

ethyloestrenol *n.* a steroid drug with *anabolic properties, used to treat conditions involving wasting of protein and

17-乙基雌烯醇 一種具有同化作用的類固醇藥物。用於治療與蛋白質和

bone, such as osteoporosis. It is administered by mouth and sometimes causes nausea, water retention, and menstrual disturbances at high doses. Trade name: **Orabolin**.

骨質消耗有關的疾病，如骨質疏鬆症。口服。有時引起噁心、水豬留。大劑量時可引起月經紊亂。

ethynodiol *n.* a synthetic female sex hormone (*see* progestogen) that is used to treat menstrual disorders and in *oral contraceptives. It is administered by mouth, usually in combination with an *oestrogen. Side-effects can include nausea, vomiting, headache, breast swelling, weight gain, fluid retention, and breakthrough bleeding.

炔諾醇 一種合成的雌性激素。用於治療月經紊亂及用作口服避孕藥。口服。常與雌激素合用。副作用有噁心、嘔吐、頭痛、乳房腫脹、體重增加、液體豬留及突發性出血。

etiology *n. see* aetiology.

病因學

etoposide (VP16-213) *n.* a *cytotoxic drug derived from an extract of the mandrake plant. It is administered intravenously or by mouth, primarily in the treatment of bronchial carcinoma and lymphomas. Side-effects include alopecia, nausea, and marrow suppression. Trade name: **Vepesid**.

表鬼臼毒吡喃葡萄糖甙（VP16－213） 從北美表鬼臼根植物中提取的一種細胞毒藥物。靜脉注射或口服。主要治療支氣管癌和淋巴瘤。副作用有脫髮、噁心及骨髓抑制。

eu- *prefix denoting* **1.** good, well, or easy. **2.** normal.

〔前綴〕 **①好，優，容易 ②正常**

eubacteria *pl. n.* a very large group of bacteria with rigid cell walls and – typically – flagella for movement. The group comprises the so-called 'true' bacteria, excluding those, such as spirochaetes and mycoplasmas, with flexible cell walls.

眞細菌 有堅硬的細胞壁，並有典型鞭毛運動的一大類細菌。這類細菌就是所謂的“眞”細菌。但不包括有柔軟細胞壁的如螺旋體和支原體之類。

eucalyptol *n.* a volatile oil that has a mild irritant effect on the mucous membranes of the mouth and digestive system. It is taken as pastilles or inhaled as vapour to relieve catarrh. Large doses may cause nausea, vomiting, and diarrhoea.

桉油醇 一種對口腔及消化道黏膜有輕微刺激作用的揮發性油。可製成錠劑服用或吸入其蒸氣，以消除卡他。大劑量時，可引起噁心、嘔吐及腹瀉。

euchromatin *n.* chromosome material (*see* chromatin) that stains most deeply during mitosis and represents the major genes. *Compare* heterochromatin.

常染色質 有絲分裂時，染色最深並代表主要基因的染色質物質。

eugenics *n.* the science that is concerned with the improvement of the

優生學 用遺傳學的原理改良人種的科學。主要是

human race by means of the principles of genetics. It is mainly concerned with the detection and, where possible, the elimination of genetic disease in man.

檢查人類遺傳病，並在可能的情况下，消除它們。

eupepsia *n.* the state of normal or good digestion: freedom from digestive symptoms.

消化正常 正常或良好的消化狀態：沒有消化道症狀。

euphoria *n.* a state of optimism, cheerfulness, and well-being. A morbid degree of euphoria is characteristic of *mania and *hypomania. *See also* ecstasy, elation.

欣快 得意、歡樂和幸福的表現。病態的歡快是躁狂的特點。

euplastic *adj.* describing a tissue that heals quickly after injury.

易於機化的 指組織損傷後很快癒合。

euploidy *n.* the condition of cells, tissues, or organisms in which there is one complete set of chromosomes or a whole multiple of this set in each cell. *Compare* aneuploidy. —**euploid** *adj.*, *n.*

整倍體 細胞、組織或生物的一種狀態。即在其每一細胞內有一整套的染色體或有整數的多套染色體。

Eustachian tube the tube that connects the middle *ear to the pharynx. It allows the pressure on the inner side of the eardrum to remain equal to the external pressure.

咽鼓管 連接中耳和咽部的管道。它使作用在鼓膜內側的壓力與外部的相等。

euthanasia *n.* the act of taking life to relieve suffering. In *voluntary euthanasia* the sufferer asks for measures to be taken to end his life. This may be accomplished by active steps, usually the administration of a drug, or by *passive euthanasia* – the deliberate withholding of treatment. In *compulsory euthanasia* society or a person acting on authority gives instructions to terminate the life of a person, such as an infant, who cannot express his wishes. In no country is either voluntary or compulsory euthanasia legal, although many societies exist to promote the cause of voluntary euthanasia.

安死術 爲除去身體的痛苦而結束生命的一種方法。自願安死術是指患者本人要求採取措施來結束其生命。可採取主動的方式，通常是用藥，或採用被動安死術——停止治療。强迫安死術是指權威性團體或個人下令來結束某人的生命，如對不能表達其願望的嬰兒。儘管在很多社會裏都存在着鼓勵採取安死術的現象，但還沒有一個國家制定出自願或强迫安死術的法律。

euthyroid *adj.* having a normally functioning thyroid gland. *Compare* hyperthyroidism, hypothyroidism. —**euthyroidism** *n.*

甲狀腺機能正常的 指有正常功能的甲狀腺。

eutocia *n.* natural uncomplicated labour and childbirth.

順產 自然的，沒有併發病的分娩。

evacuator *n.* a device for sucking fluid out of a cavity. In its simplest form it consists of a hollow rubber bulb that is attached, via a valve system, to a tube inserted into the cavity. Another valve leads to a discharge tube. Evacuators may be used to empty the bladder of unwanted material during such operations as the removal of a calculus.

排出器 從腔中吸出液體的工具。它最簡單的形式是由一個空心膠皮球和一個插入腔內的管子通過活門系統相連而組成的。另一活門在管子的排出端。排出器在手術時用於清除囊中的廢物，如在結石切除術時。

evagination *n.* the protrusion of a part or organ from a sheathlike covering or by eversion of its inner surface.

外突 某部位或器官自鞘樣結構中伸出的突起，或因內表面外翻而出現的突起。

eventration *n.* **1.** protrusion of the intestines through the abdominal wall. **2.** (of the diaphragm) abnormal elevation of part of the diaphragm due to a congenital weakness (but without true herniation), as observed by X-ray.

①**腸突出** 腸經腹壁突出。 ②**膈突出** 因先天性薄弱而部分橫膈不正常地上升（但不是真疝），X線可查出。

event sampling (in psychology) a way of recording behaviour in which the presence of a particular kind of behaviour is noted whenever it occurs. It is used for precise descriptions of behaviour and for following the course of *behaviour modification. *See also* time sampling.

事件採樣 （心理學）一種記錄行爲的方法。只要某種特殊行爲發生時，就立即把它記錄下來。本法用於準確描述行爲及跟踪行爲改變的過程。

eversion *n.* a turning outward; in *eversion of the cervix* the edges of the neck of the womb turn outward after having been torn during childbirth.

外翻 向外翻轉。在宮頸外翻中，宮頸緣在分娩時被撕裂後向外翻轉。

evisceration *n.* (in ophthalmology) an operation in which the contents of the eyeball are removed, the empty outer envelope (sclera) being left behind. *Compare* enucleation.

眼內容剜出術 （眼科）除去眼球內容物，只留下空外殼（鞏膜）的手術。

evulsion *n. see* avulsion.

撕脫

Ewing's sarcoma a highly malignant tumour of bone occurring in children and young adults. Distinguished from *osteosarcoma by J. Ewing in 1921, it commonly arises in the limbs but may

尤因氏瘤 發生於兒童和青年的高度惡化的骨腫瘤。1921年吉·尤因將此瘤與骨肉瘤區分開。此腫瘤常發生在肢體，但也可

affect any bone. It is sensitive to radiotherapy, and systemic therapy with *cytotoxic drugs has improved its prognosis.

發生於所有骨頭。對放療敏感。系統地進行細胞毒性藥物治療也可改善其預後。

ex- (exo-) *prefix denoting* outside or outer.

〔前綴〕 在……之外，外

exaltation *n. see* elation.

異常興奮

exanthem *n.* **1.** a skin rash accompanying any eruptive disease or fever. **2.** any disease characterized by a skin rash. —**exanthematous** *adj.*

①病疹 發疹性疾病或熱性病中的皮疹。 ②疹病 以皮疹爲特點的任何疾病。

excavator *n.* **1.** a spoon-shaped surgical instrument that is used to scrape out diseased tissue, usually for laboratory examination. **2.** a type of hand instrument with spoon ends used for removing decayed dentine from teeth. It may also be used as a *curette.

剜器 ①通常爲實驗室檢查而用於剜出病變組織的匙樣外科器械。 ②一種手用器械，末尾帶匙，用於從牙齒中除去腐爛牙質，也可做刮匙用。

exchange transfusion a technique for treating *haemolytic disease in newborn infants. Using a 20-ml syringe with a three-way tap, Rh positive blood is withdrawn from the baby (via the umbilical vein), ejected, and replaced by 20 ml Rh negative donor blood, without detaching the syringe. By many repetitions of this exchange, red blood cells liable to be destroyed and bilirubin released from those already destroyed are removed, while keeping the baby's blood volume and number of red cells constant.

交換輸血法 治療新生兒溶血性疾病的一種技術。用一隻帶三通接頭的20ml注射器通過臍靜脈從嬰兒體內抽出 Rh 陽性血液，不用更換注射器，再注入20mlRh 陰性血液。反覆重複這種交換，容易破壞的紅細胞及從已被破壞的紅細胞中釋放出來的膽紅素就可被除去。同時，又保持了嬰兒血容量及紅細胞數穩定不變。

excipient *n.* a substance that is combined with a drug in order to render it suitable for administration; for example in the form of pills. Excipients should have no pharmacological action themselves.

賦形劑 爲使藥物易於服用（如丸劑形式）而與其結合的物質。但其本身並沒有藥理作用。

excise *vb.* to cut out tissue, an organ, or a tumour from the body. —**excision** *n.*

切除 將組織、器官或腫瘤從體內切除。

excitation *n.* (in neurophysiology) the triggering of a conducted impulse in the membrane of a muscle cell or nerve fibre. During excitation a polarized membrane becomes momentarily depo-

興奮 （神經生理）激發肌細胞膜或神經纖維產生傳導性衝動的動因。興奮時，極化膜暫時去極化，並形成動作電位。

larized and an *action potential is set up.

excoriation *n.* the destruction and removal of the surface of the skin or the covering of an organ by scraping, the application of a chemical, or other means.

表皮脫落 因抓搔、使用化學藥品或其他方法使皮膚表面或器官外膜遭到破壞並脫落。

excrescence *n.* an abnormal outgrowth on the surface of the body, such as a wart.

贅生物 體表面不正常的生長物。如疣。

excreta *n.* any waste material discharged from the body, especially faeces.

排泄物 從體內排出的任何廢物，特別是糞便。

excretion *n.* the removal of the waste products of metabolism from the body, mainly through the action of the *kidneys. Excretion also includes the loss of water, salts, and some urea through the sweat glands and carbon dioxide and water vapour from the lungs, and the term is also used to include the egestion of faeces.

排泄 體內的代謝廢物通過腎臟的作用排出體外。但也包括水、鹽及一些尿素從汗腺排出及二氧化碳和水蒸氣從肺臟排出的過程。此術語也用來指糞便排泄。

exenteration *n.* (in ophthalmology) an operation in which all the contents of the eye socket (orbit) are removed, leaving only the bony walls intact. The bone is covered by a skin graft. This operation is sometimes necessary when there is a malignant tumour in the orbit.

眼眶內容物剜出術 除去眼眶內所有內容物，只留下完整的骨壁的手術。用移植的皮膚覆蓋骨壁。在眼眶內有惡性腫瘤有時必需施行這種手術。

exflagellation *n.* the formation and release of mature flagellated male sex cells (*see* microgamete) by the *microgametocytes of the malarial parasite (*see* Plasmodium). The process, which is completed in 10–15 minutes, occurs after the microgametocytes have been transferred from man to the stomach of a mosquito.

小配子形成 由瘧原蟲小配子母細胞形成並釋放有鞭毛的成熟雄性細胞的過程。整個過程在10～15分鐘之內完成，發生在小配子母細胞從人體轉移到蚊胃之後。

exfoliation *n.* **1.** flaking off of the upper layers of the skin. **2.** separation of a surface epithelium from the underlying tissue. **3.** the natural shedding of deciduous teeth. —**exfoliative** *adj.*

脫落 ①皮膚外層剝落。②表面上皮與皮下組織分離。 ③乳齒自然掉落。

exhalation (expiration) *n.* the act of breathing air from the lungs out through the mouth and nose. *See* breathing.

呼出 肺部的氣體從口及鼻排出的動作。

exhibitionism *n.* exposure of the genitals to another person, as a sexually deviant act. The word is often broadened to mean public flaunting of any quality of the individual.

露陰癖 向他人暴露自己的生殖器。一種不正常的性變態行爲。該詞的意思還被擴大爲公開誇耀自己的長處。

exo- *prefix. see* ex-.

〔前綴〕 **外**

exocoelom *n. see* extraembryonic coelom.

外體腔

exocrine gland a gland that discharges its secretion by means of a duct, which opens onto an epithelial surface. An exocrine gland may be *simple*, with a single unbranched duct, or *compound*, with branched ducts and multiple secretory sacs. The illustration shows some different types of these glands. Examples of exocrine glands are the sebaceous and sweat glands. *See also* secretion.

外分泌腺 通過導管排出其分泌液的腺體。導管口開向上皮表面。可分爲單管外分泌腺：只有一個不分支的導管；複管外分泌腺：有多個分支的導管和分泌囊。外分泌腺包括皮脂腺和汗腺等。下圖是這些腺體的不同類型。

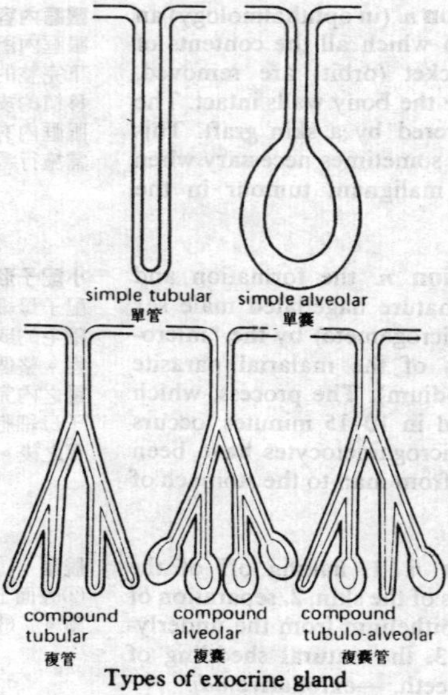

Types of exocrine gland

外分泌腺種類

exoenzyme *n.* an *enzyme that acts outside the cell that produced it. Examples of exoenzymes are the digestive enzymes.

胞外酶 在分泌細胞外發揮作用的酶。如消化酶等。

exoerythrocytic *adj.* describing those stages in the life cycle of the malarial parasite (*see* Plasmodium) that develop in the cells of the liver. Each parasite (*sporozoite) divides repeatedly to produce a schizont containing many merozoites.

紅細胞外的 指在肝細胞內生長發育的瘧原蟲生活周期中的各個階段。每一瘧原蟲又反復分裂，可產生出含有裂殖子的裂殖體。

exogenous *adj.* originating outside the body or part of the body: applied particularly to substances in the body that are derived from the diet rather than built up by the body's own processes of metabolism. *Compare* endogenous.

外原的 源於身體外或身體某部位外的。專指從飲食中得來，而不是因身體本身的代謝過程所產生的體內物質。

exomphalos *n.* an umbilical *hernia.

臍疝

exopeptidase *n.* an enzyme (e.g. *trypsin) that takes part in the digestion of proteins by splitting off the terminal amino acids of a polypeptide chain. *Compare* endopeptidase. *See also* peptidase.

肽鏈端解酶 通過分解多肽鏈終末氨基酸而參與蛋白質消化的酶（如胰蛋白酶）。

exophoria *n.* a tendency to squint in which the eye, when covered, tends to turn outwards. *See also* heterophoria.

外隱斜視 當閉眼時，眼睛向外移的斜視現象。

exophthalmic goitre (Graves's disease) *see* thyrotoxicosis.

突眼性甲狀腺腫（格雷夫斯氏病）

exophthalmometer (proptometer) *n.* an instrument for measuring the degree of protrusion of the eyeball. The distance measured is that from the rim of bone at the outer edge of the eye, forwards to the surface of the front of the cornea.

突眼計 測量眼球突出程度的儀器。測量的距離是從眼外緣的骨緣向前到角膜的前表面。

exophthalmos *n.* protrusion of the eyeballs in their sockets. This can result from injury or disease of the eyeball or socket but is most commonly associated with overactivity of the thyroid gland (*see* thyrotoxicosis).

突眼 眼球在其眼眶內突出。可因眼球及眼眶損傷或疾病引起，但主要與甲狀腺亢進有關。

exosmosis *n.* outward osmotic flow. *See also* osmosis.

外滲 體液向外滲出。

exostosis *n.* a benign cartilaginous outgrowth from a bone. *See* osteoma.

外生骨疣 生長於骨上的良性軟骨新生物。

exothermic *adj.* describing a chemical reaction in which energy is released in the form of heat. *Compare* endothermic.

放熱的 指以熱的形式釋放能量的化學反應。

exotic *adj.* describing a disease occurring in a region of the world far from where it might be expected. Thus malaria and leishmaniasis are regarded as exotic when they are diagnosed in patients in Britain.

外來的 指某地區發生了原本只發生在遠離該地區的世界某地的疾病。因此，當在英國的患者被診斷爲患瘧疾和利什曼病時，這些病就被認爲是外來的。

exotoxin *n.* a highly potent poison, often harmful to only a limited range of tissues, that is produced by a bacterial cell and secreted into its surrounding medium. It is generally unstable, being rendered inactive by heat, light, and chemicals. Exotoxins are produced by such bacteria as those causing *botulism, *diphtheria, and *tetanus. *Compare* endotoxin.

外毒素 由細菌產生，並釋放到其周圍環境的劇毒物質。通常只對組織的有限範圍有害。一般不穩定，可被熱、光、化學物質滅活。外毒素由能引起肉毒中毒、白喉及破傷風一類的細菌產生。

exotropia *n.* divergent *strabismus: a type of squint.

外斜視 散開性斜視，斜視的一種。

expectorant *n.* a drug that enhances the secretion of sputum by the air passages so that it is easier to cough up. Expectorants are used in cough mixtures; they act by increasing the bronchial secretion or make it less viscous (*see* mucolytic). Drugs such as *ipecacuanha are *stimulant expectorants* in small quantities: they irritate the lining of the stomach, which provides a stimulus for the reflex production of sputum by the glands in the bronchial mucous membrane. At higher doses they produce vomiting.

祛痰劑 促進氣道分泌痰液，使其易於咳出的藥物。用於止咳合劑中。是通過增加支氣管的分泌或使痰液稀薄而發揮作用的。小劑量的藥物如吐根屬刺激性祛痰劑：它們通過激惹胃黏膜反射地刺激支氣管黏膜內的腺體產生痰液。大劑量的吐根可導致嘔吐。

expectoration *n.* the act of spitting out material brought into the mouth by coughing.

排痰 吐出因咳嗽帶到嘴裏的東西。

expiration *n.* **1.** the act of breathing out air from the lungs: exhalation. **2.** dying.

①**呼出** 排出肺部氣體的動作。②**臨終**

explant **1.** *n.* live tissue transferred from the body (or any organism) to a suitable artificial medium for culture. The tissue grows in the artificial medium and can be studied for diagnostic or experimental purposes. Tumour growths are sometimes examined in this way. **2.** *vb.* to transfer live tissue for culture outside the body. —**explantation** *n.*

①**移出物** 從體內（或任何生物體內）移到適宜的人工培養基上進行培養的活組織。此組織在人工培養基上生長，並爲診斷或實驗的目的而對其進行研究。腫瘤生長物有時就是用這種方法進行檢查的。②**移出** 將活組織移到體外進行培養。

exploration *n.* (in surgery) an investigative operation to determine the cause of symptoms. —**exploratory** *adj.*

探查術 （外科學）爲確定症狀的原因而進行的探查性手術。

exposure *n.* (in behaviour therapy) a method of treating fears and phobias that involves confronting the individual with the situation he has been avoiding, so allowing the fears to wane by *extinction. It can be achieved gradually by *desensitization or suddenly by *flooding.

暴露療法 （行爲療法）治療害怕或恐懼的方法。讓患者親臨其曾避免遇到的現場，使懼怕心理因消退作用而消失。這種療法可通過脫敏作用而逐漸達到目的，或通過暴露於恐怖環境之中而迅速達到目的。

exsanguinate *vb.* to deprive the body of blood; for example, as a result of an accident causing severe bleeding or – very rarely – through uncontrollable bleeding during a surgical operation. —**exsanguination** *n.*

失血 體內的血液流失。如因意外事故而嚴重出血，或外科手術時不能控制的出血。後者很少見。

exsiccation *n.* drying up, as may occur in tissues deprived of an adequate supply of water during dehydration or starvation.

乾燥 缺水。常發生於脫水或飢餓時沒有充分供水的組織。

exsufflation *n.* the forcible removal of secretions from the air passages by some form of suction apparatus.

抽吸 用某種形式的抽吸器强力抽出氣道中的分泌物。

extension *n.* **1.** the act of extending or stretching, especially the muscular movement by which a limb is straightened. **2.** the application of *traction to a fractured or dislocated limb in order to restore it to its normal position.

①**伸展** 伸直或展開的動作。特別是肌肉運動，這樣可使肢體伸直。②**牽引** 用牽引的方法使骨折或錯位的肢體恢復其正常位置。

extensor *n.* any muscle that causes the straightening of a limb or other part.

伸肌 使肢體或其他部位伸直的所有肌肉。

exteriorization *n.* a surgical procedure in which an organ is brought from its normal site to the surface of the body. This may be done as a temporary or permanent measure; for example, the intestine may be brought to the surface of the abdomen (*see* colostomy). The process is also sometimes used in physiological experiments on animals.

外置術 將某器官從其正常位置移到身體表面的外科手術。可做爲暫時或永久性措施。如將腸道拉出腹壁表面。這一手術有時也用於動物的生理實驗上。

exteroceptor *n.* a sensory nerve, ending in the skin or a mucous membrane, that is responsive to stimuli from outside the body. *See also* chemoreceptor, receptor.

外感受器 末稍在皮膚或黏膜內的感覺神經。傳導體外的刺激。

extinction *n.* (in psychology) the weakening of a conditioned reflex that takes place if it is not maintained by *reinforcement. This is used as a method of treatment when undesirable behaviour (e.g. destructiveness) is reduced simply by withdrawing whatever rewards it (e.g. the fuss made by other people).

消失作用 （心理學）如果不持續强化條件，則這種條件反射會逐漸減弱。此作用可做爲一種治療方法。當發生令人不快的行爲時（如破壞行爲），只要不去理睬（如其他人大驚小怪地議論），這種行爲是會減少的。

extirpation *n.* the complete surgical removal of tissue, an organ, or a growth.

摘除 將組織、某器官或某生長物完全外科切除。

extra- *prefix denoting* outside or beyond.

〔前綴〕 **外，在……之外**

extracellular *adj.* situated or occurring outside cells; for example, *extracellular fluid* is the fluid surrounding cells.

細胞外的 位於或發生於細胞之外，如細胞外液是細胞周圍的液體。

extract *n.* a preparation containing the pharmacologically active principles of a drug, made by evaporating a solution of the drug in water, alcohol, or ether.

浸膏 具有藥物有效成分的製劑。經蒸發藥的水溶液、酒精溶液及醚溶液而製成。

extraction *n.* **1.** the surgical removal of a part of the body. Extraction of teeth is usually achieved by applying extraction *forceps to the crown or root of the tooth to dislocate it from its socket. When this is not possible, for example because the tooth or root is deeply

①**摘除術** 外科切除身體的某部位。牙齒摘除術是用拔牙鉗夾住牙冠或牙根部使其脫離牙槽而完成的。如使用這一方法不能成功，比如牙齒或牙根部深深埋入骨內，就要切除

buried within the bone, extraction is performed surgically by removing bone and dividing the tooth. **2.** the act of pulling out a baby from the body of its mother during childbirth.

牙槽骨，再分離出牙齒來完成摘除術。 ②**取出** 在分娩時，從母體內拉出嬰兒的動作。

extractor *n.* an instrument used to pull out a natural part of the body, to remove a foreign object, or to assist delivery of a baby (*see* vacuum extractor).

取出器 摘出體內某自然部分，除去異物或幫助嬰兒娩出的器械。

extradural *adj. see* epidural.

硬膜外的

extraembryonic coelom (exocoelom) the cavity, lined with mesoderm, that surrounds the embryo from the earliest stages of development. It communicates temporarily with the coelomic cavity within the embryo (peritoneal cavity). Late in pregnancy it becomes almost entirely obliterated by the growth of the *amnion, which fuses with the *chorion.

胚外體腔 最早發育期的胚胎周圍的腔。內襯以中胚層。與胚胎內體腔（腹腔）暫時相交通。妊娠後期，該腔幾乎完全被生長的與絨毛膜融合的羊膜所閉合。

extraembryonic membranes the membranous structures that surround the embryo and contribute to the placenta and umbilical cord. They include the *amnion, *chorion, *allantois, and *yolk sac. In man the allantois is always very small and by the end of pregnancy the amnion and chorion have fused into a single membrane and the yolk sac has disappeared.

胚外膜 包繞胚胎並構成胎盤和臍帶的膜樣結構。包括羊膜、絨毛膜、尿囊和卵黃囊。在人類，尿囊總是很小；而且在妊娠末期時，羊膜和絨毛膜融合在一起，形成單層膜；卵黃囊也已消失。

extrapleural *adj.* relating to the tissues of the chest wall outside the parietal *pleura.

胸膜外的 指胸膜壁層外的胸壁組織。

extrapyramidal system the system of nerve tracts and pathways connecting the cerebral cortex, basal ganglia, thalamus, cerebellum, reticular formation, and spinal neurones in complex circuits not included in the *pyramidal system. The extrapyramidal system is mainly concerned with the regulation of stereotyped reflex muscular movements.

錐體外系統 在錐體系以外的連接大腦皮層、基底神經節、丘腦、小腦網狀結構及脊神經元的神經束和傳導系統。是一套複雜的神經環路。錐體外系統主要是調節固有的肌肉運動反射。

extrasensory perception (ESP) a supposed way of perceiving that in-

超感知學 假設的不包括已知感覺的察覺方式。洞

volves none of the known senses. *Clairvoyance* is the extrasensory perception of current events; *precognition* is extrasensory perception of future events; *telepathy* is extrasensory perception of the thoughts of others.

察力就是對現實事物的超感知覺，預感就是對將來事件的超感知覺，心靈感應就是對他人想法的超感知覺。

extrasÿstole *n. see* ectopic beat.

期外收縮

extrauterine *adj.* outside the womb.

子宮外的

extravasation *n.* the leakage and spread of blood or fluid from vessels into the surrounding tissues, which follows injury, burns, inflammation, and allergy.

外滲 血液或液體從血管內滲出並擴散到周圍組織。通常發生在損傷、燒傷、炎症及過敏以後。

extraversion *n. see* extroversion.

外傾

extrinsic muscle a muscle, such as any of those controlling movements of the eyeball, that has its origin some distance from the part it acts on. *See also* eye.

外附肌 其起源與其作用部位有一定距離的肌肉。如控制眼球運動的所有肌肉。

extroversion *n.* **1.** (or **extraversion**) an enduring personality trait characterized by interest in the outside world rather than the self. People high in extroversion (*extroverts*), as measured by questionnaires and tests, are gregarious and outgoing, prefer to change activities frequently, and are not susceptible to permanent *conditioning. Extroversion was first described by Carl Jung as a tendency to action rather than thought, to scientific rather than philosophical interests, and to emotional rather than intellectual reactions. *Compare* introversion. **2.** a turning inside out of a hollow organ, such as the womb (which sometimes occurs after childbirth).

①**外傾性格** 以對外界而不是對自己感興趣爲特點的個性。以外傾性格爲主的人，經詢問和考查證明，是愛交際而且開朗的，寧願頻繁更換活動種類，也不願持續在一種恒定的環境之中生活。卡爾·容格是第一位描述外傾性格的人。他認爲：外傾性格表現爲願意活動而不願意思考；喜歡科學而不喜歡哲學；善於感情用事而不是理智地處事。
②**外翻** 某空心臟器由內翻向外。如子宮外翻（有時分娩後發生）。

extrovert *n. see* extroversion.

外傾性格者

extrusion *n.* (in dentistry) the movement of a tooth beyond its normal alignment.

上超𬌗 （牙科）超越眞牙𬌗面的牙移動。

exudation *n.* the slow escape of liquid (called the *exudate*) containing proteins and white cells through the walls of

滲出 含蛋白質和白細胞的液體（滲出液）從完整的血管緩慢溢出。通常是

intact blood vessels, usually as a result of inflammation. Exudation is a normal part of the body's defence mechanisms.

炎症的結果。滲出是身體防御機制的一部分。

eye *n.* the organ of sight: a three-layered roughly spherical structure specialized for receiving and responding to light (see illustration).
Light enters the eye through the cornea, which refracts it through the aqueous humour onto the lens. By adjustment of the shape of the lens (*see* accommodation) light is focused through the vitreous humour onto the retina. In the retina light-sensitive cells (*see* cone, rod) send nerve impulses to the brain via the optic nerve. The arrangement of the two eyes at the front of the head provides *binocular vision. Each eye is contained in an *orbit, and movement of the eye within the orbit is controlled by extrinsic eye muscles (see illustration).

眼 視覺器官。大體有三層專門接收並轉送光線的球狀結構（見圖）。
光通過角膜進入眼內，角膜又將光通過房水折射到晶體上。經晶體的調節，光通過玻璃體被集中到視網膜上。在視網膜裏，光感細胞通過視神經將神經衝動送入大腦。腦前的兩眼提供了雙眼視覺。每一眼眶裏有一隻眼，眼眶內眼的移動由眼外附肌控制。

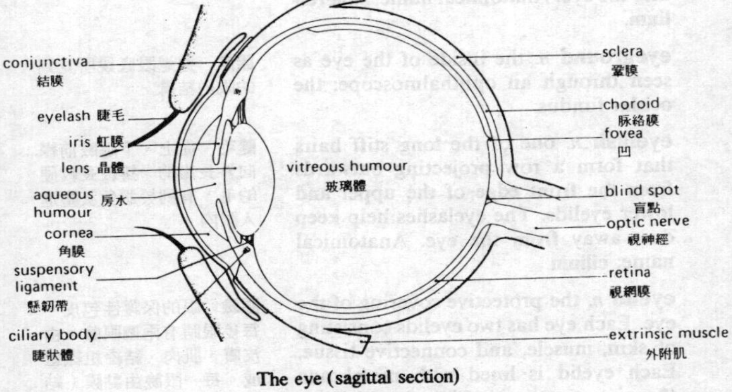

The eye (sagittal section)
眼（矢狀面）

eyeball *n.* the body of the *eye, which is roughly spherical, is bounded by the *sclera, and lies in the *orbit. It is closely associated with accessory structures – the eyelids, conjunctiva, and lacrimal (tear-producing) apparatus – and its movements are controlled by

眼球 眼的主體。近似球形，被鞏膜包繞，位於眼眶內。眼球與其附屬結構——眼瞼，結膜，淚器——密切相關，其移動由三對眼外附肌控制（見圖）。

three pairs of extrinsic eye muscles (see illustration).

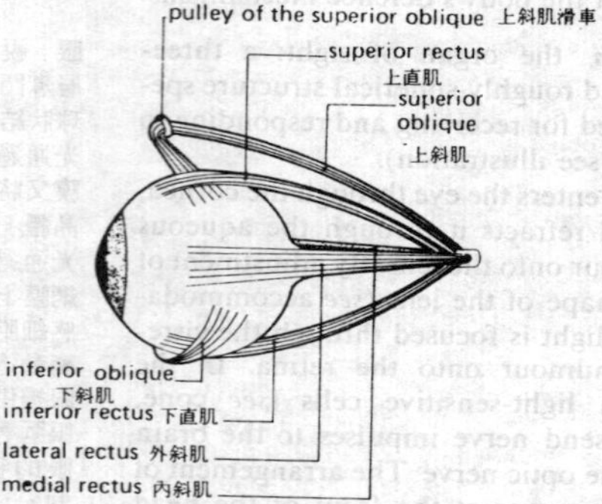

Extrinsic muscles of the eye
眼外附肌

eyebrow *n.* the small fringe of hair on the bony ridge just above the eye. It helps to prevent moisture from running into the eye. Anatomical name: **supercilium**.

眼眉 眼上方骨嵴部位上的小毛緣。可防止液體流入眼內。

eyeground *n.* the inside of the eye as seen through an ophthalmoscope; the ocular fundus.

眼底 通過眼底鏡所見到的眼內結構。

eyelash *n.* one of the long stiff hairs that form a row projecting outwards from the front edge of the upper and lower eyelids. The eyelashes help keep dust away from the eye. Anatomical name: **cilium**.

睫毛 從上、下眼瞼前緣向外長出的一排較長較硬的毛，有利於避免灰塵進入眼內。

eyelid *n.* the protective covering of the eye. Each eye has two eyelids consisting of skin, muscle, and connective tissue. Each eyelid is lined with membrane (*conjunctiva) and fringed with eyelashes. Stimulation of the pain receptors in the cornea causes the eyelids to close in a reflex action. Anatomical names: **blepharon, palpebra**.

眼瞼 眼的保護性包皮。每隻眼睛有兩個眼瞼，由皮膚、肌肉、結締組織組成。每一眼瞼由黏膜（結膜）內襯，其邊緣由睫毛裝飾。刺激角膜的疼痛感受器可引起眼瞼反射性關閉。

eyepiece *n.* the part of an optical instrument, such as a microscope, that is nearest to the eye of the examiner. *Compare* objective.

目鏡 光學儀器（如顯微鏡）中距檢查者眼睛最近的部件。

eyestrain *n.* a sense of fatigue brought on by use of the eyes for prolonged close work or in persons who have an uncorrected error of *refraction or an imbalance of the muscles that move the eyes. Symptoms are usually aching or burning of the eyes, accompanied by headache and even general fatigue if the eyes are not rested. Medical name: **asthenopia**.

眼疲勞 因長期用眼進行工作或某些人屈光不正或動眼肌不協調而引起的一種疲勞感覺。症狀有：眼疼或燒灼感；如不休息眼睛，還會發生頭痛，甚至全身疲勞。醫學術語：視覺疲勞。

F

Fabry's disease *see* angiokeratoma.

法伯瑞氏病，血管角質瘤

face-bow *n.* (in dentistry) an instrument for transferring the jaw relationship of a patient to an *articulator to allow reproduction of the lateral and protrusive movements of the lower jaw.

面弓 （牙科用語）將患者頜關係轉移到殆架上的一種器械。以複製出能夠向外或向前移動的下頜。

facet *n.* a small flat surface on a bone or tooth, especially a surface of articulation.

小平面 骨和牙齒上的小平面，特別是關節上的小平滑面。

facial nerve the seventh *cranial nerve (VII): a mixed sensory and motor nerve that supplies the muscles of facial expression, the taste buds of the front part of the tongue, the sublingual salivary glands, and the lacrimal glands. A small branch to the middle ear regulates the tension on the ear ossicles.

面神經 第四對腦神經，是感覺和運動的混合神經。分佈於面部表情肌、舌前的味蕾、舌下唾液腺及淚腺。其一小分支分佈到中耳以調節聽小骨的張力。

-facient *suffix denoting* causing or making. Example: *abortifacient* (causing abortion).

〔後綴〕 **引起，使產生** 如墮胎藥（引起流產）。

facies *n.* facial expression, often a guide to a patient's state of health as well as his emotions. The typical facies seen in adenoids is the vacant look, with the mouth drooping open. A *Hippocratic facies* is the sallow face, sagging and with listless staring eyes, that some read as the expression of approaching death.

面容 面部表情。通常是患者健康狀態及情緒的表現。增殖腺患者的典型面容是無表情並張着下垂的嘴。希波克拉底面容是面色灰黃，精神萎靡，無神而凝視的目光。有人將此面容叫做死相。

facilitation *n.* (in neurology) the phenomenon that occurs when a neurone receives, through a number of different synapses, impulses that are not powerful enough individually to start an *action potential but whose combined activity brings about some *depolarization of the membrane. In this facilitated state a small additional depolarization will suffice to trigger off an impulse in the cell.

接通作用（神經學用語）當神經元通過多種不同的突觸接受衝動時，單個的衝動如不足以引起動作電位，所有的衝動合在一起，就能引起膜的去極化。在接通期間，小量附加的去極化作用就能激發細胞內的衝動。

factitious *adj.* produced artificially, either deliberately or by accident, and therefore not to be taken into account when the results of an experiment are considered or a diagnosis is being made.

人爲的 有意或無意地人爲產生的。因此，在分析實驗結果和做出的診斷時，不予考慮。

Factory Inspectorate the largest and oldest of the statutory bodies responsible for monitoring the health and safety of factory workers. It is administered by the Department of Employment through the Health and Safety Commission under the terms of the Health and Safety at Work Act. Requirements include a routine examination of young persons and those exposed to toxic hazards (e.g. lead) and the adequate guarding of machinery. Ensuring that the atmosphere inside the factory is free from poisonous fumes and chemicals may cause conflict with local authorities, whose *Environmental Health Officers have responsibility to prevent atmospheric pollution.

工廠視察團 最大最早的負責管理工廠裏工人健康和安全的法定團體。按勞動法中健康和安全的條例要求，該視察團由雇傭部門的健康安全委員會管理。要求包括：對青年人及暴露於有害毒物（如鉛）之中的人們進行常規檢查，保證不受機器的損傷。確保廠內的空氣中無毒氣及化學物質。但這可能與當地政府相矛盾，因他們的負責防止大氣汚染的環境衞生官員也負責預防大氣汚染的工作。

facultative *adj.* describing an organism that is not restricted to one way of life. A *facultative parasite* can live either as a parasite or, in different conditions, as a nonparasite able to survive without a host. *Compare* obligate.

兼性的 指不僅限於一種生活方式的生物。兼性寄生物即可做爲寄生物生存，在不同的環境中也可不需宿主而做爲非寄生物生存。

FAD (flavin adenine dinucleotide) a *coenzyme, derived from riboflavin, that takes part in many important oxidation-reduction reactions. It consists of two phosphate groups, adenine, and ribose.

黃素腺嘌呤二核苷酸 能參與很多重要的氧化還原反應的輔酶。來於核黃素。由二個磷酸基團、腺嘌呤和核糖組成。

fading *n.* (in behaviour modification) *see* prompting.
消退　行爲矯正法用語。

faecalith *n.* a small hard mass of faeces, found particularly in the vermiform appendix: a cause of inflammation.
糞石　小硬糞便團。主要見於闌尾。可引起炎症。

faeces *n.* the waste material that is eliminated through the anus. It is formed in the *colon and consists of a solid or semisolid mass of undigested food remains (chiefly cellulose) mixed with *bile pigments (which are responsible for the colour), bacteria, various secretions (e.g. mucus), and some water. —**faecal** *adj.*
糞便　從肛門排出的廢物。形成於結腸，由未被消化的食物殘渣（主要是纖維素）與膽色素（着色物質）、細菌、各種分泌物（如黏液）及水混合而成的固體和半固體物質組成。

Fahrenheit temperature temperature expressed on a scale in which the melting point of ice is assigned a temperature of 32° and the boiling point of water a temperature of 212°. For most medical purposes the Celsius (centigrade) scale has replaced the Fahrenheit scale. The formula for converting from Fahrenheit (F) to Celsius (C) is: $C = \frac{5}{9}(F - 32)$. *See also* Celsius temperature.
華氏溫度　在溫標上以冰的融點爲32°、水的沸點爲212°表現出來的溫度。在醫學上，華氏溫標多數已被攝氏溫標所取代。換算公式是：$C=\frac{5}{9}(F-32)$。

fainting *n. see* syncope.
昏厥

falciform ligament a fold of peritoneum separating the right and left lobes of the liver and attaching it to the diaphragm and the anterior abdominal wall as far as the umbilicus.
鐮狀韌帶　分隔肝臟左右葉的腹膜皺襞。通過肝臟，上與橫膈相連，下與前腹壁臍部相連。

Fallopian tube (oviduct, uterine tube) either of a pair of tubes that conduct ova (egg cells) from the ovary to the womb (*see* reproductive system). The ovarian end opens into the abdominal cavity via a funnel-shaped structure with finger-like projections (*fimbriae*) surrounding the opening. Movements of the fimbriae at ovulation assist in directing the ovum to the Fallopian tube. The ovum is fertilized near the ovarian end of the tube.
輸卵管　將卵細胞從卵巢運送到子宮的一對管道，卵巢端通過漏斗狀結構開口於腹腔。圍繞開口處，漏斗狀結構上帶有很多指樣突起（繖）。在排卵期，繖的運動有助於卵子直接進入輸卵管。卵子在輸卵管的卵巢端附近受精。

Fallot's tetralogy *see* tetralogy of Fallot.
法樂氏四聯症

falx (falx cerebri) *n.* a sickle-shaped fold of the *dura mater that dips inwards from the skull in the midline, between the cerebral hemispheres.

大腦鐮 從顱骨突入大腦半球之間的鐮刀狀硬腦膜皺襞。

familial *adj.* describing a condition or character that is found in some families but not in others. It is often inherited.

家族的 指在同一家庭而不是其他家庭裏發現的疾病或特徵。通常是遺傳性的。

family planning 1. the use of *contraception to limit or space out the numbers of children born to a couple. **2.** provision of contraceptive methods within a community or nation.

計劃生育 ①夫妻之間通過避孕措施來限制生育或延長生育的時距。 ②在全國範圍內規定的避孕措施。

Family Practitioner Committee (FPC) (in Britain) an authority responsible for running general medical services (general practitioners, dentists, pharmacists, and opticians) for the population served by one or more District Health Authorities. Members of the FPC are appointed by the District Health Authority, local authority, local *medical committee, local dental committee, local pharmaceutical committee and local optical committee. The general practitioners have independent contracts (as distinct from salaries) with the FPC, which must approve all names included on the *medical list* (a special list of general practitioners working in the National Health Service). Such inclusion is subject to overall monitoring of the *Medical Practices Committee*, which advises the Department of Health and Social Security; similar arrangements exist for the other three services (*see* general dental services). Refusal to include a suitable registered practitioner is usually the result of there being a surplus for the population being served. However the FPC must also approve the premises and the hours of service. The committee meets regularly (e.g. every two months) and has separate subcommittees for each of the four services as

開業醫生管理委員會 （在英國）負責管理由一個或多個地段保健局管轄範圍內的所有普通醫療服務部門（包括全科醫生、牙科醫生、藥劑師、眼科醫生）的權威機構。委員會成員由地段保健局、當地政府、當地醫學委員會、當地牙科委員會、當地藥學委員會及當地眼科委員會任命。全科醫生與開業醫生管理委員會簽有獨立合同（與拿工資的醫生不同）。醫生名單（在國民保健服務制系統中工作的全科醫生的特殊名單）必須由委員會批準，再由醫學委員會全面審批。該委員會還要向保健和社會保障部門提供諮詢。其他三個醫療服務部門也有類似的規定。如果不給醫生註册登記，通常是因爲這一地區的醫生已經滿額。但開業醫生管理委員會必須規定行醫的地點及時間。委員會定期開會（如每兩月一次），並按四個醫療服務部門分成四個分會，及安排醫生的工作時間，以避免出現無人行醫的情況。委員會還

well as those concerned with vacancies, hours of availability, and allocation of patients who are refused acceptance by all general practitioners in the vicinity.

要負責分派被該地區全科醫生拒絕接受的病人。

Fanconi syndrome a disorder of the proximal kidney tubules, which may be inherited or acquired and is most common in children. It is characterized by the urinary excretion of large amounts of amino acids, glucose, and phosphates (though blood levels of these substances are normal). Symptoms may include osteomalacia, rickets, muscle weakness, and *cystinosis. Treatment is directed to the cause.

范康尼綜合征 腎臟近曲小管的疾病。可爲遺傳性或後天獲得性，最常見於兒童。特點爲從尿液中排泄出大量的氨基酸、葡萄糖及磷酸鹽（儘管這些物質在血液裏的量是正常的）。症狀有：骨軟化、佝僂病、肌無力及胱氨酸尿。針對病因治療。

fantasy (phantasy) *n.* a complex sequence of imagination in which several imaginary elements are woven together into a story. An excessive preoccupation with one's own imaginings may be symptomatic of a difficulty in coping with reality. In psychoanalytic psychology, *unconscious fantasies* are supposed to control behaviour, so that psychological symptoms can be symbols of or defences against such fantasies (*see* symbolism).

幻想 把幾種想象的情節編織成一個完整故事的複雜的幻想序列。過分沉醉於這種幻想可能是難於與現實相適應的症狀。在精神分析心理學中，潛意識的幻想被認爲能控制人的行爲，因而，心理上的症狀可能是這些幻想的象徵，也可能是對這些幻想的抵制。

farad *n.* the *SI unit of capacitance, equal to the capacitance of a capacitor between the plates of which a potential difference of 1 volt appears when it is charged with 1 coulomb of electricity. Symbol: F.

法拉 電容的國際單位。即當通入 1 庫侖電流時，兩個電壓差爲 1 伏特的電容器板之間的電容量。符號：F。

faradism *n.* the use of induced rapidly alternating electric currents to stimulate nerve and muscle activity. *See also* electrotherapy.

感應電療法 用快速感應交流電激發神經和肌肉的活性。

farcy *n. see* glanders.

馬鼻疽

farmer's lung an occupational lung disease caused by allergy to fungal spores that grow in inadequately dried stored hay. It is an allergic *alveolitis, such as also results from sensitivity to many other allergens. An acute rever-

農夫肺 一種職業性肺病。因對生長在潮濕的乾草堆裏的眞菌孢子過敏而產生。就象其他過敏原在肺部引起的結果一樣，此病是一種過敏性肺泡炎。

sible form can develop a few hours after exposure; a chronic form, with the gradual development of irreversible breathlessness, occurs with or without preceding acute attacks. Avoidance of the allergen is the main principle of treatment.

急性可逆型：接觸過敏原後數小時發病。慢性型：可在急性發作後逐漸發展成不可逆性呼吸困難，也可直接發病。主要治療原則是避免接觸過敏原。

fascia *n.* (*pl.* **fasciae**) connective tissue forming membranous layers of variable thickness in all regions of the body. Fascia surrounds the softer or more delicate organs and is divided into *superficial fascia* (found immediately beneath the skin) and *deep fascia* (which forms sheaths for muscles).

筋膜 在身體各部位形成各種厚度膜樣層的結締組織。筋膜包繞着較柔軟或較嬌嫩的器官。分爲淺筋膜（直接位於皮膚之下）和深筋膜（形成肌鞘）。

fasciculation *n.* brief spontaneous contraction of a few muscle fibres, which is seen as a flicker of movement under the skin. It is most often associated with disease of the motor neurones in the spinal cord or of the nerve fibres.

自發性收縮 少量肌纖維暫時地、自動地收縮。表現爲皮下抽動。常與脊髓中運動神經元疾病或神經纖維疾病有關。

fasciculus (fascicle) *n.* a bundle, e.g. of nerve or muscle fibres.

束 束狀物。如神經束，肌纖維束。

fasciitis *n.* inflammation of *fascia. It may result from bacterial infection or from a rheumatic disease, such as *Reiter's syndrome or ankylosing spondylitis.

筋膜炎 筋膜的炎症。可因細菌感染或風濕性疾病引起。如萊特爾氏綜合症或强直性脊椎炎。

Fasciola *n.* a genus of *flukes. *F. hepatica*, the liver fluke, normally lives as a parasite of sheep and other herbivorous animals but sometimes infects man (*see* fascioliasis).

片吸蟲屬 吸蟲的一屬。肝吸蟲在正常情況下寄生在羊及其他食草動物身上，但有時也侵犯人類。

fascioliasis *n.* an infestation of the bile ducts and liver with the liver fluke, *Fasciola hepatica*. Man acquires the infection through eating wild watercress on which the larval stages of the parasite are present. Symptoms include fever, dyspepsia, vomiting, loss of appetite, abdominal pain, and coughing; the liver may also be extensively damaged (causing *liver rot*). *Emetine and *chloroquine have been used in the treatment of fascioliasis.

片吸蟲病 肝吸蟲侵犯膽囊和肝引起的疾病。人類是通過食入附有寄生蟲幼蟲的野生水芹而感染。症狀有發熱、消化不良、嘔吐、食慾減退、腹痛及咳嗽。肝臟可有廣泛損害（肝吸蟲病）。依米丁和氯喹一直被用來治療片吸蟲病。

fasciolopsiasis *n.* a disease, common in the Far East, caused by the fluke **Fasciolopsis buski* in the small intestine. At the site of attachment of the adult flukes in the intestine there may be inflammation with some ulceration and bleeding. Symptoms include diarrhoea, and in heavy infections the patient may experience loss of appetite, vomiting, and (later) swelling of the face, abdomen, and legs. Death may follow in cases of severe ill health and malnutrition. The flukes can be removed with an anthelmintic.

布氏薑片蟲病 常見於遠東，由小腸內布氏薑片蟲引起的一種疾病。被吸蟲侵犯的小腸部位有炎症，伴有潰瘍及出血。症狀有腹瀉。嚴重感染的患者還有食慾不振，嘔吐，面部、腹部及腿部水腫（晚期）。健康狀態極差及營養不良的患者會出現死亡。驅腸蟲藥可驅除吸蟲。

Fasciolopsis *n.* a genus of large parasitic flukes widely distributed throughout eastern Asia and especially common in China. The adults of *F. buski*, the giant intestinal fluke, live in the human small intestine. Man becomes infected with the fluke on eating uncooked water chestnuts contaminated with fluke larvae and the resulting symptoms can be serious (*see* fasciolopsiasis).

薑片蟲屬 大型寄生吸蟲屬。廣泛分佈於東亞，特別是中國。布氏吸蟲的成蟲是一種大型腸道吸蟲，寄生於人類小腸。人類在食入含有幼蟲的未煮熟的荸薺後感染，並引起嚴重症狀。

fastigium *n.* the highest point of a fever.

極度 發熱的最高度。

fat *n.* a substance that contains one or more fatty acids (in the form of *triglycerides) and is the principal form in which energy is stored by the body (in *adipose tissue). It also serves as an insulating material beneath the skin (in the subcutaneous tissue) and around certain organs (including the kidneys). Much of the carbohydrate of the diet is converted to fat before it is used for providing energy. However, a certain amount of fat is necessary in the diet to provide an adequate supply of *essential fatty acids and for the efficient absorption of fat-soluble vitamins from the intestine. Excessive deposition of fat in the body leads to *obesity. *See also* brown fat, lipid.

脂肪 含有一種或多種脂肪酸（以甘油三酯的形式）的物質。是身體（在脂肪組織）貯存能量的主要形式，也可做爲皮下的絕熱物（在皮下組織），或包繞某些器官（包括腎臟）。飲食中大部分的碳水化合物在做爲能量被消耗之前要轉化成脂肪。爲獲得充分必需脂肪酸及吸收腸道內脂溶性維生素，飲食中必備一定量的脂肪。體內脂肪過分堆積可導致肥胖症。

fatigue *n.* **1.** mental or physical tiredness, following prolonged or intense

疲勞 ①在過長或緊張的活動之後，精神和體力上

activity. Muscle fatigue may be due to the waste products of metabolism accumulating in the muscles faster than they can be removed by the venous blood. Incorrect or inadequate food intake or disease may predispose a person to fatigue. **2.** the inability of an organism, an organ, or a tissue to give a normal response to a stimulus until a certain recovery period has elapsed.

的疲乏。肌疲勞是由於肌肉中代謝廢物的積累比靜脈血液清除它們的速度快而引起。飲食不當或不足或生病容易使人感到疲勞。②某生物體、器官或組織在恢復期到來以前對刺激不能產生正常反應的狀態。

fatty acid an organic acid with a long straight hydrocarbon chain and an even number of carbon atoms. Fatty acids are the fundamental constituents of many important lipids, including *triglycerides. Some fatty acids can be synthesized by the body; others, the *essential fatty acids, must be obtained from the diet. Examples of fatty acids are *palmitic acid*, *oleic acid*, and *stearic acid*. *See also* fat.

脂肪酸 帶有碳氫直長鏈和偶數碳原子的有機酸。脂肪酸是很多重要脂類，包括甘油三酯的基本成分。某些脂肪酸可在體內合成，另一些必要脂肪酸則必須從食物中獲取。脂肪酸有棕櫚酸、油酸、硬脂酸等等。

fatty degeneration deterioration in the health of a tissue due to the deposition of abnormally large amounts of fat in its cells. The accumulation of fat in the liver and heart may seriously impair their functioning. The deposition of fat may be linked with incorrect diet, excessive alcohol consumption, or a shortage of oxygen in the tissues caused by poor circulation or a deficiency of haemoglobin.

脂肪變性 某組織因其細胞內不正常地積蓄大量的脂肪而變質。肝臟和心臟脂肪積蓄可嚴重損害其功能。脂肪積蓄可與飲食不當、酗酒、或因血液循環不良或血紅蛋白不足引起的組織缺氧有關。

fauces *n.* the opening leading from the mouth into the pharynx. It is surrounded by the *glossopalatine arch* (which forms the anterior pillars of the fauces) and the *pharyngopalatine arch* (the posterior pillars).

咽門 從口腔通向咽部的開口。由舌腭弓（構成前咽弓）和咽腭弓（構成後弓）所環繞。

favism *n.* an inherited allergy to a chemical substance found in broad beans; it occurs in parts of the Mediterranean and Iran. Destruction of red blood cells may lead to severe anaemia, requiring blood transfusion.

蠶豆病 對蠶豆中某種化學物質過敏的遺傳性疾患。發生於地中海和伊朗的一些地區。紅細胞受到破壞可導致嚴重貧血。需輸血治療。

favus *n.* a type of *ringworm of the scalp, caused by the fungus *Trichophyton schoenleini*. Favus, which is rare in

黃癬 頭皮髮癬的一種。由舍恩萊因里氏髮癬菌引起。在歐洲少見。以菌絲

Europe, is typified by yellow crusts made up of the threads of fungus and skin debris, which form honeycomb-like masses.

和皮屑組成的黃痂爲特點，黃痂又形成蜂窩狀斑塊。

fear *n.* an emotional state evoked by threat of danger and usually characterized by unpleasant subjective experiences and physiological and behavioural changes. Fear is often distinguished from *anxiety in having a specific object. Physiological changes can include increases in heart rate, blood pressure, sweating, etc. Behavioural changes can include an avoidance of fear-producing objects or situations and may be extremely disabling; for example, fear of open spaces. These specific disabling fears are known as *phobias. Treatment of short-term fears, such as the fear of hearing the results of an examination, can be relieved by tranquillizers, such as diazepam.

恐懼 因受到危險威脅而引起的一種情緒狀態。通常以不愉快的主觀體驗和生理、行爲上的變化爲特點。恐懼與焦慮的區別在於：前者是針對某一對象產生的。生理上的變化包括心動過速，血壓上升，出汗增加。行爲上的變化包括離開引起恐懼的對象或環境，甚至影響正常生活能力，如曠野恐懼。這種特殊的影響正常生活能力的恐懼叫做恐怖症。對短期恐懼的治療，如對害怕聽到考試結果的患者，可使用安定藥（如安定片）治療。

febricula *n.* a fever of low intensity or short duration.

微熱 輕微或短期發熱。

febrifuge *n.* a treatment or drug that reduces or prevents fever. *See* antipyretic.

解熱藥 退熱或預防發熱的藥。

febrile *adj.* relating to or affected with fever.

發熱的 指伴有發熱的疾病。

feeblemindedness *n.* a mild degree of mental *subnormality, corresponding roughly to an *intelligence quotient of 50–70. It is usually caused by an interaction of genetic and environmental factors, the nature of the psychological environment being of much importance.

低能 一種輕度的智力低常狀態。智商爲50～70之間。通常因遺傳和環境因素的相互作用引起。心理環境的特性更爲重要。

feedback *n.* the coupling of the output of a process to the input. Feedback mechanisms are important in regulating many physiological processes; for example, hormone output and enzyme-mediated reactions. In *negative feedback*, a rise in the output of a substance (e.g. a hormone) will inhibit a further

反饋 對輸入信息發生輸出反應的全部過程。反饋機理在調節生理過程中是重要的，如激素的釋放和酶促反應。在負反饋中。某物量的上升（如激素）將直接和間接地抑制其進一步增加，在正反饋中，

increase in its production, either directly or indirectly. In *positive feedback*, a rise in the output of a substance is associated with an increase in the output of another substance, either directly or indirectly. 某物量的上升將直接或間接地促進另一物量的增加。

Fehling's solution a solution used for detecting the presence of sugar in urine. There are two components: Fehling's I (a copper sulphate solution) and Fehling's II (a solution of potassium sodium tartrate and sodium hydroxide), which are kept separate until required for use. Boiling Fehling's solution (equal amounts of Fehling's I and II) is added to an equal volume of boiling urine; a yellowish or brownish coloration indicates the presence of sugar. **費林氏溶液** 用於檢驗尿糖的溶液。有兩種成分：費林氏Ⅰ（硫酸銅溶液）和費林氏Ⅱ（酒石酸鉀鈉和氫氧化鈉溶液）。這兩種溶液要分開放置。使用時將費林氏溶液（費林氏Ⅰ和費林氏Ⅱ的量相等）加入等量的煮沸的尿液裏，若有黃或棕色出現，則表明尿中有糖。

Feingold diet a diet that purports to treat many illnesses by the elimination of artificial food colourings, preservatives, and salicylates from the diet. It is particularly recommended for the treatment of *hyperkinetic syndrome, but is of unproved value. **芬哥德飲食** 不含有人造食物色素、防腐劑和水楊酸的一種飲食，用以治療多種疾病。被特別推薦用來治療運動過度綜合症。但其效果未得到證實。

felon *n. see* whitlow. **瘭疽**

feminization *n.* the development of female secondary sexual characteristics (enlargement of the breasts, loss of facial hair, and fat beneath the skin) in the male, either as a result of an endocrine disorder or of hormone therapy. **男子女性化** 男子表現出女性的第二性徵（乳房增大、無鬍鬚、皮下脂肪增厚）。因內分泌紊亂，或激素治療引起。

femoral *adj.* of or relating to the thigh or to the femur. **股的** 指大腿和股骨。

femoral artery an artery arising from the external iliac artery at the inguinal ligament. It is situated superficially, running down the front medial aspect of the thigh. Two-thirds of the way down it passes into the back of the thigh, continuing downward behind the knee as the *popliteal artery*. **股動脉** 從腹股溝韌帶附近的髂外動脉發出的動脉。位置表淺，向下走行到大腿的前內側。在走行的三分之二處，該動脉穿入大腿的後面，改名爲膕動脉，繼續在膝後向下走行。

femoral nerve the nerve that supplies the quadriceps muscle at the front of **股神經** 支配大腿前方股四頭肌，並接收大腿前內

the thigh and receives sensation from the front and inner sides of the thigh. It arises from the second, third, and fourth lumbar nerves.

側感覺的神經。從第二、第三、第四腰神經發出。

femoral triangle (Scarpa's triangle) a triangular depression on the inner side of the thigh bounded by the sartorius and adductor longus muscles and the inguinal ligament. The pulse can be felt here as the femoral artery lies over the depression.

股三角（斯卡帕氏三角） 大腿內側面的三角形凹陷。縫匠肌、內收肌和腹股溝韌帶爲其邊界。在此三角處可摸到脉搏，因股動脉在此通過。

femur (thigh bone) *n.* a long bone between the hip and the knee (see illustration). The head of the femur articulates with the acetabulum of the *hip bone. The *greater* and *lesser trochanters* are protuberances on which

股骨 位於髖骨和膝之間的長骨（見圖）。股骨頭與髖骨的髖臼相關節。大轉子和小轉子爲股骨上的隆凸，臀肌和腰大肌分別附着於其上。外髁和內髁

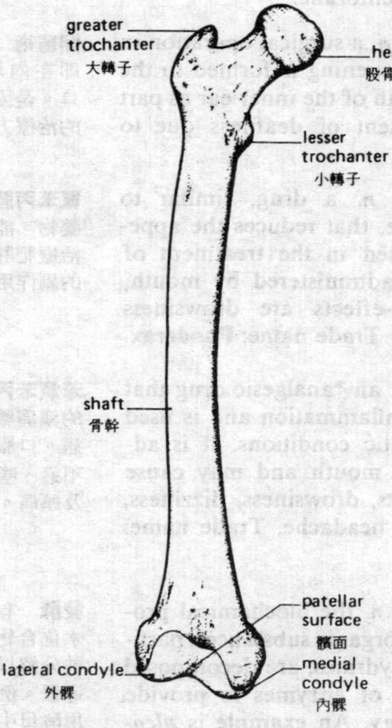

The femur (front view)
股骨（前面觀）

the gluteus and psoas major muscles, respectively, are inserted. The *lateral* and *medial condyles* articulate with the *tibia and the concave grooved *patellar surface* accommodates the kneecap (patella).

與脛骨相關節，凹陷的髕面與髕骨相接。

fenestra *n.* (in anatomy) an opening resembling a window. The *fenestra ovalis* (*fenestra vestibuli*) – the oval window – is the opening between the middle *ear and the vestibule of the inner ear. It is closed by a membrane to which the stapes is attached. The *fenestra rotunda* (*fenestra cochleae*) – the round window – is the opening between the scala tympani of the cochlea and the middle ear. Sound vibrations leave the cochlea through the fenestra rotunda which, like the fenestra ovalis, is closed by a membrane.

窗 （解剖學用語）一種類似窗戶的開口。前庭窗即卵圓窗，是中耳和內耳前庭之間的開口。該口被一層膜覆蓋，鐙骨就附着在該膜上。蝸窗爲圓形窗，是耳蝸鼓階和中耳之間的口。振動聲波從蝸窗離開耳蝸。同前庭窗一樣，蝸窗也被一層膜覆蓋。

fenestration *n.* a surgical operation in which a new opening is formed in the bony *labyrinth of the inner ear as part of the treatment of deafness due to *otosclerosis.

開窗術 一種外科手術，即在內耳骨迷路造一新口。是因耳硬化症而致聾的治療方法的一部分。

fenfluramine *n.* a drug, similar to *amphetamine, that reduces the appetite and is used in the treatment of obesity. It is administered by mouth; common side-effects are drowsiness and diarrhoea. Trade name: **Ponderax**.

氟苯丙胺 類似苯丙胺的藥物。能抑制食慾，用於治療肥胖症。口服，常見的副作用有嗜眠和腹瀉。

fenoprofen *n.* an *analgesic drug that also reduces inflammation and is used to treat arthritic conditions. It is administered by mouth and may cause digestive upsets, drowsiness, dizziness, sweating, and headache. Trade name: **Fenopron**.

苯氧苯丙酸 有消炎作用的鎮痛藥。用於治療關節病。口服。可引起消化道不適、嗜眠、暈眩、出汗及頭痛。

fermentation *n.* the biochemical process by which organic substances, particularly carbohydrates, are decomposed by the action of enzymes to provide chemical energy. An example is *alcoholic fermentation*, in which enzymes in yeast decompose sugar to form ethyl alcohol and carbon dioxide.

發酵 有機物（特別是碳水化合物）在酶的作用下被分解以提供能量的生化過程。例如：生醇發酵是用酵母中的酶將糖分解成乙醇和二氧化碳。

ferri- (ferro-) *prefix denoting* iron. 〔前綴〕 **鐵**

ferritin *n.* an iron-protein complex that is one of the forms in which iron is stored in the tissues.

鐵蛋白 鐵和蛋白的絡合物。是鐵貯存在組織裏的一種形式。

ferrous sulphate an *iron salt administered by mouth to treat or prevent iron-deficiency anaemia. There are few serious side-effects; stomach upsets and diarrhoea may be prevented by taking the drug with meals. Similar preparations used to treat anaemia include ferrous fumarate and ferrous succinate.

硫酸亞鐵 口服的一種鐵鹽。用來治療或預防缺鐵性貧血。幾乎無嚴重的副作用。若出現胃不適或腹瀉，則可在吃飯時服入藥物。治療貧血的類似製劑還有延胡索酸亞鐵、丁二酸亞鐵。

fertility rate the number of live births occurring in a year per 1000 women of child-bearing age (usually 15 to 44 years of age). A less reliable measure of fertility can be obtained from the *live birth rate* (the number of live births per 1000 of the population) or the *natural increase* (the excess of live births over deaths). More rarely quoted are the *gross reproduction rate* (the rate at which the child-bearing female population is reproducing itself) and the *net reproduction rate*, which takes into account female mortality before the age of reproduction. Other measures of fertility include the *legitimate birth rate* (the number of live births per 1000 women married once and aged 16 to 44) and the *illegitimate birth rate* (the number of illegitimate births per 1000 unmarried women and widows aged 15 to 44).

生育率 每千名育齡婦女（一般在15～44歲之間）每年生產活嬰的數量。從活嬰出生率（每千人中活嬰出生數量）或自然增長率（超過死亡數的活嬰數）中得出的生育率是不十分可靠的。粗再生率（有生育能力的婦女的繁殖率）及考慮到育齡前女性死亡率的純再生率更少使用。其它生育率的統計有婚生率（每千名16～44歲的已婚婦女中活嬰出生數）及非婚生率（每千名15～44歲的未婚婦女和寡婦中非婚生活嬰出生數）等。

fertilization *n.* the fusion of a spermatozoon and an ovum. Rapid changes in the membrane of the ovum prevent other spermatozoa from penetrating. Penetration stimulates the completion of meiosis and the formation of the second polar body. Once the male and female pronuclei have fused the zygote starts to divide by cleavage.

授精 精子和卵子融合成一體。卵細胞膜的快速變化能防止其他精子穿入。精子進入卵子能刺激減數分裂的完成和第二極體的形成。一旦精、卵原核融合爲一體，合子便開始卵裂。

festination *n.* the short tottering steps that characterize the gait of a patient with *parkinsonism.

慌張步態 短促踉蹌的步態。是帕金森氏綜合徵患者步態的特點。

fetishism *n.* sexual attraction to an inappropriate object (known as a *fetish*). This may be a part of the body (e.g. the foot or the hair), clothing (e.g. underwear or shoes), or other objects (e.g. leather handbags or rubber sheets). In all these cases the fetish has replaced the normal object of sexual love, in some cases to the point at which sexual relationships with another person are impossible or are possible only if the fetish is either present or fantasized. Treatment can involve *psychotherapy or behaviour therapy using *aversion therapy and masturbatory conditioning of desirable sexual behaviour. *See also* perversion.

戀物癖 對非性感的事物發生的性戀。戀物對象可能是身體的某些部位（如脚和體毛）或衣物（如褲衩和鞋）或其他物品（如革製手提包、膠皮床單）。在所有這類的病例中，正常的性愛對象被取代，甚至在有些病例中，患者不可能與他人有性關係，只有存在或幻想戀物對象時，才有這種可能。治療：用厭惡療法進行心理和行爲治療及用手淫法來塑造患者的性行爲。

feto- *prefix denoting* a fetus.

〔前綴〕 **胎兒**

fetor (foetor) *n.* an unpleasant smell. *Fetor oris* is bad breath (*halitosis).

臭味 令人厭惡的氣味。口臭是從口裏發出的難聞的氣味。

fetoscopy *n.* a technique in which a hollow needle is inserted through the abdomen of a pregnant woman and fetal blood is withdrawn from a blood vessel on the placenta, close to the umbilical cord. Fetoscopy, usually performed in the 18th–20th week of gestation, enables the blood of a fetus to be examined for the presence of abnormal cells and hence the *prenatal diagnosis of blood disorders (such as *thalassaemia, haemophilia, and *sickle-cell disease) and Duchenne *muscular dystrophy.

胎兒宮內觀察法 將空心針通過孕婦腹壁刺入腹腔，在臍帶附近的胎盤血管中抽出胎兒血液的一種技術。此方法通常在妊娠的第18～20週使用，以檢查血液中是否存在不正常細胞以對血液病（如地中海貧血、血友病及鐮狀細胞病）及杜興氏肌肉萎縮做出產前診斷。

fetus (foetus) *n.* a mammalian *embryo during the later stages of development within the womb. In man it refers to the products of conception from the beginning of the third month of pregnancy until birth. —**fetal** *adj.*

胎兒 在子宮內發育後期的哺乳類動物的胚胎。在人類，胎兒指從妊娠第三個月到出生這一時期的懷孕產物。

Feulgen reaction a method of demonstrating the presence of DNA in cell nuclei. The tissue section under investigation, after hydrolysis with dilute hy-

福伊爾根氏反應 檢查細胞核內 DNA 的方法。將被檢查的組織切片用稀鹽酸處理後，再用希夫氏試

drochloric acid, is treated with *Schiff's reagent. A purple coloration develops in the presence of DNA.

劑進行染色，有DNA的部位將呈現紫色。

fever (pyrexia) *n.* a rise in body temperature above the normal, i.e. above an oral temperature of 98.6°F (37°C) or a rectal temperature of 99°F (37.2°C). Fever is generally accompanied by shivering, headache, nausea, constipation, or diarrhoea. A rise in temperature above 105°F (40.5°C) may cause delirium and, in young children, *convulsions too. Fevers are usually caused by bacterial or viral infections and can accompany any infectious illness, from the common cold to *malaria. An *intermittent fever* is a periodic rise and fall in body temperature, often returning to normal during the day and reaching its peak at night, as in malaria. A *remittent fever* is one in which body temperature fluctuates out does not return to normal. *See also* relapsing fever.

發熱 身體的溫度超過正常度數。如口溫超過98.6℉（37℃）或肛溫超過99℉（37.2℃）。發熱常伴有寒顫、頭痛、噁心、便秘或腹瀉。超過105℉（40.5℃）的高燒可引起譫妄，嬰幼兒患者還可出現驚厥。發熱通常由細菌和病毒感染引起，並伴隨感冒、瘧疾等傳染病出現。間歇熱爲身體周期性發熱，通常在白天體溫恢復到正常，在夜間體溫又升到其最高度數，如在患瘧疾病時。弛張熱是一種溫度有波動但不恢復正常的發熱。

fibr- (fibro-) *prefix denoting* fibres or fibrous tissue.

〔前綴〕 **纖維，纖維組織**

fibre *n.* **1.** (in anatomy) a threadlike structure, such as a muscle cell, a nerve fibre, or a collagen fibre. **2.** (in dietetics) *see* dietary fibre. —**fibrous** *adj.*

纖維 ①（解剖學）一種線狀結構，如肌細胞、神經纖維或膠原纖維。②（飲食學）食物纖維。

fibre optics the use of fibres for the transmission of light images. Synthetic fibres with special optical properties can be used in instruments to relay pictures of the inside of the body for direct observation or photography. *See* fibrescope.

纖維光學 用纖維傳導光學形象的技術。合成的光導纖維可用在能分程傳遞體內情況的器械上，以進行直接觀察或拍照。

fibrescope *n.* an *endoscope that uses *fibre optics for the transmission of images from the interior of the body. Fibrescopes have a great advantage over the older endoscopes as they are flexible and can be introduced into relatively inaccessible cavities of the body.

纖維鏡 用光學纖維傳遞身體內部情況的內窺鏡。纖維鏡與老式內窺鏡比較有明顯的優點，它們能彎曲，而且能插入很難進入的體內腔道。

fibril *n.* a very small fibre or a constituent thread of a fibre (for example, a

原纖維 非常纖細的纖維，或組成纖維的纖維絲

*myofibril of a muscle fibre). —**fibrillar, fibrillary** *adj.*

（如肌纖維中的肌原纖維）。

fibrillation *n.* a rapid and chaotic beating of the many individual muscle fibres of the heart, which is consequently unable to maintain effective synchronous contraction. The affected part of the heart then ceases to pump blood.
Fibrillation may affect the atria or ventricles independently. *Atrial fibrillation*, a common type of *arrhythmia, results in rapid and irregular heart and pulse rates. The main causes are atherosclerosis, chronic rheumatic heart disease, and hypertensive heart disease. It may also complicate various other conditions, including chest infections and thyroid overactivity. The heart rate is controlled by the administration of *digoxin; in some cases the heart rhythm can be restored to normal by *cardioversion.
When *ventricular fibrillation* occurs the heart stops beating (*see* cardiac arrest). It is most commonly the result of *myocardial infarction.

纖維性顫動 很多心肌纖維快速、雜亂無章地跳動。其結果是心臟不能保持有效、同步的收縮。心臟受損部位停止泵血。
纖維性顫動可單獨發生在心房或心室。心房纖維性顫動是心律不齊的常見類型，可引起快速和不規則心率及脉率。主要原因是動脉粥樣硬化、慢性風濕性心臟病及高血壓性心臟病。此顫動還可發生於其它各種疾病，包括肺部感染及甲亢。服用地高辛可控制心率，對於某些病例，心律還可通過心臟復律術恢復正常。
當發生心室纖維顫動時，心臟停止跳動。最常見的原因是心肌梗死。

fibrin *n.* the final product of the process of *blood coagulation, produced by the action of the enzyme thrombin on a soluble precursor fibrinogen. The product thus formed (*fibrin monomer*) links up (polymerizes) with similar molecules to give a fibrous meshwork that forms the basis of a blood clot, which seals off the damaged blood vessel.

纖維蛋白 凝血過程中的最後產物。由凝血酶作用於可溶性纖維蛋白原而產生。所形成的物質（纖維蛋白單體）與相似的分子結合（聚合）形成纖維蛋白網，該網是形成血塊的基礎。血塊能封住損傷的血管。

fibrinogen *n.* a substance (*coagulation factor), present in blood plasma, that is acted upon by the enzyme thrombin to produce the insoluble protein fibrin in the final stage of *blood coagulation. The normal level of fibrinogen in plasma is 2–4 g/1.

纖維蛋白原 存在於血漿中的一種物質（凝血因子）。經凝血酶作用後，在凝血的最後階段產生不溶性纖維蛋白。血漿中纖維蛋白原的正常值是2～4g/ℓ。

fibrinogenopenia *n. see* hypofibrinogenaemia.

纖維蛋白原減少

fibrinoid *adj.* resembling the protein fibrin. Fibrinoid material is found in

纖維蛋白樣的 類似纖維蛋白的。纖維蛋白樣物質

the placenta in increasing amounts as pregnancy advances.

見於胎盤，隨着孕期的進展其量也在增加。

fibrinokinase *n.* one of a group of substances (activators) that convert the inactive substance plasminogen to the active enzyme *plasmin, which digests blood clots (*see* fibrinolysis). Fibrinokinase is insoluble in water and can be extracted from animal tissue.

纖維蛋白激酶 將無活性的纖維蛋白溶酶原轉化成能溶解血塊的活性纖維蛋白溶酶的一組物質（激活因子）中之一種。纖維蛋白激酶不溶於水，可從動物組織中提取。

fibrinolysin *n. see* plasmin.

纖維蛋白溶酶

fibrinolysis *n.* the process by which blood clots are removed from the circulation, involving digestion of the insoluble protein *fibrin by the enzyme *plasmin. The latter exists in the plasma as an inactive precursor (plasminogen), which is activated in parallel with the *blood coagulation process. Normally a balance is maintained between the processes of coagulation and fibrinolysis in the body; an abnormal increase in fibrinolysis leads to excessive bleeding.

纖維蛋白溶解 消除循環中的血塊，包括由纖維蛋白溶酶溶解非溶解狀態的纖維蛋白的過程。纖維蛋白溶酶的前體是無活性纖維蛋白溶酶原，存在於血漿之中，在凝血過程的同時被激活。正常情況下，體內的凝血過程和纖維蛋白溶解過程處於平衡狀態。不正常的纖維蛋白溶解過程增强，可導致大出血。

fibroadenoma *n. see* adenoma.

纖維腺瘤

fibroblast *n.* a widely distributed cell in *connective tissue that is responsible for the production of both the ground substance and of the precursors of collagen, elastic fibres, and reticular fibres.

成纖維細胞 廣泛分佈在結締組織中的細胞，是產生基質、膠原、彈力纖維及網狀纖維的前體。

fibrocartilage *n.* a tough kind of *cartilage in which there are dense bundles of fibres in the matrix. It is found in the intervertebral discs and pubic symphysis.

纖維軟骨 一種在其基質內存在着緻密纖維束的韌性軟骨。見於椎間盤和恥骨聯合。

fibrocyst *n.* a benign tumour of fibrous connective tissue containing cystic spaces. —**fibrocystic** *adj.*

囊變性纖維瘤 含有囊腔的纖維結締組織的艮性腫瘤。

fibrocystic disease of the pancreas *see* cystic fibrosis.

胰腺纖維囊性病

fibrocyte *n.* an inactive cell present in fully differentiated *connective tissue. It is derived from a *fibroblast.

纖維細胞 存在於高度分化的結締組織中的無活性的細胞。由成纖維細胞演變而來。

fibrodysplasia *n.* abnormal development affecting connective tissue.

纖維發育不良 結締組織發育不正常。

fibroelastosis *n.* overgrowth or disturbed growth of the yellow (elastic) fibres in *connective tissue, especially *endocardial fibroelastosis*, overgrowth and thickening of the wall of the heart's left ventricle.

彈力纖維組織增生 結締組織中的黃色纖維（彈力纖維）生長過度或生長紊亂。在心內膜彈力纖維組織增生病中，左心室壁增生並增厚。

fibroepithelial polyp a fibrous overgrowth covered by epithelium, often occurring in the mouth in response to chronic irritation. It is sometimes called an *epulis*.

纖維上皮息肉 纖維組織增生並由上皮覆蓋。通常發生於口腔，由慢性刺激引起。有時，此息肉也叫做齦瘤。

fibroid 1. *n.* **(fibromyoma, uterine fibroma)** a benign tumour of fibrous and muscular tissue, one or more of which may develop in the muscular wall of the womb. Fibroids often cause pain and excessive menstrual bleeding and they may become extremely large. They do not threaten life, but render pregnancy unlikely. It is usually women over 30 years of age who are affected. Fibroids can be removed surgically; in some cases removal of the womb (hysterectomy) may be necessary. If, as frequently happens, discomfort and other symptoms are absent, surgery is not required. **2.** *adj.* resembling or containing fibres.

①纖維性瘤（纖維肌瘤，子宮纖維瘤） 纖維和肌組織的良性腫瘤。生長在子宮肌壁上，單發或多發，經常引起疼痛和月經過多，並可長得很大。纖維瘤雖沒有生命危險，但却影響受孕。患此病婦女通常大於30歲。可做外科切除。有些病例則需要子宮切除（子宮切除術）。此瘤多數無不適感或其他症狀，因此無需外科手術。 **②類纖維的，含纖維的**

fibroma *n.* (*pl.* **fibromas** or **fibromata**) a nonmalignant tumour of connective tissue.

纖維瘤 結締組織的一種非惡性腫瘤。

fibromyoma *n.* a tumour of muscular and fibrous material, usually occurring in the womb (*see* fibroid).

纖維肌瘤 由肌和纖維物質構成的腫瘤。通常發生在子宮。

fibroplasia *n.* the production of fibrous tissue, occurring normally during the healing of wounds. *Retrolental fibroplasia* is the abnormal proliferation of fibrous tissue immediately behind the lens of the eye, leading to blindness. It was formerly seen in newborn premature infants due to overadministration of oxygen.

纖維組織增生 傷口癒合過程中所發生的一種正常現象。晶狀體後纖維組織增生是指直接位於眼晶狀體後的纖維組織不正常的增生，可導致失明。以前見於早產兒，因吸氧過度產生。

fibrosarcoma *n.* a malignant tumour of connective tissue, derived from *fibroblasts. Fibrosarcomas may arise in soft tissue or bone; they can affect any organ but are most common in the limbs, particularly the leg. They occur in people of all ages and may be congenital. The cells of these tumours show varying degrees of differentiation; the less well differentiated tumours containing elements of histiocytes have been recently reclassified as *malignant fibrous histiocytomas*. Tumours arising in soft tissue have a considerably better prognosis than those arising in bone.

纖維肉瘤 結締組織的惡性腫瘤。起源於成纖維細胞。可生長在軟組織和骨上。能侵犯所有器官，但常發生在肢體上，特別是腿。此病可見於任何年齡的患者，可以是先天性疾病。這些腫瘤細胞表現出不同的分化程度。分化較差的含有組織細胞成分的腫瘤，最近被重新分類爲惡性纖維組織細胞瘤。生長在軟組織的腫瘤比生長在骨上的腫瘤，相對來說預後較好。

fibrosis *n.* thickening and scarring of connective tissue, most often a consequence of inflammation or injury. *Pulmonary interstitial fibrosis* is thickening and stiffening of the lining of the air sacs (alveoli) of the lungs, causing progressive breathlessness. *See also* cystic fibrosis.

纖維化 結締組織增厚，有瘢痕形成。通常是炎症和損傷的結果。肺間質纖維化是肺泡膜增厚、僵硬，可引起進行性呼吸困難。

fibrositis *n.* inflammation of fibrous connective tissue, especially an acute inflammation of back muscles and their sheaths, causing pain and stiffness. *See also* muscular rheumatism.

纖維織炎 纖維結締組織炎症。特別是腰背部肌肉及其肌鞘的急性炎症。可引起疼痛和强直。

fibrous dysplasia a developmental abnormality in which changes occur in bony tissue, resulting in aching and a tendency to pathological fracture. In *monostotic fibrous dysplasia* one bone is affected; *polyostotic fibrous dysplasia* involves many bones.

骨纖維性結構不良 骨組織發育不正常。骨組織內的病變可引起疼痛與病理性骨折，單骨性纖維性結構不良是一個骨受損。多骨性纖維性結構不良是多個骨受損。

fibula *n.* the long thin outer bone of the lower leg. The head of the fibula articulates with the *tibia just below the knee; the lower end projects laterally as the *lateral malleolus*, which articulates with one side of the *talus.

腓骨 小腿外側的細長骨。在膝下，腓骨頭與脛骨相關節，腓骨下端外側的突起爲外踝，與距骨的一側相關節。

field of vision *see* visual field.

視野

figlu test a test for folic acid or vitamin B_{12} deficiency. A dose of the amino acid histidine, which requires the presence of folic acid or vitamin B_{12} for its

亞胺甲基穀氨酸試驗 檢驗葉酸或維生素 B_{12} 是否缺乏的試驗。口服一定量的氨基酸（組氨酸），該

complete breakdown, is given by mouth. In the absence of these vitamins, *f*orm*i*mino*glu*tamic acid (figlu) – an intermediate product in histidine metabolism – accumulates and can be detected in the urine.

酸只有在葉酸或維生素B_{12}存在時，才可完全分解。如缺乏這些維生素，組氨酸代謝的中間產物亞胺甲基穀氨酸增加，並可在尿中查出。

filament *n.* a very fine threadlike structure, such as a chain of bacterial cells. —**filamentous** *adj.*

絲 非常纖細的綫狀結構。如菌絲。

filaria *n.* (*pl.* **filariae**) any of the long threadlike nematode worms that, as adults, are parasites of the connective and lymphatic tissues of man capable of causing disease. They include the genera **Brugia*, **Loa*, **Onchocerca*, and **Wuchereria*. Filariae differ from the intestinal nematodes (*see* hookworm) in that they undergo part of their development in the body of a bloodsucking insect, e.g. a mosquito, on which they subsequently depend for their transmission to another human host. *See also* microfilaria. —**filarial** *adj.*

絲蟲 長絲狀線蟲。其成蟲寄生於人類結締組織和淋巴組織內，能夠致病。包括有：布氏絲蟲屬、羅阿絲蟲屬、盤尾絲蟲屬及吳策絲蟲屬。絲蟲與腸道線蟲不同，因爲絲蟲要在吸血性昆蟲（如蚊子）體內經歷一段發育期，並依靠這類昆蟲傳染給他人。

filariasis *n.* a disease, common in the tropics and subtropics, caused by the presence in the lymph vessels of the parasitic nematode worms *Wuchereria bancrofti* and *Brugia malayi* (*see* filaria). The worms, transmitted to man by various mosquitoes (including *Aëdes*, *Culex*, *Anopheles*, and *Mansonia*), bring about inflammation and eventual blocking of lymph vessels, which causes the surrounding tissues to swell (*see* elephantiasis). The rupture of urinary lymphatics may lead to the presence of *chyle in the urine. Filariasis is treated with the drug *diethylcarbamazine.

絲蟲病 常見於熱帶和亞熱帶地區的一種疾病。由存在於淋巴管內的班氏吳策線蟲和馬來絲蟲引起。這些絲蟲通過各種蚊子（包括伊蚊、庫蚊、按蚊和曼蚊）轉移到人體，引起淋巴管炎，並最終導致淋巴管阻塞，使其周圍組織水腫。尿道淋巴管破裂可使尿液中出現乳糜液。絲蟲病可用枸櫞酸乙胺嗪治療。

filiform *adj.* shaped like a thread; for example, the threadlike *filiform papillae* of the *tongue.

絲狀的 線樣的。如舌絲狀乳頭。

filling *n.* (in dentistry) the operation of inserting a specially prepared substance into a cavity drilled in a carious tooth. The filling may be *temporary* or *perma-*

充填 （牙科學）將特殊製備的物質填入齲齒上鑽開的洞內的手術。充填可以是暫時的也可是永久

nent, and various materials may be used (*see* amalgam, cement, composite resin, gold).

的，而且很多物質都可用做填充物。

filum *n.* a threadlike structure. The *filum terminale* is the slender tapering terminal section of the spinal cord.

絲 綫狀結構。終絲是脊髓圓椎下端的細長絲。

fimbria *n.* (*pl.* **fimbriae**) a fringe or fringelike process, such as any of the finger-like projections that surround the opening of the ovarian end of the *Fallopian tube.

繖 穗或穗樣突起。如圍繞輪卵管卵巢端開口處的指樣突起。

fingerprint *n.* the distinctive pattern of minute ridges in the outer horny layer of the skin. Every individual has his or her own unique pattern, though there are six basic fingerprint formations:

指紋 皮膚角化層上的微小皮嵴的特殊樣式。儘管每個人都有他/她自己獨特的皮紋樣式，但基本的圖樣只有 6 種：雙紋、帳

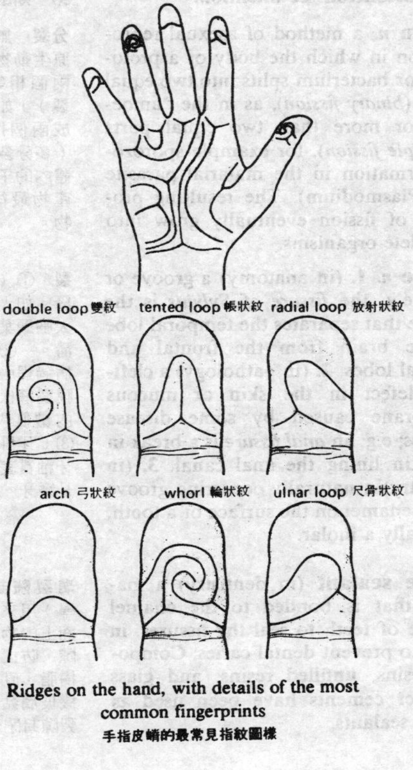

Ridges on the hand, with details of the most common fingerprints

手指皮嵴的最常見指紋圖樣

double loop, *tented loop*, *radial loop*, *arch*, *whorl*, and *ulnar loop* (see illustration). Fingerprint patterns can show the presence of inherited disorders. *See also* dermatoglyphics.

狀紋、放射狀紋、弓狀紋、輪狀紋和尺骨狀紋（見圖）。指紋的圖樣能表明是否患有遺傳病。

firedamp *n.* (in mining) an explosive mixture of gases, usually containing a high proportion of methane, occasionally encountered in pockets underground. It is distinguished from *blackdamp (chokedamp), which does not ignite.

沼氣　採礦業中遇到的一種有爆炸性的混合氣體。通常含較高比例的甲烷，偶可見於地下坑道。沼氣與礦內窒息性氣體不同，後者不能點燃。

first aid procedures used in an emergency to help a wounded or ill patient before the arrival of a doctor or admission to hospital.

急救　在醫生到來之前或在入院前，搶救傷員或患者所採取的緊急措施。

first intention *see* intention.

第一期癒合

fission *n.* a method of asexual reproduction in which the body of a protozoan or bacterium splits into two equal parts (*binary fission*), as in the *amoebae, or more than two equal parts (*multiple fission*), for example sporozoite formation in the malarial parasite (*see* Plasmodium). The resulting products of fission eventually grow into complete organisms.

分裂　無性繁殖的方式。原生動物體或細菌分裂成兩個相等的部分（二分裂），如阿米巴；或分裂成兩個以上的相等部分（多分裂），如在瘧原蟲體內的子孢子。分裂出的產物最後長成完整的生物。

fissure *n.* **1.** (in anatomy) a groove or cleft; e.g. the *fissure of Sylvius* is the groove that separates the temporal lobe of the brain from the frontal and parietal lobes. **2.** (in pathology) a cleft-like defect in the skin or mucous membrane caused by some disease process; e.g. an *anal fissure* is a break in the skin lining the anal canal. **3.** (in dentistry) a naturally occurring groove in the enamel on the surface of a tooth, especially a molar.

裂　①（解剖學）溝或縫。如大腦側裂就是分隔大腦顳葉和額葉及頂葉的溝。　②（病理學）在疾病過程中產生的皮膚和黏膜裂縫樣缺損。肛裂就是內襯肛門皮膚的撕裂。③（牙科學）自然出現在牙釉質表面上的溝，特別是磨牙。

fissure sealant (in dentistry) a material that is bonded to the enamel surface of teeth to seal the fissures, in order to prevent dental caries. Composite resins, unfilled resins, and glass ionomer cements have been used as fissure sealants.

溝裂隙封閉劑　（牙科學）用來附着在牙釉質表面上的物質，以封閉溝裂隙，防止出現齲齒。複合樹脂、直接填充樹脂和有機玻璃黏固劑都可做爲溝裂隙封閉劑。

fistula *n.* an abnormal communication between two hollow organs or between a hollow organ and the exterior. Many fistulas are due to infection or injury. For example, an *anal fistula* may develop after an abscess in the rectum has burst, creating an opening between the anal canal and the surface of the skin. Some fistulas result from malignant growths or ulceration: a carcinoma of the colon may invade and ulcerate the adjacent wall of the stomach, causing a *gastrocolic fistula*. Other fistulas develop as complications of surgery: after gall-bladder surgery, for example, bile may continually escape to the surface through the wound producing a *biliary fistula*. Fistulas may also be a form of congenital abnormality; examples include a *tracheo-oesophageal fistula* (between the windpipe and gullet) and a *rectovaginal fistula* (between the rectum and vagina).

瘻 兩個空心器官或一個空心器官與體外不正常的交通。很多瘻是由感染和損傷引起。如肛瘻可發生於直腸膿腫破裂以後，使肛管和皮膚之間出現通道。有一些瘻是由惡性腫瘤和潰瘍引起：結腸癌可侵犯或腐蝕鄰近的胃壁，導致胃結腸瘻；其他一些瘻可由手術的併發症引起。如膽囊手術後，膽汁可不斷地從刀口流出體外，形成膽瘻。瘻也可是一種先天異常，如食管支氣管瘻和陰道直腸瘻。

fit *n.* a sudden attack. The term is usually reserved for the attacks of *epilepsy but it is also used more generally, e.g. a fit of coughing.

發作 突然發病。該術語通常用來指癲癇的發病，但也普遍用來指其他疾病的發生。如咳嗽發作。

fixation *n.* **1.** (in psychoanalysis) a failure of psychological development, in which traumatic events prevent a child from progressing to the next developmental stage. This is said to be a cause of mental illness and of personality disorder. *See also* psychosexual development. **2.** a procedure for the hardening and preservation of tissues or microorganisms to be examined under a microscope. Fixation kills the tissues and ensures that their original shape and structure are retained as closely as possible. It also prepares them for sectioning and staining. The specimens can be immersed in a chemical *fixative or subjected to *freeze-drying.

①**固結** （精神分析學）心理發展受阻。即創傷性事件防礙了兒童心理繼續向下一個階段發展。這被認爲是精神上的疾病及病態人格的原因。 ②**固定** 爲進行顯微鏡下檢查而使組織或微生物變硬並將其保存起來的方法。固定是使組織失去生命力，並盡可能使組織的形狀、結構與其固定前基本相同。固定也是組織切片與染色前的準備。可將標本浸入化學固定液中或用冷凍法進行固定。

fixative (fixing agent) *n.* a chemical agent, e.g. alcohol or osmium tetroxide,

固定液 用於保護組織並使其變硬以進行顯微鏡檢

used for the preservation and hardening of tissues for microscopical study. *See* fixation (def. 2).

查的一種化學試劑。如乙醇或四氧化鋨。

flaccid *adj.* **1.** flabby and lacking in firmness. **2.** characterized by a decrease in muscle tone (e.g. flaccid *paralysis). —**flaccidity** *n.*

弛緩的 ①不結實的，不堅硬的。②肌張力下降的（如弛緩性麻痺）。

flagellate *n.* a type of *protozoan with one or more fine whiplike threads (*see* flagellum) projecting from its body surface, by means of which it is able to swim. Some flagellates are parasites of man and are therefore of medical importance. *See* Trypanosoma, Leishmania, Giardia, Trichomonas.

鞭毛蟲 原生動物的一種，其身體表面有一個或多個鞭狀線形突起，通過這種突起的作用，該蟲可以移動。有些鞭毛蟲是人類的寄生蟲，因此在醫學上有其重要性。

flagellation *n.* the act of whipping oneself or others as a means of obtaining sexual pleasure (*see* masochism, sadism). A person displaying this sexual deviation is called a *flagellant* or *flagellomane*.

鞭笞狂 在用鞭抽打自己或他人時，能獲得性滿足的一種性心理變態。具有這種性變態的人叫做鞭笞狂者。

flagellum *n.* (*pl.* **flagella**) a fine long whiplike thread attached to certain types of cell (e.g. spermatozoa and some unicellular organisms). Flagella are responsible for the movement of the organisms to which they are attached.

鞭毛 附着在某些種類細胞上的細長線樣結構（如精子及一些單細胞生物）。鞭毛能使其所附着的生物體移動。

flap *n.* **1.** (in surgery) a strip of tissue dissected away from the underlying structures but left attached at one end so that it retains its blood and nerve supply. The flap is then used to repair a defect in another part of the body. The free end of the flap is sewn into the area to be repaired and after about three weeks, when the flap has 'healed into' its new site, the other end is detached and the remainder of the flap is sewn in. Flaps are commonly used by plastic surgeons in treating patients who have suffered severe skin and tissue loss after burns or injuries not amenable to repair by split skin grafting (*see* skin graft). Skin flaps are also used to cover the end of a bone in an amputated limb. **2.** (in dentistry) a piece of mucous membrane

瓣 ①（外科學）從某部分離出的一種條形組織。一端與下面的組織相連，以保持血運及神經支配。瓣被用來修復身體其它部位的缺損。將瓣的游離端縫到要修復的部位上，約三週以後，當瓣與新組織"癒合"時，再將另一端（蒂）分離，瓣的其它部分即縫到新的部位上。瓣通常用於整形外科，以治療燒傷或損傷後皮膚或組織嚴重缺損而又不可能進行植皮修復的患者。皮瓣也用來覆蓋斷肢的骨端。②（口腔學）留有較寬蒂的一片黏膜和骨膜。將其揭開，可暴露出其下的

and periosteum attached by a broad base. It is lifted back to expose the underlying bone and enable a procedure such as surgical *extraction to be performed. It is subsequently replaced.

骨，使手術（如拔牙）能夠進行，然後再將其復位。

flare *n.* **1.** reddening of the skin that spreads outwards from a focus of infection or irritation in the skin. **2.** the red outside part of an urticarial wheal – the skin's response in an allergic or hypersensitivity reaction (*see* urticaria).

潮紅 ①感染竈或受刺激部位周圍的皮膚發紅。②蕁麻疹風塊（皮膚過敏反應）周圍的皮膚發紅。

flat-foot *n.* absence of the arching of the foot, so that the sole lies flat upon the ground. It may be present in infancy or be acquired in adult life, usually either from prolonged standing or from excessive weight. Flat feet need treatment (exercises) only if they cause pain. Medical name: **pes planus**.

扁平足 足弓缺乏。脚底着地處呈扁平形。可在嬰兒時就存在，也可在成年人時出現。通常因長期站立或身體超重引起。扁平足只有在出現疼痛時才有必要治療。

flatulence *n.* **1.** the expulsion of gas or air from the stomach through the mouth; belching. **2.** a sensation of abdominal distension. —**flatulent** *adj.*

①**噯氣** 胃內氣體從口腔內竄出。 ②**腹脹** 腹部脹氣的感覺。

flatus *n.* intestinal gas, composed partly of swallowed air and partly of gas produced by bacterial fermentation of intestinal contents. It consists of hydrogen, carbon dioxide, and methane in varying proportions.

腸氣 腸道內氣體。由吞咽的氣體和腸內容物裏的細菌發酵所產生的氣體組成。含有不同比例的氫氣、二氧化碳和甲烷。

flatworm (platyhelminth) *n.* any of the flat-bodied worms, including the *flukes and *tapeworms. Both these groups contain many parasites of medical importance.

扁蟲 身體呈扁平形的蠕蟲，包括吸蟲和絛蟲。這兩組蟲中有很多在醫學上有其重要性。

flav- (flavo-) *prefix denoting* yellow.

〔前綴〕 **黃色**

flavin adenine dinucleotide *see* FAD.

黃素腺嘌呤二核苷酸

flavin mononucleotide *see* FMN.

黃素單核苷酸

flavoprotein *n.* a compound consisting of a protein bound to either *FAD or *FMN (called *flavins*). Flavoproteins are constituents of several enzyme systems involved in intermediary metabolism.

黃素蛋白 蛋白質與黃素腺嘌呤二核苷酸或黃素單核苷酸（黃素）相結合的化合物。黃素蛋白是一些酶系統的成分，這些酶與調節代謝有關。

flea *n.* a small wingless bloodsucking insect with a laterally compressed body and long legs adapted for jumping. Adult fleas are temporary parasites on birds and mammals and those species that attack man (**Pulex*, **Xenopsylla*, and **Nosopsyllus*) may be important in the transmission of various diseases. Their bites are not only a nuisance but may become a focus of infection. *DDT and pyrethrum powders are used to destroy fleas in the home.

蚤 無翅吸血性小昆蟲。身體側向扁平，腿長以適應跳躍。蚤的成蟲可暫時寄生在鳥及哺乳類動物身上。侵襲人類的蚤（蚤屬、客蚤屬、病蚤屬）在傳播疾病方面有重要作用。蚤的刺吸不僅令人厭惡，而刺吸部位還會成爲感染病竈。滴滴涕和除蟲菊粉可消除家庭裏的蚤。

flexibilitas cerea a disorder of posture in which a patient's limbs offer a continuous mild resistance to being moved passively by the examiner and remain for long periods in the position into which the examiner has moved them. It is a feature of *catatonia. *See also* catalepsy.

蠟樣屈曲 一種姿式異常。患者肢體在被檢查者移動時，可出現持續輕度抵抗，然後，該肢體又可長時間保持被檢查者所擺放的姿式。這是緊張症的特點。

flexion *n.* the bending of a joint so that the bones forming it are brought towards each other. *Plantar flexion* is the bending of the toes (or fingers) downwards, towards the sole (or palm). *See also* dorsiflexion.

屈曲 關節彎曲。這可使形成此關節的骨互相靠攏。蹠屈是足趾（或手指）向下朝脚（或手）掌方向彎曲。

flexor *n.* any muscle that causes bending of a limb or other part.

屈肌 使肢體和其他部位彎曲的任何肌肉。

flexure *n.* a bend in an organ or part, such as the *hepatic* and *splenic flexures* of the *colon.

曲 器官或某部位的彎曲。如結腸的肝曲和脾曲。

floccillation *n. see* carphology.

摸空

flocculation *n.* a reaction in which normally invisible material leaves solution to form a coarse suspension or precipitate as a result of a change in physical or chemical conditions. Flocculation tests using serum and special reagents are useful in diagnosing liver abnormalities. *See also* agglutination.

絮凝作用 因物理和化學變化，而使溶液中正常時見不到的物質形成粗大懸浮物或沉澱物的一種反應。用血清和特殊試劑做的絮凝試驗在診斷肝臟是否異常方面很有用。

flocculus *n.* a small ovoid lobe of the *cerebellum, overhung by the posterior lobe and connected centrally with the nodulus in the midline.

絨球 位於小腦的卵圓形小葉。懸於後葉之下，其中央部與中線小結相連。

flooding *n.* **1.** excessive bleeding from the womb, as in *menorrhagia or miscarriage. **2.** (also called **implosion**) a method of treating *phobias in which the patient is exposed intensively and at length to the feared object, either in reality or fantasy. Although it is distressing and needs good motivation if treatment is to be completed, it is an effective and rapid therapy.

①**血崩** 子宮大出血。如在月經過多或流產時。②**以恐治恐法** 治療恐怖症的方法。有意讓這類患者接觸或接近可怕的事物，無論該事物是眞實的還是想象中的。儘管這種療法令患者痛苦，而且需要很好地動員患者接受這種治療方法，但如果要進行徹底治療的話，此療法確實有效且見效快。

floppy baby syndrome *see* amyotonia congenita.

小兒鬆軟綜合症 先天性肌無力。

flowmeter *n.* an instrument for measuring the flow of a liquid or gas. Anaesthetic equipment is fitted with flowmeters so that the administration of anaesthetic gases in different proportions can be controlled.

流量計 計算液體和氣體流量的儀器。麻醉設備就安有流量計，以控制患者吸入不同比例的麻醉氣體。

floxuridine *n.* a drug, similar in its action and side-effects to *fluorouracil, used to treat cancers of the digestive system. It is administered by injection.

氟苷 治療消化系統癌症的藥物。其作用與副作用與氟尿嘧啶相似。注射給藥。

fluctuation *n.* the characteristic feeling of a wave motion produced in a fluid-filled part of the body by an examiner's fingers. If fluctuation is present when a swelling is examined, this is an indication that there is fluid within and that the swelling is not due to a solid growth.

波動 檢查者的手在身體某充滿液體的部位感覺到的一種特殊的波浪震動感。當檢查腫脹部位時出現這種感覺，則表明內有液體而非固體腫物。

fludrocortisone *n.* a synthetic *corticosteroid used to treat disorders of the adrenal glands. It is administered by mouth and side-effects include muscle weakness, bone disorders, digestive and skin disorders, and fluid retention. Trade name: **Florinef**.

氟氫可地松 合成的皮質類甾醇。用於治療腎上腺疾病。口服，副作用有肌無力、骨疾病、消化道及皮膚出現異常及液體豬留。

flufenamic acid an *analgesic drug used to relieve moderate pain, such as headache, rheumatic conditions, and toothache. It is administered by mouth and may cause indigestion, nausea, and diarrhoea. Trade name: **Arlef**.

氟滅酸 解除一般疼痛（如頭痛、風濕痛及牙痛）的鎮痛藥。口服，可引起消化不良、噁心及腹瀉。

fluke *n.* any of the parasitic flatworms belonging to the group Trematoda. Adult flukes, which have suckers for attachment to their host, are parasites of man, occurring in the liver (*liver flukes*; *see* Fasciola), lungs (*see* Paragonimus), gut (*see* Heterophyes), and blood vessels (*blood flukes*; *see* Schistosoma) and often cause serious disease. Eggs, passed out with the stools, hatch into larvae called *miracidia, which penetrate an intermediate snail host. Miracidia give rise asexually to *redia larvae and finally *cercariae in the snail's tissues. The released cercariae may enter a second intermediate host (such as a fish or crustacean); form a cyst (*metacercaria) on vegetation; or directly penetrate the human skin.

吸蟲 吸蟲綱里所有的寄生性扁蟲。吸蟲成蟲具有附着於其宿主身上的吸盤，是人類的寄生蟲，寄生在肝臟（肝吸蟲）、肺臟、腸道及血管裏（血吸蟲），通常能引起嚴重疾病。同糞便一起排出的蟲卵所孵出的幼蟲叫做毛蚴，它能進入中間宿主螺類體內，並在此無性繁殖出雷蚴，最後又在螺類體內發展成尾蚴。釋放出來的尾蚴又可進入第二中間宿主（如魚或甲殼綱動物），在植物上形成後囊蚴，或直接穿透人類皮膚進入體內。

fluorescein sodium a water-soluble dye that glows with a brilliant green colour when light is shone on it. A dilute solution is used to detect defects in the surface of the cornea, since it stains areas where the *epithelium is not intact. In retinal *angiography it is injected into a vein and its circulation through the blood vessels of the retina is viewed and photographed by a special camera.

熒光素鈉 一種水溶性染料。用光照射這種染料時，能放出光芒燦爛的綠色。其稀溶液用於探查角膜表面是否有缺損。因爲它能使上皮細胞受損部位着色。在視網膜血管造影時，將該染料注射到靜脈內，就可見到視網膜的血管，及用特殊鏡頭進行拍照。

fluorescence *n.* the emission of light by a material as it absorbs radiation from outside. The radiation absorbed may be visible or invisible (e.g. ultraviolet rays or X-rays). *See* fluoroscope. —**fluorescent** *adj.*

熒光 某種物質在吸收外界的光線後所發射出來的光。所吸收的外界的光線可以是可見光，也可以是不可見光（如紫外線和X射線）。

fluoridation *n.* the addition of *fluoride to drinking water in order to reduce *dental caries. Drinking water with a fluoride ion content of one part per million is effective in reducing caries throughout life when given during the years of tooth development. *See also* fluorosis.

氟化（作用） 爲減少齲牙的發生向食用水中加入適量的氟。在牙齒發育的年齡，以百萬分之一的比例向食用水中投放氟離子，就能有效的減少人們一生的齲齒發病率。

fluoride *n.* a compound of fluorine. The incorporation of fluoride ions in the enamel of teeth makes them more

氟化物 氟的化合物。將氟離子加進牙釉質內，能使牙釉質有較强的抗齲能

resistant to *dental caries. The ions enter enamel during its formation, by surface absorption. The addition of fluoride to public water supplies is called *fluoridation. Fluoride may also be applied topically in toothpaste or by a dentist. If the water supply contains too little fluoride, fluoride salts may be given to children in the form of drops or tablets.

力。氟離子是在釉質形成時由其表面吸收到釉質內的。將適當的氟化物投放到公用飲水內叫做氟化。氟化物還可加在牙膏內或被牙科醫生使用。如果公用飲水含氟量太少，可給兒童以滴劑或片劑的形式添加氟鹽。

fluoroscope *n.* an instrument on which X-ray images may be viewed directly, without taking and developing X-ray photographs. It consists basically of a *fluorescent screen*, which is coated with chemicals that exhibit the property of *fluorescence when exposed to X-rays. Fluoroscopes are used for mass chest X-ray examinations.

熒光鏡 不用拍照和沖洗X線照片就可直接顯示出X線物像的設備。基本結構是熒光屏，其表面有一層化學物質覆蓋。當被X線照射時，這層物質能現示出特徵性的熒光。熒光鏡用於X線普查。

fluorosis *n.* the effects of high *fluoride intake. Dental fluorosis is characterized by mottled enamel, which is opaque and may be stained. Its incidence increases when the level of fluoride in the water supply is above 2 parts per million. The mottled enamel is resistant to dental caries. When the level is over 8 parts per million systemic fluorosis may occur, with calcification of ligaments.

氟中毒 服入大量氟化物的結果。牙齒氟中毒的特點是：出現斑釉色，即釉質無光澤並被着色。當公用飲水裏的氟化物超過每百萬分之二時，氟中毒的發病率就會增加。斑釉有抗齲能力。當水中氟化物超過每百萬分之八時，將發生機體氟中毒，同時伴有韌帶鈣化。

fluorouracil *n.* a drug that prevents cell growth (*see* antimetabolite) and is used in the treatment of cancers of the digestive system and breast. It is administered by mouth or injection. Side-effects, which may be severe, include digestive and skin disorders, mouth ulcers, hair loss, nail changes, and blood disorders. Fluorouracil is also applied as a cream to treat certain skin conditions, including skin cancer.

氟尿嘧啶 能防止細胞生長，用於治療消化系統和乳腺癌的藥物。口服或注射給藥。副作用很嚴重，有消化道和皮膚異常、口腔潰瘍、脫髮、指甲發生變化及血液病。該藥物也可以霜劑的形式治療某些皮膚病，包括皮膚癌。

fluphenazine *n.* a *tranquillizer used to relieve anxiety and tension and to treat nausea and vomiting following anaesthesia. It is administered by mouth or injection. High doses may cause drowsiness, restlessness, and ab-

氟奮乃靜 消除焦慮和緊張、治療痲醉後噁心和嘔吐的安定劑。口服或注射給藥。大劑量可引起嗜眠、煩躁不安及不正常肌肉運動。

normal muscular movements. Trade names: **Modecate, Moditen.**

flurazepam *n.* a sedative drug used to treat insomnia and sleep disturbances (*see* hypnotic). It is administered by mouth and sometimes causes morning drowsiness, dizziness, and muscle incoordination. Trade name: **Dalmane.**

氟胺安定 治療失眠和睡眠紊亂的鎮靜劑。口服。有時引起清晨嗜眠、眩暈及肌運動不協調。

flush *n.* reddening of the face and/or neck. *Hectic flush* occurs in such wasting diseases as pulmonary tuberculosis. A *hot flush*, accompanied by a feeling of heat, occurs in some emotional disorders and during the menopause.

潮紅 臉和/或脖子發紅。癆病性潮紅見於消耗性疾病，如肺結核。熱性潮紅伴有發熱感，見於感情失常及月經期。

fluspirilene *n.* a major *tranquillizer used to treat schizophrenia. It is administered by injection; side-effects can include fatigue, digestive upsets, and drowsiness. Trade name: **Redeptin.**

氟斯必靈 治療精神分裂症的主要藥物。注射給藥。副作用有疲乏、消化道不適和嗜眠。

flutter *n.* a disturbance of normal heart rhythm that – like *fibrillation – may affect the atria or ventricles. However, the arrhythmia is less rapid and less chaotic. The causes and treatment are similar to those of fibrillation. *See also* cardiac arrest, defibrillation.

撲動 心律紊亂的一種。類似纖維性顫動，可發生在心房或心室，但心率不如後者快及雜亂。病因及治療與纖維性顫動類似。

flux *n.* an abnormally copious flow from an organ or cavity. *Alvine flux* is *diarrhoea.

流出 器官或體腔內的大量液體不正常地溢出。拉丁文 Alvine flux 與英文 diarrhoea 同義，即腹瀉。

fly *n.* a two-winged insect belonging to a large group called the Diptera. The mouthparts of flies are adapted for sucking and sometimes also for piercing and biting. Fly larvae (maggots) may infest human tissues and cause disease (*see* myiasis).

蠅 雙翅目中的一種雙翅昆蟲。它的口器適於吸吮，有時也用來刺入及叮咬。蠅蛆可感染人體組織並致病。

FMN (flavin monucleotide) a derivative of riboflavin (vitamin B_2) that is the immediate precursor of *FAD and functions as a *coenzyme in various oxidation-reduction reactions.

黃素單核苷酸 核黃素（維生素 B_2）的衍生物。是黃素腺嘌呤二核苷酸的前體。在各種氧化還原反應中起輔酶的作用。

focal distance (of the eye) the distance between the lens and the point behind the lens at which light from a distant object is focused. In a normal-sighted person this point of focus is on the retina, but distortion of the shape of the eyeball may result in *myopia (short-sightedness) or *hypermetropia (long-sightedness).

（眼的）焦點距離 晶體和晶體後的某一點（遠處物體的光線所聚焦的那一點）之間的距離。正常視力的人，這一聚焦點在視網膜上。眼球形狀的變化可引起近視眼和遠視眼。

focus 1. *n.* the point at which rays of light converge after passing through a lens. **2.** *n.* the principal site of an infection or other disease. **3.** *vb.* (in ophthalmology) to accommodate (*see* accommodation).

①**焦點** 光線經過晶體後集中的點。 ②**病竈** 感染或其他疾病的主要部位。 ③**調節** 眼科學用語。

foetus *n. see* fetus.

胎兒

fold *n.* (in anatomy and embryology) the infolding of two surfaces of membranes.

皺襞 （解剖和胚胎學）膜表面折疊所形成的結構。

folic acid (pteroylglutamic acid) a B vitamin that is important in the synthesis of nucleic acids. The metabolic role of folic acid is interdependent with that of *vitamin B_{12} (both are required by rapidly dividing cells) and a deficiency of one may lead to deficiency of the other. A deficiency of folic acid results in the condition of megaloblastic anaemia. Good sources of folic acid are liver and vegetables. The actual daily requirement of folate is not known but the suggested daily intake is 200 μg/day for an adult, which should be doubled during pregnancy.

葉酸 一種維生素B。是形成核酸的重要物質。葉酸的代謝與維生素B_{12}的代謝互相依賴（兩者都被快速分裂的細胞所需要）。兩者缺一都可導致另一者缺乏。葉酸不足，可引起巨成紅細胞性貧血。葉酸的主要來源是肝臟和蔬菜。每日葉酸鹽的實際需要量是多少還不清楚，但有人提議：成年人每日應攝取200 μg。孕婦應加倍。

folie à deux (communicated insanity) a condition in which two people who are closely involved with each other share a system of *delusions. Sometimes one member of the pair has developed a *psychosis and has imposed it on the other by a process of suggestion; sometimes both members are schizophrenic and elaborate their delusions or hallucinations together. More than two people may be involved (*folie à trois, folie à quatre*, etc.). Treat-

二聯性精神病（感應性精神病） 兩個有血緣關係的人患有同樣妄想症狀的一種疾病。有時，其中一人發展成精神病，可通過暗示的方式使另一人發病。有時兩人同是精神分裂症患者，可同時具有同樣的妄想或幻想。此病還可出現在兩人以上的人群中（三聯性精神病，四聯性精神病）。通常的治療

ment usually involves separation of the affected people and management according to their individual requirements.

方法是將患者分開，並根據個人的需要進行處理。

folinic acid a derivative of folic acid involved in purine synthesis. Administered by mouth or by injection, it is used to reverse the biological effects of *methotrexate and so to prevent excessive toxicity. This action is termed *folinic acid rescue*. Trade name: **Leucovorin.**

亞葉酸 葉酸的衍生物。葉酸與嘌呤合成有關。口服或注射給藥。用於逆轉氨甲蝶呤的生化效應，以防止毒性過大。這一作用叫做亞葉酸解毒。

folium *n.* (*pl.* **folia**) a thin leaflike structure, such as any of the folds on the surface of the cerebellum.

葉 薄片狀結構。如小腦表面上的皺襞。

follicle *n.* a small secretory cavity, sac, or gland, such as any of the cavities in the *ovary in which the ova are formed. *See also* Graafian follicle, hair follicle. **—follicular** *adj.*

濾泡 小分泌腔、囊或腺體。如卵巢裏所有的腔，卵子就是在該腔內形成的。

follicle-stimulating hormone (FSH) a hormone (*see* gonadotrophin) synthesized and released by the anterior pituitary gland. FSH stimulates ripening of the follicles in the ovary and formation of sperm in the testes. It is administered by injection to treat sterility due to lack of ovulation, amenorrhoea, and decreased sperm production. Stimulation of ovulation by FSH may, in some cases, lead to multiple pregnancy.

促卵泡成熟激素 由前垂體腺合成並釋放出的一種激素。該激素能刺激卵巢內卵泡成熟及睾丸內精子的形成。注射給藥可治療因不排卵、閉經及精子生成過少而引起的不育症。在某些病例中，用該激素刺激排卵可導致多胎妊娠。

folliculitis *n.* inflammation of hair follicles in the skin, commonly caused by infection. *See also* sycosis.

毛囊炎 皮膚毛囊發炎。通常因感染引起。

fomentation *n. see* poultice.

罨劑

fomes *n.* (*pl.* **fomites**) any object that is used or handled by a person with a *communicable disease and may therefore become contaminated with the infective organisms and transmit the disease to a subsequent user. Common fomites are towels, bed-clothes, cups, and money.

污染物 任何被傳染病患者使用或接觸過的、並因此被感染物污染而且將疾病傳給下一個使用者的物品。常見的污染物是毛巾、牀單、口杯及貨幣。

fontanelle *n.* an opening in the skull of a fetus or young infant due to incomplete *ossification of the cranial bones and the resulting incomplete closure of the *sutures. The *anterior fontanelle* occurs where the coronal, frontal, and sagittal sutures meet; the *posterior fontanelle* occurs where the sagittal and lambdoidal sutures meet (see illustration).

囟 胎兒或嬰兒的顱骨因未完全骨化而出現的開口及由此而來的未完全閉合的骨縫。前囟是由冠狀縫、額縫、矢狀縫相滙合而形成的。後囟是由矢狀縫和人字縫滙合而成（見圖）。

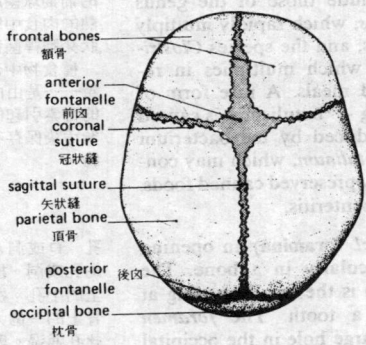

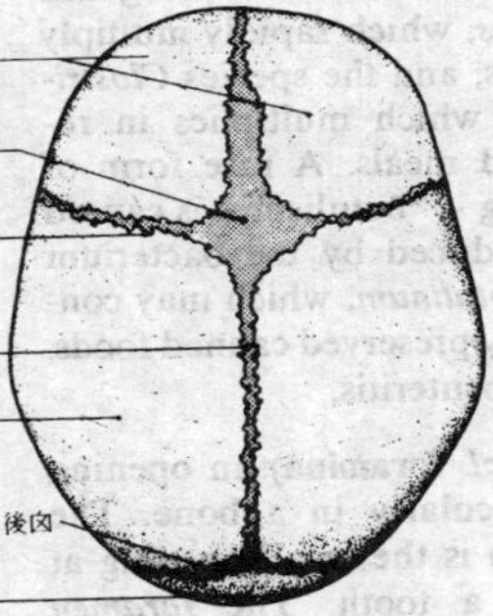

Fontanelles in the skull of a newborn infant (from above)
新生兒顱骨囟
（上面觀）

food handler a person engaged in the preparation, storage, cooking, and serving of food. Such people should be free from infectious conditions, either in the form of disease or as carriers. They may be subject to inspection to prove freedom from infection, particularly those who handle food that is either to be eaten raw or has previously been subjected to cooking (e.g. meat pies, paté)

飲食服務人員 從事食物製備、貯存、烹調、及餐廳服務人員的總稱。這樣的人應避免接觸傳染病，既不能是患者也不應是帶菌者。他們應接受檢查以證明他們未受到過傳染，特別是那些親手接觸食物（無論是生吃食物還是熟食如肉餅、餡餅）的人。

food poisoning an illness affecting the digestive system that results from eating food contaminated either by bacteria or bacterial toxins or, less commonly, by residues of insecticides (on fruit and vegetables) or poisonous chemicals such as lead or mercury. It can also be caused by eating poisonous fungi, berries, etc. Symptoms commence 1–24

食物中毒 因食入污染的食物而引起消化系統症狀的疾病。這些食物可被細菌、細菌毒素污染，偶可被殘留的殺蟲劑（如在水果上，蔬菜上）或有毒的化學物質（如鉛或汞）污染。也可因食入有毒的眞菌或槳果等引起。食入污

hours after ingestion and include vomiting, diarrhoea, abdominal pain, and nausea. Food-borne infections are caused by bacteria of the genus *Salmonella* in foods of animal origin. The disease is transmitted by human carriers who handle the food, by shellfish growing in sewage-polluted waters, or by vegetables fertilized by manure. Toxin-producing bacteria causing food poisoning include those of the genus *Staphylococcus*, which rapidly multiply in warm foods, and the species *Clostridium welchii*, which multiplies in reheated cooked meals. A rare form of food poisoning – *botulism – is caused by toxins produced by the bacterium *Clostridium botulinum*, which may contaminate badly preserved canned foods. *See also* gastroenteritis.

染物後的1～24小時開始出現症狀，包括嘔吐、腹瀉、腹痛及噁心。來於食物的感染是由產生於肉類的沙門氏菌屬引起。疾病能由處理食物的帶菌者、污水裏生長的貝殼動物或施過糞肥的蔬菜而傳染。引起食物中毒的產毒細菌包括能在熱食中快速繁殖的葡萄球菌屬和在再次加熱的肉食中繁殖的魏氏梭狀芽胞桿菌種。不常見的一種食物中毒——肉毒中毒——是由肉毒桿菌產生的毒素引起的，這種菌能夠污染保存不良的罐頭食物。

foramen *n.* (*pl.* **foramina**) an opening or hole, particularly in a bone. The *apical foramen* is the small opening at the apex of a tooth. The *foramen magnum* is a large hole in the occipital bone through which the spinal cord passes. The *foramen ovale* is the opening between the two atria of the fetal heart, which allows blood to flow from the right to the left side of the heart by displacing a membranous valve.

孔 口或洞。尤指骨頭上的孔或洞。根尖孔是牙尖上的小孔。枕骨大孔是枕骨上的一個大孔，脊髓由此孔通過。卵圓孔是胎兒心臟兩心房之間的開口，使右心房的血液衝開膜性瓣後流入左心房。

forceps *n.* a pincer-like instrument designed to grasp an object so that it can be held firm or pulled. Specially designed forceps – of which there are many varieties – are used by surgeons and dentists in operations (see illustration). The forceps used in childbirth are so designed as to fit firmly round the baby's head without damaging it. Dental *extraction forceps* are specially designed to fit the various shapes of teeth. By having long handles and short beaks they provide considerable leverage.

鉗 能牢牢夾住或拉出物體的鉗形器械。特殊設計的鉗（種類很多）用於外科和牙科手術（見圖）。用於分娩的鉗是爲能恰好夾住胎兒頭又不引起損傷而設計的。拔牙鉗是爲能適合各種牙齒形狀而特殊設計的。因爲這些鉗的柄長、嘴短，因此它們能起到重要的杠桿作用。

forebrain *n.* the furthest forward division of the *brain, consisting of the *diencephalon and the two cerebral hemispheres.

前腦 腦最前的部分，由間腦和兩側大腦半球組成。

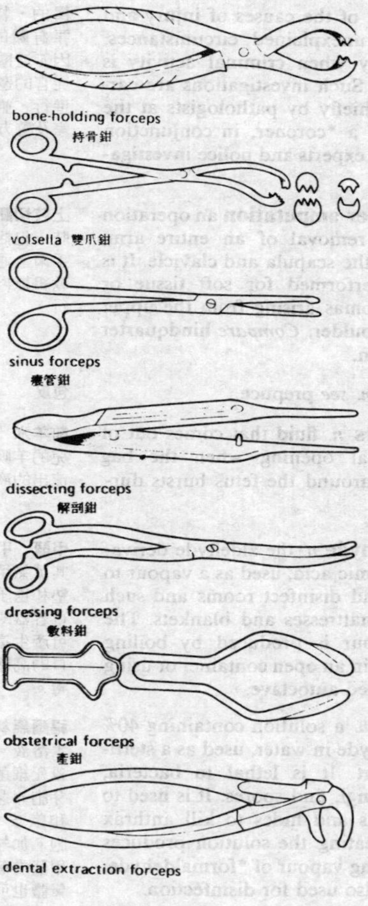

Types of forceps
鉗的種類

foregut *n.* the front part of the embryonic gut, which gives rise to the oesophagus (gullet), stomach, and part of the small intestine (from which the liver and pancreas develop).

前腸　胚腸的前部分。將生長出食道、胃和部分小腸（肝和胰就從這部分小腸中發育而成）。

forensic medicine the branch of medicine concerned with the scientific in-

法醫學　一種醫學分支。用科學的方法調查無法解

vestigation of the causes of injury and death in unexplained circumstances, particularly when criminal activity is suspected. Such investigations are carried out chiefly by pathologists at the request of a *coroner, in conjunction with other experts and police investigators.

釋的，特別是懷疑與犯罪有關的損傷和死亡原因。這種調查主要是在驗屍官的邀請下由病理學家進行，並與其他方面的專家及警方調查員相配合。

forequarter amputation an operation involving removal of an entire arm, including the scapula and clavicle. It is usually performed for soft tissue or bone sarcomas arising from the upper arm or shoulder. *Compare* hindquarter amputation.

上肢切斷術 除去全部上肢，包括肩胛骨和鎖骨的手術。通常因上肢或肩部軟組織肉瘤或骨肉瘤而施行。

foreskin *n. see* prepuce.

包皮

forewaters *n.* fluid that comes out of the vaginal opening when the bag (amnion) around the fetus bursts during labour.

前羊水 分娩時因包繞胎兒的羊膜破裂而從陰道口流出的液體。

formaldehyde *n.* the aldehyde derivative of formic acid, used as a vapour to sterilize and disinfect rooms and such items as mattresses and blankets. The toxic vapour is produced by boiling *formalin in an open container or using it in a sealed autoclave.

甲醛 甲酸的醛衍生物。其蒸氣用於消毒房間及牀墊和毯子等物件。煮沸敞口容器的福爾馬林溶液，可產生這種毒氣；或在封口的高壓消毒鍋內進行消毒。

formalin *n.* a solution containing 40% formaldehyde in water, used as a sterilizing agent. It is lethal to bacteria, viruses, fungi, and spores. It is used to treat wools and hides to kill anthrax spores. Heating the solution produces the irritating vapour of *formaldehyde, which is also used for disinfection.

福爾馬林 含40%甲醛的水溶液。做消毒劑使用可殺死細菌、病毒、眞菌和芽胞。還可用來處理羊毛和獸皮，以殺死炭疽芽胞。加熱此溶液能產生出甲醛有刺激性的氣體，該氣體也可用做消毒劑。

forme fruste an atypical form of a disease in which the usual symptoms fail to appear and its progress is stopped at an earlier stage than would ordinarily be expected.

頓挫型 疾病的非典型形式。症狀通常不表現出來，病情在早期階段即停止發展。

formication *n.* a prickling sensation said to resemble the feeling of ants crawling over the skin. It is a form of *paraesthesiae and it is sometimes a symptom of drug intoxication.

蟻走感 常被說成是類似螞蟻在皮膚上爬行感覺的一種刺激感。這是感覺異常的一種，有時是藥物中毒的症狀。

formulary *n.* a compendium of formulae used in the preparation of medicinal drugs.

處方集　用於配製醫藥的處方册。

fornix *n.* (*pl.* **fornices**) an arched or vaultlike structure, especially the *fornix cerebri*, a triangular structure of white matter in the brain, situated between the hippocampus and hypothalamus. The *fornix of the vagina* is any of three vaulted spaces at the top of the vagina, around the cervix of the womb.

穹窿　弓狀或拱頂狀結構。尤指大腦穹窿，是大腦白質的三角形結構，位於海馬和丘腦下部之間。陰道穹窿是子宮頸周圍的陰道頂部的三個拱形空間。

fossa *n.* (*pl.* **fossae**) a depression or hollow. The *cubital fossa* is the triangular hollow at the front of the elbow joint; the *iliac fossa* is the depression in the inner surface of the ilium; the *pituitary fossa* is the hollow in the sphenoid bone in which the pituitary gland is situated; a *tooth fossa* is a pit in the enamel on the surface of a tooth.

窩　一種凹陷或穴。肘窩是肘關節前面的三角形凹陷。髂窩是髂骨內表面的凹陷。垂體窩是蝶骨上的穴，垂體腺就位於此穴內。齒窩是牙齒表面釉質上的小坑。

fovea *n.* (in anatomy) a small depression, especially the shallow pit in the retina at the back of the eye. It contains a large number of *cones and is therefore the area of greatest acuity of vision: when the eye is directed at an object, the part of the image that is focused on the fovea is the part that is most accurately registered by the brain. *See also* macula (lutea).

凹　（解剖學）小凹陷。尤指眼後視網膜上的淺窩。在此窩內，含有大量視錐細胞，因此是視覺最敏感的區域。當眼睛直視物體時，聚焦在小凹上的物像部分是被大腦最精確感知到的部分。

foveola *n.* (in anatomy) a small depression.

小凹　（解剖學）小凹陷。

fracture *n.* breakage of a bone, either complete or incomplete. A *simple fracture* involves a clean break with little damage to surrounding tissues and no break in the overlying skin. If a bone end pierces the overlying skin the fracture is *compound*, and there is a risk of infection (*see* osteomyelitis). Fracture of an already diseased bone is termed a *pathological fracture* and may occur after minor injuries. Treatment of a simple fracture includes realignment of the bone ends where there is displacement, immobilization by external splints or internal fixation, followed by

骨折　骨頭完全或不完全折斷。單純性骨折指有整齊骨裂、周圍組織損傷很小、而骨折部位的皮膚無破裂的骨折。如骨折端刺破骨折部位的皮膚則爲複合骨折，有感染的危險。病骨骨折叫做病理性骨折，可發生在很輕微損傷之後。單純骨折的治療包括重新將錯位的骨折端對位，進行夾板固定或內固定，直至康復。

*rehabilitation. *See also* comminuted fracture, greenstick fracture.

fraenectomy *n.* an operation to remove the fraenum, including the underlying fibrous tissue.

繫帶切除術 去除系帶及其下方的纖維組織的手術。

fraenum (frenum, frenulum) *n.* **1.** any of the folds of mucous membrane under the tongue or between the gums and the upper or lower lips. **2.** any of several other structures of similar appearance.

繫帶 ①舌下、齦唇之間的黏膜皺襞。②所有類似皺襞的其他結構。

fragile-X syndrome an inherited cause of mental subnormality, and possibly of autism, associated with easily damaged *X chromosomes.

X染色體脆弱綜合徵 因遺傳而引起的弱智及潛在的孤獨癖。與X染色體易損傷有關。

fragilitas *n.* abnormal brittleness or fragility, for example of the hair (*fragilitas crinium*) or the bones (*fragilitas ossium*; *see* osteogenesis imperfecta).

脆弱 不正常的易碎、易斷現象。如脆髮症或脆骨症。

framboesia *n. see* yaws.

雅司病

framycetin *n.* an *antibiotic used in the form of an ointment, cream, or solution to treat skin, eye, and ear infections. It is also administered by mouth to treat gastroenteritis and food poisoning. Skin sensitivity sometimes occurs and when taken by mouth the drug may cause diarrhoea and diseases due to growth of resistant organisms. Trade names: **Framygen, Soframycin**.

新黴素B 以軟膏、乳膏劑或溶液的形式治療皮膚、眼睛、耳朵感染的抗生素。亦可口服治療胃腸炎和食物中毒，有時可出現皮膚過敏。口服此藥可引起腹瀉及因對此藥不敏感的微生物生長繁殖而引起的疾病。

fraternal twins *see* twins.

雙卵性雙胎

freckle *n.* a brown spot on the skin commonly found on the arms and face of young people with a fair complexion. Freckles, which are harmless, appear where there is excessive production of the pigment melanin in discrete areas of the skin after exposure to sunlight.

雀斑 皮膚上的小黃斑點。通常見於皮膚白晰的青年人上肢及臉部。雀斑對人體無害，是由於陽光照射後，黑色素在皮膚個別部位過量產生的結果。

free association (in *psychoanalysis) a technique in which the patient is encouraged to pursue a particular train of ideas as they enter consciousness. *See also* association of ideas.

自由聯想 （精神分析學）鼓勵病人繼續追尋其進入意識領域裏的思想序列的方法。

freeze drying a method for the *fixation of histological specimens, involving a minimum of chemical and physical change. Specimens are immersed in isopentane cooled to –190°C in liquid air. This fixes the tissue instantly, without the formation of large ice crystals (which would cause structural changes). The tissue is then dehydrated in a vacuum for about 72 hours at –32.5°C.

冷凍乾燥 固定組織標本的一種方法。此方法能使標本只發生微小的化學和物理變化。將標本浸入異戊烷內，放在－190℃的液化氣內冷凍。這種固定方法可使組織長期固定而沒有大結晶冰形成（因結晶冰可引起結構變化）。然後再將該組織在－32.5℃的眞空容器內脫水72小時。

freeze etching a technique for preparing specimens for electron microscopy. The unfixed tissue is frozen and then split with a knife and a layer of ice is sublimed from the exposed surface. The resultant image is thus not distorted by chemical fixatives.

冷凍蝕刻法 製備電子顯微鏡標本的技術。將未固定的組織冷凍，再用刀將其切成片，這樣，冰層就會從組織的切面上昇華出來。用這種方法製成的標本不會被化學固定劑所破壞。

Frei test a diagnostic test for the venereal disease *lymphogranuloma venereum. A small quantity of the virus, inactivated by heat, is injected into the patient's skin. If the disease is present a small red swelling appears at the site of injection within 48 hours.

弗萊氏試驗 性病性淋巴肉芽腫的診斷試驗。將被熱滅活的小量病毒注射到患者皮內，如患者患有此病，48小時內，注射部位有小紅腫出現。

fremitus *n.* vibrations or tremors in a part of the body, detected by feeling with the fingers or hand (*palpation) or by listening (*auscultation). The term is most commonly applied to vibrations perceived through the chest when a patient breathes, speaks (*vocal fremitus*), or coughs. The nature of the fremitus gives an indication as to whether the chest is affected by disease. For example, loss of vocal fremitus suggests the presence of fluid in the pleural cavity; its increase suggests consolidation of the underlying lung.

震顫 身體某部位震動或顫動。可用手指或手的感覺（觸診）感到，或被聽到（聽診）。此術語最常用於描述在患者呼吸、說話（語音震顫）或咳嗽時通過胸部所察覺到的震顫。震顫的特點可提示胸部是否有病，例如：語音震顫消失表明胸腔內存在液體，語顫音增强說明肺部有實變。

frenulum *n. see* fraenum.

繫帶

frenum *n. see* fraenum.

繫帶

frequency distribution (in statistics) presentation of the characteristics (*variables) of a series of individuals (e.g.

頻數分配 （統計學）以表格和直方圖的形式表現一系列個體的特點（如身

their heights, weights, or blood pressures) in tabular form or as a histogram so as to indicate the proportion of the series that have different measurements. In a *normal* or *Gaussian distribution* the number of readings and their range on either side of the *mean value is symmetrical; in a *skewed distribution* (e.g. *Poisson*) the measurements are bunched on one side of the mean and spread out over a wider range on the other.

高、體重或血壓）的方法。可表明一系列差異的比例。在正態分佈和高斯分佈中，資料上的數字和其在平均值兩側的分佈是對稱的。在偏態分佈中（如泊松分佈），測得的數字集中在平均值的一側，在另一側則分散分佈。

Freudian *adj.* relating to or describing the work and ideas of Sigmund Freud (1856–1939): applied particularly to the school of psychiatry based on his teachings (*see* psychoanalysis).

弗洛伊德氏學派的 指與西格蒙·弗洛伊德（1856～1939）工作和觀點有關的。尤指由他培養出來的精神病學派。

friction murmur (friction rub) a scratching sound, heard over the heart with the aid of the stethoscope, in patients who have *pericarditis. It results from the two inflamed layers of the pericardium rubbing together during activity of the heart.

摩擦音 用聽診器在心包炎患者心臟部位的胸壁上聽到的一種抓搔音。這是因爲在心臟活動時，心包的兩層發炎的膜互相摩擦的結果。

Friedman's test a pregnancy test in which a sample of the woman's urine is injected into an unmated female rabbit. After two days the rabbit is killed and its ovaries examined. If the woman is pregnant her urine will contain enough ovary-stimulating hormone (*chorionic gonadotrophin) to induce the development of corpora lutea in the ovaries of the rabbit.

弗里德曼氏試驗 一種妊娠試驗。將婦女尿液標本注射到未交配的母兔身上，兩天後，將兔殺死，檢查其卵巢，如果該婦女已妊娠，她的尿液含有一定量的卵巢刺激素（絨毛膜促性腺激素），能促使兔卵巢內的黃體發育。

Friedreich's ataxia *see* ataxia.

弗里德賴希氏共濟失調

frigidity *n.* lack of sexual desire or inability to reach the climax of sexual excitement. Frigidity may affect either sex, but the term is almost always applied to women only. In some cases the woman feels revulsion towards sexual activity.

性感缺失 缺乏性慾，或無能力達到性高潮。男性或女性都可患性感缺失，但該術語僅用來指女性。在某些病例中，女性對性行爲感到厭惡。

fringe medicine the various systems of healing that are not regarded as part of orthodox treatment by the medical profession. Some of these are based on

非正統醫學 不屬於專業醫學正規治療範圍的各種治療方法。其中，一些治療方法的理論在一定程度

theories that coincide to some extent with more orthodox medical ideas; others are based on ideas that bear no relation to standard medicine. Among the more reputable systems of fringe medicine are *osteopathy, *acupuncture, *homeopathy, *naturopathy, and *chiropractic.

上與正統醫學的觀點相符，另一些的觀點與標準醫學毫不相干。在非正統醫學的治療方法中，較受贊譽的是按骨術、針灸、順勢療法、自然醫術及按摩療法。

Fröhlich's syndrome a disorder of the *hypothalamus (part of the brain) affecting males: the boy is overweight with sexual development absent and disturbances of sleep and appetite. Medical name: **dystrophia adiposogenitalis**.

肥胖性生殖器退化綜合徵 男性丘腦下部（腦的一部分）疾病。男孩過度肥胖、性器官不發育及睡眠和食慾紊亂。

frontal *adj.* **1.** of or relating to the forehead (*see* frontal bone). **2.** denoting the *anterior part of a body or organ.

①**額的** ②**前面的** 指身體和器官前面的。

frontal bone the bone forming the forehead and the upper parts of the orbits; it contains several air spaces (*frontal sinuses*: *see* paranasal sinuses). At birth it consists of right and left halves, joined by a suture that usually closes during infancy. *See* skull.

額骨 形成前額及眶上部的骨。含有很多氣竇。出生時由左右兩半組成，中間為骨縫，該縫在嬰兒時閉合。

frontal lobe the anterior part of each cerebral hemisphere (*see* cerebrum), extending as far back as the deep central sulcus (cleft) of its upper and outer surface. Immediately anterior to the central sulcus lies the motor cortex, responsible for the control of voluntary movement; the area further forward – the *prefrontal lobe – is concerned with behaviour, learning, judgment, and personality.

額葉 大腦半球的前部分，向後延伸到大腦外上表面的中央溝。緊靠中央溝以前的部分是皮質運動區，負責控制自主運動。最前面的部位——前額葉——與行為、學習、判斷及個性有關。

frontal sinus *see* paranasal sinuses.

額竇

frostbite *n.* damage to the tissues caused by freezing. The affected parts, usually the nose, fingers, or toes, become pale and numb. Ice forms in the tissues, which may thus be destroyed, and amputation may become necessary. Frostbitten parts should not be rubbed, since there is no blood circulation in the tissues, but they may be

凍瘡 因受凍而引起的組織損傷。受損部位通常為鼻、手指或脚趾。表現為蒼白與麻木。如組織內有冰形成，可使組織受到破壞，必要時需截肢。凍瘡部位不能揉擦，因該部位內無血液循環，但可用溫水逐漸加溫。要特別注意

gently warmed in tepid water. Precautions must be taken against bacterial infection, to which frostbitten skin is highly susceptible.

避免細菌感染，凍瘡皮膚對細菌有極高的易感性。

frottage *n.* rubbing up against somebody (usually in a crowd) as a means of obtaining sexual pleasure. A person displaying this sexual deviation is called a *frotteur*.

摩擦淫 抵住摩擦某人（通常是在人羣中）做爲獲得性滿足的手段。表現出這種性變態的人叫做摩擦淫者。

frozen shoulder chronic painful stiffness of the shoulder joint. This may follow injury, a stroke, or *myocardial infarction or may gradually develop for no apparent reason. Treatment is by gentle stretching and exercises, sometimes combined with *corticosteroid injection into the joint. *See also* capsulitis.

凍肩 肩關節慢性疼痛性强直，可出現在外傷、腦卒中或心肌梗死之後，或無明顯原因而逐漸發展成病。治療：輕輕牽拉，做運動，有時可在肩關節內注射皮質類固醇。

fructose *n.* a simple sugar found in honey and in such fruit as figs. Fructose is one of the two sugars in *sucrose. Fructose from the diet can be used to produce energy by the process known as *glycolysis, which takes place in the liver. Fructose is important in the diet of diabetics since, unlike glucose, fructose metabolism is not dependent on insulin.

果糖 存在於蜂蜜和水果（如無花果）中的一種單糖。果糖是蔗糖中兩種單糖之一，食物中的果糖可通過在肝臟進行的糖酵解產生能量。果糖是糖尿病患者飲食中的重要成分。因它與葡萄糖不同，是不依靠胰島素代謝的。

fructosuria (levulosuria) *n.* the presence of fructose (levulose) in the urine.

果糖尿 尿里存在果糖。

frusemide *n.* a *diuretic used to treat fluid retention (oedema) associated with heart, liver, or kidney disease and also high blood pressure. It is administered by mouth or injection; common side-effects are nausea and vomiting. Trade name: **Lasix**.

速尿 治療因心臟病、肝病或腎病及高血壓引起的液體瀦留（水腫）的利尿藥。口服或注射。常見的副作用是噁心、嘔吐。

FSH *see* follicle-stimulating hormone.

促卵泡成熟激素

fuchsin (magenta) *n.* any one of a group of reddish to purplish dyes used in staining bacteria for microscopic observation and capable of killing various disease-causing microorganisms. *Acid fuchsin* (*acid magenta*) is a mixture of sulphonated fuchsins; *basic fuchsin*

品紅 用於對細菌染色、以進行顯微鏡下觀察的一種染料。顏色從紅到紫不等。品紅能殺死各種致病性微生物。酸性品紅是磺化品紅的混合物。鹼性品紅和新品紅（三甲基）是

(*basic magenta*) and *new* (*trimethyl*) *fuchsin* are basic histological dyes (basic fuchsin is also an antifungal agent).

鹼性組織染料（鹼性品紅還是一種抗眞菌劑）。

-fuge *suffix denoting* an agent that drives away, repels, or eliminates. Example: *febrifuge* (a drug that reduces fever).

〔後綴〕 有驅除、抵制或消滅作用的物質。如退熱藥（退燒藥）。

fugue *n.* a period of memory loss during which the patient leaves his usual surroundings and wanders aimlessly or starts a new life elsewhere. It is often preceded by psychological conflict and depression, and may be associated with hysteria or organic mental disease. *See also* dissociation.

神游症 患者離開他常住的環境，無目的地漫游，或在某地開始新生活。患者事後對這段時期失去記憶。患病前，患者通常有心理衝突和壓抑感，並與癔病和器質性精神病有關。

fulguration (electrodesiccation) *n.* the destruction with a *diathermy instrument of warts, growths, or unwanted areas of tissue, particularly inside the bladder. This latter operation is performed via the urethra and viewed through a cystoscope.

電灼療法 用透熱器械破壞疣、新生物或病變組織、特別是膀胱內的病變組織。此手術要通過膀胱鏡在尿道內施行。

fulminating (fulminant, fulgurant) *adj.* describing a condition or symptom that is of very sudden onset, severe, and of short duration.

暴發的 指突然發作、病情嚴重、持續期短的疾病或症狀。

fumigation *n.* the use of gases or vapours to bring about *disinfestation of clothing, buildings, etc. Sulphur dioxide, formaldehyde, and chlorine are common fumigating agents.

薰煙消毒法 一種用氣體或蒸氣消毒衣服、房屋等的方法。二氧化硫、甲醛及氯氣是常用的薰煙劑。

functional disorder a condition in which a patient complains of symptoms for which no physical cause can be found. Such a condition is frequently an indication of a psychiatric disorder. *Compare* organic disorder.

功能性疾病 從患者主訴的症狀中不能找出軀體性原因的一種疾病。這種疾病常常是心理障礙。

fundus *n.* **1.** the base of a hollow organ: the part farthest from the opening; e.g. the fundus of the stomach, bladder, or uterus. **2.** part of the interior of the eye that is situated opposite the pupil.

①**底** 空心器官的底部，距開口部最遠的部分。如胃底、膀胱底或子宮底。②**眼底** 眼睛內部與瞳孔位置相對的部位。

fungicide *n.* an agent that kills fungi. *See also* antimycotic.

殺眞菌劑

fungoid 1. *adj.* resembling a fungus. **2.** *n.* a fungus-like growth.

①蕈狀的 ②蕈樣新生物

fungus *n.* (*pl.* **fungi**) a simple plant that lacks the green pigment chlorophyll. Fungi include the *yeasts, rusts, moulds, and mushrooms. They live either as *saprophytes or as *parasites of plants and animals; some species infect and cause disease in man (*see* blastomycosis). The single-celled microscopic yeasts are a good source of vitamin B and many antibiotics are obtained from the moulds (*see* penicillin). —**fungal** *adj.*

眞菌 一種無葉綠素的簡單植物。包括酵母菌、銹菌、黴及蕈。眞菌既可做爲植物和動物的腐生物生存，也可做爲它們的寄生物生存。一些菌種還可以使人類感染致病。極微小的單細胞酵母菌是維生素B的重要來源。很多抗生素也是從黴中獲得。

funiculitis *n.* inflammation of the spermatic cord. This usually arises in association with *epididymitis and causes pain and swelling of the involved cord. Treatment is by administration of antibiotics and analgesics.

精索炎 精索炎症。通常因附睾炎而發病，受損的精索疼痛、水腫。治療：服用抗生素和鎮痛藥。

funiculus *n.* **1.** any of the three main columns of white matter found in each lateral half of the spinal cord. **2.** a bundle of nerve fibres enclosed in a sheath; a fasciculus. **3.** (formerly) the spermatic cord or umbilical cord.

①索 脊髓兩側所見到的白質中三個主要柱狀結構 ②被鞘膜包繞着的一束神經纖維。 ③精索或臍帶

funis *n.* (in anatomy) any cordlike structure, especially the umbilical cord.

索條 （解剖學）任何繩索狀結構。尤指臍帶。

furcation *n.* the place where the roots fork on a multirooted tooth.

分叉 多根牙上的牙根分支處。

furfuraceous *adj.* describing scaling of skin in which the scales resemble bran or dandruff.

皮屑狀的 指糠樣或頭皮屑樣皮膚脫屑。

furor *n.* indiscriminate violence and destructiveness, occurring especially during a period of mental confusion due to *epilepsy.

狂暴 隨意的暴力和破壞行爲，特別是發生於因癲癇而失去理智的時期。

furuncle *n. see* boil.

癤

furunculosis *n.* **1.** the occurrence of several *boils (furuncles) at the same time. **2.** the recurrence of boils in the skin over a period of weeks or months. This occurs because of persistence of the infecting bacteria (usually *Staphylo-*

癤病 ①同一時間出現多個癤腫。 ②皮膚反復出現癤腫，間隔期爲幾周或幾個月。這是因爲皮膚上始終存在着感染性細菌（通常是葡萄球菌）。治

coccus aureus) in the skin. Treatment includes thorough daily disinfection of the skin as well as antibiotic therapy.

療：每天做全身皮膚消毒，並使用抗菌素。

fusiform *adj.* spindle-shaped; tapering at both ends.

梭形的　紡錘形的，兩端呈圓錐形的。

fusion *n.* (in surgery) the joining together of two structures. For example, fusion of two or more vertebra is performed to produce a stable spine.

融合　（外科學）兩結構結合在一起。例如：將兩個或更多的脊椎融合在一起，就形成了一個牢固的脊柱。

Fusobacterium *n.* a genus of Gram-negative rodlike bacteria with tapering ends. Most species are normal inhabitants of the mouth of animals and man and produce no harmful effects, but *F. fusiformis* (*Bacteroides fusiformis*), an anaerobic species, is associated with **Borrelia vincentii* in *ulcerative gingivitis.

梭形杆菌屬　革蘭氏陰性兩端呈圓錐形的桿狀菌屬。其多數菌種正常生活在動物和人類的口腔裏，而且不產生危害。但梭狀擬桿菌（一種厭氧菌）可與奮森氏包柔氏螺旋體一起引起潰瘍性齦炎。

G

GABA *see* gamma-aminobutyric acid.

γ-氨基丁酸

Gaffkya *n.* a genus of bacteria now classified as **Micrococcus*.

加夫基氏球菌屬　細球菌屬的舊稱。

gag *n.* (in medicine) an instrument that is placed between a patient's teeth to keep his mouth open.

張口器　（醫學）放在病人牙齒之間使口保持張開的一種器械。

galact- (galacto-) *prefix denoting* **1.** milk. Example: *galactosis* (formation of). **2.** galactose.

〔前綴〕 ①**乳**　例如乳汁生成。 ②**半乳糖**

galactagogue *n.* an agent that stimulates the secretion of milk or increases milk flow.

催乳藥　刺激乳汁分泌或增加乳汁流量的藥物。

galactocele *n.* **1.** a breast tumour containing milk, caused by closure of a milk duct. **2.** an accumulation of milky liquid in the sac surrounding the testis (*see* hydrocele).

①**乳腺囊腫**　含有乳汁的乳腺腫瘤。由於輸乳管閉合所致。 ②**乳性鞘膜積液**　陰囊內積聚乳狀液體。

galactorrhoea *n.* **1.** abnormally copious milk secretion. **2.** secretion of milk after breast feeding has been stopped.

乳溢 ①乳汁分泌異常豐富。②母乳餵養停止後的乳汁分泌。

galactosaemia *n.* an inborn inability to utilize the sugar galactose, which in consequence accumulates in the blood. Untreated, affected infants fail to thrive and become mentally retarded, but if galactose is eliminated from the diet growth and development may be normal.

半乳糖血症 一種不能利用半乳糖的先天性疾患。其結果導致半乳糖蓄積於血內。如不治療，患兒不能茁壯成長，智力發育遲緩；但飲食中消除了半乳糖，生長發育可以恢復正常。

galactose *n.* a simple sugar and a constituent of the milk sugar *lactose. Galactose is converted to glucose in the liver. The enzyme necessary for this conversion is missing in infants with a rare inherited metabolic disease called *galactosaemia.

半乳糖 一種單糖。乳糖的一種成分。半乳糖在肝內轉變爲葡萄糖。半乳糖血症是嬰兒的一種少見的遺傳性代謝病。是由於體內缺少半乳糖轉變爲葡萄糖所必需的酶所致。

galea *n.* **1.** a helmet-shaped part, especially the *galea aponeurotica*, a flat sheet of fibrous tissue (*see* aponeurosis) that caps the skull and links the two parts of the *epicranius muscle. **2.** a type of head bandage.

①**帽狀腱膜** 顱頂肌的頭盔狀腱膜。大片腱膜覆蓋於顱頂上，前後各與顱頂肌的額腹和枕腹相連。
②**帽狀綳帶** 爲頭部綳帶的一種類型。

galenical *n.* a pharmaceutical preparation of a drug of animal or plant origin.

蓋侖氏製劑 一種以動物或植物爲原料的藥物製劑。

gallamine *n.* a drug administered by injection to produce muscle relaxation during anaesthesia (*see* muscle relaxant). It is also used in a diagnostic test for *myasthenia gravis. Trade name: **Flaxedil**.

加拉明 一種注射用的肌肉弛緩藥。痲醉時使用。亦用於對重症肌無力的診斷試驗。商品名：弛肌碘。

gall bladder a pear-shaped sac (7–10 cm long), lying underneath the right lobe of the liver, in which *bile is stored (see illustration). Bile passes (via the hepatic duct) to the gall bladder from the liver, where it is formed, and is released into the duodenum (through the common bile duct) under the influence of the hormone *cholecystokinin-pancreozymin, which is secreted when food is present in the duodenum.

膽囊 一個貯存膽汁的梨形囊。位於肝右葉下面（見圖）。在肝內生成的膽汁（經肝管）進入膽囊貯存。當食物進入十二指腸，即刺激分泌縮膽囊素——促胰酶素；這種激素引起膽囊收縮，使膽汁（經膽總管）排入十二指腸。

gallstone *n.* a hard mass composed of bile pigments, cholesterol, and calcium

膽石 一種由不同比例的膽色素、膽固醇和鈣鹽組

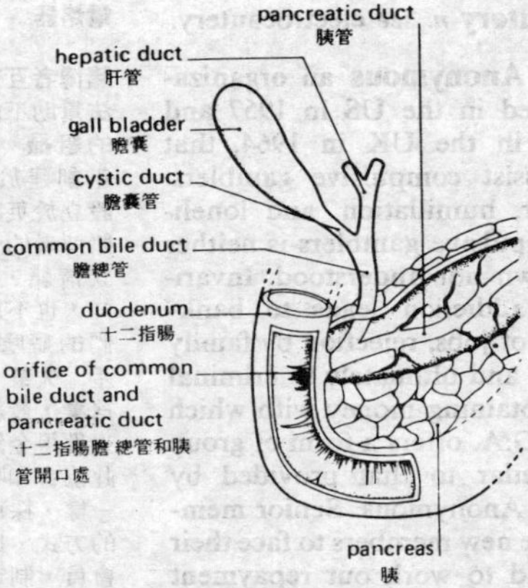

The gall bladder and pancreas and their associated ducts
膽囊和胰及其導管

salts, in varying proportions, that can form in the gall bladder. The formation of gallstones (*cholelithiasis*) occurs when the physical characteristics of bile alter so that cholesterol is less soluble, though chronic inflammation of the gall bladder (*see* cholecystitis) may also be a contributory factor. Gallstones may exist for many years without causing symptoms. However, they may cause severe pain (*see* biliary colic) or they may pass into the common bile duct and cause obstructive *jaundice or *cholangitis. Gallstones containing calcium may be seen as a plain X-ray (opaque stones), but if their calcium content is low they can be seen only by *cholecystography. Cholelithiasis is treated by surgical removal of the gall bladder or the stones themselves.

成的硬的凝結物。膽石可於膽囊內形成。當膽汁發生物理特性改變時，膽固醇的溶解度減低，導致膽石形成。慢性膽囊炎也是引起膽石形成的一個因素。膽石可存在許多年而並不出現症狀。膽石可引起劇烈疼痛，或因進入膽總管而導致阻塞性黃疸或膽囊炎。含鈣質的膽石可於 X 線平片上顯影（不透明膽石），但如其所含鈣的量少，則只能見於膽囊造影。治療：手術摘除膽囊，或從膽囊取出膽石。

galvanism *n.* (formerly) any form of medical treatment using electricity. *Interrupted galvanism* is a form of *electrotherapy in which direct current, in impulses lasting for 30 to 100 milliseconds, is used to stimulate the activity of nerves or the muscles they supply. *See also* faradism.

電療法　（舊稱）採用任何形式的電流進行治療的醫療方法。斷續電療是電療法的一種形式。這種電療採用持續 30 至 100 毫秒的直流電脉衝，刺激神經及其所支配的肌肉。

galvanocautery *n. see* electrocautery.

電烙器

Gamblers Anonymous an organization, founded in the US in 1957 and established in the UK in 1964, that seeks to assist compulsive gamblers. The despair, humiliation, and loneliness of compulsive gamblers is neither widely known nor understood. Invariably their addiction leads to bankruptcy, loss of jobs, rejection by family and friends, and ultimately to criminal means of obtaining money with which to gamble. G.A. offers a form of group therapy similar to that provided by *Alcoholics Anonymous. Senior members help the new members to face their creditors and to work out repayment budgets that will eventually free them from their obligations. The sister organization, Gam-Anon, provides advice and encouragement for the families of compulsive gamblers.

賭博者互戒協會　一個設法幫助不能自拔的賭博者的組織。這個組織 1957 年創建於美國，1964 年設立於英國。不能自拔的賭博者的失望、羞辱、孤立情緒，是旣不爲人所知，也不爲人理解的。他們的癖嗜肯定會導致破產、失業、被家庭和朋友捨棄，最終用犯罪的手段去獲得金錢，再去賭博。此協會和嗜酒者互戒協會一樣，採用一種集體治療的方式，以老會員幫助新會員，制定向債權人償還債務的計劃，最終使他們從債務中擺脫出來。與此協會配合的婦女組織對不能自拔的賭博者的家屬進行勸告和鼓勵。

gamete *n.* a mature sex celi: the *ovum of the female or the *spermatozoon of the male. Gametes are haploid, containing half the normal number of chromosomes.

配子　一種成熟的性細胞。如女子的卵子或男子的精子。配子是單倍體的，含有正常數一半的染色體。

gametocide *n.* a drug that kills *gametocytes. Drugs such as *primaquine destroy gametocytes of the malaria parasite (*see* Plasmodium), so interrupting the life cycle and preventing infection of the mosquito.

殺配子〔體〕劑　一種殺滅配子體的藥物。例如破壞瘧原蟲配子體的藥物伯氨喹啉，能使瘧原蟲的生活周期被中斷，防止蚊蟲感染。

gametocyte *n.* any of the cells that are in the process of developing into gametes by undergoing *gametogenesis. *See also* oocyte, spermatocyte.

配子體　在配子形成過程中發育成爲配子的細胞。

gametogenesis *n.* the process by which spermatozoa and ova are formed. In both sexes the precursor cells undergo *meiosis, which halves the number of chromosomes. However, the timing of events and the size and number of gametes produced are very different in the male and female. *See* oogenesis, spermatogenesis.

配子形成　精子和卵子形成的過程。精子和卵子的母細胞進行減數分裂，使其染色體數目減少一半。而雄性和雌性配子形成時間的長短、大小和數目是極不相同的。

gamma aminobutyric acid (GABA) an amino acid found in the central nervous system, predominantly in the brain, where it acts as an inhibitory *neurotransmitter.

γ-氨基丁酸 一種氨基酸。存在於中樞神經系統，主要在腦內。起着抑制神經遞質的作用。

gamma benzene hexachloride a drug used in creams, lotions, solutions, or shampoos to treat infestations caused by scabies, mites, and lice (including head lice). Mild skin reactions occasionally occur. Trade names: **Lorexane, Quellada**.

γ-六氯化苯 一種用以治療由疥螨和蝨（包括頭蝨）引起的感染的藥物。可用作乳劑、洗劑、溶液劑或洗髮劑。偶有輕微的皮膚反應。商品名：丙體六六六。

gamma camera a piece of apparatus for taking photographs of parts of the body into which radioactive isotopes that give off *gamma rays have been introduced as *tracers.

γ照相機 一種拍攝γ射線的照相機。所拍攝的γ射線係由置入體內作爲示踪物的放射性核素釋出的。

gamma globulin any of a class of proteins, present in the blood *plasma, identified by their characteristic rate of movement in an electric field (*see* electrophoresis). Almost all gamma globulins are *immunoglobulins. *See also* globulin.

γ球蛋白 存在於血漿中的一類蛋白質。此類蛋白質根據其在電場內特定的移動速度來測定。幾乎所有的γ球蛋白都是免疫球蛋白。

gamma rays electromagnetic radiation of wavelengths shorter than X-rays, given off by certain radioactive substances. Gamma rays have greater penetration than X-rays; they are harmful to living tissues and can be used to sterilize certain materials. Carefully controlled doses are used in *radiotherapy.

γ射線 一種電磁輻射的波長短於X線的射線。由某些放射性物質所釋放。γ射線有較X線更强的穿透力，對活組織有危害，可用於消毒某些用具。嚴格控制劑量的γ射線可用於放射治療。

gamo- *prefix denoting* marriage.

〔前綴〕 **婚配**

gangli- (ganglio-) *prefix denoting* a ganglion.

〔前綴〕 **神經節**

ganglion *n.* (*pl.* **ganglia**) **1.** (in neurology) any structure containing a collection of nerve cell bodies and often also numbers of synapses. In the *sympathetic nervous system chains of ganglia are found on each side of the spinal cord, while in the *parasympathetic system ganglia are situated in or nearer to the organs innervated. Swellings in

①**神經節** （神經病學）含有神經細胞胞體集團，並常有許多突觸的結構。在交感神經系統，神經節鏈排於脊柱兩旁；而在副交感系統，神經節位於所支配的器官內或其附近。含有感覺纖維的脊神經後根的膨大部也稱爲神經

the posterior sensory *roots of the spinal nerves are termed ganglia; these contain cell bodies but no synapses. Within the central nervous system certain well-defined masses of nerve cells are called ganglia (or *nuclei*); for example, the *basal ganglia. **2.** an abnormal but harmless swelling (cyst) that sometimes forms in tendon sheaths, especially at the wrist.

節。這些神經節有細胞胞體而無突觸。在中樞神經系統內某些清晰的神經團也稱爲神經節（或核）。例如，基底神經節。② **腱鞘囊腫** 一種異常但無危害的腫塊（囊腫）。有時見於腱鞘內，尤其在腕部。

ganglioside *n.* one of a group of *glycolipids found in the brain, liver, spleen, and red blood cells (they are particularly abundant in nerve cell membranes). Gangliosides are chemically similar to *cerebrosides but contain additional carbohydrate groups.

神經節苷脂 爲糖脂類的一種。見於腦、肝、脾和紅細胞（在神經細胞膜中尤其豐富）。神經節苷脂和腦苷脂在化學結構上近似，但前者額外有一個糖基。

gangosa *n.* a lesion that occasionally appears in the final stage of *yaws, involving considerable destruction of the tissues of both the hard palate and the nose.

毁形性鼻咽炎 在雅司病末期偶爾出現的一種損害。硬腭和鼻的組織都遭到相當的破壞。

gangrene *n.* death and decay of part of the body due to deficiency or cessation of blood supply. The causes include disease, injury, or *atheroma in major blood vessels, frostbite or severe burns, and diseases such as *diabetes mellitus and *Raynaud's disease. *Dry gangrene* is death and withering of tissues caused simply by a cessation of local blood circulation. *Moist gangrene* is death and putrefactive decay of tissue caused by bacterial infection. *See also* gas gangrene.

壞疽 由於血液供應缺乏或停止而使身體的一個部分壞死和腐爛。其病因包括損傷、大血管粥樣化、凍瘡或嚴重燒傷，以及糖尿病、雷諾氏病等疾病。乾性壞疽係單純由於局部血管的循環停止所致，組織壞死和乾枯。濕性壞疽係由於細菌感染所致，組織壞死並腐爛。

Ganser state (pseudodementia) a syndrome characterized by *approximate answers*, i.e. the patient gives grossly and absurdly false replies to questions, but the reply shows that the question has been understood. For example, the question "What colour is snow?" may elicit the reply "Green". This can be accompanied by odd behaviour or episodes of *stupor. The condition is due to *hysteria or to conscious malingering.

甘塞氏狀態（假性痴呆） 一種以似是而非的回答爲特徵的綜合徵。病人對問題做出粗俗、荒謬的錯誤回答，但從回答中可以看出他對所提的問題是理解的。例如，問"雪是甚麼顏色？"回答"藍色。"答話時伴有古怪的舉止或木僵發作。這種病態是由於癔病所致，或者是詐病。

gargoylism *n. see* Hurler's syndrome.

脂肪軟骨營養不良

gas gangrene death and decay of wound tissue infected by the soil bacterium *Clostridium welchii*. Toxins produced by the bacterium cause putrefactive decay of connective tissue with the generation of gas. Treatment is usually by surgery.

氣性壞疽 由土壤中魏氏梭狀芽胞桿菌感染傷口組織所致的壞死和腐爛。桿菌的毒素引起結締組織腐爛，產生氣體。常用外科治療。

Gasterophilus *n.* a genus of widely distributed non-bloodsucking beelike flies. The parasitic maggots normally live in the alimentary canal of horses but, rarely, can also infect man and cause an inflamed itching eruption of the skin (*see* creeping eruption).

胃蠅屬 一種廣泛分佈的蜜蜂狀非吸血蠅屬。其蛆正常寄生於馬的消化道中，但偶爾也能感染人，引起瘙癢的炎性皮疹。

gastr- (gastro-) *prefix denoting* the stomach. Examples: *gastralgia* (pain in); *gastrocolic* (relating to the stomach and colon).

〔前綴〕 **胃** 例如：胃痛，胃結腸的。

gastrectasia *n.* dilatation of the stomach. This may be caused by *pyloric stenosis or it may occur as a complication of abdominal operations or trauma.

胃擴張 胃的擴張。可由幽門狹窄引起，或是腹部手術或創傷的合併症。

gastrectomy *n.* a surgical operation in which the whole or a part of the stomach is removed. *Total gastrectomy*, in which the oesophagus is joined to the duodenum, is usually performed for stomach cancer but occasionally for the *Zollinger-Ellison syndrome. In *partial* (or *subtotal*) *gastrectomy* the upper third or half of the stomach is joined to the duodenum or small intestine (*gastroenterostomy*): an operation usually carried out in severe cases of *peptic ulcers. After gastrectomy capacity for food is reduced, sometimes leading to weight loss. Other complications of gastrectomy include *dumping syndrome, anaemia, and *malabsorption.

胃切除術 一種全部或部分切除胃的外科手術。在全胃切除術中，將食管與十二指腸吻合，此手術常用於胃癌，偶爾也用於卓-艾二氏綜合徵。在部分（或次全）胃切除術中，將上端⅓或½的胃與十二指腸或小腸吻合（胃腸吻合術）。此手術常用於嚴重的胃潰瘍。施行胃切除術後食物的容量減小，有時導致體重下降。胃切除術的其他合併症有傾倒綜合徵、貧血和吸收障礙。

gastric *adj.* relating to or affecting the stomach.

胃的 與胃有關的，或侵襲胃的。

gastric glands tubular glands that lie in the mucous membrane of the sto-

胃腺 胃黏膜上的管狀腺。胃腺有三種：賁門

mach wall. There are three varieties: the *cardiac*, *fundic* (*oxyntic*), and *pyloric glands*, and they secrete *gastric juice.

腺、胃底腺（胃酸腺）和幽門腺。這些腺體分泌胃液。

gastric juice the liquid secreted by the *gastric glands of the stomach. Its main digestive constituents are hydrochloric acid, mucin, *rennin, and pepsinogen. The acid acts on pepsinogen to produce *pepsin, which functions best in an acid medium. The acidity of the stomach contents also kills unwanted bacteria and other organisms that have been ingested with the food. Gastric juice also contains *intrinsic factor, which is necessary for the absorption of vitamin B_{12}.

胃液 胃腺分泌的液體。其主要的具有消化功能的成分有鹽酸、黏蛋白、凝乳酶和胃蛋白酶原。鹽酸作用於胃蛋白酶，其功能在酸性介質中最强。胃內容物的酸度也能殺死隨食物攝入的有害的細菌或其他微生物。胃液尚含有爲吸收維生素 B_{12} 所必需的內因子。

gastric ulcer an ulcer in the stomach, caused by the action of acid, pepsin, and bile on the stomach lining (mucosa). The output of stomach acid is not usually increased. Symptoms include vomiting and pain in the upper abdomen soon after eating, and such complications as bleeding, *perforation, and obstruction due to scarring may occur. Symptoms are relieved by antacid medicines, but surgery may be required if the ulcer persists. Since stomach cancer may mimic a gastric ulcer, all gastric ulcers should be examined by a *gastroscope to aid in their differentiation.

胃潰瘍 胃部的潰瘍。由於胃酸、胃蛋白酶和膽汁作用於胃黏膜所致。胃酸的分泌量不一定增加。胃潰瘍的症狀包括進食後不久即發生嘔吐和上腹部疼痛。可發生出血、穿孔或由於瘢痕形成所致的梗阻等合併症。服用抗酸藥物可使症狀緩解；但如潰瘍持久不癒，則需手術治療。由於胃癌的症狀與胃潰瘍極相似，因此所有胃潰瘍患者都應做胃鏡檢查，以資鑑別。

gastrin *n.* a hormone produced in the mucous membrane of the pyloric region of the *stomach. Its secretion is stimulated by the presence of food. It is circulated in the blood to the rest of the stomach, where it stimulates the production of *gastric juice.

促胃液素 胃幽門區黏膜產生的一種激素。此激素受食物的刺激而分泌，通過血液循環至胃的其餘部分，刺激胃液的產生。

gastritis *n.* inflammation of the lining (mucosa) of the stomach. *Acute gastritis* is caused by ingesting excess alcohol or other irritating or corrosive substances and causes vomiting. *Chronic gastritis* is associated with smoking and chronic alcoholism and may be caused by bile entering the stomach from the duo-

胃炎 胃黏膜的炎症。急性胃炎由於飲酒過多或攝入其他刺激性或腐蝕性物質所致，可引起嘔吐。慢性胃炎與吸煙和慢性酒精中毒有關，並可能由膽汁從十二指腸返流於胃內引起。慢性胃炎缺乏特異性

denum. It has no definite symptoms, but the patient is liable to develop gastric ulcers. *Atrophic gastritis*, in which the stomach lining is atrophied, may succeed chronic gastritis but may occur spontaneously as an *autoimmune disease. Dyspeptic symptoms such as nausea, vomiting, loss of appetite, and abdominal discomfort, popularly ascribed to gastritis, are not due to inflammation of the stomach.

症狀，但易發展爲胃潰瘍。萎縮性胃炎的胃黏膜有萎縮改變，可能是慢性胃炎續發的，或可能是一種特發的自體免疫性疾病。一般認爲屬於萎縮性胃炎的消化不良症狀，如噁心、嘔吐、食慾不佳和上腹部不適，並非由於胃的炎症所致。

gastrocele *n.* a *hernia of the stomach.

胃膨出 胃疝。

gastrocnemius *n.* a muscle that forms the greater part of the calf of the leg (see illustration). It flexes the knee and foot (so that the toes point downwards).

腓腸肌 一塊佔有大部分小腿肚子的肌肉（見圖）。腓腸肌使膝和足彎曲（致使脚趾向下）。

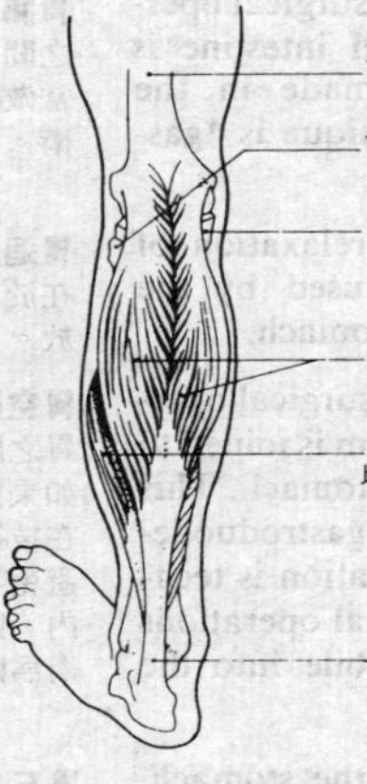

Gastrocnemius and soleus muscles
腓腸肌和比目魚肌

gastrocolic reflex a wave of peristalsis produced in the colon by introducing food into a fasting stomach.

胃結腸反射 空腹進食時引起結腸的蠕動波。

gastroduodenostomy *n.* a surgical operation in which the *duodenum (usually the third or fourth part) is joined to an opening made in the stomach in order to bypass an obstruc-

胃十二指腸吻合術 在十二指腸（通常在⅓或¼處）與胃之間造一通道的手術。此手術使胃梗阻（如幽門梗阻）有旁道相

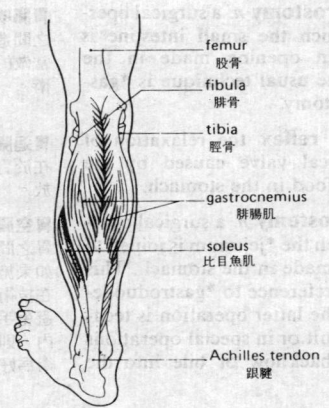

tion (such as *pyloric stenosis) or to facilitate the exit of food from the stomach after vagotomy. *See also* duodenostomy.

通，或者便於施行迷走神經切斷術後胃內食物的排空。

gastroenteritis *n.* inflammation of the stomach and intestine. It is usually due to acute infection by viruses or bacteria or to food-poisoning toxins and causes vomiting and diarrhoea. The illness usually lasts 3–5 days. Fluid loss is sometimes severe, especially in infants, and intravenous fluid replacement may be necessary.

胃腸炎 胃和腸的炎症。常由於細菌或病毒的急性感染或食物中毒所致，引起嘔吐和腹瀉。病程通常爲3～5天。有時體液喪失嚴重，尤其在嬰兒，可能需要靜脈注射補充液體。

gastroenterology *n.* the study of gastrointestinal disease, which includes disease of any part of the digestive tract and also of the liver, biliary tract, and pancreas.

胃腸病學 研究胃腸疾病的學科。包括消化道任何部位的疾病，也包括肝、膽道和胰的疾病。

gastroenterostomy *n.* a surgical operation in which the small intestine is joined to an opening made in the stomach. The usual technique is *gastroduodenostomy.

胃腸吻合術 在小腸與胃之間造一通道的手術。通常做的是胃十二指腸吻合術。

gastroileac reflex the relaxation of the *ileocaecal valve caused by the presence of food in the stomach.

胃迴腸反射 由於食物存在於胃中引起的迴盲瓣開放。

gastrojejunostomy *n.* a surgical operation in which the *jejunum is joined to an opening made in the stomach. This is done in preference to *gastroduodenostomy if the latter operation is technically difficult or in special operations to avoid a backflow of bile into the stomach.

胃空腸吻合術 在空腸與胃之間造一通道的手術。如果施行胃十二指腸手術在技術上有困難，或者要避免手術後膽汁返流到胃內，則以施行胃空腸吻合術爲好。

gastrolith *n.* a stone in the stomach, which usually builds up around a *bezoar.

胃石 胃內的石塊。常由糞石形成。

gastro-oesophagostomy *n.* a surgical operation in which the *oesophagus (gullet) is joined to the stomach, bypassing the natural junction when this is obstructed by *achalasia, *stricture (narrowing) of the oesophagus, or cancer. This operation is rarely performed, because gastric juices entering the oesophagus through the artificial junction cause inflammation and stricture.

胃食管吻合術 食管與胃之間繞過自然連接處相連接的手術。施行於賁門失弛緩症、食管狹窄或食管癌。此手術已較少施行，因爲胃液會通過人工接連處進入食管，引起炎症和狹窄。

gastropexy *n.* surgical attachment of the stomach to the abdominal wall.

胃固定術 將胃附着於腹壁的手術。

gastroplasty *n.* surgical treatment of a deformity of the stomach, e.g. a deformity due to peptic ulcers.

胃成形術 胃變形的外科治療。例如因胃潰瘍引起的變形。

gastroptosis *n.* a condition in which the stomach hangs low in the abdomen. Although the diagnosis was once used to explain various abdominal complaints, it is now known that the stomach may assume various anatomical positions without causing any symptoms.

胃下垂 胃向下腹移位。胃下垂的診斷曾用於解釋種種腹部病痛，而現在認爲胃可以有不同的解剖位置，而不引起任何症狀。

gastrorrhoea *n.* excessive secretion of gastric juice. *See* hyperchlorhydria.

胃液溢 胃液分泌過多。

gastroscope *n.* an illuminated optical instrument used to inspect the interior of the stomach. For many years these were rigid or semi-rigid instruments affording only limited views, but modern fully flexible *fibreoptic instruments allow all areas of the stomach to be seen and photographed and specimens taken for microscopic examination. As the same instruments can usually be introduced into the duodenum they are also known as *gastroduodenoscopes* or *oesophagogastroduodenoscopes*. —**gastroscopy** *n.*

胃鏡 一種用於檢查胃內部的光學照明器械。多年來採用的胃鏡管是硬質的或半硬質的，只能用以看到有限的胃區，而現代使用十分柔軟的光學纖維管，可以看到胃的各個部分，並可攝影和採取標本做顯微鏡檢查。因此鏡亦可用以檢查十二指腸，故也稱爲胃十二指腸鏡或食管胃十二指腸鏡。

gastrostaxis *n.* an old term for *haematemesis (bleeding from the stomach).

胃滲血 嘔血的舊稱（胃出血）。

gastrostomy *n.* a surgical operation in which the stomach is brought through the abdominal wall and an opening made into it. It is usually performed to allow food and fluid to be poured directly into the stomach when swallowing is impossible because of disease or obstruction of the oesophagus. Sometimes it is used temporarily after operations on the oesophagus, until healing has occurred.

胃造口術 在胃與腹壁間造一瘻管通至體外的手術。當因食管疾患或阻塞而不能吞嚥時，常施行此手術以便把食物直接灌入胃中。有時在施行食管手術後暫時用此方法，直至食管癒合爲止。

gastrotomy *n.* a procedure during abdominal surgery in which the sto-

胃切口術 切開胃壁的手術。常用於檢查胃內部

mach is opened, usually to allow inspection of the interior (e.g. to find a point of bleeding), to remove a foreign body, or to allow the oesophagus to be approached from below (e.g. to pull down a tube through a constricting growth).

（尋找出血點），或去除胃內異物，或從下端接近食管（例如，穿過腫瘤狹窄處將導管拉下來）。

gastrula *n.* an early stage in the development of many animal embryos. It consists of a double-layered ball of cells formed by invagination and movement of cells in the preceding single-layered stage (blastula) in the process of *gastrulation*. It contains a central cavity, the *archenteron, which opens through the *blastopore* to the outside. True gastrulation only occurs in the embryos of amphibians and certain fish, but a similar process occurs in the embryonic disc in other vertebrates, including man.

原腸胚 爲許多動物胚胎發育中的早期階段。在原腸胚形成的過程中，由單層的囊胚泡內陷和移動而形成兩層的細胞球。原腸胚含有一個中心腔，即原腸，開口於胚孔。眞性的原腸胚形成僅發生於兩棲類和某些魚類的胚胎；但其他脊椎動物（包括人類）的胚盤形成，也有類似的過程。

Gaucher's disease an inborn chemical defect causing accumulation of fatty compounds (*cerebrosides) in the liver, spleen, lymph nodes, and nervous system. The disease is fatal in infancy; a less severe form may become apparent only in adult life.

高雪氏病 一種先天的代謝障礙性疾病。引起肝、脾、淋巴結和神經系統內的脂類化合物（腦苷脂）蓄積。此病在嬰兒是致命的，在成人偶可以較輕的形式出現。

gauss *n.* a unit of magnetic flux density equal to 1 maxwell per square centimetre. 1 gauss = 10^{-4} tesla.

高斯 磁場强度單位。每個單位等於每平方厘米 1 麥克斯威。1 高斯＝10^{-4}特斯拉。

Gaussian distribution *see* frequency distribution, significance.

高斯氏分佈

gauze *n.* thin open-woven material used in several layers for the preparation of dressings and swabs.

紗布 細薄的稀疏織品。用幾層紗布可製成敷料或拭子。

gavage *n.* forced feeding: any means used to get an unwilling or incapacitated patient to take in food by mouth, especially via a stomach tube.

管飼法 强制餵養的方法。使不願意或無能力進食的病人進食。常使用胃管餵飼。

gel *n.* a colloidal suspension that has set to form a jelly. Some insoluble drugs are administered in the form of gels.

凝膠 一種混懸膠體。放置後形成膠凍。有些不溶解的藥物常採用凝膠劑型。

gelatin *n.* a jelly-like substance formed when tendons, ligaments, etc. containing *collagen (a protein) are boiled in water. Gelatin has been used in medicine as a source of protein in the treatment of malnutrition, in pharmacy for the manufacture of capsules and suppositories, and in bacteriology for preparing culture media.

明膠 一種膠凍狀物質。當肌腱、韌帶等含有膠原（一種蛋白質）的物質在水中煮沸後即形成明膠。明膠在醫學中作爲蛋白質的一種來源用以治療營養不良；在製藥中用以製造膠囊和栓劑；在細菌學中用以配製培養基。

gemmule *n.* one of the minute spines or surface extensions of a *dendrite, through which contact is made with another neurone at a *synapse.

樹突棘 神經細胞樹突表面許多細刺狀突起或棘。通過樹突棘與另一個神經元的突觸相接觸。

gene *n.* the basic unit of genetic material, which is carried at a particular place on a *chromosome. Originally it was regarded as the unit of inheritance and mutation but is now usually defined as a piece of *DNA or *RNA that acts as the unit controlling the formation of a single polypeptide chain (*see* cistron). In diploid organisms, including man, genes occur as pairs of *alleles. Various kinds of gene have been discovered: *structural genes* determine the biochemical makeup of the proteins; *regulator genes* control the rate of protein production (*see* operon). *Architectural genes* are responsible for the integration of the protein into the structure of the cell, and *temporal genes* control the time and place of action of the other genes and largely control the *differentiation of the cells and tissues of the body.

基因 遺傳物質的基本單位。位於染色體的特定位置上。原先認爲基因是遺傳和突變的生物單位，而現在常把基因看作是一種脫氧核糖核酸或核糖核酸，是控制形成一條多肽鏈的功能單位。在二倍體的生物，包括人類在內，基因以成對的等位基因出現。已發現有很多種的基因：結構基因，決定蛋白質的生物化學組成；調節基因，控制蛋白質生成的速度；建築基因，負責把蛋白質整合於細胞結構中去；時間基因，控制其他基因作用的時間和地點，並很大程度上控制身體的細胞和組織的分化。

general dental services a part of the NHS dental service. Dentists are included on the dental list of the appropriate *Family Practitioner Committee and are independent contractors. They are paid by item of service and the contract with a patient is for a course of treatment only. They are entirely responsible for the financial management of their own practices.

普通牙醫服務所 從屬於國民保健服務系統牙醫服務部。牙醫在所屬的家庭醫師委員會牙醫花名册上登記，單獨與患者簽訂合同。他們由病人按所服務的項目支酬，僅與病人簽訂一個療程的合同。他們完全自負盈虧。

general paralysis of the insane (GPI) a late consequence of syphilitic

麻痺性痴呆 梅毒感染的晚期後果。具有痴呆病人

infection. The symptoms are those of a *dementia and spastic weakness of the limbs. Deafness, epilepsy, and *dysarthria (defective pronunciation) may occur. The infecting organism can be detected in the brain cells and the *Wasserman reaction is usually positive in blood and cerebrospinal fluid. When the symptoms are combined with those of *tabes dorsalis, the condition is called *tabo-paresis*. Vigorous treatment with procaine penicillin is required.

的症狀和肢體强直性無力。並可有耳聾、癲癇、發音困難。腦細胞中可檢出梅毒螺旋體，血液和腦脊液中乏色曼氏反應常呈陽性。如合併有脊髓痨症狀時，則稱爲脊髓痨性麻痺性痴呆。需用大劑量普魯卡因青黴素治療。

general practitioner (GP) a doctor who is the main agent of *primary medical care*, through whom patients make first contact with health services for a new episode of illness or fresh developments of chronic diseases. Advice and treatment are provided for those who do not require the expertise of a consultant or other specialist services of hospitals (*secondary medical care*). In the British *National Health Service patients on the practice list of a GP receive care without payment on an open-access basis. A practitioner may have private patients in addition to NHS patients; a few have exclusively private practices. No NHS patient may be charged for a NHS prescription or for a medical certificate; conversely no private patient may receive a NHS prescription. Two or more practitioners may form a partnership sharing fees and work loads, including cross-cover for each other's NHS patients. When they share premises, secretarial help, and other resources this constitutes a *group practice* and the premises from which they operate may be privately owned or may be a publicly owned *health centre. Remuneration of GPs is based on a quarterly capitation fee for each registered patient (higher for those over 65 years of age) regardless of the number of consultations; however, additional claims can be made for a few services (e.g. antenatal care and household calls during sleeping hours).

全科醫師 承擔一級衞生保健工作的主要醫師。病人初患新病或其慢性病有新的變化，首先通過他們與衞生保健機構接觸。如果病人不需要邀請專家會診或轉送其他醫院專科治療（二級衞生保健），即由他們進行診治。在英國參加國民保健服務制的病人，接受全科醫師的衞生保健服務不需要支付費用。全科醫師除了爲參加國民保健服務制的病人服務外，還可以有自己的病人。有一小部分全科醫師只私人開業。參加國民保健服務制的病人不需要負擔國民保健服務制的處方或醫療證明的費用；相反，沒有參加國民保健服務制的病人則不能取得國民保健服務制的處方。兩個或兩個以上的全科醫師可以結成同伴合作共事和分享收入，並可互相交換診治各自所屬的國民保健服務制的病人。當他們有共同的房產、辦事人員和其他資源時，即組成一個聯合診所。其辦公的房產可以是私人擁有的，也可以是一個公有的衞生保健中心。全科醫師的報酬來自每個登記參加國民保健服務制的病人每季交付的保健稅（65 歲以上的病人交付較多），而與其求治的次數無關。有些服務則需收額外的費用（例如產前衛生保健服務和夜間出診）。

generic *adj.* of or relating to a *genus.

屬的 屬的，或有關屬的。

-genesis *suffix denoting* origin or development. Example: *spermatogenesis* (development of spermatozoa).

〔後綴〕 **起源，發生** 例如：精子發生。

genetic code the information carried by *DNA and *messenger RNA that determines the sequence of amino acids in every protein and thereby controls the nature of all proteins made by the cell. The genetic code is expressed by the sequence of *nucleotide bases in the nucleic acid molecule, a unit of three consecutive bases (a *codon*) coding for each amino acid. The code is translated into protein at the ribosomes (*see* transcription, translation). Changes in the genetic code result in the insertion of incorrect amino acids in a protein chain, giving a *mutation.

遺傳密碼 由脫氧核糖核酸和信使核糖核酸傳遞的遺傳信息。它決定每個蛋白質中的氨基酸順序，並控制細胞所有蛋白質的性能。遺傳密碼是由核酸分子中的核苷酸鹼基的順序來表示的，每個氨基酸的密碼字母都是連續的三個核苷酸（密碼子）的組合。密碼被翻譯到蛋白質的核糖體上。遺傳密碼的改變造成蛋白質鏈內插入錯誤的氨基酸，從而引起突變。

genetic drift the tendency for variations to occur in the genetic composition of small isolated inbreeding populations by chance. Such populations become genetically rather different from the original population from which they were derived.

遺傳漂變 遺傳成分的隨機變異。這種變異傾向出現於與外界隔離的近親婚配的小羣體中。這種羣體與他們由來的原先羣體在遺傳學上變得頗爲不同。

genetics *n.* the science of inheritance. It attempts to explain the differences and similarities between related organisms and the ways in which characters are passed from parents to their offspring. *Human* and *medical genetics* are concerned with the study of inherited diseases. *See also* cytogenetics, Mendel's laws.

遺傳學 遺傳的科學。這門科學企圖解釋有關的生物之間的不同點和相似點，以及雙親的特徵傳給其後代的各種方式。人類遺傳學和醫學遺傳學對遺傳性疾病進行研究。

geni- (genio-) *prefix denoting* the chin.

〔前綴〕**頦**

-genic *suffix denoting* **1.** producing. **2.** produced by.

〔後綴〕 ①**產生的** ②**被產生的**

genicular *adj.* relating to the knee joint: applied to arteries that supply the knee.

膝的 有關膝關節的。以動脉爲例：供應膝的動脉。

geniculum *n.* a sharp bend in an anatomical structure, such as the bend in the facial nerve in the medial wall of the middle ear.

膝 强度彎曲的解剖學結構。例如中耳內側壁的面神經的膝狀神經節。

genion *n.* (in *craniometry) the tip of the protuberance of the chin.

頦尖 （顱測量法）頦的隆凸尖端。

genioplasty *n.* an operation performed in plastic surgery to build up the cheek bone with grafted bone, cartilage, or artificial material.

頦成形術 一種整形外科手術。用移植的骨、軟骨或人工材料重建面頰骨。

genital *adj.* relating to the reproductive organs or to reproduction.

生殖的 有關生殖器的，或有關生殖的。

genital herpes *see* herpes.

生殖器疱疹

genitalia *pl. n.* the reproductive organs of either the male or the female. However, the term is usually used in reference to the external parts of the reproductive system. *See also* vulva.

生殖器 生殖的器官。有男性的或女性的。此名詞常用以表達生殖系統的外面部分。

genito- *prefix denoting* the reproductive organs. Examples: *genitoplasty* (plastic surgery of); *genitourinary* (relating to the reproductive and excretory systems).

〔前綴〕 **生殖器** 例如：生殖器成形術，泌尿生殖的。

genogram *n.* a technique of family *psychotherapy, in which a family tree and family history are constructed in view of the whole family to help them understand each other better.

遺傳圖象 一種家庭心理治療採用的方法。把家譜和家庭史編出來，以幫助所有家庭成員更好地相互瞭解。

genome *n.* the basic *haploid set of chromosomes of an organism. Man has a genome of 23 chromosomes.

染色體組 一個生物的基本的單倍體染色體組。人類具有 23 個染色體的染色體組。

genotype *n.* **1.** the genetic constitution of an individual or group, as determined by the particular set of genes it possesses. **2.** the genetic information carried by a pair of alleles, which determines a particular characteristic. *Compare* phenotype.

①**遺傳型** 個體或羣體的遺傳組成。這是由其特有的基因組決定的。 ②**基因型** 由一對等位基因傳遞的遺傳信息，決定一種獨特的特徵。

gentamicin *n.* an *antibiotic used to treat infections caused by a wide range of bacteria. It can be administered by injection or applied in a cream to the skin or in drops to the ears and eyes. Kidney and ear damage may occur at high doses. Trade names: **Cidomycin**, **Genticin**.

慶大黴素 一種抗生素。用於治療許多種細菌的感染。可注射用，或以乳膏用於皮膚，或製成滴耳劑、滴眼劑。用大劑量時可有腎臟和耳的損害出現。

gentian violet 1. *see* crystal violet. **2.** *see* methyl violet.

①**龍膽紫** ②**甲紫**

genu *n.* **1.** the knee. **2.** any bent anatomical structure resembling the knee. —**genual** *adj.*

膝 ①膝蓋。②任何彎曲的形狀像膝的解剖學結構。

genus *n.* (*pl.* **genera**) a category used in the classification of animals and plants. A genus consists of several closely related and similar species; for example the genus *Canis* includes the dog, wolf, and jackal.

屬 動物和植物分類的類目。一個屬由一些密切相關的或近似的種組成。

genu valgum abnormal in-curving of the legs, resulting in excessive separation of the feet when the knees are in contact. *See* knock-knee.

膝外翻 大腿異常內曲，造成兩膝靠攏，兩脚過度分開。

genu varum abnormal outward curving of the legs, resulting in separation of the knees. *See* bow-legs.

膝內翻 大腿異常外曲，造成兩膝分開。

geo- *prefix denoting* the earth or soil.

〔前綴〕 **土，地**

geophagia *n.* the eating of dirt. *See* pica.

食土癖 吃髒物。

ger- (gero-, geront(o)-) *prefix denoting* old age.

〔前綴〕 **老年**

geriatrics *n.* the branch of medicine concerned with the diagnosis and treatment of disorders that occur in old age and with the care of the aged. *See also* gerontology.

老年病學 醫學的一個分支。研究老年期發生的疾病的診斷和治療，以及對老年人的衛生保健。

germ *n.* any microorganism, especially one that causes disease. *See also* infection.

微生物 任何微小的生物。尤指致病的微生物。

German measles a mild highly contagious virus infection, mainly of childhood, causing enlargement of lymph

風疹 一種症狀較輕而有高度傳染性的病毒傳染病。主要見於兒童，有頸

nodes in the neck and a widespread pink rash. The disease is spread by close contact with a patient. After an incubation period of 2–3 weeks a headache, sore throat, and slight fever develop, followed by swelling and soreness of the neck and the eruption of a rash of minute pink spots, spreading from the face and neck to the rest of the body. The spots disappear within seven days but the patient remains infectious for a further 3–4 days. An infection usually confers immunity. As German measles can cause fetal malformations during early pregnancy, girls should be immunized against the disease before puberty. Medical name: **rubella**. *Compare* scarlet fever.

部淋巴結腫大和廣泛的淺紅色皮疹出現。此病通過與病人緊密接觸而傳播。經2～3星期的潛伏期後出現頭痛、咽喉痛和輕微發燒，繼而出現頸部腫塊和疼痛以及淺紅色的細小斑點狀皮疹，從面頸部擴散至全身。皮疹在7天內消失，但其後3～4天內仍有傳染性。通常一次感染就獲得免疫。由於在妊娠早期感染風疹可導致胎兒畸形，因而女孩在青春期前就應該接受免疫接種以預防此病。

germ cell (gonocyte) any of the embryonic cells that have the potential to develop into spermatozoa or ova. The term is also applied to any of the cells undergoing gametogenesis and to the gametes themselves.

生殖細胞 任何能夠發育成為精子或卵子的胚細胞。此詞亦指任何經歷配子形成的細胞或配子本身。

germicide *n.* an agent that destroys microorganisms, particularly those causing disease. *See* antibiotic, antimycotic, antiseptic, disinfectant.

殺菌劑 一種消滅微生物的製劑。尤指消滅致病微生物的製劑。

germinal *adj.* **1.** relating to the early developmental stages of an embryo or tissue. **2.** relating to a germ.

①**生發的** 有關胚胎或組織早期發育的。 ②**病菌的** 有關致病菌的。

germinal epithelium the epithelial covering of the ovary, which was formerly thought to be the site of formation of *oogonia. It is now thought that oogonia persist in a dormant state from the prenatal period until required in reproductive life.

生殖上皮 覆蓋於卵巢的上皮。先前認為是卵原細胞生成的場所。現在認為卵原細胞自出生前直到育齡時長期處於休眠狀態。

germinal vesicle the nucleus of a mature *oocyte, prior to fertilization. It is considerably larger than the nucleus of other cells.

生發泡 一個成熟的卵母細胞受精前的核。此核要比其他細胞的核大得多。

germ layer any of the three distinct types of tissue found in the very early stages of embryonic development (*see*

胚層 在胚胎發育最早期見到的三層清晰的組織。在整個胚胎發育期間能找

ectoderm, endoderm, mesoderm). The germ layers can be traced throughout embryonic development as they differentiate to form the entire range of body tissues.

見三胚層分化形成身體各組織的全部過程。

germ plasm the substance postulated by 19th century biologists (notably Weismann) to be transmitted via the gametes from one generation to the next and to give rise to the body cells.

胚質，種質 19 世紀生物學家（著名的魏斯曼）的假說，認爲有一種通過生殖細胞代代相傳的種質。體細胞就是由種質產生的。

gerontology *n.* the study of the changes in the mind and body that accompany ageing and the problems associated with them.

老人學 研究老年人心理和身體改變及其有關問題的學科。

Gerstmann's syndrome a group of symptoms that represent a partial disintegration of the patient's recognition of his *body image. It consists of an inability to name the individual fingers, misidentification of the right and left sides of the body, and inability to write or make mathematical calculations (*see* acalculia, agraphia). It is caused by disease in the association area of the left parietal lobe of the brain.

格斯特曼氏綜合徵 病人對其身體某部分的形象不能分辨的一組症狀。包括手指認識不能、左右失認、失寫、計算不能。此綜合徵由大腦左側頂葉聯合區的病竈引起。

gestaltism *n.* a school of psychology that regards mental processes as wholes (*gestalts*) that cannot be broken down into constituent parts. From this was developed *gestalt therapy*, which aims at achieving a suitable gestalt within the patient that includes all facets of functioning.

完形心理學 一種心理學學說。認爲整體（完形）的心理過程不能細分爲各個組成部分。由此觀點而發展爲完形心理療法。旨在使病人獲得一個適宜的，包括適合各方面功能活動的完形心態。

gestation *n.* the period during which a fertilized egg cell develops into a baby that is ready to be delivered. Gestation averages 266 days in humans (or 280 days from the first day of the last menstrual period). *See also* pregnancy.

妊娠 受精卵細胞發育成爲即將出生的嬰兒的過程。人的妊娠期平均爲 266 天（或者自最後一次月經的第一天算起爲 280 天）。

Ghon's focus the lesion produced in the lung of a previously uninfected person by tubercle bacilli. It is a small focus of granulomatous inflammation, which may become visible on a chest X-

岡氏病竈 一個先前未曾受過結核桿菌感染的人的肺部結核性損害。是一個小的肉芽腫性炎症病竈。當其長得足夠大或者鈣化

ray if it grows large enough or if it calcifies. A Ghon focus usually heals without further trouble, but in some patients tuberculosis spreads from it via the lymphatics, the air spaces, or the bloodstream.

時，可在胸部 X 線透視中見到。一個岡氏病竈通常癒合而無進一步病變發生；但在某些病人結核由此病竈經淋巴管、氣管或血流擴展開來。

giant cell any large cell, such as a *megakaryocyte. Giant cells may have one or many nuclei.

巨細胞 任何巨大的細胞。如巨核細胞。巨細胞可有一個或多個細胞核。

giant-cell arteritis *see* arteritis.

巨細胞性動脉炎

Giardia *n.* a genus of parasitic pear-shaped protozoa inhabiting the small intestine of man. They have four pairs of *flagella, two nuclei, and two sucking discs used for attachment to the intestinal wall. *Giardia* is usually harmless but may occasionally cause diarrhoea (*see* giardiasis).

賈第蟲屬 寄生於人的小腸內的一種梨形原蟲屬。具有四對鞭毛，兩個細胞核，以及兩個用以吸附於腸黏膜上的吸盤。賈第蟲一般不致病，但偶可引起腹瀉。

giardiasis (lambliasis) *n.* a disease caused by the parasitic protozoan *Giardia lamblia* in the small intestine. Man becomes infected by eating food contaminated with cysts containing the parasite. Symptoms include diarrhoea, nausea, bellyache, flatulence, and the passage of pale fatty stools (steatorrhoea). Large numbers of the parasite may interfere with the absorption of food through the gut wall. The disease occurs throughout the world and is particularly common in children; it responds well to oral doses of quinacrine and *metronidazole.

賈第蟲病（蘭伯氏鞭毛蟲病） 由寄生的原蟲蘭伯氏賈第蟲引起的一種疾病。人吃了染有此寄生蟲包囊的食物而感染。症狀有腹瀉、噁心、腹痛、腹脹，並排出帶有脂肪的灰白色糞便（脂肪瀉）。爲數很多的寄生蟲可使腸壁吸收受阻。此病發生於世界各地，兒童尤爲常見。口服喹那克林（阿的平）和甲硝唑（滅滴靈）治療有效。

gibbus (gibbosity) *n.* a sharply angled curvature of the backbone, resulting from collapse of a vertebra. Infection with tuberculosis was a common cause.

駝背 脊柱呈銳角形彎曲。由脊椎萎陷所致。結核感染爲其常見病因。

Giemsa's stain a mixture of *methylene blue and *eosin, used for distinguishing different types of white blood cell and for detecting parasitic microorganisms in blood smears. It is one of the *Romanowsky stains.

吉姆薩氏染劑 一種亞甲藍和曙紅的混合液。用以區分白細胞的不同類型，並用於寄生微生物的血塗片檢驗。這種染劑是羅曼諾夫斯基氏染劑的一種。

gigantism *n.* abnormal growth causing excessive height, most commonly due to oversecretion during childhood of

巨人症 身體異常生長，導致長得過分高大。大多由於兒童時期垂體生長激

*growth hormone (somatotrophin) by the pituitary gland. In *eunuchoid gigantism* the tall stature is due to delayed puberty, which results in continued growth of the long bones before their growing ends (epiphyses) fuse. *See also* acromegaly.

素分泌過多所致。在無睾性巨人症，其身材高大是由於青春期延遲引起。病人青春期延遲，導致長骨在其生長端（骺）融合前繼續增長。

Gilbert's syndrome familial unconjugated hyperbilirubinaemia: a condition due to an inherited congenital deficiency of the enzyme UDP glucuronyl transferase in the liver cells. Patients become mildly jaundiced, especially if they fast or have some minor infection. Occasionally they have mild abdominal discomfort. The jaundice can be diminished by small doses of phenobarbitone, which stimulates enzyme activity. The condition is harmless.

吉伯特氏綜合徵 家族性非結合型高膽紅素血症。是肝細胞中缺乏二磷酸尿苷葡萄糖醛酸轉移酶的一種先天性遺傳性疾患。病人有輕度黃疸，尤其在他們空腹或有輕度感染時，並偶可有輕度胃腸道不適。使用小劑量苯巴比妥可刺激酶的活力而使黃疸消失。本病預後良好。

Gilles de la Tourette syndrome a condition of severe and multiple *tics, including vocal tics and involuntary obscene speech (*coprolalia). The patient may also involuntarily repeat the words or imitate the actions of others (*see* palilalia). The condition usually starts in childhood and becomes chronic; the causes are unknown. Drug treatment (for example, with *haloperidol) is sometimes successful.

圖雷特氏綜合徵 一種嚴重的多發性抽搐疾患。其症狀包括爆發性發聲和不隨意的猥褻言語（穢褻言語）。病人也可不隨意地重複他人的言語和模倣他人的動作。常於兒童時期發病，並轉爲慢性。病因未明。藥物治療（如用氟哌啶醇）有時見效。

gingiv- (gingivo-) *prefix denoting* the gums. Example: *gingivoplasty* (plastic surgery of).

〔前綴〕 **齦** 指齒齦。例如齦成形術。

gingiva *n.* (*pl.* **gingivae**) the gum: the layer of dense connective tissue and overlying mucous membrane that covers the alveolar bone and necks of the teeth. —**gingival** *adj.*

齦 齒齦。包被牙槽骨和牙頸的一層結締組織，外面有黏膜覆蓋。

gingivectomy *n.* the surgical removal of excess gum tissue.

齦切除術 手術除去多餘的齦組織。

gingivitis *n.* inflammation of the gums (*see* gingiva) caused by *plaque on the surfaces of the teeth at their necks. The gums are swollen and bleed easily. *Chronic gingivitis* is an early stage of

齦炎 齒齦的炎症。由牙頸表面的菌斑引起。齒齦腫脹並容易出血。慢性齦炎是牙周病的早期階段，但如注意口腔衞生，可以

*periodontal disease but is reversible with good oral hygiene. *Ulcerative gingivitis is painful and destructive.

復原。潰瘍性齦炎是疼痛的，並是破壞性的。

ginglymus (hinge joint) *n.* a form of *diarthrosis (freely movable joint) that allows angular movement in one plane only, increasing or decreasing the angle between the bones. Examples are the knee joint and the elbow joint.

滑車關節（屈戌關節） 動關節（可自由活動的關節）的一種類型。這種關節只能在一個平面上轉動，使兩骨間的角度增大或減小。如膝關節和肘關節。

girdle *n.* (in anatomy) an encircling or arching arrangement of bones. *See also* pelvic girdle, shoulder girdle.

帶 （解剖學）環形或半圓形的骨性支架。

glabella *n.* the smooth rounded surface of the *frontal bone in the middle of the forehead, between the two eyebrows.

眉間 兩眉的中間部分。額中央圓而光滑的額骨面。

gladiolus *n.* the middle and largest segment of the *sternum.

胸骨體 胸骨中間的最大節塊。

gland *n.* an organ or group of cells that is specialized for synthesizing and secreting certain fluids, either for use in the body or for excretion. There are two main groups of glands: the *exocrine glands, which discharge their secretions by means of ducts, and the *endocrine glands, which secrete their products – hormones – directly into the bloodstream. *See also* secretion.

腺 專門合成和分泌某種體液的一種器官或一團細胞。這種體液或被身體利用，或被排出體外。腺體有兩大類：外分泌腺，有腺管排出其分泌物；內分泌腺，其分泌的激素直接流入血循環。

glanders (equinia) *n.* an infectious disease of horses, donkeys, and mules that is caused by the bacterium *Actinobacillus mallei* and can be transmitted to man. Symptoms include fever and inflammation (with possible ulceration) of the lymph nodes (a form of the disease known as *farcy*), skin, and nasal mucous membranes. In the untreated acute form death may follow in 2–20 days. In the more common chronic form, many patients survive without treatment. Administration of sulphonamides or streptomycin is usually effective.

鼻疽（馬鼻疽） 馬、騾和驟的一種傳染病。由鼻疽放線桿菌引起，能傳播於人。症狀有發燒以及淋巴結（一種稱爲馬皮疽的疾病）、皮膚和鼻黏膜炎症（可能形成潰瘍）。未經治療的急性病人可能於2～20天內死亡。較爲常見的慢性病人大多不經治療也可存活。用磺胺類藥物或鏈黴素治療常有效。

glandular fever an infectious disease, thought to be caused by the Epstein-Barr virus, that affects the lymph nodes

腺熱 一種傳染病。一般認爲係由埃-巴二氏病毒所致。病變累及頸部、腋

in the neck, armpits, and groin; it mainly affects adolescents and young adults. After an incubation period of up to seven weeks, symptoms commence with swelling and tenderness of the lymph nodes, fever, headache, a sore throat, and loss of appetite. In some cases the liver is affected, causing *hepatitis, or the spleen is enlarged. Glandular fever is diagnosed by the presence of large numbers of *monocytes in the blood. Complications are rare but symptoms may persist for weeks before recovery. Medical name: **infectious mononucleosis**.

窩和腹股溝淋巴結，主要感染青少年。經過接近七個星期的潛伏期後，開始出現淋巴結腫大和觸痛、發燒、頭痛、咽喉痛和食慾不佳。有的病例累及肝臟，引起肝炎，或有脾臟腫大。腺熱的診斷由血液中存在大量單核白細胞確定。很少有合併症，但在恢復前症狀可持續數周。醫學名稱：傳染性單核細胞增多症。

glans (glans penis) *n.* the acorn-shaped end part of the *penis, formed by the expanded end of the corpus spongiosum (erectile tissue). It is normally covered by the prepuce (foreskin), unless this has been removed by circumcision. The term glans is also applied to the end of the *clitoris.

陰莖頭 陰莖的橡子狀末端。由尿道海綿體（勃起組織）末端的膨大部分組成。正常有包皮覆蓋，除非施行包皮環切術將其切除。陰莖頭的名稱亦用於陰蒂的末端部分。

glaucoma *n.* a condition in which loss of vision occurs because of an abnormally high pressure in the eye. In most cases there is no other ocular disease. This is known as *primary glaucoma* and there are two pathologically distinct types: *acute congestive glaucoma*, in which a sudden rise in pressure is accompanied by pain and marked blurring of vision; and *chronic simple glaucoma*, in which the pressure increases gradually, usually without producing pain, and the visual loss is insidious. The same type of visual loss may occur in eyes with a normal pressure: this is called *low-tension glaucoma*. Primary glaucoma occurs increasingly with age and is an important cause of blindness. *Secondary glaucoma* may occur when other ocular disease impairs the normal circulation of the aqueous humour and causes the intraocular pressure to rise.

In all types of glaucoma the eventual problem is to reduce the intraocular pressure. Drops are put into the eye at

青光眼 眼內壓異常升高的病變。引起視力喪失。在大多數病例無其他眼疾存在，稱爲原發性青光眼。原發性青光眼在病理學上有兩個不同的類型：急性充血性青光眼，眼壓突然升高，伴有眼痛和顯著的視力模糊；慢性單純性青光眼，眼壓逐漸升高，常無眼痛，視力喪失是隱襲的。同樣的視力喪失可發生於眼壓正常的眼睛，稱爲低眼壓性青光眼。原發性青光眼隨年齡增長而增多，是失明的重要病因。繼發性青光眼由於眼的其他疾患引起。因眼的疾患破壞房水的正常循環而導致眼內壓升高。所有類型的青光眼其根本的治療措施是降低眼內壓。使用眼藥水按規定間隔滴入眼內以增加房水引流，以及使用眼藥水和內服藥（如利尿劑）以減少

regular intervals to improve the outflow of aqueous humour from the eye, and drops and tablets (e.g. diuretics) are used to reduce the production of aqueous humour. If this treatment is inadequate surgery may be performed to make an accessory channel through which the aqueous humour may drain from the eye in sufficient quantities to allow the pressure to return to normal. Such operations are known as *drainage* or *fistularizing operations*.

房水的產生。如治療無效，可施行手術，造一輔助的通道使有足夠量的房水流出，以恢復正常眼內壓。這種手術稱爲引流手術或造瘻手術。

gleet *n.* a discharge of purulent mucus from the penis or vagina resulting from chronic *gonorrhoea.

後淋 自陰莖或陰道排出的膿性黏液。係由慢性淋病引起。

glenohumeral *adj.* relating to the glenoid cavity and the humerus: the region of the shoulder joint.

盂肱的 有關關節盂和肱骨的。在肩關節部位。

glenoid cavity (glenoid fossa) the socket of the shoulder joint: the pear-shaped cavity at the top of the *scapula into which the head of the humerus fits.

關節盂（關節窩） 肩關節臼。肩胛骨頂端的梨形盂，適合肱骨頭置於其中。

gli- (glio-) *prefix denoting* **1.** glia. **2.** a glutinous substance.

〔前綴〕 **膠質** ①神經膠質。②膠狀物質。

glia (neuroglia) *n.* the special connective tissue of the central nervous system, composed of different cells, including the *oligodendrocytes, *astrocytes, ependymal cells (*see* ependyma), and *microglia, with various supportive and nutritive functions (see illustration). Glial cells outnumber the neurones by between five and ten to one, and make up some 40% of the total volume of the brain and spinal cord. —**glial** *adj.*

神經膠質 中樞神經系統特殊的結締組織。由不同的細胞組成，包括少突膠質細胞、星形膠質細胞、室管膜細胞和小膠質細胞。這些細胞具有不同的支持功能和營養作用（見圖）。神經膠質細胞的數量爲神經元的5～10倍，約佔腦和脊髓全部體積的40%。

gliadin *n.* a protein, soluble in alcohol, that is obtained from wheat. It is one of the constituents of *gluten.

麥膠蛋白 一種從小麥中獲得的蛋白質。溶於酒精。是麩質的一個部分。

glibenclamide *n.* a drug that reduces the level of sugar in the blood and is used to treat diabetes. It is administered by mouth. Side-effects include mild digestive upsets and skin reactions. Trade name: **Daonil, Euglucon**.

優降糖 降低血糖水平的藥物。用於治療糖尿病。口服。副作用包括輕度胃腸不適和皮膚過敏。

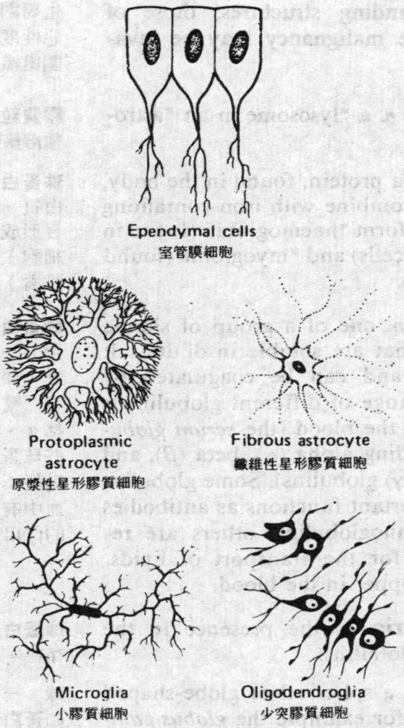

Types of glia
神經膠質細胞的類型

gliding joint *see* arthrodic joint.

摩動關節

glioblastoma (spongioblastoma) *n.* the most malignant type of brain tumour derived from non-nervous (glial) tissue (*see* astrocytoma). Its rapid enlargement destroys normal brain cells, with a progressive loss of function, and raises the intracranial pressure, causing headache, vomiting, and drowsiness.

成膠質細胞瘤 最惡性的一型腦瘤。由非神經的（神經膠質的）組織所衍生。腦瘤迅速擴大，破壞正常腦細胞，使腦功能逐漸喪失，腦壓增高，引起頭痛、嘔吐和倦眠。

glioma *n.* any tumour of non-nervous cells (*glia) in the nervous system. The term is sometimes used for all tumours that arise in the central nervous system, including *astrocytomas, *oligodendrogliomas, medulloblastomas, and ependymomas. Tumours of low-grade malignancy produce symptoms by pressure

神經膠質瘤 神經系統中各種非神經細胞的（神經膠質的）腫瘤。此詞有時用於中樞神經系統發生的所有腫瘤，包括星形細胞瘤、少突膠質細胞瘤、成神經管細胞瘤和室管膜細胞瘤。惡性度低的腫瘤產

on surrounding structures; those of high-grade malignancy may be invasive.

生周圍結構受壓的症狀，惡性度高的腫瘤可侵犯周圍組織。

gliosome *n.* a *lysosome in an *astrocyte.

膠質粒 星形細胞內的一種溶酶體。

globin *n.* a protein, found in the body, that can combine with iron-containing groups to form *haemoglobin (found in red blood cells) and *myoglobin (found in muscle).

珠蛋白 人體內的一種蛋白質。能與含鐵的基團結合形成血紅蛋白（見於紅細胞）和肌紅蛋白（見於肌肉）。

globulin *n.* one of a group of simple proteins that are soluble in dilute salt solutions and can be coagulated by heat. A range of different globulins is present in the blood (the *serum globulins*, including alpha (α), beta (β), and *gamma (γ) globulins). Some globulins have important functions as antibodies (*see* immunoglobulin); others are responsible for the transport of lipids, iron, or copper in the blood.

球蛋白 一類單純蛋白質中的一種。能溶於稀鹽溶液，加熱後凝結。血液中有一羣不同的球蛋白，包括 α 、β 和 γ 球蛋白。有些球蛋白具有抗體的重要功能；另外一些球蛋白在血中有運載脂類、鐵或銅的作用。

globulinuria *n.* the presence in the urine of globulins.

球蛋白尿 尿內有球蛋白存在。

globus *n.* a spherical or globe-shaped structure; for example the *globus pallidus*, part of the lenticular nucleus in the brain (*see* basal ganglia).

球 一種球形的結構。例如蒼白球，是大腦豆狀核的一部分。

glomangioma *n.* a harmless but often painful tumour usually occurring in the skin at the ends of the fingers and toes. It arises from nerve tissue in the blood vessels.

血管球瘤 一種並無危害而常有疼痛的腫瘤。通常發生於手指或足趾末端的皮膚內。係起源於血管的神經組織。

glomerulitis *n.* any one of a variety of lesions of the glomeruli (*see* glomerulus) associated with acute or chronic kidney disease. Such lesions are recognized by electron microscopic examination, using immunofluorescent staining techniques, of kidney biopsy specimens taken during the course of the disease.

腎小球炎 急性或慢性腎疾病引起的腎小球的某種損害。在發病過程中取腎的活組織標本，採用熒光免疫染色技術和電子顯微鏡檢查，可以發現這種損害。

glomerulonephritis *n.* a disease of the kidneys resulting in the syndrome of *acute nephritis*: the passage of blood in the urine and occasionally fluid retention and swelling (*see* oedema). The

腎小球腎炎 導致急性腎炎症狀的一種腎臟疾病。有血尿，並偶有尿瀦留和浮腫。急性腎小球腎炎的確切病因尚不明；但在大

exact cause of acute glomerulonephritis is obscure, but in most cases it is thought to represent an abnormal allergic response following a streptococcal sore throat. The acute form of the disease usually settles completely, with rapid return to normal kidney function. Occasionally, it progresses to chronic glomerulonephritis and kidney failure, sometimes via the *nephrotic syndrome.

多數病例，認爲係由鏈球菌咽炎引起的一種異常過敏反應所致。急性腎小球腎炎常可完全痊癒，腎功能迅速恢復正常，偶可發展爲慢性腎小球腎炎和腎功能衰竭，有時轉爲腎病綜合徵。

glomerulus *n.* (*pl.* **glomeruli**) **1.** the network of blood capillaries contained within the cuplike end (*Bowman's capsule*) of a *nephron. It is the site of primary filtration of waste products from the blood into the kidney tubule. **2.** any other small rounded mass.

①**腎小球**　包含在一個腎單位的杯狀囊（鮑曼氏囊）內的毛細血管網。是血液中的廢物以原尿形式濾入腎小管的場所。②**小球**　任何其他小圓球狀物。

glomus *n.* (*pl.* **glomera**) a small communication between a tiny artery and vein in the skin of the limbs. It is concerned with the regulation of temperature. Occasionally its malformation and overgrowth produces a small painful tender red swelling (*glomus tumour*). This may be cauterized or removed surgically.

血管球　肢體皮膚內細小動脈和靜脈間的一個小的脈絡球，與溫度調節有關。偶爾其畸變或過度生長而形成一個有觸痛的小紅塊（血管球瘤）。此腫塊可能需要施行手術烙除或切除。

gloss- (glosso-) *prefix denoting* the tongue. Examples: *glossopharyngeal* (relating to the tongue and pharynx); *glossoplasty* (plastic surgery of).

〔前綴〕**舌**　例如：舌咽的，舌成形術。

glossa *n. see* tongue.

舌

glossectomy *n.* surgical removal of the tongue, an operation usually carried out for cancer in this structure.

舌切除術　切除舌的手術。常用於治療舌癌。

Glossina *n. see* tsetse.

舌蠅屬

glossitis *n.* inflammation of the tongue. This can be caused by anaemia, candidiasis, vitamin deficiency, or lichen planus.

舌炎　舌的炎症。可因貧血、念珠菌病、維生素缺乏或扁平苔蘚引起。

glossolalia *n.* nonsense speech that mimics normal speech in that it is appropriately formed into an imitation of syllables, words, and sentences. It can be uttered in *trance states and during sleep.

癔語　毫無意義的言語。患者模仿近乎正常的音節、單詞和句子說話，但不可理解。這種言語能在恍惚狀態和睡眠時說出來。

glossopharyngeal nerve the ninth *cranial nerve (IX), which supplies motor fibres to part of the pharynx and to the parotid salivary glands and sensory fibres to the posterior third of the tongue and the soft palate.

舌咽神經 第九腦神經(Ⅸ)。其運動纖維佈於部分咽部和腮腺，感覺纖維佈於舌的後三分之一部分和軟腭。

glossoplegia *n.* paralysis of the tongue.

舌癱瘓 舌麻痺。

glottis *n.* the space between the two *vocal cords. The term is often applied to the vocal cords themselves or to that part of the larynx associated with the production of sound.

聲門 兩條聲帶之間的空隙。此詞亦常指聲帶本身或指喉的發聲部分。

gluc- (gluco-) *prefix denoting* glucose. Example: *glucosuria* (urinary excretion of).

〔前綴〕 **糖** 指葡萄糖。例如糖尿。

glucagon *n.* a hormone, produced by the pancreas, that causes an increase in the blood sugar level and thus has an effect opposite to that of *insulin. Glucagon is administered by injection to counteract diabetic *hypoglycaemia.

高血糖素 由胰臟產生的一種激素。導致昇高血糖水平，因而具有與胰島素相反的作用。高血糖素用於對抗糖尿病的血糖過少。注射用。

glucocorticoid *n. see* corticosteroid.

糖皮質激素

glucokinase *n.* an enzyme, found in the liver, that catalyses the conversion of glucose to glucose-6-phosphate. This is the first stage of *glycolysis.

葡萄糖激酶 肝內的一種酶。催化葡萄糖轉變爲6-磷酸葡萄糖。這是糖酵解的第一個步驟。

gluconeogenesis *n.* the biochemical process in which glucose, an important source of energy, is synthesized from non-carbohydrate sources, such as amino acids. Gluconeogenesis occurs mainly in the liver and kidney and meets the needs of the body for glucose when carbohydrate is not available in sufficient amounts in the diet.

糖原異生 由非糖物質(如氨基酸)合成葡萄糖(能量的一個重要來源)的生化過程。糖原異生主要在肝和腎內進行，在遇到飲食中缺少足夠量的糖類，而體內需要葡萄糖時發生。

glucosamine *n.* the amino sugar of glucose, i.e. glucose in which the hydroxyl group is replaced by an amino group. Glucosamine is a component of *mucopolysaccharides and *glycoproteins: for example, hyaluronic acid, a mucopolysaccharide found in synovial fluid, and *heparin.

葡糖氨 氨基葡萄糖。係葡萄糖的羥基被氨基所替代。葡糖氨是黏多糖和糖蛋白的一個成分，如透明質酸(在滑液中見到的一種黏多糖)和肝素。

glucose (dextrose) *n.* a simple sugar containing six carbon atoms (a hexose). Glucose is an important source of energy in the body and the sole source of energy for the brain. Free glucose is not found in many foods (grapes are an exception); however, glucose is one of the constituents of both sucrose and starch, both of which yield glucose after digestion. Glucose is stored in the body in the form of *glycogen. The concentration of glucose in the blood is maintained at around 5 mmol/l by a variety of hormones, principally *insulin and *glucagon. If the blood-glucose concentration falls below this level neurological and other symptoms may result (*see* hypoglycaemia). Conversely, if the blood-glucose level is raised above its normal level, to 10 mmol/l, the condition of *hyperglycaemia develops. This is a symptom of *diabetes mellitus.

葡萄糖（右旋糖） 一種含有六個碳原子的糖（己糖）。葡萄糖是身體能量的重要來源，並是腦能量的唯一來源。在許多食物內並無游離的葡萄糖（葡萄例外），但葡萄糖是蔗糖和澱粉的一個成分，當它們被消化後即產生葡萄糖。葡萄糖以糖原的形式貯存於體內。血液中葡萄糖的濃度受幾種激素——主要是胰島素和高血糖素調節，維持在5mmol/l左右。血糖濃度低於此水平會出現神經方面的或其他的症狀。相反，如血糖濃度高於此水平到達10 mmol/l，則將呈現高血糖症。這是糖尿病的一種症狀。

glucose tolerance test a test used in the diagnosis of *diabetes mellitus. A quantity of glucose is given to the patient by mouth, after a period of fasting, and the concentration of sugar in the blood and urine is estimated at regular intervals during the next few hours. These readings indicate the ability of the patient's body to utilize glucose.

葡萄糖耐量測驗 一種用於診斷糖尿病的試驗。在禁食一段時間後給病人口服一定量的葡萄糖，在服後數小時內每隔規定的時間測量血和尿中的糖濃度，所得的曲線代表病人體內利用葡萄糖的能力。

glucoside *n. see* glycoside.

葡萄糖苷

glucuronic acid a sugar acid derived from glucose. Glucuronic acid is an important constituent of *chondroitin sulphate (found in cartilage) and *hyaluronic acid (found in synovial fluid).

葡萄糖醛酸 由葡萄糖衍生的一種糖酸。葡萄糖醛酸是硫酸軟骨素（見於軟骨中）和透明質酸（見於滑液中）的重要成分。

glutamate dehydrogenase (glutamic acid dehydrogenase) an important enzyme involved in the *deamination of amino acids.

穀氨酸脫氫酶 催化氨基酸脫氨基作用的一種重要的酶。

glutamic acid (glutamate) *see* amino acid.

穀氨酸

glutamic oxaloacetic transaminase (GOT) an enzyme involved in the

穀氨酸草醯乙酸轉氨酶（穀草轉氨酶） 催化氨

*transamination of amino acids. This enzyme is present in blood serum (*serum GOT, SGOT*); measurement of SGOT may be used in the diagnosis of acute *myocardial infarction and acute liver disease.

基酸氨基轉移的一種酶。這種酶存在於血漿中（血漿穀草轉氨酶），測量其在血漿中的濃度以診斷急性心肌梗塞和急性肝病。

glutamic pyruvic transaminase (GPT) an enzyme involved in the *transamination of amino acids. High levels of this enzyme are found in the liver, and measurement of GPT in the serum (*serum GPT, SGPT*) is of use in the diagnosis and study of acute liver disease.

穀氨酸丙酮酸轉氨酶（穀丙轉氨酶） 催化氨基酸氨基轉移的一種酶。這種酶在肝內的濃度高。測量血漿中穀丙轉氨酶的濃度，用以診斷和研究急性肝病。

glutaminase *n.* an enzyme, found in the kidney, that catalyses the breakdown of the amino acid glutamine to ammonia and glutamic acid: a stage in the production of urea.

穀氨醯胺酶 在腎內見到的一種酶。這種酶催化穀氨醯胺分解爲氨和穀氨酸。這是產生尿素的一個步驟。

glutamine *n. see* amino acid.

穀氨醯胺

glutathione *n.* a peptide containing the amino acids glutamic acid, cysteine, and glycine. It functions as a *coenzyme in several oxidation-reduction reactions.

穀胱甘肽 含有穀氨酸、半胱氨酸和甘氨酸的一種肽。在某幾種氧化-還原反應中起輔酶作用。

glutelin *n.* one of a group of simple proteins found in plants and soluble only in dilute acids and bases. An example is *glutenin*, found in wheat (*see* gluten).

穀蛋白 植物中一類單純蛋白質的一種。僅溶於稀酸和稀鹼中。如小麥中的麥穀蛋白。

gluten *n.* a mixture of the two proteins *gliadin* and *glutenin*. Gluten is present in wheat and rye and is important for its baking properties: when mixed with water it becomes sticky and enables air to be trapped and dough to be formed. Sensitivity to gluten leads to *coeliac disease in children.

麸質 丙種蛋白質——麥膠蛋白和麥穀蛋白的混合物。麸質存在於小麥和黑麥中，它有一種重要特性：用水混合後即成爲黏性的、含有空氣的麵團，故適於烘烤。對麸質敏感的兒童可致腹部疾患。

glutethimide *n.* a drug used to treat insomnia and other sleep disturbances (*see* hypnotic). It is administered by mouth. Side-effects can include nausea, mental excitement, and skin rashes, and prolonged use may lead to dependence of the *barbiturate type. Trade name: **Doriden**.

格魯米特 一種用於治療失眠或其他睡眠障礙的藥物。口服。副作用有噁心、精神興奮和皮疹。長期使用可導致與巴比妥類藥物同樣的賴藥性。商品名：導眠能。

gluteus *n.* one of three paired muscles of the buttocks (*gluteus maximus*, *gluteus medius* and *gluteus minimus*). They are responsible for movements of the thigh. **—gluteal** *adj.*

臀肌 臀部三對肌肉之一（臀大肌、臀中肌、臀小肌）。臀肌司大腿的運動。

glyc- (glyco-) *prefix denoting* sugar.

〔前綴〕 **糖**

glyceride *n.* a *lipid consisting of glycerol (an alcohol) combined with one or more fatty acids. *See also* triglyceride.

甘油酯 由甘油（一種醇）與一個或多個脂肪酸結合成的一種脂。

glycerin (glycerol) *n.* a clear viscous liquid obtained by hydrolysis of fats and mixed oils and produced as a by-product in the manufacture of soap. It is used as an *emollient in many skin preparations, as a laxative (particularly in the form of *suppositories), and as a sweetening agent in the pharmaceutical industry.

甘油 由脂肪或混合的油水解獲得的一種清澈的黏性液體。是製造肥皂過程中產生的副產品。在許多皮膚製劑中用作潤滑劑。或用作輕瀉劑（特別是製成栓劑）。在製藥工業中用作甜味劑。

glyceryl trinitrate (nitroglycerin) a drug that dilates blood vessels and is used to prevent and treat angina (*see* vasodilator). It is administered by mouth and large doses may cause flushing, headache, and fainting. Trade names: **Nitrocontin, Sustac.**

三硝酸甘油酯 一種擴張血管的藥物。用於預防和治療心絞痛。含服。大劑量可引起面部潮紅、頭痛和昏厥。

glycine *n. see* amino acid.

甘氨酸

glycocholic acid *see* bile acids.

甘氨膽酸

glycogen *n.* a carbohydrate consisting of branched chains of glucose units. Glycogen is the principal form in which carbohydrate is stored in the body: it is the counterpart of starch in plants. Glycogen is stored in the liver and muscles and may be readily broken down to glucose.

糖原 由許多葡萄糖單位的支鏈組成的碳水化合物。糖原是體內貯存糖的主要形式。糖原與植物中的澱粉極類似。糖原貯存於肝和肌肉內，可隨時分解爲葡萄糖。

glycogenesis *n.* the biochemical process, occurring chiefly in the liver and in muscle, by which glucose is converted into glycogen.

糖原生成 葡萄糖轉變爲糖原的生化過程。主要發生於肝和肌肉內。

glycogenolysis *n.* a biochemical process, occurring chiefly in the liver and in muscle, by which glycogen is broken

糖原分解 糖原分解爲1磷酸葡萄糖的生化過程。主要發生於肝和肌肉內。

down into glucose-1-phosphate. Glycogenolysis forms the first stage of *glycolysis.

糖原分解是糖酵解的第一個步驟。

glycolipid *n.* a *lipid containing a sugar molecule (usually galactose or glucose). The *cerebrosides are examples of glycolipids.

糖脂 一種含有糖分子（常是半乳糖或葡萄糖）的脂類。如腦苷脂。

glycolysis *n.* the conversion of glucose, by a series of ten enzyme-catalysed reactions, to lactic acid. Glycolysis takes place in the cytoplasm of cells and the first nine reactions (converting glucose to pyruvate) form the first stage of cellular *respiration. The process involves the production of a small amount of energy (in the form of ATP), which is used for biochemical work. The final reaction of glycolysis (converting pyruvate to lactic acid) provides energy for short periods of time when oxygen consumption exceeds demand; for example, during bursts of intense muscular activity. *See also* lactic acid.

糖酵解 葡萄糖轉變爲乳糖的過程。糖酵解的全過程包括十種酶促反應。糖酵解在細胞的胞漿中進行，其前九種反應（葡萄糖轉變爲丙酮酸）是細胞呼吸的第一個階段。在此過程中產生的少量能量（以三磷酸腺苷的形式），用於生化反應的消耗。糖酵解最後一種反應（丙酮酸轉變爲乳酸），是爲在短促的時間內氧耗急劇增加而供氧不足時提供能量。例如在肌肉劇烈活動時。

glycoprotein *n.* one of a group of compounds consisting of a protein combined with a carbohydrate (such as galactose or mannose). Examples of glycoproteins are certain enzymes, hormones, and antigens.

糖蛋白 由蛋白質和糖（如半乳糖或甘露糖）結合組成的一類化合物。例如某些酶、激素和抗原都是糖蛋白。

glycoside *n.* a compound formed by replacing the hydroxyl (–OH) group of a sugar by another group. (If the sugar is glucose the compound is known as a *glucoside*.) Glycosides found in plants include some pharmacologically important products (such as *digitalis). Other plant glycosides are natural food toxins, present in cassava, almonds, and other plant products, and may yield hydrogen cyanide if the plant is not prepared properly before eating.

糖苷 糖的羥基（—OH）被其他基團替代而形成的一種化合物。（如果此糖是葡萄糖，其形成的化合物稱爲葡萄糖苷。）在植物中發現的糖苷包括某些有重要藥理作用的製品（如毛地黃）。其他植物糖苷是天然的食物毒素，存在於木薯、杏仁或其他植物產品中，如在食用前不加以適當處理，可產生氰化氫。

glycosuria *n.* the presence of glucose in the urine in abnormally large amounts. Only very minute quantities

糖尿 尿內有異常大量的葡萄糖。在正常情況下尿內只能見到極微量的葡萄

of this sugar may be found normally in the urine. Higher levels may be associated with diabetes mellitus, kidney disease, and some other conditions.

糖。高濃度糖尿可能與糖尿病、腎病或某些其他疾病有關。

glymidine *n.* a drug that reduces the level of sugar in the blood and is used to treat diabetes. It is administered by mouth; the commonest side-effects are digestive upsets and skin reactions. Trade name: **Gondafon**.

苯磺嘧啶 一種降低血糖水平的藥物。用於治療糖尿病。口服，最常見的副作用有胃腸道不適和皮疹。

gnath- (gnatho-) *prefix denoting* the jaw. Example: *gnathoplasty* (plastic surgery of).

〔前綴〕 **頜** 如頜成形術

gnathion *n.* the lowest point of the midline of the lower jaw (mandible).

頜下點 下頜骨中線的最下點。

Gnathostoma *n.* a genus of parasitic nematodes. Adult worms are commonly found in the intestines of tigers, leopards, and dogs. The presence of the larval stage of *G. spinigerum* in man, who is not the normal host, causes a skin condition called *creeping eruption.

腭口屬 一屬寄生性線蟲。其成蟲常見於虎、豹和狗的腸內。棘腭口線蟲的正常宿主不是人類；其幼蟲侵入人的皮膚所造成的損害稱爲匐形疹。

gnotobiotic *adj.* describing germ-free conditions or a germ-free animal that has been inoculated with known microorganisms.

無菌生物的 描述處於無菌狀態的生物，或者描述接種了已知微生物的無菌動物。

goblet cell a column-shaped secretory cell found in the *epithelium of the respiratory and intestinal tracts. Goblet cells secrete the principal constituents of mucus.

杯狀細胞 一種柱形的分泌細胞。見於呼吸道和腸道的上皮內。杯狀細胞分泌黏液的主要成分。

goitre *n.* a swelling of the neck due to enlargement of the thyroid gland. This may be due to lack of dietary iodine, which is necessary for the production of thyroid hormone: the gland enlarges in an attempt to increase the output of hormone. This was the cause of *endemic goitre*, formerly common in regions where the diet lacked iodine. *Sporadic goitre* may be due to simple overgrowth (hyperplasia) of the gland or to a tumour. In *exophthalmic goitre* (Gra-

甲狀腺腫 由於甲狀腺腫大引起的頸部腫塊。可因飲食內缺乏生產甲狀腺激素所必需的碘所致。甲狀腺增大是爲了增加激素排出量。地方性甲狀腺腫以往常發生於飲食中缺碘的地區。散發性甲狀腺腫可由於腺體單純肥大（增生）或由於腫瘤所致。突眼性甲狀腺腫（格雷夫斯氏病）的腺體腫大，與腺

ves's disease) the swelling is associated with overactivity of the gland and is accompanied by other symptoms (*see* thyrotoxicosis).

體過度活動有關，並伴有其他症狀。

gold *n.* **1.** a bright yellow metal that is very malleable. In dentistry pure gold is occasionally used as a filling. Alloys are used extensively for *crowns, *inlays, and *bridges, either alone or veneered with a tooth-coloured material. Gold alloys are now only rarely used as the metal framework for partial dentures, *cobalt-chromium alloys being used instead. **2.** (in pharmacology) any of several compounds of the metal gold, used in the treatment of rheumatoid arthritis. It is administered by injection. Common side-effects include mouth ulcers, itching, blood disorders, skin reactions, and inflammation of the colon and kidneys. Trade name: **Myocrisin**.

金 ①一種延展性很强的發亮的黃色金屬。在口腔醫學，純金偶爾用作填料；其合金廣泛用作套冠、嵌體和橋體，可單獨使用，或覆蓋一層天然牙色的材料。金合金已很少用作部分托牙的金屬構架，現已用鈷-鉻合金替代。 ②（藥理學）有幾種金的化合物都可用以治療類風濕性關節炎。注射用。常見的副作用包括口腔潰瘍、瘙癢、血液病、皮膚反應以及結腸和腎的炎症。商品名：硫代蘋果酸金鈉。

Golgi apparatus a collection of vesicles and folded membranes in a cell, usually connected to the *endoplasmic reticulum. It stores and later transports the proteins manufactured in the endoplasmic reticulum. The Golgi apparatus is well developed in cells that produce secretions, e.g. pancreatic cells producing digestive enzymes.

高爾基氏體 細胞內一羣囊泡和褶膜的複合體。常與內質網相連接。在內質網內製造的蛋白質經由高爾基氏體貯存並轉運。高爾基氏體在產生分泌物的細胞（例如產生消化酶的胰細胞）內發育良好。

Golgi cells types of *neurones (nerve cells) within the central nervous system. *Golgi type I neurones* have very long axons that connect different parts of the system; *Golgi type II neurones*, also known as *microneurones*, have only short axons or sometimes none.

高爾基氏細胞 中樞神經系統內的各型神經元（神經細胞）。高爾基氏 I 型神經元具有很長的軸突，與中樞神經系統各部分相連接。高爾基氏 II 型神經元又稱爲小神經元，僅有短的軸突，或有的沒有軸突。

Golgi tendon organ *see* tendon organ.

高爾基氏腱器

Gomori's method a method of staining for the demonstration of enzymes, especially phosphatases and lipases, in histological specimens.

果莫里氏法 一種顯示組織學標本中的酶的染色法。特別是用於顯示磷酸酶和脂酶。

gomphosis *n.* a form of *synarthrosis (immovable joint) in which a conical process fits into a socket. An example is the joint between the root of a tooth and the socket in the jawbone.

釘狀嵌合 不動關節的一種形式。這種關節由一個圓錐形突起插在一個臼窩內組成。例如牙根與下頜骨牙槽之間的關節。

gonad *n.* a male or female reproductive organ, which produces the gametes. *See* ovary, testis.

性腺 產生配子的雄性或雌性生殖器官。

gonadotrophin (gonadotrophic hormone) *n.* any of several hormones synthesized and released by the pituitary gland that act on the testes or ovaries (gonads) to promote production of sex hormones and either sperm or ova. The main gonadotrophins are *follicle-stimulating hormone and *luteinizing hormone. They may be given by injection to treat infertility. *See also* chorionic gonadotrophin.

促性腺激素 作用於睾丸或卵巢（性腺）促使其產生性激素和精子或卵子的幾種激素。這些激素由垂體合成並釋放。最主要的促性腺激素是促卵泡激素和促黃體激素，可用來注射，治療不育症。

gonagra *n.* gout in the knee.

膝痛風 膝關節痛風。

goni- (gonio-) *prefix denoting* an anatomical angle or corner.

角 指解剖學的角或角度。

goniometer *n.* an instrument for measuring angles, such as those made in joint movements.

測角計 一種測量角度的儀器。如測量關節移動的測角計。

gonion *n.* the point of the angle of the lower jawbone (mandible).

下頜骨點 下頜骨角的尖端。

goniopuncture *n.* an operation for congenital glaucoma (*see* buphthalmos) to enable fluid to be drawn from the eye. Using a fine knife, an incision is made from within the eye into Schlemm's canal, at the junction of the cornea and sclera, and continued outwards until the knife appears beneath the conjunctiva. This creates a pathway for fluid to drain from the anterior chamber of the eye to the subconjunctival tissue. The tip of the knife within the eye is observed through a special contact lens.

前房角穿刺術 一種治療先天性青光眼的手術。此手術使房水得以從眼內流出。在角膜和鞏膜結合處用鋒利小刀在眼內作一切口，進入施累姆氏管，繼而向外直至刀口出現於結膜下面。這樣就建造了一個通道，使房水得以從眼的前房流入結膜下組織。手術時用一種特殊的接觸鏡片來觀察眼內的刀尖。

gonioscope *n.* a special lens used for viewing the structures around the edge of the anterior chamber of the eye (in front of the lens). These structures are

前房角鏡 一種用以觀察眼前房角周圍結構（在晶體前面）的特殊鏡片。這些結構隱藏於鞏膜後面，

hidden behind the sclera just beyond the edge of the cornea and are not accessible to direct viewing.

恰好在角膜緣之外，不易直接觀察到。

goniotomy (trabeculotomy) *n.* an operation for congenital glaucoma (*see* buphthalmos) in which a fine knife is used to make an incision into Schlemm's canal from within the eye. It is the first stage of *goniopuncture.

前房角切開術（小樑切開術） 一種用於治療先天性青光眼的手術。用一把鋒利小刀向眼內作一切口進入施累姆氏管。這是前房角穿刺的第一個步驟。

gonococcus *n.* (*pl.* **gonococci**) the causative agent of gonorrhoea: the bacterium **Neisseria gonorrhoeae*. —**gonococcal** *adj.*

淋球菌 淋病的致病菌。即淋病奈瑟氏菌。

gonocyte *n. see* germ cell.

生殖母細胞

gonorrhoea *n.* a venereal disease, caused by the bacterium *Neisseria gonorrhoeae*, that affects the genital mucous membranes of either sex. Symptoms develop about a week after infection and include pain on passing water and discharge of pus (known as *gleet*) from the penis (in men) or vagina (in women); some infected women, however, experience no symptoms. If a pregnant woman has gonorrhoea, her baby's eyes may become infected during passage through the birth canal (*see* ophthalmia neonatorum). In untreated cases, the infection may spread throughout the reproductive system, causing sterility; severe inflammation of the urethra in men can prevent passage of water (a condition known as *stricture*). Later complications include arthritis, inflammation of the heart valves (*endocarditis), and infection of the eyes, causing conjunctivitis. Treatment with sulphonamides, penicillin, or tetracycline in the early stages of the disease is usually effective. *Compare* syphilis.

淋病 由淋病奈瑟氏菌引起的一種性病。累及兩性的生殖器黏膜，感染後約一星期出現症狀，包括尿時疼痛並從陰莖（在男子）或從陰道（在女子）排膿（稱爲後淋），但也有些被感染的婦女未感到有症狀。如孕婦患有淋病，其嬰兒的眼睛可在出生時通過產道而受感染。在未經治療的病例，感染可遍及整個生殖系統而導致不育。男子的尿道有嚴重炎症時可使排尿困難（尿道狹窄）。晚期合併症包括關節炎、心臟瓣膜炎（心內膜炎），以及眼受感染引起的結膜炎。在患病早期用磺胺類藥物、青黴素或四環素治療往往奏效。

good neighbour scheme (in Britain) a voluntary experimental scheme organized by Social Service Departments of local authorities to bridge the gap in the care of the elderly between total inde-

睦鄰組合 （在英國）由地方當局社會服務部組織的一種志願的試驗性組合。這種組合爲解決老年人的照管問題，在完全可

pendence and the provision of a home help. *See also* social services.

以自理生活和需要家庭幫助的鄰居之間搭起橋樑。

goose flesh the reaction of the skin to cold or fear. The blood vessels contract and the small muscle attached to the base of each hair follicle also contracts, causing the hairs to stand up: this gives the skin an appearance of plucked goose skin. Medical name: **cutis anserina**.

鷄皮疙瘩 對冷或驚恐的皮膚反應。血管收縮，附於每個毛囊底部的細小肌肉也收縮，導致毛髮豎立，皮膚的外貌如同拔了毛的鷄（鵝）皮。醫學名：鷄（鵝）皮現象。

gorget *n.* an instrument used in the operation for removal of stones from the bladder. It is a *director or guide with a wide groove.

有槽導子 用於膽結石摘除手術的一種器械。是一種具有寬闊槽溝的導子。

gouge *n.* a curved chisel used in orthopaedic operations to cut and remove bone (see illustration).

圓鑿 骨科手術中用以切割和去除骨的一種彎曲形鑿子（見圖）。

A gouge
圓鑿

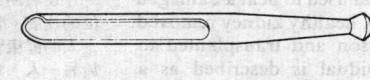

goundou (anákhré) *n.* a condition following an infection with *yaws in which the nasal processes of the upper jaw bone thicken (*see* hyperostosis) to form two large bony swellings, about 7 cm in diameter, on either side of the nose. The swellings not only obstruct the nostrils but also interfere with the field of vision. Initial symptoms include persistent headache and a bloody purulent discharge from the nose. Early cases can be treated with injections of neosalvarsan; otherwise surgical removal of the growths is necessary. Goundou occurs in central Africa and South America.

根度病（鼻骨增殖性骨膜炎） 感染雅司病後的一種病損。上頜骨的鼻突增厚，形成鼻兩側骨性腫大，直徑約 7 cm。腫塊不僅堵塞鼻孔，而且干擾視野。最初的症狀包括持續頭痛和流帶血的膿性鼻涕。早期病例可注射新胂凡納明治療，否則需要外科切除腫塊。根度病發生於中非洲和南美洲。

gout *n.* a disease in which a defect in uric acid metabolism causes an excess of the acid and its salts (urates) to accumulate in the bloodstream and the joints. It results in attacks of acute gouty arthritis and chronic destruction of the joints and deposits of urates (*tophi*) in the skin and cartilage, espe-

痛風 一種尿酸代謝紊亂的疾病。在血流和關節內有過多尿酸和尿酸鹽蓄積，導致急性痛風性關節炎發作和慢性關節組織破壞，以及皮膚、軟骨、特別是耳的軟骨內尿酸鹽（痛風石）沉積。過多的

cially of the ears. The excess of urates also damages the kidneys, in which stones may form. Treatment with drugs that increase the excretion of urates (*uricosuric drugs) or with *allopurinol, which slows their formation, has largely controlled the disease. *See also* podagra.

尿酸鹽亦使腎臟受損，形成腎結石。治療：用加快尿酸鹽排泄的藥物（促尿酸尿藥物）或減慢尿酸鹽形成的藥物——別嘌呤醇，能有效地控制痛風。

Graafian follicle a mature follicle in the ovary prior to ovulation, containing a large fluid-filled cavity that distends the surface of the ovary. The *oocyte develops inside the follicle, attached to one side.

格雷夫氏卵泡 在排卵前卵巢內的一種成熟卵泡。含有一個充滿液體的大囊腔，使卵巢表面膨脹。卵母細胞在卵泡內發育，附着於卵泡的一邊。

graft 1. *n.* any organ, tissue, or object used for *transplantation to replace a faulty part of the body. A *skin graft is a piece of skin cut from a healthy part of the body and used to heal a damaged area of skin. A healthy kidney removed from one person and transplanted to another individual is described as a *kidney* (or *renal*) *graft*. Corneal grafts are taken from the eye of a recently dead individual to repair corneal opacity (*see* keratoplasty). Artificial valve grafts are used to replace faulty heart valves. **2.** *vb.* to transplant an organ or tissue.

①移植物 任何用來移植以替代身體受損部分的器官、組織或物體。皮膚移植是割取身體健康部分的一片皮膚用來癒合受損部位的皮膚。腎移植是切除一人的健康腎臟用來移植於另一人。角膜移植是從新近死亡的人身上取下的眼角膜用來醫治角膜混濁。人工瓣膜移植物用來替換受損的心臟瓣膜。**②移植** 移植一個器官或一種組織。

graft-versus-host disease a condition that occurs following bone marrow transplantation, in which lymphocytes from the grafted marrow reject the host tissues. The skin, gut, and liver are the most severely affected. Drugs that suppress the immune reaction, such as steroids and *cyclosporin A, reduce the severity of the rejection.

移植物抗宿主病 骨髓移植術後發生的一種疾病。由於供者骨髓的淋巴細胞排斥宿主的組織所致。皮膚、腸和肝受累最爲嚴重。抑制免疫反應的藥物，如固醇類化合物和環孢菌素 A，可減輕排斥的嚴重程度。

grain *n.* a unit of mass equal to 1/7000 of a pound (avoirdupois). 1 grain = 0.0648 gram.

釐 質量的一種單位。等於 1/7000 磅（英衡制）。1 釐=0.0648 克。

gram *n.* a unit of mass equal to one thousandth of a kilogram. Symbol: g.

克 質量的一種單位。等於千分之一公斤。符號：g。

-gram *suffix denoting* a record; tracing. Example: *electrocardiogram* (record of an electrocardiograph).

〔後綴〕 **圖，像** 表示一種記錄或描記。例如心電圖（心電描記器的記錄）。

gramicidin *n.* an *antibiotic that acts against a wide range of bacteria. It is used alone or in combination with other antibiotics or antiseptics in ointments, solutions, or sprays for the treatment of infected ulcers, wounds, and burns.

短桿菌肽　一種具有廣泛抗菌作用的抗生素。單獨使用，或與其他抗生素或防腐劑聯合使用。用作軟膏、溶液劑或噴霧劑，以治療受感染的潰瘍、創傷和燒傷。

Gram's stain a method of staining bacterial cells, used as a primary means of identification. A film of bacteria spread onto a glass slide is dried and heat-fixed, stained with a violet dye, treated with decolourizer (e.g. alcohol), and then counterstained with red dye. *Gram-negative* bacteria lose the initial stain but take up the counterstain, so that they appear red microscopically. *Gram-positive* bacteria retain the initial stain, appearing violet microscopically. These staining differences are based on variations in the structure of the cell wall in the two groups.

革蘭氏染色法　染細菌細胞的一種方法。係用於鑑別細菌的一種主要手段。將細菌標本置於載玻片上塗成薄膜，晾乾並加熱固定，用紫色染料染色，經脫色劑（如酒精）處理後再用紅色染料復染。革蘭氏陰性細菌失去最初的染劑而攝取復染劑，故在顯微鏡下呈現紅色。革蘭氏陽性細菌保留最初的染劑而在顯微鏡下呈現紫色。這兩種染色差別是根據兩類不同的細胞壁結構決定的。

grand mal (major epilepsy) an epileptic fit, sometimes called the *tonic-clonic fit*. At the onset the patient falls to the ground unconscious with his muscles in a state of spasm. The lack of any respiratory movement results in a bluish discoloration of the skin and lips (cyanosis). This – the tonic phase – is replaced by convulsive movements, when the tongue may be bitten and urinary incontinence may occur (the clonic phase). Movements die away and the patient may rouse in a state of confusion, complaining of headache, or he may fall asleep. *See also* epilepsy.

癲癇大發作　一種癲癇發作。有時稱爲强直-陣攣性發作。發作時病人失去知覺，跌倒在地，肌肉處於痙攣狀態。呼吸運動受阻時，皮膚和脣變爲青紫色（發紺）。這種狀態（强直期）被抽搐運動替代（陣攣期），此時舌可被咬破，並可發生小便失禁。抽搐停止後，病人從意識模糊狀態中清醒過來，感到頭痛，或又入睡。

granular cast a cellular *cast derived from a kidney tubule. In certain kidney diseases, notably acute *glomerulonephritis, abnormal collections of renal tubular cells are shed from the kidney, often as a cast of the tubule. The casts can be observed on microscopic examination of the centrifuged deposit of a

顆粒管型　來自腎小管的一種細胞管型。在某些腎臟疾病，特別是急性腎小球腎炎，從腎小管脫落的異常積聚物，常像一種小管的模型。可用尿標本離心後取沉渣作顯微鏡檢查，以觀察管型。尿內出

specimen of urine. Their presence in the urine indicates continued activity of the disease.

現管型表示疾病在繼續活動。

granulation *n.* the growth of small rounded outgrowths, made up of small blood vessels and connective tissue, on the healing surface of a wound (when the edges do not fit closely together) or an ulcer. Granulation is a normal stage in the healing process.

肉芽 由許多小血管和結締組織構成的小圓肉團。生長於傷口癒合面（當其邊緣不能合攏時）或潰瘍上。肉芽發生是癒合的一個正常步驟。

granulocyte *n.* any of a group of white blood cells that, when stained with *Romanowsky stains, are seen to contain granules in their cytoplasm. They can be subclassified on the basis of the colour of the stained granules into *neutrophils, *eosinophils, and *basophils.

粒細胞 用羅曼諾夫斯基氏染劑可見到細胞質內含有顆粒的任何一類白細胞。粒細胞按其所染顆粒的顏色可分爲中性、嗜酸性和嗜鹼性三類。

granulocytopenia *n.* a reduction in the number of *granulocytes (a type of white cell) in the blood. *See* neutropenia.

粒細胞減少 血液中粒細胞（白細胞的一種類型）的數目減少。

granuloma *n.* (*pl.* **granulomata** or **granulomas**) a mass of *granulation tissue produced in response to chronic infection, inflammation, a foreign body, or to unknown causes. Infections giving rise to granulomata include tuberculosis, syphilis, *granuloma inguinale, *Wegener's granuloma, leprosy, and some fungal diseases, such as coccidiodomycosis. Granulomata may occur as reactions to such foreign bodies as starch and talc following surgical procedures or to some metals, such as beryllium and zirconium. Sarcoidosis and Crohn's disease are granulomatous diseases of which the causes are not known. A granuloma may occur around the apex of a tooth root as a result of inflammation or infection of its pulp. —**granulomatous** *adj.*

肉芽腫 由肉芽組織形成的腫塊。係因慢性感染、炎症或異物引起，有的病因不明。由感染引起的肉芽腫包括結核、梅毒、腹股溝肉芽腫、韋格內肉芽腫、痲瘋和某些黴菌病，如球孢子菌病。肉芽腫可由於外科處置後的澱粉或滑石粉等異物，或由於諸如鈹、鋯等金屬所引起的反應所致。肉樣瘤病和克羅恩氏病是病因未明的肉芽腫性疾病。肉芽腫可發生於牙根尖端的周圍，係由於牙髓的炎症或感染所致。

granuloma inguinale an infectious disease caused by the bacterium *Donovania granulomatis*, usually transmitted during sexual intercourse. It is marked by a pimply rash on and around the

腹股溝肉芽腫 由肉芽腫杜諾凡氏菌引起的一種感染性疾病，通常經性交傳佈。在外生殖器周圍皮膚上出現膿疱性丘疹，並形

genital organs, which develops into a granulomatous ulcer. The disease responds to treatment with tetracyclines and streptomycin.

成肉芽腫性潰瘍。本病用四環素族抗生素和鏈黴素治療有效。

granulomatosis *n.* any condition marked by multiple widespread *granulomas.

肉芽腫病 以蔓延的多發性肉芽腫爲特徵的任何一種疾患。

granulopoiesis *n.* the process of production of *granulocytes, which normally occurs in the blood-forming tissue of the *bone marrow. Granulocytes are ultimately derived from a *haemopoietic stem cell, but the earliest precursor that can be identified microscopically is the *myeloblast. This divides and passes through a series of stages of maturation termed respectively *promyelocyte, *myelocyte, and *metamyelocyte, before becoming a mature granulocyte. *See also* haemopoiesis.

粒細胞生成 粒細胞產生的過程。正常發生於骨髓的造血組織。粒細胞淵源於造血幹細胞，但在顯微鏡下可辨認的最早的前體是原粒細胞。由原粒細胞經過一系列的成熟期，分別稱爲早幼粒細胞、中幼粒細胞和晚幼粒細胞，而分化演變爲成熟的粒細胞。

graph- (grapho-) *prefix denoting* handwriting.

〔前綴〕 **書寫的** 表示與書寫有關的。

-graph *suffix denoting* an instrument that records. Example: *electrocardiograph* (instrument recording heart activity).

〔後綴〕 **描記器** 表示一種記錄儀器。例如：心電描記器（記錄心臟活動的儀器）。

graphology *n.* the study of the characteristics of handwriting to obtain indications about a person's psychological make-up or state of health. It is possible to detect certain signs of physical disease, such as fine nervous tremors or irregularity of the pulse.

筆體學 研究書寫特徵以獲得人的心理氣質或健康狀態特徵的科學。根據筆體來察知軀體疾病的某些體徵是可能的，諸如細微的神經性震顫或不整脉。

grattage *n.* the process of brushing or scraping the surface of a slowly healing ulcer or wound to stimulate healing. Grattage removes *granulation tissue, which – though a stage in the healing process – sometimes overgrows or becomes infected and therefore delays healing.

刷除術 用刷除或刮除緩慢癒合的潰瘍或傷口的表面以刺激其癒合的方法。採用刷除術去除肉芽組織。肉芽組織的發生雖然是癒合過程的一個步驟，但其有時過度生長或受感染時，可延遲癒合。

gravel *n.* small stones formed in the urinary tract. The stones usually consist of calcareous debris or aggregations of other crystalline material. The passage of gravel from the kidneys is usually

尿沙 在泌尿道內形成的小石子。這些石子常由石灰質的碎屑或其他晶體物質的聚集體組成。尿沙從腎內排出時常伴有劇痛

associated with severe pain (*ureteric colic*) and may cause blood in the urine. *See also* calculus.

（輸尿管絞痛），並可導致血尿。

Graves's disease (exophthalmic goitre) *see* thyrotoxicosis.

格雷夫斯氏病（突眼性甲狀腺腫）

gravid *adj.* pregnant.

妊娠的 懷孕的。

Grawitz tumour *see* hypernephroma.

格雷維次氏瘤

gray *n.* the *SI unit of absorbed dose of ionizing radiation, being the absorbed dose when the energy per unit mass imparted to matter by ionizing radiation is 1 joule per kilogram. It has replaced the rad. Symbol: Gy.

戈瑞 國際單位制的電離輻射吸收劑量單位。電離輻射給予物體的能量爲每千克 1 焦耳的吸收劑量時，即爲 1 戈瑞。此單位已替代拉德單位。符號：Gy。

green monkey disease *see* Marburg disease.

綠猴病

greenstick fracture an incomplete break in a long bone occurring in children, whose bones have greater flexibility. *See also* fracture.

青枝骨折 一種不完全骨折。發生於兒童的長骨。因兒童長骨有較大的韌性。

grey matter the darker coloured tissues of the central nervous system, composed mainly of the cell bodies of neurones, branching dendrites, and glial cells (*compare* white matter). In the brain grey matter forms the *cerebral cortex and the outer layer of the cerebellum; in the spinal cord the grey matter lies centrally and is surrounded by white matter.

灰質 中樞神經系統的顏色較深的組織（與白質相比)。主要由神經元的細胞體，分支的樹突和神經膠質細胞組成。在腦內的灰質形成大腦皮質和小腦外層；在脊髓內灰質居於中央，四周被白質包圍。

gripe *n.* severe abdominal pain (*see* colic).

腸絞痛 嚴重的腹痛。

griseofulvin *n.* an *antibiotic administered by mouth to treat fungal infections of the hair, skin, and nails, such as ringworm. Mild and temporary side-effects such as headache, skin rashes, and digestive upsets may occur. Trade names: **Fulcin, Grisovin**.

灰黃黴素 一種治療頭髮、皮膚和指甲的黴菌感染（如癬菌病）的口服抗生素。可有暫時的輕微副作用，如頭痛、皮疹和胃腸道不適。

groin *n.* the external depression on the front of the body that marks the junction of the abdomen with either of the thighs. *See also* inguinal.

腹股溝 在身體前面腹部與兩側大腿相接處呈現的外表凹陷。

grommet *n.* a double-cuffed tube that is inserted in the eardrum to allow drainage of fluid from the middle ear in secretory *otitis media (glue ear).

通氣管　一種雙套囊的管子。用以插入鼓膜內引流分泌性中耳炎的液體。

ground substance the matrix of *connective tissue, in which various cells and fibres are embedded.

基質　結締組織的細胞間質。在其中包埋着各種細胞和纖維。

group practice *see* general practitioner.

聯合診所

group therapy 1. (group psychotherapy) *psychotherapy involving at least two patients and a therapist. The patients are encouraged to understand and analyse their own and one another's problems. *See also* encounter group, psychodrama. **2.** therapy in which people with the same problem, such as *alcoholism, meet and discuss together their difficulties and possible ways of overcoming them.

集體治療　①（集體心理治療）至少有兩個病人和一個治療師在一起進行的心理治療。鼓勵病人互相瞭解和分析自已的和他人的問題。②對病情相同（如酒精中毒）的病人在一起進行的治療。病人聚在一起討論他們的困難和克服困難的可能途徑。

growth hormone (GH, somatotrophin) a hormone, synthesized and stored in the anterior pituitary gland, that promotes growth of the long bones in the limbs and increases protein synthesis. Excessive production of growth hormone results in *gigantism before puberty and *acromegaly in adults. Lack of growth hormone in children causes *dwarfism.

生長激素（GH）　在垂體前葉內合成並貯藏的一種激素。此激素促進四肢長骨的生長和增加蛋白質的合成。生長激素產生過多導致青春期前的巨人症和成人的肢端巨大症。在兒童時缺少生長激素會引起侏儒症。

grumous *adj.* coarse; lumpy; clotted; often used to describe the appearance of the centre of wounds or diseased cells or the surface of a bacterial culture.

凝塊的　粗糙的，結塊的，凝結的。常用於描述創傷或患病細胞中央部分，或細菌培養基表面的外貌。

guaiphenesin *n.* an *expectorant used in cough mixtures and tablets.

癒創木酚甘油醚　一種祛痰劑。用作止嗽合劑或片劑。

guanethidine *n.* a drug that is used to reduce high blood pressure (*see* sympatholytic). It is administered by mouth; common side-effects are diarrhoea, faintness, and dizziness. Trade name: **Ismelin**.

胍乙啶　一種降血壓藥物。口服。副作用：常有腹瀉、乏力和暈眩。

guanine *n.* one of the nitrogen-containing bases (*see* purine) that occurs in the nucleic acids DNA and RNA.

鳥嘌呤 含氮鹼基中的一種。存在於脫氧核糖核酸和核糖核酸的核酸中。

guanosine *n.* a compound containing guanine and the sugar ribose. *See also* nucleotide.

鳥苷 一種含有鳥嘌呤和核糖的化合物。

gubernaculum *n.* (*pl.* **gubernacula**) either of a pair of fibrous strands of tissue that connect the gonads to the inguinal region in the fetus. In the male they guide and possibly move the testes into the scrotum before birth. In the female the ovaries descend only slightly within the abdominal cavity and the gubernacula persist as the round ligaments connecting the ovaries and uterus (womb) to the abdominal wall.

引帶 在胚胎期連接生殖腺於腹股溝區的一對索狀纖維組織。在男性出生前引帶引導睾丸並可能牽拉睾丸進入陰囊中。在女性卵巢於腹腔內僅稍微下降，其引帶成爲連接卵巢和子宮於腹壁的圓韌帶。

Guillain-Barré syndrome a disease of the peripheral nerves in which there is numbness and weakness in the limbs. It usually develops 10–20 days after a respiratory infection that provokes an allergic response in the peripheral nerves. A rapidly progressive form of the disease is called *Landry's paralysis*. *See* polyradiculitis.

格-巴二氏綜合徵 周圍神經的一種疾病。具有四肢麻木無力的症狀。常在某次呼吸系統感染後10～20天發生，係感染引起周圍神經的一種變態反應。此病的一種急進性形式稱爲蘭德里氏麻痹。

guillotine *n.* a surgical instrument used for removing the tonsils. It is loop-shaped and contains a sliding knife blade (see illustration).

鍘除刀 用於切除扁桃體的一種外科器械，圈環狀，並裝有滑動的刀片（見圖）。

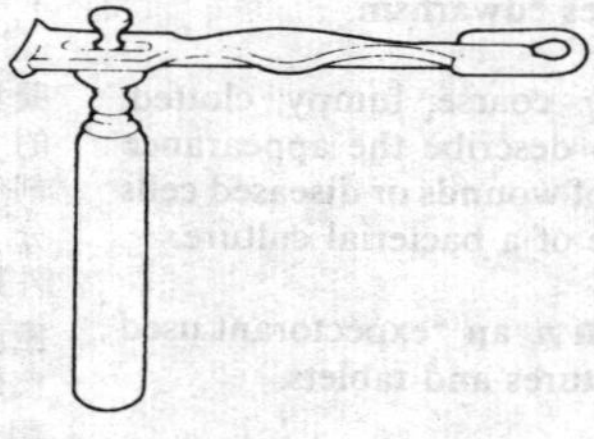

A tonsil guillotine
扁桃體鍘除刀

guinea worm a nematode worm, *Dracunculus medinensis*, that is a parasite of man. The white threadlike adult female, 60–120 cm long, lives in the

幾內亞蟲 麥地那龍線蟲。是人類的一種寄生蟲。線狀的白色雌性成蟲長60～120 cm，寄生於皮

connective tissues beneath the skin. It releases its larvae into a large blister on the legs or arms; when the limbs are immersed in water the larvae escape and are subsequently eaten by tiny water fleas (*Cyclops*), in which their development continues. The disease *dracontiasis results from drinking water contaminated with *Cyclops*.

下結締組織內，其幼蟲在小腿或手臂上形成一個大型疱狀突起。當人的肢體浸入水中時，幼蟲即逸出，繼而被小的水蚤（劍水蚤）吞食，並在其體內繼續發育。麥地那龍線蟲病係飲了受劍水蚤污染的水所致。

gullet *n.* *see* oesophagus.

食管

gum *n.* (in anatomy) *see* gingiva.

齦 （解剖學）

gumboil *n.* the opening on the surface of the gum of a chronic abscess associated with the roots of a tooth. It may be accompanied by varying degrees of swelling, pain, and discharge and is more often related to deciduous than to permanent teeth.

齦膿腫 開口於牙齦表面與牙根相通的慢性膿腫。有不同程度的腫脹和疼痛，膿溢也多少不等。在乳齒較在恒齒更爲常見。

gumma *n.* a small soft tumour, characteristic of the tertiary stage of *syphilis, that occurs in connective tissue, the liver, brain, testes, heart, or bone.

梅毒瘤，樹膠樣腫 一種小的軟瘤。爲第三期梅毒的特徵。發生於結締組織、肝、腦、睪丸、心和骨內。

gumshield *n.* a soft flexible cover that fits over the teeth for protection in contact sports. The best type is specially made to fit the individual.

護齒 一種柔軟的套在牙齒上的掩護物。在交手運動項目中作保護用。最好的護齒是爲適合個人而特製的。

gustation *n.* the sense of taste or the act of tasting.

味覺 味道的感覺或嚐味。

gustatory *adj.* relating to the sense of taste or to the organs of taste.

味覺的 有關味覺或味覺器官的。

gut *n.* **1.** *see* intestine. **2.** *see* catgut.

①腸 ②腸線

Guthrie test examination of blood obtained from a heel stab to exclude the presence of *phenylketonuria. This rare metabolic disorder (estimated incidence 1/20,000) has severe consequences in terms of mental handicap unless the child receives a special diet from an early age.

加斯里氏試驗 排除苯丙酮尿症的試驗。用針刺足後跟採血檢查。這種罕見的代謝缺陷（估計發生率爲 1/20 000）能產生嚴重精神障礙。在幼年時給兒童一種特殊的飲食即可避免。

gutta *n.* (*pl.* **guttae**) (in pharmacy) a drop. Drops are the form in which medicines are applied to the eyes and ears.

滴 （調劑學）一種滴劑。在醫藥上滴劑是用於眼和耳的一種劑型。

gutta percha the juice of an evergreen Malaysian tree, which is hard at room temperature but becomes soft and elastic when heated in boiling water. On cooling gutta percha will retain any deformity imparted to it when hot; thus it was used in dentistry as an impression material and as a temporary filling material. It has been superseded by better materials but is still used as the core of *root fillings.

馬來乳膠 馬來西亞的一種常綠樹的膠汁。這種乳膠在室溫時是堅硬的，而在沸水中加熱則變得柔軟而有彈性。乳膠冷却後保持其加熱時所具有的形狀，這樣就可用於口腔醫學作爲印模材料和暫時充塡的材料。這種乳膠現已被更好的材料所替代，但仍用於作爲根管充塡的塡料。

guttate *adj.* describing lesions in the skin that are shaped like drops.

滴狀的 描述形狀如滴狀的皮膚損害。

gyn- (gyno-, gynaec(o)-) *prefix denoting* women or the female reproductive organs.

〔前綴〕 **女性** 表示女子或女性生殖器官。

gynaecology *n.* the study of diseases of women and girls, particularly those affecting the female reproductive system. *Compare* obstetrics. **—gynaecological** *adj.* **—gynaecologist** *n.*

婦科學 研究婦女和少女的疾病，特別是累及女性生殖系統的疾病的學科。

gynaecomastia *n.* enlargement of the breasts in the male, due either to hormone imbalance or to hormone therapy.

男子女性型乳房 男子乳房增大。若不是由於激素失衡所致，就是由於激素治療所致。

gypsum *n. see* plaster of Paris.

石膏

gyr- (gyro-) *prefix denoting* **1.** a gyrus. **2.** a ring or circle.

〔前綴〕 ①**回** 腦回。
②**環** 圓環或圈。

gyrus *n.* (*pl.* **gyri**) a raised convolution of the *cerebral cortex, between two sulci (clefts).

腦回 大腦皮層兩條裂溝（裂口）之間高起的回旋。

H

habituation *n.* (in pharmacology) the condition of being psychologically dependent on a drug, following repeated consumption, marked by a craving for the drug if it is withdrawn. *See also* dependence.

習慣性 在藥理學中，指反復使用某種藥物後，在生理上產生依賴性的狀態。以一旦停藥時就渴望得到該藥爲特徵。

habitus *n.* an individual's general physical appearance, especially when this is associated with a constitutional tendency to a particular disease.

體型 一個人身體的一般外貌。尤指與患某種病的體質有聯繫者。

haem *n.* an iron-containing compound (a *porphyrin) that combines with the protein globin to form *haemoglobin, found in the red blood cells.

血紅素 一種含鐵化合物，與珠蛋白結合形成血紅蛋白。見於紅細胞中。

haem- (haema-, haemo-, haemat(o)-) *prefix denoting* blood. Examples: *haematogenesis* (formation of); *haemophobia* (fear of).

〔前綴〕 **血** 例如：造血（血的形成），血恐怖（對血的恐懼）。

haemangioblastoma (Lindau's tumour) *n.* a tumour of the brain or spinal cord arising in the blood vessels of the meninges or brain. It is often associated with *phaeochromocytoma and *syringomyelia. *See also* von Hippel-Lindau disease.

成血管細胞瘤 發生於腦膜或腦血管的腦脊髓腫瘤。常伴有嗜鉻細胞瘤和脊髓空洞症。

haemangioma *n.* a benign tumour of blood vessels. It often appears on the skin as a type of birthmark (*see* naevus). For example, a *strawberry haemangioma* is seen in newborn babies and infants, usually on the face; it is red and may attain a very large size, but usually disappears spontaneously within the first year of life. *Senile haemangiomas* occur in the elderly. *See also* angioma.

血管瘤 一種血管的良性腫瘤。常見於皮膚上，爲胎痣的一種類型。例如：草莓狀血管瘤，常見於新生兒及嬰兒面部，色紅，可極大，但在生後一年內往往自行消失。老年性血管瘤發生於較年長者。

Haemaphysalis *n.* a genus of hard *ticks. Certain species transmit tick *typhus in the Old World; *H. spinigera* transmits the virus causing *Kyasanur Forest disease in India.

血蜱屬 硬蜱的一屬。在歐洲，其某些種可傳播蜱傳性傷寒。在印度，距刺血蜱可傳播病毒，引起夸賽納森林病。

haemarthrosis *n.* joint pain and swelling caused by bleeding into a joint. This may follow injury or may occur spontaneously in a disease of the blood, such as *haemophilia. Treatment is by immobilization, cold compresses, and correction of the blood disorder (if present). Removal of blood from the joint may relieve the pain.

關節積血 因出血血液進入關節內所致的關節疼痛和腫脹。本病可發生於損傷後，在血液病中也可自然發生，如血友病時。治療包括固定關節、冷敷，有血液病者治療該病。排除關節中積血可減輕疼痛。

haematemesis *n.* the act of vomiting blood. The blood may have been swallowed (e.g. following nosebleed or tonsillectomy) but more often arises from bleeding in the oesophagus, stomach, or duodenum. Common causes are gastric and duodenal ulcers, gastritis brought on by irritating food or drink, and varicose veins in the oesophagus. If much blood is lost, it is usually replaced by blood transfusion.

嘔血 嘔吐血液的動作。血液可被吞嚥（例如：鼻出血或扁桃體切除後），而食道、胃或十二指腸出血時較常發生嘔血。常見的原因有胃和十二指腸潰瘍、飲食刺激引起的胃炎以及食道靜脈曲張。如失血過多，往往需予輸血。

haemathidrosis (haematidrosis) *n. see* haematohidrosis.

血汗症

haematin *n.* a chemical derivative of *haemoglobin formed by removal of the protein part of the molecule and oxidation of the iron atom from the ferrous to the ferric form.

高鐵血紅素 血紅蛋白的化學衍生物。通過去掉血紅蛋白分子中的蛋白部分，以及將鐵原子由亞鐵氧化成高鐵所形成。

haematinic *n.* a drug that increases the amount of *haemoglobin in the blood, e.g. ferrous sulphate and other iron-containing compounds. Haematinics are used, often in combination with vitamins and *folic acid, to prevent and treat anaemia due to iron deficiency. They are used particularly to prevent anaemia during pregnancy. Digestive disturbances sometimes occur with haematinics.

補血藥 增加血液中血紅蛋白含量的藥物。例如硫酸亞鐵以及其他含鐵化合物。補血藥通常與維生素類及葉酸聯合使用，用於預防和治療缺鐵性貧血。本藥尤多用於預防妊娠期貧血。服用補血藥有時可發生消化紊亂。

haematocoele *n.* a swelling caused by leakage of blood into a cavity, especially that of the membrane overlying the front and sides of the testis. A *parametric* (*pelvic*) *haematocoele* is a swelling near the womb formed by the escape of blood, usually from a Fallopian tube in ectopic pregnancy.

體腔積血（鞘膜積血） 血液漏入腔內引起的一種腫脹。尤其指睾丸鞘膜的積血。子宮旁（盆腔）積血，通常是由於輸卵管異位妊娠，血液漏出，在子宮附近形成的一種腫脹。

haematocolpos *n.* the accumulation of menstrual blood in the vagina because the hymen at the entrance to the vagina lacks an opening. *See* cryptomenorrhoea.

陰道積血 由於陰道入口處的處女膜閉鎖，月經血積聚於陰道內所致。

haematocrit *n. see* packed cell volume.

紅細胞壓積

haematocyst *n.* a cyst containing blood.

血囊腫 內含血液的囊腫。

haematogenous (haematogenic) *adj.* **1.** relating to the production of blood or its constituents; haematopoietic. **2.** produced by, originating in, or carried by the blood.

①**生血的** 與血或血液成分的產生有關的。 ②**血源性的** 由血產生的，起源於血的或經血流的。

haematohidrosis (haemathidrosis, haematidrosis) *n.* the secretion of sweat containing blood.

血汗症 排出含血的汗液。

haematology *n.* the study of blood and blood-forming tissues and the disorders associated with them. —**haematological** *adj.* —**haematologist** *n.*

血液學 研究血液和造血組織及其疾病的學科。

haematoma *n.* an accumulation of blood within the tissues that clots to form a solid swelling. Injury, disease of the blood vessels, or a clotting disorder of the blood are the usual causative factors. An *intracranial haematoma* causes symptoms by compressing the brain and by raising the pressure within the skull. Injury to the head may tear the middle meningeal artery, giving rise to a rapidly accumulating *extradural haematoma* requiring urgent surgical treatment. In elderly people a relatively slight head injury may tear the veins where they cross the space beneath the dura, giving rise to a *subdural haematoma.* Excellent results are obtained by surgical treatment. An *intracerebral haematoma* may be a consequence of severe head injury but is more often due to *atherosclerosis of the cerebral arteries and high blood pressure. *See also* perianal haematoma.

血腫 血液在組織內蓄積，凝結成一固性腫塊。血管病、凝血障礙是引起本病的常見因素。顱內血腫能引起腦受壓和顱內壓升高的症狀。頭部損傷可撕破腦膜中動脉，迅速引起血液積聚而形成硬膜外血腫。本病需要緊急外科治療。對老年人，相對輕度的頭部損傷，可撕破穿過硬腦膜下部的靜脉，引起硬腦膜下血腫。外科治療可獲顯效。顱內血腫可能是嚴重的頭部外傷的結果。但較常見的是由於腦動脉硬化和高血壓。

haematometra *n.* **1.** accumulation of menstrual blood in the womb. **2.** abnormally copious bleeding in the womb.

子宮積血 ①月經血蓄積於子宮內。 ②子宮內異常的大量出血。

haematomyelia *n.* bleeding into the tissue of the spinal cord. This has been thought to be the cause of acutely developing symptoms that mimic *syringomyelia.

脊髓出血 出血時血液進入脊髓組織內。現認爲本病是假性脊髓空洞症症狀急性發展的原因。

haematopoiesis *n. see* haemopoiesis.

血細胞生成

haematoporphyrin *n.* a type of *porphyrin produced during the metabolism of haemoglobin.

血卟啉 卟啉的一種類型。產生於血紅蛋白代謝過程中。

haematosalpinx (haemosalpinx) *n.* the accumulation of menstrual blood in the *Fallopian tubes.

輸卵管積血 經血蓄積於輸卵管內。

haematoxylin *n.* a colourless crystalline compound extracted from logwood (*Haematoxylon campechianum*) and used in various histological stains. When oxidized haematoxylin is converted to *haematein*, which imparts a blue colour to certain parts of cells, especially cell nuclei. *Heidenhain's iron haematoxylin* is used to stain sections that are to be photographed, since it gives great clarity at high magnification.

蘇木精 一種無色的晶狀化合物。由洋蘇木提取，用於各種組織學染色。蘇木精可氧化成氧化蘇木精，它可使細胞的某些部分染成藍色，尤其是細胞核部分。由於海登海恩氏鐵蘇木精在高倍放大下呈現高的清晰度，故常用於染攝影用的切片。

haematuria *n.* the presence of blood in the urine. The blood may come from the kidneys, one or both ureters, the bladder, or the urethra, as a result of injury or disease.

血尿 尿中存有血液。血液可來自腎、一側或兩側輸尿管、膀胱或尿道，因損傷或疾病所致。

haemin *n.* a chemical derivative of haemoglobin formed by removal of the protein part of the molecule, oxidation of the iron atom, and combination with an acid to form a salt (*compare* haematin). *Chlorohaemin* forms characteristic crystals, the identification of which provides the basis of a chemical test for blood stains.

氧化血紅素 血紅蛋白的化學衍生物。通過去掉血紅蛋白分子中的蛋白部分，使鐵原子氧化，以及與酸結合成鹽形成的。氯化血紅素形成有特徵性的晶體，辨認其晶體特徵爲血痕（法醫）化驗的基礎。

haemo- *prefix. see* haem-.

〔前綴〕 **血**

haemochromatosis (bronze diabetes, iron-storage disease) *n.* a hereditary disorder in which there is excessive absorption and storage of iron. This leads to damage and functional impairment of many organs, including the liver, pancreas, and endocrine glands. The main features are a bronze colour of the skin, diabetes, and liver failure. Iron may be removed from the body by blood letting or an iron *chelating agent may be administered. *Compare* haemosiderosis.

血色素沉着症（青銅色糖尿病，鐵貯積病） 鐵貯積過多的一種遺傳性疾病。它可引起許多器官包括肝、胰和內分泌腺損傷和功能降低。本症的主要特徵是：青銅色皮膚、糖尿病和肝功能衰竭。可通過放血或給予鐵螯合劑使鐵從體內排出。

haemoconcentration *n.* an increase in the proportion of red blood cells relative to the plasma, brought about by a decrease in the volume of plasma. Haemoconcentration may occur in any condition in which there is a severe loss of water from the body. *Compare* haemodilution.

血濃縮 由於血漿容量下降，造成紅細胞與血漿之比相對增加。血濃縮可發生於任何身體失水的情况。

haemocytoblast *n. Obsolete.* a type of cell, found in the bone marrow, that was thought by early microscopists to be the ultimate precursor from which all blood cells were derived. *See also* haemopoietic stem cell.

成血細胞 （廢用詞）見於骨髓中的一種類型的細胞。早期的組織學者認爲，它是最原始的血母細胞，由它衍生出所有的血細胞。

haemocytometer *n.* a special glass chamber of known volume into which diluted blood is introduced. The numbers of the various blood cells present are then counted visually, through a microscope. Haemocytometers have been largely replaced by electronic cell counters.

血細胞計數器 已知容積的特製玻璃池。將稀釋的血液滴入池內，各種血細胞的數目就可顯示出來，而後通過顯微鏡，以目視計數。血細胞計數器已基本被電子計數器所取代。

haemodialysis *n.* a technique of removing waste materials or poisons from the blood using the principle of *dialysis. Haemodialysis is performed on patients whose kidneys have ceased to function; the process takes place in an *artificial kidney*, or *dialyser*. A stream of blood taken from an artery is circulated through the dialyser on one side of a semipermeable membrane, while a solution of similar electrolytic composition to the patient's blood circulates on the other side. Water and waste products from the patient's blood filter through the membrane, whose pores are too small to allow passage of blood cells and proteins. The purified blood is then returned to the patient's body through a vein.

血液透析 運用透析的原理排除血中廢物和毒物的一種技術。血液透析用於兩側腎已喪失功能的病人，透析通過人工腎或透析器進行。方法是引出一動脉血流，使在透析器中半透膜的一側循環，而與病人的血液電解質成分類似的溶液，在半透膜的另一側循環。病人血中的水分和廢物通過此膜濾過。由於膜孔很小，血細胞和蛋白質不能通過，然後純淨的血經靜脉回流至病人體內。

haemodilution *n.* a decrease in the proportion of red blood cells relative to the plasma, brought about by an increase in the total volume of plasma. This may occur in a variety of conditions, including pregnancy and enlarge-

血液稀釋 由於血漿總容量的增加，血細胞與血漿之比相對下降。血液稀釋可發生於各種情況，包括妊娠和脾腫大。

ment of the spleen. *Compare* haemoconcentration.

haemoglobin *n.* a substance contained within the red blood cells (*erythrocytes) and responsible for their colour, composed of the pigment *haem* (an iron-containing *porphyrin) linked to the protein *globin*. Haemoglobin has the unique property of combining reversibly with oxygen and is the medium by which oxygen is transported within the body. It takes up oxygen as blood passes through the lungs and releases it as blood passes through the tissues. Blood normally contains 12–18 g/dl of haemoglobin. *See also* oxyhaemoglobin.

血紅蛋白 存在於紅細胞內，決定紅細胞顏色的一種物質。它由血色素（一種含鐵卟啉）與珠蛋白結合組成。血紅蛋白具有獨特的性質，即與氧呈可逆性結合，在體內作爲輸送氧的媒介。當血流通過肺部時血紅蛋白即吸取氧，而當通過組織時則將氧釋放出來。正常血紅蛋白含量爲12～18*g*/dℓ。

haemoglobinometer *n.* an instrument for determining the concentration of *haemoglobin in a sample of blood, which is a measure of its oxygen-carrying power.

血紅蛋白計 測定血標本中血紅蛋白濃度的儀器，也是測定血紅蛋白攜氧能力的儀器。

haemoglobinopathy *n.* any of a group of inherited diseases, including *thalassaemia and *sickle-cell disease, in which there is an abnormality in the production of haemoglobin.

血紅蛋白病 爲一組遺傳性疾病。包括地中海貧血、鐮狀細胞病等。本組疾病中血紅蛋白生成異常。

haemoglobinuria *n.* the presence in the urine of free haemoglobin. Haemoglobinuria occurs if haemoglobin, released from disintegrating red blood cells, cannot be taken up rapidly enough by blood proteins. The condition sometimes follows strenuous exercise. It is also associated with certain infectious diseases (such as blackwater fever), ingestion of certain chemicals (such as arsenic), and injury.

血紅蛋白尿 指尿中出現游離的血紅蛋白。當血紅蛋白從破壞的紅細胞中大量釋放出來，而且不能快速地與足夠的血漿蛋白結合時，即可發生血紅蛋白尿。這種病症有時發生於劇烈的鍛煉以後。也可伴發於某些傳染病（如黑尿熱）、攝入某些化學製品（如砷）和損傷等。

haemogram *n.* the results of a routine blood test, including an estimate of the blood haemoglobin level, the *packed cell volume, and the numbers of red and white blood cells (*see* blood count). Any abnormalities seen in microscopic examination of the blood are also noted.

血像 血常規檢驗的結果。包括血紅蛋白值的測定、血細胞壓積以及白細胞計數。並記錄血液顯微鏡檢查中發現的任何異常情況。

haemolysin *n.* a substance capable of bringing about destruction of red blood cells (*haemolysis). It may be an antibody or a bacterial toxin.

溶血素 能引起紅細胞破壞的一種物質。它可能是一種抗體或一種毒素。

haemolysis *n.* the destruction of red blood cells (*erythrocytes). Within the body, haemolysis may result from defects within the red cells or from poisoning, infection, or the action of antibodies in mismatched blood transfusions and it leads to anaemia. Haemolysis of blood specimens may result from unsatisfactory collection or storage or be brought about intentionally as part of an analytical procedure (*see* laking).

溶血 紅細胞的破壞。體內溶血可由於紅細胞本身的缺陷，或因中毒、感染，或因輸血配血不當時抗體的作用引起，均可導致貧血。血標本溶血可由採集或貯存不當造成，或爲了作化驗分析而故意造成的。

haemolytic *adj.* causing, associated with, or resulting from destruction of red blood cells (*erythrocytes). For example, a *haemolytic antibody* is one that causes destruction of red cells; a *haemolytic anaemia* is due to red-cell destruction (*see* anaemia).

溶血的 引起、伴有或造成紅細胞的破壞。例如溶血性抗體是引起紅細胞溶血的一種物質，溶血性貧血是由紅細胞的破壞引起的。

haemolytic disease of the newborn the condition resulting from destruction (haemolysis) of the red blood cells of the fetus by antibodies in the mother's blood passing through the placenta. This most commonly happens when the red blood cells of the fetus are Rh positive (i.e. they have the *rhesus factor) but the mother's red cells are Rh negative. The fetal cells are therefore incompatible in her circulation and evoke the production of antibodies. This may result in very severe anaemia of the fetus, leading to heart failure with oedema (*hydrops foetalis) or stillbirth. When the anaemia is less severe the fetus may reach term in good condition, but the accumulation of the bile pigment bilirubin from the destroyed cells causes severe jaundice after birth, which may require *exchange transfusion. If untreated it may cause serious brain damage (*see* kernicterus).

新生兒溶血性疾病 胎兒紅細胞破壞（溶血）引起的病症。由母血中的抗體通過胎盤進入胎兒血循環所致。當胎兒紅細胞是 Rh 陽性（即血紅細胞具有獼因子），而母親紅細胞是 Rh 陰性時極易發生本病。胎兒的血細胞在母親的血循環中不相適應而引起抗體的產生。本病可造成胎兒的嚴重貧血，進而導致心力衰竭與水腫（胎兒水腫）或死胎。當貧血不太嚴重時，胎兒可足月順產，但當紅細胞破壞引起的膽汁色素（膽紅素）積集時，胎兒出生後可發生嚴重黃疸，可能需予換血。如未予治療，可引起嚴重的腦損傷。姙娠早期做血液檢查能檢測母血中的抗體，進而採用各種預防措施，以保證

A blood test early in pregnancy enables the detection of antibodies in the mother's blood and the adoption of various precautions for the infant's safety. Some cases of predictably very severe haemolytic disease have been successfully treated by intrauterine transfusion. The incidence of the disease has been greatly reduced by preventing the formation of antibodies in a Rh negative mother. If fetal cells are detected in a woman's blood soon after delivery or after an abortion (using the *Kleihauer technique*), she is given an injection of Rh antibody (anti-D immunoglobulin). This rapidly destroys any Rh positive fetal cells so that they do not remain long enough to stimulate antibody production in her blood (which could affect her next pregnancy).

嬰兒的安全。某些預示嚴重的溶血性疾病的病例，通過子宮內輸血已治療成功。通過預防 Rh 陰性母體內抗體的形成，本病的發病率已大爲減少。如一個婦女在分娩後或流產後在母血中立即測出胎兒 Rh 陽性血細胞（用克萊豪爾氏技術），這位婦女應予注射 Rh 抗體（抗-D 免疫球蛋白）。此抗體能迅速地破壞 Rh 陽性胎兒細胞，以致 Rh 陽性胎兒細胞不能長時間存在，不能在該婦女血中刺激抗體的產生（此種抗體可影響母親下次妊娠）。

haemolytic uraemic syndrome a condition in which sudden rapid destruction of red blood cells (*see* haemolysis) causes acute renal failure due partly to obstruction of small arteries in the kidneys. The haemolysis also causes a reduction in the number of platelets, which can lead to severe haemorrhage. The syndrome may occur as a result of septicaemia, eclamptic fits in pregnancy (*see* eclampsia), or as a reaction to certain drugs. There may also be small sporadic outbreaks of the condition without any obvious cause.

溶血性尿毒症綜合徵 血細胞突然迅速地破壞，腎內小動脉部分梗阻，引起急性腎功能衰竭的一種病症。這種溶血也引起血小板計數減少，導致嚴重出血。本綜合徵可因敗血症、妊娠子癇發作或某些藥物反應而發生。有些輕度散發病例沒有明顯的原因。

haemopericardium *n.* the presence of blood within the membranous sac (pericardium) surrounding the heart, which may result from injury, tumours, rupture of the heart (e.g. following myocardial infarction), or a leaking aneurysm. The heart is compressed (*cardiac tamponade*) and the circulation impaired; a large fall in blood pressure and cardiac arrest may result. Surgical drainage of the blood may be life saving.

心包積血 指包繞心臟的膜性囊（心包）內積有血液。本病可由損傷、腫瘤、心臟破裂（例如心肌梗塞後）或漏血性動脉瘤引起。心臟受壓（心臟塡塞）和循環受阻，可引起血壓下降和心搏停止。血液外科引流可挽救患者生命。

haemoperitoneum *n.* the presence of blood in the peritoneal cavity, between

腹腔積血 腹腔內存有血液。血液存於腹部或骨盆

the lining of the abdomen or pelvis and the membrane covering the organs within.

內面的腹膜與臟器表面的腹膜之間。

haemophilia *n.* a hereditary disorder in which the blood clots very slowly, due to a deficiency of one of the *coagulation factors (*antihaemophilic factor* or *Factor VIII*). The patient may experience prolonged bleeding following any injury or wound, and in severe cases there is spontaneous bleeding into muscles and joints. Bleeding in haemophilia may be treated by transfusions of plasma (which contains Factor VIII). Alternatively concentrated preparations of Factor VIII, obtained by freezing fresh plasma, may be administered (*see* cryoprecipitate). Haemophilia is controlled by a *sex-linked gene, which means that it is almost exclusively restricted to males: women can carry the disease – and pass it on to their sons – without being affected themselves.

血友病　一種遺傳性疾病。本病因缺乏一種凝血因子（抗血友病因子或凝血因子Ⅷ），血液凝固極爲緩慢。病人可能有損傷或創傷後出血延長的病史。嚴重病例可有自發性出血，血液進入肌肉和關節中。血友病出血可用輸血漿（其中含因子Ⅷ）來治療。亦可給予由冷凍新鮮血漿獲得的凝血因子Ⅷ濃縮製劑。血友病是由伴性基因控制。發病者幾乎全部只限於男性，而女性可攜帶本病基因，並將本病基因傳給她們的子女，而她們自己並不發病。

Haemophilus *n.* a genus of Gram-negative aerobic nonmotile parasitic rodlike bacteria frequently found in the respiratory tract. They can grow only in the presence of certain factors in the blood and/or certain coenzymes: they are cultured on fresh blood *agar. Most species are pathogenic: *H. aegyptius* causes conjunctivitis, and *H. ducreyi* soft sore (chancroid). *H. influenzae* is associated with acute and chronic respiratory infections and is a common secondary cause of influenza infections.

嗜血桿菌屬　革蘭氏陰性需氧型桿菌的一屬。無活動能力，屬寄生菌，常見於呼吸道。它只能生長於存有一定因子的血液及/或一定的輔酶時。可培養於新鮮血液瓊脂。其多數種是致病性的：結膜炎嗜血桿菌引起結膜炎；杜克雷氏嗜血桿菌引起軟下疳；流感嗜血桿菌引起急性和慢性呼吸道感染，而且是流感繼發感染的常見原因。

haemophthalmia *n.* bleeding into the *vitreous humour of the eye.

眼球積血　血液進入眼的玻璃體中。

haemopneumothorax (pneumohaemothorax) *n.* the presence of blood and air in the pleural cavity, usually as a result of injury. Both must be drained out to allow the lung to expand normally. *See also* haemothorax.

血氣胸　胸膜腔中存有血液及氣體。往往係損傷的結果。必須將血液及氣體自胸膜腔引流出，使肺能正常地擴張。

haemopoiesis *n.* the process of production of blood cells and platelets

血生成　血細胞和血小板的產生過程。這個過程持

which continues throughout life, replacing aged cells (which are removed from the circulation). In healthy adults, haemopoiesis is confined to the *bone marrow, but in embryonic life and in early infancy, as well as in certain diseases, it may occur in other sites (*extramedullary haemopoiesis*). *See also* erythropoiesis, leucopoiesis, thrombopoiesis. —**haemopoietic** *adj.*

續終身，以淘汰老的細胞（從血液循環中排除）。在健康的成人中，血生成限於骨髓中，而在胚胎期、幼小嬰兒以及某些疾病中，血生成則可發生於其他部位（骨髓外造血）。

haemopoietic stem cell the cell from which all classes of blood cells are derived. It cannot be identified microscopically, although some workers believe that it is identical in appearance with a *lymphocyte. It can be demonstrated by *tissue culture of the blood-forming tissue of the bone marrow, as well as in certain other sites. *See also* haemopoiesis.

造血幹細胞　衍生所有各級血細胞的原始造血細胞。儘管有些人認爲，其外觀與淋巴細胞完全相同，在顯微鏡下兩者無法區分，但通過骨髓以及某些其他部位造血組織的培養可證明它們是不相同的。

haemoptysis *n.* the coughing up of blood. This symptom should always be taken seriously, however small the amount. In some patients the cause is not serious; in others it is never found. But it should always be reported to a doctor.

咯血　咳出血液。無論出血量多少，對這種症狀應取認眞的態度。儘管有些病人出血的原因是不嚴重的，甚至有些病人未找到原因，然一旦發現，必須向醫生報告。

haemorrhage (bleeding) *n.* the escape of blood from a ruptured blood vessel, externally or internally. Arterial blood is bright red and emerges in spurts, venous blood is dark red and flows steadily, while damage to minor vessels may produce only an oozing. Rupture of a major blood vessel such as the femoral artery can lead to the loss of several litres of blood in a few minutes, resulting in *shock, collapse, and death, if untreated. *See also* haematemesis, haematuria, haemoptysis.

出血　血液從破裂的血管向體外或體內漏出。動脈血鮮紅，是涌出的；靜脈血暗紅，是緩緩流出的。當傷及小血管時，可引起滲血。大血管一如股動脈出血，可在幾分鐘內丟失幾升血液，如未經治療可造成休克、虛脫及死亡。

haemorrhagic *adj.* associated with or resulting from blood loss. (*See* haemorrhage.) For example, *haemorrhagic anaemia* is due to blood loss (*see* anaemia).

出血的　與失血有關的或失血引起的。例如，出血性貧血是失血所致。

haemorrhoidectomy *n.* the surgical operation for removing *haemorrhoids,

痔切除術　切除痔的外科手術。手術時先將痔核結

which are tied and then excised. Possible complications are bleeding or, later, anal stricture (narrowing). The operation is usually performed only for second- or third-degree haemorrhoids.

紮，然後再予切除。可能的併發症是出血，或晚期的肛門狹窄。這種手術往往只用於第二或第三度痔。

haemorrhoids (piles) *pl. n.* enlarged (varicose) veins in the wall of the anus (*internal haemorrhoids*), usually a consequence of prolonged constipation or, occasionally, diarrhoea. They most commonly occur at three main points equidistant around the circumference of the anus. Uncomplicated haemorrhoids are seldom painful; pain is usually caused by a *fissure. The main symptom is bleeding, and in *first-degree haemorrhoids*, which never appear at the anus, bleeding at the end of defaecation is the only symptom. *Second-degree haemorrhoids* protrude beyond the anus as an uncomfortable swelling but return spontaneously; *third-degree haemorrhoids* remain outside the anus and need to be returned by pressure. First- and second-degree haemorrhoids may respond to bowel regulation using a high-fibre diet with faecal softening agents. If bleeding persists, an irritant fluid (a sclerosing agent) may be injected around the swollen veins to make them shrivel up. Forceful dilation of the anus under general anaesthesia is also effective. Third-degree haemorrhoids often require surgery (*see* haemorrhoidectomy), especially if they become *strangulated (producing severe pain and further enlargement). *External haemorrhoids* are either prolapsed internal haemorrhoids or – more often – *perianal haematomas or the residual skin tags remaining after a perianal haematoma has healed.

痔 肛門壁擴張（曲張）的靜脈（內痔）。往往繼發於長期便秘，或偶爾繼發於腹瀉。內痔最常發生於圍繞肛周等距離的三個主要點。沒有合併症的痔少有疼痛，疼痛往往是肛裂所致。其主要症狀爲出血。第一度痔肛門內還未出現痔核時，排便後出血是唯一的症狀；第二度痔在肛一側凸出，並有不舒適的腫脹感，但能自行回復；第三度痔脫出於肛門外，並需用壓力托回。第一及第二度痔，用高纖維軟食及潤滑劑，以使有規律地排便，可能是有效的。如持續出血，可圍繞腫脹的靜脉注入一種刺激性液體（一種硬化劑），使痔萎縮。在全身麻醉下做肛門强行擴張術也是有效的。第三度痔，往往需行外科手術治療，尤其如痔形成絞窄時（造成劇烈疼痛並進一步增大）。外痔或者是脫出的內痔，或者（較常見的）是肛周血腫癒合後餘留的殘餘皮贅。

haemosalpinx *n. see* haematosalpinx.

輸卵管積血

haemosiderin *n.* a substance composed of a protein shell containing iron salts which may be present inside certain cells, being one of the forms in which iron is stored within the body. It

含鐵血黃素 由含鐵鹽蛋白殼組成的物質。它可存於某些細胞內，是鐵貯存於人體內的一種形式。它是不可溶的，在經過適當

is insoluble and may be demonstrated microscopically in suitably stained tissue preparations.

染色的組織標本中，可在顯微鏡下顯示出。

haemosiderosis *n.* a disorder caused by excessive deposition of iron, which in turn results from excessive intake or administration of iron, usually in the form of blood transfusions. It results in damage to various organs, including the heart and liver. *Compare* haemochromatosis.

含鐵血黃素沉積症 鐵沉積過多引起的疾患。本病是由於攝取或投予鐵過多引起，且通常是以輸血的形式輸入。本症可導致各種器官一包括心和肝的損傷。

haemostasis *n.* the arrest of bleeding, involving the physiological processes of *blood coagulation and the contraction of damaged blood vessels. The term is also applied to various surgical procedures (for example the application of *ligatures or *diathermy to cut vessels) used to stop bleeding.

止血 出血停止。包括血凝固和損傷血管收縮的生理過程。此術語也適用於各種手術操作（例如結紮或燒灼血管）。

haemostatic (styptic) *n.* an agent that stops or prevents haemorrhage; for example, *phytomenadione and *thromboplastin. Haemostatics are used to control bleeding due to various causes and may be used in treating bleeding disorders, such as haemophilia.

止血劑 止住或預防出血的製劑。例如維生素 K_1 及凝血激酶。止血劑不僅用於控制各種原因引起的出血，而且還可用於治療各種出血性疾病，例如血友病。

haemothorax *n.* blood in the pleural cavity, usually due to injury. If the blood is not drained dense fibrous *adhesions occur between the pleural surfaces, which can impair the normal movement of the lung. The blood may also become infected (*see* empyema).

血胸 血液存於胸膜腔中。通常由損傷引起。如血液不引流出來，胸膜表面之間就會發生緻密的纖維黏連，可損害肺的正常運動。血液也可受感染。

haemozoin *n.* an iron-containing pigment present in the organisms that cause malaria (**Plasmodium* species).

瘧原蟲色素 存在於瘧疾的病原體內的含鐵色素。

hair *n.* a threadlike keratinized outgrowth of the epidermis of the *skin. It develops inside a tubular *hair follicle*. The part above the skin consists of three layers: an outer *cuticle*; a *cortex*, forming the bulk of the hair and containing the pigment that gives the hair its colour; and a central core (*medulla*), which may be hollow. The

毛髮 表皮上線樣的角質化生出物。它在管狀的毛囊內發育。皮膚上面的部分由三層組成：外面有一層小皮；中層是皮質，構成毛髮的主體，並含有色素，使毛髮呈特有的顏色；核心（髓質）可以是中空的。毛根位於皮膚表

root of the hair, beneath the surface of the skin, is expanded at its base to form the *bulb*, which contains a matrix of dividing cells. As new cells are formed the older ones are pushed upwards and become keratinized to form the root and shaft. A hair may be raised by a small erector muscle in the dermis, attached to the hair follicle.

面下，在其基部膨大，形成毛球，球內含有分裂細胞的母質。當新的細胞形成時，老的細胞則被上推，然後角質化，形成毛根和毛幹。一根毛髮可通過眞皮內的、附着於毛囊上的、小的立毛肌將其豎起。

hair follicle a sheath of epidermal cells and connective tissue that surrounds the root of a *hair.

毛囊 圍繞毛根的表皮細胞及結締組織鞘。

hair papilla a projection of the dermis that is surrounded by the base of the hair bulb. It contains the capillaries that supply blood to the growing *hair.

毛乳頭 被毛球基底面圍繞着的眞皮突起。其中含有許多毛細血管，對毛髮的生長提供血液。

hairy cell an abnormal white blood cell that has the appearance of an immature lymphocyte with fine hairlike cytoplasmic projections around the perimeter of the cell. It is found in a rare form of leukaemia most commonly occurring in young men.

毛狀細胞 一種不正常的白細胞。它具有不成熟淋巴細胞的外形以及圍繞細胞周邊的細毛髮樣的胞漿突起。這種細胞主要見於年輕人的罕見型的白血病。

halfway house a residential home for a group of people where some professional supervision is available. It is used as a stage in the rehabilitation of the mentally ill, usually when they have just been discharged from hospital and are able to work but are not yet ready for independent life.

重返社會訓練所 爲一羣人而設的、可獲得專業性管理的住所。它用於精神病人的康復階段，當病人剛出院，雖能做一些事，但不能獨立生活時。

halitosis *n.* bad breath. Causes of temporary halitosis include recently eaten strongly flavoured food, such as garlic or onions, and drugs such as paraldehyde. Other causes include mouth breathing, *periodontal disease, and infective conditions of the nose, throat, and lungs (especially *bronchiectasis). Constipation, indigestion, and some liver diseases may also cause the condition.

口臭 呼出難聞的氣味。一時性口臭的原因包括新近食入濃味食物，如蒜頭或洋葱，以及藥物如副醛。其他原因包括口呼吸、牙周病以及鼻、咽和肺（特別是支氣管擴張）的感染性疾病。便秘、消化不良以及某些肝病也可引起本症。

hallucination *n.* a false perception of something that is not really there. Hallucinations may be visual, auditory, tactile, gustatory (of taste), or olfactory

幻覺 一種並非眞實存在的事物的虛假知覺。幻覺可以是視覺的、聽覺的、觸覺的、味覺的或者是嗅

(of smell). They may be provoked by psychological illness (such as *schizophrenia) or physical disorders in the brain (such as temporal lobe *epilepsy) or they may be caused by drugs or sensory deprivation. Hallucinations should be distinguished from dreams and from *illusions (since they occur at the same time as real perceptions).

覺的。這些幻覺可由精神病（如精神分裂症）或腦的器質性疾患（如顳葉癲癇）或者由藥物或感覺喪失引起。幻覺應與夢和錯覺相區別（因這些錯覺與眞實知覺同時發生）。

hallucinogen *n.* a drug that produces hallucinations, e.g. *cannabis and *lysergic acid diethylamide. Hallucinogens were formerly used to treat certain types of mental illness. —**hallucinogenic** *adj.*

致幻劑 引起幻覺的一種藥劑。例如：大麻、麥角醯二乙胺等。過去致幻藥用於治療某些類型的精神病。

hallux *n.* (*pl.* **halluces**) the big toe.

踇 即大趾。

haloperidol *n.* a *tranquillizer used to relieve anxiety and tension in the treatment of schizophrenia and other psychiatric disorders. It is administered by mouth or injection; muscular incoordination and restlessness are common side-effects. Trade names: **Haldol**, **Serenace**.

氟哌啶醇 在治療精神分裂症和其它精神病中，用於減輕焦慮及緊張的一種安定藥。口服或注射。最常見的副作用有肌共濟失調和不安。

halophilic *adj.* requiring solutions of high salt concentration for healthy growth. Certain bacteria are halophilic. —**halophile** *n.*

嗜鹽的 需要有高濃度鹽溶液才能正常生長的。某些細菌是嗜鹽的。

halos *pl. n.* coloured rings seen around lights by people with acute congestive glaucoma and sometimes by people with cataract.

暈 急性充血性青光眼患者看到的圍繞燈光的彩色環。白內障患者有時亦有此症狀。

halothane *n.* a potent general *anaesthetic administered by inhalation, used for inducing and maintaining anaesthesia in all types of surgical operations. Reduced blood pressure and irregular heartbeat may occur during halothane anaesthesia. Trade name: **Fluothane**.

氟烷 有效的吸入性全身麻醉藥。在所有類型外科手術中用於誘導和維持麻醉。氟烷麻醉過程中可發生血壓下降與心律不齊。

hamartoma *n.* an overgrowth of mature tissue in which the elements show disordered arrangement and proportion in comparison to normal. The overgrowth is benign but malignancy may

錯構瘤 一種過度生長的成熟組織。與正常組織比較，其成分在排列及比例上顯得混亂。這種過度的生長物是良性的。但其中

occur in any of the constituent tissue elements.

任何一種組織成分均可發生惡性變。

hamate bone (unciform bone) a hook-shaped bone of the wrist (*see* carpus). It articulates with the pisiform and triquetral bones behind and with the fourth and fifth metacarpal bones in front.

鈎骨 腕的鈎狀骨。其後與豆骨及三角骨相關節，前與第四及第五掌骨相關節。

hammer *n.* (in anatomy) *see* malleus.

錘骨

hammer toe a deformity of a toe, most often the second, caused by fixed flexion of the first joint. A corn often forms over the deformity, which may be painful. If severe pain does not respond to strapping or corrective footwear, it may be necessary to perform *arthrodesis at the affected joint.

錘狀趾 足趾的一種畸形。最常見於第二趾骨，因第一趾關節固定於屈曲位所致。在畸形處常形成鷄眼而致疼痛，貼絆創膏或穿矯正鞋無效的話，有必要做患關節的關節固定術。

hamstring *n.* any of the tendons at the back of the knee. They attach the *hamstring muscles* (the biceps femoris, semitendinosus, and semimembranosus) to their insertions in the tibia and fibula.

膕繩肌腱 膝後的任何肌腱。它們連接膕繩肌羣（股二頭肌、半腱肌及半膜肌）至脛骨與腓骨的附着處。

hamulus *n.* (*pl.* **hamuli**) any hooklike process, such as occurs on the hamate, lacrimal, and sphenoid bones and on the cochlea.

鈎 任何鈎形的突起。例如發生於鈎骨的、淚骨的、蝶骨的以及耳蝸的。

handicap *n.* partial or total inability to perform a social, occupational, or other activity. It reflects the extent to which an individual is disadvantaged by some partial or total *disability* when compared with those in a peer group who have no such disability. A handicap is usually related to an identifiable structural *impairment*, often based on a range of two standard deviations from the *mean observation obtained from studying a large number of apparently healthy subjects. It may also reflect functional impairment, which may be unsuspected by the individual and discovered by clinical observation or testing. The alternative terms *abnormality*, *defect*, or *malformation* (for impair-

缺陷 部分或完全不能履行社會職務或者其他方面的活動。它反映某個人當與那些沒有同樣缺陷的同等人羣比較時，由於某些方面的部分或完全缺陷而不能利用其有利條件的程度。缺陷通常是涉及到某一明顯的結構上的損害，是在大量調查明顯健康的人獲得的平均數（觀測值）兩個標準差範圍以上者。缺陷也可反映功能性的損傷，本人可能沒有覺察到，而是通過臨床觀察和測試才發現的。其他作者有用異常、缺損、畸形（對損傷）及功能障礙

ment) and *malfunction* (for disability) are used by many authorities but this may sometimes cause confusion.
（對喪失勞動力）等替換的術語，但有時可引起混亂。

Hand-Schüller-Christian disease *see* reticuloendotheliosis.
漢-許-克三氏病（網狀內皮肉芽腫）

Hansen's bacillus *see* Mycobacterium.
漢森氏桿菌（痲風桿菌）

haploid (monoploid) *adj.* describing cells, nuclei, or organisms with a single set of unpaired chromosomes. In man the gametes are haploid following *meiosis. *Compare* diploid, triploid. —**haploid** *n.*
單倍的 描述細胞、核或生物體具有單套不成對的染色體。在人類生殖細胞減數分裂後的精子和卵子是單倍的。

hapt- (hapto-) *prefix denoting* touch.
〔前綴〕 **接觸**

hapten *n. see* antigen.
半抗原

haptoglobin *n.* a protein present in blood plasma that binds with free haemoglobin to form a complex that is rapidly removed from the circulation. Depletion of plasma haptoglobin is a feature of anaemias in which red blood cells are destroyed inside the circulation with the release of haemoglobin into the plasma.
結合珠蛋白 血漿中存在的一種蛋白。與游離的血紅蛋白結合，形成一種複合物，很快離開血循環。血漿結合珠蛋白的缺失是多種貧血的特徵，此類貧血是血循環中紅細胞破壞，將血紅蛋白釋放到血漿中，與結合珠蛋白結合所致。

harara *n.* a severe and itchy inflammation of the skin occurring in people continuously subjected to the bites of the *sandfly *Phlebotomus papatasii*. The incidence of this allergic skin reaction, prevalent in the Middle East, may be checked by controlling the numbers of sandflies.
白蛉皮炎 一種嚴重且發癢的皮膚炎症。發生於經常遭受巴氏白蛉叮咬的人。這種在中東流行的變應性皮膚反應，可通過控制白蛉的數量來阻止。

harelip *n.* the congenital deformity of a cleft in the upper lip, on one or both sides of the midline. It occurs when the three blocks of embryonic tissue that go to form the upper lip fail to fuse and it is often associated with a *cleft palate. Medical name: **cheiloschisis**.
唇裂 上唇發生裂口的先天性畸形。發生於中線的一側或兩側。在胚胎時期形成上唇的三塊組織不能融合時可發生本病症。醫學上的名稱：Cheiloschisis。

Harrison's sulcus a depression on both sides of the chest wall of a child between the pectoral muscles and the lower margin of the ribcage. It is caused
哈里遜氏溝（胸廓下溝） 小兒兩側胸壁上，在胸肌與肋骨下緣之間的一種凹陷。當吸氣時以及發生呼

by exaggerated suction of the diaphragm when breathing in and develops in conditions in which the airways are partially obstructed or when the lungs are abnormally congested due to some congenital abnormality of the heart.

吸道部分受阻的情況時，或肺異常充血（由於某些心臟先天性異常）時，因膈肌過度牽引胸壁所致。

Hartnup disease a hereditary defect in the metabolism of the amino acid tryptophan, leading to mental retardation, thickening and roughening of the skin, and lack of muscular coordination.

哈特納普氏病 一種遺傳性色氨酸代謝缺陷。可致精神發育不全，皮膚增厚、粗糙，以及肌共濟失調。

harvest mite *see* Trombicula.

秋蟎

Hashimoto's disease chronic inflammation of the thyroid gland (*thyroiditis*) due to the formation of antibodies against normal thyroid tissue (autoantibodies). Its features include a firm swelling of the thyroid and partial or total failure of secretion of thyroid hormones; often there are autoantibodies to other organs, such as the stomach.

橋本氏病 甲狀腺的慢性炎症（甲狀腺炎）。由於形成抗正常甲狀腺組織的抗體（自身抗體）引起。其特徵包括甲狀腺硬性腫大、甲狀腺激素的分泌部分或完全停止，往往對其他器官如胃也有自身抗體。

hashish *n. see* cannabis.

大麻

haustrum *n.* one of the pouches on the external surface of the *colon.

袋 結腸外表面上的一種囊。

Haversian canal one of the small canals (diameter about 50 μm) that ramify throughout compact *bone. *See also* Haversian system.

哈弗氏管 貫穿密質骨並成網狀的一種小管（直徑約50μm）。

Haversian system one of the cylindrical units of which compact *bone is made. A *Haversian canal* forms a central tube, around which are alternate layers of bone matrix (*lamellae*) and *lacunae* containing bone cells. The lacunae are linked by minute channels (*canaliculi*).

哈弗氏系統 組成密質骨的圓柱形骨單位。即以哈弗氏管爲中心，繞以一層一層的骨基質（板）以及含骨細胞的腔隙。這些腔隙由許多小管把它們貫通起來。

hay fever a form of *allergy due to the pollen of grasses, trees, and other plants, characterized by inflammation of the membrane lining the nose and

枯草熱 一型由草、樹木以及其它植物引起的變態反應。以鼻炎爲特徵，有時有結膜炎。打噴嚏、

sometimes of the conjunctiva. The symptoms of sneezing, running or blocked nose, and watering eyes are due to histamine release and often respond to treatment with *antihistamines. If the allergen is identified, it may be possible to undertake *desensitization. Medical name: **allergic rhinitis.**

流鼻涕或鼻塞以及流淚等症狀是由於組織胺釋放之故。用抗組胺類藥物治療往往有效。如能鑑定其變應原，就有可能做脫敏治療。

HCG *see* chorionic gonadotrophin.

人絨〔毛〕膜促性腺激素

head *n.* **1.** the part of the body that contains the brain and the organs of sight, hearing, smell, and taste. **2.** the rounded portion of a bone, which fits into a groove of another to form a joint; for example, the head of humerus or femur.

頭 ①包含腦以及視、聽、味與嗅覺等器官的人體的一部分。 ②骨的圓形部。它的形狀適宜於進入另一相應的窩，以形成關節，例如肱骨或股骨的頭。

headache *n.* pain felt deep within the skull. Most headaches are caused by emotional stress or fatigue but some are symptoms of serious intracranial disease. *See also* migraine.

頭痛 顱內疼痛。多數由情緒緊張或疲乏引起，但有些是顱內嚴重疾患的症狀。

health centre (in Britain) a building, owned or leased by a District Health Authority, that houses personnel and/or services from one or several sections of the National Health Service (e.g. general practitioners, *community nurses, dentists, *child health clinics, and facilities for X-rays, laboratory tests, and electrocardiography). Services provided by local authorities, such as social services, chiropody, and child psychology, may also operate from such a centre.

衛生院 在英國指地段保健局自已所有或由該局租賃的一種機構。該機構的工作人員及/或設施（例如全科醫師，公共保健護士，牙科醫生，兒童保健站，以及X線、實驗室檢查、心電描記技術設備等）來自國民保健服務制的一個或幾個部門。由地方當局提供的服務項目，如社會服務、手足醫術以及小兒心理諮詢等也可由衛生院承擔。

health education persuasive methods used to encourage people (either individually or collectively) to adopt life styles that the educators believe will improve health and to reject habits regarded as harmful to health or likely to shorten life expectancy. The term is also used in a broader sense to include instruction about bodily function, etc., so that the public is better informed about health issues.

衛生宣傳教育 用說服教育的方法鼓勵人們（單個的或集體的）採納教育家認爲會增進健康的生活方式，並拋棄那些有害健康或很可能縮短預期壽限的習性。此術語廣義上也包括講授有關人體的功能等，以便使民衆了解有關的健康常識。

health service commissioner (ombudsman) an official responsible to Parliament and appointed to protect the interests of patients in relation to administration of the *National Health Service. He can investigate complaints and allegations of maladministration but not of professional negligence.

衛生事業專員（政府官員） 一種對國會負責的官員，其任務是維護病人在國民保健服務系統中應享受的利益。他可調查有關行政管理不當方面的投訴和陳述，但不過問技術事故。

health visitor a trained nurse with experience in midwifery and special training in preventive medicine (including health education). The training usually takes place at a technical college over three academic terms, the course being approved by the *United Kingdom Central Council for Nursing, Midwifery, and Health Visiting.* All births are notified to the appropriate health visitor, most of whose work is concerned with routine visiting of selected preschool children (though the elderly and chronic sick also receive routine visits). Health visitors do not carry out practical nursing care but seek to educate parents or relatives how best to care for their charges, in particular by drawing attention to unmet needs in terms of health care and those of the social services likely to improve health. A few health visitors have specialist roles (e.g. handicapped children, the elderly, or the tuberculous). Many belong to a professional body known as the *Health Visitors Association* but membership is not obligatory.

保健員 一種受過預防醫學（包括衛生宣傳）特別訓練、對助產有經驗的護士。通常在技校培訓三個學期。課程由聯合王國護士、助產士和保健員委員會提供。所有出生的嬰兒向相應的保健員報告。多數保健員的工作是定期訪問經選擇的學齡前兒童（儘管是年齡較大的以及慢性疾患的兒童也可受到定期訪問）。保健員不做實際的護理工作，而是力求做好對雙親或家庭成員的宣傳教育，指導他們如何很好地負起責任，特別要引起他們注意，在保健方面，以及增進健康的社會服務方面，哪些需要沒有得到滿足。少數保健員具有專業任務（例如對老年人，殘疾兒童或結核病患者的照顧）。許多保健員屬於專業團體保健員協會的成員，但不是一律都要加入協會。

hearing aid an electronic device to enable a deaf person to hear, consisting of a miniature sound receiver, an amplifier, and either an earpiece or a vibrator to transfer the amplified sound to the ear. The earpiece fits into the ear; the vibrator (used in cases of conductive *deafness) fits behind the ear and transmits through the bone directly to the inner ear. The aid is powered by a battery, and the whole unit is usually small enough to fit behind the ear inconspicuously.

助聽器 一種能使聾人聽到聲音的電子儀器。它由小型的聲音接受器、放大器和耳機（或振動器）組成。耳機將放大的聲音傳入耳內。耳機置於耳內，振動器（用於傳導性耳聾的病例）置於耳後，使聲音通過骨直接傳入內耳。助聽器由電池啟動，其總的體積往往很小，可裝在耳後而不致顯眼。

heart *n.* a hollow muscular cone-shaped organ, lying between the lungs, with the pointed end (*apex*) directed downwards, forwards, and to the left. The heart is about the size of a closed fist. Its wall consists largely of *cardiac muscle (myocardium), lined and surrounded by membranes (*see* endocardium, pericardium). It is divided by a *septum* into separate right and left halves, each of which is divided into an upper *atrium and a lower *ventricle (see illustration). Deoxygenated blood from the *venae cavae passes through the right atrium to the right ventricle. This contracts and pumps blood to the lungs via the *pulmonary artery. The newly oxygenated blood returns to the left atrium via the pulmonary veins and passes through to the left ventricle. This forcefully contracts, pumping blood out to the body via the *aorta. The direction of blood flow within the heart is controlled by *valves.

心　中空的圓錐形肌性器官。位於兩肺之間，尖端向左前下方。心臟約有握拳大小。心壁大體上由心肌、心內膜以及心臟外面的心包組成。它由一間隔分成左右兩個部分。每一半側心又分成上面的心房和下面的心室。脫氧血由腔靜脈經右心房到右心室。右心室收縮將血經肺動脈泵入肺內。攜氧血經肺靜脈重新回到左心房，然後到左心室。左心室有力地收縮，將血泵出，通過主動脈輸送到全身。心臟內血流的方向是由瓣膜來控制的。

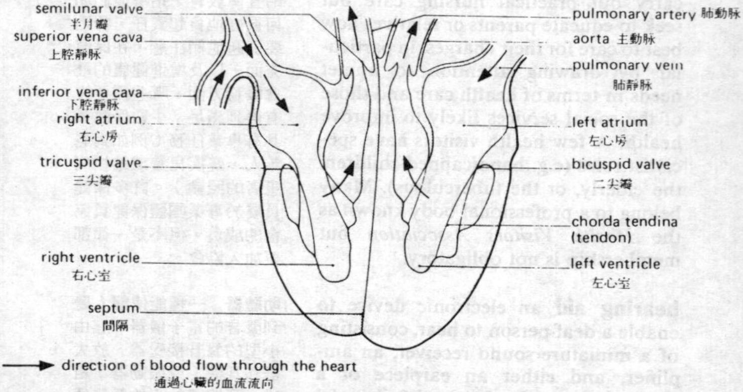

Vertical section through the heart
心臟的垂直切面

heart attack *see* myocardial infarction.

心臟驟停

heart block a condition in which conduction of the electrical impulses generated by the natural pacemaker of

心傳導阻滯　一種心臟疾患。由於心臟自然起搏點發出的電衝動的傳導受到

the heart (the *sinoatrial node) is impaired, so that the pumping action of the heart is slowed down. In *partial* or *incomplete heart block* conduction between atria and ventricles is delayed (*first degree heart block*) or not all the impulses are conducted from the atria to the ventricles (*second degree heart block*). In *third degree* or *complete heart block* no impulses are conducted and the ventricles beat at their own slow intrinsic rate (20–40 per minute).
Heart block may be congenital or it may be due to heart disease, including myocardial infarction, myocarditis, cardiomyopathy, and disease of the valves. It is most frequently seen in the elderly as the result of chronic degenerative scarring around the conducting tissue. There may be no symptoms, but when very slow heart and pulse rates occur the patient may develop heart failure or *Stokes-Adams syndrome. Symptoms may be abolished by the use of an artificial *pacemaker.

損害，以致其泵血作用減緩。部分或不完全傳導阻滯是心房和心室之間的傳導延遲（Ⅰ度心傳導阻滯）或不能傳導所有從心房到心室的衝動（Ⅱ度心傳導阻滯）。Ⅲ度或完全心傳導阻滯是不能傳導衝動，心室以其自身緩慢的固有心率（20-40 次/分）搏動。心傳導阻滯可以是先天性的，也可能是由於心臟病（包括心肌梗塞、心肌炎、心肌病以及瓣膜病）引起。心傳導阻滯最常見於較年長者，這是由於傳導組織周圍慢性退行性變化的結果。本病可無症狀，但當心率和脈搏非常緩慢時可出現症狀，病人可發生心力衰竭或阿-斯二氏綜合徵。可使用人工起搏器消除症狀。

heartburn (pyrosis) *n.* discomfort or pain, usually burning in character, that is felt behind the breastbone and often appears to rise from the abdomen towards or into the throat. It may be accompanied by the appearance of acid or bitter fluid in the mouth and is usually caused by regurgitation of the stomach contents into the gullet or by *oesophagitis.

胃灼熱 以燒灼感爲特徵的胃部不適或疼痛。燒灼感位於胸骨後，從腹部上升到咽喉部，可伴有吐酸水或苦水，這往往是由於胃內容物反流到食管或食管炎引起。

heart failure a condition in which the pumping action of the ventricle of the heart is inadequate. This results in back pressure of blood, with congestion of the lungs and liver. The veins in the neck becomed engorged and fluid accumulates in the tissues (*see* oedema). There is a reduced flow of arterial blood from the heart, which in extreme cases results in peripheral circulatory failure (cardiogenic shock). Heart failure may result from any condition that overloads, damages, or reduces the

心力衰竭 心室的泵血作用不足的一種狀態。可引起血壓下降、肺和肝充血。頸靜脈充盈，液體蓄積於組織內（水腫）。來自心臟的動脈血流量減少，在嚴重病例中導致周圍循環衰竭（心源性休克）。心力衰竭可由任何情況如負荷過重、損傷、心肌效力下降等引起。常見的原因是冠狀動脈血栓形成、高血壓、慢性瓣膜

efficiency of the heart muscle. Common causes are coronary thrombosis, hypertension, chronic disease of the valves, and arrhythmias. The patient experiences breathlessness, even when lying flat, and oedema of the legs.
Treatment consists of rest, a low salt diet, diuretic drugs (e.g. frusemide), and digitalis derivatives (e.g. digoxin). Structural abnormalities, such as defective valves, may be corrected surgically.

疾患以及心律不齊。病人有喘息（甚至在平臥時）以及腿腫。
治療包括休息、低鹽飲食、服利尿藥（例如速尿）以及洋地黃毒甙。結構上的異常，如瓣膜疾患，可用外科方法糾正。

heart-lung machine an apparatus for taking over temporarily the functions of both the heart and the lungs during heart surgery. It incorporates a pump, to maintain the circulation, and equipment to oxygenate the blood. Blood is taken from the body by tubes inserted into the superior and inferior venae cavae, and the oxygenated blood is returned under pressure into a large artery, such as the femoral artery. The surgeon is therefore able to undertake the repair or replacement of heart valves or perform other surgical operations involving the heart and great blood vessels.

心肺機 心肺手術時用於暫時替代心肺功能的一種器械。它把用於維持循環的泵和用於充氧的器械結合起來。血液是通過插進上下腔靜脈的小管引出身體，而含氧血在壓力下返回大動脈，例如股動脈。因此，外科醫生就可着手作心瓣膜的修復或置換手術，或者做其他外科手術，包括心臟或大血管的手術。

heat exhaustion fatigue and collapse due to the low blood pressure and blood volume that result from loss of body fluids and salts after prolonged or unaccustomed exposure to heat. It is most common in new arrivals in a hot climate and is treated by giving drinks or intravenous injections of salted water.

中暑虛脫 由血壓低和血容量下降引起的疲勞和虛脫。是長期或不習慣暴露於熱環境後體液和鹽份丢失造成的。本病最常見於新到熱帶的人。可予飲水或靜脈注射鹽水治療。

heat rash *see* prickly heat.

熱疹（痱子）

heatstroke (sunstroke) *n.* raised body temperature (pyrexia), absence of sweating, and eventual loss of consciousness due to failure or exhaustion of the temperature-regulating mechanism of the body. It is potentially fatal unless treated immediately: the body should be cooled by applying damp cloths and body fluids restored by giving drinks or intravenous injections of salted water.

中暑（日射病） 由體溫調節機制衰竭引起的體溫升高、不出汗以及最終意識喪失。如不及時治療，可能致死。治療：披蓋濕布使身體涼下來，並給予飲水或靜脈注射鹽水，使體液恢復。

hebephrenia *n.* a form of *schizophrenia. It is typically a chronic condition, and the most prominent features are disordered thinking; inappropriate emotions with thoughtless cheerfulness, apathy, or querulousness; and silly behaviour. It typically starts in adolescence or young adulthood. Social and occupational rehabilitation are the most important therapies for most patients; drugs such as the *phenothiazines or butyrophenones can also help. —**hebephrenic** *adj.*

青春期痴呆 精神分裂症的一個類型。它是一種典型的慢性疾患。其突出的特徵是：思維紊亂，不適當的感情以及無思想內容的高興、冷淡、發牢騷和愚蠢行為。本病典型的發病始於青春期或年輕的成年人。對多數患者來講，恢復正常的社會生活和職業是最重要的治療方法，藥物如吩噻嗪類或丁醯苯類可能也是有幫助的。

Heberden's node a lump of cartilage-covered bone arising at the terminal joint of a finger in *osteoarthritis. It is often inherited.

希伯登氏結 覆蓋軟骨的一種腫塊。骨關節炎時發生於指關節末端。本病通常是遺傳性的。

hebetude *n.* apathy and emotional dullness. This is not a symptom specific to any one condition; extreme degrees are found in *schizophrenia and *dementia.

精神遲鈍 冷淡和感情遲鈍。它不是某一疾病特有的症狀。程度最嚴重的見於精神分裂症和痴呆。

hectic *adj.* occurring regularly. A *hectic fever* typically develops in the afternoons, in cases of pulmonary tuberculosis.

潮式的 有規律發生的。潮熱，在肺結核病中，典型的發生於下午。

hecto- *prefix denoting* a hundred.

〔前綴〕 **百**

heel *n.* the part of the foot that extends behind the ankle joint, formed by the *heel bone* (*see* calcaneus).

〔足〕跟 足的一部分，由跟骨形成，延伸到踝關節後。

Hegar's sign an indication of pregnancy that may be detectable during the second and third months. If fingers of one hand are inserted into the vagina and those of the other are placed over the pelvic cavity, the lower part of the womb, including the neck, can easily be compressed between the two hands. *See also* Jacquemier's sign.

黑加氏徵 妊娠的一種象徵。妊娠第二、三個月時可查出。將一隻手的手指插入陰道內，另一隻手的手指置於盆腔上面，子宮的下端（包括子宮頸）可容易地被兩手指壓縮。

helc- (helco-) *prefix denoting* an ulcer.

〔前綴〕 **潰瘍**

helcoplasty *n.* the surgical repair of ulcers by skin grafting. *See* skin graft.

潰瘍成形術 用植皮修復潰瘍的手術。

helicotrema *n.* the narrow opening between the scala vestibuli and the

蝸孔 耳蝸尖端前庭階和鼓階之間的狹窄開口。

scala tympani at the tip of the *cochlea in the ear.

helio- *prefix denoting* the sun. 〔前綴〕 日〔光〕

heliotherapy *n.* the use of sunlight to promote healing; sunbathing.
日光療法 利用陽光促進治癒；日光浴。

helix *n.* the outer curved fleshy ridge of the *pinna of the outer ear.
耳輪 外耳耳廓外部的曲線形肉質緣。

Heller's syndrome (disintegrative psychosis) a rare mental illness of childhood. Abnormalities of behaviour may be the only sign at first but the condition progresses to psychotic manifestations, such as *stereotypies and hallucinations, and ultimately to dementia. Nearly always a physical cause can be found. The illness progresses to severe incapacity or death.
海勒氏綜合徵（分裂型精神病） 小兒罕見的一種精神病。初起時，行爲異常可能是唯一的徵候，而後發展到精神病的表現，如有刻板動作及幻覺，終至痴呆。幾乎總能找到軀體性病因。本病可發展到嚴重的能力喪失或死亡。

Heller's test a test for the presence of protein (albumin) in the urine. A quantity of urine is carefully poured onto the same quantity of pure nitric acid in a test tube. A white ring forms at the junction of the liquids if albumin is present. However, a similar result may be obtained if the urine contains certain drugs or is very concentrated. A dark brown ring indicates the presence of an abnormally high level of potassium indoxyl sulphate in the urine (*see* indicanuria).
海勒氏試驗 檢查尿中蛋白（白蛋白）的一種試驗。將一定的尿量倒入同量純硝酸的試管中。如尿中含有白蛋白，在兩種液體接觸面形成一白色環。然而，如尿中含有某些藥物或尿液是很濃縮的，也可獲得同樣結果。深棕色環表明尿中有異常高濃度的硫酸吲哚酚鉀鹽。

Helly's fluid a mixture of potassium bichromate, sodium sulphate, mercuric chloride, formaldehyde, and distilled water, used in the preservation of bone marrow.
海利氏液 重鉻酸鉀、硫酸鈉、氯化汞、甲醛和蒸餾水的混合物。用於保存骨髓。

helminth *n.* any of the various parasitic worms, including the *flukes, *tapeworms, and *nematodes.
蠕蟲 體內寄生蟲的一種。包括吸蟲類、絛蟲類和線蟲類。

helminthiasis *n.* the diseased condition resulting from an infestation with parasitic worms (helminths).
蠕蟲病 感染寄生性蠕蟲造成的疾病。

helminthology *n.* the study of parasitic worms.
蠕蟲學 研究寄生性蠕蟲的學科。

heloma *n.* a *callosity or *corn on the foot or hand.

雞眼 手上或腳上的一種胼胝或皮膚硬結。

hemeralopia *n. see* day blindness.

夜盲症

hemi- *prefix denoting* (in medicine) the right or left half of the body. Example: *hemianaesthesia* (anaesthesia of one side of the body).

〔前綴〕 **偏（單）側** 醫學中指人體的右或左半側。例如：偏側感覺缺失（人體的一側感覺缺失）。

hemiachromatopsia *n.* loss of colour appreciation in one half of the visual field.

偏〔側〕色盲 視野的一半不能識別顏色。

hemianopia *n.* absence of half of the normal field of vision. The commonest type is *homonymous hemianopia*, in which the same half (right or left) in lost in both eyes. Sometimes the inner halves of the visual field are lost in both eyes, producing a *binasal hemianopia*, while in others the outer halves are lost, producing a *bitemporal hemianopia*. Very rarely both upper halves or both lower halves are lost, producing an *altitudinal hemianopia*.

偏盲 正常視野的一半缺失。最常見的類型是同側偏盲，即兩眼的同一半側（右或左）偏盲。有時是兩眼視野的內半部缺失，產生鼻側偏盲；而外半部視野缺失，則產生顳側偏盲。罕見的兩眼上半或下半視野缺失，產生上下側偏盲。

hemiballismus *n.* a violent involuntary movement usually restricted to one arm and primarily involving the proximal muscles. It is a symptom of disease of the *basal ganglia.

偏身顫搐 一種強烈的不隨意的運動。通常只限於某一手臂，而且首先侵犯附近的肌肉。本症是基底神經節疾患的一種症狀。

hemicolectomy *n.* surgical removal of about half the *colon (large intestine), usually the right section (*right hemicolectomy*) with subsequent joining of the *ileum to the transverse colon. This is performed for disease of the terminal part of the ileum (such as *Crohn's disease) or of the caecum or ascending colon (such as cancer or Crohn's disease).

結腸部分切除術 外科切除約 1/2 的結腸（大腸）。通常是結腸右部（右結腸部分切除術），將回腸與橫結腸相連。這種手術可用於回腸末端疾患（例如克羅恩氏病），或盲腸端及升結腸疾患（例如癌或克羅恩氏病）。

hemicrania *n.* **1.** a headache affecting only one side of the head, usually *migraine. **2.** absence of half of the skull in a developing fetus.

①**偏側頭痛** 只侵犯一側頭部的一種頭痛。通常是指偏頭痛。 ②**半無腦〔畸形〕** 在胎兒發育中，頭顱的一半缺失。

hemimelia *n.* congenital absence or gross shortening (aplasia) of the distal

半肢畸形 手臂或腿的遠側部先天性缺失或短粗

portion of the arms or legs. Sometimes only one of the two bones of the distal arm (radius and ulna) or leg (tibia and fibula) may be affected. *See also* ectromelia.

（發育不全）。有時只有前臂骨（橈骨與尺骨）或小腿骨（脛骨與腓骨）中的一個缺失。

hemiparesis *n. see* hemiplegia.

輕偏癱

hemiplegia (hemiparesis) *n.* paralysis of one side of the body. Movements of the face and arm are often more severely affected than those of the leg. It is caused by disease of the opposite (contralateral) hemisphere of the brain.

偏癱　身體一側癱瘓。面部與手臂的運動通常比腿部受累較爲嚴重。本病由對側大腦半球疾患引起。

hemisacralization *n.* fusion of the fifth lumbar vertebra to one side only of the sacrum. *See* sacralization.

〔第五腰椎〕半骶化　第五腰椎只一側與骶骨融合。

hemisphere *n.* one of the two halves of the *cerebrum, not in fact hemispherical but more nearly quarter-spherical.

半球　大腦的（左側或右側）一半。事實上並非半球狀的，而是呈 1/4 球面狀。

hemizygous *adj.* describing genes that are carried on an unpaired chromosome, for example the genes on the X chromosome in man. —**hemizygote** *n.*

半合子的　描述具有不成對染色體的基因。例如男性 X 染色體上的基因。

hemlock *n.* the plant *Conium maculatum*, found in Britain and central Europe. It is a source of the poisonous alkaloid *coniine.

毒茴類毒草　毒茴植物。見於不列顛及中歐。它是有毒生物鹼歐毒芹鹼的來源。

hemp *n. see* cannabis.

大麻

Henle's loop the part of a kidney tubule that forms a loop extending towards the centre of the kidney. It is surrounded by blood capillaries, which reabsorb water and selected soluble substances back into the bloodstream.

漢勒氏襻（細尿管襻）　腎小管的一部分。它形成一襻狀，伸向腎中心。襻周圍有毛細血管圍繞，其功能是重吸收水分，選擇性地使某些可溶性物質返回血流中。

henry *n.* the *SI unit of inductance, equal to the inductance of a closed circuit with a magnetic flux of 1 weber per ampere of current. Symbol: H.

亨〔利〕　電感的 SI 國際單位。等於在閉合電路中每安〔培〕電流產生 1 韋〔伯〕磁通量的電感。符號：H。

Hensen's node (primitive knot) the rounded front end of the embryonic *primitive streak.

亨森氏結（原結）　胚胎原條前端的圓形結節。

heparin *n.* an *anticoagulant produced in liver cells, some white blood cells, and certain other sites, which acts by inhibiting the action of the enzyme *thrombin in the final stage of *blood coagulation. An extracted purified form of heparin is widely used for the prevention of blood coagulation both in patients with thrombosis and similar conditions and in blood collected for examination. The drug is usually administered by injection and the most important side-effect is bleeding.

肝素 在肝細胞、某些白細胞以及其它部位產生的抗凝血物質。其作用是抑制血液凝固最後階段的酶（凝血酶）的活動。提純的肝素廣泛用於治療血栓形成和類似的疾患，以及實驗採血時用作抗凝劑。治療用時通常是注射給藥，其最主要的副作用是出血。

hepat- (hepato-) *prefix denoting* the liver. Examples: *hepatopexy* (surgical fixation of); *hepatorenal* (relating to the liver and kidney).

〔前綴〕 **肝** 例如：肝固定術（外科固定肝的手術），肝腎的（與肝及腎有關的）。

hepatalgia *n.* pain in or over the liver. It is caused by liver inflammation (especially an abscess) or swelling (as in cardiac failure).

肝痛 肝內或肝區疼痛。可由肝臟的炎症（尤其是膿腫）或腫大（如心力衰竭時）引起。

hepatectomy *n.* the operation of removing the liver. *Partial hepatectomy* is the removal of one or more lobes of the liver; it may be carried out after severe injury or to remove a tumour localized in one part of the liver.

肝切除術 切除肝的手術。部分肝切除術是切除一葉或一葉以上肝臟；肝損傷後可行這種手術，局限於肝臟某一部位的腫瘤可用這種手術切除。

hepatic *adj.* relating to the liver.

肝的 與肝有關的。

hepatic duct *see* bile duct.

肝管

hepatic encephalopathy (portosystemic encephalopathy) a condition in which brain function is impaired by the presence of toxic substances, absorbed from the colon, which are normally removed or detoxified by the liver. It occurs when the liver is severely damaged (as in cirrhosis) or bypassed. Symptoms include drowsiness, confusion, difficulty in performing tasks (e.g. writing), and coma. Treatment consists of stopping protein intake and giving antibiotics (to prevent bacterial production of toxins) and enemas and cathartics (to remove colonic toxins).

肝性腦病（門體靜脈性腦病） 由於毒性物質的存在使大腦功能損害的一種疾病。這些毒性物質從結腸中吸收，在正常情況下是通過肝排除或解毒的。當肝嚴重損傷（如肝硬化）或側枝循環形成時可發生本病。症狀包括倦睡、精神錯亂、難於完成某些任務(如寫字)以及昏迷。治療：限制蛋白質攝入，給予抗生素（預防細菌性毒素產物），灌腸以及瀉藥(排除結腸毒素)。

hepatic flexure the bend in the *colon, just underneath the liver, where the ascending colon joins the transverse colon.

結腸右曲 結腸的右側彎曲。正好在肝的下面。在該處升結腸連接橫結腸。

hepaticostomy *n.* a surgical operation in which a temporary or permanent opening is made into the main duct carrying bile from the liver.

肝管造口術 在膽總管處做一暫時性的或持久性開口的外科療法，以從肝臟運送膽汁。

hepatic vein one of several short veins originating within the lobes of the liver as small branches, which unite to form the hepatic veins. These lead directly to the inferior vena cava, draining blood from the liver.

肝靜脉 幾條短靜脉中的一條。其小分支起於肝葉內，而後合併成肝靜脉。這些肝靜脉直接通入下腔靜脉，從肝臟引流血液。

hepatitis *n.* inflammation of the liver due to a virus infection or such diseases as amoebic dysentery and lupus. *Infectious hepatitis* (*epidemic hepatitis, epidemic jaundice*) is transmitted by food or drink contaminated by a carrier or patient and commonly occurs where sanitation is poor. After an incubation period of 15–40 days, the patient develops fever and sickness. Yellow discoloration of the skin (*see* jaundice) appears about a week later and persists for up to three weeks. The patient may be infectious throughout this period. Serious complications are unusual and an attack often confers immunity. Injection of *gamma globulin provides temporary protection.

Serum hepatitis is transmitted by infected blood or blood products contaminating hypodermic needles, blood transfusions, or tattooing needles: it often occurs in drug addicts. Symptoms, which develop suddenly after an incubation period of 1–6 months, include headache, fever, chills, general weakness, and jaundice. Most patients make a gradual recovery but the mortality rate is 5–20%. Patients may be detected by identification of the *Australia antigen in their blood.

肝炎 由病毒感染或某些疾病（如阿米巴痢疾或狼瘡）引起的肝臟炎症。傳染性肝炎（流行性肝炎）是通過被帶病毒者或病人污染的食物或飲水傳播的。常見於缺少衛生條件的地區。潛伏期15-40天，然後病人出現發熱和噁心、嘔吐。經一周後，皮膚發黃，而且持續到3周。在這期間，病人可能有傳染性。嚴重的併發症是不常見的，一旦發病後常產生免疫力。注射丙種球蛋白可提供暫時性預防。

血清性肝炎是通過感染的血或血製品污染皮下注射針頭、輸血、或皮膚刺紋針（它常發生於嗜毒者）傳染的。症狀在潛伏期1-6個月後突然發生，包括頭痛、發熱、寒戰、虛弱和黃疸。多數病人可逐漸恢復，死亡率是5～20。通過鑑定病人血中的澳大利亞抗原可查明本病。

hepatization *n.* the conversion of lung tissue, which normally holds air, into a

肝樣變 肺組織轉變成肝樣的。在正常情況下肺組

solid liver-like mass during the course of acute lobar pneumonia.

纖含有氣體，在急性大葉性肺炎的過程中，則變爲實質性的肝樣團塊。

hepato- *prefix. see* hepat-.

〔前綴〕 **肝**

hepatoblastoma *n.* a malignant tumour of the liver occurring in children, made up of embryonic liver cells. It is often confined to one lobe of the liver; such cases may be treated by partial *hepatectomy.

肝胚細胞瘤 一種肝的惡性腫瘤。發生於小兒。由胚胎的肝細胞組成。它通常局限於肝的一個葉，這樣的病例可通過部分肝切除術治療。

hepatocellular *adj.* relating to or affecting the cells of the liver.

肝細胞的 與肝細胞有關的或影響肝細胞的。

hepatocyte *n.* the principal cell type in the *liver: a large cell with many metabolic functions, including synthesis, storage, detoxification, and bile production.

肝細胞 肝的主要細胞類型：一種大型的具有許多代謝功能（包括合成、貯存、解毒和產生膽汁）的細胞。

hepatoma *n.* a malignant tumour of the liver, originating in mature liver cells. In Western countries it is rare in normal livers, but often develops in patients with cirrhosis. In Africa and other tropical countries it is frequent, possible causes including fungi (*see* aflatoxin) and other ingested toxins. Hepatomas often synthesize *alpha-fetoprotein, which circulates in the blood and is a useful indicator of these tumours.
The term hepatoma is often, though incorrectly, used to include malignant tumours arising in the bile duct (*cholangiocarcinomas*).

肝細胞癌 一種肝的惡性腫瘤。起源於成熟的肝細胞。在西方國家裏，本病在正常肝中是很少見的，但常發生於肝硬化患者。本病常見於非洲和其它熱帶國家，其可能原因包括黴菌和其它攝入的毒素。這些肝細胞癌往往合成甲胎蛋白，在血中循環，因而它是診斷這種腫瘤有用的標誌。肝細胞癌這術語常常（不正確地）包括發生於膽管的惡性腫瘤（膽管癌）。

hepatomegaly *n.* enlargement of the liver to such an extent that it can be felt below the rib margin. This may be due to congestion (as in heart failure), inflammation, infiltration (e.g. by fat), or tumour.

肝大 肝臟增大，達到可在肋緣下觸及的程度。本症可由充血（如心力衰竭時）、炎症、脂肪浸潤或腫瘤引起。

hepatotoxic *adj.* damaging or destroying liver cells. Drugs such as *paracetamol and *phenacemide can cause liver damage at high doses or with prolonged use.

肝細胞毒的 損傷或破壞肝細胞的。一些藥物如撲熱息痛、苯乙醯脲，在高劑量和長期應用的情況下，可引起肝損害。

hept- (hepta-) *prefix denoting* seven.

〔前綴〕 **七，庚**

heptabarbitone *n.* a *barbiturate administered by mouth to treat insomnia. A common side-effect is drowsiness, and prolonged use can lead to dependence. Trade name: **Medomin**.

庚巴比妥 治療失眠症的口服巴比妥。常見的副作用有倦眠，長期應用可導致賴藥性。

hereditary *adj.* transmitted from parents to their offspring; inherited.

遺傳的 由父母傳給他們的子女的。

heredity *n.* the process that causes the biological similarity between parents and their offspring. *Genetics is the study of heredity.

遺傳 決定父母與子女之間生物學相似性的過程。遺傳學是研究遺傳的學科。

heredo- *prefix denoting* heredity.

〔前綴〕 **遺傳**

hermaphrodite *n.* an individual in which both male and female sex organs are present or in which the sex organs contain both ovarian and testicular cells. Human hermaphrodites are very rare. —**hermaphroditism** *n.*

兩性體 出現男性和女性兩性器官，或性器官含有卵巢細胞和睾丸細胞的人。人類兩性體是很少見的。

hernia *n.* the protrusion of an organ or tissue out of the body cavity in which it normally lies. An *inguinal hernia* (or *rupture*) occurs in the lower abdomen; a sac of peritoneum, containing fat or part of the bowel, bulges through a weak part (*inguinal canal*) of the abdominal wall. It may result from physical straining or coughing. A *scrotal hernia* is an inguinal hernia so large that it passes into the scrotum; a *femoral hernia* is similar to an inguinal hernia but protrudes at the top of the thigh, through the point at which the femoral artery passes from the abdomen to the thigh. A *diaphragmatic hernia* is the protrusion of an abdominal organ through the diaphragm into the chest cavity; the most common type is the *hiatus hernia*, in which the stomach passes partly or completely into the chest cavity through the hole (*hiatus*) for the oesophagus (gullet). An *umbilical hernia*, most common in young children, appears as a bulge at the navel.

疝 某一器官或組織從體腔的正常位置向外突出。腹股溝疝發生於下腹部；為一腹膜囊，內含脂肪或一部分腸，經腹壁的薄弱部（腹股溝管）膨出。它可因全身用力或咳嗽引起。陰囊疝是由於腹股溝疝過大，以致通入陰囊內；股疝與腹股溝疝類似，不同的是經過股動脈從腹部到大腿通過的點突出至大腿上部。膈疝是某一腹部器官經膈肌突入胸腔內；最常見的類型是裂孔疝，它是胃的一部分或全部經食管裂孔突入胸腔。臍疝最常見於幼小兒童，表現為臍部膨出。

這些疝有時因不能回復到它們正常的位置（不能還原的）而變得複雜化，增大，且固定於其囊內（箝頓性的），或失去血液供應，出現疼痛，終至壞死（絞窄性的）。這種疝最

Hernias may be complicated by becoming impossible to return to their normal site (*irreducible*); swollen and fixed within their sac (*incarcerated*); or cut off from their blood supply, becoming painful and eventually gangrenous (*strangulated*). The best treatment for hernias, especially if they are painful, is surgical repair (*see* hernioplasty).

好的治療方法——尤其如有疼痛時——是外科修補術。

hernio- *prefix denoting* a hernia.

〔前綴〕 疝

hernioplasty *n.* the surgical operation to repair a hernia, in which the abnormal opening is sewn up and/or the weakness strengthened with suture material.

疝根治術 修補疝的外科手術。即縫合疝的異常開口，及/或用縫線加强薄弱部位。

herniorrhaphy *n.* surgical repair of a hernia.

疝縫合術 疝的外科修補術。

heroin (diamorphine) *n.* a white crystalline powder derived from *morphine but with a shorter duration of action. Like morphine it is a powerful narcotic analgesic whose continued use leads to *dependence.

海洛因（二乙醯嗎啡） 由嗎啡衍生的白色結晶形粉劑。但作用時間比嗎啡短。和嗎啡一樣，它是强的痲醉鎮痛劑，長期應用可導致賴藥性。

herpangina *n.* a viral infectious disease of sudden onset that causes fever, blisters, and ulceration of the soft palate and tonsillar area.

疱疹性咽峽炎 突然發作的病毒感染性疾病。它引起發熱、水疱和軟腭與扁桃體區的潰瘍。

herpes *n.* inflammation of the skin caused by viruses and characterized by collections of small blisters. *Herpes simplex* (*cold sore*) can cause an acute *conjunctivitis or inflammation of the mouth or vagina, but many people contract the virus without showing any symptoms. The disease may recur. *Genital herpes*, caused by herpes simplex II virus, is a sexually transmitted disease characterized by painful blisters in the genital region. It is recurrent and extremely contagious as the blisters burst to release viruses that infect the sexual partner. *Herpes zoster* (*shingles*) usually starts with pain along the distribution of a nerve (often in the face, chest, or abdomen), followed by the development of vesicles. The disease subsides in about three weeks, though some-

疱疹 病毒引起的皮膚炎症。以成堆的小水疱爲特徵。單純疱疹（感冒瘡）可引起結膜炎或口腔與陰道的炎症，但許多人感染這種疾病而不表現任何症狀。本病可復發。生殖器疱疹由Ⅱ型單純疱疹病毒引起，是一種性傳染病，以生殖器部位的疼痛性水疱爲特徵。它是反復發作性的，而且當水疱破裂釋放病毒時，極易傳染其配偶。帶狀疱疹往往以沿神經分佈（常見於面、胸或腹部）的疼痛開始，隨後發生水疱。受侵神經的區域有時疼痛嚴重，可持續數月，但本病一般約於3周內消退。引起帶狀疱疹

times severe pain may persist for many months in the area of the affected nerve. The virus that causes herpes zoster can also cause chickenpox in children. *See also* Ramsay Hunt syndrome.

的這種病毒，在小兒也可引起水痘。

herpesvirus *n.* one of a group of DNA-containing viruses causing latent infections in man and animals. The herpesviruses are the causative agents of *herpes and chickenpox. The group also includes the *cytomegalovirus and *Epstein-Barr virus. *Herpesvirus simiae* (*virus B*) causes an infection in monkeys similar to herpes simplex, but when transmitted to man it can produce fatal encephalitis.

疱疹病毒 含DNA病毒羣的一種。在人類和動物引起潛伏性感染。疱疹病毒是疱疹和水痘的病因。這病毒羣也包括巨細胞病毒和埃-巴二氏病毒（非洲淋巴瘤病毒）。猿猴B病毒在猿猴中引起與單純疱疹相同的一種感染，但傳到人類時則可發生致死性的腦炎。

hertz *n.* the *SI unit of frequency, equal to one cycle per second. Symbol: Hz.

赫〔兹〕 頻率的國際標準單位。等於每秒一周。符號：Hz。

heter- (hetero-) *prefix denoting* difference; dissimilarity.

〔前綴〕 **異**

heterochromatin *n.* chromosome material (*see* chromatin) that stains most deeply when the cell is not dividing. It is thought not to represent major genes but may be involved in controlling these genes, and also in controlling mitosis and development. *Compare* euchromatin.

異染色質 細胞不分裂時染色體中染色最深的物質。現認爲，它不代表多數基因，但它可參與控制這些基因，而且也控制有絲分裂和發育。

heterochromia *n.* colour difference in the iris of the eye, which is usually congenital but is occasionally secondary to inflammation of the iris. In *heterochromia iridis* one iris differs in colour from the other; in *heterochromia iridum* one part of the iris differs in colour from the rest.

異色性 指眼虹膜的顏色不同。它往往是先天性的，但偶爾是虹膜炎症的繼發感染。一眼虹膜異色是一眼虹膜的顏色與另一眼不同；兩眼虹膜異色是兩眼虹膜某一部分的顏色與其餘部分不同。

heterogametic *adj.* describing the sex that produces two different kinds of gamete, which carry different *sex chromosomes, and that therefore determines the sex of the offspring. In humans men are the heterogametic sex: the sperm cells carry either an X or a Y chromosome. *Compare* homogametic.

異型配子的 描述產生兩種不同類型配子的性別的。即帶有不同的性染色體，因而確定子女的性別。在人類男性是異型配子性別：其精子細胞帶一個X或一個Y染色體。

heterograft (xenograft) *n.* a living tissue graft that is made from one animal species to another. For example, attempts have been made to graft animal organs into humans.

異種移植物 從一種動物移到另一種動物的活組織移植物。例如將動物器官移植到人類。

heterophoria *n.* a tendency to squint. Under normal circumstances both the eyes work together and look at the same point simultaneously, but if one eye is covered it will move out of alignment with the object the other eye is still viewing. When the cover is removed the eye immediately returns to its normal position. Most people have a small degree of the type of heterophoria known as *exophoria,* in which the covered eye turns outwards, away from the nose (*compare* esophoria). Heterophoria often produces eyestrain because of the unconscious effort required to keep the two eyes coordinated. *See also* strabismus.

隱斜視 一種斜眼的傾向。在正常情況下，兩眼一起動作，同時看到物體的同一點上，但如遮着一隻眼，此眼的視線就離開物體，而另一眼則仍注視着物體。當將遮蔽物移去時，該眼即回到正常的位置。多數人都有點外隱斜視（隱斜視的一型），此型隱斜視，被遮住的眼球離鼻側向外轉動。隱斜視時，由於需要無意識的用力，以使兩眼協調，因此常引起眼疲勞。

Heterophyes *n.* a genus of small parasitic *flukes occurring in Egypt and the Far East. Adult flukes of the species *H. heterophyes* live in the small intestine of man and other fish-eating animals; in man the flukes can produce serious symptoms (*see* heterophyiasis). The fluke has two intermediate hosts, a snail and a mullet fish.

異形吸蟲屬 發生於埃及和遠東的小型寄生性吸蟲的一屬。異形吸蟲的成蟲寄生於人和其他食魚類動物的小腸中，在人體可引起嚴重症狀。這種吸蟲有兩個中間宿主，即蝸牛和鯔魚。

heterophyiasis *n.* an infestation of the small intestine with the parasitic fluke **Heterophyes heterophyes*. Man becomes infected on eating raw or salted fish that contains the larval stage of the fluke. The presence of adult flukes may provoke symptoms of abdominal pain and diarrhoea; if the eggs reach the brain, spinal cord, and heart (via the bloodstream) they produce serious lesions. *Tetrachloroethylene is used in treatment of the infection.

異形吸蟲病 由寄生性吸蟲“異形吸蟲”引起的小腸感染。人因食進生的或醃過的魚（含有吸蟲的幼蟲階段）而感染。吸蟲成蟲的存在可引起腹痛和腹瀉症狀；其蟲卵移行至大腦、脊髓和心臟（經血流）時可引起該部位的嚴重損害。可用四氯乙烯治療。

heteroplasty *n.* the grafting of tissue from an animal of one species to another.

異種移植術 把某一個種的動物組織移植到另一個種。

heteropsia *n.* different vision in each eye.

雙眼不等視 每隻眼的視力不相同。

heterosexuality *n.* the pattern of sexuality in which sexual behaviour and thinking are directed towards people of the opposite sex. It includes both normal and deviant forms of sexual activity. —**heterosexual** *adj.*, *n.*

異性性慾 性慾的類型。其性行爲和思維針對着相反性別的人。它包括正常和變態型性慾。

heterosis *n.* hybrid vigour: the increased sturdiness, resistance to disease, etc., of individuals whose parents are of different races or species compared both with their parents and with the offspring of genetically similar parents.

雜種優勢 雜種生物的活力增强：父母是不同族或不同種，其子女的個體，與他們的父母比，或者與遺傳學上相同的父母所生子女比較時顯得更加健壯，抗病力强。

heterotopia (heterotopy) *n.* the displacement of an organ or part of the body from its normal position.

異位 人體某一器官或部位離開其正常位置。

heterotrophic (organotrophic) *adj.* describing organisms (known as heterotrophs) that use complex organic compounds to synthesize their own organic materials. Most are *chemoheterotrophic*, i.e. they use the organic compounds as an energy source. This group includes the majority of bacteria and all animals and fungi. *Compare* autotrophic.

異養的（器官營養的） 指用複雜的有機化合物合成自身有機物的生物體（通稱異養生物）。多數是化學異養的，即它們用有機化合物作爲能量的來源。這羣生物包括多數細菌、所有動物和黴菌。

heterotropia *n. see* strabismus.

斜視

heterozygous *adj.* describing an individual in whom the members of a pair of genes determining a particular characteristic are dissimilar. *See* allele. *Compare* homozygous. —**heterozygote** *n.*

雜合的 決定某一個體某一性狀的一對基因互不相同。

hex- (hexa-) *prefix denoting* six.

〔前綴〕 六，己

hexacanth *n. see* oncosphere.

六鈎蚴

hexachlorophane *n.* a disinfectant similar to *phenol, formerly used in soaps and creams to treat skin disorders. Its use in medicinal products was limited by law in 1973 because of the toxic effects it might produce when absorbed into the body.

雙三氯酚 與酚相同的一種消毒劑。過去用其肥皂類和乳劑類以治療皮膚疾患。由於當本藥吸收進入人體時可能產生毒性作用，因此其醫藥產品的應用，已受 1973 年的法令限制。

hexachromia *n.* the ability to distinguish only six of the seven colours of the spectrum, the exception being indigo. Most people cannot distinguish indigo from blue or violet.

六色症 只能分辨七色光譜中六色的能力（排除靛藍）。多數人不能分辨藍色和紫色。

hexamine (methenamine) *n.* an *antiseptic with a wide range of antibacterial activity, used to treat infections and inflammation of the urinary tract, such as cystitis. High doses may cause irritation of the stomach or bladder. Trade names: **Hiprex, Mandelamine.**

烏洛托品 抗菌效力廣泛的一種抗菌劑。用於治療泌尿道感染和炎症，如膀胱炎。大劑量可引起胃和膀胱的刺激作用。

hexobarbitone *n.* an intermediate-acting *barbiturate administered by mouth to treat insomnia. Prolonged use can lead to dependence.

環己巴比妥 口服用中效巴比妥。用於治療失眠症。長期使用可引起賴藥性。

hexokinase *n.* an enzyme that catalyses the conversion of glucose to glucose-6-phosphate. This is the first stage of *glycolysis.

己糖〔磷酸〕激酶 催化葡萄糖轉化爲 6-磷酸葡萄糖的一種酶。是糖酵解的第一階段。

hexosamine *n.* the amino derivative of a *hexose sugar. The two most important hexosamines are *glucosamine and galactosamine.

己糖胺 己糖的氨基衍生物。兩種最重要的己糖胺類是氨基葡萄糖和氨基半乳糖。

hexose *n.* a simple sugar with six carbon atoms. Hexose sugars are the sugars most frequently found in food. The most important hexose is *glucose.

己糖 含六個碳原子的單糖，是食物中最多見的糖類，其中最重要的是葡萄糖。

hiatus *n.* an opening or aperture. For example, the diaphragm contains hiatuses for the oesophagus and aorta.

裂孔 一種開口或孔。如膈肌上的食管裂孔和主動脉裂孔。

hiatus hernia *see* hernia.

裂孔疝

hiccup *n.* abrupt involuntary lowering of the diaphragm and closure of the sound-producing folds at the upper end of the trachea, producing a characteristic sound as the breath is drawn in. Hiccups, which usually occur repeatedly, may be caused by indigestion or more serious disorders, such as alcoholism. Medical name: **singultus.**

呃逆 膈肌突然不自主地下降和氣管上端的聲帶皺襞突然關閉，產生一種獨特的如呼吸頓止的聲音。呃逆往往反復發生，可因消化不良或更嚴重的疾病（如酒精中毒）引起。

hidr- (hidro-) *prefix denoting* sweat. Example: *hidropoiesis* (formation of).

〔前綴〕 **汗** 例如汗生成。

hidradenitis (hidrosadenitis) *n.* inflammation of the sweat glands, usually occurring when the glands become blocked. This may occur in the armpit, around the nipple or umbilicus, or in the groin; if infection develops the condition is called *hidradenitis suppurativa.*

汗腺炎 汗腺的炎症。常發生於汗腺堵塞時。本病可發生於腋窩、乳頭、臍周圍或腹股溝。如感染進一步發展，這種情況就稱之爲化膿性汗腺炎。

hidroa *n. see* hydroa.

①水疱 ②水疱病

hidrosis *n.* **1.** the excretion of sweat. **2.** excessive sweating.

①出汗 ②多汗

hidrotic *n.* an agent that causes sweating. *Parasympathomimetic drugs are hidrotics.

發汗藥 引起發汗的一種藥。擬副交感神經藥是發汗藥。

hilus *n.* (*pl.* **hila**) a hollow situated on the surface of an organ, such as the kidney or spleen, at which structures such as blood vessels, nerve fibres, and ducts enter or leave it.

門 位於某一器官（如腎或脾）表面的凹洞。該器官的血管、神經以及管道等結構由此進出。

hindbrain *n.* the part of the *brain comprising the cerebellum, pons, and medulla oblongata. The pons and medulla contain the nuclei of many of the cranial nerves, which issue from their surfaces, and the reticular formation. The fluid-filled cavity in the midline is the fourth *ventricle.

菱腦 由小腦、腦橋以及延髓組成的腦的一部分。腦橋和延髓內含有許多腦神經核（腦神經由其外面發出）和網狀結構。位於其中線上充滿液體的腔隙是第四腦室。

hindgut *n.* the back part of the embryonic gut, which gives rise to part of the large intestine, the rectum, bladder, and urinary ducts. *See also* cloaca.

後腸 胚胎腸的後部。由此發生大腸的一部分、直腸、膀胱和尿道。

hindquarter amputation an operation involving removal of an entire leg and part or all of the pelvis associated with it. It is usually performed for soft tissue or bone sarcomas arising from the upper thigh, hip, or buttock. *Compare* forequarter amputation.

髂腹間切斷術 包括切除整個大腿以及部分或全部骨盆在內的一種手術。在股、髂或臀上部發生軟組織或骨肉瘤時往往可行此術。

hinge joint *see* ginglymus.

屈戌關節

hip *n.* the region of the body where the thigh bone (femur) articulates with the *pelvis: the region on each side of the pelvis.

髖部 股骨與骨盆形成關節連接的人體的部位。此部位在骨盆兩側。

hip bone (innominate bone) a bone formed by the fusion of the ilium, ischium, and pubis. It articulates with the femur by the *acetabulum*, a deep socket into which the head of the femur fits. Between the pubis and ischium, below and slightly in front of the acetabulum, is a large opening – the *obturator foramen*. The right and left hip bones form part of the *pelvis.

髖骨 由髂骨、坐骨和耻骨融合形成的骨。通過髂臼與股骨形成關節連接（即股骨頭進入髂臼窩）。耻骨與坐骨間、髂臼下稍前方是一大的開口——閉孔，左，右側髂骨形成骨盆的一部分。

hip girdle *see* pelvic girdle.

髖帶

Hippelates *n.* a genus of small flies. The adults of *H. pallipes* are suspected of transmitting *yaws in the West Indies. Other species of *Hippelates* may be involved in the transmission of conjunctivitis.

潛蠅屬 小蠅的一屬。在西印度羣島，淡色潛蠅可能傳播雅司疹。潛蠅屬的其它蟲種參與傳播結膜炎。

hippocampal formation a curved band of cortex lying within each cerebral hemisphere: in evolutionary terms one of the brain's most primitive parts. It forms a portion of the *limbic system and is involved in the complex physical aspects of behaviour governed by emotion and instinct.

海馬結構 位於每側大腦半球內的皮質的彎曲帶。從進化的觀點來看，是腦最古老的部分之一。它形成邊緣系統的一部分，由情緒和本能所控制的行爲，其複雜的生理活動與此結構有關。

hippocampus *n.* a swelling in the floor of the lateral *ventricle of the brain. It contains complex foldings of cortical tissue and is involved, with other connections of the *hippocampal formation, in the workings of the *limbic system. —**hippocampal** *adj.*

海馬 大腦的側腦室底的一隆突。此隆突內含有皮質組織的複雜皺褶，與海馬有關的其它結構聯繫在一起，參與邊緣系統的種種活動。

Hippocratic oath the oath taken by a doctor that binds him to observe the code of behaviour and practice followed by the Greek physician Hippocrates (460–370 BC), called the 'Father of Medicine', and the students of the medical school in Cos where he taught.

希波克拉底誓言 醫生用以約束自己的誓言。醫生立誓要按照醫學之父希臘醫生希波克拉底（公元前460～370）及他任教的科斯島醫學校的學生們的行醫準則行事。

hippus *n.* abnormal rhythmical variations in the size of the pupils, independent of the intensity of the light falling on the eyes. It is occasionally seen in various diseases of the nervous system.

虹膜震顫 瞳孔大小發生異常的節律性的變化。與進入眼中的光的強度無關。偶爾見於各種神經系統疾病。

Hirschsprung's disease a congenital condition in which the rectum and sometimes part of the lower colon have failed to develop a normal nerve network. The affected portion does not expand or conduct the contents of the bowel, which accumulate in and distend the upper colon. Symptoms, which are usually apparent in the first weeks of life, are abdominal pain and swelling and severe or complete constipation. Diagnosis is by X-ray and by microscopic examination of samples of the bowel wall, which shows the absence of nerve cells. Treatment is by surgery to remove the affected segment and join the remaining (normal) colon to the anus. *See also* megacolon.

赫希施普龍氏病 一種先天性疾病：在胚胎發育中直腸和部分下段結腸未形成正常的神經網。受累部位不能擴張或輸送腸內容物，以致腸內容物在腸內聚積，而其上段結腸擴張。其症狀往往在生後幾週內出現，有腹痛、腹脹以及嚴重便秘或完全不能排便。通過X線以及腸壁標本的顯微鏡檢查來診斷，顯微鏡檢查顯示神經細胞缺失。通過外科手術治療，切除受累腸段，將剩餘的結腸（正常的）接到肛門上。

hirsutism *n.* excessive hairiness, particularly in women. Rarely, the cause may be a disturbance of the hormone systems but usually the cause is not known.

多毛症 毛髮過多，尤其是婦女。少見，其原因往往不明。

hirudin *n.* an *anticoagulant present in the salivary glands of leeches and in certain snake venoms, that prevents *blood coagulation by inhibiting the action of the enzyme *thrombin.

水蛭素 存在於水蛭腮腺和某些蛇毒液中的抗凝血劑。它通過抑制凝血酶的作用以預防血液凝固。

hist- (histio-, histo-) *prefix denoting* tissue

〔前綴〕 **組織**

histaminase *n.* an enzyme, widely distributed in the body, that is responsible for the inactivation of histamine.

組胺酶 廣泛分佈於體內的一種酶。它能滅活組織胺。

histamine *n.* a compound derived from the amino acid histidine. It is found in nearly all tissues of the body, associated mainly with the *mast cells. Histamine has pronounced pharmacological activity, causing dilation of blood vessels and contraction of smooth muscle (for example, in the lungs). It is an important mediator of inflammation and is released in large amounts after skin damage (such as that due to animal venoms and toxins),

組織胺 由氨基酸（組氨酸）衍生的一種化合物。它幾乎見於人體的所有組織，主要與肥大細胞有關。組織胺有顯著的藥理學作用，引起血管擴張和平滑肌（例如肺中）收縮。組織胺是炎症的一種重要介質，皮膚損傷後（例如由於動物毒液和毒素）大量釋放，產生獨特的皮膚反應（由潮紅、風

producing a characteristic skin reaction (consisting of flushing, a flare, and a wheal). Histamine is also released in anaphylactic reactions and allergic conditions, including asthma, and gives rise to some of the symptoms of these conditions. *See also* anaphylaxis.

疹塊組成）。在過敏反應和變態反應病（包括哮喘）中也釋放出組織胺，能引發此類疾病的某些症狀。

histamine acid phosphate a derivative of *histamine used to test for acid secretion in the stomach in conditions involving abnormal gastric secretion, such as *Zollinger-Ellison syndrome. It is administered by injection and can cause headache, wheezing, rapid heart beat, disturbed vision, and digestive upsets.

磷酸組織胺 組織胺的一種衍生物。用於包括胃分泌異常（例如佐-埃二氏綜合徵——促胃泌素瘤）等疾病的胃酸分泌試驗。注射給藥，可引起頭痛、喘鳴、心跳加快、視力模糊以及消化紊亂。

histidine *n.* an *amino acid from which *histamine is derived.

組氨酸 一種氨基酸。組織胺由其衍生。

histiocyte *n.* a fixed *macrophage, i.e. one that is stationary within connective tissue.

組織細胞 一種在結締組織內靜止不動的巨噬細胞。

histiocytoma *n.* a tumour that contains *macrophages or *histiocytes, large cells with the ability to engulf foreign matter and bacteria. *See also* fibrosarcoma (malignant fibrous histiocytoma).

組織細胞瘤 一種含有巨噬細胞或組織細胞的腫瘤。大的細胞具有吞噬異物和細菌的能力。

histiocytosis *n.* any of a group of diseases in which there are abnormalities in certain large phagocytic cells (*histiocytes), leading to biochemical defects, such as abnormal storage of fats (as in *Gaucher's disease), and other poorly understood conditions, such as Letterer-Siwe disease and Hand-Schüller-Christian disease (*see* reticuloendotheliosis).

組織細胞增生症 某種大吞噬細胞（組織細胞）發生異常的一組疾病。可導致生化方面的缺陷，例如脂肪異常貯積（高歇氏病），以及其它病因不明的疾病，例如累-賽二氏病和漢-許-克三氏病。

histochemistry *n.* the study of the identification and distribution of chemical compounds within and between cells, by means of stains, indicators, and light and electron microscopy. —**histochemical** *adj.*

組織化學 以染劑、指示劑以及光學顯微鏡和電子顯微鏡檢查，研究細胞內或細胞間化合物的成分和分佈的科學。

histocompatibility *n.* the form of *compatibility that depends upon tissue

組織相容性 與組織成分（主要是細胞膜內特異性

components, mainly specific glycoprotein antigens in cell membranes. A high degree of histocompatibility is necessary for a tissue graft or organ transplant to be successful. —**histocompatible** *adj.*

糖蛋白）相容的性質。爲使組織移植或器官移植成功，需要高度的組織相容性。

histogenesis *n.* the formation of tissues.

組織發生 組織的形成。

histogram *n.* a form of statistical graph in which values are plotted in the form of rectangles on a chart; a bar-chart.

直方圖 統計圖的一種類型。其值以長方形繪製於圖表上；直條圖。

histoid *adj.* **1.** resembling normal tissue. **2.** composed of one type of tissue.

①**組織樣的** 類似正常組織的。 ②**單一組織的** 由一種類型的組織構成的。

histology *n.* the study of the structure of tissues by means of special staining techniques combined with light and electron microscopy. —**histological** *adj.*

組織學 以特別的染色技術以及光學顯微鏡和電子顯微鏡檢查研究組織結構的學科。

histone *n.* a simple protein that combines with a nucleic acid to form a *nucleoprotein.

組蛋白 一種單純蛋白。與核酸結合，形成一種核蛋白。

Histoplasma *n.* a genus of parasitic yeastlike fungi. The species *H. capsulatum* causes the respiratory infection *histoplasmosis.

組織胞漿菌屬 寄生性酵母菌的一屬。該菌屬的莢膜組織胞漿菌能引起的呼吸道感染，即組織胞漿菌病。

histoplasmin *n.* a preparation of antigenic material from a culture of the fungus *Histoplasma capsulatum*, used to test for the presence of the disease *histoplasmosis by subcutaneous injection.

莢膜組織胞漿菌素 由眞菌——莢膜組織胞漿菌培養出的抗原性物質的一種製劑。通過皮下注射，用於測驗組織胞漿菌病的存在。

histoplasmosis *n.* an infection caused by inhaling spores of the fungus *Histoplasma capsulatum*. The primary pulmonary form usually produces no symptoms or harmful effects and is recognized retrospectively by X-rays and positive *histoplasmin skin testing. Occasionally, progressive histoplasmosis, which resembles tuberculosis, develops. Symptomatic disease is treated with intravenous amphotericin-B. The

組織胞漿菌病 通過吸入眞菌——莢膜組織胞漿菌的孢子引起的一種感染。起初的肺型往往不引起症狀或有危害的後果，通過X線和陽性莢膜組織胞漿菌素皮膚試驗作追溯性的診斷。偶爾，進行性組織胞漿菌病類似活動性肺結核。有症狀的組織胞漿菌病可用靜脉注射二性

spores are found in soil contaminated by faeces, especially from chickens and bats. The disease is endemic in the northern and central US, Argentina, Brazil, Venezuela, and parts of Africa.

黴素B治療。孢子見於被糞便（尤其是鷄類和蝙蝠類）汚染的土壤。本病流行於美國北部和中部、阿根廷、巴西、委內瑞拉以及非洲部分地區。

histotoxic *adj.* poisonous to tissues: applied to certain substances and conditions.

組織毒的 對組織有毒的：描述某些物質和狀況。

hives *n. see* urticaria.

蕁麻疹

HL-A system histocompatibility lymphocyte-A system: a group of eight antigens that are the most important of the 20 or more antigens responsible for *histocompatibility. Successful tissue transplantation requires a minimum number of HL-A differences between donor's and recipient's tissues.

人白細胞抗原系 組織相容性淋巴細胞A位點系：對組織相容性起作用的20種以上抗原中最重要的一組（8種）抗原。成功的組織移植要求供者與受者之間的人白細胞抗原的差別很小才行。

hobnail liver the liver of a patient with cirrhosis, which has a knobbly appearance caused by regenerating nodules separated by bands of fibrous tissue.

結節樣肝臟 肝硬變病人的肝臟。由於纖維組織索將再生的小結分隔開，故肝臟具有結節樣外觀。

Hodgkin's disease a malignant disease of lymphatic tissues, usually characterized by painless enlargement of one or more groups of lymph nodes in the neck, armpits, groin, chest, or abdomen; the spleen, liver, bone marrow, and bones may also be involved. Apart from the enlarging glands, there may also be weight loss, fever, profuse sweating at night, and itching (known as *B symptoms*). Treatment depends on the extent of disease and may include surgery, radiotherapy, drug therapy, or a combination of these. Drugs used in the treatment of the disease include nitrogen mustard, vincristine, procarbazine, prednisone, chlorambucil, and vinblastine. Many patients can be cured; in the early stages of the disease this may be in the order of 85% or more.

何傑金氏病 淋巴組織的惡性疾病。往往以頸、腋、腹股溝、胸或腹部的單個或多羣淋巴結的無痛性腫大爲特徵，脾、骨髓和骨也受累。除腺體腫大外，也可有體重下降、發熱、夜間大量出汗以及瘙癢（通稱B症狀）。按疾病的蔓延範圍，治療可包括外科手術、放射治療、藥物治療，或這些療法的聯合應用。用以治療本病的藥物包括氮芥、長春新鹼、甲基苄肼、强的松、苯丁酸氮芥以及長春鹼。許多病人是可以治癒的：在疾病的早期階段，其治癒率可爲85%或更高。

holistic *adj.* describing an approach to patient care in which the physical, mental, and social factors in the pa-

機能整體性的 描述照料病人的一種思路：應考慮病人的肉體、精神以及社

tient's condition are taken into account, rather than just the diagnosed disease. 會等各方面因素，而不是僅僅考慮經診斷的疾病。

Holmes-Adie syndrome *see* Adie's syndrome. **霍-艾二氏綜合徵**

holo- *prefix denoting* complete or entire. 〔前綴〕 **完全，全部**

holocrine *adj.* describing a gland or type of secretion in which the entire cell disintegrates when the product is released. **全〔漿分〕泌的** 描述腺體或分泌的形式。當釋放其產物時，整個的細胞發生解體。

home help *see* social services. **家庭服務**

home nurse (district nurse) (in Britain) a trained nurse with special training in *domiciliary services. Formerly all home nurses were State Registered, but in recent years increasing numbers of State Enrolled Nurses are working in this field. Prior to 1974 they were employed either by voluntary agencies on repayment from local health authorities or by these authorities directly. The home nursing service is now the responsibility of District Health Authorities; normally day care only is provided but under special circumstances out of hours nursing can be arranged. Formerly each nurse was allocated to a geographic district and doctors requiring the services for their patients had to contact the local headquarters. However, it is now common for nurses to be allocated to a designated general practice, an arrangement sometimes known as *attachment*. **家庭護士（地段護士）**（在英國）在家庭服務部門受過專門訓練的護士。過去所有的家庭護士都是國家註册護士，近幾年來國家錄用護士逐步增加。1974 年以前他們或是由地方保健局付報酬的志願機構來僱用，或是由這些保健局直接僱用。家庭護理工作目前是地段保健局負責；正常情況下只提供日間護理，在特殊情況下可安排超時護理。過去，每一護士被分配到一定的地段，當醫生要求爲他們的病人提供服務時，必須與地方總部聯系。但現在通常是分配護士從事指定的護理工作，這種安排稱之爲附加護理。

homeo- (homoeo-) *prefix denoting* similar; like. 〔前綴〕 **相同，類似**

homeopathic (homoeopathic) *adj.* **1.** of or relating to *homeopathy. **2.** infinitesimally small, as applied to the dose of a drug. **①順勢療法的** 與順勢療法有關的。 **②極小的** 指藥物劑量。

homeopathy (homoeopathy) *n.* a system of medicine based on the theory that 'like cures like'. The patient is treated with extremely small quantities of drugs that are themselves capable of producing symptoms of his particular disease. The system was founded by Samuel Hahnemann (1755–1843) at the end of the 18th century and is followed by a minority of doctors in the UK. There is a Royal London Homeopathic Hospital. *See also* fringe medicine. —**homeopathist** *n.*

順勢療法 根據"通因通用"理論的一種醫學體系。即用極小的藥量治療病人，該藥有可能使病人產生與所患疾病相同的症狀。此體系於 18 世紀末由塞繆爾·哈曼（1755～1843）創立，在英國只有少數醫生沿用，並設有倫敦皇家順勢療法醫院。

homeostasis *n.* the physiological process by which the internal systems of the body (e.g. blood pressure, body temperature, *acid-base balance) are maintained at equilibrium, despite variations in the external conditions. —**homeostatic** *adj.*

內環境穩定 儘管外界條件不斷變化，仍能使身體的內部系統（例如血壓、體溫、酸鹼度）維持於平衡狀態的生理過程。

homo- *prefix denoting* the same or common.

〔前綴〕**同**

homoeopathy *n. see* homeopathy.

順勢療法

homogametic *adj.* describing the sex that produces only one kind of gamete, which carries the same *sex chromosome, and that therefore does not determine the sex of the offspring. In humans women are the homogametic sex: each egg cell carries an X chromosome. *Compare* heterogametic.

同型配子的 描述只能產生一種類型的配子的性別。這種配子帶有同樣的性染色體，因而不能決定子女的性別。在人類，婦女是同型配子性染色體：即每一卵細胞都帶有一個 X 染色體。

homogenize *vb.* to reduce material to a uniform consistency, e.g. by crushing and mixing. Organs and tissues are homogenized to determine their overall content of a particular enzyme or other substance. —**homogenization** *n.*

勻化 使物質變得均一。例如壓碎和混合。器官和組織經勻化，可以確定它們的特殊酶或其他物質的總含量。

homogentisic acid a product formed during the metabolism of the amino acids phenylalanine and tyrosine. In normal individuals homogentisic acid is oxidized by the enzyme *homogentisic acid oxidase*. In rare cases this enzyme is lacking and a condition known as *alcaptonuria, in which large amounts of homogentisic acid are excreted in the urine, results.

尿黑酸 氨基酸（苯丙氨酸和酪氨酸）代謝過程中形成的一種代謝產物。在正常人，尿黑酸由尿黑酸氧化酶氧化。在少數病例中，缺乏尿黑酸氧化酶，因而引起稱之爲尿黑酸尿的一種疾患。此症患者生成大量的尿黑酸從尿中排出。

homograft (allograft) *n.* a living tissue or organ graft between two members of the same species; for example, a heart transplant from one person to another. Such grafts will not survive unless the recipient is treated to suppress his body's automatic rejection of the foreign tissue.

同種移植物（異體移植物） 兩個同種生物體之間的活的組織或器官移植物。例如，某個人的心臟移植到另一個人的體內。這類移植物活的時間不會長，除非接受者經某種處理，以抑制體內對異物的自動排斥反應。

homoiothermic *adj.* warm-blooded: able to maintain a constant body temperature independently of, and despite variations in, the temperature of the surroundings. Mammals (including man) and birds are homoiothermic. *Compare* poikilothermic. —**homoiothermy** *n.*

恒溫的 溫血的。能自主地維持恒定體溫的，儘管周圍的溫度是變化着的。哺乳動物類（包括人）以及鳥類是恒溫的。

homolateral *adj. see* ipsilateral.

同側的

homologous *adj.* **1.** (in anatomy) describing organs or parts that have the same basic structure and evolutionary origin, but not necessarily the same function or superficial structure. *Compare* analogous. **2.** (in genetics) describing a pair of chromosomes of similar shape and size and having identical gene loci. One member of the pair is derived from the mother; the other from the father.

①**同種的** （解剖學）用於描述具有同樣基本結構和進化起源的器官或部位，但不一定有同一的功能或淺表結構。 ②**同源的** （遺傳學）用於描述具有同樣形狀和大小以及相同的基因位點的一對染色體。一對染色體之一是由母親帶來的，另一個則由父親帶來。

homoplasty *n.* surgical repair of defective or damaged tissues or organs with a *homograft.

同種移植術 以同種移植物來修復缺陷或損傷組織或器官的外科手術。

homosexuality *n.* the condition of being sexually attracted, covertly or overtly, by members of one's own sex: it can affect either sex (*see also* lesbianism). The cause of homosexuality remains unclear, although explanations in terms of either a deviant family structure or an environment with limited opportunities for heterosexual contacts are increasingly accepted. Homosexuality is no longer generally regarded as a psychological disorder but therapy may be offered to individuals wishing to change their sexual orienta-

同性性慾（同性戀） 同性之間隱蔽地或公開地產生性的吸引的情況，兩種性別均可發生。關於同性性慾的原因尚不清楚，儘管以家庭結構異常或其環境接觸異性機會受限等解釋日益為人們所接受。一般已不再認為同性性慾是一種心理上的紊亂，但對希望改變他們的性指向的人，可以提供治療。沒有有效的藥物來改變其性指向，儘管有可能抑制其性

tion. There are no drugs available for changing sexual orientation, although it is possible to depress the sexual drive. Treatment consists of psychotherapy or specific *behaviour therapy designed to eliminate homosexual behaviour and fantasy and to increase heterosexual behaviour. Persons seeking help for their homosexuality may benefit from *counselling to reduce their anxiety and guilt, rather than trying to change their sexual behaviour. —**homosexual** *adj.*, *n.*

衝動。治療包括心理療法或特殊的行爲療法（以消除同性戀行爲和幻想，並增强異性戀行爲）。對要求得到幫助的同性戀者，可通過勸告他們減少焦慮和罪惡感而獲效，而不是力圖改變他們的性行爲。

homozygous *adj.* describing an individual in whom the members of a pair of genes determining a particular characteristic are identical. *See* allele. *Compare* heterozygous. —**homozygote** *n.*

純合的 決定個體某種特徵的一對基因是完全相同的。

homunculus *n.* **1.** **(manikin)** a dwarf with no deformity or abnormality other than small size. **2.** **(manikin)** a small jointed anatomical model of a man. **3.** (in early biological theory) a miniature human being thought to be contained within each of the reproductive cells.

①**矮人** 沒有畸形或發育異常、只是身材矮小的人。②**人體模型** 指小型的可拆卸的人體解剖模型。③**小人** 早期的生物學理論，認爲是存在於每個生殖細胞內的微小的人。

hook *n.* a surgical instrument with a bent or curved tip, used to hold, lift, or retract tissue at operation.

鈎 尖端彎曲的一種外科器械。手術中用於把持組織、抬舉組織或將組織拉開。

hookworm *n.* either of two nematode worms, **Necator americanus* or **Ancylostoma duodenale*, which live as parasites in the intestine of man. Both species, also known as the New and Old World hookworms respectively, are of great medical importance (*see* hookworm disease).

鈎蟲 美洲板口線蟲或十二指腸鈎蟲。此類鈎蟲作爲寄生物生活於人的腸道中。這兩種蟲，稱爲新大陸線蟲和舊大陸線蟲，是醫學中極爲重要的兩種線蟲。

hookworm disease a condition resulting from an infestation of the small intestine by hookworms. Hookworm larvae live in the soil and infect man by penetrating the skin. The worms travel to the lungs in the bloodstream and from there pass via the windpipe and

鈎蟲病 由小腸受鈎蟲感染引起的一種疾患。鈎蟲幼蟲生活於土壤中，穿過人的皮膚感染人體。鈎蟲隨血流運行到肺部，然後由此經氣管及食管達到小腸。大量的鈎蟲感染可引

gullet to the small intestine. Heavy hookworm infections may cause considerable damage to the wall of the intestine, leading to a serious loss of blood; this, in conjunction with malnutrition, can provoke severe anaemia. Symptoms include abdominal pain, diarrhoea, debility, and mental inertia. The disease occurs throughout the tropics and subtropics and is prevalent in areas of poor personal hygiene and sanitation. Bephenium hydroxynaphthoate, reliable and easy to administer, is used in treatment.

起嚴重的腸壁損傷，導致嚴重失血以及營養不良，可造成嚴重貧血。症狀包括腹痛、腹瀉、虛弱以及精神不振。本病發生於整個熱帶和亞熱帶地區，流行於個人衞生和環境衞生條件差的地方。治療可用療效可靠、給藥方便的羥萘酸苄酚寧。

hordeolum *n. see* stye.

瞼腺炎

hormone *n.* a substance that is produced in one part of the body (by an *endocrine gland, such as the thyroid, adrenal, or pituitary), passes into the bloodstream and is carried to other (distant) organs or tissues, where it acts to modify their structure or function. Examples of hormones are corticosteroids (from the adrenal cortex), growth hormone (from the pituitary gland), and androgens (from the testes).

激素 身體的某一部分產生的一種物質（由內分泌腺，例如甲狀腺、腎上腺或垂體產生），進入血液後被帶到其它（遠隔）器官或組織，從而改變該器官或組織的結構和功能。例如有皮質類固醇（由腎上腺皮質產生）、生長激素（由垂體產生）以及雄激素（由睾丸產生）等激素。

horn *n.* (in anatomy) a process, outgrowth, or extension of an organ or other structure. It is often paired. In the spinal cord crescent-shaped areas of grey matter (seen in cross section) are known as the dorsal and ventral horns.

角 （解剖學）指器官或其它結構向外生長或延伸的一種突起。通常是成對的。脊髓中月牙形的灰質區（見於横切面）稱之爲〔灰質〕後角和〔灰質〕前角。

Horner's syndrome a group of symptoms that are due to a disorder of the sympathetic nerves in the cervical (neck) region. The syndrome consists of a constricted pupil, drooping of the upper eyelid (*ptosis), and an absence of sweating over the affected side of the face.

霍納氏綜合徵 由頸交感神經紊亂引起的症候羣。綜合徵包括瞳孔縮小、眼瞼下垂以及患側面部無汗等。

horseshoe kidney an anatomical variation in kidney development whereby the lower poles of both kidneys are

蹄鐵形腎 腎在發育過程中解剖學上的改變。即兩側腎的下極結合在一起，

joined together. This usually causes no trouble but it may be associated with impaired drainage of urine from the kidney by the ureters, which cross in front of the united lower segment.

形如蹄鐵。這種情况往往不引起任何不適，但可伴有從腎到輸尿管的排尿障礙（輸尿管橫過兩腎聯結下段的前方）。

hospice *n.* an institution that specializes in the care of terminally ill patients, using narcotic drugs in carefully controlled doses for the relief of pain.

臨終病室 爲看護臨終病人特設的一種機構。在謹愼控制藥物劑量的情况下使用麻醉藥，以減輕疼痛。

hospital *n.* an institution offering residential, investigatory, and/or therapeutic care regarded as too complex or specialized for provision as a *domiciliary service. Such care may be residential (in-patient), including the care of patients for a whole day and their return home at night (*day hospital*). Out-patient services include consultation with designated specialists by prior appointment, X-rays, laboratory tests, physiotherapy, and accident and emergency services for those requiring urgent care. Most Health Districts have a *general hospital* (*DGH*), which provides sufficient basic services for the population of the District. Some larger hospitals have resources that are more highly specialized, to meet the needs of a wider population, providing so-called *regional* or *supra-regional* (*national*) services. Such hospitals often provide training for medical students (*teaching* or *university hospitals*) and for postgraduate education. Some smaller hospitals – known as *community hospitals* – are staffed mainly or exclusively by general practitioners and are intended for patients for whom home care is impracticable on social grounds.

醫院 一種提供留住、觀察及/或治療看護的機構。這種機構可提供像家庭那樣的服務，只是更複雜、更專門化。有的需要留住（住院病人），有的全日看護病人，而夜晚回家（晝間醫院）。門診病人的服務項目包括預先安排的指定專家診治、X線檢查、實驗室檢查、理療，以及急症的照看和處理。多數責任地段擁有綜合醫院，對該地區人口提供足夠的、基本的服務項目。一些較大的醫院具有更高度專業化的條件，以滿足更廣大人口的需要，提供所謂地區性的或跨地區性的（全國性的）服務項目。有些醫院往往爲醫學生（教學醫院或大學醫院）和研究生教學提供訓練。有些較小的醫院稱之爲社區醫院，主要或全部的工作人員是全科醫生，其所收治的是由於社會經濟條件不能進行家庭護理的病人。

Hospital Activity Analysis *see* Hospital In-patient Enquiry.

醫院活動分析

hospital fatality ratio *see* case fatality ratio.

住院病死率

Hospital In-patient Enquiry (in Britain) a statistical review, organized

住院病人調查 在英國由保健部、社會保障部以

jointly by the *Department of Health and Social Security and the *Office of Population Censuses and Surveys, providing information about in-patients treated in National Health Service hospitals. The data, based on a sample of episodes of illness (as distinct from individual patients), include diagnosis on discharge or death, duration on the waiting list, and length of stay. More detailed information, including aspects of therapy while in the hospital, are included in *Hospital Activity Analysis*. *Compare* record linkage.

及人口普查局共同組織的一種統計學調查。提供在國民保健服務制醫院治療的住院病人的信息。根據疾病抽樣（不同於個別病人）得到的資料，內容包括出院或死亡診斷、等候入院時間的長短以及住院的時間長短。更詳細的信息（包括住院期間治療方面的信息）包括在醫院工作分析中。

host *n.* an animal or plant in or upon which a *parasite lives. An *intermediate host* is one in which the parasite passes its larval or asexual stages; a *definitive* host is one in which the parasite develops to its sexual stage.

宿主 寄生物寄生於其內（或其上）的動物或植物。中間宿主是寄生蟲的幼蟲或無性生殖階段暫時寄生之處，終宿主則供寄生蟲發育至其有性生殖階段。

hourglass contraction constriction of an organ at its centre as a result of abnormal muscular contraction. Hourglass contraction may be a complication of labour, tending to trap the placenta in the upper part of the constricted womb and possibly leading to excessive blood loss after delivery.

葫蘆狀收縮 由於器官中肌肉的異常收縮，使其中間部分縮窄，形如葫蘆。葫蘆狀收縮可能是分娩的一種併發症，使縮窄的子宮上部的胎盤滯留，可能會導致產後失血過多。

housemaid's knee a fluid-filled swelling of the bursa in front of the kneecap, often resulting from frequent kneeling. Treatment – and prevention – is by avoidance of kneeling. *See also* bursitis.

髕前囊炎 髕骨前囊的一種充液性腫脹。往往因頻繁下跪所致。防治方法是避免下跪。

house physician/surgeon *see* doctor.

住院內科醫生/外科醫生

humectant 1. *n.* a substance that is used for moistening. **2.** *adj.* causing moistening.

①**致濕劑** 用於引起潮濕的物質。 ②**致濕的** 引起潮濕的。

humerus *n.* the bone of the upper arm. The *head* of the humerus articulates with the *scapula at the shoulder joint. At the lower end of the shaft the *trochlea* articulates with the *ulna and part of the radius. The radius also articulates with a rounded protuber-

肱骨 上臂骨。肱骨頭在肩關節處與肩胛骨相關節。肱骨體下端滑車與尺骨和部分橈骨相關節。橈骨也與圓形的肱骨突起（肱骨小頭）在滑車附近相關節。當屈曲或伸直上

ance (*capitulum*) close to the trochlea. Depressions (*fossae*) at the front and back of the humerus accommodate the ulna and radius, respectively, when the arm is flexed or straightened.

臂時，肱骨的前後兩個凹陷（窩）分別與尺骨和橈骨相適應。

humour *n.* a body fluid. *See* aqueous humour, vitreous humour.

液 體液。

Hurler's syndrome an inborn defect of metabolism causing the accumulation of mucopolysaccharides and lipids in the cells of the body. This leads to mental retardation, enlargement of the liver and spleen, deformities of the bones, and coarsening and thickening of the features (*gargoylism*).

胡爾勒氏綜合徵 一種新生兒代謝缺陷。可引起黏多糖類和脂肪類在體內的聚積。本綜合徵可致精神發育不全、肝脾腫大、骨畸形以及臉面粗糙和增厚（脂肪軟骨營養不良）。

Hutchinson's teeth narrowed and notched permanent incisor teeth: a sign of congenital *syphilis.

郝秦生氏牙 狹小而有切口的恒切牙：先天梅毒的一種體徵。

hyal- (hyalo-) *prefix denoting* **1.** glassy; transparent. **2.** hyalin. **3.** the vitreous humour of the eye.

〔前綴〕 **①玻璃狀的，透明的 ②透明蛋白 ③眼的水狀液（眼房水）**

hyalin *n.* a clear glassy material produced as the result of degeneration in certain tissues, particularly connective tissue and epithelial cells.

透明蛋白 一種清澈的玻璃樣物質。由某些組織，特別是結締組織和上皮細胞變性所致。

hyaline cartilage the most common type of *cartilage: a bluish-white elastic material with a matrix of chondroitin sulphate in which fine collagen fibrils are embedded.

透明軟骨 最常見的軟骨類型；一種具有軟骨素硫酸鹽基質的藍白色彈性物質。其中嵌有纖細的膠原纖維。

hyaline membrane disease *see* respiratory distress syndrome.

透明膜病

hyalitis *n.* inflammation of the *vitreous body of the eye. *Asteroid hyalitis* is a degenerative condition (rather than an inflammation), in which the vitreous contains many small white opacities.

玻璃體炎 眼的玻璃體炎症。星狀玻璃體炎是一種變性疾患（非炎症），玻璃體內含有許多小的白濁斑。

hyaloid artery a fetal artery lying in the *hyaloid canal of the eye and supplying the lens.

玻璃體動脉 胎兒動脉。位於眼的玻璃管內，並供給晶狀體血液。

hyaloid canal a channel within the vitreous humour of the *eye. It extends from the centre of the optic disc, where

玻璃體管 眼玻璃體內一種小管。它由視神經乳頭的中央（在該處與視神經

it communicates with the lymph spaces of the optic nerve, to the posterior wall of the lens.

的淋巴間隙相通）延伸至晶狀體後壁。

hyaloid membrane the transparent membrane that surrounds the *vitreous humour of the eye, separating it from the retina.

玻璃體膜 圍繞眼玻璃體的透明膜，使玻璃體與視網膜分隔開。

hyaluronic acid an acid *mucopolysaccharide that acts as the binding and protective agent of the ground substance of connective tissue. It is also present in the synovial fluid around joints and in the vitreous and aqueous humours of the eye.

透明質酸 一種酸性黏多糖。在結締組織基質中起黏合劑和保護劑的作用。此酸也存在於關節的滑液中以及眼的玻璃體和房水中。

hyaluronidase *n.* an enzyme that depolymerizes *hyaluronic acid and therefore increases the permeability of connective tissue. Hyaluronidase is found in the testes, in semen, and in other tissues.

透明質酸酶 能使透明質酸解聚，因而增加結締組織通透性的酶。透明質酸酶見於睾丸、精子以及其他組織中。

hybrid *n.* the offspring of a cross between two genetically unlike individuals. A hybrid, whose parents are usually of different species or varieties, is often sterile.

雜種 基因不同的個體之間交配所生下來的後代。其雙親往往是不同的種或變種。雜種通常是不育的。

hydatid *n.* a bladder-like cyst formed in various human tissues following the growth of the larval stage of an **Echinococcus* tapeworm. *E. granulosus* produces a single large fluid-filled cyst, called *unilocular hydatid*, which gives rise internally to smaller daughter cysts. The entire hydatid is bound by a fibrous capsule. *E. multilocularis* forms aggregates of many smaller cysts with a jelly-like matrix, called an *alveolar hydatid*, and enlarges by budding off external daughter cysts. Alveolar hydatids are not delimited by fibrous capsules and produce malignant tumours, which invade and destroy human tissues. *See also* hydatid disease.

棘球蚴囊 棘球屬絛蟲的幼蟲階段在人體的各種組織生長後形成的球狀囊。細粒棘球絛蟲產生單一的、大的充滿液體的囊，叫單房性棘球蚴囊，在囊內發生較小的子囊。完整的棘球蚴囊由纖維性被膜包繞。多房型棘球絛蟲形成內含膠狀基質的許多較小蚴囊的集結，叫泡狀棘球蚴囊，它向外萌發子囊而增大。泡狀棘球幼囊不以纖維性被膜爲界，而且產生惡性腫瘤，此瘤侵入和破壞人體組織。

hydatid disease (hydatidosis, echinococciasis, echinococcosis) a condition resulting from the presence in the liver, lungs, or brain of the *hydatid

棘球蚴病 由於棘球蚴囊存於肝、肺或腦而引起的一種疾患。多房型棘球絛蟲的棘球蚴囊形成惡性腫

cysts. The cysts of *Echinococcus multilocularis* form malignant tumours; those of *E. granulosus* exert pressure as they grow and thereby damage surrounding tissues. The presence of hydatids in the brain may result in blindness and epilepsy, and the rupture of any cyst can cause severe allergic reactions including fever and *urticaria. Treatment may necessitate surgical removal of the cysts. Spread of hydatid disease, particularly common in sheep-raising countries, can be prevented by the deworming of dogs.

瘤；細粒棘球絛蟲的棘球蚴囊生長時可產生壓力，而且繼之損傷周圍組織。棘球蚴囊存於腦中可導致失明和癲癇，而且任何蚴囊的破裂均可引起嚴重的變態反應，包括發熱和蕁麻疹。治療須行手術切除蚴囊。棘球蚴病的傳播在養羊的國家尤爲常見，可通過爲狗驅蟲來預防。

hydatidiform mole (hydatid mole, vesicular mole) a collection of fluid-filled sacs that develop when the membrane (chorion) surrounding the embryo degenerates in early pregnancy. These sacs give the placenta the appearance of a bunch of grapes. The embryo dies, the womb enlarges, and there is a discharge of pinkish liquid and cysts from the vagina. A malignant condition may subsequently develop (*see* chorionepithelioma).

水泡狀胎塊（葡萄胎） 妊娠早期，當圍繞胚胎的膜（絨毛膜）變性時，發生的充滿液體的囊狀物聚集。這些囊使胎盤的外觀有如一串葡萄。胎盤和子宮增大，有粉紅色的液體和囊自陰道流出。惡性疾患可相繼發生。

hydatidosis *n. see* hydatid disease.

棘球蚴病

hydr- (hydro-) *prefix denoting* water or a watery fluid.

〔前綴〕 **水，水樣液**

hydraemia *n.* the presence in the blood of more than the normal proportion of water.

稀血症 水在血中的比例較正常爲大。

hydragogue *n.* an agent that produces a watery discharge, particularly a laxative that produces watery stools.

水瀉劑 使產生水樣排出物的製劑。尤指排出水樣便的輕瀉劑。

hydrallazine *n.* a drug that lowers blood pressure and is used, usually in conjunction with *diuretics, to treat hypertension. It is given by mouth or injection; side-effects, including rapid heart rate, headache, faintness, and digestive upsets, can occur, especially at high doses. Trade name: **Apresoline**.

肼苯噠嗪 一種降壓藥。通常與利尿藥聯合使用治療高血壓。口服或注射給藥。副作用包括心率增快、頭痛、暈厥、消化紊亂，尤其大劑量應用時更易發生。

hydramnios (hydramnion) *n.* the presence of an abnormally large amount of *amniotic fluid surrounding

羊水過多 從妊娠約5個月出現異常大量的羊水圍繞胎兒。子宮變大，以致

the fetus from about the fifth month of pregnancy. The womb becomes swollen, which causes breathlessness, excess fluid in the body tissues, and other symptoms in the woman, and there may be a difficult birth. Most cases of hydramnios are associated with twin pregnancies.

引起呼吸困難、人體組織內液體過多以及婦女其他症狀，而且可能有難產。多數羊水過多病例伴有雙胎妊娠。

hydrargaphen *n.* a mercury-containing drug with antibacterial and antifungal activity, used to treat skin and ear infections. It is applied in a cream, solution, dusting powder, or pessary and has the toxic effects of *mercury.

萘磺汞 具有抗菌和抗眞菌效能的含汞藥物。用於治療皮膚和耳部感染。用其乳劑、溶液、撲粉劑或陰道栓劑。本藥具有汞的毒性副作用。

hydrargyria *n. see* mercurialism.

汞中毒

hydrarthrosis *n.* swelling at a joint caused by excessive synovial fluid. The condition usually involves the knees and may be recurrent. Often no cause is apparent; in some cases rheumatoid arthritis develops later.

關節積水 滑膜液過多引起的關節腫脹。本病症往往侵犯膝部，而且可復發。通常無明顯的病因，有些病例以後發生類風濕性關節炎。

hydroa (hidroa) *n.* an eruption of small blisters accompanied by intense itching, occurring (usually in preadolescent boys) on skin surfaces exposed to sunlight. Hydroa is a severe form of light-sensitive dermatitis, described as *polymorphic light eruptions.*

水疱病 伴劇癢的小水疱疹。發生於（通常見於青春期前男孩）暴露日光下的皮膚表面。水疱病是一種嚴重型的光敏性皮炎，又稱多形性光疹。

hydrocele *n.* the accumulation of watery liquid in a sac, usually the sac surrounding the testes. This condition is characterized by painless enlargement of the scrotum; it is treated surgically, by drainage of the fluid or removal of the sac.

鞘膜積液（陰囊水囊腫） 水樣液在囊內（通常是圍繞睾丸的囊）聚積的情況。本病症以陰囊無痛性增大爲特徵，可行排液或囊腫切除的外科治療。

hydrocephalus *n.* an abnormal increase in the amount of cerebrospinal fluid within the ventricles of the brain. In childhood, before the sutures of the skull have fused, hydrocephalus makes the head enlarge. In adults, because of the unyielding nature of the skull, hydrocephalus raises the intracranial pressure with consequent drowsiness and vomiting. Hydrocephalus may be

腦積水 腦脊液量在腦室內異常增加的情況。在兒童期，顱骨縫未閉合以前，腦積水可使頭部增大。在成人，由於顱骨的形狀不易變形，腦積水可引起顱內壓增高，伴隨而來的是倦睡和嘔吐。腦積水可由腦脊液自腦室流出受阻或再吸收到大腦靜脈

caused by obstruction to the outflow of cerebrospinal fluid from the ventricles or a failure of its reabsorption into the cerebral sinuses. *Spina bifida is commonly associated with hydrocephalus.

竇障礙引起，脊柱裂通常伴有腦積水。

hydrochloric acid a strong acid present, in a very dilute form, in gastric juice. The secretion of excess hydrochloric acid by the stomach results in the condition *hyperchlorhydria.

鹽酸 以極爲稀釋的形式存在於胃內的一種强酸。胃內鹽酸分泌過多可致胃酸過多症。

hydrochlorothiazide *n.* a *diuretic used to treat fluid retention (oedema) and high blood pressure. It is administered by mouth, and side-effects can include digestive upsets, skin reactions, and dizziness. Trade names: **Direma, Esidrex, Hydrosaluric**.

雙氫克尿塞 用於治療體液豬留（水腫）和高血壓的一種利尿劑。口服給藥。副作用包括消化紊亂、皮膚反應、頭暈等。商品名：雙氫氯噻嗪。

hydrocolpos *n.* a cyst containing watery liquid or mucus formed in the vagina.

陰道積水 在陰道內形成的內含水狀液體或黏液的一種囊。

hydrocortisone (cortisol) *n.* a steroid hormone: the major glucocorticoid synthesized and released by the human adrenal cortex (*see* corticosteroid). It is important for normal carbohydrate metabolism and for the normal response to any stress. Hydrocortisone is used to treat adrenal failure (*Addison's disease) and inflammatory, allergic, and rheumatic conditions (including rheumatoid arthritis, colitis, and eczema). It may be given by mouth, by injection, or in the form of a cream or ointment. Possible side-effects of hydrocortisone therapy include peptic ulcers, bone and muscle damage, suppression of growth in children, and the signs of *Cushing's syndrome.

氫化可的松（皮質醇） 類固醇激素：由人腎上腺皮質合成和分泌的重要糖皮質激素。氫化可的松對正常碳水化合物代謝和來自任何刺激的正常應答都是重要的。它用於治療腎上腺衰竭（阿狄森氏病）以及炎性、變態反應性、以及風濕性疾患（包括風濕性關節炎、結腸炎與濕疹）。本藥可口服、注射或以乳劑或軟膏劑的形式用藥。氫化可的松治療可能產生的副作用包括消化性潰瘍、骨和肌肉損害、小兒生長受抑以及柯興氏綜合徵的體徵。

hydrocyanic acid (prussic acid) an intensely poisonous volatile acid that can cause death within a minute if inhaled. It smells of bitter almonds. *See* cyanide.

氫氰酸 毒性極强的揮發性酸。吸入後幾分鐘內可引起死亡。它有苦扁桃味。

hydroflumethiazide *n.* a *diuretic used to treat fluid retention (oedema) and high blood pressure. It is adminis-

雙氫氟噻嗪 用於治療體液豬留（水腫）和高血壓的利尿藥。口服給藥。可

tered by mouth and may cause skin reactions, digestive upsets, dizziness, and weakness. Trade name: **Hydrenox**.

引起皮膚反應、消化紊亂、頭暈以及虛弱。

hydrogenase *n.* an enzyme that catalyses the addition of hydrogen to a compound in reduction reactions.

氫化酶 在還原反應中催化某化合物加氫作用的一種酶。

hydrogen bond a weak electrostatic bond formed by linking a hydrogen atom between two electronegative atoms (e.g. nitrogen or oxygen). The large number of hydrogen bonds in proteins and nucleic acids are responsible for maintaining the stable molecular structure of these compounds.

氫鍵 由兩個負電荷原子（例如氮或氧）以氫原子連接起來形成的一種較弱的靜電結合鍵。蛋白質或核酸中大量的氫鍵能維持這些化合物穩定的分子結構。

hydrogen peroxide a colourless liquid used as a disinfectant for cleansing wounds and, diluted, as a deodorant mouthwash or as ear drops for removing wax. Strong solutions irritate the skin.

過氧化氫 一種無色液體。用於清潔傷口的消毒劑，其稀釋液作爲漱口藥的除臭劑或排除耵聹的滴耳劑。其濃溶液刺激皮膚。

hydrolase *n.* an enzyme that catalyses the hydrolysis of compounds. Examples are the *peptidases.

水解酶 催化化合物水解的酶。例如肽酶。

hydroma *n. see* hygroma.

水囊瘤

hydromyelia *n.* a dilatation of the central canal of the spinal cord (which is a continuation of the ventricular system of the brain). It has been suggested that the canal is distended by a rise in the pressure of the ventricular cerebrospinal fluid caused by a blockage to its normal outflow to the surface of the brain. The patient's symptoms are those of *syringomyelia.

脊髓積水 脊髓的中央管（與腦室系統相連續）擴張。有人認爲，中央管擴張是由於腦脊液的正常流出受阻，引起腦脊液壓力升高所致。患者具有脊髓空洞症的症狀。

hydronephrosis *n.* distension and dilatation of the pelvis of the kidney. This is due to an obstruction to the free flow of urine from the kidney. An obstruction at or below the neck of the bladder will cause hydronephrosis of both kidneys. The term *primary pelvic hydronephrosis* is used when the obstruction, usually functional, is at the junction of the renal pelvis and ureter. Surgical relief by *pyeloplasty is advisable to

腎盂積水 腎盂膨脹和擴張。本病症是由於尿從腎中自由流出發生梗阻。如梗阻發生於膀胱頸或其以下部位，會引起兩側腎盂積水。當梗阻是在腎盂和輸尿管的連接處（通常是功能性的）時，可用原發性腎盂積水這一術語。可行腎盂成形術來緩解腎盂積水，以避免返壓性腎萎

avoid the back pressure atrophy of the kidney and the complications of infection and stone formation. —**hydronephrotic** *adj.*

縮、感染性合併症以及結石形成。

hydropericarditis *n. see* hydropericardium.

積水性心包炎

hydropericardium *n.* accumulation of a clear serous fluid within the membranous sac surrounding the heart. It occurs in many cases of *pericarditis (*hydropericarditis*). If the heart is compressed the fluid is withdrawn (aspirated) via a needle inserted into the pericardial sac through the chest wall (*pericardiocentesis*). *See also* hydropneumopericardium.

心包積液 一種清澈的漿液在圍繞心臟的膜性囊內積聚。本病症發生於許多心包炎（積水性心包炎）的病例中。如有液體擠壓心臟，可通過胸壁將針刺入心包囊中抽吸液體（心包穿刺術）。

hydroperitoneum *n. see* ascites.

腹水

hydrophobia *n. see* rabies.

狂犬病

hydrophthalmos *n. see* buphthalmos.

水眼

hydropneumopericardium *n.* the presence of air and clear fluid within the pericardial sac around the heart, which is most commonly due to entry of air during pericardiocentesis (*see* hydropericardium). The presence of air does not affect the management of the patient.

水氣心包 空氣和清澈液體積於心包囊內。本病症最常見的原因是由於行心臟穿刺時空氣進入心包內。空氣的存在不影響對患者的治療。

hydropneumoperitoneum *n.* the presence of fluid and gas in the peritoneal cavity. This may be due either to the introduction of air through an instrument being used to remove the fluid; because a perforation in the digestive tract has allowed the escape of fluid and gas; or because gas-forming bacteria are growing in the peritoneal fluid.

水氣腹 液體與氣體積於腹腔內。可能由於腹腔抽液時通過器械將空氣引入；亦可由於消化道穿孔使液體和空氣漏入；或產氣細菌在腹水中生長。

hydropneumothorax (pneumohydrothorax) *n.* air and fluid in the pleural cavity. If the patient is shaken the fluid makes a splashing sound (called a *succussion splash*). An *effusion of serous fluid commonly complicates a *pneumothorax, and must be drained.

水氣胸 空氣和液體積於胸腔內。當搖動病人時液體可產生擊水聲（振蕩音）。漿液性滲漏液常常合併水氣胸，應予引流。

hydrops foetalis the state of certain infants severely affected by *haemolytic disease. Fluid accumulates in the body cavities, especially in the peritoneal and pleural cavities (*see* oedema, ascites) and the liver becomes enlarged: these are features of chronic heart failure due to profound anaemia. Repeated intrauterine transfusions into the fetal peritoneum during pregnancy have saved some infants in whom hydrops foetalis was predicted.

胎兒水腫 某些患有嚴重溶血性疾病的嬰兒的狀態。液體積聚於體腔，尤其是在腹腔與胸腔內，而且肝臟變得腫大。這些都是由於嚴重貧血引起的慢性心力衰竭的特徵。當診斷出有胎兒水腫時，在妊娠期反復向母體子宮內行胎兒腹膜腔內輸血，曾挽救過一些嬰兒。

hydrorrhoea *n.* a watery discharge. *Hydrorrhoea gravidarum* occurs during pregnancy: excessive secretion by the glands of the womb leads to a discharge from the vagina.

液溢 排出水樣液體。妊娠子宮液溢發生於妊娠時，子宮腺體的過度分泌，導致液體從陰道內溢出。

hydrosalpinx (hydrops tubae) *n.* the accumulation of watery fluid in one of the *Fallopian tubes, which becomes swollen. In *intermittent hydrosalpinx* so much fluid accumulates that some of it is forced into the womb.

輸卵管積水 水樣液在輸卵管內蓄積。可引起輸卵管腫脹。間歇性（外溢性）輸卵管積水時，由於大量積水，致使一些液體被迫流入子宮內。

hydrotherapy *n.* the use of water in the treatment of disorders: today restricted in orthodox medicine to exercises in remedial swimming pools for the *rehabilitation of arthritic or partially paralysed patients.

水療法 用水治療疾病。在正統醫學中現今只限用於爲關節炎或部分癱瘓病人康復治療，病人在治療用游泳池內進行鍛煉。

hydrothorax *n.* fluid in the pleural cavity. *See also* hydropneumothorax.

胸腔積水 液體在胸腔內蓄積。

hydroureter *n.* an accumulation of urine in one of the tubes (ureters) leading from the kidneys to the bladder. The ureter becomes swollen and the condition usually results from obstruction of the ureter by a stone or a misplaced artery.

輸尿管積水 尿液在輸尿管（尿液從腎導入膀胱的管道）積聚。輸尿管腫脹。這種病症通常由輸尿管結石梗阻或動脉異位引起。

hydrovarium *n.* the accumulation of watery fluid in an ovary.

卵巢積水 水樣液在卵巢內積聚。

hydroxocobalamine *n.* a cobalt-containing drug administered by injection to treat conditions involving vitamin B_{12} deficiency, such as pernicious anaemia. Trade names: **Cobalin-H**, **Neo-Cytamen**.

羥鈷胺 一種含鈷藥物。注射給藥。用以治療維生素 B_{12} 缺乏症，如惡性貧血。

hydroxyamphetamine *n.* a *sympathomimetic drug used in solution or sprays for the relief of nasal symptoms such as congestion, inflammation, and sinusitis. It is also used to dilate the pupil of the eye for eye examinations. Side-effects can include headache, nausea, vomiting, and palpitations.

羥苯丙胺 一種擬交感神經藥。用其溶液或噴霧劑以減輕鼻部症狀，例如充血、炎症以及鼻竇炎。檢查眼睛時也用於散瞳。副作用包括頭痛、噁心、嘔吐以及心悸。

hydroxychloroquine *n.* a drug similar to *chloroquine, used mainly to treat lupus erythematosus and rheumatoid arthritis. Side-effects such as skin reactions, hair loss, and digestive upsets may occur and prolonged use can lead to eye damage. Trade name: **Plaquenil**.

羥氯喹 和氯喹相似的一種藥。主要用於治療紅斑狼瘡以及類風濕性關節炎。副作用有皮膚反應、脫髮以及消化紊亂等。長期應用可致眼部損害。

hydroxyprogesterone *n.* a synthetic female sex hormone (*see* progestogen) administered by injection to prevent miscarriage and to treat menstrual disorders. There may be pain at the injection site, and progestogens taken by mouth are often preferred. Trade name: **Primolut**.

17-羥孕酮 一種合成的女性激素。注射給藥，以預防流產和治療月經病。注射部位可有疼痛，因而往往寧願口服。

hydroxyproline *n.* a compound, similar in structure to the *amino acids, found only in *collagen.

羥脯氨酸 結構與氨基酸相同的一種化合物。只見於膠原組織中。

hydroxystilbamidine *n.* a drug used to treat infections caused by fungi and protozoa, such as blastomycosis. It is administered by injection and may cause dizziness, headache, nausea, and fainting if injected too quickly.

羥乙磺酸羥芪咪 一種治療眞菌和原蟲感染（例如芽生病菌）的藥物。注射給藥。如注射太快可引起頭暈、頭痛、噁心以及暈厥等。

hydroxytryptamine *n. see* serotonin.

5-羥色胺

hydroxyurea *n.* a drug that prevents cell growth and is used to treat some types of leukaemia. It is administered by mouth. Hydroxyurea may lower the white cell content of the blood due to its effects on the bone marrow. Trade name: **Hydrea**.

羥基脲 一種阻止細胞生長的藥物。用於治療某些類型白血病。口服給藥。由於羥基脲對骨髓的抑制作用，可使血中白細胞數減少。

hydroxyzine *n.* an *antihistamine drug with sedative properties, used to relieve anxiety, tension, and agitation and to treat nausea and vomiting. It is

羥嗪 具有鎮靜作用的抗組胺藥。用於解除焦慮、緊張和激動，而且用於治療噁心和嘔吐。口服給

administered by mouth and may cause drowsiness, headache, dry mouth, and itching. Trade name: **Atarax**.

藥。可引起倦睡、頭痛、口乾和瘙癢。商品名：安泰樂。

hygiene *n.* the science of health and the study of ways of preserving it, particularly by promoting cleanliness.

衛生學 研究健康和保護健康方法的學科。尤其是促進清潔衛生以保護健康。

hygr- (hygro-) *prefix denoting* moisture.

〔前綴〕 **濕** 指潮濕。

hygroma (hydroma) *n.* a type of cyst. It may develop from a *lymphangioma (*cystic hygroma*) or from the liquified remains of a subdural *haematoma (*subdural hygroma*).

水囊瘤 一種類型的囊腫。此囊可由淋巴管瘤（水囊狀淋巴管瘤），或由硬膜下血腫的遺留物液化（硬膜下水囊瘤）而發生。

hymen *n.* the membrane that covers the opening of the vagina at birth but usually perforates spontaneously before puberty. If the initial opening is small it may tear, with slight loss of blood, at the first occasion of sexual intercourse.

處女膜 出生時覆蓋陰道口的膜。在青春期前往往自然穿孔。如原來的口小，在第一次性交時可穿孔，且有少量出血。

Hymenolepis *n.* a genus of small widely distributed parasitic tapeworms. The dwarf tapeworm, *H. nana*, only 40 mm in length, lives in the human intestine. Fleas can be important vectors of this species, and children in close contact with flea-infested dogs are particularly prone to infection. *H. diminuta* is a common parasite of rodents; man occasionally becomes infected on swallowing stored cereals contaminated with insect pests – the intermediate hosts for this parasite. Symptoms of abdominal pain, diarrhoea, loss of appetite, and headache are obvious only in heavy infections of either species. Treatment involves a course of *anthelmintics.

膜殼〔絛蟲〕屬 廣泛分佈的小型寄生性絛蟲的一屬。其中短小的絛蟲——短膜殼絛蟲只有40毫米長，寄生於人的小腸中。蚤可能是這種蟲的重要媒介，兒童與帶有受染蚤的狗密切接觸時，特別容易感染。長膜殼絛蟲是嚙齒動物常見的寄生蟲；當人吞食被受染昆蟲（這種寄生蟲的中間宿主）汚染的久貯穀類時，偶爾能引起感染。其症狀是腹痛、腹瀉、食慾減退，而頭痛僅見於其中的重度感染者。治療包括抗蠕蟲療法。

hymenorrhaphy *n.* a tissue-grafting operation on the hymen at the entrance to the vagina in order to partially or completely close the vagina.

處女膜縫合術 在陰道入口處的處女膜組織移植術，以部分或完全地關閉陰道。

hymenotomy *n.* incision of the hymen at the entrance to the vagina. This

處女膜切除術 陰道入口處處女膜的切開手術。年

operation may be performed on a young girl if the membrane completely closes the vagina and thus impedes the flow of menstrual blood.

輕姑娘如其處女膜完全將陰道關閉，以致阻礙經血流出時，可行這種手術。

hyo- *prefix denoting* the hyoid bone. Example: *hyoglossal* (relating to the hyoid bone and tongue).

〔前綴〕 **舌骨** 例如舌骨舌的（與舌骨和舌有關的）。

hyoglossus *n.* a muscle that serves to depress the tongue. It has its origin in the hyoid bone.

舌骨舌肌 使舌下降的肌肉。此肌起點在舌骨上。

hyoid bone a small isolated U-shaped bone in the neck, below and supporting the tongue. It is held in position by muscles and ligaments between it and the styloid process of the temporal bone.

舌骨 在頸部的一個小而孤立的 U 形骨。在舌下支撑着舌。舌骨通過它和顳骨莖突之間的肌肉和韌帶保持其位置。

hyoscine (scopolamine) *n.* a drug that prevents muscle spasm (*see* parasympatholytic). It is used in the treatment of gastric or duodenal ulcers, spasm in the digestive system, and difficult or painful menstruation and also to relax the womb in labour. It can also be used to calm excitement in some psychiatric conditions, for preoperative medication, for travel sickness, and to dilate the pupil and paralyse the muscles of the eye for examination. It is administered by mouth or injection. Side-effects are rare but can include dry mouth, blurred vision, difficulty in urination, and increased heart rate. Trade names: **Buscospan**, **Pamine.**

東莨菪鹼 防止肌痙攣的一種藥。此藥用於治療胃或十二指腸潰瘍、消化系統痙攣以及月經困難或痛經，分娩時也用於鬆弛子宮。對某些精神病也可用於鎮靜，對暈車可作事前給藥，而且驗眼時可用於散瞳和麻痹眼肌。口服或注射給藥。副作用少見，可有口乾、視力模糊，排尿困難以及心率加快。

hyoscyamine *n.* a drug with similar activity to *hyoscine, used, often in mixtures, to treat muscle spasm. It is administered by mouth. Trade name: **Peptard**.

莨菪鹼 與東莨菪鹼有同樣活性的一種藥。常用其合劑，用於治療肌痙攣。口服給藥。

hyp- (hypo-) *prefix denoting* **1.** deficiency, lack, or small size. Example: *hypognathous* (having a small lower jaw). **2.** (in anatomy) below; beneath. Example: *hypoglossal* (under the tongue).

〔前綴〕 ①**缺乏，不足，過小** 例如下頜突出的（下頜骨過小）。②**下** 例如舌下的（在舌的下面）。

hypalgesia *n.* an abnormally low sensitivity to pain.

痛覺減退 對疼痛的敏感性降低。

hyper- *prefix denoting* **1.** excessive; abnormally increased. **2.** (in anatomy) above.	〔前綴〕①過多，異常增加 ②上
hyperacusis *n.* abnormally acute hearing or painful sensitivity to sounds.	**聽覺過敏** 異常靈敏的聽覺或對聲音產生疼痛的敏感性。
hyperadrenalism *n.* overactivity of the adrenal glands. *See* Cushing's syndrome.	**腎上腺機能亢進** 腎上腺的活動過度。
hyperaemia *n.* the presence of excess blood in the vessels supplying a part of the body. In *active hyperaemia* (*arterial hyperaemia*) the arterioles are relaxed and there is an increased blood flow. In *passive hyperaemia* the blood flow from the affected part is obstructed.	**充血** 供應人體某一部位的血管內存有過多的血液。在主動性充血中（動脈性充血），小動脈擴張，而且血流量增加。在被動性充血中，血自患部流出受阻。
hyperaesthesia *n.* excessive sensibility, especially of the skin.	**感覺過敏** 過度的敏感性，尤指皮膚。
hyperalgesia *n.* an abnormal state of increased sensitivity to painful stimuli.	**痛覺過敏** 對疼痛刺激敏感性增加的異常狀態。
hyperbaric *adj.* at a pressure greater than atmospheric pressure.	**高壓的** 壓力較大氣壓大的。
hyperbaric oxygenation a technique for exposing a patient to oxygen at high pressure. It is used to treat carbon monoxide poisoning, gas gangrene, and acute breathing difficulties. It is also used in some cases during heart surgery.	**高壓氧療法** 將病人暴露於高壓氧的一種技術。用於治療一氧化碳中毒、氣性壞疽以及急性呼吸困難。也可用於某些心臟手術時。
hypercalcaemia *n.* the presence in the blood of an abnormally high concentration of calcium. *Idiopathic hypercalcaemia*, which affects infants who have received too much vitamin D, leads to mental disorder. *Compare* hypocalcaemia.	**高鈣血症** 血中鈣的濃度異常增高。原發性高鈣血症發生於接受過量維生素D的嬰兒，可致精神紊亂。
hypercalcinuria (hypercalcuria) *n.* the presence in the urine of an abnormally high concentration of calcium.	**高鈣尿症** 尿中鈣的濃度異常增高。
hypercapnia (hypercarbia) the presence in the blood of an abnormally high concentration of carbon dioxide.	**高碳酸血症** 血中二氧化碳的濃度異常增高。

hyperchloraemia *n.* the presence in the blood of an abnormally high concentration of chloride.

高氯血症 血中氯化物的濃度異常增高。

hyperchlorhydria *n.* a greater than normal secretion of hydrochloric acid by the stomach, usually associated with a *duodenal ulcer. Extremely high levels of acid secretion are found in the *Zollinger-Ellison syndrome.

胃酸過多症 胃中分泌的鹽酸較正常的爲多。通常伴有十二指腸潰瘍。胃酸分泌濃度極高者見於佐-埃二氏綜合徵（胰源性潰瘍綜合徵）。

hyperchromatism *n.* the property of the nuclei of certain cells (for example, those of tumours) to stain more deeply than normal. —**hyperchromatic** *adj.*

着色過度 某些細胞（例如腫瘤細胞）核的染色較正常爲深。

hyperdactylism (polydactylism) *n.* the condition of having more than the normal number of fingers or toes. The extra digits are commonly undersized (rudimentary) and are usually removed surgically shortly after birth.

多指（趾） 具有較正常人多的手指或足趾。多出的指（趾）一般要比正常的小（發育不完全），生後往往即行外科切除。

hyperdynamia *n.* excessive activity of muscles.

肌力過度 肌活動過度。

hyperemesis *n.* severe vomiting. *Hyperemesis gravidarum* affects pregnant women: the stomach contents and bile are vomited, and the acidity of the arterial blood increases. If the vomiting is allowed to continue for a long time, liver disease may develop. If rest, restriction of liquid intake, controlled diet, and drugs aimed at stopping the vomiting fail to cure the condition, it may be necessary to terminate the pregnancy. *Hyperemesis lactentium* is vomiting by babies at the breast-feeding stage.

劇吐 嚴重嘔吐。妊娠劇吐影響孕婦健康：吐出胃內容物和膽汁，因而動脉血酸度增加。如任其長時間繼續嘔吐，可發生肝病。如休息，限制液體攝入，控制飲食，服用止吐藥等治療無效，可能要終止妊娠。乳兒劇吐是嬰兒哺乳階段發生嘔吐。

hyperextension *n.* excessive and forceful extension of a limb beyond the normal limits, usually as part of an orthopaedic procedure to correct deformity.

伸展過度 肢體超過正常限度的伸展和過度用力。通常作爲矯形方法的一部分，以矯正畸形。

hyperglycaemia *n.* an excess of glucose in the bloodstream. It may occur in a variety of diseases, most notably in *diabetes mellitus, due to insufficient insulin in the blood and excessive

高血糖症 血中葡萄糖過多。本症發生於各種疾病中，最值得注意的是糖尿病，由於血中胰島素不足以及攝取過多糖類所致。

intake of carbohydrates. Untreated it may progress to diabetic coma.

如不治療可發展爲糖尿病性昏迷。

hyperidrosis (hyperhidrosis) *n.* excessive sweating, which may occur in certain diseases, such as fevers or thyrotoxicosis, or following the use of certain drugs.

多汗〔症〕 過度出汗。可發生於某些疾病，例如發熱性疾病、甲狀腺毒症或使用某些藥物以後。

hyperinsulinism *n.* **1.** excessive secretion of the hormone insulin by the islet cells of the pancreas. **2.** metabolic disturbance due to administration of too much insulin.

①**胰島素分泌過多** 胰腺中的胰島細胞分泌過多的胰島激素。 ②**胰島素過多症** 由於給予過多的胰島素而引起的代謝紊亂。

hyperinvolution (superinvolution) *n.* **1.** excessive shrinkage of the womb and associated structures after childbirth. The condition may become extreme if breast-feeding continues for a very long time or if the reproductive tract becomes seriously infected shortly after delivery. **2.** excessive reduction in the size of any organ after it has attained an extremely large size.

復舊過度 ①產後子宮及有關結構過度收縮。如母乳哺育繼續很長時間，或產後不久生殖道受到嚴重感染，這種情況可變得嚴重。②任何器官達到極大程度後，其大小過度回縮。

hyperkalaemia *n.* the presence in the blood of an abnormally high concentration of potassium. *See* electrolyte.

高鉀血症 血中鉀的濃度異常增高。

hyperkeratosis *n.* thickening of the outer horny layer of the skin. It may occur as an inherited disorder, affecting the palms and soles. Another inherited disorder in which hyperkeratosis occurs is *ichthyosis.

角化過度〔症〕 皮膚外部的角化層增厚。本症可以是一種遺傳病，侵犯掌及蹠部。其它遺傳性疾病發生的角化過度〔症〕是魚鱗癬。

hyperkinesia *n.* a state of overactive restlessness in children. *See* hyperkinetic syndrome. —**hyperkinetic** *adj.*

運動過度 小兒過度活動不安的狀態。

hyperkinetic syndrome a mental disorder, usually of children, characterized by a grossly excessive level of activity and a marked impairment of the ability to attend. Learning is impaired as a result, and behaviour is disruptive and may be defiant or aggressive. The syndrome is most common in the intellectually subnormal, the epileptic, and the brain-damaged. Treatment usually involves drugs (such as amphetamines

運動過度綜合徵 小兒常見的精神病。以活動度明顯超過正常情況以及注意力明顯不集中爲特徵。結果學習受到影響，而且舉止異常，可能是挑衅性的或者是進攻性的。這種綜合徵在智力低下、癲癇以及腦損傷性疾病中是極爲常見的。治療通常包括藥物（例如苯異丙胺類或氟

or haloperidol) and behaviour therapy; the family usually needs advice.

哌啶醇）以及行爲療法；通常需要向家屬提出建議（諮詢意見）。

hyperlipaemia *n.* the presence in the blood of an abnormally high concentration of fats.

高脂血症 血中脂肪類的濃度異常增高。

hyperlipoproteinaemia *n.* the presence in the blood of abnormally high concentrations of *lipoproteins.

高脂蛋白血症 血中脂蛋白的濃度異常增高。

hypermetropia (long-sightedness) *n.* the condition in which parallel light rays are brought to a focus behind the retina when the *accommodation is relaxed (see illustration). Objects closer than six metres from the eye appear blurred, and objects further than six metres from the eye are not seen clearly but in many cases can be made sharp by an effort of accommodation. Normal vision can be restored by wearing spectacles with convex lenses. *Compare* emmetropia, myopia.

遠視 當眼調節弛緩時，平行光線集中到視網膜最後的一焦點上。物體距眼近於 6 米時，就顯得模糊，而物體距眼遠於 6 米時，兩眼也不易看清，但許多情況下通過調節尚可看清。可戴凸透鏡恢復眼的正常視力。

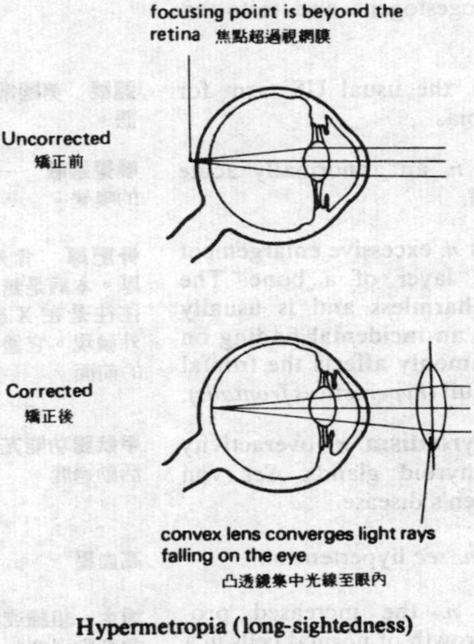

Hypermetropia (long-sightedness)
遠視

hypermotility *n.* excessive movement or activity, especially of the stomach or intestine.

運動過强 過度的運動或活動。尤指胃或腸的運動。

hypernatraemia *n.* the presence in the blood of an abnormally high concentration of *sodium. *See also* electrolyte.

高鈉血症 血中鈉的濃度異常增高。

hypernephroma (Grawitz tumour, renal cell carcinoma) *n.* a malignant tumour of kidney cells, so called because it is said to resemble part of the adrenal gland and at one time was thought to originate from this site. It may be present for some years before giving rise to symptoms, which include fever, loin pain, and blood in the urine. Treatment is by surgery but tumours are apt to recur locally. The tumour spreads via the bloodstream and can often be seen growing along the renal vein. Secondary growths from a renal cell carcinoma in the lung have a characteristic 'cannon-ball' appearance. These tumours are relatively insensitive to radiotherapy and cytotoxic drugs but some respond to such hormones as progestogens and testosterone.

腎上腺樣瘤（格臘維次氏瘤，腎細胞瘤） 一種腎細胞的惡性腫瘤。因據稱與腎上腺的結構類似，而且一度認爲此腫瘤是起源於腎上腺，故稱。在出現症狀（包括發熱、腰痛以及血尿）以前，可能已存在數年。可用外科方法治療，但腫瘤易於局部復發。腫瘤通過血流蔓延，而且常常可發現沿腎靜脈生長。肺中來自腎細胞癌的繼發性腫物，具有特殊的"炮彈"樣外觀。這些腫瘤對放射治療和細胞毒藥物相對來說是不敏感的，但某些激素如黃體酮和睾酮可獲一定療效。

hyperopia *n.* the usual US term for *hypermetropia.

遠視 美國常用的遠視術語。

hyperosmia *n.* an abnormally acute sense of smell.

嗅覺過敏 一種異常敏銳的嗅覺。

hyperostosis *n.* excessive enlargement of the outer layer of a bone. The condition is harmless and is usually recognized as an incidental finding on X-ray. It commonly affects the frontal bone of the skull (*hyperostosis frontalis*).

骨肥厚 骨外層過度增厚。本病是無害的，而且往往是在 X 線檢查中意外發現。它通常侵犯顱骨的前面。

hyperparathyroidism *n.* overactivity of the parathyroid glands. *See* von Recklinghausen's disease.

甲狀腺功能亢進 甲狀腺活動過度。

hyperpiesia *n. see* hypertension.

高血壓

hyperplasia *n.* the increased production and growth of normal cells in a tissue or organ. The affected part be-

增生 組織或器官中的正常細胞過度生長。增生部位變大，但仍保持其正常

comes larger but retains its normal form. During pregnancy the breasts grow in this manner. *Compare* hypertrophy, neoplasm.

類型。妊娠時乳房以這種形式生長。

hyperpnoea *n.* an increase in the rate of breathing that is proportional to an increase in metabolism; for example, on exercise. *Compare* hyperventilation.

呼吸過度 呼吸頻率增加。它與代謝增加成正比，例如鍛煉時。

hyperpraxia *n.* excessive motor activity, such as is seen in *mania and the *hyperkinetic syndrome.

活動過度 運動活動過度。如見於躁狂和運動過度綜合徵。

hyperpyrexia *n.* a rise in body temperature above 106°F (41.1°C). *See* fever.

高熱 體溫升高到 106℉（41.1℃）以上。

hypersensitive *adj.* prone to respond abnormally to the presence of a particular antigen, which may cause a variety of tissue reactions ranging from *serum sickness to an allergy (such as hay fever) or, at the severest, to anaphylactic shock (*see* anaphylaxis). It is thought that when the normal antigen-antibody defence reaction is followed by tissue damage this may be due to an abnormality in the working of the *complement system. *See also* allergy, immunity. —**hypersensitivity** *n.*

過敏的 對某種特異抗原有異常反應傾向的。它可引起各種組織反應，從血清病到變態反應（例如枯草熱）不等，最嚴重的可致過敏性休克。一般認爲，如在正常的抗原-抗體防禦性反應之後發生組織損傷，則可能是由於補體系統功能的異常。

hypersomnia *n.* sleep lasting for exceptionally long periods, as occurs in some cases of brain inflammation.

睡眠過度 異常長時間地持續睡眠。如發生於某些大腦炎症性病例。

hypersplenism *n.* a decrease in the numbers of red cells, white cells, and platelets in the blood resulting from destruction or pooling of these cells by an enlarged spleen. Hypersplenism may occur in any condition in which there is enlargement of the spleen (*see* splenomegaly).

脾功能亢進 由於脾腫大致使紅細胞、白細胞和血小板破壞和鬱積，從而引起這些細胞在血液中數量減少。本病可發生於任何有脾腫大的時候。

hypersthenia *n.* an abnormally high degree of strength or physical tension in all or part of the body.

體力過盛 全身或身體的某部分力量異常增强或緊張過度。

hypertension *n.* high *blood pressure, i.e. elevation of the arterial blood pressure above the normal range expected in a particular age group. Hypertension may be of unknown cause (*essential*

高血壓 血壓增高。即動脉血壓升高到某特定年齡組預期的正常值以上。血壓高的原因可能是不明的（特發性高血壓或高血壓

hypertension or *hyperpiesia*). It may also result from kidney disease, including narrowing (stenosis) of the renal artery (*renal hypertension*), endocrine diseases (such as Cushing's disease or phaeochromocytoma) or disease of the arteries (such as coarctation of the aorta), when it is known as *secondary* or *symptomatic hypertension.*

病）。它也可由腎臟疾患（例如庫興氏病或嗜鉻細胞瘤），或動脉疾患（例如主動脉縮窄）引起，這時即稱之爲繼發性或症狀性高血壓。

Complications that may arise from hypertension include atherosclerosis, heart failure, cerebral haemorrhage, and kidney failure, but treatment may prevent their development. Hypertension is symptomless until the symptoms of its complications develop. Some cases of hypertension may be cured by eradicating the cause. Most cases, however, depend upon long-term drug therapy to lower the blood pressure and maintain it within the normal range. The drugs used include thiazide *diuretics, *beta blockers, *methyldopa, *guanethidine, and many others. Combinations of drugs may be needed to obtain optimum control. *See also* portal hypertension, pulmonary hypertension.

由高血壓引起的併發症包括動脉粥樣硬化、心力衰竭、腦出血和腎衰竭，只有治療高血壓才能預防其發生。高血壓可從無症狀直至出現併發症的症狀。有些高血壓可通過根除病因而治癒。然而，多數病例須依賴長期的藥物治療來降低血壓和維持血壓在正常範圍內。所用的藥物包括噻嗪類、利尿藥類、β受體阻滯類、甲基多巴、胍乙啶以及許多其它藥。爲使高血壓獲得良好的控制，聯合用藥可能是需要的。

hyperthermia (hyperthermy) *n.* **1.** exceptionally high body temperature (about 41°C or above). *See* fever. **2.** treatment of disease by inducing fever. *Compare* hypothermia.

高溫 ①體溫異常升高（約 41℃ 或 41℃ 以上）。 ②通過促使發熱來治療疾病。

hyperthyroidism *n.* overactivity of the thyroid gland, either due to a tumour, overgrowth of the gland, or Graves's disease. *See* thyrotoxicosis.

甲狀腺功能亢進 甲狀腺活動過度。或因腫瘤、腺體過度生長，或因格雷夫斯氏病（突眼性甲狀腺腫）引起。

hypertonia (hypertonicity) *n.* exceptionally high tension in muscles.

張力過高 肌張力異常增高。

hypertonic *adj.* **1.** describing a solution that has a greater osmotic pressure than another solution. *See* osmosis. **2.** describing muscles that demonstrate an abnormal increase in *tonicity.

高張的 ①描述比其它溶液具有較高滲透壓的。②描述肌緊張性變得異常增高的。

hypertrichosis *n.* excessive growth of hair (*see* hirsutism).

多毛症 毛髮過度生長。

hypertrophy (hypertrophia) *n.* increase in the size of a tissue or organ brought about by the enlargement of its cells rather than by cell multiplication (as during normal growth and tumour formation). Muscles undergo this change in response to increased work. *Compare* hyperplasia.

肥大 由於細胞本身增大而不是細胞數增多（如正常的生長或腫瘤形成時）引起的組織或器官增大。肌肉負荷增加時肌肉可出現這種變化。

hypertropia *n. see* strabismus.

上斜肌

hyperuricaemia (lithaemia) *n.* the presence in the blood of an abnormally high concentration of uric acid. *See* gout.

高尿酸血症 血中尿酸的濃度異常增高。

hyperuricuria (lithuria) *n.* the presence in the urine of an abnormally high concentration of uric acid.

高尿酸尿症 尿中尿酸的濃度異常增高。

hyperventilation *n.* breathing at an abnormally rapid rate at rest. This can be done deliberately and causes unconsciousness by lowering the carbon dioxide concentration in the blood. It occurs clinically if the carbon dioxide level is abnormally high as a result of impaired gas exchange in the lungs, which occurs, for example, in pneumonia.

換氣過度 靜止時，呼吸速度異常增快。這種情況可故意產生。因血中二氧化碳濃度下降，可引起意識喪失。在臨床上，如因肺內氣體交換過程障礙，例如肺炎時，二氧化碳在血中濃度異常增高，就可發生換氣過度。

hypervitaminosis *n.* the condition resulting from excessive consumption of vitamins. This is not serious in the case of water-soluble vitamins, when any intake in excess of requirements is easily excreted in the urine. However, fat-soluble vitamins A and D are toxic if taken in excessive amounts.

維生素過多症 攝取過多維生素類引起的病症。水溶性維生素過多的病例並不嚴重，因超出人體需要量的維生素易從尿中排出。然而，脂溶性維生素類（維生素 A 及 D）如攝取過量，可出現毒性。

hypervolaemia *n.* an increase in the volume of circulating blood.

血量增多 循環血的容量增加。

hyphaema *n.* bleeding into the chamber of the eye that lies in front of the lens.

眼前房積血 血液進入位於晶狀體前方的眼房內。

hyphedonia *n.* a lower than normal capacity for achieving enjoyment.

快感減小 得到快感的能力較正常人爲低。

hypn- (hypno-) *prefix denoting* **1.** sleep. **2.** hypnosis.

〔前綴〕 ①**睡眠** ②**催眠**

hypnagogic *adj. see* imagery.

接近入眠的

hypnopompic *adj. see* imagery.

半醒的

hypnosis *n.* a sleeplike state, artificially induced in a person by a *hypnotist*, in which the mind is more than usually receptive to suggestion and memories of past events – apparently forgotten – may be elicited by questioning. Hypnotic suggestion has been used for a variety of purposes in medicine, for example as a cure for addiction and in other forms of *psychotherapy.

催眠狀態 類似睡眠的一種狀態。由催眠術士人爲地誘發某人睡眠。此時受催眠的人通常較易接受暗示，而且對過去事物的記憶，即使顯然已經忘掉的，也可通過提問來引出。催眠暗示在醫學中用於各種目的，例如用於治療嗜毒以及用於其他各種心理療法。

hypnotic (soporific) *n.* a drug that produces sleep by depressing brain function. Hypnotics include *barbiturates, *chloral hydrate, *methaqualone, and *nitrazepam. Hypnotics are used for insomnia and sleep disturbances, especially in mental illnesses and in the elderly. They often cause hangover effects in the morning and the barbiturate hypnotics can lead to *dependence.

催眠藥 通過抑制大腦功能促使睡眠的一種藥物。催眠藥包括巴比妥類、水合氯醛以及硝基安定。本藥用於失眠症以及睡眠紊亂，尤多用於精神病以及年長者。催眠藥往往引起早起感覺不舒服，且巴比妥類催眠藥類可導致賴藥性。

hypnotism *n.* the induction of *hypnosis.

〔前綴〕 **下，低，少，減退，不足**

hypo- *prefix. see* hyp-.

〔前綴〕 **下，低，少，減退，不足**

hypoaesthesia *n.* a condition in which the sense of touch is diminished; uncommonly this may be extended to include other forms of sensation.

感覺減退 觸覺減低的一種情況。有時此概念可擴大到包括其它類型的感覺減退。

hypobaric *adj.* at a pressure lower than that of the atmosphere.

低壓的 壓力低於大氣壓的。

hypobulia *n.* mild deficiency of will power. *See* abulia.

意志薄弱 缺乏意志。

hypocalcaemia *n.* the presence in the blood of an abnormally low concentration of calcium. *See* tetany. *Compare* hypercalcaemia.

低鈣血症 血中鈣的濃度異常減低。

hypocapnia *n.* the presence in the blood of an abnormally low concentration of carbon dioxide.

低碳酸血症 血中二氧化碳的濃度異常減低。

hypochloraemia *n.* the presence in the blood of an abnormally low concentration of chloride.

低氯血症 血中氯化物的濃度異常減低。

hypochlorhydria *n.* reduced secretion of hydrochloric acid by the stomach. *See* achlorhydria.

胃酸過少症 胃分泌鹽酸減少。

hypochondria *n.* preoccupation with the physical functioning of the body and with fancied ill health. It may amount to a handicapping neurosis and dominate a person's life. In the most severe form there are delusions of ill health, usually due to underlying *depression. Treatment with reassurance, *antidepressant drugs, and/or psychotherapy is usual, but the condition is often chronic. —**hypochondriac** *adj., n.*

疑病（症） 過分關注身體的功能，幻想有病。本症是可使人致殘的神經症，能控制一個人的生活。最嚴重情況有不健康妄想，通常是由於潛在的壓抑引起的。治療通常以消除疑慮，用抗抑鬱藥及/或心理療法，但病程往往是慢性的。

hypochondrium *n.* the upper lateral portion of the *abdomen, situated beneath the lower ribs. —**hypochondriac** *adj.*

季肋部 腹部的上外側部。位於肋弓的下面。

Hypoderma *n.* a genus of non-bloodsucking beelike insects – the warble flies – widely distributed in Europe, North America, and Asia. Cattle are the usual hosts for the parasitic maggots, but rare and accidental infections of man have occurred (*see* myiasis), especially in farm workers. The maggots migrate beneath the skin surface, producing an inflamed linear lesion similar to that of *creeping eruption.

皮下蠅屬 非吸血性蜜蜂樣昆蟲的一屬。皮蠅廣泛分佈於歐洲、北美和亞洲。牛是其寄生性蛆的常見宿主，但已發現人類有少見的偶然感染，尤其是農業工人。其蛆移行於皮表下面，產生一種炎性線形病變，如同匐行疹。

hypodermic *adj.* beneath the skin: usually applied to subcutaneous *injections. The term is also applied to the syringe used for such injections, and sometimes – loosely – to any injection.

皮下的 在皮膚下面的。此術語通常指皮下注射，也指皮下注射器，廣義指各種注射。

hypodermoclysis *n.* the continuous infusion under the skin of saline or other medicated solution to clean away blood, pus, and foreign matter from a wound.

皮下灌注術 持續將鹽水以及其它藥用溶液輸入皮下，以清除傷口中的血液、膿液以及異物。

hypodontia *n.* a reduction in the normal number of teeth through congenital absence.

牙發育不全 因先天性缺失，牙的正常數目減少。

hypofibrinogenaemia (fibrinogenopenia) *n.* a deficiency of the clotting factor *fibrinogen in the blood, which results in an increased tendency to

血纖維蛋白原過少 血中凝血因子纖維蛋白原缺乏。本病症可增加出血的傾向性。它可以是一種遺

bleed. It may occur as an inherited disorder in which either production of fibrinogen is impaired or the fibrinogen produced does not function in the normal way (*dysfibrinogenaemia*). Alternatively, it may be acquired.

傳性疾病，或因纖維蛋白原的產生發生障礙，或因產生的纖維蛋白原不能發揮其正常作用（血纖維蛋白原異常）。也可以是後天性的。

hypogammaglobulinaemia *n.* a deficiency of the protein *gamma globulin in the blood. It may occur in a variety of inherited disorders or as an acquired defect, as in certain *lymphomas. Since gamma globulin consists mainly of defensive antibodies (*immunoglobulins), hypogammaglobulinaemia results in an increased susceptibility to infections.

血丙種球蛋白減少 血中的丙種球蛋白缺乏。本病症可發生於各種先天性疾病，或是一種後天性缺陷，如某些淋巴組織瘤類。由於丙種球蛋白大部分是防禦性抗體（免疫球蛋白），血丙種球蛋白減少可導致易感性的增加。

hypogastrium *n.* that part of the central *abdomen situated below the region of the stomach. —**hypogastric** *adj.*

下腹 中腹的一部分。位於胃區的下面。

hypogeusia *n.* a condition in which the sense of taste is abnormally weak. *See also* hypoaesthesia.

味覺減退 味覺異常差的一種情況。

hypoglossal nerve the twelfth *cranial nerve (XII), which supplies the muscles of the tongue and is therefore responsible for the movements of talking and swallowing.

舌下神經 第十二對腦神經。分佈於舌肌，因而對說話和吞嚥活動起作用。

hypoglycaemia *n.* a deficiency of glucose in the bloodstream, causing muscular weakness and incoordination, mental confusion, and sweating. If severe it may lead to *hypoglycaemic coma*. Hypoglycaemia most commonly occurs in *diabetes mellitus, as a result of insulin overdosage and insufficient intake of carbohydrates. It is treated by administration of glucose, by injection if the patient is in a coma; by mouth otherwise. —**hypoglycaemic** *adj.*

血糖過少 血中缺少葡萄糖。可引起肌肉軟弱無力和共濟失調、精神混亂及出汗。如嚴重，可引起低血糖性昏迷。血糖過少最常發生於糖尿病，由使用胰島素過量以及攝取糖類不足引起。治療可用葡萄糖，如病人昏迷時，注射給藥，否則可口服用藥。

hypogonadism *n.* impaired function of the testes or ovaries, causing absence or impairment of the *secondary sexual characteristics.

性腺機能減退 睾丸或卵巢功能發生障礙。可引起第二性徵缺失或不明顯。

hypoidrosis (hypohidrosis) *n.* the production of an abnormally small amount of sweat relative to the environmental temperature, bodily activity, or other relevant circumstances.

少汗 與環境溫度、身體活動度或其他情况不相適應的汗量異常少的情况。

hypoinsulinism *n.* a deficiency of insulin due either to inadequate secretion of the hormone by the pancreas or to inadequate treatment of diabetes mellitus.

胰島素分泌過少 因胰腺分泌激素不足或因糖尿病治療不當引起的胰島素缺乏。

hypokalaemia *n.* the presence of abnormally low levels of potassium in the blood: occurs in dehydration. *See* electrolyte.

低鉀血症 血中鉀的濃度異常減低。發生於失水。

hypomania *n.* a mild degree of *mania. Elated mood leads to faulty judgment; behaviour lacks the usual social restraints and the sexual drive is increased; speech is rapid and animated; the individual is energetic but not persistent and tends to be irritable. The abnormality is not so great as in mania and the patient may appear normal and 'a bit of a character' to those who do not know him (*see* elation, euphoria). Treatment follows the same principles as for mania, and it may be difficult to prevent an individual from damaging his own interests with extravagant behaviour. —**hypomanic** *adj.*, *n.*

輕躁狂症 一種輕度的躁狂症。洋洋自得的心境引起判斷失誤，行爲缺乏起碼的社會約束，而且性慾增强，説話快且生動，個別的人顯得精力旺盛，但不持久，而且易激動。這種異常不如躁狂症嚴重，病人可表現正常以及不易識別的一些特徵。治療原則和躁狂症相同，但約束患者的放蕩行爲可能有困難。

hypomenorrhoea *n.* the release of an abnormally small quantity of blood at menstruation. The duration of bleeding may be normal or less than normal.

月經過少 行經時排出的血量異常減少。出血時間正常或較正常爲短。

hyponatraemia *n.* the presence in the blood of an abnormally low concentration of *sodium: occurs in dehydration. *See* electrolyte.

低鈉血症 血中鈉的濃度異常減低。發生於失水時。

hypoparathyroidism *n.* subnormal activity of the parathyroid glands, causing a fall in the blood concentration of calcium and muscular spasms (*see* tetany).

甲狀旁腺機能減退 甲狀旁腺的活動異常低下。引起血鈣濃度下降以及肌痙攣。

hypophysectomy *n.* the surgical removal or destruction of the pituitary gland (hypophysis) in the brain. The operation may be conducted by opening the skull or by inserting special needles that produce a very low temperature (*see* cryosurgery).

垂體切除術 外科切除或破壞大腦垂體。這種手術可通過開顱或插入特製的針（產生很低的溫度）來操作。

hypophysis *n. see* pituitary gland.

垂體

hypopiesis *n.* abnormally reduced blood pressure in the absence of organic disease (*see* hypotension).

低血壓 在不存在器質性疾病時血壓異常地降低。

hypopituitarism *n.* subnormal activity of the pituitary gland, causing *dwarfism in childhood and a syndrome of impaired sexual function, pallor, and premature ageing in adult life (*see* Simmond's disease).

垂體機能減退 垂體的活動低於正常。在小兒引起侏儒症，在成人則引起性功能障礙綜合徵、蒼白以及早老。

hypoplasia *n.* underdevelopment of an organ or tissue. *Dental hypoplasia* is the defective formation of parts of a tooth due to illnesses such as measles or starvation while the tooth is being formed. It is marked by transverse lines of brown defective enamel, which define the date of the illness.

發育不良 器官或組織的發育低下。牙發育不良是由於當牙齒萌出時，患麻疹或飢餓引起部分牙的萌出障礙。以棕色缺損的牙釉質橫線為特徵，此線可表明患病的日期。

hypopnoea *n.* a decrease in breathing rate which indicates that the body is attempting to compensate for metabolic disturbances due to disease in nonrespiratory organs by retaining acid in the form of carbon dioxide.

呼吸不足 呼吸頻率減少。這說明身體企圖代償由於非呼吸器官疾病引起的代謝紊亂（以二氧化碳的形式保留體內的酸）。

hypopraxia *n.* **1.** a condition of diminished and enfeebled activity. **2.** a lack of interest in, or a disinclination for, activity; listlessness.

活動減退 ①活動減少且虛弱的一種情況。②缺乏興趣或不願活動，懶洋洋。

hypoproteinaemia *n.* a decrease in the quantity of protein in the blood. It may result from malnutrition, impaired protein production (as in liver disease), or increased loss of protein from the body (as in the *nephrotic syndrome). It results in swelling (*oedema), because of the accumulation of fluid in the tissues, and increased susceptibility to

低蛋白血症 血中的蛋白量減少。可由營養不良、蛋白產生發生障礙（如患肝病時），或從體內蛋白丟失增加（如腎變病綜合徵時）。由於液體在組織內積聚，可引起水腫，而且增加對感染的易感性。

infections. *See also* hypogammaglobulinaemia.

hypoprothrombinaemia *n.* a deficiency of the clotting factor *prothrombin in the blood, which results in an increased tendency to bleed. It may occur as an inherited defect, as the result of liver disease, vitamin K deficiency, or anticoagulant treatment.

低凝血酶原血症 血中缺乏凝血因子——凝血酶原。可增加出血的傾向。本症可以是一種遺傳性缺陷，也可以是肝病、維生素 K 缺乏或抗凝治療的結果。

hypopyon *n.* pus in the chamber of the eye that lies in front of the lens.

眼前房積膿 膿液積存於晶狀體前的眼房。

hyposensitive *adj.* less than normally responsive to the presence of antigenic material. *Compare* hypersensitive. —**hyposensitivity** *n.*

敏感減輕的 對存在的抗原性物質的反應低於正常的。

hyposensitization *n. see* desensitization.

減敏作用

hyposmia *n.* a condition in which the sense of smell is exceptionally weak. *See also* hypoaesthesia.

嗅覺減退 嗅覺異常差的一種情況。

hypospadias *n.* a congenital abnormality in which the opening of the *urethra is on the underside of the penis: either on the glans penis (*glandular hypospadias*), at the junction of the glans with the shaft (*coronal hypospadias*), or on the shaft itself (*penile hypospadias*). All varieties can be treated surgically, and neither micturition nor sexual function need be impaired.

尿道下裂 一種先天性異常。其尿道的開口在陰莖的下側，或者在陰莖頭上（腺狀尿道下裂），或在陰莖頭及陰莖體連接處（冠狀尿道下裂），或在陰莖體本身（陰莖部尿道下裂）。各種尿道下裂可用外科方法治療，既不會有排尿困難，也不會發生性功能障礙。

hypostasis *n.* accumulation of fluid or blood in a dependent part of the body, under the influence of gravity, in cases of poor circulation. Hypostatic congestion of the lung bases may be seen in debilitated patients who are confined to bed. It predisposes to pneumonia (hypostatic pneumonia) but may be prevented by careful nursing and physiotherapy. A similar condition affects the dependent parts of the body after death. —**hypostatic** *adj.*

墜積 在循環不良的一些病例中，在重力的影響下，液體或血液積聚於人體的下垂部位。肺底的墜積性充血可見於臥床的虛弱病人。這情況易患肺炎（墜積性肺炎），但可通過精心護理和物理療法來預防。同樣的情況常發生於死後人體的下垂部位。

hyposthenia *n.* a state of physical weakness or abnormally low muscular tension.

衰弱 身體虛弱或肌張力異常低下的狀態。

hyposthenuria *n.* the secretion of urine of low specific gravity. The inability to concentrate the urine occurs in patients at the final stage of chronic renal failure.

低滲尿 排出低比重的尿。不能濃縮尿液。見於慢性腎功能衰竭的晚期。

hypotension *n.* a condition in which the arterial *blood pressure is abnormally low. It occurs after excessive fluid loss (e.g. through diarrhoea, burns, or vomiting) or following severe blood loss (haemorrhage) from any cause. Other causes include myocardial infarction, pulmonary embolism, severe infections, allergic reactions, arrhythmias, acute abdominal conditions (e.g. pancreatitis), Addison's disease, and drugs (e.g. an overdose of the drugs used to treat hypertension).
Some people experience a temporary fall in blood pressure when rising from a horizontal position (*orthostatic hypotension*). Temporary hypotension may result in a simple faint (sýncope). The patient becomes light-headed, sweats, and may develop impaired consciousness. In severe cases peripheral circulatory failure (cardiogenic shock) develops, with unrecordable blood pressure, weak pulses, and suppression of urine production. The patient is placed flat, with legs elevated, and given oxygen. Fluid and blood are replaced by an intravenous infusion as required. Specific treatment of the cause is provided (e.g. corticosteroids in Addison's disease).

低血壓 動脉血壓異常低的一種情况。低血壓發生於大量失水後（例如腹瀉、燒傷或嘔吐後）或任何原因的嚴重失血（出血）後。其它原因包括心肌梗塞、肺栓塞、嚴重感染、變態反應、心律失常、急性腹部疾患（例如胰腺炎）、阿狄森氏病以及用藥不當（例如治療高血壓用藥過量）。
有些人當從水平位起立時發生暫時性的血壓下降（起立性低血壓）。暫時性低血壓可引起單純性暈厥。患者有輕度頭痛、出汗，而且可發生意識障礙。在嚴重病例中可發生周圍循環衰竭（心原性休克）、血壓不能測出、脉搏細弱以及尿量減少。此時應使患者平臥，腿抬高，給氧。必要時靜脉輸注液體和血液。針對病因作特殊治療（例如阿狄森氏病時用皮質類固醇）。

hypothalamus *n.* the region of the forebrain in the floor of the third ventricle, linked with the thalamus above and the *pituitary gland below (*see* brain). It contains several important centres controlling body temperature, thirst, hunger, and eating, water balance, and sexual function. It is also

丘腦下部 位於前腦第三腦室底部的一個區域。它上與丘腦相接，下與垂體相接。丘腦下部包含幾個重要的神經中樞，控制人體的體溫、渴、飢餓、吃飯、水平衡和性功能。也與情緒活動和睡眠密切相

closely connected with emotional activity and sleep and functions as a centre for the integration of hormonal and autonomic nervous activity through its control of pituitary secretions (*see* neuroendocrine system, pituitary gland). —**hypothalamic** *adj.*

關，而且通過它控制垂體分泌的作用，發揮着激素和自主神經活動整合中樞的功能。

hypothenar *adj.* describing or relating to the fleshy prominent part of the palm of the hand below the little finger. *Compare* thenar.

小魚際的 描述手掌小指下部的肉質隆起部，或與此有關的。

hypothermia *n.* **1.** accidental reduction of body temperature below the normal range in the absence of protective reflex actions, such as shivering. Often insidious in onset, it is particularly liable to occur in babies and the elderly if they are living in poorly heated homes and have inadequate clothing. **2.** deliberate lowering of body temperature for therapeutic purposes. This may be done during surgery, in order to reduce the patient's requirement for oxygen.

①**低溫** 體溫偶然低於正常範圍，而沒有發生保護性反射作用（如發抖）。常是隱伏發生，尤其容易發生於嬰兒和年長者，如他們是住在不暖和的屋內而且衣服不夠時。 ②**降溫** 爲了治療，有意識地降低體溫。手術時，爲了降低病人對氧的需要量，可進行降溫。

hypothymia *n.* a diminished intensity of emotional response. It is a feature of *asthenic personalities, of some chronic schizophrenics, and of some depressives.

情感減退 情緒反應强度減低。它是無力型人格、某些慢性精神分裂症以及某些抑鬱症者的特徵。

hypothyroidism *n.* subnormal activity of the thyroid gland. If present at birth and untreated it leads to *cretinism. In adult life it causes mental and physical slowing, undue sensitivity to cold, slowing of the pulse, weight gain, and coarsening of the skin (*myxoedema*). The condition can be treated by administration of thyroxine.

甲狀腺機能減退 甲狀腺的活動低於正常。如出生時就存在，而且不經治療時可致克汀病。在成人可引起精神和身體活動遲鈍，對寒冷過度敏感，脉搏緩慢，體重增加以及皮膚粗糙（黏液性水腫）。本病可用甲狀腺素治療。

hypotonia *n.* a state of reduced tension in muscle.

張力減退 肌張力降低的一種狀態。

hypotonic *adj.* **1.** describing a solution that has a lower osmotic pressure than another solution. *See* osmosis. **2.** describing muscles that demonstrate diminished *tonicity.

①**低滲的** 比其他溶液滲透壓低的。 ②**低張的** 肌緊張性降低的。

hypotrichosis *n.* a condition in which less hair develops than normal.

毛髮稀少 毛髮生長比正常少的一種情況。

hypotropia *n. see* strabismus.

下斜視

hypoventilation *n.* breathing at an abnormally slow rate, which results in an increased amount of carbon dioxide in the blood.

肺換氣不足 以異常緩慢的速度呼吸。可引起血二氧化碳量增加。

hypovitaminosis *n.* a deficiency of a vitamin caused either through lack of the vitamin in the diet or from an inability to absorb or utilize it.

維生素缺少症 飲食中維生素不足或不能吸收和利用維生素引起的病症。

hypovolaemia (oligaemia) *n.* a decrease in the volume of circulating blood. *See* shock.

血容量減少 即循環血容量減少。

hypoxaemia *n.* the presence in the blood of an abnormally low concentration of oxygen, usually as a result of inadequate uptake of oxygen in the lungs because of lung disease. *See also* anoxia.

低氧血症 血中氧濃度異常低的情況。通常因肺部疾患攝取氧氣不足引起的。

hypoxia *n.* a deficiency of oxygen in the tissues. *See also* anoxia, hypoxaemia.

氧不足 即組織中缺氧。

hypsarrhythmia *n.* an abnormal and chaotic pattern of brain activity, demonstrated by *encephalography, that is usually associated with *infantile spasms.

嚴重腦電節律失常 腦電活動波型的異常和混亂。可由腦電描記術證實。本病常伴隨嬰兒痙攣發生。

hyster- (hystero-) *prefix denoting* **1.** the womb. **2.** hysteria.

〔前綴〕 ①**子宮** ②**癔病**

hysteralgia (hysterodynia, uteralgia) *n.* pain in the womb.

子宮痛 即子宮疼痛。

hysterectomy *n.* the surgical removal of the womb, either through an incision in the abdominal wall or through the vagina. *Subtotal hysterectomy* involves removing the body of the womb but leaving the neck (cervix); in *total hysterectomy* (*panhysterectomy*) the entire womb is removed. The operation is most commonly performed if the womb contains large *fibroids; other cases requiring hysterectomy include cervical

子宮切除術 經腹壁或經陰道切除子宮的手術。次全子宮切除術包括切除子宮體，但保留子宮頸，全子宮切除術則全部切除子宮。如子宮長有大的子宮肌瘤時，最常見的是做這種手術；其他需要做子宮切除術的病例包括子宮頸癌，子宮的惡性腫瘤或癌前細胞，或剖腹產後子宮

cancer, malignant tumours or precancerous cells in the womb, or severe damage to the womb following a *Caesarean section. Although pregnancy is no longer possible, hysterectomy does not affect sexual desire or activity.

嚴重損傷。儘管手術後再無妊娠的可能性，子宮切除術並不影響性慾或性活動。

hysteria *n.* **1.** a neurosis whose principal features consist of emotional instability, repression, *dissociation, physical symptoms, and vulnerability to suggestion. Freud postulated that hysteria arose as the result of frustrated libidinous impulses. Two types are usually described: *conversion hysteria*, characterized mainly by physical symptoms, such as paralysis; and *dissociative hysteria*, in which patients show changes in thinking, such as multiple personality states or amnesia. There is doubt as to whether hysteria constitutes a clinical entity. Patients with such symptoms are usually treated with psychotherapy. *See also* hysterical. **2.** a state of great emotional excitement.

①**癔病**　一種神經官能症。其主要特徵是情緒不穩定，壓抑，分裂，易接受暗示以及出現某些軀體症狀等。弗洛伊德氏認爲，癔病的發生是由性慾衝動受到挫折引起的。常被描述的有兩種類型：轉換性癔病，主要以軀體症狀（如癱瘓）爲特徵；分裂性癔病，患者顯示思維變化，如：多重人格狀態或遺忘症。關於癔病是否已構成一個獨立疾病，仍有疑問。有這樣症狀的病人通常用心理療法治理。②**歇斯底里**　情緒非常激動的一種狀態。

hysterical *adj.* **1.** describing a symptom that is not due to organic disease, is produced unconsciously, and from which the individual derives some gain. For example paralysis can be a hysterical symptom. **2.** describing a kind of *personality disorder characterized by instability and shallowness of feelings and by superficiality and a tendency to manipulate in personal relationships.

①**癔病的**　描述非因器質性疾病引起的一種症狀，雖是無意識發生的，但患者却有某些目的。例如癱瘓可能是癔病的一種症狀。　②**歇斯底里的**　描述一種人格障礙。其特徵是情緒不穩定和容易動感情，在人與人的關係上是淺薄的，有假情假意的傾向。

hysterocele (uterocele) *n.* hernia (rupture) of the womb, usually during pregnancy.

子宮疝　子宮的膨出（由裂孔）。通常發生於妊娠期。

hysterocleisis *n.* surgical closure of the passage from the womb to the vagina at the mouth of the womb.

子宮閉合術　在子宮口上以外科手術關閉從子宮到陰道的通路。

hysteropexy *n.* stitching the womb to the abdominal wall to prevent its downward displacement. *See* prolapse.

子宮固定術　將子宮縫到腹壁上，以防止子宮向下移位。

hysterorrhaphy *n.* stitching the womb. *See also* hysteropexy.

子宮縫合術 縫合子宮。

hysterorrhexis (metrorrhexis) *n.* rupture of the womb.

子宮破裂

hysterosalpingography *n. see* utero-salpingography.

子宮輸卵管攝影術

hysteroscope (uteroscope) *n.* a tubular instrument with a light source for observing the interior of the womb. *See also* endoscope.

子宮鏡 一種帶有光源的管狀器械。用於觀察子宮內部。

hysterotomy *n.* incision of the womb, either through the abdominal wall or the vagina. *See* Caesarean section.

子宮切開術 經腹壁或陰道行子宮切開術。

I

I

-iasis *suffix denoting* a diseased condition. Example: *leishmaniasis* (disease caused by *Leishmania* species).

〔後綴〕 **病** 指一種疾病的狀態。例如：利什曼病（利什曼原蟲屬引起的某種疾病）。

iatro- *prefix denoting* **1.** medicine. **2.** doctors.

〔前綴〕 ①**醫學** ②**醫生**

iatrogenic *adj.* describing a condition that has resulted from treatment, as either an unforeseen or inevitable side-effect

醫原性的 描述由於治療引起的某種情況。這種情況或者是不可預料的，或者是不可避免的副作用。

ibuprofen *n.* an *analgesic that relieves inflammation, used in the treatment of arthritic conditions. It is administered by mouth and sometimes causes skin rashes and digestive upsets. Trade name: **Brufen**.

異丁苯丙酸 一種緩解炎症的鎮痛藥。用於治療關節疾患。口服用藥，有時可引起皮疹和胃腸道不適。商品名：布洛芬。

ichor *n.* a watery material oozing from wounds or ulcers.

敗液 由傷口或潰瘍面滲出的水樣物質。

ichthyosis *n.* a congenital condition, usually present at birth, in which the skin is dry, rough, and scaly because of a defect in *keratinization. Ichthyosis

魚鱗癬 一種先天性疾病。往往在出生時就存在。由於皮膚角化方面的缺陷，致皮膚發乾、粗

varies in severity from slight skin dryness to a severe condition in which an infant is born, usually dead, with skin like armour plate.

糙，似魚鱗。本病嚴重程度不同，輕者皮膚發乾，重者嬰兒出生時往往死亡，皮膚似披有盔甲。

ICSH (interstitial-cell-stimulating hormone) *see* luteinizing hormone.

促間細胞激素

icterus *n. see* jaundice.

黃疸

ictus *n.* a stroke or any sudden attack. The term is often used for an epileptic fit, stressing the suddenness of its onset.

突發　卒中或者任何突然發作。此術語常用於癲癇發作，强調其發病的突然性。

id *n.* (in psychoanalysis) a part of the unconscious mind governed by the instinctive forces of *libido and the death wish. These violent forces seek immediate release in action or in symbolic form. The id is therefore said to be governed by the pleasure principle and not by the demands of reality or of logic. In the course of individual development some of the functions of the id are taken over by the *ego.

伊德　在精神分析中指部分潛意識心理。由性欲和死亡願望的本能來控制。這種强大的力量試圖立即以行動或符號形式釋放出來。因此，所謂伊德是由求樂原則控制的，而不出於現實的或邏輯的需要。在個體發育的過程中，伊德的某些功能由自我來控制。

-id *suffix denoting* relationship or resemblance to. Example: *spermatid* (a stage of sperm formation).

〔後綴〕**形狀**　指與…有關或相似。例如：精子細胞（精子形成的一個階段）。

ideation *n.* the process of thinking or of having *imagery or ideas.

思想作用　思維或意象或思想的過程。

identical twins *see* twins.

單卵性雙胎

identification *n.* (in psychological development) the process of adopting other people's characteristics more or less permanently. Identification with a parent is important in personality formation, and has been especially implicated in the development of a moral sense and of an appropriate sex role.

認同　在心理發育中指或多或少永久地承認他人特徵與自己的特徵相似的過程。與父母相認同，對個性的形成是重要的，認同和道德觀念和相應的由性角色的發展的關係尤爲密切。

ideo- *prefix denoting* **1.** the mind or mental activity. **2.** ideas.

〔前綴〕 **①精神或心理活動　②觀念**

ideomotor *adj.* describing or relating to a motor action that is evoked by an idea. *Ideomotor apraxia* is the inability to translate the idea of a complex behaviour into action.

意念動作的　描述一種運動行爲是由某種觀念引起的或與該種運動有關的。意念動作失用症是不能把複雜的行爲觀念轉化爲行動。

idio- *prefix denoting* peculiarity to the individual.

〔前綴〕**自體，自發，特異** 指與個體特性有關的。

idiocy *n.* a profound degree of intellectual *subnormality in which the affected individual can do nothing for himself and cannot speak. The term is now obsolete, but roughly corresponds to an *intelligence quotient of less than 20. There are usually associated physical handicaps and there is always physical damage of the brain.

白痴 極度的智力低常狀態。患者生活不能自理，不能說話。此術語現已廢棄，大致相當於智商低於20者。往往伴有體格上的障礙以及大腦的器質性損傷。

idiopathic *adj.* denoting a disease or condition the cause of which is not known or that arises spontaneously. —**idiopathy** *n.*

特（自）發性 指原因未明或自然發生的疾病或狀態。

idiosyncrasy *n.* an unusual and unexpected sensitivity exhibited by an individual to a particular drug or food. —**idiosyncratic** *adj.*

特異反應性 某一個體對某種特定的藥物或食物顯出異常或不可預料的敏感性。

idiot savant an individual whose overall functioning is at the level of mental *subnormality but who has one or more special intellectual abilities that are advanced to a high level. Musical ability, calculating ability, and rote memory are examples of abilities that may be highly developed. Many such individuals suffer from *autism.

低能特才者 其個體的精神功能雖處於全面低常狀態的水平，但有一種或數種智能達到高度發展水平的人。如音樂才能、計算才能以及死記硬背的能力等。許多這樣的個體患有孤獨症。

idioventricular *adj.* affecting or peculiar to the ventricles of the heart. The term is most often used to describe the very slow beat of the ventricles under the influence of their own natural subsidiary pacemaker (*idioventricular rhythm*).

心室自主的 影響心室或心室特有的。這術語最常用於描述緩慢的心室搏動（心室自主節律）。此心搏是心室本身產生的一種輔助性節律。

idoxuridine *n.* an iodine-containing drug that inhibits the growth of viruses and is used to treat viral infections of the eye (such as keratitis). It is administered in eye drops or ointment and may cause irritation and stinging on application. Trade names: **Dendrid, Kerecid.**

碘苷 一種含碘的藥物。本藥可抑制病毒生長，用於治療眼的病毒感染（如角膜炎）。以滴眼劑或軟膏形式給藥，在使用中可引起刺激作用和刺痛。商品名：疱疹凈。

ifosfamide *n.* a *cytotoxic drug used in the treatment of malignant disease,

異環磷醯胺 一種細胞毒類病。用於治療惡性疾

particularly sarcomas, testicular tumours, and lymphomas. It is administered intravenously by injection or infusion. Side-effects include nausea, vomiting, alopecia, and haemorrhagic cystitis; concommitant administration of *mesna is recommended to prevent cystitis. Trade name: **Mitoxana.**

病，尤用於肉瘤、睪丸腫瘤以及淋巴瘤。以靜脉注射或滴注給藥。副作用包括噁心、嘔吐、脫髮以及出血性膀胱炎；建議同時給予巰乙磺酸鈉以預防膀胱炎。

ile- (ileo-) *prefix denoting* the ileum. Examples: *ileocaecal* (relating to the ileum and caecum); *ileocolic* (relating to the ileum and colon).

〔前綴〕**回腸** 例如：回盲腸炎的（與回腸和盲腸有關的）；回結腸的（與回腸和結腸有關的）。

ileal conduit a segment of small intestine (ileum) used to convey urine from the ureters to the exterior into an appliance. The ureters are implanted into an isolated segment of bowel, usually ileum but sometimes sigmoid colon, one end of which is brought through the abdominal wall to the skin surface. This end forms a spout, or *stoma*, which projects into a suitable urinary appliance. The ureters themselves cannot be used for this purpose as they tend to narrow and retract if brought through the skin. The operation is performed if the bladder has to be removed or bypassed; for example, because of cancer.

回腸導水管 小腸（回腸）的一段。用於運送尿液，將尿從輸尿管引到體外一容器中。將輸尿管植入游離的腸段（通常是回腸，但有時是乙狀結腸），將腸的一末端拉到腹壁皮膚表面，並做成一個出水口（孔），此口將尿液引到相應的尿容器中。輸尿管本身不能用於這一目的，因爲如把輸尿管拉出皮膚外，易發生狹窄和回縮。這種手術常用於必須切開膀胱或膀胱改道時，如癌手術。

ileectomy *n.* surgical removal of the ileum (small intestine) or part of the ileum.

回腸切除術 回腸（小腸）或部分回腸的外科切除術。

ileitis *n.* inflammation of the ileum (small intestine). It may be caused by *Crohn's disease, tuberculosis, or typhoid or it may occur in association with ulcerative *colitis (when it is known as *backwash ileitis*).

回腸炎 回腸（小腸）的炎症。本病可由克羅恩氏病、結核病或傷寒引起，也可與潰瘍性結腸炎（如衆所周知的返流性回腸炎）同時發生。

ileocaecal valve a valve at the junction of the small and large intestines consisting of two membranous folds that close to prevent the backflow of food from the colon and caecum to the ileum.

回盲瓣 由兩個膜性皺襞組成的、位於小腸與大腸接連處的瓣膜。它關閉時可防止食物由結腸和盲腸返流到回腸。

ileocolitis *n.* inflammation of the ileum and the colon (small and large

回腸結腸炎 回腸和結腸（小腸和大腸）的炎症。

intestines). The commonest causes are *Crohn's disease and tuberculosis.

最常見的原因爲克羅恩氏病和結核病。

ileocolostomy *n.* a surgical operation in which the ileum is joined to some part of the colon. It is usually performed when the right side of the colon has been removed or if it is desired to bypass either the terminal part of the ileum or right side of the colon.

回腸結腸吻合術 把回腸接到結腸某部分的外科手術。這種手術最常在右側結腸已被切除或需要做回腸末端與右側結腸的改道手術時施行。

ileoproctostomy (ileorectal anastomosis) *n.* a surgical operation in which the ileum is joined to the rectum, usually after surgical removal of the colon (*see* colectomy).

回腸直腸吻合術 將回腸接到直腸的外科手術。往往是在結腸切除手術後做這種手術。

ileostomy *n.* a surgical operation in which the ileum is brought through the abdominal wall to create an artificial opening (*stoma*) through which the intestinal contents can discharge, thus bypassing the colon. Various types of bag may be worn to collect the effluent. The operation is usually performed in association with *colectomy; or to allow the colon to rest and heal in cases of colitis; or following injury or surgery to the colon.

回腸造口術 將回腸通過腹壁拉出以塑造一個人工開口的外科手術。由此造口排出腸內容物，因而繞過結腸。各種類型的袋子都可用於收集流出物。這種手術通常與結腸切除手術同時進行，或在結腸炎病例中（使結腸得到休息），或在結腸損傷或結腸手術後施行。

ileum *n.* the lowest of the three portions of the small *intestine. It runs from the jejunum to the *ileocaecal valve. —**ileal**, **ileac** *adj.*

回腸 小腸三個部分中最下一部分。它由空腸延至回盲瓣。

ileus *n.* intestinal obstruction, usually obstruction of the small intestine (ileum). *Paralytic* or *adynamic ileus* is functional obstruction of the ileum due to loss of intestinal movement (peristalsis), which may be caused by abdominal surgery (*see* laparotomy), spinal injuries, deficiency of potassium in the blood (hypokalaemia), or peritonitis. Treatment consists of intravenous administration of fluid and nutrients and removal of excess stomach secretions by tube until peristalsis returns. If possible, the underlying condition is treated. Mechanical obstruction of the ileum may be caused by a gallstone

腸梗阻 腸梗阻通常是指小腸（回腸）的梗阻。麻痹性或無動力性腸梗阻是小腸不能運動（蠕動）的功能性腸梗阻，它可由腹部手術、脊髓損傷、血中缺鉀（低鉀血症）或腹膜炎引起。治療包括靜脉輸液與輸注營養物質，以及用吸管排出過多的胃分泌物，直至恢復蠕動。如可能，治療原發的疾病。機械性腸梗阻可由於膽石通過瘻管或擴大的膽道進入腸內（膽石性腸梗阻）；有囊性纖維化遺傳病的新

entering the bowel through a fistula or widened bile duct (*gallstone ileus*); thickened *meconium in newborn babies with *cystic fibrosis (*meconium ileus*); or intestinal worms, usually the threadworm *Enterobius vermicularis* (*verminous ileus*).

生兒粘稠的胎糞（胎糞性腸梗阻）；或腸道蠕蟲，通常是線蟲——蠕蟲引起（蠕蟲性腸梗阻）。

ili- (ilio-) *prefix denoting* the ilium.

〔前綴〕**髂** 指髂骨。

iliac arteries the arteries that supply most of the blood to the lower limbs and pelvic region. The right and left *common iliac arteries* form the terminal branches of the abdominal aorta. Each branches into the *external iliac artery* and the smaller *internal iliac artery*.

髂動脉 供給下肢和盆骨區大部分血液的動脉。左、右髂骨總動脉形成髂總動脉的終末支。每支分爲髂外動脉和較小的髂內動脉。

iliacus *n.* a flat triangular muscle situated in the area of the groin. This muscle acts in conjunction with the *psoas muscle to flex the thigh.

髂肌 位於腹股溝區的扁平三角形肌肉。此肌肉連接腰大肌，屈曲大腿。

iliac veins the veins draining most of the blood from the lower limbs and pelvic region. The right and left *common iliac veins* unite to form the inferior vena cava. They are each formed by the union of the *internal* and *external iliac veins*.

髂靜脉 從下肢與盆骨區引流大部分血液的靜脉。左、右髂骨總靜脉聯合形成下腔靜脉。每條髂總靜脉由內外髂靜脉聯合形成的。

iliopsoas *n.* a composite muscle made up of the *iliacus and *psoas muscles, which have a common tendon.

髂腰肌 由髂肌和腰大肌組成的複合肌。它們有一共有的肌腱。

ilium *n.* the haunch bone: a wide bone forming the upper part of each side of the *hip bone (*see also* pelvis). There is a concave depression (*iliac fossa*) on the inside of the pelvis; the right iliac fossa provides space for the vermiform appendix. **—iliac** *adj.*

髂骨 俗稱胯骨。形成每邊髂骨上部的一寬骨頭。在盆骨的內側面有一凹窩（髂窩），右髂窩爲闌尾提供空間。

illusion *n.* a false perception due to misinterpretation of the stimuli arising from an object. For example, a patient may misinterpret the conversation of others as the voices of enemies conspiring to destroy him. Illusions can occur in quite normal people, when they are

錯覺 由於對某一事物所產生的刺激發生誤解而造成的一種失眞知覺。例如病人可把他人的談話誤解爲敵人圖謀要傷害他的聲音。錯覺可發生於極正常的人，但往往自然地得到

usually spontaneously corrected. They may also occur in almost any psychiatric syndrome, especially *depression. *Compare* hallucination.
Optical illusions are perceptions that do not agree with the actual object in the external world. They are produced by deceptive qualities of the stimulus and are in no way pathological.

糾正。本症幾乎也可發生於任何精神病的綜合徵中，特別是抑鬱症。視錯覺是與外界眞實的事物不一致的知覺，是由易使人誤解的事物的刺激產生的，絕不是病理現象。

imagery *n.* the production of vivid mental representations by the normal processes of thought. *Hypnagogic imagery* occurs just before falling asleep, and the images are often very distinct. *Hypnopompic imagery* occurs in the state between sleep and full wakefulness. Like hypnagogic imagery, the experiences may be very vivid. *Eidetic imagery*, commoner in children than adults, is the production of images of exceptional clarity, which may be recalled long after being first experienced.

意象活動 通過正常的思維過程產生逼眞的心理現象。催眠意象發生於正要睡眠前，而這種意象往往很清晰。覺醒前意象發生於睡眠和完全覺醒之間的狀態中。和催眠意象一樣，這種體驗可能是很逼眞的。小兒較成人多見，是異常清晰意象的產物，它可在第一次體驗後經過很長時間回憶起來。

imago *n.* (in psychoanalysis) the internal unconscious representation of an important person in the individual's life, particularly a parent.

潛意識理想化表象 在精神分析中指在一個人的生活中，對某一重要的人（特別是父母）產生的內在的無意識表象。

imbecility *n.* a moderate to severe degree of intellectual *subnormality that falls short of *idiocy. The term is now obsolete, but roughly corresponds to an *intelligence quotient of between 20 and 50. It is almost always caused by physical damage to the brain, and affected individuals usually require help and supervision throughout their lives.

痴愚 不到白痴程度的中到重度智力低常狀態。此術語現已廢棄，約相當於智商在20～50之間。本病幾乎都是由腦的器質性損傷所致，患者終身需要別人幫助和監督。

imipramine *n.* a drug administered by mouth or injection to treat depression (*see* antidepressant). Its effects may be slow to develop; common side-effects include dry mouth, blurred vision, constipation, sweating, and rapid heart beat. Trade names: **Berkomine**, **Dimipressin**, **Tofranil**.

丙咪嗪 治療抑鬱症藥。可口服或注射給藥。其作用可能緩慢地產生。最常見的副作用包括口乾、視力模糊、便祕、出汗和心動過速。

imitation *n.* acting in the same way as another person, either temporarily or

模仿 暫時的或持久地採取與他人同樣形式的動

permanently. This is one of the mechanisms of *identification. It can be used in therapy (*see* modelling).

作。這是認同機制的一種。它可用於治療。

immersion foot *see* trench foot.

漫泡足

immobilization *n.* the procedure of making a normally movable part of the body, such as a joint, immovable. This helps an infected, diseased, or injured tissue (bone, joint, or muscle) to heal. Immobilization may be temporary (for example, by means of a plaster of Paris cast on a limb) or it may be permanent. Permanent immobilization of a joint is achieved by the operation of *arthrodesis.

固定術 使身體正常活動的部位（如關節）不活動。這種辦法可助感染、患病或損害的組織（骨、關節或肌肉）痊癒。固定術可能是暫時性的（例如用煆石膏貼於肢體上），也可能是永久性的。關節的永久固定可由關節固定術來完成。

immune *adj.* protected against a particular infection by the presence of specific antibodies against the organisms concerned. *See* immunity.

免疫的 通過抗有關微生物的特異抗體的出現，防禦特異感染。

immunity *n.* the body's ability to resist infection, afforded by the presence of circulating *antibodies and white blood cells. Antibodies are manufactured specifically to deal with the antigens associated with different diseases as they are encountered. *Active immunity* arises when the body's own cells produce, and remain able to produce, appropriate antibodies following an attack of a disease or deliberate stimulation (*see* immunization). *Passive immunity*, which is only short-lived, is provided by injecting ready-made antibodies in *antiserum taken from another person or animal already immune. Babies have passive immunity, conferred by antibodies from the maternal blood and *colostrum, to common diseases for several weeks after birth.

免疫性 人體抵抗感染的能力。通過循環性抗體和白細胞的出現產生。抗體是機體爲對付其所遭受各種疾病的相關抗原特別地製造的。自動免疫是機體突然發病或接受緩慢刺激後，機體自身細胞不斷產生相應的抗體。被動免疫維持的時間短，是由注射製備的抗體提供的免疫。這種抗體存在於已獲得免疫的其他人或動物的抗血清中。嬰兒在生後幾週內從母血和初乳中獲得抗體，從而對常見病產生被動免疫。

immunization *n.* the production of *immunity by artificial means. Passive immunity, which is temporary, may be conferred by the injection of an *antiserum, but the production of active immunity calls for the use of treated antigens, to stimulate the body to produce its own antibodies: this is the

免疫 用人工方法產生的免疫。被動免疫是暫時性的，可由注射一種抗血清獲得，而自動免疫的產生則需要用處理過的抗原，刺激機體產生自身抗體，這過程叫預防接種（也稱預防注射）。用於免疫的

procedure of *vaccination (also called *inoculation*). The material used for immunization (the *vaccine) may consist of live bacteria or viruses so treated that they are harmless while remaining antigenic or completely dead organisms or their products (e.g. toxins) chemically or physically altered to produce the same effect.

物質（疫苗）是經過處理的活細菌或病毒，使其無害但仍保留抗原性；或者是完全減活的或其產物（如毒素）經由化學的或物理學的作用而變爲具有同樣免疫效果的產品。

immuno- *prefix denoting* immunity or immunological response.

〔前綴〕**免疫** 指免疫性或免疫應答。

immunoelectrophoresis *n.* a technique for identifying antigenic fractions in a serum. The components of the serum are separated by *electrophoresis and allowed to diffuse through agar gel towards a particular antiserum. Where the antibody meets its antigen, a band of precipitation occurs. *See also* precipitin.

免疫電泳 用來鑑定血清中抗原組分的一種技術。通過電泳使血清中的成分被分開，並通過瓊脂凝膠使其向特異的抗血清擴散。在瓊脂中抗體遇到其抗原，即產生一沉澱區帶。

immunofluorescence *n.* a technique for observing the amount and/or distribution of antibody or antigen in a tissue section. The antibodies are labelled (directly or indirectly) with a fluorescent dye (e.g. fluorescein) and applied to the tissue, which is observed through an ultraviolet microscope. In *direct immunofluorescence* the antibody is labelled before being applied to the tissue. In *indirect immunofluorescence* the antibody is labelled after it has bound to the antigen, by means of fluorescein-labelled anti-immunoglobulin serum. —**immunofluorescent** *adj.*

免疫熒光法 觀察組織切片上抗體或抗原量及／或分佈的一種技術。抗體直接或間接地標有熒光染劑（如熒光素）後用於組織中，通過紫外線顯微鏡觀察。直接免疫熒光法是先將抗體標上熒光素，再用於組織中；間接免疫熒光法是抗體與抗原結合後才用熒光素標記（係用熒光素標記過的抗免疫球蛋白血清）。

immunoglobulin (Ig) *n.* one of a group of structurally related proteins (gamma *globulins) that act as antibodies. Several classes of Ig with different functions are distinguished – IgA, IgD, IgE, IgG, and IgM. They can be separated by *immunoelectrophoresis. *See* antibody.

免疫球蛋白 在結構上相關的一組蛋白的一種（丙種球蛋白）。起抗體的作用。依不同的功能區分爲幾種——免疫球蛋白A、免疫球蛋白D、免疫球蛋白E、免疫球蛋白G和免疫球蛋白M。可通過免疫電泳把它們分開。

immunological tolerance a failure of the body to distinguish between materials that are 'self', and therefore to be

免疫耐受性 機體缺乏鑑別自身物質（可耐受的）與非自身物質（對該物質

tolerated, and those that are 'not self', against which antibodies are produced. For example, the body fails to produce antibodies against foreign materials if an antigen has previously been introduced into the body before the antibody-producing system is mature; apparently the presence of antigen within the growing cells inhibits antibody formation.

產生抗體）的能力。例如，如果產生抗體的系統成熟前，抗原就預先進入體內，機體就不能產生抗體以抵禦異物；顯然是生長細胞中存在的抗原抑制抗體形成。

immunology *n.* the study of *immunity and all of the phenomena connected with the defence mechanisms of the body. —**immunological** *adj.*

免疫學 研究免疫性及所有與機體防禦機制有關的現象的學科。

immunophoresis *n.* a technique, relying upon the *precipitin reaction, for identifying an unknown antigen or testing for an antibody in a serum. Antibody and antigen are allowed to diffuse towards each other in agar gel.

免疫滲透 一種有賴於沉澱素反應的技術。用於鑑定某一未知抗原或檢驗血清中某一抗體。使抗原和抗體在瓊脂凝膠中彼此互相擴散。

immunosuppressive *n.* a drug, such as *azathioprine or *cyclophosphamide, that reduces the body's resistance to infection and other foreign bodies by suppressing the immune system. Immunosuppressives are used to maintain the survival of organ and tissue transplants and to treat various *autoimmune diseases, including rheumatoid arthritis. Because immunity is lowered during treatment with immunosuppressives, there is an increased risk of infection.

免疫抑制劑 通過抑制免疫系統減少機體抗感染和排斥其他異物功能的一種藥。例如硫唑嘌呤或環磷醯胺。免疫抑制劑用於維持器官和組織移植的存活，以及治療各種自身免疫性疾病，包括類風濕性關節炎。由於在用免疫抑制劑治療的過程中免疫力下降，因而增加了感染的危險性。

immunotherapy *n.* the prevention or treatment of disease using agents that may modify the immune response. It is a largely experimental approach, studied most widely in the treatment of cancer.

免疫療法 運用可改變免疫反應的製劑以預防和治療疾病。主要是一種實驗性的方法，極廣泛地用於癌症治療的研究。

immunotransfusion *n.* the transfusion of an *antiserum to treat or give temporary protection against a disease.

免疫製劑輸入法 輸入一種抗血清以治療或暫時預防疾病。

impacted *adj.* firmly wedged. An *impacted tooth* (usually a wisdom tooth) is one that cannot erupt into a normal position because it is obstructed by

嵌入（阻生，嵌塞）的 固定楔入的。阻生牙（往往是智牙）是不能在其平常位置萌出的牙，由於其

other tissues. *Impacted faeces* are so hard and dry that they cannot pass through the anus without special measures being taken (*see* constipation). An *impacted fracture* is one in which the bone ends are driven into each other. —**impaction** *n.*

它內組織將其阻塞所致。嵌塞糞便是由於糞便太硬、太乾，以致如不採取特殊的措施，糞便就不能通過肛門。嵌入骨折是骨頭的末端嵌入另一段骨裏。

impairment *n. see* handicap.

損害

impalpable *adj.* describing a structure within the body that cannot be detected (or that can be detected only with difficulty) by feeling with the hand.

不可觸知的 描述人體內部的某種結構用手觸摸不能查清的（或難於查明的）。

imperforate *adj.* lacking an opening. Occasionally girls at puberty are found to have an *imperforate hymen* (a fold of membrane close to the vaginal orifice), which impedes the flow of menstrual blood.

閉鎖的 缺乏某種開口的。偶爾發現，一些青春期少女的處女膜是閉鎖的（膜的皺襞接近陰道口），因此阻礙經血的流出。

imperforate anus (proctatresia) partial or complete obstruction of the anus: a condition, discovered at birth, due to failure of the anus to develop normally in the embryo. There are several different types of imperforate anus, including *developmental anal stenosis*, *persistent anal membrane*, and *covered anus* (due to fused genital folds). If the anal canal fails to develop, the rectum ends blindly above the muscles of the perineum. Most mild cases of imperforate anus can be treated by a simple operation. If the defect is extensive a temporary opening is made in the colon (*see* colostomy), with later surgical reconstruction of the rectum and anus.

肛門閉鎖 肛門的部分或完全梗阻。是出生時發現的一種疾患。胚胎時期肛門的正常發育發生障礙所致。肛門閉鎖有不同的類型，包括肛門發育不全、肛膜未破及隱蔽肛門（由於生殖褶襞融合）。如肛管停止發育，直腸就在會陰肌上成一個盲端。多數輕度肛門閉鎖的病例可通過簡單的手術治療。如這種缺陷是廣泛性的，可行暫時性結腸造口，以後再行直腸與肛門的重建手術。

impetigo *n.* a bacterial skin infection usually caused by staphylococci, though occasionally by streptococci. Impetigo is particularly common in babies and children, occurring mainly on the face and limbs. The infection, which spreads quickly over the body, starts as a red patch and develops into small pustules that join together, forming crusty yellow sores. Impetigo is very

膿疱症 往往由葡萄球菌引起的細菌性皮膚感染。不過偶爾由鏈球菌引起。膿疱病常見於嬰兒和兒童，主要發生於面部與四肢。這種感染很快蔓延至全身，開始如紅斑，進而發展成融合在一起的小膿疱，形成痂性黃瘡。膿疱病極易接觸感染，尤其是

contagious, especially in communities of children, being readily spread by contact and via towels and face cloths. The condition usually responds to treatment with antibiotics, applied locally, within 7 to 10 days. Impetigo of the newborn is rare today but an outbreak may spread rapidly in a maternity unit.

在兒童團體中很快通過接觸、毛巾和面巾蔓延。本病局部採用抗生素治療7-10天往往是有效的。現在新生兒膿疱病已很少見，但在產院內可很快暴發蔓延。

implant *n.* **1.** a substance (such as a drug) or a tissue graft inserted into the skin. **2.** (in dentistry) a rigid structure that is embedded in bone or under its periosteum to provide support for replacement teeth on a *denture or a *bridge. Another type protrudes through the end of a shortened tooth root to stabilize it.

植入物 ①埋入皮膚的物質（如藥物）或組織移植物。 ②牙科中指包埋在骨中或骨膜下的堅硬結構，爲托牙或橋基上的義齒提供支撐。另一種類是從縮短了的牙根末端伸出來以固定義齒的結構。

implantation *n.* **1.** (*or* **nidation**) the attachment of the early embryo to the lining of the womb, which occurs at the *blastocyst stage of development, six to eight days after ovulation. The site of implantation determines the position of the placenta. **2.** the placing of a substance (e.g. a drug) or an object (e.g. an artificial pacemaker) within a tissue. **3.** the surgical replacement of damaged tissue with healthy tissue (*see* transplantation).

①**着牀** 早期胚胎附着在子宮內膜。它發生於排卵（卵子受精）6-7天後胚泡發育階段。其植入的部位決定了胎盤的位置。
②**植入** 將某一種物質（如藥物）或某物體（如起搏器）埋於組織內。
③**移植** 用健康組織行損傷組織的外科置換手術。

implosion *n.* *see* flooding.

血崩

impotence *n.* inability in a man to have sexual intercourse. Impotence may be *erectile*, in which the penis does not become firm enough to enter the vagina, or *ejaculatory*, in which penetration occurs but there is no ejaculation of semen (orgasm). Either kind of impotence may be due to a physical disease, such as diabetes (*organic*) or to a psychological or emotional problem (*psychogenic*).

陽萎 指男性性交不能。有一種陽萎是陰莖勃起不夠堅硬，以致不能進入陰道內（勃起性陽萎）；另一種是陰莖雖能插入陰道，但沒有精液射出（性慾高潮時），即射精性陽萎。任何一種陽萎可能是由於全身性疾病，如糖尿病（器質性的），或是心理、情緒的問題引起。

impression *n.* (in dentistry) an elastic mould made of the teeth and surrounding soft tissues or of a toothless jaw. A soft impression material is placed over

印模 口腔科內指按牙齒及其周圍組織或無牙頜取得的彈性模子（鑄型）。將一種軟的印模材料覆蓋

the teeth or jaw and sets within several minutes. After removal from the mouth a plaster model is made; on this are constructed *restorations of teeth, *dentures, or *orthodontic appliances.

於牙齒或頜骨上，置數分鐘。從口腔中取下後即可造石膏模型。按此模型可製造牙的修復體、托牙，或口腔正畸矯正器。

imprinting *n.* (in animal behaviour) a rapid and irreversible form of learning that takes place in some animals during the first hours of life. Animals attach themselves in this way to members of their own species, but if they are exposed to creatures of a different species during this short period, they become attached to this species instead.

印刻（銘記） 動物的行爲。一些動物出生後數小時中發生的一種迅速而不可逆的學習形式。動物借此依附於本種的成員。但如在這短暫的時間內暴露於不同種的動物中，它們就會依附於該種動物。

impulse *n.* (in neurology) *see* nerve impulse.

衝動 指神經衝動。

in- (im-) *prefix denoting* **1.** not. **2.** in; within; into.

〔前綴〕①**不** ②**內** 在…內，進入到。

inanition *n.* a condition of exhaustion caused by lack of nutrients in the blood. This may arise through starvation, malnutrition, or intestinal disease.

營養不足 由於血中缺乏營養引起的消耗性疾病。本病可因飢餓、營養不良或腸道疾病而發生。

inappetence *n.* lack of desire, usually for food.

食慾不振 通常缺乏對食物的欲望。

in articulo mortis Latin: at the moment of death.

臨終時 拉丁語：在死亡的瞬間。

inbreeding *n.* the production of offspring by parents who are closely related; for example, who are first cousins or siblings. The amount of inbreeding in a population is largely controlled by culture and tradition. *Compare* outbreeding.

近親交配 有密切血統關係的配偶之間生育後代。如堂（表）兄妹之間或親兄妹之間。近親交配在人口中的數量主要受文化和傳統的制約。

incarcerated *adj.* confined or constricted so as to be immovable: applied particularly to a type of *hernia.

箝閉的 受限制或絞窄以致不能活動的。特指疝的一種。

incidence rate (inception rate) a measure of morbidity based on the number of new episodes of illness arising in a population over an estimated period. It can be expressed in terms of sick persons or episodes per 1000 individuals at risk. *Compare* prevalence rate.

發病率 根據一定時期內某一人羣中新發某病的例數，來衡量患病情況的指標。它可用每年每1000人口中的病人數或發病數來表示。

incision *n.* **1.** the surgical cutting of soft tissues, such as skin or muscle, with a knife or scalpel. **2.** the cut so made.

①**切開** 用刀或解剖刀行外科破開軟組織（皮膚或肌肉）的方法。 ②**切口**

incisor *n.* any of the four front teeth in each jaw, two on each side of the midline. *See also* dentition.

切牙 每一頜骨中的四個前牙，中線每側各兩個。

incisure *n.* (in anatomy) a notch, small hollow, or depression.

切迹 解剖學上指小的凹痕或缺口。

inclusion bodies particles occurring in the nucleus and cytoplasm of cells usually as a result of virus infection. Their presence can sometimes be used to diagnose such an infection.

包涵體 發生於細胞核和細胞漿的微粒。通常是病毒感染的結果。它們的存在有時可用於診斷某些感染。

incompatibility *n. see* compatibility.

不相容性

incompetence *n.* impaired function of the valves of the heart or veins, which allows backward leakage of blood. *See* aortic regurgitation, mitral incompetence, varicose veins.

關閉不全 心臟或靜脈瓣膜的功能損傷，致使血液反流。

incontinence *n.* **1.** the inappropriate involuntary passage of urine, resulting in wetting. *Stress incontinence* is the leak of urine on coughing and straining. It is common in women in whom the muscles of the pelvic floor are weakened after childbirth. *Overflow incontinence* is leakage from a full bladder, which occurs most commonly in old men with bladder outflow obstruction or in patients with neurological conditions affecting bladder control. *Urge incontinence* is leakage of urine that accompanies an intense desire to pass water with failure of restraint. *See also* enuresis. **2.** inability to control bowel movements (*faecal incontinence*).

失禁 ①不適宜的、不隨意的排尿，造成尿濕。壓迫性尿失禁是咳嗽、緊張時尿液漏出。常見於產後盆骨底肌肉衰弱的婦女。溢流性尿失禁是尿液從充滿的膀胱漏出，最常見於膀胱排尿梗阻的老人或膀胱神經失控的患者。尿意性尿失禁是有强烈尿慾而對排尿不能控制所引起的尿液漏出。 ②不能控制排便（大便失禁）。

incoordination *n.* (in neurology) an impairment in the performance of precise rapid movements. These are dependent upon the normal function of the whole nervous system, and incoordination may result from a disorder in any part of it. *See* apraxia, ataxia, dyssynergia.

共濟失調 神經病學中指完成準確、快速運動的能力障礙。這些運動是依靠完整的神經系統的正常功能完成的。神經系統任何部位的疾患均可造成共濟失調。

incubation *n.* **1.** the process of development of an egg or a culture of bacteria. **2.** the care of a premature baby in an *incubator.

①**孵育** 卵或細菌培養的發育過程。 ②**保溫** 把早產兒放在恒溫箱中護理。

incubation period (latent period) 1. the interval between exposure to an infection and the appearance of the first symptoms. **2.** (in bacteriology) the period of development of a bacterial culture.

潛伏期 ①暴露於感染和第一次出現症狀之間的時期。 ②細菌學中指細菌培養的發育時期。

incubator *n.* a transparent container for keeping premature babies in controlled conditions and protecting them from infection. Other forms of incubator are used for cultivating bacteria in Petri dishes and for hatching eggs.

保溫箱 用於控制早產兒的生活條件（溫度等）和預防早產兒感染的透明容器。其它形式的保溫箱是用於陪替氏培養皿的細菌培養及孵蛋。

incudectomy *n.* surgical removal of the second ear ossicle, the incus, as in the treatment of chronic middle ear infection (*otitis media).

砧骨切除術 第二聽小骨——砧骨的外科切除術。做爲慢性中耳感染（中耳炎）的治療。

incus *n.* a small anvil-shaped bone in the middle *ear that articulates with the malleus and the stapes. *See* ossicle.

砧骨 中耳內的小鐵砧樣骨頭。其關節與錘骨和鐙骨連接。

Inderal *n. see* propranolol.

心得安

indican *n.* a compound excreted in the urine as a detoxification product of *indoxyl. Indican is formed by the conjugation of indoxyl with sulphuric acid.

尿藍母 尿中排泄的一種化學物。是吲哚酚的解毒產物。尿藍母由吲哚酚與硫酸結合生成。

indicanuria *n.* the presence in the urine of an abnormally high concentration of *indican. This may be a sign that the intestine is obstructed.

尿藍母尿 尿中出現的不正常高濃度的尿藍母。它可能是腸梗阻的一種體徵。

indication *n.* (in medicine) a strong reason for believing that a particular course of action is desirable. In a wounded patient, the loss of blood, which would lead to circulatory collapse, is an indication for blood transfusion. *Compare* contraindication.

適應症 指這樣一種情況（或疾病）：有充分的理由確信，採取某種特殊的措施是符合需要的。如某一患者外傷失血而可能導致循環衰竭時，就是輸血的適應症。

indigestion *n. see* dyspepsia.

消化不良

indole *n.* a derivative of the amino acid tryptophan, excreted in the urine and faeces. Abnormal patterns of urinary

吲哚 氨基酸（色氨酸）的代謝產物。由尿和糞中排出。某些精神上受到壓

indole excretion are found in some mentally retarded patients.

抑的患者，其尿中吲哚排出異常。

indolent *adj.* describing a disease process that is failing to heal or has persisted. The term is applied particularly to ulcers of skin or mucous membrane.

難癒合的 描述一種不能治癒或持續不癒的過程。此術語特別用於皮膚或黏膜潰瘍。

indomethacin *n.* an *analgesic that relieves inflammation, used in the treatment of arthritic conditions. It is administered by mouth or in suppositories; common side-effects are headache, dizziness, and digestive upsets. Trade names: **Imbrilon**, **Indocid**.

消炎痛 一種緩解炎症的鎮痛藥。用於治療關節疾患。口服給藥或用於栓劑。最常見的副作用是頭痛、頭暈以及消化系統紊亂。

indoxyl *n.* an alcohol derived from *indole by bacterial action. It is excreted in the urine as *indican.

吲哚酚 通過細菌作用，由吲哚產生的一種醇。它變成尿藍母，從尿中排出。

induction *n.* **1.** (in obstetrics) the artificial starting of childbirth. Labour can often be reduced by giving the pregnant woman a warm bath followed by an enema. If necessary the muscles of the womb may be stimulated to contract by injections of *oxytocin or by puncturing the sac surrounding the baby to release some of the amniotic fluid in which it is bathed. Induction of labour is attempted if pregnancy has continued considerably beyond the expected date of birth or if there is a risk to the health of mother or infant. If induction is not successful it may be necessary to perform a *Caesarean section. **2.** (in anaesthetics) initiation of *anaesthesia. General anaesthesia is usually induced by injecting certain drugs, usually barbiturates, into the bloodstream. In acupuncture, anaesthesia is induced by the manipulation of needles in a specified area of skin. **3.** (in embryology) the process by which a chemical released from one part of an embryo causes another part to develop in a particular way. Also called: **evocation**.

①**引產** 產科學中指人工引起分娩。可通過給孕婦洗溫水浴後灌腸來促進分娩。必要時，可通過注射催產素或穿刺圍繞嬰兒的羊膜囊來減少浸浴嬰兒的羊水，刺激子宮肌肉收縮。如妊娠持續下去，大大超過預產期或對母親或嬰兒的健康有危險性，可行引產。如不成功，做剖腹產術是必要的。②**誘導麻醉** 麻醉學中，指開始麻醉。全身麻醉往往通過注射一定的藥物（通常是巴比妥酸鹽類）進入血液來誘導。針刺麻醉是通過在特殊皮膚區域的針刺手術來誘導。③**誘導** 胚胎學中指從胚胎的一個部分釋放的化學物質引起另一部分的特殊發育。也稱啓發。

induration *n.* abnormal hardening of a tissue or organ. *See also* sclerosis.

硬結 不正常的、變硬的組織或器官。

indusium *n.* a thin layer of grey matter covering the upper surface of the *corpus callosum between the two cerebral hemispheres.

被蓋 覆蓋在兩個大腦半球之間，胼胝體表面上薄層灰質。

industrial disease *see* occupational disease.

工業病

inertia *n.* (in physiology) sluggishness or absence of activity in certain smooth muscles. In *uterine inertia* the muscular wall of the womb fails to contract adequately during labour, making the process excessively long. This inertia may be present from the start of labour or it may develop because of exhaustion following strong contractions.

無力 生理學中指某些平滑肌活動遲緩或消失。在子宮無力的病例中，因分娩時子宮壁肌肉不能適當地收縮，使生產延長。這種無力分娩開始就可出現，或因强烈收縮後肌力耗竭而發生。

in extremis Latin: at the point of death.

瀕死 行將死亡的時候。

infant *n.* a child incapable of any form of independence from its mother: a child under one year of age, especially a premature or newborn child. In legal use the term denotes a child up to the age of seven years.

嬰兒 離開母體無任何獨立生活能力的小兒。指一歲以下的小兒，尤指早產兒或新生兒。在法律上，此術語表示七歲以下的小兒。

infanticide *n.* (in Britain) under the terms of the Infanticide Act (1938), the felony of child destruction by the natural mother within 12 months of birth when the balance of her mind is disturbed because she has not fully recovered from childbirth and/or lactation. Under such circumstances a charge that would have been one of murder is reduced to manslaughter.

殺嬰罪 根據英國1938年禁止殺嬰法令，在孩子出生12個月內，母親尚未完全從分娩及／或哺乳中恢復過來而出現精神失常時，殺死嬰兒的犯罪行爲。此時，將被指控的謀殺罪減輕爲過失殺人。

infantile *adj.* **1.** denoting conditions occurring in adults that are recognizable in childhood, e.g. poliomyelitis (*infantile paralysis*) and *infantile scurvy*. **2.** of, relating to, or affecting infants.

嬰兒的 ①指成人中發生的某些常見於兒童期的疾病，如脊髓灰質炎（嬰兒癱）以及嬰兒壞血病。②與嬰兒有關的、或嬰兒好發的。

infantile spasms a serious brain disorder of infants, usually beginning under the age of six months. The spasms are involuntary flexing movements of the arms, legs, neck, and trunk; each spasm lasts 1–3 seconds and is associated with flushing of the face, and runs

嬰兒痙攣 嬰兒嚴重的大腦疾病。首次發病通常是在6個月以內。這種痙攣是臂、腿、頸和軀幹的不隨意的屈曲運動。每次痙攣持續1～3秒鐘，而且伴有面部潮紅。一連重復發

of spasms occur over a period of several minutes. The baby fails to respond to human contact and development is profoundly slowed. An EEG pattern of *hypsarrhythmia is sometimes seen. Interpretation of the spasms as wind has often delayed diagnosis, but immediate recognition and treatment with corticosteroids and ACTH offers a chance of arresting the disease.

生的痙攣要經數分鐘。嬰兒對人們的撫摸無反應，而且發育非常緩慢。有時發現嚴重腦節律失常的腦電圖型。將痙攣誤診爲小兒驚風，往往會延緩診斷，而及早發現，並用皮質類固醇和ACTH治療，有終止發作的可能性。

infantilism *n.* persistence of childlike physical or psychological characteristics into adult life.

幼稚型 直到成人仍保留類似小兒的體格和心理特徵。

infant mortality rate (IMR) the number of deaths of infants under one year of age per 1000 live births in a given year. Included in the IMR are the *neonatal death rate* (calculated from deaths occurring in the first four weeks of life) and *postneonatal death rate* (from deaths in the remainder of the first year). Neonatal deaths are further subdivided into *early* (first week) and *late* (second, third, and fourth weeks). In prosperous countries neonatal deaths account for about two-thirds of infant mortalities, the majority being in the first week. The IMR is usually regarded more as a measure of social affluence than a measure of the quality of antenatal and/or obstetric care; the latter is more truly reflected in the *perinatal mortality rate* (the sum of stillbirths and first-week or neonatal deaths per 1000 total births).

嬰兒死亡率 在指定的一年內每1000個活產中1歲以內嬰兒的死亡數目。嬰兒死亡率包括新生兒死亡率（計算生後頭四週內死亡者）及新生兒期後死亡率（只計算生後頭一年，除去生後頭四週的死亡者。）新生兒死亡進一步分爲早期（第一週）及後期（第二、三及四週）。在一些發達國家中，新生兒死亡率約佔嬰兒死亡數的⅔，而且主要是在第一週內死亡。一般來說，嬰兒死亡率與其看作出生前護理及／或產時護理質量的評價指標，不如把它看作爲社會富裕程度的指標。而護理質量更眞實地反映在圍產期死亡率上（統計每1000次分娩中的死產數及產後第一週或新生兒期死亡數）。

infarct *n.* see infarction.

梗塞

infarction *n.* the death of part or the whole of an organ that occurs when the artery carrying its blood supply is obstructed by a blood clot (thrombus) or an *embolus. For example, *myocardial infarction, affecting the muscle of the heart, follows coronary thrombosis. A small localized area of dead tissue

梗塞 某器官的一部分或全部死亡。發生於當對它供血的動脉被血凝塊（血栓）或栓子阻淤時，例如心肌梗塞，是隨冠狀動脉血栓形成而發生的。小區域的組織壞死（即所謂梗塞）是供血不充分產生的。

produced as a result of an inadequate blood supply is known as an *infarct*.

infection *n.* invasion of the body by harmful organisms (pathogens), such as bacteria, fungi, protozoa, rickettsiae, or viruses. The infective agent may be transmitted by a patient or *carrier in airborne droplets expelled during coughing and sneezing or by direct contact, such as kissing or sexual intercourse (*see* venereal disease); by animal or insect *vectors; by ingestion of contaminated food or drink; or from an infected mother to the fetus during pregnancy or birth. Pathogenic organisms present in soil, organisms from animal intermediate hosts, or those living as *commensals on the body can also cause infections. Organisms may invade via a wound or bite or through mucous membranes. After an *incubation period symptoms appear, usually consisting of either localized inflammation and pain or more remote effects. Treatment with drugs is usually effective against all but the viral infections (there is no specific treatment for most of the common viral infections, including the common cold and influenza).

傳染 人體受致病微生物（病原體）如細菌、眞菌、原蟲、立克次氏體或病毒的侵入。傳染的發生可能通過患者或帶菌者咳嗽或打噴嚏排出的由空氣傳播的微粒，或直接接觸如接吻或性交；或通過動物或昆蟲的媒介；或由被汚染的食物與飲水通過消化道傳播；或者在妊娠或分娩時由感染的母親傳給胎兒。致病性微生物存在於土壤中，通過動物中間宿主，或那些生活在機體上的共生體，也可以傳染。微生物可通過傷口、咬傷或通過黏膜侵襲人體。潛伏期後出現症狀，通常或爲局部炎症及疼痛，或爲遠隔部位的反應。用藥物治療，除病毒外對所有微生物通常是有效的。對大多數病毒感染，包括常見的感冒和流感尙無特殊的療法。

infectious disease *see* communicable disease.

梗塞性疾病

infectious mononucleosis *see* glandular fever.

傳染性單核細胞增多症

inferior *adj.* (in anatomy) lower in the body in relation to another structure or surface.

下的 解剖學中指人體內對於其他結構或表面而言是下部的。

inferior dental block a type of injection to anaesthetize the inferior *dental nerve. Inferior dental block is routinely performed to allow dental procedures to be carried out on the lower teeth on one side of the mouth.

下牙阻滯 爲麻醉下牙神經的一種注射方法。下牙阻滯是常見的麻醉，可使口腔一側的下牙手術得以進行。

inferior dental canal a bony canal in the *mandible on each side. It carries

下牙管 每側下頸的骨性管。下牙神經和血管通過

the inferior *dental nerve and vessels and for part of its length its outline is visible on a radiograph.

此管，而其外形長度的一部分在X線片上可見到。

inferiority complex 1. an unconscious and extreme exaggeration of feelings of insignificance or inferiority, which is shown by behaviour that is defensive or compensatory (such as aggression). **2.** (in psychoanalysis) a *complex resulting from the conflict between Oedipal wishes (*see* Oedipus complex) and the reality of the child's lack of power. This gives rise to repressed feelings of personal inferiority.

①**自卑情結** 一種自覺低微或卑下的感覺被無意識地極端誇大。它通過行爲表現出來，爲防衛性的或補償性的（如攻擊）。②**自卑情綜** 在精神分析中，指戀母情綜的願望與孩子缺乏力量的現實相抵觸而產生的情綜。

infertility *n.* inability in a woman to conceive or in a man to induce conception. Female infertility may be due to failure to ovulate, to obstruction of the *Fallopian tubes, or to disease of the lining of the uterus (endometrium). Male infertility may be due to spermatozoa in the ejaculate being defective either in motility (necrospermia) or in numbers (*see* oligospermia) or to a total absence of sperm (*see* azoospermia).

不孕症 婦女不能懷孕或男人不能促使懷孕。婦女不孕症可因不能排卵、輸卵管梗阻或子宮內膜疾患引起。男人不孕症可由射精時精子缺乏活動力（死精症）或精子的各類數目或總數缺乏。

infestation *n.* the presence of animal parasites either on the skin (for example ticks) or inside the body (for example tapeworms).

寄生 動物性寄生蟲在皮膚上（如蜱）或體內（如絛蟲）存在。

infiltration *n.* **1.** the abnormal entry of a substance (*infiltrate*) into a cell, tissue, or organ. Examples of infiltrates are blood cells, cancer cells, fat, starch, or calcium and magnesium salts. **2.** the injection of a local anaesthetic solution into the tissues to cause local *anaesthesia. Infiltration anaesthesia is routinely used to anaesthetize upper teeth to allow dental procedures to be carried out.

浸潤 ①某種物質不正常地進入細胞、組織或器官中，例如血細胞、癌細胞、脂肪、澱粉或鈣及鎂鹽等浸潤。②局部注射麻醉劑使組織局部麻木。浸潤麻醉常規地用於麻木下牙以使牙的手術操作得以完成。

inflammation *n.* the body's response to injury, which may be acute or chronic. *Acute inflammation* is the immediate defensive reaction of tissue to any injury, which may be caused by infection, chemicals, or physical agents. It involves pain, heat, redness, swelling,

炎症 人體對損傷的反應。這種反應可以是急性的或慢性的。急性炎症是組織對任何損傷的即刻防禦性反應，它可由感染、化學藥物或物理因素引起。可有紅、腫、熱、

and loss of function of the affected part. Blood vessels near the site of injury are dilated, so that blood flow is locally increased. White blood cells enter the tissue and begin to engulf bacteria and other foreign particles. Similar cells from the tissues remove and consume the dead cells, sometimes with the production of pus, and the process of healing commences. In certain circumstances healing does not occur and *chronic inflammation* ensues.

痛，而且受影響的部位失去功能。靠近損傷部位的血管擴張，以致局部血流增加。白細胞進入組織中，並且開始吞噬細菌以及其他外來的微粒。組織中與白細胞相似的細胞把死亡的細胞清除掉，有時伴有濃液產生，然後開始痊癒的過程。在某些情況下損傷不能痊癒，而變成慢性炎症。

influenza *n.* a highly contagious virus infection that affects the respiratory system. The viruses are transmitted by coughing and sneezing. Symptoms commence after an incubation period of 1–4 days and include headache, fever, loss of appetite, weakness, and general aches and pains. They may continue for about a week. After bed rest and aspirin most patients recover, but a secondary infection of the lungs is a common serious complication. An infection – and immunization too – provides protection only against the specific strain of virus concerned.

流行性感冒　一種具有高度傳染性的病毒傳染病。可感染呼吸系統。這種病毒通過咳嗽和打噴嚏傳播。在潛伏期1-4天後開始出現症狀，包括頭痛、發熱、食慾減退、虛弱以及全身疼痛。這些症狀可持續約一週。經臥床休息及服用阿司匹林，多數病人可恢復。但肺部的繼發感染是最常見的嚴重併發症。感染（以及免疫）只能對特異株的病毒提供預防作用。

infra- *prefix denoting* below.

〔前綴〕**下**　指在…下面。

infrared radiation the band of electromagnetic radiation that is longer in wavelength than the red of the visible spectrum. Infrared radiation is responsible for the transmission of radiant heat. It may be used in physiotherapy to warm tissues, reduce pain, and improve circulation, but is not as effective as *diathermy for deep structures. Special photographic film sensitive to infrared radiation is used in *thermography.

紅外線照射　波長比可見光譜紅光長的電磁輻射帶。紅外線照射能傳導輻射熱。它可用於理療以溫暖組織，減少疼痛並改善循環，但對深部結構不如透熱療法有效。對紅外線照射敏感的特別攝影膠片常用於溫度記錄法。

infundibulum *n.* any funnel-shaped channel or passage, particularly the hollow conical stalk that extends downwards from the hypothalamus and is continuous with the posterior lobe of the pituitary gland.

漏斗　任何漏斗狀的管或通道。尤指從丘腦下部向下延伸的空心的圓錐形柄。此柄與垂體後葉相連。

infusion *n.* **1.** a slow injection of a substance (e.g. saline or dextrose) into a vein or subcutaneous tissue. **2.** the process whereby the active principles are extracted from plant material by steeping it in water that has been heated to boiling point (as in the making of tea). **3.** the solution produced by this process.

①**輸注** 緩慢注射某種物質（如鹽或糖）進入靜脉或皮下組織。 ②**浸出** 通過浸出的原理，從浸泡在水（已加熱至沸點，如泡茶）中的植物性原料提取的過程。 ③**浸劑** 通過浸出過程產生的液體。

ingesta *pl. n.* food and drink that is taken into the alimentary canal through the mouth.

飲食物 經口腔攝入消化道的食物和飲料。

ingestion *n.* **1.** the process by which food is taken into the alimentary canal. It involves chewing and swallowing. **2.** the process by which a phagocytic cell takes in solid material, such as bacteria.

①**攝食** 攝取食物進入消化道的過程。這種過程包括咀嚼和吞咽。 ②**吞噬** 吞噬細胞攝取固體物質如細菌的過程。

ingravescent *adj.* gradually increasing in severity.

漸重的 嚴重性逐漸增加的。

inguinal *adj.* relating to or affecting the region of the groin (inguen).

腹股溝的 與腹股溝有關的，影響腹股溝區的。

inguinal canal either of a pair of openings that connect the abdominal cavity with the scrotum in the male fetus. The inguinal canals provide a route for the descent of the testes into the scrotum, after which they normally become obliterated.

腹股溝管 在男性胎兒中，其兩端的開口分別與腹腔和陰囊相連的管。腹股溝管爲睾丸降入陰囊提供通道。正常情况下，睾丸下降後，此開口閉合。

inguinal hernia *see* hernia.

腹股溝疝

inguinal ligament (Poupart's ligament) a ligament in the groin that extends from the anterior superior iliac spine to the pubic tubercle. It is part of the *aponeurosis of the external oblique muscle of the abdomen.

腹股溝韌帶（普帕氏韌帶） 由髂前上棘延伸到耻骨結節的韌帶。它是腹外斜肌腱膜的一部分。

INH *see* isoniazid.

異煙肼

inhalation *n.* **1.** (*or* **inspiration**) the act of breathing air into the lungs through the mouth and nose. *See* breathing. **2.** a gas, vapour, or aerosol breathed in for the treatment of conditions of the respiratory tract.

①**吸入** 經口、鼻把空氣吸進肺內的動作。 ②**吸入劑** 吸進用於治療呼吸道疾患的氣體、蒸氣或氣霧劑等。

inhibition *n.* **1.** (in physiology) the prevention or reduction of the function-

抑制 ①生理學中指通過一定的神經衝動，使器

ing of an organ, muscle, etc., by the action of certain nerve impulses. **2.** (in psychoanalysis) an inner command that prevents one from doing something forbidden. Some inhibitions are essential for social adjustment, but excessive inhibitions can severely restrict one's life. **3.** (in psychology) a tendency not to carry out a specific action, produced each time the action is carried out.

官、肌肉等的功能受阻或減少。 ②精神分析中指內在的克制，以阻止某人做某事。某些抑制對社會的調節是必須的，但過分的抑制可嚴重地約束一個人的生活。 ③心理學中指每當產生一定的動作時，就產生一種抵制這個特殊動作的傾向。

inhibitor *n.* a substance that prevents the occurrence of a given process or reaction. *See also* MAO inhibitor.

抑制劑 阻止特定過程或反應出現的物質。

inion *n.* the projection of the occipital bone that can be felt at the base of the skull.

枕外隆突 在顱骨底可被觸摸到的枕骨的突起。

injection *n.* introduction into the body of drugs or other fluids by means of a syringe, usually drugs that would be destroyed by the digestive processes if taken by mouth. Common routes for injection are into the skin (*intracutaneous* or *intradermal*); below the skin (*subcutaneous*), e.g. for insulin; into a muscle (*intramuscular*), for drugs that are slowly absorbed; and into a vein (*intravenous*), for drugs to be rapidly absorbed. *Enemas are also regarded as injections.

注射 將藥物或其他液體用注射器注進體內。通常是口服時經消化過程會被破壞的藥物。注射常用的方法是皮內（眞皮）、皮下（如用於注射胰島素），肌肉內（用於需吸收緩慢的藥物）。靜脉內注射用於需快速吸收的藥物。各種灌腸也被看做爲注射。

inlay *n.* **1.** a substance or piece of tissue inserted to replace a defect in a tissue. For example, a bone graft may be inlaid into an area of missing or damaged bone. **2.** (in dentistry) a rigid restoration inserted into a tapered cavity in a tooth. It is held in place with a cement *lute. The material most widely used is cast gold.

嵌體 ①將其插入以替代缺失組織的一種物質或組織塊。例如骨移植物可插入缺失或損傷的骨的某一區域。 ②牙科中，指將一堅固的修復物插入上大下小（圓椎形）的牙洞中，再用黏固粉將其封住。應用最廣的修復材料是合金。

inlet *n.* an aperture providing the entrance to a cavity, such as that of the pelvis.

入口 通入洞腔的口。如盆骨的入口。

innate *adj.* describing a condition or characteristic that is present in an individual at birth and is inherited from his parents. *See also* congenital.

先天 描述某個人生來就有的，由父母遺傳的某種疾患或特徵。

inner ear *see* labyrinth.

內耳

innervation *n.* the nerve supply to an area or organ of the body, which can carry either motor impulses to the structure or sensory impulses away from it towards the brain.

神經支配　神經支配到人體的某一區或器官。它可向一定的組織結構傳出運動衝動或從組織結構向腦傳入感覺衝動。

innocent *adj.* (of a tumour) benign; not malignant.

良性的　非惡性的（指腫瘤）。

innominate artery (brachiocephalic artery) a short artery originating as the first large branch of the *aortic arch, passing upwards to the right, and ending at the lower neck near the right sternoclavicular joint. Here it divides into the right common carotid and the right subclavian arteries.

無名動脉（頭臂動脉）　起於主動脉弓第一大分支的一短動脉。向右上方上升，止於下頸部近右胸鎖關節處。在此處分爲右頸總動脉和鎖骨下動脉。

innominate bone *see* hip bone.

髂骨

innominate vein (brachiocephalic vein) either of two veins, one on each side of the neck, formed by the junction of the external jugular and subclavian veins. The two veins join to form the superior vena cava.

無名靜脉（頭臂靜脉）　由頸外靜脉和鎖骨下靜脉滙合而成的，分別位於每側頸部的兩條靜脉。這兩條靜脉滙成上腔靜脉。

ino- *prefix denoting* **1.** fibrous tissue. **2.** muscle.

〔前綴〕　**①纖維組織　②肌**

inoculation *n.* the introduction of a small quantity of vaccine in the process of *immunization: a more general name for *vaccination.

接種　免疫過程中將少量疫（菌）苗注入體內。較爲通用的名稱爲 vaccination（預防接種）。

inoculum *n.* any material that is used for inoculation.

接種物　用做接種的任何物質。

inositol *n.* a compound similar to a hexose sugar. Inositol is present in many foods, in particular in the bran of cereal grain. It is sometimes classified as a vitamin but it can be synthesized by most animals and there is no evidence that it is essential to man.

肌醇　與己糖相似的一種化合物。它存於多種食物中，特別是在穀糠中。有時將肌醇歸爲一種維生素，但多數動物能合成這種肌醇，而且無證據表明它是人體所必需的。

inotropic *adj.* affecting the contraction of heart muscle. Drugs such as *digitalis have positive inotropic action, stimulating heart muscle contractions and causing the heart rate to increase. *Beta-blocker drugs, such as *propra-

變力性的　即影響心肌收縮力的。例如洋地黃類藥物有正性變力作用，它增强心肌收縮力，並致心率加快。β-受體阻滯劑類藥物，例如心得安，則有

nolol, have negative inotropic action, reducing heart muscle contractions and causing the heart rate to decrease.

負性變力作用，它減弱心肌收縮力，並致心率減慢。

in-patient *n.* a patient who is admitted to a bed in a hospital ward and remains there for a period of time for treatment, examination, or observation. *Compare* out-patient.

住院病人 收容入醫院病房某一床位，並留住一段時間做檢查、治療或觀察的病人。

inquest *n* an official judicial enquiry into the cause of a person's death: carried out when the death is sudden or takes place under suspicious circumstances. The results of medical and legal investigations that have been carried out are considered by a *coroner, sitting with or without a jury, and made publicly known. *See also* autopsy.

驗屍 在職司法人員調查某人死亡的原因：當死亡是突然發生的或發生可疑的情況下做此項檢查。醫學和法律的調查結果由驗屍官來考慮，並在開庭期在有或無陪審團的情況下公佈於衆。

insanity *n.* a degree of mental illness such that the affected individual is not responsible for his actions or is not capable of entering into a legal contract. The term is used in legal rather than medical contexts.

精神病 某種程度的精神疾患，以致患者對他的行動不能負責或不可能接受法律上的約束。這術語除用於法律方面，還用於醫學文獻中。

insect *n.* a member of a large group of mainly land-dwelling *arthropods. The body of the adult is divided into a head, thorax, and abdomen. The head bears a single pair of sensory antennae; the thorax bears three pairs of legs and, in most insects, wings (these are absent in some parasitic groups, such as lice and fleas). Some insects are of medical importance. Various bloodsucking insects transmit tropical diseases, for example the female *Anopheles* mosquito transmits malaria and the tsetse fly transmits sleeping sickness. The bites of lice can cause intense irritation and, secondarily, bacterial infection. The organisms causing diarrhoea and dysentery can be conveyed to food on the bodies of flies. *See also* myiasis.

昆蟲 主要指生活在陸地中的一大類節肢動物。成蟲身體分頭、胸和腹三部。頭部具有一對觸角，胸部有三對足，多數昆蟲有翅（在某些寄生性羣中，如蝨、蚤等是無翅的）。某些昆蟲對醫學是重要的。各種吸血昆蟲傳播熱帶病，例如雌性按蚊傳播瘧疾，彩彩蠅傳播睡眠病。蝨叮咬可引起强的刺激作用，繼而引起細菌感染。能引起腹瀉和痢疾的微生物可藉蒼蠅運送到食物中。

insecticide *n.* a preparation used to kill destructive or disease-carrying insects. Ideally, an insecticide should have no toxic effects when ingested by human beings or animals, but modern

殺昆蟲藥 用於殺死有害的或帶病昆蟲的一種製劑。一種理想的殺蟲藥當被人類或動物誤食時應是無害的，但近年强有力的

powerful compounds have inherent dangers and have caused fatalities. Some insect powders contain organic phosphorus compounds and fluorides; when ingested accidentally they may cause damage to the nervous system. The use of such compounds is generally under strict control. *See also* DDT, dieldrin.

化合物均具有危險性，並曾引起死亡。一些殺昆蟲的粉劑包括有機磷化合物和氟化物類，如偶爾被誤食，可能引起神經系統的損傷。一些化合物的應用通常在嚴格的控制下。

insemination *n.* introduction of semen into the vagina. *See also* artificial insemination.

授精 引精子進入陰道。

insertion *n.* (in anatomy) the point of attachment of a muscle (e.g. to a bone) that is relatively movable when the muscle contracts. *Compare* origin.

附着 解剖學中指某一肌肉的附着點（例如附於骨）。當肌肉收縮時，此點相對來說是可移動的。

insight *n.* (in psychology) knowledge of oneself. The term is applied particularly to a patient's recognition that he has psychological problems; in this sense absence of insight is a feature of psychosis. The term is also applied to the patient's accuracy of understanding the development of his personality and his problems; in this sense insight is enhanced by psychotherapy.

自知力 對自己的認識。這個術語特別用於病人對自己有無精神疾病的認識。在這意義上，沒有自知力是精神病的一種特徵。這術語也用於病人理解自己的個性和問題的準確性。在這意義上，通過心理治療可增進自知力。

insolation *n.* exposure to the sun's rays. *See also* heatstroke.

日射 暴露於陽光下。

insomnia *n.* inability to fall asleep or to remain asleep for an adequate length of time, so that tiredness is virtually permanent. Insomnia may be associated with disease, particularly if there are painful symptoms, but is more often caused by worry.

失眠〔症〕 不能入睡或不能持續睡到足夠長的時間，以致實際上是持久的疲勞。失眠〔症〕可能與疾病有關，特別是如有疼痛症狀時。但較常見的由煩惱引起。

inspiration *n. see* inhalation.

吸氣

instillation *n.* **1.** the application of liquid medication drop by drop, as into the eye. **2.** the medication, such as eye drops, applied in this way.

①**滴注法** 一滴一滴液體的投藥法，如把藥液滴入眼中。 ②**滴劑** 按此投藥法應用的藥物，如滴眼劑。

instinct *n.* **1.** a complex pattern of behaviour innately determined, which is characteristic of all individuals of the

本能 ①先天確定的複雜的行爲方式。它是同種所有個體的特徵。這種行爲

same species. The behaviour is released and modified by environmental stimuli, but its pattern is relatively uniform and predetermined. **2.** an innate drive that urges the individual towards a particular goal (for example, *libido in psychoanalytic psychology).

可因環境的刺激而產生和改變，但其方式相對來說是無變化的，是預先確定的。②個體先天存在的某種本能要求（例如，精神分析心理學中的里比多，即性力）。

institutionalization *n.* a condition produced by residence in an unstimulating impersonal institution (such as some mental hospitals and orphanages). The individual adapts to the behaviour characteristic of the institution to such an extent that he is handicapped in other environments. The features often include apathy, dependence, and a lack of personal responsibility. Some symptoms, such as *stereotypy, are commoner in the institutionalized.

收容所症　由於居住在缺乏刺激的、無人情味的機構（如精神病院和孤兒院）引起的一種狀態。這種人已適應這種機構所特有的行爲方式，以致到其他環境中就要發生障礙。常見的特徵包括感情淡漠、依賴性、缺乏自理能力。有些症狀如刻板症等是收容中較常見的。

insufficiency *n.* inability of an organ or part, such as the heart or kidney, to carry out its normal function.

功能不全　某器官或部位（如心臟或腎臟）不能行使其正常功能。

insufflation *n.* the act of blowing gas or a powder, such as a medication, into a body cavity.

吹入　把氣體或粉末（例如某種藥劑）吹進體腔的動作。

insula *n.* an area of the *cerebral cortex that is overlapped by the sides of the deep lateral sulcus (cleft) in each hemisphere.

腦島　大腦皮質的一個區域。它爲每側大腦半球外側裂的深面所覆蓋。

insulin *n.* a protein hormone, produced in the pancreas by the beta cells of the *islets of Langerhans, that is important for regulating the amount of sugar (glucose) in the blood. Insulin secretion is stimulated by a high concentration of blood sugar. Lack of this hormone gives rise to *diabetes mellitus, in which large amounts of sugar are present in the blood and urine. This condition may be treated successfully by insulin injections.

胰島素　一種蛋白質激素。在胰腺內由郎罕氏島的β細胞所產生。它對調節血糖量起重要作用。高濃度的血糖可促進胰島素分泌。胰島素缺乏可發生糖尿病，血及尿中出現大量的糖。糖尿病可以注射胰島素治療而獲顯效。

insulinase *n.* an enzyme, found in such tissues as the liver and kidney, that is responsible for the normal breakdown of insulin in the body.

胰島素酶　見於一些組織如肝與腎等一種酶。它能破壞體內正常的胰島素。

insulinoma *n.* an insulin-producing tumour of the beta cells in the *islets of Langerhans of the pancreas. Symptoms include sweating, faintness, episodic loss of consciousness, and other features of *hypoglycaemia. Single tumours can be removed surgically. Multiple very small tumours scattered throughout the pancreas cannot be treated by surgery but do respond to drugs that poison the beta cells, including *diazoxide.

胰島素瘤 胰腺郎罕氏島中產生胰島素的β細胞瘤。症狀包括出汗、暈厥、發作性的意識喪失以及低血糖等其他特徵。單一的胰島素瘤可手術切除。播散整個胰腺的多發性細小腫瘤不能用外科方法治療，而用破壞β細胞的藥物包括二氮嗪是很有效的。

Intal *n. see* cromolyn sodium.

色甘酸鈉

integration *n.* the blending together of the *nerve impulses that arrive through the thousands of synapses at a nerve cell body. Impulses from some synapses cause *excitation, and from others *inhibition; the overall pattern decides whether an individual nerve cell is activated to transmit a message or not.

整合作用 通過成千突觸達到某一神經細胞體的神經衝動互相混合（而產生協同效應）。來自一些突觸的衝動引起興奮，來自其他突觸的衝動則引起抑制；而整合的類型決定於該神經細胞是否被激活而能傳遞信息。

integument *n.* **1.** the skin. **2.** a membrane or layer of tissue covering any organ of the body.

①皮 **②包膜** 覆蓋人體任何器官的一種組織膜或組織層。

intelligence quotient (IQ) an index of intellectual development. In childhood and adult life it represents intellectual ability relative to the rest of the population; in children it can also represent rate of development (*mental age as a percentage of chronological age). Most *intelligence tests are constructed so that the resulting intelligence quotients in the general population have a *mean of about 100 and a *standard deviation of about 15.

智商 智力發展的一種指數。在小兒及成人的生活中，它是和人羣中其他人的智能的比較中得出的。在兒童中它也可表明發育速度（代表智力年齡，爲實足年齡的百分數）。多數智力測驗都是以智商的結果在一般人羣中平均數約爲100，而且約有15的標準差。

intelligence test a standardized assessment procedure for the determination of intellectual ability. The score produced is usually expressed as an *intelligence quotient. Most tests present a series of different kinds of problems to be solved. The best known are the Wechsler Adult Intelligence Scale (WAIS), the Wechsler Intelli-

智力測驗 評定智力的標準化方法。其得分通常是以智商表示。多數測驗提出必須解答的一系列不同類型的問題。最常用的有魏克斯勒成人智力量表（WAIS）、魏克斯勒小兒智力量表（WISC）以及斯坦福比內特智力量

gence Scale for Children (WISC), and the Stanford Binet Intelligence Scale. Scores on intelligence tests are used for such purposes as the diagnosis of *subnormality and the assessment of intellectual deterioration.

表。智力測驗的得分用於診斷低常狀態以及評價智力衰退。

intention *n.* a process of healing. Healing by *first intention* is the natural healing of a wound or surgical incision when the edges are brought together under aseptic conditions and *granulation tissue forms.

癒合 傷口長好的過程。第一期癒合是在無菌情況下傷口或手術切口的自然癒合，此時創緣合攏在一起並有肉芽組織形成。

intention tremor *see* tremor.

意向震顫

inter- *prefix denoting* between. Examples: *intercostal* (between the ribs); *intertrochanteric* (between the trochanters).

〔前綴〕 **兩者之間** 例如肋間的（在兩肋之間），轉子間的（在兩轉子之間）。

intercalated *adj.* describing structures, tissues, etc., that are inserted or situated between other structures.

插入的 描述結構、組織等被插進或置於其他兩結構之間。

intercellular *adj.* situated or occurring between cells.

細胞間的 位於或發生於細胞之間的。

intercostal muscles muscles that occupy the spaces between the ribs and are responsible for controlling some of the movements of the ribs. The superficial *external intercostals* lift the ribs during inspiration; the deep *internal intercostals* draw the ribs together during expiration.

肋間肌 佔據兩肋之間的肌肉。它能支配一些肋骨的活動。吸氣時淺外側肋間肌抬起肋骨，呼氣時深內側肋間肌一起拉下肋骨。

intercurrent *adj.* going on at the same time: applied to an infection contracted by a patient who is already suffering from an infection or other disease.

間發的 同時進行的，指已感染或已患病的患者又得另一種新感染。

interferon *n.* a substance that is produced by cells infected with a virus and has the ability to inhibit viral growth. Interferon is active against many different viruses, but particular interferons are effective only in the species that produces them. Attempts are being made to produce human interferon in large quantities in bacterial host cells.

干擾素 由受病毒感染並有抑制病毒生長能力的細胞產生的物質。干擾素對許多不同的病毒是有效的，但特殊的干擾素只對產生該干擾素的種有效。現在試圖在細菌寄生細胞中生產大量人類干擾素。

interkinesis *n.* **1.** the resting stage between the two divisions of *meiosis. **2.** *see* interphase.

分裂間期 兩期減數分裂之間的靜止期。

intermittent claudication *see* claudication.

間歇性跛行

intermittent fever a fever that rises, subsides, then returns again. *See* malaria.

間歇熱 升高、降退、然後又重復的一種熱型。

intern *n. see* Doctor.

實習醫生

International Classification of Diseases a list of all known diseases and syndromes published by the World Health Organization every ten years (approximately). Diseases are grouped either according to system (e.g. cardiovascular, respiratory) or type (e.g. malignant growths, accidents); each is allocated a three-digit number for computerization and hence comparison of mortality and morbidity rates, both regionally and nationally. Agreed simplified groupings exist, and some rubrics are subdivided by the use of a fourth digit.

國際疾病分類 所有已公認的疾病和綜合徵的一種編目。約每10年由世界衞生組織出版。這些病根據系統（例如心血管系、呼吸系）或類型（例如惡性腫瘤、事故）分類；每一分類給予三位數字編號以便輸入計算機，借此可以比較地區性的以及全國性的死亡率與患病率。建立了一些一致同意的簡化分類法，還有一些按第四位數字格式的詳細分類。

interneurone *n.* a neurone in the central nervous system that acts as a link between the different neurones in a *reflex arc. It usually possesses numerous branching processes (dendrites) that make possible extensive and complex circuits and pathways within the brain and spinal cord.

中間神經元 中樞神經系統的一種神經元。其作用是在反射弧中作爲不同神經元之間的環節。它通常具有許多分支樣突起（樹突），這種樹突使大腦與脊髓內有可能形成廣泛而複雜的環路和通路。

internode *n.* the length of *axon covered with a myelin sheath. Internodes are separated by nodes of Ranvier, where the sheath is absent.

結間部 被覆髓鞘的軸索，在其全長中被郎飛氏結分隔成結間部。在郎飛氏結處髓鞘消失。

interoceptor *n.* any *receptor organ composed of sensory nerve cells that respond to and monitor changes within the body, such as the stretching of muscles or the acidity of the blood.

內感受器 由感覺神經細胞組成的，能反應與監測體內變化（例如肌肉的伸展或血的酸度）的任何感受器官。

interparietal bone (inca bone, incarial bone) the bone lying between the *parietal bones, at the back of the skull.

頂間骨 位於兩頂骨間的骨，在頭顱後部。

interpeduncular *adj.* situated between the peduncles of the cerebrum or cerebellum.

腦脚間的　位於大腦脚或小腦脚之間的。

interphase (interkinesis) *n.* the period when a cell is not undergoing division (mitosis), during which activities such as DNA synthesis occur.

分裂間期　細胞未發生有絲分裂的時期。在這時期，像合成DNA這樣一些活動在進行。

intersex *n.* an individual who shows anatomical characteristics of both sexes. *See* hermaphrodite, pseudohermaphroditism. —**intersexuality** *n.*

雌雄間體　顯示兩種性別解剖特徵的某個人。

interstice *n.* a small space in a tissue or between parts of the body. —**interstitial** *adj.*

小間隙　人體組織內或兩部之間的小空隙。

interstitial cells (Leydig cells) the cells interspersed between the seminiferous tubules of the *testis. They secrete *androgens in response to stimulation by *luteinizing hormone from the anterior pituitary gland.

間質細胞（萊廸希氏細胞）　散在於睪丸的生精小管之間的細胞。它們在垂體前葉黃體激素的刺激下能分泌雄性激素類。

interstitial-cell-stimulating hormone *see* luteinizing hormone.

促間質細胞激素

intertrigo *n.* superficial inflammation (dermatitis) of two skin surfaces that are in contact, such as between the thighs or under the breasts, particularly in obese people. The dermatitis is caused by friction, warmth, moisture, and sweat and is often aggravated by infection.

擦爛　兩個互相接觸的皮膚表面的淺表炎症（皮炎）。例如兩個大腿之間或兩側乳房下面，多見於肥胖的人。這種皮炎由摩擦、溫熱、濕氣以及汗液所致，常因感染而加重。

intervention study a comparison of the outcome between two or more groups of patients that are deliberately subjected to different regimes (usually of treatment but sometimes of a preventive measure, such as vaccination). Wherever possible those entering the trial should be allocated to their respective groups by means of random numbers, and one such group (*controls*) should have no active treatment (*randomized controlled trial*). Ideally neither the patient nor the person assessing the outcome should be aware of which therapy is allocated to which patient

防治實驗研究　對兩組或兩組以上病人之間的觀察結果所做的一種比較。這些病人均經受不同的措施（通常是治療方面的，但有時是預防措施）。應盡可能將受試者進行隨機分組，並以其中一個組（對照）不做積極處理（隨機對照試驗）。最理想的是，既不讓病人以及評價試驗結果的人瞭解給予病人的治療方法（單盲試驗），也不讓負責治療的醫生瞭解（雙盲試驗）。

(*blind trial*), nor should the doctor responsible for treatment (*double-blind trial*), and groups should exchange treatment after a prearranged period (*cross-over trial*).

而且，經過預先安排的一段時期以後，各組間做交換治療（交叉試驗）。

intervertebral disc the flexible plate of fibrocartilage that connects any two adjacent vertebrae in the backbone. At birth the central part of the disc – the *nucleus pulposus* – consists of a gelatinous substance, which becomes replaced by cartilage with age. The intervertebral discs account for one quarter of the total length of the backbone; they act as shock absorbers, protecting the brain and spinal cord from the impact produced by running and other movements. *See also* prolapsed intervertebral disc.

椎間盤　在脊柱內連接着任何兩個相鄰椎骨的柔韌的纖維軟骨板。出生時椎間盤的中心部分——髓核由膠狀物質構成，隨年齡的增長即爲軟骨所代替。所有椎間盤總計爲脊柱總長度的¼，其作用是減輕外來的震動，預防來自跑步和其他運動對大腦與脊髓的衝擊。

intestinal flora bacteria normally present in the intestinal tract. Some are responsible for the synthesis of *vitamin K. By producing a highly acidic environment in the intestine they may also prevent infection by pathogenic bacteria that cannot tolerate such conditions.

腸內菌叢　腸道內正常存在的細菌。有些細菌能合成維生素K。在腸道內有這些細菌產生的高濃度的酸性環境，也可防止那些不能耐受這種條件的致病菌的感染。

intestinal juice *see* succus entericus.

腸液

intestine (bowel, gut) *n.* the part of the *alimentary canal that extends from the stomach to the anus. It is divided into two main parts – the small intestine and the large intestine. The *small intestine* is divided into the *duodenum, *jejunum, and *ileum. It is here that most of the processes of digestion and absorption of food take place. The surface area of the inside of the small intestine is increased by the presence of finger-like projections called *villi* (see illustration). Glands in the mucous layer of the intestine secrete digestive enzymes and mucus. The *large intestine* consists of the *caecum, vermiform *appendix, *colon, and *rectum. It is largely concerned with the absorption of water from the material passed from the small intestine. The contents of the

腸　消化道的一部分。其範圍由口至肛門。它分爲兩個主要部分——小腸及大腸。小腸又分爲十二指腸、空腸和迴腸。食物消化和吸收的主要過程在小腸內進行。小腸內具有指狀突起的絨毛使得小腸內的表面增加面積。小腸黏膜層的腺體分泌消化酶和黏液。大腸由盲腸、蠕蟲樣的闌尾、結腸和直腸組成。大腸基本上是與水分吸收有關，而水分是來自小腸和經過小腸的物質。借助於腸肌有規律的收縮，腸內容物被推向前進。

intestines are propelled forwards by means of rhythmic muscular contractions (*see* peristalsis). —**intestinal** *adj.*

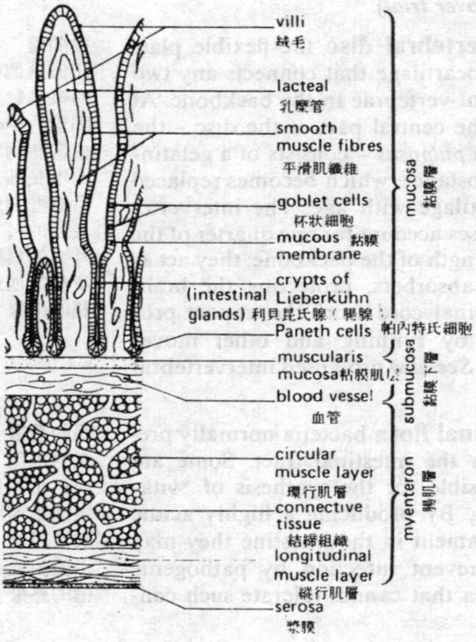

Longitudinal section through the ileum

迴腸縱切面

intima (tunica intima) *n.* **1.** the inner layer of the wall of an *artery or *vein. It is composed of a lining of endothelial cells and an elastic membrane. **2.** the inner layer of various other organs or parts.

內膜 ①動脈或靜脈壁的內層。它由襯里的內皮細胞與彈力膜構成。 ②各種其他器官或部位的內層。

intolerance *n.* the inability of a patient to tolerate a particular drug, manifested by various adverse reactions.

不耐性 即病人不能耐受特殊的藥物。以出現各種副反應爲特徵。

intoxication *n.* the symptoms of poisoning due to ingestion of any toxic material, including alcohol and heavy metals.

中毒 由於攝入任何有毒物（包括酒精與重金屬）引起的一些中毒症狀。

intra- *prefix denoting* inside; within. Examples: *intralobular* (within a lobule); *intrauterine* (within the womb).

〔前綴〕**內的** 例如小葉內的，子宮內的。

intracellular *adj.* situated or occurring inside a cell or cells.

細胞內的，細胞間的 位於或發生於細胞內或細胞間的。

intracranial *adj.* within the skull.

顱內的 在頭顱內的。

intradermal *adj.* within the skin. An *intradermal injection* is made into the skin.

皮內的 在皮膚內的。皮內注射即在皮膚內注射。

intramuscular *adj.* within a muscle. An *intramuscular injection* is made into a muscle.

肌內的 在某一肌肉內的。肌肉注射即肌肉內注射。

intraocular *adj.* of or relating to the area within the eyeball.

眼內 在眼球內的或與眼球內有關的。

intrathecal *adj.* within the *meninges of the spinal cord. An *intrathecal injection* is made into the meninges.

鞘內的 在脊髓膜內的。鞘內注射即在脊膜內注射。

intrauterine device *see* IUD.

宮內避孕器

intravenous *adj.* into or within a vein. An *intravenous injection* is made into a vein.

靜脉內的 進入靜脉的或在靜脉內的。靜脉注射即在靜脉內注射。

intravenous pyelogram (IVP) a succession of X-ray films of the urinary tract following the injection into a vein of an iodine-containing substance (which is opaque to X-rays). This material is concentrated and excreted by the kidneys, and the IVP reveals details of the kidneys, the ureters, and subsequently the bladder. An IVP tests kidney function and reveals the presence of stones in the kidneys or ureters and other abnormalities of the urinary tract. *See also* pyelography.

靜脉腎盂造影片 靜脉注射一種含碘物質（它不透X光線）後攝取的泌尿道連續X線片。這種物質由腎濃縮和排泄，因而靜脉腎盂造影片能顯示腎、輸尿道以及膀胱的詳細情況。這種造影可檢測腎功能，顯示腎或輸尿道結石以及泌尿道的其他異常。

intraversion *n. see* introversion.

牙弓狹窄

intra vitam Latin: during life.

生活期間

intrinsic factor a glycoprotein secreted in the stomach. The secretion of intrinsic factor is necessary for the absorption of *vitamin B_{12}; a failure of secretion of intrinsic factor leads to a deficiency of the vitamin and the condition of *pernicious anaemia.

〔造血〕內因子 胃內分泌的一種糖蛋白。內因子的分泌對維生素B_{12}的吸收是必要的。內因子分泌不足，可導至維生素B_{12}缺乏發生惡性貧血。

intrinsic muscle a muscle that is contained entirely within the organ or part it acts on. For example, there are intrinsic muscles of the tongue, whose contractions change the shape of the tongue.

內附肌 完全被包圍在器官內或器官的一部分，並對該器官起作用的一種肌肉。例如舌中具有的內附肌，其收縮可改變舌的形狀。

intro- *prefix denoting* in; into.

〔前綴〕**在內，入內**

introitus *n.* (in anatomy) an entrance into a hollow organ or cavity.

入口 解剖學中指進入空腔器官或腔洞的一種入口。

introjection *n.* (in psychoanalysis) the process of adopting, or of believing that one possesses, the qualities of another person. This can be a form of *defence mechanism. *See also* identification.

內向投射 精神分析學中指某人採納或相信具有他人品質的過程。這過程可以是一種防禦機制。

intromission *n.* the introduction of one organ or part into another, e.g. the penis into the vagina.

插入 某一器官或器官的一部分插入其他器官內，例如陰莖插入陰道。

introversion *n.* **1.** (*or* **intraversion**) an enduring personality trait characterized by interest in the self rather than the outside world. People high in introversion (*introverts*), as measured by questionnaires and psychological tests, tend to have a small circle of friends, like to persist in activities once they have started, and are highly susceptible to permanent *conditioning. Introversion was first described by Carl Jung as a tendency to distancing oneself from others, to philosophical interests, and to reserved defensive reactions. *Compare* extroversion. **2.** a turning inwards of a hollow organ (such as the womb) on itself.

①**內向** 一種以自我欣賞而對外界不感興趣爲特徵的內傾性格特徵。內向性高的人如用調查表和心理學測驗來檢測，顯示交遊不廣、固執以及極不適應不斷變化的環境。卡爾•榮格首先將內向描述成一種與他人疏遠、熱衷於哲學問題以及保留防禦性反應的性格傾向。 ②**內翻** 空腔臟器（如子宮）向內翻轉。

introvert *n. see* introversion.

①**內向** ②**內向者**

intubation *n.* the introduction of a tube into part of the body for the purpose of diagnosis or treatment. Thus *gastric intubation* may be performed to remove a sample of the stomach contents for analysis or to administer drugs directly into the stomach.

插管〔法〕 將一個管子插入人體的某一部位以診斷和治療疾病。因此，爲取胃內容物作標本作分析，或向胃內直接給藥，可做胃插管。

intumescence *n.* a swelling or an increase in the volume of an organ.

腫大 某一器官的腫大或體積增加。

intussusception *n.* the telescoping (*invagination*) of one part of the bowel into another: most common in young children under the age of four. As the contents of the intestine are pushed onwards by muscular contraction more and more intestine is dragged into the invaginating portion, resulting in obstruction. Symptoms include intermittent pain, vomiting, and the passing of red jelly with the stools; if the condition does not receive prompt surgical treatment, shock from gangrene of the bowel may result.

腸套疊 腸的一個部分套入另一個部分。最常見於4歲以下幼小兒童。由於肌肉收縮，腸內容物被向前推進，腸即越來越被曳入套疊部，最後導致梗阻。症狀包括間歇性疼痛、嘔吐以及一時性紅色肉凍樣便，本病如不即時進行外科治療，可導致休克（因腸壞死所致）。

inulin *n.* a carbohydrate with a high molecular weight, used in a test of kidney function called *inulin clearance*. Inulin is filtered from the bloodstream by the kidneys. By injecting it into the blood and measuring the amount that appears in the urine over a given period, it is possible to calculate how much filtrate the kidneys are producing in a given time.

菊粉 一種高分子碳水化合物。用於腎功能試驗，即菊粉攝清率試驗。菊粉從血流中經腎濾過。通過將菊粉注入血中，然後測定經一段時間後出現於尿中的菊粉量，即可計算在一段時間內腎的濾過量是多少。

inunction *n.* the rubbing in with the fingers of an ointment or liniment.

塗擦法 用手指塗擦軟膏或擦劑。

invagination *n.* **1.** the infolding of the wall of a solid structure to form a cavity. It occurs in some stages of embryonic development. **2.** *see* intussusception.

①**凹入** 實心結構的壁凹陷折疊而成為一種腔。它發生於胎盤發育的某些階段。②**〔腸〕套疊**

inversion *n.* **1.** the turning inwards or inside-out of a part or organ: commonly applied to the state of the womb after childbirth when its upper part is pulled through the cervical canal. **2.** a chromosome mutation in which a block of genes within a chromosome are in reverse order, due to that section of the chromosome becoming inverted. The centromere may be included in the inverted segment (*pericentric inversion*) or not (*paracentric inversion*).

①**內翻** 某器官或器官的一部分向內翻轉或由內向外翻出，常用於描述產後子宮上部經宮頸管牽拉出的狀態。②**倒位** 染色體畸變。指一條染色體內的一組基因順序顛倒，這是由於該段染色體倒轉所致。着絲粒可包括在倒轉的段內（臂間倒位）或不包括在內（臂內倒位）。

invertebrate 1. *n.* an animal without a backbone. The following are invertebrate groups of medical importance:

①**無脊椎動物** 一種沒有脊椎的動物。醫學上重要的無脊椎動物如下：昆蟲

*insects, *ticks, *nematodes, *flukes, *protozoans, and *tapeworms. **2.** *adj.* not possessing a backbone.

類、線蟲類、吸蟲類、原蟲類以及絛蟲類。 ②**無脊椎的** 不具有脊椎的。

in vitro Latin: describing biological phenomena that are made to occur outside the living body (traditionally in a test-tube).

在活體外 描述在活的生物體外人工產生的生物現象（傳統是在試管內）。

in vitro fertilization *see* test-tube baby.

試管內授精

in vivo Latin: describing biological phenomena that occur or are observed occurring within the bodies of living organisms.

在活體內 描述在活的生物體內發生或觀察到的生物學現象。

involucrum *n.* a growth of new bone, formed from the *periosteum, that sometimes surrounds a mass of infected and dead bone in osteomyelitis.

包殼 一種生長的新骨。由骨膜形成。在骨髓炎中，這種包殼有時包繞一感染的死骨塊。

involuntary muscle muscle that is not under conscious control, such as the muscle of the gut, stomach, blood vessels, and heart. *See also* cardiac muscle, smooth muscle.

不隨意肌 不受意識控制的肌肉，例如腸、胃、血管以及心臟的肌肉。

involution *n.* **1.** the shrinking of the womb to its normal size after childbirth. **2.** atrophy of an organ in old age.

①**復舊** 產後子宮退縮到其正常大小。 ②**退化** 老年人某一器官萎縮的現象。

involutional melancholia a severe *depression, usually psychotic, appearing for the first time in the involutional period of middle life (approximately 40–55 for women, 50–65 for men). Such an illness classically has characteristic features, including agitation; delusions of ill-health, poverty, sin, and sometimes of the nonexistence of the world; and preoccupations with death and loss. However, the features are not always classical, and many authorities do not regard the condition as a clinical entity separate from depressive psychosis. *See* manic-depressive psychosis.

更年期憂鬱症 更年期（大約女40～55歲，男50～65歲）開始出現一種嚴重的憂鬱症，通常屬精神憂鬱。其典型特徵是情緒激動，有不適、貧窮、罪惡以及虛無等妄想，死亡和損失等占先狀態。然而這種特徵往往是不典型的，而且許多專家認爲，這種病徵在臨床實際是不能與憂鬱性精神病鑑別的。

iodine *n.* an element required in small amounts for healthy growth and development. An adult body contains about 30 mg of iodine, mostly concentrated in

碘 機體健康成長和發育所需要的一種微量元素。成人機體約有30毫克碘，主要在甲狀腺內濃縮。甲

the thyroid gland: this gland requires iodine to synthesize *thyroid hormones. A deficiency of iodine leads to *goitre. The daily requirement of iodine in an adult is thought to be about 150 μg per day; dietary sources of iodine are sea food and vegetables grown in soil containing iodide and also iodized table salt. Radioactive isotopes of iodine (usually iodine-131), which are *radio-opaque, are used in the diagnosis and treatment of diseases of the thyroid gland. Iodine is also used as an antiseptic.

狀腺需碘以合成甲狀腺激素，碘缺乏可導致甲狀腺腫。成人每日碘的需要量約爲100微克；碘的食物來源是海產品類、生長於含碘土壤的一些蔬菜以及加碘的食鹽。碘的放射性同位素（通常是^{131}碘）用於診斷和治療甲狀腺疾病。碘也用做抗菌劑。

iodipamide *n.* a *radio-opaque iodine-containing compound used as a *contrast medium in radiography.

膽影酸 一種不透射線的含碘化合物。在放射攝影中做爲一種造影劑。

iodism *n.* iodine poisoning. The main features are a characteristic staining of the mouth and odour on the breath. Vomited material may be yellowish or bluish. There is pain and burning in the throat, intense thirst, and diarrhoea, with dizziness, weakness, and convulsions. Emergency treatment includes administration of starch or flour in water and lavage with sodium thiosulphate solution.

碘中毒 主要特徵爲口腔特別的着色以及特有的呼吸氣味。嘔吐物可能是淺黃或淺藍色的。有咽痛和燒灼感，劇渴及腹瀉，並伴有頭暈、虛弱和驚厥。緊急處理包括給予溶於水中的澱粉或面粉，並用硫代硫酸鈉溶液灌洗。

iontophoresis *n.* the technique of introducing through the skin, by means of an electric current, charged particles of a drug, so that it reaches a deep site. The method has been used to transfer salicylate ions through the skin in the treatment of deep rheumatic pain. *See also* cataphoresis.

電離子透入療法 用電流經過皮膚導入帶電荷的藥物離子使之達到人體深部的一種技術。在治療深部風濕性疼痛中，用此法經皮膚透入水楊酸鹽離子。

iopanoic acid *n.* a *radio-opaque iodine-containing compound used in radiography to outline the gall bladder (*see* cholecystography). Given by intravenous injection, the iopanoic acid is concentrated in the bile by the liver and thus shows up the gall bladder clearly during X-ray examination.

碘泛諾酸 一種不透射線的含碘化合物。在放射攝影中用於顯示膽囊裏的輪廓，由靜脉注射後，碘泛諾酸經肝濃集於膽汁中，因此，在做X線檢查時可清晰地顯示出膽囊。

iophendylate *n.* a *radio-opaque iodine-containing compound that is

碘苯酯 一種不透射線的含碘化合物，有時也在放

sometimes used in radiography to show up the spinal canal (*see* myelography). It is injected through a *lumbar puncture needle.

射攝影中用於顯示椎管。此葯用腰穿針注入。

ipecacuanha *n.* a plant extract used in small doses, usually in the form of tinctures and syrups, as an *expectorant to relieve coughing and to induce vomiting. Ipecacuanha irritates the digestive system, and high doses may cause severe digestive upsets.

吐根 小劑量應用的植物提取物。通常以酊劑和糖漿的形式做爲一種祛痰劑，以減輕咳嗽和誘發嘔吐。吐根刺激消化系統，大劑量可引起嚴重的消化紊亂。

iprindole *n.* a drug administered by mouth for the treatment of depression (*see* antidepressant). Response may take place gradually, and side-effects, such as dry mouth, blurred vision, constipation, and sweating, may occur. Trade name: **Prondol**.

胺丙吲哚 治療憂鬱症的一種口服藥。藥效逐漸發生，可有口乾、視力模糊、便秘以及出汗等副作用。

iproniazid *n.* a drug administered by mouth to treat all types of depression (*see* antidepressant). Side-effects may include constipation, dizziness, difficulty in urination, insomnia, headaches, and impotence. Trade name: **Marsilid**.

異丙異煙肼 治療各種憂鬱症的一種口服藥。副作用包括便秘、頭暈、排尿困難、失眠、頭痛以及陽萎等。

ipsilateral (ipselateral, homolateral) *adj.* on or affecting the same side of the body: applied particularly to paralysis (or other symptoms) occurring on the same side of the body as the brain lesion that caused them. *Compare* contralateral.

同側的 在人體的同一側或影響人體的同一側的。尤用於大腦損傷引起的發生於人體同側的癱瘓（或其他症狀）。

IQ *see* intelligence quotient.

智商

irid- (irido-) *prefix denoting* the iris.

〔前綴〕 **虹膜**

iridectomy *n.* an operation on the eye in which a part of the iris is removed.

虹膜切除術 切除部分虹膜的一種眼科手術。

iridencleisis *n.* an operation for *glaucoma in which a small incision is made into the eye, beneath the *conjunctiva and close to the cornea, and part of the iris is drawn into it. The iris acts like a wick and keeps the incision open for the drainage of fluid from the front

虹膜嵌頓術 青光眼的一種手術治療。這種手術在結膜下靠近角膜處向眼內做一小切口，將一部分虹膜拖入切口內。這虹膜就起如同燈心的作用，而且保持切口開放，使液體從

chamber of the eye to the tissue beneath the conjunctiva.

眼前方引流到結膜下組織。

iridocyclitis *n.* inflammation of the iris and ciliary body of the eye. *See* uveitis.

虹膜睫狀體炎 眼內虹膜和睫狀體的炎症。

iridodialysis *n.* a tear, caused by injury to the eye, in the attachment of the iris to the ciliary body. Usually a black crescentic gap is seen at the edge of the iris where the tear has occurred, and the pupil is displaced away from the site of the tear.

虹膜脫離 眼損傷引起的虹膜與睫狀體附着處撕裂。往往在撕裂處虹膜的邊緣見到黑色新月型的裂隙，而瞳孔從撕裂處偏移。

iridodonesis *n.* tremulousness of the iris when the eye is moved. It is due to absence of support from the lens, against which the iris normally lies, and occurs when the lens is absent or dislocated from its normal position.

虹膜震顫 眼運動時虹膜發生顫動。此病症是由於失去晶狀體的支持（虹膜靠晶狀體保持正常狀態），當晶狀體缺乏或從其他正常位置脫位時即可發生此症。

iridoplegia *n.* paralysis of the iris, which is usually associated with *cycloplegia and results from injury, inflammation, or the use of drugs in the eye. In the case of injury, the pupil is usually larger than normal and moves little, if at all, in response to light and drugs.

虹膜麻痹 虹膜的麻痹。本病症通常伴有睫狀肌麻痹，由損傷、炎症或由使用眼藥所致。在損傷的病例中，瞳孔較正常大，而且即使對光線與藥物有反應的話，變化也是小的。

iridotomy *n.* an operation on the eye in which an incision is made in the iris.

虹膜切開術 一種眼科手術。在虹膜內做一切口。

iris *n.* the part of the eye that regulates the amount of light that enters. It forms a coloured muscular diaphragm across the front of the lens; light enters through a central opening, the *pupil*. A ring of muscle round the margin contracts in bright light, causing the pupil to become smaller (*see* pupillary reflex). In dim light a set of radiating muscles contract and the constricting muscles relax, increasing the size of the pupil. The outer margin of the iris is attached to the *ciliary body.

虹膜 眼的一部分。其作用是調節進入眼內的光量。它形成一着色的肌性隔膜橫過晶狀體前；光線經中央孔（即瞳孔）進入眼內。圍繞虹膜邊緣的環形肌，遇亮光時即收縮，引起瞳孔變小。在暗光時一羣放射狀肌收縮，且環行肌鬆馳，瞳孔增大。虹膜外緣附着於睫狀體。

iris bombé an abnormal condition of the eye in which the iris bulges forward towards the cornea. It is due to pressure from the aqueous humour behind the

虹膜膨起 虹膜向前（朝角膜）鼓起的一種眼的異常狀態。這是由於房水經瞳孔到眼前房的通路受阻

iris when its passage through the pupil to the anterior chamber of the eye is obstructed. 時，虹膜後房水形成的壓力引起的。

iritis *n.* inflammation of the iris. *See* uveitis. **虹膜炎**

iron *n.* an element essential to life. The body of an adult contains on average 4 g of iron, over half of which is contained in *haemoglobin in the red blood cells, the rest being distributed between myoglobin in muscles, *cytochromes, and iron stores in the form of *ferritin and *haemosiderin. Iron is an essential component in the transfer of oxygen in the body. The absorption and loss of iron is very finely controlled. A good dietary source is meat, particularly liver. The recommended daily intake of iron is 10 mg per day for men and 12 mg per day for women during their reproductive life. A deficiency of iron may lead to *anaemia.
Many preparations of iron are used to treat iron-deficiency anaemia. These include preparations taken by mouth, such as *ferrous sulphate, and those administered by injection, such as *iron dextran.

鐵 生命不可缺少的一種元素。成年人平均有4克鐵。半數人以上的鐵存在於紅細胞的血紅蛋白中，其餘則分佈於肌肉的肌紅蛋白、細胞色素之內，鐵以含鐵蛋白及含鐵血黃素的形式貯存起來。鐵在人體運送氧中是一種不可缺少的組成部分。鐵的吸收和排出受到極爲嚴密的控制。鐵的食物來源是肉，尤其是肝。建議每日鐵的攝取量：男性每日10毫克，生育女性每日12毫克。鐵缺乏可導致貧血。

iron dextran a drug containing *iron and *dextran, administered by intramuscular or intravenous injection to treat iron-deficiency anaemia. Side-effects can include pain at the site of injection, rapid beating of the heart, and allergic reactions. Trade name: **Imferon**.

葡聚糖鐵 含鐵及葡聚糖的一種藥物。肌肉或靜脈注射給藥，以治療缺鐵性貧血。副作用有注射部位疼痛、心跳加速以及變態反應。

iron lung *see* respirator. **鐵肺**

iron-storage disease *see* haemochromatosis. **鐵沉着病**

irradiation *n.* the therapeutic application of electromagnetic radiation (usually alpha, beta, gamma, or X-rays) to a particular structure. *See* radiotherapy.

照射〔法〕 電磁輻射（通常是α、β、γ或X線）對特殊組織的治療應用。

irreducible *adj.* unable to be replaced in a normal position: applied particularly to a type of *hernia.

不能還原的 不能回復到正常的位置。特別指疝的一種類型。

irrigation *n.* the process of washing out a wound or hollow organ with a continuous flow of water or medicated solution.

冲洗法 用流水或藥液洗淨傷口或空腔器官的過程。

irritability *n.* (in physiology) the property of certain kinds of tissue that enables them to respond in a specific way to outside stimuli. Irritability is shown by nerve cells, which can generate and transmit electrical impulses when stimulated appropriately, and by muscle cells, which contract when stimulated by nerve impulses.

應激性 生理學中指某些組織或細胞的特性。可使該組織（或細胞）能以特殊的方式對外界刺激發生反應。顯示應激性的有神經細胞（給予適當刺激時能產生和傳導電衝動）和肌肉細胞（當受到神經刺激時能發生收縮）。

irritable bowel syndrome (spastic colon, mucous colitis) a common condition in which recurrent abdominal pain with constipation and/or diarrhoea continues for years without any general deterioration in health. There is no detectable structural disease; the symptoms are caused by abnormal muscular contractions in the colon. The cause is unknown, but the condition is often associated with stress or anxiety and may follow severe infection of the intestine.

應激性腸綜合徵（痙攣性結腸，粘液性結腸炎） 一種常見的腸道疾患。以復發性腹痛伴有便祕及／或腹瀉持續數年而無任何健康上的衰退爲特徵。在組織結構上無病變可尋，症狀是因結腸異常的肌肉收縮引起的。本徵病因未明，但往往與緊張或焦慮有關，而且可在嚴重腸道感染後發病。

irritant *n.* any material that causes irritation of a tissue, ranging from nettles (causing pain and swelling) to tear gas (causing watering of the eyes). Chronic irritation by various chemicals can give rise to *dermatitis.

刺激物 能刺激組織的任何物質。從蕁蔴類（引起疼痛的腫脹）直至催淚氣（引起流淚）。由各種化學物品引起的慢性刺激可發生皮炎。

isch- (ischo-) *prefix denoting* suppression or deficiency.

〔前綴〕**抑制，缺乏**

ischaemia *n.* an inadequate flow of blood to a part of the body, caused by constriction or blockage of the blood vessels supplying it. Ischaemia of heart muscle produces *angina pectoris.

局部缺血 人體某一部分的血流不足。由供應該組織的血管收縮或阻滯所致。心肌局部缺血可產生心絞痛。

ischi- (ischio-) *prefix denoting* the ischium.

〔前綴〕**坐骨**

ischiorectal abscess an abscess in the space between the sheet of muscle that assists in control of the rectum (levator ani) and the pelvic bone. It may occur

坐骨直腸窩膿腫 參與控制直腸的大片肌（直腸提肌）和骨盆之間的膿腫。它可以是自發的，但往往

spontaneously, but is often secondary to an anal fissure, thrombosed *haemorrhoids, or other disease of the anus. Symptoms are severe throbbing pain near the anus with swelling and fever. Pus is drained from the abscess by surgical incision.

繼發於肛裂、血栓性痔或其他肛門疾病。症狀有接近肛門的搏動痛，伴有腫脹和發熱。可通過手術切開將膿液從膿腫處引流。

ischium *n.* a bone forming the lower part of each side of the *hip bone (*see also* pelvis). —**ischiac, ischial** *adj.*

坐骨 形成每側髖骨下部的骨骼。

ischuria *n.* retention or suppression of the urine. *See* anuria, retention.

尿閉 尿豬留或受阻。

island *n.* (in anatomy) an area of tissue or group of cells clearly differentiated from surrounding tissues.

島 解剖學中指組織的某一區域或與其周圍組織明顯不同的細胞羣。

islet *n.* (in anatomy) a small group of cells that is structurally distinct from the cells surrounding it.

小島 解剖學指結構上與其周圍的細胞有明顯區別的一小羣細胞。

islets of Langerhans small groups of cells, scattered through the material of the *pancreas, that secrete the hormones *insulin and *glucagon. There are three main histological types of cells: alpha (α), beta (β), and D-cells (α_1). The alpha and beta cells produce glucagon and insulin, respectively.

郞格罕氏島（胰島） 散在胰腺組織間的一小羣細胞。它分泌的激素有胰島素及胰高血糖素。組織學上有三種主要類型的細胞：α、β 及 α_1 細胞。α 細胞與 β 細胞分別產生胰高血糖素及胰島素。

iso- *prefix denoting* equality, uniformity, or similarity.

〔前綴〕**相等，均勻，類同**

isoagglutinin (isohaemagglutinin) *n.* one of the antibodies occurring naturally in the plasma that cause *agglutination of red blood cells of a different group.

同種凝集素（同種血細胞凝集素） 血漿中生來就有的一種抗體。它可使不同型的血細胞發生凝集。

isoagglutinogen *n.* one of the *antigens naturally occurring on the surface of red blood cells that is attacked by an isoagglutinin in blood plasma of a different group, so causing *agglutination.

同種凝集素原 紅細胞表面生來就有的一種抗原。它受不同血型血漿中的同種凝集素的作用而致凝集。

isoaminile *n.* a drug administered in capsules and linctuses to suppress coughs (*see* antitussive). Rarely, it may cause dizziness, nausea, constipation, and diarrhoea. Trade name: **Dimyril**.

異丙苯戊腈 由膠囊和舐劑給藥以抑制咳嗽的一種藥（鎮咳藥）。少數情況下本藥可引起頭暈、噁心、便祕和腹瀉。商品名：咳得平。

isoantibody *n.* an *antibody that occurs naturally against the components of foreign tissues from an individual of the same species.

同種抗體 自然存在的一種抗體。抗同種不同個體的組織成分。

isoantigen *n.* an antigen that forms a natural component of an individual's tissues. Thus the antigens of the *HL-A system are isoantigens, as are the agglutinogens of the different *blood groups.

同種抗原 形成個體組織天然成分的一種抗原。例如，同種白細胞抗原系統（HL-A）、不同血型的凝集原，都是同種抗原。

isodactylism *n.* a congenital defect in which all the fingers are the same length.

指等長 所有各指均有同等長度的一種先天性缺陷。

isoenzyme (isozyme) *n.* a physically distinct form of a given enzyme. Isoenzymes catalyse the same type of reaction but have slight physical and immunological differences. Isoenzymes of dehydrogenases, oxidases, transaminases, phosphatases, and proteolytic enzymes are known to exist.

同功酶 同一種酶的物理性質各有不同的類型。同功酶能催化同一形式的反應，但有輕微的物理學和免疫學的差別。已知下列的酶有同功酶：脫氫酶、氧化酶、轉氨酶、磷酸酶及蛋白水解酶。

isograft (isogenic graft, syngraft) *n.* a *graft of tissue from one identical twin to another or between animals that are genetically identical.

同基因移植物 同卵雙胎之間或同系動物（基因相同）之間的組織移植物。

isohaemagglutinin *n.* *see* isoagglutinin.

同種血凝素

isoimmunization *n.* the development of antibodies (*isoantibodies*) within an individual against antigens from another individual of the same species.

同種免疫作用 某一個體內針對同種的另一個體抗原產生抗體（同種抗體）的作用。

isolation *n.* **1.** the separation of a person with an infectious disease from noninfected people. *See also* quarantine. **2.** (in surgery) the separation of a structure from surrounding structures by the use of instruments.

①**隔離** 指將已患感染性疾病的人與未受感染的人分開。②**分離** 外科中，指用器械將某一組織結構與其周圍的組織結構分開。

isoleucine *n.* an *essential amino acid. *See also* amino acid.

異亮氨酸 一種必需氨基酸。

isomerase *n.* any one of a group of enzymes that catalyse the conversion of one isomer of a compound into another.

異構酶 催化某化合物的一異構物轉變爲另一異構物的一組酶的任何一種。

isometric exercises (isometrics) a system of exercises based on the princi-

等長收縮鍛煉 根據肌肉等長收縮原理的一種鍛煉

ple of *isometric contraction* of muscles. This occurs when the fibres are called upon to contract and do work, but despite an increase in tension do not shorten in length. It can be induced in muscles that are used when a limb is made to pull or push against something that does not move. The exercises increase fitness and build muscle.

系統。當肌纖維收縮和做工時，儘管其緊張度增加而長度不縮短時可發生此情況。當使用某一肢體推拉某種不同的物體時，可在肌肉內產生等長收縮。這種鍛煉可使身體健康，肌肉發達。

isometropia *n.* an equal power of *refraction in both eyes.

屈光相等 兩眼屈光度相等。

isomorphism *n.* the condition of two or more objects being alike in shape or structure. It can exist at any structural level, from molecules to whole organisms. —**isomorphic**, **isomorphous** *adj.*

同形 兩個或兩個以上物體在形狀或結構上相同的情況。這種情況出現於任何結構水平，從分子水平直至完整的生物體。

isoniazid (isonicotinic acid hydrazide, INH) *n.* a drug used in the treatment of tuberculosis, usually taken by mouth. Because tuberculosis bacteria soon become resistant to isoniazid, it is usually given in conjunction with streptomycin or PAS. Occasional side-effects include digestive disturbances and dry mouth; high doses or prolonged treatment may cause inflammation of the nerves, which can be countered by including pyridoxine (vitamin B_6) in the preparation.

異煙肼 用於治療結核病的一種藥物。常口服給藥。由於結核菌很快對異煙肼形成抗藥性，故通常與鏈霉素或對氨水楊酸聯合應用。偶見的副作用包括消化紊亂和口乾，大劑量或長期治療可引起神經炎。包括吡哆醇（維生素 B_6）在內的制劑對神經炎有效。

isoprenaline *n.* a *sympathomimetic drug used to dilate the air passages in asthma and other bronchial conditions. It also stimulates the heart and is used to treat some heart conditions involving reduced heart activity. It is administered by inhalation, by mouth, by injection, or in suppositories. Side-effects such as increased heart rate, palpitations, chest pain, dizziness, and fainting may occur. Trade names: **Aleudrin**, **Lomupren**, **Medihaler-Iso**, **Prenomiser**.

異丙腎上腺素 一種擬交感神經藥。用於哮喘時擴張氣道以及用於其他支氣管疾病。它也興奮心臟而用於治療某種心臟病，包括心臟功能減退。以吸入、口服、注射或栓劑給藥。副作用有心率加速、心悸、胸痛、頭暈以及無力等。

isopropamide *n.* a *parasympatholytic drug that prevents muscle spasm in the digestive system and helps to reduce acid secretion in the stomach. It is administered by mouth for the treat-

異丙醯銨 一種預防消化系肌肉痙攣並有助於減少胃酸分泌的副交感神經阻滯藥。口服給藥。用於治療胃及十二指腸潰瘍。副

ment of stomach and duodenal ulcers. Side-effects can include dry mouth, disturbed vision, increased heart rate, difficulty in urination, and constipation.

作用有口乾、視力模糊、心率增快、排尿困難及便祕等。

isosthenuria *n.* inability of the kidneys to produce either a concentrated or a dilute urine. This occurs in the final stages of renal failure.

等滲尿 即兩側腎不能產生濃縮尿或稀釋尿，此病症發生於腎功能衰竭晚期。

isotonic *adj.* **1.** describing solutions that have the same osmotic pressure. *See* osmosis. **2.** describing muscles that have equal *tonicity.

①**等滲的** 描述具有同等滲透壓的溶液。 ②**等張** 描述具有同等緊張性的肌肉。

isotope *n.* any one of the different forms of an element, possessing the same number of protons (positively charged particles) in the nucleus, and thus the same atomic number, but different numbers of neutrons. Isotopes therefore have different atomic weights. Radioactive isotopes decay into other isotopes or elements, emitting alpha, beta, or gamma radiation. Some radioactive isotopes may be produced artificially by bombarding elements with neutrons. These are known as *nuclides* and are used extensively in *radiotherapy for the treatment of cancer.

同位素 具有與某種元素相同的質子數和原子序數，而中子數不同的任何元素（質子、中子都是原子核內的粒子）。因此各種同位素具有不同的原子量。放射性同位素衰變成其他同位素或元素，放射出α、β或γ射線。用中子轟擊元素可人工產生某些放射性同位素。這些衆所周知的核素廣泛用於癌腫的放射治療。

isoxuprine *n.* a drug that dilates blood vessels and is used to improve blood flow in such conditions as cerebrovascular disease and arteriosclerosis and to inhibit contractions in premature labour. It is administered by mouth or injection and rarely it may cause flushing, increased heart rate, dizziness, and nausea. Trade names: **Duvalidan, Defencin.**

苯氧丙酚胺 一種血管擴張藥。在一些疾病中如腦血管疾病和動脈硬化用於改善血流量，並用於抑制習慣性流產時的子宮收縮。可口服或注射給藥。少數情況下可引起潮紅、心率增快、頭暈以及噁心。

isozyme *n. see* isoenzyme.

同功酶

isthmus *n.* a constricted or narrowed part of an organ or tissue, such as the band of thyroid tissue connecting the two lobes of the thyroid gland.

峽 某一器官或組織的縮窄或狹小部。例如連接甲狀腺左右兩葉的甲狀腺峽部。

itch *n.* **1.** local discomfort or irritation of the skin, prompting the sufferer to

①**癢** 促使患者去抓或去搔患部的局部不適或皮膚

scratch or rub the affected area. *See* pruritus. **2.** a rarely used common name for *scabies.

刺激。 ②疥瘡　罕用的通俗名稱。

itch mite *see* Sarcoptes.

疥螨

-itis *suffix denoting* inflammation of an organ, tissue, etc. Examples: *arthritis* (of a joint); *peritonitis* (of the peritoneum).

〔後綴〕炎　指某一器官或組織的炎症。例如：關節炎，腹膜炎。

IUD (intrauterine device) a plastic or metal coil, spiral, or other shape, about 25 mm long, that is inserted into the cavity of the womb to prevent conception. Its exact mode of action is unknown but it is thought to interfere with implantation of the embryo. Early IUDs (such as the *Lippes loop*) were made of plastic; later variants (such as the *Gravigard*) are covered with copper, which slowly dissolves and augments the contraceptive action. Devices such as the *Progestasert* release small amounts of a contraceptive hormone drug. About one-third of women fitted with an IUD find the side-effects (heavy menstrual bleeding or back pain) unacceptable, but most have no complaints. The unwanted pregnancy rate is about 2 per 100 woman-years. If pregnancy should occur there is normally no need to remove the device (it may, however, become detached spontaneously).

宮內避孕器　用於阻止妊娠的物體。係一種塑料環或金屬圈，也有螺旋形或其他形的物體，長約25毫米，插入宮腔內。其確切的作用方式未明，現認爲是干擾胚胎植入。早期的宮內避孕器（如利帕氏環）是由塑料製作的，以後的改良型（如格雷維加德氏環）是包以金屬銅，它緩慢溶解，增加避孕效果。一些避孕器如黃體酮釋放式宮內避孕器釋放小量避孕激素。約⅓上了避孕器的婦女出現難以忍受的副作用（經血過多或腰痛），但多數沒有什麼不適。帶環妊娠率約爲2%人-年。如發生妊娠，正常情況下不需要除去避孕器（它可自行脫離）。

IVP *see* intravenous pyelogram.

靜脉造影照片

Ixodes *n.* a genus of widely distributed parasitic ticks. Several species are responsible for transmitting the diseases *tularaemia, Queensland tick typhus, and *Russian spring-summer encephalitis. The bite of a few species can give rise to a serious paralysis, caused by a toxin in the tick's saliva.

硬蜱屬　一屬分佈廣的寄生蜱。有幾個種能傳播土拉菌病、昆士蘭蜱傳傷寒、蘇聯春夏型腦炎等病。有幾個種其唾液中含有一種毒素，叮咬後可引起嚴重麻痹。

ixodiasis *n.* any disease caused by the presence of *ticks.

蜱病　由於蜱的存在而引起的任何疾病。

Ixodidae *n.* a family of *ticks.

硬蜱科　蜱類的一科。

J

J

Jacksonian epilepsy *see* epilepsy.

傑克遜氏癲癇

Jacquemier's sign (Spiegelberg's sign) a bluish or purplish coloration of the membrane lining the vagina: a possible indication of pregnancy.

傑克米埃士徵（施皮格爾伯格氏徵） 襯附於陰道的淺藍色或淺紫色的膜：可能爲妊娠的象徵。

jactitation *n.* restless tossing and turning of a person suffering from a severe disease, frequently one with a high fever.

輾轉不安 患嚴重疾病的人不安地翻來覆去。患者常有高熱。

jamais vu one of the manifestations of temporal lobe *epilepsy, in which there is a sudden feeling of unfamiliarity with everyday surroundings.

舊事如新症 顳葉癲癇的表現之一。患者對日常生活的環境突然感到陌生。

jaundice *n.* a yellowing of the skin or whites of the eyes, indicating excess bilirubin (a bile pigment) in the blood. Jaundice is classified into three types. *Obstructive jaundice* occurs when bile made in the liver fails to reach the intestine due to obstruction of the *bile ducts (e.g. by gallstones) or to *cholestasis. The urine is dark, the faeces pale, and the patient may itch. *Hepatocellular jaundice* is due to disease of the liver cells, such as *hepatitis, when the liver is unable to utilize the bilirubin, which accumulates in the blood. The urine may be dark but the faeces retain their colour. *Haemolytic jaundice* occurs when there is excessive destruction of red cells in the blood (*see* haemolysis). Urine and faeces retain their normal colour. Medical name: **icterus**.

黃疸 皮膚或眼白發黃。表明血中膽紅素（一種膽色素）過多。黃疸可分爲三種類型。梗阻性黃疸：其原因是肝臟中生成的膽汁，由於膽道梗阻（例如結石）或膽汁淤積而不能到達腸道之故。尿色深，糞便色白，患者可覺瘙癢。肝細胞性黃疸：是由於肝細胞疾病（如肝炎）引起，此時肝臟不能利用膽紅素，膽紅素就聚積於血中。尿色深，而糞便顏色不變。溶血性黃疸：當血中紅細胞破壞過多時可發生。尿及糞便保持其正常顏色。

jaw *n.* either the *maxilla (upper jaw) or the *mandible (lower jaw). The jaws form the framework of the mouth and provide attachment for the teeth.

頜 指上頜骨（上頜）或下頜骨（下頜）。上、下頜骨形成口的骨架，也做爲牙齒的附着處。

jejun- (jejuno-) *prefix denoting* the jejunum.

〔前綴〕 **空腸**

jejunal biopsy removal of a piece of the lining (mucosa) of the upper small intestine. This can be done by a surgical operation but is usually performed by a

空腸活〔組織〕檢〔查〕 切一塊上部小腸的粘膜以資檢查。可通過外科手術獲得，但常用的辦法是由患

special metal capsule, swallowed by the patient. When the capsule is in the *jejunum a small knife within it is triggered by suction on an attached tube, cutting off a small piece of mucosa. The specimen may be examined microscopically to assist in the diagnosis of *coeliac disease or intestinal infections, or its enzyme content may be measured chemically to detect, for example, *lactase deficiency.

者吞入一種特製的金屬囊來獲取。當金屬囊進入空腸時，通過安裝在側管內的抽吸裝置，啓動囊內的小刀，切取一小塊粘膜。標本可在顯微鏡下檢查，以協助腹腔疾病或腸道感染的診斷，或者用化學方法測定標本中的酶含量，例如乳糖酶缺乏時。

jejunal ulcer *see* peptic ulcer, Zollinger-Ellison syndrome.

空腸潰瘍

jejunectomy *n.* surgical removal of the jejunum or part of the jejunum.

空腸切除術 空腸或部分空腸的外科切除術。

jejunoileostomy *n.* an operation in which the jejunum is joined to the ileum (small intestine), when either the end of the jejunum or the beginning of the ileum has been removed or is to be bypassed. It is usually performed for intestinal disease (e.g. Crohn's disease) but sometimes for the treatment of obesity.

空腸迴腸吻合術 把空腸與迴腸連接的一種手術。用於空腸末端或迴腸起始段已被切除時，或可能患小腸疾病（例如克羅恩氏病）時，但有時是爲了治療肥胖症。

jejunostomy *n.* a surgical operation in which the jejunum is brought through the abdominal wall and opened.

空腸造口術 將空腸經腹壁拉出，並做開口的一種外科手術。

jejunotomy *n.* a surgical incision into the jejunum in order to inspect the interior or remove something from within it.

空腸切開術 爲了檢查空腸內部或從空腸內取出某物，而在空腸施行的一種外科切開術。

jejunum *n.* part of the small *intestine. It comprises about two-fifths of the whole small intestine and connects the duodenum to the ileum. —**jejunal** *adj.*

空腸 小腸的一部分。它約佔整個小腸的2/5，上接十二指腸，下與迴腸相接。

jerk *n.* the sudden contraction of a muscle in response to a nerve impulse. The *knee jerk* (*see* patellar reflex) is the reflex kicking movement produced by contraction of the quadriceps muscle of the thigh after it has been stretched by tapping the tendon below the knee. Eliciting this and other jerks, such as the ankle and elbow jerks, is a means of testing the nerve pathways, via the

反射 肌肉爲應答神經衝動引起的突然收縮。膝反射是一種踢腿反射，其產生是通過敲膝下肌腱，使股四頭肌收縮，大腿伸直。引出膝反射和其他反射如踝、肘反射等，是檢查神經通路的辦法。這些神經通路是通過脊髓參與各種反射活動的。

spinal cord, which are involved in *reflexes.

jigger *n. see* Tunga.

恙螨

joint *n.* the point at which two or more bones are connected. The opposing surfaces of bone are lined with cartilaginous, fibrous, or soft (synovial) tissue. The three main classes of joint are *diarthrosis (freely movable), *amphiarthrosis (slightly movable), and *synarthrosis (immovable).

關節 指兩個或較多骨骼的連接。相對的骨面襯有軟骨、纖維、軟組織（滑膜）等。關節的三種主要類型是：動關節（自由活動的），微動關節（輕度活動的），不動關節（不活動的）。

joule *n.* the *SI unit of work or energy, equal to the work done when the point of application of a force of 1 newton is displaced through a distance of 1 metre in the direction of the force. In electrical terms the joule is the work done per second when a current of 1 ampere flows through a resistance of 1 ohm. Symbol: J. *See also* calorie.

焦耳 功或能的國際單位，等於用一牛頓的力將某物沿力的方向移動1米的距離所作的功。在電學術語中指1安培的電流通過1歐姆的電阻每秒鐘所作的功。

jugular *adj.* relating to or supplying the neck or throat.

頸的 與頸部或喉部有關的，或供應頸部咽喉部的。

jugular vein any one of several veins in the neck. The *internal jugular* is a very large paired vein running vertically down the side of the neck and draining blood from the brain, face, and neck. It ends behind the sternoclavicular joint, where it joins the subclavian vein. The *external jugular* is a smaller paired vein running superficially down the neck to the subclavian vein and draining blood from the face, scalp, and neck. Its tributary, the *anterior jugular*, runs down the front of the neck.

頸靜脉 頸部的任何一條或幾條靜脉。頸內靜脉是很大的成對靜脉，沿頸的一側垂直向下，引流來自腦、面部及頸部的血液。它止於胸鎖關節下，在該處連接鎖骨下靜脉。頸外靜脉是較小的成對靜脉，沿頸部淺表向下至鎖骨下靜脉，引流來自面部、頭皮或頸部的血液。其分支頸前靜脉沿頸前向下。

jugum *n.* (in anatomy) a ridge or furrow that connects two parts of a bone.

軛 解剖學中指連接骨骼兩個部分的嵴或溝。

junction *n.* (in anatomy) the point at which two different tissues or structures are in contact. *See also* neuromuscular junction.

接點 解剖學中指兩種不同的組織或結構相接觸的點。

juxta- *prefix denoting* proximity to. Example: *juxta-articular* (near a joint).

〔前綴〕**近** 指與…接近。例如：近關節的（靠近關節）。

K

Kahn reaction a test for syphilis, in which antibodies specific to the disease are detected in a sample of the patient's blood by means of a *precipitin reaction. The test is not as reliable as the *Wassermann reaction, but is useful as confirmation.

康氏反應 用於檢查梅毒的一種試驗。以沉澱反應的方法，從病人的血標本中可測得梅毒特異性抗體。本試驗不如華氏反應可靠，但作爲進一步確診是有用的。

kala-azar (visceral leishmaniasis, Dumdum fever) *n.* a tropical disease caused by the parasitic protozoan **Leishmania donovani*. The parasite, transmitted to man by *sandflies, invades the cells of the lymphatic system, spleen, and bone marrow. Symptoms include enlargement and subsequent lesions of the liver and spleen; anaemia; a low *leucocyte count; weight loss; and irregular fevers. The disease occurs in Asia, South America, the Mediterranean area, and Africa. Drugs containing antimony are used in the treatment of this potentially fatal disease.

黑熱病（內臟利什曼病） 由寄生性原蟲杜諾凡氏利什曼原蟲引起的一種熱帶病。這種寄生蟲通過白蛉傳播給人，侵犯淋巴系統的細胞、脾和骨髓。症狀包括肝、脾腫大以及繼發性的損害，貧血，白細胞計數減少，體重減輕，以及不規則發熱。本病發生於亞洲、南美、地中海地區以及非洲。銻劑可用於治療這種可能致死的疾病。

kallidin *n.* a naturally occurring polypeptide consisting of ten amino acids. Kallidin is a powerful vasodilator and causes contraction of smooth muscle; it is formed in the blood under certain conditions. *See* kinin.

卡里定（緩激肽，血管舒緩素） 天然存在的多肽。由10種氨基酸組成。卡里定是一種强的血管舒張藥，可引起平滑肌收縮。在一定條件下，它可在血中形成。

kallikrein *n.* one of a group of enzymes found in the blood and body fluids that act on certain plasma globulins to produce bradykinin and kallidin. *See* kinin.

激肽釋放酶（激肽原酶） 見於血液和體液的一組酶的一種。這些酶作用於某種血球蛋白，以產生緩激肽及卡里定。

kanamycin *n.* an *antibiotic used to treat a wide range of bacterial infections. It is administered mainly by injection but is given by mouth for infections of the intestine and by inhalation for respiratory infections. Mild side-effects sometimes occur, including skin rashes, fever, headache, nausea, vomiting, and tingling sensations. Trade name: **Kantrex**.

卡那黴素 用於治療細菌感染的廣譜抗生素。主要注射給藥，但腸道感染時可口服，呼吸道感染時可通過吸入給藥。有時可發生輕度副作用，包括皮疹、發熱、頭痛、噁心、嘔吐以及麻刺感。商品名：硫酸卡那黴素。

kaolin *n.* a white clay that contains aluminium and silicon and is purified and powdered for use as an adsorbent. It is taken by mouth to treat the diarrhoea and vomiting due to food poisoning and other digestive disorders. Kaolin is also used in dusting powders and poultices.

白陶土 一種白黏土。含有鋁和硅。將其精製並研成粉末，可用作吸附劑。白陶土口服可治療由於食物中毒和其他消化系統疾病引起的腹瀉和嘔吐。白陶土也可用於撲粉和泥罨劑。

Kaposi's sarcoma a malignant tumour usually arising in the skin. It is common in Africa but rare in the western world, except in patients with *AIDS. The tumour evolves slowly; radiotherapy is the treatment of choice but chemotherapy may be of value in metastatic disease.

卡波濟氏肉瘤 常發生於皮膚上的一種惡性腫瘤。這種腫瘤常見於非洲，而西方罕見，除非病人患有艾滋病。本病發病緩慢，可先用放射線治療，而化學療法對轉移性疾病可能有效。

kary- (karyo-) *prefix denoting* a cell nucleus.

〔前綴〕**核** 細胞核。

karyokinesis *n.* division of the nucleus of a cell, which occurs during cell division before division of the cytoplasm (*cytokinesis*). *See* mitosis.

〔間接〕核分裂 細胞的分裂。發生於細胞漿分裂（細胞質變動）以前的細胞分裂期間。

karyolysis *n.* the breakdown of the cell nucleus in mitosis.

核溶解 有絲分裂時細胞核崩潰。

karyoplasm *n. see* nucleoplasm.

核質

karyosome *n.* the dense mass of *chromatin found in the cell nucleus, which is composed mainly of chromosomes.

核粒 見於細胞核中濃稠的染色質團。它主要由染色體組成。

karyotype *n.* **1.** the *chromosome set of an individual or species described in terms of both the number and structure of the chromosomes. **2.** the representation of the chromosome set in a diagram.

核型 ①描述某一個體或某物體的染色體組數目或結構特徵的術語。 ②以圖表來表示染色體組織型。

katathermometer *n.* a thermometer used to measure the cooling power of the air surrounding it, having its bulb covered with water-moistened material. The instrument is brought to a steady temperature of 100°F and then exposed to the air. The time taken for the temperature recorded by the thermometer to fall to 95°F gives an index of the air's cooling power.

乾濕球溫度計 用以測定乾濕球周圍空氣冷却力的一種溫度計（溫度計的球部蓋有用水浸濕的材料）。先使溫度計的溫度穩定在100°F，而後暴露於空氣中。溫度計上記錄到的溫度降至95°F的時間，作爲空氣冷却力的指數。

Kayser-Fleischer ring a brownish-yellow ring in the outer rim of the cornea of the eye. It is a deposit of copper granules and is diagnostic of *Wilson's disease. When well developed it can be seen by unaided observation, but faint Kayser-Fleischer rings may only be detected by specialized ophthalmological examination.

凱-費二氏環 眼角膜外面的棕黃色環。它是一種銅粒的沉着物，是威爾遜氏病（肝豆狀核變性）的診斷依據。當充分發展時可用肉眼觀察到，而輕微的凱-費二氏環只能用專門的眼科檢查來檢定。

keloid (cheloid) *n.* hard prominent irregular scar tissue in the skin that often increases in size. It often forms where healing injuries, burns, or surgical incisions are under tension; for example, on the back or neck.

瘢痕疙瘩（瘢痕瘤） 在皮膚內硬而突起的、不規則的疤痕組織。常可增大，往往在損傷、燒傷癒合處形成，或在低張力的外科切口處形成，例如在背部或頸部。

kelvin *n.* the *SI unit of temperature, formally defined as the fraction 1/273.16 of the temperature of the triple point of water. A temperature in kelvins is equal to a Celsius temperature plus 273.15°C. Symbol: K.

開〔爾文〕 溫度的國際標準單位。正式規定爲水三相點溫度的1/273.16。開〔爾文〕溫度等於攝氏溫度加273.15℃。符號：K。

kerat- (kerato-) *prefix denoting* **1.** the cornea. Example: *keratopathy* (disease of). **2.** horny tissue, especially of the skin.

〔前綴〕①**角膜** 例如：角膜病。 ②**角質組織** 尤其指皮膚的角質層。

keratalgia *n.* pain arising from the cornea.

角膜痛 起因於角膜的疼痛。

keratectasia *n.* bulging of the cornea at the site of scar tissue (which is thinner than normal corneal tissue).

角膜突出 疤痕組織處的角膜膨出（它比正常的角膜組織要薄）。

keratectomy *n.* an operation in which a part of the cornea is removed, usually a superficial layer.

角膜切除術 切除部分角膜的一種手術。通常切除一淺表層。

keratin *n.* a fibrous protein that forms the body's horny tissues, such as fingernails. It is also found in the skin and hair.

角蛋白 形成人體角質組織（例如指甲）的一種纖維蛋白。它也可見於皮膚和毛髮。

keratinization (cornification) *n.* the process by which cells become horny due to the deposition of *keratin within them. It occurs in the *epidermis of the skin and associated structures (hair, nails, etc.), where the cells become

角〔質〕化 由於角蛋白在細胞內沉積，使細胞成角質的過程。角化發生於皮膚表皮和有關的結構（毛髮、指甲等）。該處細胞變扁平，失去細胞核，而

flattened, lose their nuclei, and are filled with keratin as they approach the surface.

且在近外表面處充滿角蛋白。

keratitis *n.* inflammation of the *cornea of the eye. The eye waters and is very painful and vision is blurred. It may be due to physical or chemical agents (abrasions, exposure to dust, vapours, ultraviolet light, etc.) or result from infection. Keratitis not due to infection usually responds to keeping the eyes covered until the corneal surface has healed; infections often require specific drug treatment, e.g. with antibiotics.

角膜炎 眼角膜的炎症。流淚、眼劇痛及視力模糊。可由物理的或化學的因素（擦傷，暴露於塵土、蒸氣、紫外線等）或感染引起。非感染引起的角膜炎，遮蓋患眼至角膜表面癒合，往往是有效的。感染性的角膜炎需用特殊藥物治療，例如用抗生素。

keratoacanthoma (molluscum sebaceum) *n.* a firm nodule, appearing singly on the skin and growing to around 2 cm across in about six weeks, gradually disappearing during the next few months. Men are affected more often than women, commonly between the ages of 50 and 70. Keratoacanthomas occur on the nose, face, hands and fingers and sometimes on the scalp or neck. The cause is not known. Although the nodules disapppear spontaneously they may leave an unsightly scar, therefore treatment by curettage, cautery, or excision and suture is often carried out.

角化棘皮瘤（觸染性軟疣） 出現於皮膚上的單個硬結。約經6周，可長成圓形，直徑2cm，在以後的幾個月內逐漸消失。男性患者往往較女性多，常發生於50～70歲之間的中老年人。本病發生於鼻部、面、手及手指，有時在頭皮或頸部。發病原因未明。儘管這種硬結可自行消失，但可留有難看的疤痕；因此，往往要做刮除術、燒灼術或切除術等。

keratocele (descemetocele) *n.* outward bulging of the base of a deep ulcer of the cornea. The deep layer of the cornea (Descemet's membrane) is elastic and very resistant to ulceration; it therefore bulges when the overlying cornea has been destroyed.

角膜深〔彈性〕層突出 角膜的深度潰瘍，其基底層向外膨出。角膜深層（德斯密氏膜）是有彈性的，而且不易形成潰瘍，因此當角膜外層被破壞時，角膜深層即可突出。

keratoconjunctivitis *n.* combined inflammation of the cornea and conjunctiva of the eye.

角膜結膜炎 眼角膜和結膜的合併發炎。

keratoconus *n.* conical cornea: an abnormal condition of the eye in which the cornea, instead of having a regular curvature, comes to a rounded apex towards its centre. The 'cone' tends to become sharper with age. It is usually

圓錐形角膜 即成圓錐形的角膜：眼的異常狀態。此眼角膜的曲度不正，其中心呈圓頂狀態。年老時這種"圓錐"變得明顯。本病症是角膜的中心先天

due to a congenital weakness of the centre of the cornea, but may not produce symptoms until later childhood.

性缺陷所致，但幼年時，可不產生症狀。

keratoglobus (megalocornea) *n.* a congenital disorder of the eye in which the whole cornea bulges forward in a regular curve. *Compare* keratoconus.

球形角膜 眼部的一種先天性疾病。整個角膜以整齊的曲度向前凸出。

keratoma *n. see* keratosis.

角化病

keratomalacia *n.* a progressive disease of the eye due to vitamin A deficiency. The cornea softens and may become perforated. This condition is very serious and blindness is usually inevitable. *See also* xerophthalmia.

角膜軟化 因維生素A缺乏引起眼的進行性疾患。角膜變軟，而且可致穿孔。本病症極爲嚴重，往往不可避免地導致失明。

keratome *n.* any instrument designed for cutting the cornea. The simplest type has a flat triangular blade attached at its base to a handle, the other two sides being very sharp and tapering to a point. Power-driven keratomes have oscillating or rotating blades.

角膜刀 供切開角膜用的任何器械。最簡單的類型是具有扁三角形刀刃，其底連接於手柄，另外兩邊極鋭，而且其頭部漸漸變尖。驅動式角膜刀具有擺動或旋轉的刀口。

keratometer (ophthalmometer) *n.* an instrument for measuring the radius of curvature of the cornea. It is used for assessing the degree of abnormal curvature of the cornea in *astigmatism. Usually the vertical and horizontal curvatures are measured. All keratometers work on the principle that the size of the image of an object reflected from a convex mirror (in this case, the cornea) depends on the curvature of the mirror. The steeper the curve, the smaller the image. —**keratometry** *n.*

角膜曲度計 用於測量角膜彎曲半徑的一種儀器。即用於評價散光時的角膜異常曲度。通常要測出角膜垂直及水平曲度。各種角膜曲度計的工作原理是：從凸的鏡面（假設是角膜）上反映出的物像的大小取决於鏡面的曲度。曲度越大，物像越小。

keratoplasty (corneal graft) *n.* an eye operation in which any diseased parts of the cornea are replaced by clear corneal tissue from a donor. All layers of the cornea may be replaced (*penetrating keratoplasty*) or only some of its layers, the deeper layer remaining (*lamellar keratoplasty*). In the latter case the thickness of the replacement cornea is correspondingly reduced.

角膜成形術（角膜移植術） 用來自供體的透明角膜組織替代任一患病部位的角膜的眼科手術。可替換全層角膜，或只替換角膜的某些層，保留其深層（板層角膜成形術）。在後者的情況下，應適當減少換角膜的厚度。

keratoscope (Placido's disc) *n.* an instrument for detecting abnormal curvature of the cornea. It consists of a black disc, about 20 cm in diameter, marked with concentric white rings. The examiner looks through a small lens in the centre at the reflection of the rings in the patient's cornea. A normal cornea will reflect regular concentric images of the rings; a cornea that is abnormally curved (for example in *keratoconus) or scarred reflects distorted rings.

角膜鏡（普拉西多氏盤） 一種用於檢查角膜異常曲度的儀器。該鏡是一個黑色圓盤，直徑約20cm，標有白色的同心圓。檢查者通過鏡中心的小凸透鏡觀察同心環在患者角膜上的成像；而異常曲度的角膜（例如圓錐形角膜）或疤痕化的角膜，則呈歪歪曲曲的環。

keratosis (keratoma) *n.* any horny growth of the skin. There are two common types. *Actinic keratosis* is a well-defined red or skin-coloured warty growth, usually occurring in middle or old age, caused by overexposure to the sun. *Seborrhoeic keratosis* (or *warts*) are yellow or brown oval spots with clearly marked perimeters and raised surfaces, developing in middle age.

角化病 任何皮膚的角質增加。有兩種常見的類型：光化性角化病是一種界限清楚的紅色或肉色的疣狀增生，常見於中老年人，由於過多暴露於陽光下引起。皮脂溢性角化病（或疣）是黃色或棕色的卵圓形斑塊，周邊清楚，高出皮面，發生於中年人。

keratotomy *n.* an incision into the cornea.

角膜切開術

kerion *n.* a soft inflammatory swelling covered with pustules, caused by a ringworm fungus infection.

膿癬 有膿疱覆蓋的軟的炎性腫脹。由一種癬菌感染引起。

kernicterus *n.* staining and subsequent damage of the brain by bile pigment (bilirubin), which may occur in severe cases of *haemolytic disease of the newborn. Immature brain cells in the *basal ganglia are affected, and as brain development proceeds a pattern of *cerebral palsy emerges at about six months, with uncoordinated movements, deafness, disturbed vision, and feeding and speech difficulties.

核黃疸 由膽色素（膽紅素）引起着色的、繼發的腦損傷。本病可發生於嚴重的新生兒溶血的病例。基底神經節中未成熟的腦細胞受累，並且隨着腦的發育，在約6個月的時間就會出現某種大腦性麻痹，可有運動不協調、耳聾、視力障礙以及攝食和說話困難。

Kernig's sign a symptom of *meningitis in which the hamstring muscles in the legs are so stiff that the patient is unable to extend his legs at the knee when the thighs are held at a right angle to the body.

克尼格氏徵 腦膜炎的一種體徵。此徵因腿部膕繩肌腱僵直，以致當患者大腿與身體成直角時，膝部不能伸直。

ketogenesis *n.* the production of *ketone bodies. These are normal products of lipid metabolism and can be used to provide energy. The condition of *ketosis can occur when excess ketone bodies are produced.

酮生成 產生酮體。酮體是脂肪代謝的正常產物，而且能用於提供能量。當人體產生過多的酮體時，則可發生酮病狀態。

ketogenic diet a diet that promotes the formation of *ketone bodies in the tissues. A ketogenic diet is one in which the principal energy source is fat rather than carbohydrate.

生酮飲食 能促使酮體在組織內形成的飲食。生酮飲食是主要能源之一，其來源是脂肪，而不是碳水化合物。

ketonaemia *n.* the presence in the blood of *ketone bodies.

酮血〔症〕 血中出現酮體。

ketone *n.* any member of a group of organic compounds consisting of a carbonyl group (=CO) flanked by two alkyl groups. The ketones acetoacetic acid, acetone, and β-hydroxybutyrate (known as *ketone* (or *acetone*) *bodies*) are produced during the metabolism of fats. *See also* ketosis.

酮 羰基兩側各接連着一個烴基構成的一種有機化合物。酮類（乙醯乙酸、丙酮以及 β-羥丁酸）通稱酮或酮體，是脂肪代謝的產物。

ketonuria (acetonuria) *n.* the presence in the urine of *ketone (acetone) bodies. This may occur in diabetes mellitus, starvation, or after persistent vomiting and results from the partial oxidation of fats. Ketone bodies may be detected by adding a few drops of 5% sodium nitroprusside solution and a solution of ammonia to the urine; the gradual development of a purplish-red colour indicates their presence.

酮尿〔症〕 尿中存有酮體〔丙酮〕。本症可發生於糖尿病、飢餓或持續嘔吐等，以及脂肪不全氧化時。在尿中加幾滴5%亞硝基鐵氰化鈉及氨液可測出酮體：逐漸出現淺紫紅色，表明有酮體存在。

ketoprofen *n.* an *analgesic that reduces inflammation, administered by mouth to treat various arthritic and rheumatic diseases. Side-effects are rare, but indigestion sometimes occurs. Trade name: **Orudis**.

苯酮苯丙酸 緩解炎症的一種鎮痛藥。口服用藥，治療各種關節疾病和風濕病。副作用少見，但有時可發生消化不良。

ketose *n.* a simple sugar that terminates with a keto group (–C=O); for example, *fructose.

酮糖 分子中有酮基（-C=O）的單糖。例如果糖。

ketosis *n.* raised levels of *ketone bodies in the body tissues. Ketone bodies are normal products of fat metabolism and can be oxidized to produce

酮病 酮體在人體組織內的含量升高。酮體是脂肪代謝的正常產物，可被氧化，產生能量。當脂肪代

energy. Elevated levels arise when there is an imbalance in fat metabolism, such as occurs in diabetes mellitus or starvation. Ketosis may result in severe *acidosis. *See also* ketonuria.

謝失衡，例如發生糖尿病或飢餓時，酮體濃度升高。酮病可導致嚴重的酸中毒。

kidney *n.* either of the pair of organs responsible for the excretion of nitrogenous wastes, principally urea, from the blood (see illustration). The kidneys are situated at the back of the abdomen, below the diaphragm, one on each side of the spine; they are supplied with blood by the renal arteries. Each kidney is enclosed in a fibrous capsule and is composed of an outer *cortex* and an inner *medulla*. The active units of the kidney are the *nephrons, within the cortex and medulla, which filter the blood under pressure and then reabsorb water and selected substances back into the blood. The *urine thus formed is conducted from the nephrons via the renal tubules into the *renal pelvis* and from here to the ureter, which leads to the bladder.

腎 專司排出血中含氮廢物（主要是尿素）的一對器官（見圖）。腎位於腹部的後面，在膈肌下，分別位於脊柱的兩側，由腎動脈供給血液。每側腎由纖維性囊包繞。腎由外面的皮質和裏面的髓質組成。腎的功能單位是腎單位（在皮質和髓質內），在壓力影響下將血濾過，然後重吸收水分及經選擇的物質回到血液中。這樣形成的尿，經腎單位的通路腎小管進入腎盂，再由此經輸尿管，導入膀胱。

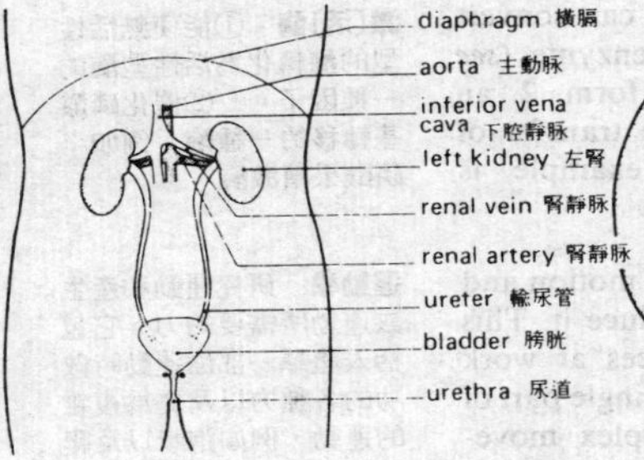

Position of the kidneys
腎的位置

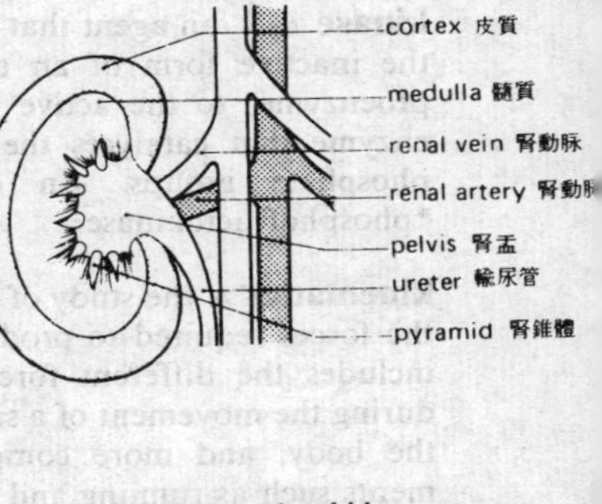

Section through a kidney
腎的切面

kilo- *prefix denoting* a thousand.

〔前綴〕**千** 一千。

kilocalorie *n.* one thousand calories. *See* calorie.

千卡 一千卡。

kilogram *n.* the *SI unit of mass equal to 1000 grams and defined in terms of the international prototype (a cylinder

千克 質量等於1000克，並且由國際原器（鉑-銥合金的圓柱，此器存於巴

of platinum-iridium alloy) kept at Sèvres, near Paris. Symbol: kg.

黎附近的塞夫勒）規定的國際標準單位。符號kg。

kin- (kine-) *prefix denoting* movement.

〔前綴〕**活力，運動**

kinaesthesia *n.* the sense that enables the brain to be constantly aware of the position and movement of muscles in different parts of the body. This is achieved by means of *proprioceptors, which send impulses from muscles, joints, and tendons. Without this sense, coordinated movement would be impossible with the eyes closed.

運動覺 指人腦總是能意識到人體不同部位肌肉的位置和活動的感覺。這種感覺是通過從肌肉、關節和肌腱發出衝動的本體感受器獲得的。沒有這種感覺，閉眼時則不可能產生協調的運動。

kinaesthesiometer *n.* an instrument for measuring a patient's awareness of the muscular and joint movements of his own body: used during the investigation of nervous and muscular disorders and certain forms of brain damage.

肌動覺測量器 測量患者本身肌肉和關節運動知覺的一種儀器。在神經和肌肉疾患以及某些類型腦損傷的調查研究中使用。

kinanaesthesia *n.* inability to sense the positions and movements of parts of the body, with consequent disordered physical activity.

運動感覺缺失 不能感覺人體各部位的位置和運動，以及隨之發生的身體活動障礙。

kinase *n.* **1.** an agent that can convert the inactive form of an enzyme (*see* proenzyme) to the active form. **2.** an enzyme that catalyses the transfer of phosphate groups. An example is *phosphofructokinase.

激〔活〕酶 ①能使無活性型的酶轉化爲活性型酶的一種因子。 ②催化磷酸基轉移的一種酶。例如：磷酸果糖激酶。

kinematics *n.* the study of motion and the forces required to produce it. This includes the different forces at work during the movement of a single part of the body, and more complex movements such as running and climbing.

運動學 研究運動和產生該運動所需要的力。它包括人體單一部位運動時做功的各種力以及更爲複雜的運動，例如跑步以及爬山。

kineplasty *n.* a method of amputation in which the muscles and tendons of the affected limb are arranged so that they can be integrated with a specially made artificial replacement. This enables direct movement of the artificial hand or limb by the muscles.

運動整形截肢術 截肢術的一種方法。術中，修整患肢的肌肉和肌腱，使肌肉和肌腱能與特製人工裝置結合成一整體。這樣就可通過肌肉使人工手或人工肢體直接活動。

-kinesis *suffix denoting* movement.

〔後綴〕**運動**

kinetochore *n. see* centromere.

着絲點

kinin *n.* one of a group of naturally occurring polypeptides that are powerful *vasodilators, which lower blood pressure, and cause contraction of smooth muscle. The kinins *bradykinin* and *kallidin* are formed in the blood by the action of proteolytic enzymes (*kallikreins*) on certain plasma globulins (*kininogens*). Kinins are not normally present in the blood, but are formed under certain conditions; for example when tissue is damaged or when there are changes in the pH and temperature of the blood. They are thought to play a role in inflammatory response.

激肽 一組天然存在的多肽的一種。它是强有力的血管擴張劑，可降低血壓，並引起平滑肌收縮。激肽類緩激肽和卡里定是通過蛋白水解酶（激肽釋放酶）對血漿球蛋白（激肽原）的作用在血中形成的。在平常情況下激肽不存於血液中，而是在一定的條件下形成的：例如當組織損傷或者當血的酸鹼度和溫度有變化時。據認爲，激肽在炎症反應中起作用。

kiss of life emergency *artificial respiration, performed mouth-to-mouth, by blowing air into the victim's lungs to inflate them and then allowing exhalation to occur automatically. The operator should aim to produce roughly 20 cycles of respiration per minute, or more for a younger victim.

口對口復甦法 口對口進行的緊急人工呼吸。即通過將空氣吹入患者肺內，使肺膨脹，然後使其自動呼出。術者應有目的地使其產生約每分鐘20次的呼吸，如爲較年輕的患者則應超過20次。

Klebsiella *n.* a genus of Gram-negative rodlike nonmotile mostly lactose-fermenting bacteria found in the respiratory, intestinal, and urinogenital tracts of animals and man. The species *K. aerogenes* is associated with human urinary infections; *K. pneumoniae* is associated with pneumonia and other respiratory infections. The species *K. rhinoscleromatis* causes *rhinoscleroma, a chronic infection of the nose and pharynx.

克雷伯氏桿菌屬 一類革蘭氏陰性桿狀菌。爲不動型細菌，大部分能使乳糖發酵。見於動物及人的呼吸道、腸道以及泌尿生殖道。有些菌種，如產氣克雷伯氏桿菌與人泌尿道感染有關；肺炎桿菌與肺炎及其他呼吸道感染有關；而鼻硬結克雷伯氏桿菌則引起鼻硬結〔症〕及鼻咽的慢性感染。

Klebs-Loeffler bacillus *see* Corynebacterium.

克-呂二氏桿菌（白喉桿菌）

klepto- *prefix denoting* stealing.

〔前綴〕 **偷竊**

kleptomania *n.* a pathologically strong impulse to steal, often in the absence of any desire for the stolen object(s). It is sometimes associated with *depression.

偷竊狂 一種病態的强烈的偷竊衝動，往往並不是眞正想要偷東西。本病有時伴有抑鬱症。

Klinefelter's syndrome a genetic disorder in which there are three sex

克萊恩費爾特氏綜合徵 一種遺傳性疾病。本徵有

chromosomes, XXY, rather than the normal XX or XY. Affected individuals are apparently male, but are tall and thin, with small testes, failure of normal sperm production (azoospermia), enlargement of the breasts (gynaecomastia), and absence of facial and body hair.

三個性染色體（XXY），而不是正常的XX或XY。患病的個體外表雖然是男性，但體瘦細高，睾丸小，無正常精子產生（精子缺乏），乳房增大（男子女性型乳房），面及身體無毛。

Klumpke's paralysis a partial paralysis of the arm caused by injury to a baby's *brachial plexus during birth. This may result from an obstetric manoeuvre in which the arm is raised at the shoulder to an extreme degree, which damages the lower cervical (neck) and upper thoracic (chest) nerve roots of the spinal cord. It results in weakness and wasting of the muscles of the hand.

克隆普克氏麻痹 本病可由助產時過度抬肩，損傷下頸部和上胸部脊神經根引起。可導致手部肌肉軟弱和消瘦。

kneading *n. see* petrissage.

揉捏法

knight's-move thought a form of thought disorder, characteristic of *schizophrenia, in which the *associations of ideas are bizarre and tortuous.

騎士思維 思維紊亂的一個類型。乃精神分裂症的特徵。本病患者有古怪和離奇的觀點。

knock-knee *n.* abnormal in-curving of the legs, resulting in a gap between the feet when the knees are in contact. In severe cases there is stress on the knee, ankle, and foot joints, resulting eventually in degenerative arthritis. The condition may be corrected by *osteotomy. Medical name: **genu valgum**.

膝外翻 腿的異常彎曲。當兩膝接觸時，導致兩足之間形成一間隙。在嚴重病例中，有膝、踝以及足關節的壓迫感，最終造成退行性關節炎。本病可通過切骨術糾正。

Koch's bacillus *see* Mycobacterium.

郭霍氏桿菌（結核桿菌）

Köhler's disease inflammation of the *navicular bone of the foot (*see* osteochondritis). It occurs in children, causing pain and limping, and is treated by strapping the foot.

科勒氏病 足的舟狀骨的炎症。發生於兒童，引起疼痛和軟弱無力。可用橡皮膏貼足來治療。

koilonychia *n.* the development of thin (brittle) concave (spoon-shaped) nails, a common disorder that can occur with anaemia due to iron deficiency, though the cause is not known. Treatment is by treating any underlying disease.

反甲 異常薄（脆）、凹陷（匙狀）的指甲。病因不明，可能發生於缺鐵性貧血，是一種常見疾患。治療方法是治療其原發性疾病。

Koplik's spots small red spots with bluish-white centres that often appear on the mucous membranes of the mouth in *measles.

科潑力克氏徵（斑） 中心是淡藍色發白的小紅斑。出現於痲疹患者的口腔黏膜。

koro *n.* a state of acute anxiety, seen only in certain cultures (such as that of the Chinese of SE Asia), characterized by a sudden belief that the penis is shrinking into the abdomen and will disappear. Occasionally women have a similar belief that their breasts are disappearing into their body. It is usually treated with tranquillizing drugs and reassurance.

柯羅病（縮陰） 一種急性焦慮的狀態。只見於具有某些文化背景的人羣（例如東南亞的華裔）。其特徵是突然相信其陰莖縮入腹部內，並會消失。偶爾，婦女也有同樣的信念，認爲其乳房縮入體內而消失。本病通常用安定藥和再建立信心來治療。

Korsakoff's syndrome (Korsakoff's psychosis) an organic disorder affecting the brain that results in a memory defect in which new information fails to be learnt although events from the past are still recalled; *disorientation for time and place; and a tendency to invent material to fill memory blanks (*see* confabulation). The commonest cause of the condition is alcoholism, especially when this has led to deficiency of thiamin (vitamin B_1). Large doses of thiamin are given as treatment. The condition often becomes chronic.

科爾薩科夫氏綜合徵（科爾薩科夫精神病） 影響大腦的一種器質性疾病。導致記憶喪失。儘管過去的事件還能回想起來，但不能學到新的信息，不能判定時間及空間；傾向於虛構素材以填滿記憶的空白。本病最常見的原因是酒精中毒，尤其是當已引起硫胺（維生素 B_1）缺乏時。可予大劑量硫胺來治療。本病常變爲慢性。

kraurosis *n.* shrinking of a body part, usually the vulva in elderly women (*kraurosis vulvae*).

乾皺 身體某一部分皺縮。通常指老年婦女的外陰。

Krebs cycle (citric acid cycle) a complex cycle of enzyme-catalysed reactions, occurring within the cells of all living animals, in which acetate, in the presence of oxygen, is broken down to produce energy in the form of *ATP (via the *electron transport chain) and carbon dioxide. The cycle is the final step in the oxidation of carbohydrates, fats, and proteins; some of the intermediary products of the cycle are used in the synthesis of amino acids.

克雷布氏循環（三羧酸循環） 一種酶促反應的複雜循環。發生於所有活的動物細胞內。乙酸化合物參加此循環中，在有氧存在的情況下被分解，產生ATP形式的能量（通過電子轉移鏈）和二氧化碳。此循環是糖類、脂肪類以及蛋白質氧化的最後步驟。循環的中間產物用於合成氨基酸。

Krukenberg tumour a rapidly developing malignant growth in one or (more often) both ovaries: a type of

克魯肯伯格氏瘤 在一側或兩側（更常見）卵巢內迅速發展的一種惡性腫

*fibrosarcoma. The tumour usually arises following the development of a similar growth in the stomach or intestine.

瘤。纖維肉瘤的一種類型。此瘤通常繼發於胃或腸的同樣的腫瘤之後。

krypton-81m *n.* a radioactive gas that is the shortest-lived isotope in medical use (half-life 13 seconds). It can be used to investigate the function of the lungs. The patient breathes a small quantity of the gas, the arrival of which in different parts of the lungs is recorded by means of a *gamma camera. *See also* rubidium-81.

氪-81m　一種放射性氣體。是醫學上用的壽命最短的（半衰期13秒）放射性同位素。它可用於肺功能的研究。患者呼出的少量氣體（從肺的不同部位呼出的）用γ照相機記錄。

Kupffer's cells phagocytic cells that line the sinusoids of the *liver (*see* macrophage). They are particularly concerned with the formation of *bile and are often seen to contain fragments of red blood cells and pigment granules derived from the breakdown of haemoglobin.

枯否氏細胞（星狀細胞） 位於肝竇狀隙內的吞噬細胞。尤其與膽汁的形成有關。常發現此種細胞內含有紅細胞碎片以及由血紅蛋白分解產生的色素顆粒。

kuru (trembling disease) *n.* a disease that affects only members of the Fore tribe of New Guinea. It involves a progressive degeneration of the nerve cells of the central nervous system, particularly in the region of the brain that controls movement. Muscular control becomes defective and shiver-like tremors occur in the trunk, limbs, and head. Kuru affects mainly women and children and usually proves fatal within 9–12 months. It is thought to be caused by a virus and transmitted by cannibalism.

庫魯病（顫抖病） 只侵襲新幾內亞富爾部族居民的一種病。本病包括中樞神經細胞進行性變性，尤其是控制大腦的運動區域的細胞。由於肌肉失控，在軀幹、四肢和頭部發生顫抖樣震顫。庫魯病主要侵犯婦女和兒童，而且在9～12個月內造成死亡。人們認爲，本病是由一種病毒引起，通過同類相食傳播。

kwashiorkor *n.* a form of malnutrition due to a diet deficient in protein and energy-producing foods, common among certain African tribes. Kwashiorkor develops when, after prolonged breast feeding, the child is weaned onto an inadequate traditional family diet. The diet is such that it is physically impossible for the child to consume the required quantity in order to obtain sufficient protein and energy. Kwashiorkor is most common in children

夸希奧科病（惡性營養不良病） 營養不良的一種類型。由於食物中缺乏蛋白質和產能食物。常見於非洲某些部族中。本病發生於哺乳時間過長、小兒斷乳後喂以不適宜的傳統家族飲食時。這種飲食不可能供給小兒的生理需要量，因而小兒不可能獲得足夠的蛋白質和能量。本病最常見於1～3歲小兒。

between the ages of one and three years. The symptoms are *oedema, loss of appetite, diarrhoea, general discomfort, and apathy; the child fails to thrive and there is usually associated gastrointestinal.

症狀是水腫、食慾減退、腹瀉、全身不適和淡漠；小兒不能茁壯成長，而且伴有胃腸感染。

Kyasanur Forest disease a tropical disease, common in southern India, caused by a virus transmitted to man through the bite of the forest-dwelling tick *Haemaphysalis spinigera*. Symptoms include fever, headache, muscular pains, vomiting, conjunctivitis, exhaustion, bleeding of nose and gums and, subsequently, internal bleeding and the *necrosis of various tissues. General therapy, in the absence of specific treatment, involves relief of dehydration and loss of blood; analgesics are given to alleviate pain.

夸賽納森林病 一種熱帶病。常見於印度南部，由一種病毒引起，通過居住在森林的蜱（距刺血蜱）的叮咬傳給人。症狀包括發熱、頭痛、肌肉疼痛、嘔吐、結膜炎、疲憊、鼻和牙齦出血，以及相繼的內出血和各種組織壞死。在還沒有特殊療法的情況下，一般療法包括減輕脫水和失血；給予鎮痛藥以減輕疼痛。

kymograph *n.* an instrument for recording the flow and varying pressure of the blood within blood vessels. —**kymography** *n.*

記波器 用於記錄血管內的血流和血壓的變化。

kypho- *prefix denoting* a hump.

〔前綴〕**駝背**

kyphos *n.* a sharply localized forward angulation of the spine, resulting in the appearance of a lump (the deformity of the traditional hunchback). The deformity is due to collapse of the anterior part of a vertebra, usually caused by osteoporosis, a secondary malignant deposit, or tuberculosis.

脊柱後凸 脊柱的局部明顯地向前成角。其結果是出現一隆突（傳統的駝背畸形）。這種畸形是由於椎骨的前部萎縮。通常由骨質疏鬆症、繼發性惡性變或結核病引起。

kyphoscoliosis *n.* abnormal curvature of the spine both forwards and sideways: *kyphosis combined with *scoliosis. The deformity may occur during growth for no apparent reason (*idiopathic kyphoscoliosis*) or may result from any of several diseases involving the vertebrae and spinal muscles. Special braces can reduce the extent of the deformity; *osteotomy of the backbone may be required to correct severe deformity.

脊柱後側凸 脊柱的異常彎曲：脊柱後凸合併脊柱側凸。這種畸形發生於成長期間，無明顯原因（原發性後側凸）或由某些疾病侵襲脊柱和棘肌造成的。特製的支撐物可減少畸形擴大，糾正嚴重畸形需要行脊柱切骨術。

kyphosis *n.* excessive outward curvature of the spine, causing hunching of the back. A *mobile kyphosis* may be caused by bad posture or muscle weakness or may develop to compensate for another condition, such as hip deformity. A *fixed kyphosis* may result from collapse of the vertebrae (as in senile *osteoporosis), from *osteochondritis in the young, or from ankylosing *spondylitis. Lesser degrees of fixed kyphosis may be balanced by *lordosis (inward curvature) in another part of the spine. Treatment depends on the cause, and may include physiotherapy, bracing, and spinal *osteotomy in severe cases. *See also* kyphos, kyphoscoliosis.

脊柱後凸 脊柱過度向外彎曲，引起駝背。可動性脊柱後凸由不良的姿勢或肌肉衰弱引起，或是因其他疾病（例如髂畸形）產生的代償性變化。不動性脊柱後凸可由脊柱萎陷（如老年性骨質疏鬆）、年輕人骨軟骨炎、或强直性脊柱炎引起。較輕的不動性脊柱後凸可通過脊柱其他部分的脊柱前凸（向內彎曲）使其平衡。治療：視病因而定，包括理療，支撐，嚴重病例可行脊椎切骨術。

L

L

labial *adj.* **1.** relating to the lips or to a labium. **2.** designating the surface of a tooth adjacent to the lips.

唇的 ①與唇有關的。②指與唇相鄰的牙齒表面。

labio- *prefix denoting* the lip(s).

〔前綴〕唇

labiomancy *n.* lip-reading.

唇讀 視唇動而知內容。

labioplasty (cheiloplasty) *n.* surgical repair of injury or deformity of the lips.

唇成形術 對唇外傷或缺損進行的外科修復手術。

labium *n.* (*pl.* **labia**) a lip-shaped structure, especially either of the two pairs of skin folds that enclose the *vulva. The larger outer pair are known as the *labia majora* and the smaller inner pair the *labia minora*.

唇 唇樣結構，尤指遮閉外陰的兩邊皮膚褶。外面的一對較大，稱大陰唇，裏面的一對較小，稱小陰唇。

labour *n.* the sequence of actions by which a baby and the afterbirth are expelled from the womb at childbirth. The process usually starts spontaneously about 280 days after conception, but it may be started by artificial means (*see* induction). In the first stage the muscular wall of the womb begins

分娩 出生時嬰兒和胎盤從子宮排出的全過程。此過程通常於妊娠約280天時自動發生，但可用人工手段引起。第一產程時，子宮壁肌肉開始收縮而子宮頸肌纖維鬆弛，因而宮頸擴張。包繞胎兒的部分

contracting while the muscle fibres of the cervix (neck of the womb) relax so that the cervix expands. A portion of the membranous sac (amnion) surrounding the baby is pushed into the opening and bursts under the pressure, releasing *amniotic fluid to the exterior. In the second stage the baby's head appears at the cervix and the contractions of the womb strengthen. The passage of the infant through the vagina is assisted by contractions of the abdominal muscles and conscious pushing by the mother. When the top of the baby's head appears at the vaginal opening the whole infant is eased clear of the vagina, and the umbilical cord is cut. If the emergence of the head is impeded a cut may be made in the surrounding tissue (*see* episiotomy). In the final stage the placenta and membranes are pushed out by the continuing contraction of the womb, which eventually returns to its unexpanded state. The average duration of labour is about 13 hours in first pregnancies and about 8 hours in subsequent pregnancies. Labour pains can be lessened by previous training of the abdominal muscles and by the use of drugs. *See also* Caesarean section.

羊膜突入子宮頸口，胎膜在壓力下破裂，羊水流出。第二產程時，胎兒露出宮頸，子宮收縮加强。藉助於母親的腹肌收縮和有意識的娩出動作，嬰兒得以通過陰道。在胎頭先露部露出陰道口時，整個胎兒便可順利娩出，剪斷臍帶。若胎頭娩出受阻，可施行外陰切開術。第三產程時，子宮持續收縮使胎盤和胎膜娩出，子宮最終恢復至不擴張狀態。分娩平均持續時間初產婦爲13小時，經產婦爲8小時。預先鍛煉腹肌及使用藥物可減輕分娩疼痛。

labrum *n.* (*pl.* **labra**) a lip or liplike structure; occurring, for example, around the margins of the articulating socket (acetabulum) of the hip bone.

唇 唇或唇樣結構，例如髖臼的關節盂邊緣。

labyrinth (inner ear) *n.* a convoluted system of cavities and ducts comprising the organs of hearing and balance. The *membranous labyrinth* is a series of interconnected membranous canals and chambers consisting of the *semicircular canals, *utricle, and *saccule (concerned with balance) and the central cavity of the *cochlea (concerned with hearing). (See illustration.) It is filled with a fluid – *endolymph*. The *bony labyrinth* is the system of the bony canals and chambers that surround the

迷路（內耳） 由組成聽覺和平衡器官的一些管道和腔室形成的螺旋狀系統。膜迷路指一系列相聯繫的管道和腔室，包括半規管、橢圓囊、球囊（與平衡覺有關）和蝸管的中央腔（與聽覺有關）。管道和腔內充滿液體——內淋巴。骨迷路指圍繞在膜迷路外面的骨質管道和腔室系統。位於顳骨岩部，充滿液體（外淋巴）。

membranous labyrinth. It is embedded in the petrous part of the *temporal bone and is filled with fluid (*perilymph*).

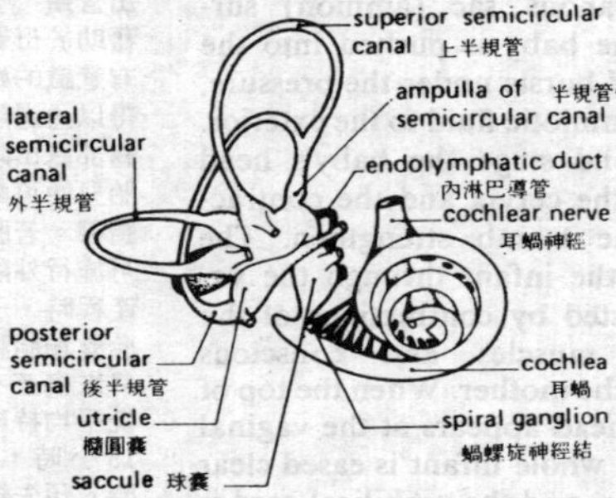

Membranous labyrinth of the right ear
右耳膜迷路

labyrinthitis (otitis interna) *n.* inflammation of the inner ear (labyrinth). *See* otitis.

迷路炎（內耳炎） 內耳（迷路）的炎症。

laceration *n.* a tear in the flesh producing a wound with irregular edges.

撕裂 軟組織撕裂造成的邊緣不規則的傷口。

lacertus *n.* a band of fibres or a tendon-like structure.

纖維束 一束纖維組織或腱樣結構。

lacrimal apparatus the structures that produce and drain away fluid from the eye (see illustration). The *lacrimal gland* secretes *tears, which drain away through small openings (*puncta*) at the inner corner of the eye into two *lacrimal canaliculi*. From there the tears pass into the nasal cavity via the *lacrimal sac* and the *nasolacrimal duct.

淚器 眼內產生並排出液體的結構（見圖）。淚腺分泌淚液，淚液經眼內眥的淚點流入兩條淚小管，再經淚囊和鼻淚管入鼻腔。

lacrimal bone the smallest bone of the face: either of a pair of rectangular bones that contribute to the orbits. *See* skull.

淚骨 顏面最小的骨，是構成眼眶（兩側各一）的長方形骨。

lacrimation *n.* the production of excess tears; crying. *See also* lacrimal apparatus.

流淚 大量淚液生成；哭泣。

lacrimator *n.* an agent that irritates the eyes, causing excessive secretion of tears.

催淚劑 刺激眼引起大量淚液分泌的製劑。

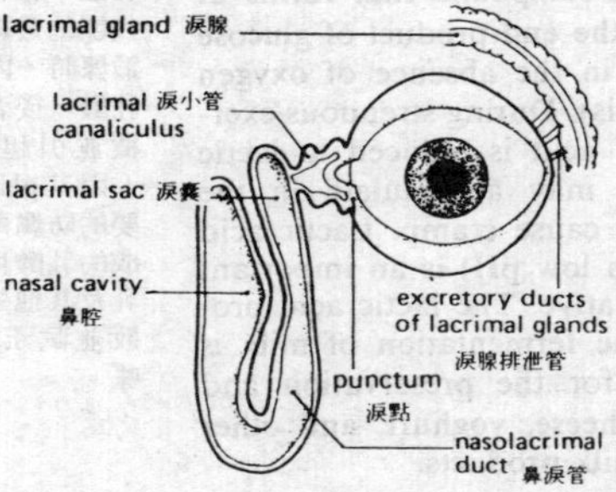

The lacrimal apparatus
淚器

lact- (lacti-, lacto-) *prefix denoting* **1.** milk. **2.** lactic acid.

〔前綴〕①乳 ②乳酸

lactalbumin *n.* a milk protein present in milk at a lower concentration than *casein. Unlike casein, it is not precipitated from milk under acid conditions; it is therefore a constituent of cheese made from whey rather than curd.

乳白蛋白 乳汁中的一種蛋白質，其濃度低於酪蛋白。乳蛋白不同於酪蛋白的原因是：不是乳汁在酸性環境中沉澱下來；而是用乳清（而非凝乳）製成的乳酪的成分。

lactase *n.* an enzyme, secreted by the glands of the small intestine, that converts lactose (milk sugar) into glucose and galactose during digestion.

乳糖酶 小腸腺分泌的一種酶。在消化過程中可將乳糖分解爲葡萄糖和半乳糖。

lactation *n.* the secretion of milk by the *mammary glands of the breasts, which usually begins at the end of pregnancy. A fluid called *colostrum is secreted before the milk is produced; both secretions are released in response to the sucking action of the infant on the nipple. Lactation is controlled by hormones (*see* prolactin, oxytocin); it stops when the baby is no longer fed at the breast.

泌乳 乳腺分泌乳汁的過程。通常在妊娠末期開始泌乳。在乳汁生成前分泌的液體稱初乳。嬰兒吸吮乳頭反射地引起初乳和乳汁分泌。泌乳過程受激素控制。嬰兒斷奶後，泌乳隨着停止。

lacteal *n.* a blind-ended lymphatic vessel that extends into a villus of the small *intestine. Digested fats are absorbed into the lacteals.

乳糜管 伸入小腸絨毛中的盲端淋巴管。脂肪消化後被吸收進入乳糜管。

lactic acid a compound that forms in the cells as the end-product of glucose metabolism in the absence of oxygen (*see* glycolysis). During strenuous exercise pyruvic acid is reduced to lactic acid, which may accumulate in the muscles and cause cramp. Lactic acid (owing to its low pH) is an important food preservative. The lactic acid produced by the fermentation of milk is responsible for the preservation and flavour of cheese, yoghurt, and other fermented milk products.

乳酸 細胞內葡萄糖無氧代謝的最終產物。在緊張鍛煉時，丙酮酸被分解爲乳酸，後者可在肌肉內蓄積並引起肌痙攣。乳酸（因其pH低）是一種重要的防腐劑。牛乳發酵生成的乳酸可防止乳酪、酸乳及其他牛奶發酵製品腐敗並賦予這類食物以美味。

lactiferous *adj.* transporting or secreting milk, as the *lactiferous ducts* of the breast.

輸乳的 輸送或分泌乳汁的，例如乳腺的輸乳管。

lactifuge *n.* a drug that reduces the secretion of milk. Oestrogenic drugs, such as *chlorotrianisene and *dienoestrol, have this effect and are used to suppress milk production in mothers not breast feeding.

回乳劑 減少乳汁分泌的藥物。雌激素類藥物如三對甲氧苯氯乙烯和乙二烯雌酚均有回乳作用。斷奶的母親常用此類藥物抑制乳汁分泌。

Lactobacillus *n.* a genus of Gram-positive nonmotile rodlike bacteria capable of growth in acid media and of producing lactic acid from the fermentation of carbohydrates. They are found in fermenting animal and plant products, especially dairy products, and in the alimentary tract and vagina. They are responsible for the souring of milk. The species *L. acidophilus* is found in milk and is associated with dental caries. It occurs in very high numbers in the faeces of breast- or bottle-fed infants.

乳桿菌屬 一屬革蘭染色陰性、無活動能力的桿菌。能在酸性培養基中生活，使碳水化合物發酵生成乳酸，在動植物性發酵食物——尤其是乳製品中，以及在消化道和陰道內均可發現此菌。本菌是牛乳變酸的原因。嗜酸乳桿菌可見於牛乳中，並與齲齒有關。母乳餵養和人工餵養嬰兒的糞便中有大量乳桿菌存在。

lactogenic hormone *see* prolactin.

生乳激素

lactose *n.* a sugar, consisting of one molecule of glucose and one of galactose, found only in milk. Lactose is split into its constituent sugars by the enzyme *lactase, which is secreted in the small intestine. This enzyme is missing or is of low activity in certain people of some Eastern and African races. This leads to the inability to absorb lactose, known as *lactose intolerance*.

乳糖 由一分子葡萄糖和一分子半乳糖組成的糖。僅存在於乳中。乳糖經小腸分泌的乳糖酶分解爲其組成成分單糖。有些東方和非洲種族的人缺乏乳糖酶或酶活性低，結果導致不能吸收乳糖，即所謂乳糖耐受不良。

lactosuria *n.* the presence of milk sugar (*lactose) in the urine. This often occurs during pregnancy and breast-feeding or if the milk flow is suppressed.

乳糖尿 尿中出現乳糖。常發生於妊娠和哺乳或乳汁分泌受阻時。

lacuna *n.* (*pl.* **lacunae**) (in anatomy) a small cavity or depression; for example, one of the spaces in compact bone in which a bone cell lies.

腔隙，陷窩 （解剖學）小的腔隙或凹窩。例如密質骨內容納骨細胞的腔隙。

laetrile *n.* a cyanide-containing compound extracted from peach stones. It has been used, despite the lack of evidence for its therapeutic value, in the treatment of various forms of cancer.

扁桃苷製劑 一種從桃仁製取的含氰化物的化合物。一直用於治療多種癌症，儘管療效不能肯定。

laevo- *prefix. see* levo-.

〔前綴〕**左**

laevocardia *n.* the normal position of the heart, in which its apex is directed towards the left. *Compare* dextrocardia.

左位心 心臟的正常位置，心尖指向左方。

lagaena (lagena) *n.* the closed end of the spiral *cochlea. This term is more commonly used to describe the structure homologous to the cochlea in primitive vertebrates.

壺 螺旋蝸管的盲端。此詞更常用於指低等脊椎動物與耳蝸類似的結構。

lagophthalmos *n.* any condition in which the eye does not close completely. It may lead to corneal damage from undue exposure.

兔眼 指眼不能完全閉合的狀態。兔眼患者可因暴露過久而發生眼角膜損害。

laking *n.* the physical or chemical treatment of blood to abolish the structure of the red cells and thus form a homogeneous solution. Laking is an important preliminary step in the analysis of haemoglobin or enzymes present in red cells.

紅細胞溶解 用物理或化學方法處理血液，破壞紅細胞結構從而使血液變成勻質溶液。紅細胞溶解是進行紅細胞內血紅蛋白和酶成分分析的首要步驟。

-lalia *suffix denoting* a condition involving speech.

〔後綴〕**言語** 指與說話有關的狀況。

lallation (lalling) *n.* **1.** unintelligible speech-like babbling, as heard from infants. **2.** the immature substitution of one consonant for another (e.g. *l* for *r*).

嬰兒樣語 ①說話難懂，像嬰兒咿啞學語。 ②**輔音混淆** 例如將 ℓ 發作 r。

lambda *n.* the point on the skull at which the lambdoidal and sagittal *sutures meet.

人字縫尖 顱骨上人字縫的滙合點。

lambdoidal suture *see* suture (def. 1). 人字縫

lambliasis *n. see* giardiasis. **蘭氏鞭毛蟲病**

lamella *n.* (*pl.* **lamellae**) **1.** a thin layer, membrane, scale, or plate-like tissue or part. In *bone tissue, lamellae are thin bands of calcified matrix arranged concentrically around a Haversian canal. **2.** a thin gelatinous medicated disc used to apply drugs to the eye. The disc is placed on the eyeball; the gelatinous material dissolves and the drug is absorbed.

①**板** 薄層膜，鱗片或板狀組織或結構。在骨組織中，骨板是圍繞哈弗管呈向心排列的鈣化基質薄板。 ②**眼片** 眼部用藥時使用的一種凝膠藥物薄片。將眼片貼在眼球上，凝膠溶解，藥物被吸收。

lamina *n.* (*pl.* **laminae**) a thin membrane or layer of tissue.

板 薄膜或薄層組織。

laminectomy (rachiotomy) *n.* surgical cutting into the backbone to obtain access to the spinal cord. The surgeon excises the rear part (the posterior arch) of one or more vertebrae. The operation is performed to remove tumours, to treat injuries to the spine, such as prolapsed intervertebral (slipped) disc (in which the affected disc is removed), or to relieve pressure on a spinal nerve.

椎板切除術 手術切開椎骨以形成通達脊髓的通路。外科醫師切開一個或幾個椎骨的後部（後弓），以切除腫瘤，治療脊髓損傷如椎間盤脫出（將受累的椎間盤切除），或解除對脊神經的壓迫。

lanatoside *n.* a drug similar to *digitalis, used in the treatment of heart failure. It is administered by mouth or injection. High doses may cause loss of appetite, nausea, vomiting, headache, disturbed vision, and abnormal heart activity. Trade name: **Cedilanid**.

毛花甙 類似洋地黃的藥物。用於治療心力衰竭。口服或注射。大劑量可引起食慾喪失、噁心、嘔吐、頭痛、視力障礙及心臟活動異常。

Lancefield classification a classification of the **Streptococcus* bacteria based on the presence or absence of antigenic carbohydrate on the cell surface. Species are classified into the groups A–P. Most species causing disease in man belong to group A.

蘭斯菲爾德分類法 一種鏈球菌分類法。根據鏈球菌表面是否存在抗原性糖類分類。將鏈球菌分爲A-P組。引起人類疾病的主要是A組鏈球菌。

lancet *n.* a broad two-edged surgical knife with a sharp point.

柳葉刀 一種尖頭寬雙刃手術刀。

lancinating *adj.* describing a sharp stabbing or cutting pain.

刺割樣的 描述尖銳的戳刺或刀割樣疼痛。

Landry's paralysis a rapidly progressive form of the *Guillain-Barré syndrome.

蘭德里氏麻痹 格-巴二氏綜合徵的急性速進展型。

Lange curve a method of detecting excess globulins in the protein of the cerebrospinal fluid. It is useful in the diagnosis of neurosyphilis and multiple sclerosis.

蘭奇曲線 一種檢測腦脊液內球蛋白過多的方法。用於診斷神經梅毒和多發性硬化。

lanugo *n.* fine hair covering the body and limbs of the human fetus. It is most profuse at about the seventh month of gestation and is shed in the ninth month.

胎毛 覆蓋人胎軀體和四肢的毳毛。胎兒於妊娠7個月左右最多，至9個月時脫落。

laparo- *prefix denoting* the loins or abdomen.

〔前綴〕 **腰，腹**

laparoscope (peritoneoscope) *n.* a surgical instrument (a type of *endoscope) comprising an illuminated viewing tube that is inserted through the abdominal wall to enable the surgeon to view the organs in the abdomen (*see* laparoscopy).

腹腔鏡 一種外科器械（內窺鏡的一種），由一根帶照明的觀察管組成。外科醫師將此管經腹壁插入腹腔，得以觀察腹腔器官。

laparoscopy (peritoneoscopy, abdominoscopy) *n.* examination of the abdominal structures (which are contained within the peritoneum) by means of an illuminated tubular instrument (*laparoscope) passed through a small incision in the wall of the abdomen. Laparoscopy is often used for examining the ovaries and Fallopian tubes as well as for performing one method of sterilization.

腹腔鏡檢查 將一根有照明裝置的管狀器械（腹腔鏡）經腹壁小切口插入腹腔檢查腹腔內結構。常用於檢查卵巢和輸卵管及絕育手術。

laparotomy *n.* a surgical incision into the abdominal cavity. The operation is done to examine the abdominal organs as a help to diagnosis; for example, to establish the spread of a growth (*exploratory laparotomy*) or as a prelude to major surgery.

剖腹術 切開腹腔的手術。用於檢查腹部器官以輔助診斷，例如確定腫物是否擴散（剖腹探查）或作爲腹部大手術的開始步驟。

lardaceous *adj.* resembling lard: often applied to tissue infiltrated with the starchlike substance amyloid (*see* amyloidosis).

豚脂性的 豬油樣的，常用以描述澱粉樣物質浸潤的組織。

larva *n.* (*pl.* **larvae**) the preadult or immature stage hatching from the egg of some animal groups, e.g. insects and nematodes, which may be markedly different from the sexually mature adult and have a totally different way of life. For example, the larvae of some flies are parasites of animals and cause disease whereas the adults are free-living. —**larval** *adj.*

幼蟲 某些動物，例如昆蟲和線蟲從卵孵出到成蟲前的未成熟狀態。幼蟲可明顯區別於性成熟的成蟲，而且生活方式也完全相異。例如，某些蠅的幼蟲是動物的寄生蟲並能引起疾病，而成蟲則是非寄生性的。

larva migrans *see* creeping eruption.

游走性幼蟲病

laryng- (laryngo-) *prefix denoting* the larynx.

〔前綴〕**喉**

laryngeal reflex a cough produced by irritating the larynx.

喉反射 刺激喉引起咳嗽。

laryngectomy *n.* surgical removal of the whole or a part of the larynx, as in the treatment of laryngeal carcinoma.

喉切除術 切除全部或部分喉的外科手術，用於治療喉癌。

laryngismus *n.* closure of the vocal cords by sudden contraction of the laryngeal muscles, followed by a noisy indrawing of breath. It occurs in young children and was in the past associated with low-calcium rickets. Now it occurs when the larynx has been irritated following administration of anaesthetic, when a foreign body has lodged in the larynx, or in *croup.

喉痙攣 由喉肌突然收縮引起的聲帶關閉，隨後發生一個帶聲音的吸氣。發生於年幼兒童，過去多與低鈣佝僂病同時存在。現在可見於下述情況：喉受麻醉藥刺激，異物堵在喉內，白喉。

laryngitis *n.* inflammation of the larynx and vocal cords, due to infection by bacteria or viruses or irritation by gases, chemicals, etc. The cords lose their vibrance (owing to swelling) and the voice becomes husky or is lost completely; breathing is harsh and difficult (*see* stridor); and the cough is painful and honking. Obstruction of the airways may occasionally be serious, especially in children (*see* croup). The patient should rest his voice and remain in a warm moisture-laden atmosphere; steam inhalations for 15–20 minutes every 2–3 hours are traditionally beneficial. The patient should avoid cold air or fog and smoking.

喉炎 喉和聲帶的炎症，係由細菌或病毒感染，或氣體、化學劑等刺激所致。聲帶因水腫而不能振動，聲音沙啞甚至完全失聲，呼吸困難並發出粗糙的聲音，咳嗽時疼痛，聲音像雁鳴。氣道阻塞（特別是兒童）偶可引起嚴重後果。病人須讓聲帶休息，生活在溫暖而濕度高的環境中，每2～3小時作15～20分鐘蒸氣吸入通常有益。應避免接觸冷空氣、霧和煙。

laryngocele *n.* a developmental defect in which an air sac communicates with the larynx. The sac forms a swelling in the neck that dilates on coughing or straining.

喉囊腫 一種發育缺陷，爲一個與喉通連的含氣囊腫。囊腫引起頸部腫脹，當咳嗽或使勁時擴大。

laryngofissure *n. see* laryngotomy.

喉切開術

laryngology *n.* the study of diseases of the larynx and vocal cords.

喉科學 研究喉和聲帶疾病的學科。

laryngopharynx *n.* the part of the pharynx that lies below the hyoid bone.

喉咽 咽的一部分，位於舌骨下。

laryngoscope *n.* an instrument for examining the larynx. There are several types, the simplest consisting of a curved blunt metal blade, used to press the tongue out of the line of vision, and a small light to illuminate the field.

喉鏡 用於檢查喉的器械。有幾種類型，最簡單的一種是彎曲的鈍緣金屬板，用以壓迫舌使之不擋住視線，並有一小燈照明視野。

laryngospasm *n.* closure of the larynx, obstructing the flow of air to the lungs. It usually occurs as part of an allergic reaction, such as *angioneurotic oedema.

喉痙攣 喉關閉阻塞出肺的氣流。常作爲變應性反應（如血管神經性水腫）的一部分而發生。

laryngotomy (laryngofissure) *n.* surgical incision of the larynx. *Inferior laryngotomy*, in which an incision is made in the cricothyroid membrane beneath the larynx, is a life-saving operation when there is obstruction to breathing at or above the larynx. *See* tracheostomy.

喉切開術 切開喉的外科手術。喉下部切開術是在緊靠喉下環甲膜作切開，爲喉或喉以上發生呼吸阻塞時施行的急救手術。

laryngotracheobronchitis *n.* a severe infection of the respiratory tract, especially of young children, in whom there may be a dangerous degree of obstruction either at the larynx (*see* croup) or main air passages (bronchi) due to the thickness and stickiness of the fluid (exudate) produced by the inflamed tissues. Treatment: as for *laryngitis, with *tracheostomy if necessary and bronchoscopy in addition, during which it may be possible to clear the obstructing exudate by bronchial lavage and suction.

喉氣管支氣管炎 呼吸道的一種嚴重感染。幼兒多見，當喉部主氣道（支氣管）因炎症組織產生的液體（滲出液）變稠而阻塞時，可危及生命。治療：同喉炎，必要時作氣管切開，還可作支氣管鏡檢查，以便施行支氣管灌洗和抽吸以清除阻塞的滲出液。

larynx *n.* the organ responsible for the production of vocal sounds, also serv-

喉 發聲器官，也是空氣由咽入肺的通道。位於頸

ing as an air passage conveying air from the pharynx to the lungs. It is situated in the front of the neck, above the trachea. It is made up of a framework of nine cartilages (see illustration) – the epiglottis, thyroid, cricoid, arytenoid (two), corniculate (two), and cuneiform (two) – bound together by ligaments and muscles and lined with mucous membrane. Within are a pair of *vocal cords, which function in the production of voice. —**laryngeal** *adj.*

前部氣管上方。由9塊軟骨（見圖）藉韌帶和肌肉連成的支架所構成，內面襯有黏膜。9塊軟骨是：會厭軟骨、甲狀軟骨、環狀軟骨、杓狀軟骨（2塊）、角狀軟骨（2塊）和楔狀軟骨（2塊）。喉內有一對聲帶，其功能爲發聲。

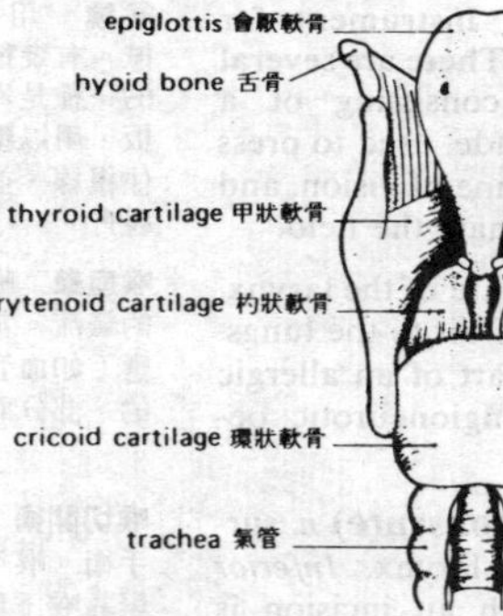

Cartilages of the larynx
喉的軟骨

laser *n.* a device that produces a very thin beam of light in which high energies are concentrated. In surgery lasers can be used to operate on small areas of abnormality (for example, in the retina of the eye) without damaging delicate surrounding tissue.

激光器 產生集中了高能量的極細光束的裝置。在外科中激光器可用作小範圍病變（例如眼視網膜）的手術而不損傷周圍緊鄰的組織。

Lasix *n. see* frusemide.

速尿

Lassa fever a serious virus disease confined to Central West Africa. After an incubation period of 3–21 days, headache, high fever, and severe muscular pains develop; difficulty in swallowing often arises. Death from kidney or heart failure occurs in over 50% of cases. Treatment with plasma from recovered patients is the best therapy.

拉沙熱 一種嚴重的病毒性疾病，發生於中西非。在3～21天的潛伏期後，出現頭痛、高熱和劇烈的肌肉痛，常有吞嚥困難，50%以上的病例心腎功能衰竭。用恢復期病人血漿治療效果最佳。

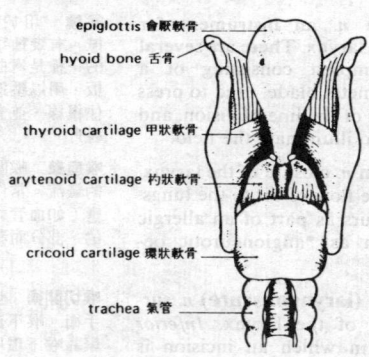

latah *n.* a pattern of behaviour seen only in certain cultures, such as that of Malaysia. After a psychological shock the affected individual becomes very anxious and very suggestible and shows excessive obedience and pathological imitation of the actions of another person (echopraxia).

拉他 見於馬來西亞等國家的一種獨特性的行爲方式。在受到强烈精神刺激以後，患者變得焦躁不安，易受暗示影響，表現出過分的順從和病態地模倣他人的動作（模倣行動）。

latent period (in neurology) the pause of a few milliseconds between the time that a nerve impulse reaches a muscle fibre and the time that the fibre starts to contract.

潛伏期 （神經病學）神經衝動達到肌纖維和肌纖維開始收縮之間的幾個毫秒的時間間隔。

lateral *adj.* **1.** situated at or relating to the side of an organ or organism. **2.** (in anatomy) relating to the region or parts of the body that are furthest from the *median plane. **3.** (in radiology) in the *sagittal plane.

①**側的** 指位於器官或機體側方的。②（解剖學）**外側的** 指離正中斷面最遠的區域或身體部分。③**矢狀面** 放射學用語。

lateroversion *n.* a turning or displacement of an organ, for example the womb (*uterine lateroversion*) to one side.

側傾 器官轉位或移位。例如子宮傾向一側。

lathyrism *n.* a disease, characterized by muscular weakness and paralysis, found among people whose staple diet consists mostly of large quantites of *Lathyrus sativus*, a kind of chick pea, and/or vetches and pulses related it. Except in mild cases complete recovery does not occur, despite administration of an adequate diet and physiotherapy.

山黧豆中毒 一種以肌肉無力和麻痹爲特徵的疾病，見於以大量草香豌豆（鷹嘴豆的一種）和／或野豌豆及有關豆類爲主食的人羣。除輕病例外，即使改用適宜的飲食和採用理療，均不能完全恢復正常。

laudanum *n.* a hydroalcoholic solution containing 1% morphine, prepared from macerated raw opium. It was formerly widely used as a narcotic analgesic, taken by mouth.

阿片酊 含1％嗎啡的酊劑，用生阿片浸製而成。曾廣泛用於麻醉止痛，口服。

laughing gas *see* nitrous oxide.

笑氣

lavage *n.* washing out a body cavity, such as the colon or stomach, with water or a medicated solution.

灌洗 用水或藥物溶液冲洗體腔（如結腸、胃）。

laxative (cathartic, purgative) *n.* a drug used to stimulate or increase the frequency of bowel evacuation, or to encourage a softer or bulkier stool. The

輕瀉藥 用於刺激結腸增加排便次數，或使大便軟化或體積增加的藥物。常用的輕瀉藥有蓖麻油、球

common laxatives are the irritants castor oil and jalop; senna and its derivatives; magnesium sulphate and other mineral salts; and methylcellulose and other bulking agents.

根牽牛、番瀉葉及其衍化物、硫酸鎂及其他礦物鹽、甲基纖維素及其他增加大便體積的藥物。

LD_{50} the dose of a toxic compound that causes death in 50% of a group of experimental animals to which it is administered: used as a measure of the toxicity of drugs.

半數致死量（LD_{50}）毒性化合物其能使50%實驗動物死亡的劑量。用以測量藥物的毒性。

L-dopa *n. see* levodopa.

左旋多巴

lead[1] *n.* a soft bluish-grey metallic element that forms several poisonous compounds. Acute lead poisoning, which may follow inhalation of lead fumes or dust, causes abdominal pains, vomiting, and diarrhoea, with paralysis and convulsions and sometimes *encephalitis. In chronic poisoning a characteristic bluish marking of the gums ('lead line') is seen and the peripheral nerves are affected; there is also anaemia. Treatment is with *EDTA. The use of lead in paints is now strictly controlled. Symbol: Pb.

鉛 藍灰色軟性金屬元素，可形成數種中毒性化合物。急性鉛中毒可發生於吸入鉛蒸氣或鉛塵後，病人出現腹痛、嘔吐和腹瀉，伴有麻痹和抽搐，有時發生腦炎。慢性鉛中毒時牙齦可見典型的藍色標記（“鉛線”），周圍神經受累，並有貧血。治療用乙二胺四乙酸。現時已嚴格控制在顏料中使用鉛。符號Ｐｂ。

lead[2] *n.* a portion of an electrocardiographic record that is obtained from a single electrode or a combination of electrodes placed on a particular part of the body (*see* electrocardiogram, electrocardiography). In the conventional ECG, 12 leads are recorded. Each lead represents the electrical activity of the heart as 'viewed' from a different position on the body surface and may help to localize myocardial damage.

導程 將單個電極或一組電極置於身體特定部位獲得的心電描記記錄。常規心電描記記錄採用12個導程。每一導程作爲“可見的圖像”，反映了從體表不同部位得到的心電活性，有助於確定心肌損害的部位。

lecithin *n.* one of a group of *phospholipids that are important constituents of cell membranes and are involved in the metabolism of fat by the liver. An example is *phosphatidylcholine*.

卵磷脂 磷脂族中的一種，是細胞膜的重要組成成分，參與肝的脂肪代謝。例如磷脂醯膽鹼。

lecithinase *n.* an enzyme from the small intestine that breaks *lecithin down into its constituents (i.e. glycerol, fatty acids, phosphoric acid, and choline).

卵磷脂酶 小腸分泌的一種酶，能將磷脂分解爲其組成成分即甘油、脂肪酸、磷酸和膽鹼。

Ledermycin *n. see* demethylchlortetracycline.

去甲金黴素

leech *n.* a type of worm that possesses suckers at both ends of its body. Leeches occur in tropical forests and grasslands and in water. Certain parasitic species suck blood from animals and man, and their bites cause irritation and, occasionally, infection. Rarely, leeches are taken in with foul drinking water and pass from the mouth to the nose, where they provoke headache and nose bleeds. A leech can be detached from its host either by applying salt or by touching it with a lighted cigarette. Calamine lotion eases the irritation of the bites. Leeches were formerly used in bloodletting.

水蛭 一種身體兩端有吸盤的蠕蟲。常見於熱帶森林、草地或水中。某些種爲寄生性，吸吮動物和人血，其叮咬可引起刺激，有時可導致感染。偶見因飲用污染水而誤食水蛭，水蛭經口入鼻，引起頭痛和鼻衄。用鹽或點燃的香煙可將水蛭驅離宿主。爐甘石洗劑可減輕水蛭叮咬的刺激。水蛭過去曾用於放血。

Legg-Calvé-Perthes disease (Perthes disease, pseudocoxalgia) inflammation of the heads of the femurs (thighbones), resulting in loss of the blood supply and death of the outer layer of bone (avascular necrosis) (*see* osteochondritis). It occurs most commonly in boys between the ages of 5 and 10, and causes aching and a limp. Unless early and effective treatment by bed rest and calipers is carried out, deformity, shortening, and secondary osteoarthritis of the bones result.

萊-卡-佩三氏病（萊格氏病，假性關節炎） 股骨頭的炎症。係由供血障礙和骨膜壞死（無血管性壞死）所致。最常發生於5～10歲男孩。造成疼痛和跛行。如不在早期給予有效治療，如臥牀休息和用矯正器，則會發生骨變形、骨短和繼發性骨關節炎。

legionnaires' disease a bacterial infection of the lungs, named after an outbreak of 182 cases at the American Legion convention in Pennsylvania in 1976. Symptoms appear after an incubation period of about seven days: malaise and muscle pain are succeeded by a fever, dry cough, chest pain, and breathlessness. There is loss of protein in the urine and impaired kidney function. X-ray of the lungs shows patchy consolidation. Erythromycin provides the most effective therapy.

軍團病 一種肺的細菌性感染，係由於1976年美國賓夕法尼亞的美國軍團代表大會上暴發182個病例而得名。在約7天的潛伏期後出現症狀：先是不適和肌肉疼痛，接看發熱、乾咳、胸痛、呼吸困難。尿中出現蛋白，腎功能受損。肺X線檢查見實變斑塊。紅黴素療效最佳。

leio- *prefix denoting* smoothness. Example: *leiodermia* (abnormal smoothness of the skin).

〔前綴〕**平滑** 例如滑澤皮（皮膚異常光滑）。

leiomyoma *n.* a benign tumour of smooth muscle. Such tumours occur most commonly in the uterus (*see* fibroid) but can also arise in the digestive tract, walls of blood vessels, etc. They may undergo malignant change (*see* leiomyosarcoma).

平滑肌瘤 平滑肌的良性腫瘤。最常見於子宮，但亦可在消化道、血管壁等處發生。平滑肌瘤可發生惡變。

leiomyosarcoma *n.* a malignant tumour of smooth muscle, most commonly found in the womb, stomach, small bowel, and at the base of the bladder. It is the second most common *sarcoma of soft tissues. This tumour is rare in children, occurring most commonly in the bladder, prostate, and stomach.

平滑肌肉瘤 平滑肌的惡性腫瘤。最常見於子宮、胃、小腸及膀胱底部。是第二位最常見的軟組織肉瘤。在兒童少見，其最常發生部位是膀胱、前列腺和胃。

Leishman-Donovan body *see* Leishmania.

黑熱病小體，利-杜小體

Leishmania *n.* a genus of parasitic flagellate protozoans, several species of which cause disease in man (*see* leishmaniasis). The parasite assumes a different form in each of its two hosts. In man, especially in *kala-azar patients, it is a small rounded structure, with no flagellum, called a *Leishman-Donovan body*, which is found within the cells of the lymphatic system, spleen, and bone marrow. In the insect carrier it is long and flagellated.

利什曼原蟲屬 一屬有鞭毛的寄生原蟲，其中一些種能引起人類疾病。該寄生蟲在兩種宿主體內以不同的形式存在。在人體內，尤其在黑熱病患者體內，爲小的圓形結構，無鞭毛，稱爲黑熱病小體，見於淋巴系統、脾和骨髓的細胞內，在昆蟲體內則爲長形並有鞭毛。

leishmaniasis *n.* a disease, common in the tropics and subtropics, caused by parasitic protozoans of the genus *Leishmania*, which are transmitted by the bite of sandflies. There are two principal forms of the disease: *visceral leishmaniasis*, in which the cells of various internal organs are affected (*see* kala-azar); and *cutaneous leishmaniasis*, which affects the tissues of the skin. Cutaneous leishmaniasis itself has several different forms, depending on the region in which it occurs and the species of *Leishmania* involved. In Asia it is common in the form of *oriental sore. In America there are several forms of leishmaniasis (*see* chiclero's ulcer,

黑熱病，利什曼病 一種熱帶和亞熱帶的常見病，由利什曼原蟲屬的一些寄生原蟲引起，通過白蛉的叮咬傳播。本病有兩種主要類型：內臟利什曼病，不同的內臟器官的細胞均可受侵襲；皮膚利什曼病，皮膚組織受累。皮膚利什曼病又可根據發生的區域及種的不同而分爲幾種類型。在亞洲常見的是東方瘡。在美洲有幾類（樹膠樣潰瘍、鼻黏膜利什曼病）。治療利什曼病用含銻的藥物。

espundia). Leishmaniasis is treated with drugs containing antimony.

lemniscus *n.* a ribbon-like tract of nerve tissue conveying information from the spinal cord and brainstem upwards through the midbrain to the higher centres. On each side a *medial lemniscus* acts as a pathway from the spinal cord, while an outer *lateral lemniscus* commences higher up and is mainly concerned with hearing.

丘系 從脊髓和腦幹向上經中腦向更高級的中樞傳遞信息的帶狀神經束。每側的內側丘系是傳遞來自脊髓的信息的通道，而外側丘系則起始於較高部位，主要與聽覺有關。

lens *n.* **1.** (in anatomy) the transparent crystalline structure situated behind the pupil of the eye and enclosed in a thin transparent *capsule*. It helps to refract incoming light and focus it onto the *retina. *See also* accommodation. **2.** (in optics) a piece of glass shaped to refract rays of light in a particular direction. *Convex lenses* converge the light, and *concave lenses* diverge it; they are worn to correct faulty eyesight. *See also* bifocal lenses, contact lenses, trifocal lenses.

①**晶狀體** （解剖學）眼瞳孔後方包在一薄層透明囊膜內的透明水晶狀結構。使進入的光線折射而聚焦於網膜上。 ②**鏡片** （光學）使光線向特定方向折射的一定形狀的玻璃片。凸透鏡使光線會聚，凹透鏡則使光線分散。戴用此類鏡片以矯正視力異常。

lenticonus *n.* a condition in which the central part of the front surface of the lens of the eye (or sometimes, the back) has a much steeper curvature than normal and bulges forwards in a blunted cone. It is usually congenital.

錐狀晶狀體 一種眼病，表現為眼晶狀體前表面（有時為後表面）中央部分的曲度遠較正常為大，呈鈍圓錐形向前突出。通常為遺傳性。

lenticular nucleus (lentiform nucleus) *see* basal ganglia.

豆狀核

lentigo *n.* a brown roundish flat spot on the skin caused by excess development of melanin. Commoner in old people, lentigo sometimes turns into a slow-growing skin cancer.

着色斑 由於黑色素過多而在皮膚上形成的棕色圓形扁平斑。較常見於老年人，有時轉變為生長緩慢的皮膚癌。

leontiasis *n.* overgrowth of the skull bones, said to resemble the appearance of a lion's head: a rare feature of untreated *Paget's disease. Medical name: **leontiasis ossea**.

骨性獅面 顱骨過度生長，呈有如獅頭的外觀。為未經治療的佩吉特氏病的罕見表現。

lepidosis *n.* any skin eruption that causes scaling.

脫屑疹 產生鱗屑的任何皮疹。

lepra reaction an aggravation of lumps on the skin caused by *leprosy, accompanied by fever and malaise.

痲瘋反應 痲瘋所致的皮膚結節病變惡化現象，伴有發熱和不適。

leproma *n.* a lump on the skin characteristic of *leprosy.

痲瘋結節 痲瘋特有的皮膚腫塊。

lepromin *n.* a chemical prepared from lumps on the skin caused by lepromatous *leprosy.

痲瘋菌素 從瘤型痲瘋的皮膚結節中提取的化學物質。

leprosy (Hansen's disease) *n.* a chronic disease, caused by the bacterium *Mycobacterium leprae*, that affects the skin, mucous membranes, and nerves. It is confined mainly to the tropics and is transmitted by direct contact. After an incubation period of 1–30 years, symptoms develop gradually and mainly involve the skin and nerves. *Lepromatous leprosy* is a contagious steadily progressive form of the disease characterized by the development of widely distributed lumps on the skin, thickening of the skin and nerves, and in serious cases by severe numbness of the skin, muscle weakness, and paralysis leading to disfigurement and deformity. Tuberculosis is a common complication. *Tuberculoid leprosy* is a benign, often self-limiting, form of leprosy causing discoloration and disfiguration of patches of skin (sparsely distributed) associated with localized numbness. *Indeterminate leprosy* is a form of the disease in which skin manifestations represent a combination of the two main types. Leprosy can be controlled, but not cured, by prolonged treatment with *sulphone drugs.

痲瘋（漢森氏病） 由痲瘋分枝桿菌引起的慢性疾病，侵犯皮膚、黏膜和神經。主要發生於熱帶，藉直接接觸傳染，經過1-30年的潛伏期後，逐漸出現症狀，主要為皮膚和神經症狀。瘤型痲瘋是本病的傳染性持續進展型，特徵是廣泛發生皮膚結節，皮膚變厚，神經增粗，重症病例發生嚴重的皮膚痲木、肌肉無力、痲痺，進展為毀形和畸形，常併發結核病。結核樣型痲瘋是一種良性的常為自限性的痲瘋類型，皮膚有稀散分佈的斑塊和退色和毀形，伴有局部痲木感。未定型痲瘋是上述兩種主要類型和皮膚病混合存在的痲瘋類型。長期使用碸類藥物可控制痲瘋發展，但不能治癒。

lept- (lepto-) *prefix denoting* **1.** slender; thin. **2.** small. **3.** mild; slight.

〔前綴〕①**細，薄** ②**小** ③**輕度，輕微**

leptocyte *n.* a red blood cell (*erythrocyte) that is abnormally thin. Leptocytes are seen in certain types of anaemia.

薄紅細胞 一種異常薄的紅細胞，見於某些類型的貧血。

leptomeninges *pl. n.* the inner two *meninges: the arachnoid and pia mater.

柔腦(脊)膜 內面的兩層腦膜，即蛛網膜和軟腦膜。

leptomeningitis *n.* inflammation of the inner membranes (the *pia mater and *arachnoid) of the brain and spinal cord. *See also* meningitis.

柔腦(脊)膜炎 腦和脊髓內層腦膜（軟腦膜和蛛網膜）的炎症。

leptophonia *n.* weakness of the voice.

聲弱 聲音微弱。

Leptospira *n.* a genus of spirochaete bacteria, commonly bearing hooked ends. They are not visible with ordinary light microscopy and are best seen using dark-ground microscopy. The parasitic species *L. icterohaemorrhagiae* is the main causative agent of *leptospirosis (Weil's disease), but many closely related species cause similar symptoms.

鈎端螺旋體屬 一種螺旋體菌，通常兩端呈鈎形。在普通光學顯微鏡下不可見，而在暗視野下看得最爲清楚。寄生性的出血性黃疸鈎端螺旋體是引起鈎端螺旋體病（魏爾氏病）的主要致病菌，但許多近緣種也能引起類似的症狀。

leptospirosis (Weil's disease) *n.* an infectious disease, caused by bacteria of the genus *Leptospira*, that occurs in rodents, dogs, and other mammals and may be transmitted to people whose work brings them into contact with these animals. The disease begins with a fever and may affect the liver (causing jaundice) or meninges (resulting in meningitis); in some cases the kidneys are involved.

鈎端螺旋體病（魏爾氏病） 由鈎端螺旋體屬細菌引起的傳染病，發生於嚙齒動物、狗和其他哺乳類動物以及人。可由動物傳播給因工作與此等動物接觸的人。以發熱起病，可累及肝臟（引起黃疸）或腦膜（引起腦膜炎），有些病例侵及腎臟。

leptotene *n.* the first stage in the first prophase of *meiosis, in which the chromosomes become visible as single long threads.

細線期 減數分裂第一期的第一階段，此時染色體變爲可見，呈單個長線形。

leresis *n.* rambling speech, immature both in syntax and pronunciation. It is a feature of dementia.

兒稚樣語言 說話雜亂無章，發音和句法均顯幼稚。爲痴獃的一種表現。

lesbianism *n.* the condition in which a woman is sexually attracted to, or engages in sexual behaviour with, another woman (*see also* homosexuality). Treatment for lesbianism varies: many therapists prefer to reduce the anxiety and guilt associated with the condition rather than try to change it directly. —**lesbian** *adj.*, *n.*

女子同性戀 一女性對另一女性發生性愛，或與其發生性行爲的狀況。對女子同性戀有不同的治療方法。許多醫生傾向於設法減輕伴隨同性戀而來的焦慮和內疚感，而不是試圖直接改變這種病態。

lesion *n.* a zone of tissue with impaired function as a result of damage by

損害 由疾病或外傷造成的伴有功能障礙的組織部

disease or wounding. Apart from direct physical injury, examples of primary lesions include abscesses, ulcers, tumours; secondary lesions (such as crusts and scars) are derived from primary ones.

位。除直接的物理性損傷外，屬於原發性損害的有：膿腫，潰瘍，腫瘤；由原發性損害派生的爲繼發性損害，如結痂和瘢痕。

lethal gene a gene that, under certain conditions, causes the death of the individual carrying it. Lethal genes are usually *recessive: an individual will die only if both his parents carry the gene. If only one parent is affected, the lethal effects of the gene will be masked by the dominant *allele inherited from the normal parent.

致死性基因 一種在一定條件下能引起攜帶該基因的個體死亡的基因。致死性基因通常爲隱性，只有父母雙方均攜帶此種基因的子代才會死亡。如果僅父母之一方攜帶此基因，則其致死作用將被從正常父或母遺傳而來的顯性等位基因所掩蓋。

lethargy *n.* mental and physical sluggishness: a degree of inactivity and unresponsiveness approaching or verging on the unconscious. The condition results from disease (such as sleeping sickness) or hypnosis.

昏睡，嗜睡 精神和體力的遲鈍狀態，即達到或瀕臨喪失意識前的某種程度的無活動和無反應狀態。疾病（如睡眠症）或催眠可造成此種狀態。

Letterer-Siwe disease *see* reticuloendotheliosis.

萊-賽二氏病 網狀內皮細胞增多症。

leuc- (leuco-, leuk-, leuko-) *prefix denoting* **1.** lack of colour; white. **2.** leucocytes.

〔前綴〕 ①**無色，白** ②**白細胞**

leucine *n.* an *essential amino acid. *See also* amino acid.

亮氨酸 一種必需氨基酸。

leucocidin *n.* a bacterial *exotoxin that selectively destroys white blood cells (leucocytes).

殺白細胞素 一種選擇性破壞白細胞的細菌外毒素。

leucocyte (white blood cell) *n.* any blood cell that contains a nucleus. In health there are three major subdivisions: *granulocytes, *lymphocytes and *monocytes, which are involved in protecting the body against foreign substances and in antibody production. In disease, a variety of other types may appear in the blood, most notably immature forms of the normal red or white blood cells.

白細胞 指一切有核的血細胞。健康人的白細胞包括三個主要類型：粒細胞、淋巴細胞和單核細胞，它們參與機體對異物的防禦和抗體生成過程。疾病時血中可出現各種其他類型的細胞，最值得注意的是正常紅細胞和白細胞的幼稚型。

leucocytosis *n.* an increase in the number of white blood cells (leucocytes) in the blood. *See* basophilia, eosinophilia, lymphocytosis, monocytosis.

白細胞增多 血中白細胞數量增多。

leucoderma *n. see* vitiligo.

白斑病

leucolysin *n. see* lysin.

白細胞溶素

leucoma *n.* a white opacity in the cornea. Most leucomas result from scarring after corneal inflammation or ulceration. Congenital types may be associated with other abnormalities of the eye.

角膜白斑 角膜的白色混濁物。多數角膜白斑爲角膜炎症或潰瘍後瘢痕形成的後果。先天性角膜白斑可伴有眼的其他異常。

leuconychia *n.* white discoloration of the nails, which may be total or partial. The cause is unknown.

白甲病 部分或整個指甲變成白色。病因不明。

leucopenia *n.* a reduction in the number of white blood cells (leucocytes) in the blood. *See* eosinopenia, lymphopenia, neutropenia.

白細胞減少 血中白細胞數減少。

leucoplakia (leukoplakia) *n.* thickened white patches on mucous membranes, such as the mouth lining or vulva, due to an overgrowth of the tissues. Some leucoplakia may be caused by excessive smoking or alcohol or by certain infections; occasionally it can become malignant.

黏膜白斑病 黏膜上厚的白色斑塊，如口腔黏膜和陰唇上的白斑，係因組織過度生長所致。有些黏膜白斑病可由過度抽煙或飲酒或某些感染所致；偶可惡變。

leucopoiesis *n.* the process of the production of white blood cells (leucocytes), which normally occurs in the blood-forming tissue of the *bone marrow. *See also* granulopoiesis, haemopoiesis, lymphopoiesis, monoblast.

白細胞生成 白細胞生成的過程。正常時白細胞在骨髓造血組織內生成。

leucorrhoea (whites) *n.* a whitish or yellowish discharge of mucus from the vaginal opening. It may occur normally at all times, the quantity increasing before and after menstruation. An abnormally large discharge may indicate infection of the lower reproductive tract, e.g. by the protozoan *Trichomonas vaginalis* (*see* vaginitis).

白帶 陰道口流出的白色或淺黃色的黏液。正常時任何時候均可有白帶，月經前後量增多。異常大量白帶可能是下生殖道感染的表現，如陰道毛滴蟲感染。

leucotomy *n.* the surgical operation of interrupting the pathways of white nerve fibres within the brain: it is the most common procedure in *psychosurgery. In the original form, *prefrontal leucotomy* (*lobotomy*), the operation involved cutting through the nerve fibres connecting the *frontal lobe with the *thalamus and the association fibres of the frontal lobe. This was often successful in reducing severe emotional tension but had serious side-effects, including epilepsy and changes in the personality towards apathy and irresponsibility.
Modern procedures use *stereotaxy and make selective lesions in smaller areas of the brain. Side-effects are uncommon and the operation is used for intractable pain, severe depression, obsessional neurosis, and chronic anxiety, where very severe emotional tension has not been relieved by other treatments.

腦白質切斷術 切除腦內白色神經纖維通路的外科手術，是精神外科學中最常用的手術。其原型爲前額葉腦白質切斷術（葉切除術），手術是切斷聯結額葉和丘腦的神經纖維以及額葉的聯絡纖維。過去常可成功地減輕嚴重的情緒緊張，但也有嚴重的副作用，如癲癇、性格改變爲淡漠和無責任感。現在的做法是採用立體定位法在腦的細小範圍內造成選擇性損傷。副作用不常見。手術用於頑固性疼痛、嚴重抑鬱症、强迫性神經症和慢性焦慮症時嚴重的情緒緊張用其他治療均未能奏效者。

leukaemia *n.* any of a group of malignant diseases in which the bone marrow and other blood-forming organs produce increased numbers of certain types of white blood cells (*leucocytes). Overproduction of these white cells, which are immature or abnormal forms, suppresses the production of normal white cells, red cells, and platelets. This leads to increased susceptibility to infection (due to *neutropenia), *anaemia, and bleeding (due to *thrombocytopenia). Other symptoms include enlargement of the spleen, liver, and lymph nodes.
Leukaemias are classified into *acute* or *chronic* varieties depending on the rate of progression of the disease. They are also classified according to the type of white cell that is proliferating abnormally; for example *lymphoblastic leukaemia* (*see* lymphoblast) and *acute myeloblastic leukaemia* (*see* myeloblast). (*See also* myeloid leukaemia.) Leukaemias are treated with radiother-

白血病 一組惡性疾病，表現爲骨髓和其他造血器官生成大量某型白細胞。由於白細胞（幼稚型或異常型）過量生成，抑制了正常細胞、紅細胞和血小板的生成，導致易發生感染（由於中性白細胞減少）、貧血和出血（由於血小板減少）。其他還有脾、肝和淋巴結腫大。
白血病根據疾病進展速度，區分爲急性和慢性；也可根據異常增殖的白細胞類型分型，如淋巴母細胞性白血病、急性原粒細胞白血病。治療白血病採用放射治療或細胞毒藥物，目的是抑制異常細胞生成。

apy or *cytotoxic drugs, which are aimed at suppressing the reproduction of the abnormal cells.

leukoplakia *n. see* leucoplakia.

黏膜白斑病

leukotaxine *n.* a chemical, present in inflammatory exudates, that attracts white blood cells (leucocytes) and increases the permeability of blood capillaries. It is probably produced by injured cells.

白細胞趨化素 存在於炎性滲出物中的一種化學物質，能吸引白細胞和增加血管通透性。可能是受損細胞產生的。

levallorphan *n.* a drug that counteracts the depression in breathing caused by narcotic analgesics such as morphine without affecting their pain-relieving effects. It is administered by injection, usually before or at the same time as the analgesic. Trade name: **Lorfan**.

l-N-丙烯基-3-羥基嗎啡烷 一種能對抗麻醉性鎮痛藥（如嗎啡）所引起的呼吸抑制而不影響鎮痛效果的藥物。注射，通常在給鎮痛藥之前或同時給予。

levator *n.* **1.** a surgical instrument used for levering up displaced bone fragments in a depressed fracture of the skull. **2.** any muscle that lifts the structure into which it is inserted; for example, the *levator scapulis* helps to lift the shoulder blade.

①**起子** 用於顱骨凹陷骨折時撬起錯位的骨折片的外科器械。 ②**提肌** 能將它們所附着的結構提升的肌肉，例如肩胛提肌協助提升肩胛骨。

levo- (laevo-) *prefix denoting* **1.** the left side. **2.** (in chemistry) levorotation.

〔前綴〕 ①**左側** ②**左旋**（化學）

levodopa (L-dopa) *n.* a naturally occurring amino acid administered by mouth to treat *parkinsonism. Common side-effects are nausea, vomiting, loss of appetite, and involuntary facial movements; high doses may cause weakness, faintness, and dizziness. Trade names: **Berkdopa**, **Brocadopa**, **Larodopa**, **Veldopa**.

左旋多巴 一種天然存在的氨基酸。口服，用於治療帕金森氏病。常見副作用有噁心、嘔吐、食慾喪失、不隨意面部運動，大劑量可引起無力、暈厥和頭暈。

levorphanol *n.* a narcotic analgesic, similar to *morphine, used to relieve severe pain. It is administered by mouth or injection and may cause nausea, vomiting, loss of appetite, constipation, and confusion. Dependence may develop. Trade name: **Dromoran**.

左嗎南 一種類似嗎啡的麻醉性鎮痛藥。用於解除劇烈疼痛。口服或注射。可引起噁心、嘔吐、食慾喪失和神經錯亂。可產生賴藥性。

levulosuria *n. see* fructosuria.

果糖尿

Leydig cells *see* interstitial cells.

萊廸希氏細胞

LH *see* luteinizing hormone.

黃體生成素

Lhermitte's sign a tingling shocklike sensation passing down the arms or trunk when the neck is flexed. It is a nonspecific indication of disease in the cervical (neck) region of the spinal cord.

萊爾米特氏徵 當屈頸時產生一種突然的電震樣感覺，沿手臂或軀幹傳導。爲脊髓頸段疾病的非特異性徵候。

libido *n.* the sexual drive: the term is often used to refer to the intensity of sexual desires. In psychoanalytic theory, the libido (like the death instinct) is one of the fundamental sources of energy for all mental life. The normal course of development (*see* psychosexual development) can be altered by fixation at one level and by regression.

性慾 性衝動。此術語常用於表示强烈的性要求。在精神分析理論中，性慾（猶如死亡本能一樣）乃是全部精神生活的基本能源之一。正常的性發育過程可以停滯在某一水平或發生倒退。

Librium *n. see* chlordiazepoxide.

利眠寧

lice *pl. n. see* louse.

蝨

lichen *n.* any of several types of skin disease in which small round hard lesions occur close together. For example, *lichen planus* is an inflammatory condition in which wide flat mauve pimples are found mainly on the forearms, neck, and between the thighs. It may occur in the mouth and often causes symptomless white patches; occasionally it forms painful erosions.

苔蘚 皮膚上出現密集的小圓形發硬的損害的一類皮膚病。例如，扁平苔蘚是一種炎性疾病，主要在前臂、頸、大腿內側可見大片平坦的紫紅色丘疹。也可發生於口腔，形成無症狀的白色斑，偶爾可因發生糜爛而疼痛。

lichenification *n.* the thickening of certain cell layers in the epidermis causing brown or violet patches in the skin with exaggeration of the normal creases. A criss-cross appearance results, containing lozenge-shaped flat-topped shiny areas. The cause is abnormal scratching or rubbing of the skin.

苔蘚化 表皮內幾層細胞增厚，使皮膚內形成棕色或紫色斑，伴有正常皮紋增粗。結果形成一些呈十字交叉的表面平坦光滑的菱形小區。係由於搔抓和摩擦皮膚所致。

lichenoid *adj.* describing any skin disease that resembles *lichen.

苔蘚樣的 指任何類似苔蘚的皮膚病變。

Lieberkuhn's glands (crypts of Lieberkuhn) simple tubular glands in the mucous membrane of the *intestine. In the small intestine they lie between the villi. They are lined with columnar *epithelium in which various types of secretory cells are found. In the large intestine Lieberkuhn's glands are lon-

利貝昆氏腺，腸腺（利貝昆氏隱窩） 腸黏膜內的單管腺，在小腸內位於絨毛之間。腸腺與含有各種類型分泌細胞的柱狀上皮相伴行。大腸內腸腺較長，含有較多的黏液分泌細胞。

ger and contain more mucus-secreting cells.

lien *n. see* spleen.
脾

lien- (lieno-) *prefix denoting* the spleen. Example: *lienopathy* (disease of).
〔前綴〕 **脾** 例如脾病。

lientery *n.* diarrhoea with the passage of undigested food in the faeces. This may indicate simply rapid transit of food through the digestive tract or some form of *malabsorption.
消化不良性腹瀉 糞便內含有未消化食物的腹瀉。這種腹瀉表明可能只是食物過快地通過消化道，也可能是某種類型的吸收障礙。

life table an actuarial presentation of the ages at which a group of males and/or females will die and from which mean *life expectancy* at any age can be estimated, based on the assumption that mortality patterns current at the time of preparation of the table will continue to apply.
壽命表 表示一組男性和／或女性將來死亡的年齡和保險計算表格，據此可以推算任何年齡時的平均預期壽限。製訂此表時假設死亡率形式持續不變。

ligament *n.* **1.** a tough band of white fibrous connective tissue that links two bones together at a joint. Ligaments are inelastic but flexible; they strengthen the joint and limit its movements to certain directions. **2.** a sheet of peritoneum that supports or links together abdominal organs.
韌帶 ①將兩塊骨連結於關節處的一條白色堅韌的纖維結締組織索帶。韌帶無彈性但可彎曲，它對關節起强固作用，並限制關節只能向特定的方向活動。②支持或連結腹腔器官的由腹膜形成的片狀物。

ligation *n.* the application of a *ligature.
結紮 用線結紮。

ligature *n.* any material – for example, nylon, silk, catgut, or wire – that is tied firmly round a blood vessel to stop it bleeding or around the base of a structure (such as the *pedicle of a growth) to constrict it.
結紮線 任何結紮用的材料。如尼龍線、絲線、腸線或金屬線，用以緊紮血管以止血或某結構的基部（如生長物的蒂）使之縮小。

light adaptation reflex changes in the eye to enable vision either in normal light after being in darkness or in very bright light after being in normal light. The pupil contracts (*see* pupillary reflex) and the pigment in the *rods is bleached. *Compare* dark adaptation.
光適應 從暗處轉入正常光線下或從正常光線下轉入極明亮處時，眼睛為了能夠視物發生的反射變化。瞳孔縮小，視桿細胞內的色素退色。相反的為暗適應。

lightening *n.* the descent of the womb into the pelvic cavity at a late stage of pregnancy, usually two to three weeks before labour begins but sometimes, in women who have given birth previously, not until the onset of labour. Lightening occurs when the head of the fetus turns down towards the vagina.

（孕腹）輕鬆感 妊娠晚期子宮降入骨盆所致的輕鬆感。通常始於分娩前2～3周，在經產婦有時直至分娩時才出現。輕鬆感發生於胎頭下降接近陰道時。

light reflex *see* pupillary reflex.

光反射

lignocaine *n.* a widely used local *anaesthetic administered by injection for minor surgery and dental procedures. It can also be applied directly to the eye, throat, and mouth as it is absorbed through mucous membranes. Lignocaine is also injected to treat conditions involving abnormal heart rhythm, particularly myocardial infarction. When used as a local anaesthetic, side-effects are rare. Trade names: **Xylocaine**, **Xylotox**.

利多卡因 一種廣泛用於外科小手術和口腔科手術的注射用局部麻醉藥。也可直接外用於眼、喉和口腔內，因其可經黏膜吸收。利多卡因注射還用於治療某種心律失常的疾病，特別是心肌梗塞。用作局部麻醉藥時，副作用少見。

limbic system a complex system of nerve pathways and networks in the brain, involving several different nuclei, that is involved in the expression of instinct and mood in activities of the endocrine and motor systems of the body. Among the brain regions involved are the *amygdala, *hippocampal formation, and *hypothalamus. The activities of the body that are governed are those concerned with self-preservation (e.g. searching for food, fighting) and preservation of the species (e.g. reproduction and the care of offspring), the expression of fear, rage, and pleasure, and the establishment of memory patterns. *See also* reticular activating system.

邊緣系統 大腦內由神經通路、網絡以及一些不同的核團構成的複雜系統。此系統與本能的表達以及機體內分泌和運動系統的功能活動方式有關。參與邊緣系統的大腦區域有杏仁核、海馬結構和下丘腦。受其控制的機體活動有：保存自體的（如尋覓食物、搏鬬）和保存種系的活動（如繁殖和養育後代）、懼怕、發怒和高興的表情，以及記憶模式的建立。

limbus *n.* (in anatomy) an edge or border; for example, the *limbus sclerae* is the junction of the cornea and sclera of the eye.

緣 （解剖學）邊緣或邊界。例如鞏膜緣指眼角膜與鞏膜的接合部。

limen *n.* (in anatomy) a border or boundary. The *limen nasi* is the boundary between the bony and cartilaginous parts of the nasal cavity.

閾 （解剖學）邊界或分界線。鼻閾指鼻腔骨部與軟骨部的分界處。

liminal *adj.* (in physiology) relating to the threshold of perception.

閾的 （生理學）指知覺閾。

limosis *n.* abnormal hunger or an excessive desire for food.

善饑症 異常的饑餓或强烈的進食慾望。

lincomycin *n.* an *antibiotic used to treat infections caused by a narrow range of bacteria, including osteomyelitis. It is administered by mouth or injection and occasionally causes diarrhoea, nausea, and stomach pains. Trade names: **Lincocin**, **Mycivin**.

林肯黴毒 一種抗生素，用於治療由爲數有限的幾種細菌所致的感染，如骨髓炎。口服或注射，偶可引起腹瀉、噁心和胃痛。

linctus *n.* a syrupy liquid medicine, particularly one used in the treatment of irritating coughs.

舔膏劑 一種糖漿型藥物。主要用於治療刺激性咳嗽。

Lindau's tumour *see* haemangioblastoma.

林道氏瘤

linea *n.* (*pl.* **lineae**) (in anatomy) a line, narrow streak, or stripe. The *linea alba* is a tendinous line, extending from the xiphoid process to the pubic symphysis, where the flat abdominal muscles are attached.

線 （解剖學）細的線形紋理或條紋。白線是從劍突到耻骨聯合的一條腱，爲扁平腹肌所附着。

linear accelerator (linac) a machine that accelerates particles to produce high-energy radiation, used in the treatment of malignant disease.

直線加速器 一種可加速粒子使產生高能射線的機器。用於治療惡性腫瘤。

lingual *adj.* relating to, situated close to, or resembling the tongue (lingua). The lingual surface of a tooth is the surface adjacent to the tongue.

舌的 指舌、位於舌附近或舌樣的。牙的舌面指與舌相貼近的牙表面。

lingula *n.* **1.** the thin forward-projecting portion of the anterior lobe of the cerebellum, in the midline. **2.** a small section of the upper lobe of the left lung, extending downwards in front of the heart. **3.** a bony spur on the inside of the mandible, above the angle of the jaw. **4.** a small backward-pointing projection on each side of the sphenoid bone.

小舌 ①**小腦舌** 小腦前葉正中線上向前突出的菲薄部分。②**左肺小舌** 左肺上葉的一小部分，向前下方延伸到心臟前方。③**下頜小舌** 下頜內面下頜角上方的骨突。④**蝶骨小舌** 蝶骨兩側向後方的小突起。

liniment *n.* a medicinal preparation that is rubbed onto the skin or applied on a surgical dressing. Liniments often contain camphor and alcohol.

搽劑 塗搽皮膚或抹在外科敷料上的藥劑。搽劑常含樟腦或乙醇。

linin *n.* the lightly staining material surrounding the much more deeply staining *chromatin in the nucleus of a cell not undergoing division.

核絲 細胞未分裂時胞核內圍繞在深染的染色質周圍的淺染物質。

lining *n.* (in dentistry) a protective layer placed in a prepared tooth cavity before a restoration is inserted.

襯料 （牙料）在製備好的牙洞內，於塡入修復體之前置入的一層保護性的物質。

linkage *n.* the situation in which two or more genes lie close to each other on a chromosome and are therefore very likely to be inherited together. The further two genes are apart the more likely they are to be separated by *crossing over during meiosis and to come to lie on different homologous chromosomes.

連鎖 兩個或兩個以上基因在同一染色體內緊密相鄰的狀態。因此這些基因很可能一起遺傳。兩個基因距離越遠，它們在減數分裂期間越是可能通過交叉而分離，連到不同的同源染色體上。

linoleic acid *see* essential fatty acid.

亞油酸

linolenic acid *see* essential fatty acid.

亞麻酸

lint *n.* a material used in surgical dressings, made of scraped linen or a cotton substitute. It is usually fluffy one side and smooth the other.

絨布 作外科敷料用的材料。用刮擦過的亞麻布或棉質代用品做成。通常一面呈絨毛狀，另一面光滑。

liothyronine *n.* a hormone produced by the thyroid gland that is similar to *thyroxine and used to treat conditions of thyroid deficiency. It is administered by mouth or injection and has a rapid but short-lived effect.

三碘甲狀腺氨酸 甲狀腺製造的一種類似甲狀腺素的激素。用於治療甲狀腺機能不足的疾病。口服或注射。顯效快但維持時間短。

lip- (lipo-) *prefix denoting* **1.** fat. **2.** lipid.

〔前綴〕 ①**脂肪** ②**脂質**

lipaemia *n.* the presence in the blood of an abnormally large amount of fat, such as *cholesterol.

脂血症 血液中存在異常大量脂肪，如膽固醇。

lipase (steapsin) *n.* an enzyme, produced by the pancreas and the glands of the small intestine, that breaks down fats into glycerol and fatty acids during digestion.

脂酶（胰脂酶） 胰腺和小腸腺製造的一種酶，在消化過程中能將脂肪分解爲甘油和脂肪酸。

lipid *n.* one of a group of naturally occurring compounds that are soluble in solvents such as chloroform or alcohol, but insoluble in water. Lipids are

脂質，脂類 一族天然存在的化合物。溶於氯仿或乙醇之類的溶媒，不溶於水。脂類是膳食的重要成

important dietary constituents, not only because of their high energy value but also because certain vitamins and essential fatty acids are associated with them. The group includes *fats, *steroids, *phospholipids, and *glycolipids.

分，它們不僅具有很高的能量價值，還有些維生素和必需脂肪酸是伴隨脂類存在的。屬於這一族的有脂肪、固醇、磷脂和甘油脂。

lipidosis (lipoidosis) *n.* (*pl.* -ses) any disorder of lipid metabolism within the cells of the body. The *brain lipidoses* (*see* Gaucher's disease, Hurler's syndrome, Tay-Sachs disease) are inborn defects causing the accumulation of lipids within the brain.

脂沉積 機體細胞內的脂肪代謝障礙。大腦脂沉積症是一種引起脂質在大腦內蓄積的先天性缺陷。

lipochondrodystrophy *n.* multiple congenital defects affecting lipid (fat) metabolism, cartilage and bone, skin, and the major internal organs, leading to mental retardation, dwarfism, and deformities of the bones.

脂肪軟骨營養不良 一種多發性先天性缺陷。本病可累及脂肪代謝、軟骨、骨、皮膚及主要內臟器官，導致精神發育遲滯、侏儒症和骨變形。

lipochrome *n.* a pigment that is soluble in fat and therefore gives colour to fatty materials. An example is *carotene, the pigment responsible for the colour of egg yolks and butter.

脂色素 一種溶解於脂肪因而使脂肪物質着色的色素。胡蘿蔔素即爲一例，該色素使蛋黃和黃油着色。

lipodystrophy *n.* any disturbance of fat metabolism or of the distribution of fat in the body. In *inferior lipodystrophy* fat is absent from the legs; in *insulin lipodystrophy*, sometimes occurring in diabetics, it disappears from the areas at which insulin is injected.

脂肪營養不良 脂肪代謝障礙或體內脂肪分佈異常。下肢脂肪營養不良表現爲兩腿無脂肪；糖尿病時有時可有胰島素性脂肪營養不良，胰島素注射部位脂肪消失。

lipofuscin *n.* a brownish pigment staining with certain fat stains. It is most common in the cells of heart muscle, nerves, and liver and is normally contained within the *lysosomes.

脂褐質 一種被脂肪色素染成褐色的色素。最常存在於心肌、神經和肝細胞內，正常情況下含於溶酶體內。

lipogenesis *n.* the process by which glucose and other substances, derived from carbohydrate in the diet, are converted to *fatty acids in the body.

脂肪生成 食物中的葡萄糖和其他碳水化合物的衍生物在體內轉變爲脂肪酸的過程。

lipogranulomatosis *n.* an abnormality of lipid metabolism causing deposition of yellowish nodules in the skin.

脂肪肉芽腫病 一種脂肪代謝障礙引起皮膚內黃色小結節沉積的疾病。

lipoic acid a sulphur-containing compound that can be readily interconverted to and from its reduced form, *dihydrolipoic acid*. Lipoic acid functions in carbohydrate metabolism as one of the *coenzymes in the oxidative decarboxylation of pyruvate and other α-keto acids.

硫辛酸 一種含硫化合物，它與其還原形式——二氫硫辛酸之間，可以容易地互相轉換。硫辛酸在碳水化合物代謝中起輔酶作用，催化丙酮酸鹽及其它α-酮酸的氧化脫羧過程。

lipoid factor one of the substances involved in the clotting of blood, important for the activation of plasma *thromboplastin.

脂樣因子 一種參與血液凝固、在血漿凝血致活酶的激活中起主要作用的物質。

lipoidosis *n. see* lipidosis.

脂沉積症

lipolysis *n.* the process by which lipids, particularly triglycerides in fat, are broken down into their constituent fatty acids in the body by the enzyme *lipase. —**lipolytic** *adj.*

脂肪分解 體內脂類，特別是脂肪中的三酸甘油酯，在脂酶作用下分解爲其組成成分脂肪酸的過程。

lipoma *n.* a common benign tumour composed of well-differentiated fat cells. It is doubtful whether malignant change ever occurs.

脂肪瘤 一種常見的良性腫瘤，由分化良好的脂肪構成。能否發生惡變尚屬可疑。

lipomatosis *n.* **1.** the presence of an abnormally large amount of fat in the tissues. **2.** the presence of multiple *lipomas.

①**脂肪過多症** 組織內有異常大量脂肪。 ②**脂肪瘤病** 多發性脂肪瘤。

lipopolysaccharide *n.* a complex molecule containing both a lipid and a polysaccharide component. Lipopolysaccharides are constituents of the cell walls of Gram-negative bacteria and are important in determining the antigenic properties of these bacteria.

脂多糖 含有脂質和多糖成份的復合分子。爲革蘭陰性菌細胞壁的組成成分，對於決定這些細菌的抗原性物質有重要意義。

lipoprotein *n.* one of a group of proteins, found in blood plasma and lymph, that are combined with fats or other lipids (such as cholesterol). Lipoproteins are important for the transport of lipids in the blood and lymph.

脂蛋白 存在於血漿和淋巴內的一組蛋白質。它與脂肪或其他脂質（如膽固醇）結合在一起，在血液和淋巴的脂質轉運中起重要作用。

liposarcoma *n.* a malignant tumour of fat cells. It is most commonly found in the thigh and is rare under the age of 30 years. There are four main histological types: *well-differentiated*, *myxoid*, *pleo-*

脂肉瘤 一種脂肪細胞惡性腫瘤。最常發生於大腿，30歲以前少見。可分爲4個主要組織學類型：分化良好型、黏液樣型、

morphic, and *round-cell liposarcomas*, the first two of which are the most sensitive to treatment.

多形型、圓細胞型。第一、二型對治療最敏感。

liposome *n.* a microscopic spherical membrane-enclosed vesicle or sac (20–30 nm in diameter) made artificially in the laboratory by the addition of an aqueous solution to a phospholipid gel. The membrane resembles a cell membrane and the whole vesicle is similar to a cell organelle. Liposomes can be incorporated into living cells and are used to transport relatively toxic drugs into diseased cells, where they can exert their maximum effects. For example, liposomes containing *methotrexate can be injected into the patient's blood. The cancerous organ is heated to a temperature higher than body temperature, so that when the liposome passes through its blood vessels the membrane melts and the drug is released.

脂質體　一種顯微鏡下可見的球形有膜包裹的泡或囊（直徑20～30mm），係實驗室中將水溶液加於磷脂凝膠中所人工造成。膜與細胞膜類似，整個囊泡則與細胞器類似。脂質體可嵌入活細胞內，故被用於運載有較大毒性的藥物進入病變細胞，使藥物在細胞內發揮最大作用。例如可將含氨甲喋呤的脂質體注入病人血內。將患癌的器官加溫到高出體溫，當脂質通過該器官的血管時，囊膜融化，將藥物釋出。

lipotrophin *n.* a hormone-like substance from the anterior pituitary gland that stimulates the transfer of fat from the body stores to the bloodstream.

促脂激素　垂體前葉分泌的一種激素類物質，刺激脂肪從體內脂庫進入血流。

lipotropic *adj.* describing a substance that promotes the transport of fatty acids from the liver to the tissues or accelerates the utilization of fat in the liver itself. An example of such a substance is the amino acid methionine.

促脂肪的　指一種能促進脂肪酸從肝臟轉運到組織和加速肝臟本身利用脂肪的物質。甲硫氨酸則爲此類物質之一例。

lipping *n.* overgrowth of bone as seen in X-rays near a joint margin. This is a characteristic sign of degenerative or inflammatory joint disease and occurs most frequently and prominently in osteoarthrosis. *See also* osteophyte.

唇樣變　X線檢查時見於關節緣附近的骨質過度生長。爲關節變性或炎性病變的典型徵象，主要見於骨關節病。

lipuria *n.* the presence of fat or oil droplets in the urine.

脂肪尿　尿中出現脂肪或油滴。

liquor *n.* (in pharmacy) any solution, usually an aqueous solution.

液　（藥劑學）各種溶液。通常指水溶液。

Listeria *n.* a genus of Gram-positive aerobic motile rodlike bacteria that are parasites of warm-blooded animals.

李司忒氏菌屬　一屬革蘭陽性需氧有活力的桿狀菌。寄生於溫血動物體

The single species, *L. monocytogenes*, infects many domestic and wild animals and, on transmission to man, causes *meningoencephalitis and occasionally infection of the womb.

內。單核細胞增多性李司忒氏菌單株能感染許多家畜和野生動物，傳染人時引起腦膜腦炎，偶可引起子宮感染。

lith- (litho-) *prefix denoting* a calculus (stone). Example: *lithogenesis* (formation of).

〔前綴〕**結石** 例如結石形成。

-lith *suffix denoting* a calculus (stone). Example: *faecalith* (a stony mass of faeces).

〔後綴〕**結石** 例如糞石。

lithaemia *n. see* hyperuricaemia.

尿酸鹽血症

lithagogue *n.* an agent that promotes the removal of stones (calculi), such as kidney stones in the urine or gallstones from the gall bladder.

驅石劑 促使結石排出的藥物。例如促使腎結石隨尿排出或者膽結石從膽囊排出。

lithiasis *n.* formation of stones (*see* calculus) in an internal organ, such as the gall bladder (*see* gallstone), urinary system, pancreas, or appendix.

結石病 內臟器官（如膽囊、泌尿系統、胰腺或闌尾）內結石形成。

lithium (lithium carbonate) *n.* a drug given by mouth to prevent manic-depressive psychosis or to treat mania. Side-effects include tremor, weakness, nausea, thirst, and excessive urination. Thyroid function can be interfered with, and changes in the kidney can appear after long-term treatment. Excessive doses can cause an *encephalopathy and even death. The levels of lithium in the blood are therefore usually checked during long-term therapy. Trade names: **Camcolit**, **Priadel**.

鋰劑（碳酸鋰） 一種預防躁狂抑鬱性精神病或治療躁狂症的口服藥。副作用有：震顫、無力、噁心、口渴和多尿。甲狀腺機能可能受累，長期治療可能出現腎臟的改變。劑量過大可能引起腦病甚至死亡。因此，長期治療時通常須測定血鋰的水平。

litholapaxy (lithotripsy) *n.* the operation of crushing a stone in the bladder, using an instrument called a *lithotrite*. The small fragments of stone can then be removed by irrigation and suction.

碎石術 使用稱爲碎石器的器械壓碎膀胱內結石的手術，小的結石碎片可通過冲洗和抽吸除去。

lithonephrotomy *n.* surgical removal of a stone from the kidney. *See* nephrolithotomy, pyelolithotomy.

腎石切除術 從腎內取出結石的手術。

lithopaedion *n.* a fetus that has died in the womb or abdominal cavity and has become calcified (stony).

胎兒石化 胎兒在子宮內或腹腔內死亡並發生鈣化（石化）。

lithotomy *n.* the surgical removal of a stone (calculus) from the urinary tract. *See* nephrolithotomy, pyelolithotomy, ureterolithotomy.

腎石切除術 從泌尿道內取出結石的手術。

lithotripsy *n. see* litholapaxy.

碎石術

lithotrite *n.* a surgical instrument used for crushing a stone in the bladder. *See* litholapaxy.

碎石器 用以壓碎膀胱內的結石的外科器械。

lithotrophic *adj. see* autotrophic.

自營的

lithuresis *n.* the passage of small stones or *gravel in the urine.

石尿症 小結石或沙礫隨尿排出。

lithuria *n. see* hyperuricuria.

尿酸鹽尿症

litre *n.* a unit of volume equal to the volume occupied by 1 kilogram of pure water at 4°C and 760 mmHg pressure. In *SI units the litre is treated as a special name for the cubic decimetre, but is not used when a high degree of accuracy is required (1 litre = 1.0000028 dm^3). For approximate purposes 1 litre is assumed to be equal to 1000 cubic centimetres (cm^3), therefore 1 millilitre (ml) is often taken to be equal to 1 cm^3. This practice is now deprecated.

升 體積單位。相當於1㎏純水在4℃760㎜Hg壓力下所佔的體積。在國際單位中，升（L）作爲$1dm^3$的專門術語使用，但當要求高度精確時則不適用，因爲$1\ell = 1.0000028\ dm^3$。爲了取近似值，將1ℓ看作等於$1000cm^3$因而1mℓ通常當作$1cm^3$。這種做法現時已遭到反對。

Little's disease a form of *cerebral palsy involving both sides of the body and affecting the legs more severely than the arms.

李特爾氏病，痙攣性雙癱 一種大腦性痲痺，累及身體兩側，對兩腿的影響重於兩臂。

livedo *n.* a discoloured area or spot on the skin, often caused by local congestion of the circulation.

青斑 皮膚上的變色區或斑點。通常由局部血管充血引起。

liver *n.* the largest gland of the body, weighing 1200–1600 g. Situated in the top right portion of the abdominal cavity, the liver is divided by fissures (*fossae*) into four lobes: the *right* (the largest lobe), *left*, *quadrate*, and *caudate lobes*. It is connected to the diaphragm and abdominal walls by five ligaments: the membranous *falciform* (which separates the right and left lobes), *coronary*, and *right* and *left triangular ligaments* and the fibrous *round ligament*, which is

肝 機體最大的腺體，重1200～1600ｇ，位於腹腔右上方。肝藉裂隙分爲4葉：右葉（最大）、左葉、方形葉及尾形葉。藉5條韌帶：膜狀的鐮狀韌帶（將肝區分爲左右葉）、冠狀韌帶、左和右三角韌帶以及纖維性的肝圓韌帶（由胚胎期的臍靜脈演化而成）與膈及腹壁相連。已經消化的食物隨

derived from the embryonic umbilical vein. Venous blood containing digested food is brought to the liver in the *hepatic portal vein* (*see* portal system). Branches of this vein pass in between the lobules and terminate in the *sinusoids* (see illustration). Oxygenated blood is supplied in the *hepatic artery*. The blood leaves the liver via a central vein in each lobule, which drains into the *hepatic vein. The liver is supplied by parasympathetic nerve fibres from the vagus nerve, and by sympathetic fibres from the solar plexus. The liver has a number of important functions. It synthesizes *bile, which drains into the *gall bladder before being released into the duodenum. The liver is an important site of metabolism of carbohydrates, proteins, and fats. It regulates the amount of blood sugar, converting excess glucose to *glycogen; it removes excess amino acids by breaking them down into ammonia and finally *urea; and it stores and meta-

靜脈血經肝靜脈進入肝內，門靜脈的分支在小葉間行進，最後終於肝竇（見圖）。氧合血由肝動脈供應。血液經每個小葉的中央靜脈離開肝臟，流入肝靜脈內。肝臟的副交感神經纖維來自迷走神經，交感神經纖維來自太陽叢。肝臟具有多種重要機能。肝合成膽汁，膽汁引流入膽囊，然後排入十二指腸。肝是進行碳水化合物、蛋白質和脂肪代謝的主要部位。肝參與調節血糖含量，使過剩的葡萄糖轉化為糖原，過剩的氨基酸在肝內分解為氨，最終成為尿素。肝又是脂肪貯存和代謝的場所。肝還合成纖維蛋白原、凝血酶原（主要的凝血物質）和肝素（抗凝劑）。胚胎期肝生成紅細胞，並且是製造血漿蛋白的場所。肝在

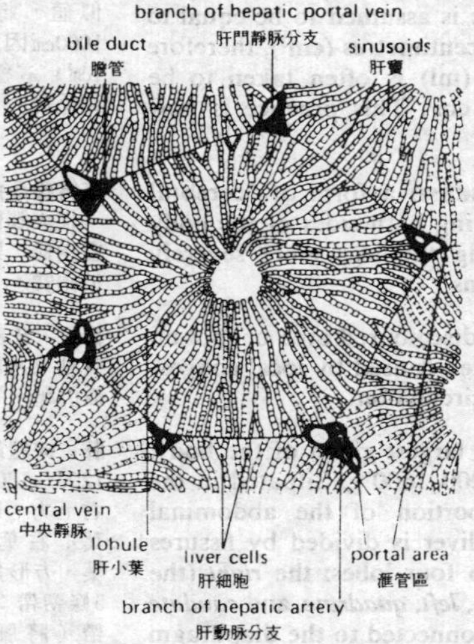

The microscopic structure of the liver
肝的顯微結構

bolizes fats. The liver also synthesizes *fibrinogen and *prothrombin (essential blood-clotting substances) and *heparin, an anticoagulant. It forms red blood cells in the fetus and is the site of production of plasma proteins. It has an important role in the detoxification of poisonous substances and it breaks down worn out red cells and other unwanted substances, such as excess oestrogen in the male (*see also* Kupffer's cells). The liver is also the site of *vitamin A synthesis; this vitamin is stored in the liver, together with vitamins B_{12}, D, and K.

毒性物質的解毒過程中起重要作用，衰老的紅細胞以及其他無用物質（如男性體內過多的雌激素）在肝內分解。肝還是維生素A的合成部位，維生素A以及維生素B_{12}、維生素D和維生素K均貯存在肝內。

liver spot a local brown discoloration on the skin known medically as senile *lentigo. The term is sometimes also used for *chloasma and some medical sources also apply the term to *pityriasis versicolor* – a mild chronic infection of the skin, caused by the fungus *Malassezia furfur*, that produces discrete depigmented areas on the body.

雀斑 皮膚上的部分棕色變色區，醫學上稱爲老年斑。此術語有時指褐黃斑，有些醫學文獻中用於指花斑糠疹——由糠秕馬拉色黴菌引起的一種輕型慢性感染，在體表形成稀疏的無色素區。

livid *adj.* denoting a bluish colour of the skin, such as that produced locally by a bruise or of the general complexion in *cyanosis.

青紫的 指皮膚帶藍色。如挫傷所致的局部青紫，或紫紺時全身的皮膚色調。

Loa *n.* a genus of parasitic nematode worms (*see* filaria). The adult eye worm, *L. loa*, lives within the tissues beneath the skin, where it causes inflammation and swelling (*see* loiasis). The motile embryos, present in the blood during the day, may be taken up by bloodsucking *Chrysops* flies. Here they develop into infective larvae, ready for transmission to a new human host.

羅阿絲蟲屬 一屬寄生性線蟲。眼絲蟲（羅阿絲蟲）的成蟲寄生於皮下組織內，引起炎症和水腫。晝間存在於血內的能活動的蟲胚，可被吸血斑虻吸取，在虻體內發育爲有感染力的幼蟲，以傳給新的人宿主。

lobe *n.* a major division of an organ or part of an organ, especially one having a rounded form and often separated from other lobes by fissures or bands of connective tissue. For example, the brain, liver, and lung are divided into lobes. —**lobar** *adj.*

葉 某一器官的一級分部或由某一器官分出來的（尤指圓形的）部分。葉與葉之間常藉裂隙或結締組織索帶隔開。例如腦、肝、肺均分爲葉。

lobectomy *n.* the surgical removal of a lobe of an organ or gland, such as the lung, thyroid, or brain. Lobectomy of the lung may be performed for cancer or other disease of the lung.

葉切除術 手術切除器官（如肺、腦）或腺體（如甲狀腺）的一葉。肺癌或肺的其他疾病時可施行肺葉切除術。

lobeline *n.* a drug administered by injection to stimulate breathing or given by mouth as a smoking deterrent Side-effects can include nausea, vomiting, coughing, headache, tremors, and dizziness.

山梗菜鹼 一種興奮呼吸的注射藥物。口服可作爲戒煙藥。副作用有噁心、震顫和頭暈。

lobotomy (prefrontal leucotomy) *see* leucotomy.

葉切斷術（前額葉白質切斷術）

lobule *n.* a subdivision of a part or organ that can be distinguished from the whole by boundaries, such as septa, that are visible with or without a microscope. For example, the *lobule of the liver* is a structural and functional unit seen in cross-section under a microscope as a column of cells drained by a central vein and bounded by a branch of the portal vein. The *lung lobule* is a practical subdivision of the lung tissue seen macroscopically in lung slices as outlined by incomplete septa of fibrous tissue. It is made up of three to five lung *acini.

小葉 器官或結構部分的二級分部，藉隔之類的分界從整體上區分出來。分界有時肉眼可見，有的則需用顯微鏡。例如，肝小葉是肝的結構和機能單位，顯微鏡下可見切片上的肝小葉爲一細胞柱，由一條中央靜脉供引流，藉門靜脉分支與其他小葉分界。肺小葉是肺組織的實際二級分部，在肺切片上肉眼可見，由不完整的纖維組織隔構成輪廓。3～5個肺泡囊組成一個肺小葉。

lochia *n.* the material eliminated from the womb through the vagina after the completion of labour. The first discharge, *lochia rubra* (*lochia cruenta*), consists largely of blood. This is followed by *lochia serosa*, a brownish mixture of blood and mucus, and finally *lochia alba* (*lochia purulenta*), a yellowish or whitish discharge containing microbes and cell fragments. Each stage may last for several days. —**lochial** *adj.*

惡露 分娩後從子宮經陰道排出的物質。最初排出的是含有大量血液的紅色惡露；接着是漿液性惡露，爲血和黏液組成的褐色混合物；最後是白色惡露，呈淡黃色或白色，內含細菌和細胞碎片。每種惡露可持續數日。

lockjaw *n. see* tetanus.

牙關緊閉

locomotor ataxia *see* tabes dorsalis.

運動性共濟失調

loculus *n.* (in anatomy) a small space or cavity.

小腔 （解剖學）小的空間或腔室。

locum tenens a doctor who stands in temporarily for a colleague who is absent or ill and looks after the patients in his practice. Often shortened to **locum**.

代理醫師 暫時代替因病或其他原因缺席的同事照料其病人的醫師。

locus *n.* **1.** (in anatomy) a region or site. The *locus ceruleus* is a small pigmented region in the floor of the fourth ventricle of the brain. **2.** (in genetics) the region of a chromosome occupied by a particular gene.

部位 ①（解剖學）指區域或位置。藍斑爲第四腦室底的一小塊含色素的區域。 ②（遺傳學）特定基因在染色體上所佔的區域。

log- (logo-) *prefix denoting* words; speech.

〔前綴〕 **詞，言語**

logopaedics *n.* the scientific study of defects and disabilities of speech and of the methods used to treat them; speech therapy.

言語矯正學 研究語言缺陷及其治療方法的專門學科；言語療法。

logorrhoea *n.* a rapid flow of voluble speech, often with incoherence, such as is encountered in *mania.

多言症 口若懸河，但常是語無倫次，此種情況可見於躁狂症。

-logy (-ology) *suffix denoting* field of study. Example: *cytology* (study of cells).

〔後綴〕 **學** 指學術的領域。例如細胞學（關於細胞的學問）。

loiasis *n.* a disease, occurring in West and Central Africa, caused by the eye worm **Loa loa*. The adult worms live and migrate within the skin tissues, causing the appearance of transitory *calabar* swellings. These are probably an allergic reaction to the worms' waste products, and they sometimes lead to fever and itching. Worms often migrate across the eyeball just beneath the conjunctiva, where they cause irritation and congestion. Loiasis is treated with *diethylcarbamazine, which kills both the adults and larval forms.

羅阿絲蟲病 一種發生於中非和西非，由眼絲蟲（羅阿絲蟲）引起的疾病。成蟲在皮膚內寄居並游走，引起短暫的卡拉巴絲蟲腫。後者可能是對蟲排泄物的變應反應，有時可引起發熱和瘙癢。蟲常在結膜下游走，穿過眼球，在所過之處引起刺激和充血。治療：用海羣生可殺死成蟲和幼蟲。

loin *n.* the region of the back and side of the body between the lowest rib and the pelvis.

腰 身體後面和兩側最下位肋骨與盆骨之間的區域。

long-sightedness *n. see* hypermetropia.

遠視

loop *n.* **1.** a bend in a tubular organ, e.g. *Henle's loop in a kidney tubule. **2.**

襻 ①管狀器官的彎曲部，如腎小管的亨利氏

one of the patterns of dermal ridges in *fingerprints.

襻。②指紋中的一種皮嵴類型。

lorazepam *n.* a *tranquillizer used to relieve moderate or severe anxiety and tension and to treat insomnia. It is administered by mouth and may cause drowsiness, dizziness, blurred vision, and nausea. Trade name: **Ativan**.

氯羥安定 安定藥。用以緩解中度或嚴重焦慮症和緊張，還用於治療失眠。口服。可引起倦怠、頭暈、視物模糊和噁心。

lordosis *n.* inward curvature of the spine. A certain degree of lordosis is normal in the lumbar and cervical regions of the spine: loss of this is a sign of ankylosing *spondylitis. Exaggerated lordosis may occur in adolescence, through faulty posture or as a result of disease affecting the vertebrae and spinal muscles. *Compare* kyphosis.

脊柱前凸 脊柱向前彎曲。脊柱腰段和頸段一定程度前凸是正常現象，失去前凸倒是强直性脊柱炎的體徵。過度的脊柱前凸可發生於青春期，由於姿勢不正確或是疾病影響脊柱和脊肌所致。

lotion *n.* a medicinal solution for washing or bathing the external parts of the body. Lotions usually have a cooling, soothing, or antiseptic action.

洗液 用於洗浴身體外部的藥物溶液。通常有涼爽、舒適或抗菌的作用。

loupe *n.* a small magnifying hand lens used for examining the front part of the eye. It is usually used with a pocket torch to provide illumination.

角膜放大鏡 小型袖珍放大鏡，用於檢查眼球前部。使用時通常用手電提供照明。

louse *n.* (*pl.* **lice**) a small wingless insect that is an external parasite of man. Lice attach themselves to hair and clothing using their well-developed legs and claws. Their flattened leathery bodies are resistant to crushing and their mouthparts are adapted for sucking blood. Lice thrive in overcrowded and unhygienic conditions and they may transmit disease. *See also* Pediculus, Phthirus.

蝨 一種無翅昆蟲。寄生於人體外部。蝨藉其發達的腿和爪貼附在頭髮和衣服上。其平坦、堅韌的身體可抵禦壓榨，其口器則適於吸血。蝨在人羣密集和不衞生環境中大量繁殖，並可傳播疾病。

lozenge *n.* a medicated tablet containing sugar. Lozenges should dissolve slowly in the mouth so that the medication is applied to the mouth and throat.

錠劑（糖錠） 含糖的藥片。錠劑在口內緩慢溶解，適用於口腔和咽喉疾痛。

LSD *see* lysergic acid diethylamide.

麥角醯二乙胺

lubb-dupp *n.* a representation of the normal heart sounds as heard through the stethoscope. Lubb (the first heart

路布-杜普 對用聽診器聽到的正常心音的模倣音。路布（第一心音）在

sound) coincides with closure of the mitral and tricuspid valves; dupp (the second heart sound) is due to closure of the aortic and pulmonary valves.

二尖瓣和三尖瓣關閉時出現，杜普（第二心音）發生於主動脈瓣和肺動脈瓣關閉時。

Ludwig's angina severe inflammation caused by infection of both sides of the floor of the mouth, resulting in massive swelling of the neck. If untreated, it may obstruct the airways, necessitating tracheostomy.

路德維希氏咽峽炎 口底兩側感染引起嚴重炎症，導致頸部廣泛水腫。若不治療，可阻塞氣道而需行氣管切開術。

lues *n.* a serious infectious disease such as syphilis.

梅毒 一種嚴重的傳染性疾病。

lumbago *n.* low backache, of any cause or description. Severe lumbago, of sudden onset while bending or lifting, can be due either to a slipped disc or to a strained muscle or ligament. When associated with *sciatica it is probably due to a slipped disc.

腰痛 各種原因引起的形形色色的背下部疼痛。發作於彎腰或提物時的嚴重腰痛，可能是由於椎間盤脫出或者肌肉或韌帶拉傷所致。若伴有坐骨神經痛，則多半是椎間盤脫出。

lumbar *adj.* relating to the loin.

腰的 與腰有關的。

lumbar puncture a procedure in which cerebrospinal fluid is withdrawn by means of a hollow needle inserted into the *subarachnoid space in the region of the lower back (usually between the third and fourth lumbar vertebrae). The fluid thus obtained is examined for diagnostic purposes. The procedure is usually without risk to the patient, but in patients with raised intracranial pressure it may be hazardous and the optic fundi must be examined for the presence of *papilloedema. *See also* Queckenstedt test.

腰椎穿刺 在腰部（通常是第三與第四腰椎之間）用一根空芯針刺入蛛網膜下腔抽出腦脊液的操作。對得到的體液進行檢查以作診斷。此操作對病人一般無危險，但在顱壓高的病人可能有害，故須檢查眼底觀察有無乳頭水腫。

lumbar vertebrae the five bones of the *backbone that are situated between the thoracic vertebrae and the sacrum, in the lower part of the back. They are the largest of the unfused vertebrae and have stout processes for attachment of the strong muscles of the lower back. *See also* vertebra.

腰椎 胸椎和骶椎之間的5塊椎骨，位於脊柱腰部。是不融合的椎骨中最大的，有粗的突起，為腰部强大的肌肉所附着。

lumbo- *prefix denoting* the loin; lumbar region.

〔前綴〕 **腰，腰部**

lumbosacral *adj.* relating to part of the spine composed of the lumbar vertebrae and the sacrum.

腰骶的　指由腰椎和骶椎組成的脊柱部分。

lumen *n.* **1.** the space within a tubular or sac-like part, such as a blood vessel, the intestine, or the stomach. **2.** the *SI unit of luminous flux, equal to the amount of light emitted per second in unit solid angle of 1 steradian by a point source of 1 candela. Symbol: lm.

①腔　管道或囊腔樣結構內的空間，諸如血管腔、腸腔或胃腔。　②流明　國際單位制中的光通量單位，相當於1坎德拉的點光源每秒經1球面度單位立體角發出的光量。符號：lm。

lunate bone a bone of the wrist (*see* carpus). It articulates with the capitate bone in front and with the radius and ulna behind.

月骨　腕骨之一。前方與頭骨成關節，後方與橈骨和尺骨成關節。

lung *n.* one of the pair of organs of *respiration, situated in the chest cavity on either side of the heart and enclosed by a serous membrane (*see* pleura). The lungs are fibrous elastic sacs that are expanded and compressed by movements of the rib cage and diaphragm during *breathing. They communicate

肺　成對的呼吸器官，位於胸腔內心臟兩側，外包一層漿膜。肺是有彈性的囊袋，呼吸時隨肋骨架和膈的運動而被擴張和壓縮。肺通過開口於咽的氣管與大氣相溝通。氣管分支爲二條支氣管，支氣管

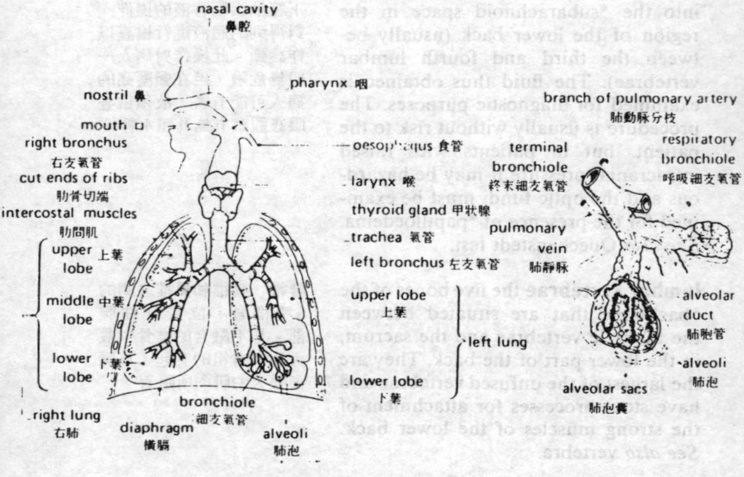

The lungs and main air-passages, with details of the alveoli
肺和主要氣管，附肺泡細部

with the atmosphere through the *trachea, which opens into the pharynx. The trachea divides into two bronchi (*see* bronchus), which enter the lungs and branch into *bronchioles. These divide further and terminate in minute air sacs (*see* alveolus), the sites of gaseous exchange. (See illustration.) Atmospheric oxygen is absorbed and carbon dioxide from the blood of the pulmonary capillaries is released into the lungs; in each case down a concentration gradient (*see* pulmonary circulation). The total capacity of the lungs in an adult male is about 5.5 litres, but during normal breathing only about 500 ml of air is exchanged (*see also* residual volume). Other functions of the lung include water evaporation: an important factor in the fluid balance and heat regulation of the body.

進入肺內並分支爲細支氣管。後者繼續分支，最終成爲細小的肺泡——氣體交換的場所（見圖）。大氣中的氧被吸收，來自肺毛細血管的二氧化碳被釋放入肺，兩者均按濃度梯度進行。成年男子的肺總氣量約爲5.5升，而正常呼吸時僅有約500mℓ空氣交換。肺的另一機能是蒸發水分，這是維持體液平衡和調節體溫的重要因素。

lung cancer cancer arising in the epithelium of the air passages (*bronchial cancer*) or lung. It is a very common form of cancer, particularly in Britain, and is strongly associated with cigarette smoking and exposure to industrial air pollutants (including asbestos). There are often no symptoms in the early stages of the disease, when diagnosis is made on X-ray examination. Treatment includes surgical removal of the affected lobe or lung (20% of cases are suitable for surgery), radiotherapy, and chemotherapy.

肺癌 起自氣道上皮或肺的癌瘤。前者稱爲支氣管癌。是一種極爲常見的癌瘤類型，尤其是在英國，與吸煙和工業大氣汚染（如石棉）有密切關係。本病早期常無症狀，須依靠X線檢查作出診斷。治療包括手術和切除受累的肺葉或一肺（20%病例適於手術）、放射治療和化學治療。

lunula *n.* the whitish crescent-shaped area at the base of a *nail.

弧影 指甲基部色發白的新月形區域。

lupus *n.* any of several chronic skin diseases. Used alone, lupus generally refers to tuberculosis of the skin (*lupus vulgaris). *See also* lupus erythematosus, lupus verrucosus.

狼瘡 一種慢性皮膚病。狼瘡一詞單用一般指皮膚結核（尋常狼瘡）。

lupus erythematosus (LE) a chronic inflammatory disease of connective tissue, affecting the skin and various internal organs. Typically, there is a red

紅斑狼瘡 一種侵犯皮膚和不同內臟器官的慢性結締組織炎性疾病。典型表現有：面部紅色脫屑性皮

scaly rash on the face, affecting the nose and cheeks; arthritis; and progressive damage to the kidneys. Often the heart, lungs, and brain are also affected by progressive attacks of inflammation followed by the formation of scar tissue (fibrosis). In a milder form of the disease only the skin is affected. LE is regarded as an *autoimmune disease and can be diagnosed by the presence of abnormal antibodies in the bloodstream, most easily detected by a test that reveals characteristic white blood cells (*LE cells*). The disease is treated with corticosteroids.

疹，位於鼻和兩頰；關節炎；進行性腎臟損害。心、肺和腦也反復遭受炎症侵襲，繼而有瘢痕組織形成（纖維化）。輕型時僅皮膚受侵。本病被認爲是一種自身免疫性疾病，可根據血內出現異常抗體作出診斷，最簡單的辦法是查出特徵性的白細胞（狼瘡細胞試驗）。本病用皮質類固醇治療。

lupus verrucosus a tuberculous infection of the skin – commonly the arm or hand – typified by warty lesions. It occurs in those who have been reinfected with tuberculosis.

疣狀狼瘡 一種皮膚結核性感染，常發生於臂和手，以疣狀損害爲特徵。本病見於再次感染結核的病人。

lupus vulgaris tuberculous infection of the skin, usually due to direct inoculation of the tuberculosis bacillus into the skin. This type of lupus often starts in childhood, with dark red patches on the nose or cheek. Unless treated lupus vulgaris spreads, ulcerates, and causes extensive scarring. Treatment is with antituberculous drugs.

尋常狼瘡 皮膚的結核性感染，通常由於結核桿菌直接侵犯皮膚所致。此型狼瘡常起於兒童期，在鼻或頰部出現暗紅色斑，若不治療，可播散，形成潰瘍，導致廣泛的瘢痕。治療用抗結核藥。

lute *n.* (in dentistry) a thin layer of cement inserted into the minute space between a prepared tooth and a crown or inlay to hold it permanently in place.

密封 （牙科學）將一薄片黏固劑塡入已製備好的牙和牙冠之間的微小腔洞內，使之永久固定在原位。

lutein *n.* **1.** *see* xanthophyll. **2.** the yellow pigment of the corpus luteum.

①葉黃素 ②黃體素 黃體的黃色色素。

luteinizing hormone (LH) a hormone (*see* gonadotrophin), synthesized and released by the anterior pituitary gland, that stimulates ovulation, *corpus luteum formation, progesterone synthesis by the ovary (*see also* menstrual cycle), and androgen synthesis by the interstitial cells of the testes. Also called: **interstitial cell stimulating hormone (ICSH).**

促黃體生成激素 垂體前葉合成和分泌的一種激素，能刺激排卵、黃體形成、卵巢合成孕酮和睾丸間質細胞合成睾酮。又名間質細胞刺激素。

luteo- *prefix denoting* **1.** yellow. **2.** the corpus luteum.

〔前綴〕 **①黃色 ②黃體**

luteotrophic hormone (luteotrophin) *see* prolactin.
促黃體激素 催乳激素。

lux *n.* the *SI unit of intensity of illumination, equal to 1 lumen per square metre. This unit was formerly called the metre candle. Symbol: lx.
勒〔克司〕 國際單位制中照明强度單位，等於每平方米1流明。此單位過去稱爲米燭光。符號：lx。

luxation *n. see* dislocation.
脫位

lyase *n.* one of a group of enzymes that catalyse the linking of groups by double bonds.
裂解酶 一組能裂解以雙鍵連結的基團的酶。

lycanthropy *n.* a very rare symptom of mental disorder in which an individual believes that he can change into a wolf.
變狼妄想 一種極罕見的精神障礙症狀。病人相信他會變成狼。

lymph *n.* the fluid present within the vessels of the *lymphatic system. It consists of the fluid that bathes the tissues, which is derived from the blood and is drained by the lymphatic vessels. Lymph passes through a series of filters (*lymph nodes) and is ultimately returned to the bloodstream via the *thoracic duct. It is similar in composition to plasma, but contains less protein and some cells, mainly *lymphocytes.
淋巴 淋巴系統的淋巴管內的液體。來自血液的組織液進入淋巴管內組成淋巴。淋巴通過一系列濾過器（淋巴結），最終經胸導管反回血流。淋巴的成分與血漿相似，但所含蛋白質和某些細胞較少，主要含淋巴細胞。

lymphaden- (lymphadeno-) *prefix denoting* lymph node(s).
〔前綴〕 **淋巴結**

lymphadenectomy *n.* surgical removal of lymph nodes, an operation commonly performed when a cancer has invaded nodes in the drainage area of an organ infiltrated by a malignant growth.
淋巴結切除術 手術切除淋巴結。當惡性腫瘤浸潤某器官的淋巴引流區以致侵及淋巴結時，通常施行淋巴結切除術。

lymphadenitis *n.* inflammation of lymph nodes, which become swollen, painful, and tender. Some cases may be chronic (e.g. tuberculous lymphadenitis) but most are acute and localized adjacent to an area of infection. The most commonly affected lymph nodes are those in the neck, in association with tonsillitis. The lymph nodes help to contain and combat the infection. Occasionally generalized lymphadeni-
淋巴結炎 淋巴結的炎症。淋巴結腫脹、疼痛、變硬。有時呈慢性經過（如結核性淋巴炎），但多數爲急性，局限於與感染部位毗鄰的淋巴結。最常受累的是頸部淋巴結，伴發於扁桃體炎。淋巴結參與抑制和抵抗感染。病毒感染時偶見全身性淋巴結炎。針對病因治療。

tis occurs as a result of virus infections. The treatment is that of the cause.

lymphadenoma *n.* an obsolete term for *lymphoma.

淋巴組織瘤 淋巴瘤的舊稱，已廢用。

lymphagogue *n.* an agent that stimulates the secretion of lymph.

利淋巴藥 刺激淋巴分泌的藥物。

lymphangi- (lymphangio-) *prefix denoting* a lymphatic vessel.

〔前綴〕 **淋巴管**

lymphangiectasis *n.* dilatation of the lymphatic vessels, which is usually congenital and produces enlargement of various parts of the body (e.g. the leg in Milroy's disease). It may also be caused by obstruction of the lymphatic vessels (*see* lymphoedema).

淋巴管擴張 淋巴管的擴張。通常爲先天性，引起身體不同部位腫大（如米爾羅依氏病的腿腫）。本病也可由淋巴管阻塞引起。

lymphangiography *n.* X-ray examination of the lymphatic vessels and lymph nodes after a contrast medium has been injected into them (*see* angiography). Its main uses are in the investigation of the extent and spread of cancer of the lymphatic system and in the investigation of lymphoedema.

淋巴管造影術 將造影劑注入淋巴管和淋巴結後，對兩者進行X線檢查。主要用於檢查淋巴系統癌瘤的範圍和蔓延程度以及檢查淋巴水腫。

lymphangioma *n.* a localized collection of distended lymphatic vessels, which may result in a large cyst in the neck or armpit (*cystic hygroma*). This can be removed surgically.

淋巴管瘤 局限性的擴張的淋巴管集羣。可在頸部或腋窩形成一個大囊腫（囊性水瘤）。外科手術切除。

lymphangiosarcoma *n.* a malignant tumour of the lymphatic vessels. It is most commonly seen in the chronically swollen (oedematous) arms of women who have had a mastectomy for breast cancer.

淋巴管肉瘤 淋巴管惡性腫瘤。最常見於因乳腺癌行乳房切除術後發生慢性上臂水腫的婦女。

lymphangitis *n.* inflammation of the lymphatic vessels, which can be seen most commonly as red streaks in the skin adjacent to a focus of streptococcal infection. Occasionally a more chronic form results in *lymphoedema. The infected part is rested and the infection can be eliminated by an antibiotic (e.g. penicillin).

淋巴管炎 淋巴管的炎症。最常見於鏈球菌感染病竈附近的皮膚，表現爲一條紅線。偶可以較慢性形式，導致淋巴水腫。治療：患部休息，使用抗生素（如青黴素）消除感染。

lymphatic 1. *n.* a lymphatic vessel. *See* lymphatic system. **2.** *adj.* relating to or transporting lymph.

①淋巴管 ②淋巴的 輸送淋巴的。

lymphatic system a network of vessels that conveys electrolytes, water, proteins, etc. – in the form of *lymph – from the tissue fluids to the bloodstream (see illustration). It consists of fine blind-ended lymphatic capillaries, which unite to form lymphatic vessels. At various points along the lymphatic vessels are *lymph nodes. Lymph drains into the capillaries and passes

淋巴（管）系統 以淋巴的形式，將電解質、水、蛋白質等自組織液運送到血液的管道網絡（見圖）。由盲端的毛細淋巴管和由之滙合而成的淋巴管組成。沿淋巴管走行在不同部位有淋巴結。淋巴被引入毛細淋巴管，再進入淋巴管，淋巴管內有瓣

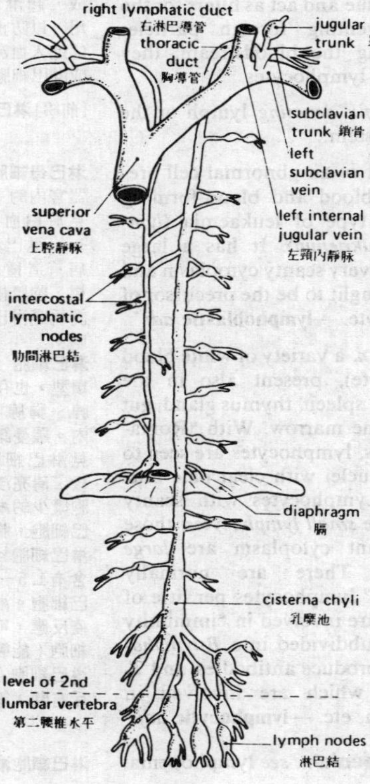

The lymphatic system
淋巴系統

into the lymphatic vessels, which have valves to prevent backflow of lymph. The lymphatics lead to two large channels – the *thoracic duct* and the *right lymphatic duct* – which return the lymph to the bloodstream via the innominate veins.

膜防止淋巴逆向流動。淋巴管滙成兩條大管道——胸導管和左淋巴導管，兩者通過無名靜脉將淋巴輸回血流。

lymph node one of a number of small swellings found at intervals along the lymphatic system. Groups of nodes are found in many parts of the body; for example, in the groin and armpit and behind the ear. They are composed of lymphoid tissue and act as filters for the lymph, preventing foreign particles from entering the bloodstream; they also produce lymphocytes.

淋巴結　沿淋巴管系統走行可間隔地見到的一些小型膨大物。在身體的一些部位，如腹股溝、腋窩和耳後，可查見成組的結節。淋巴結由淋巴組織構成，起淋巴濾過器的作用，以防止異物從入侵部位進入血流。淋巴結還生成淋巴細胞。

lympho- *prefix denoting* lymph or the lymphatic system.

〔前綴〕**淋巴，淋巴系統**

lymphoblast *n.* an abnormal cell present in the blood and blood-forming organs in a type of leukaemia (*lymphoblastic leukaemia*). It has a large nucleus with very scanty cytoplasm and was once thought to be the precursor of the lymphocyte. —**lymphoblastic** *adj.*

淋巴母細胞　血液和造血器官內的一種異常細胞，見於白血病的一種類型——淋巴母細胞性白血病。這種細胞有一個大核，胞漿極少，曾一度被認爲是淋巴細胞的前體細胞。

lymphocyte *n.* a variety of white blood cell (leucocyte), present also in the lymph nodes, spleen, thymus gland, gut wall, and bone marrow. With *Romanowsky stains, lymphocytes are seen to have dense nuclei with clear pale-blue cytoplasm. Lymphocytes with scanty cytoplasm are *small lymphocytes*; those with abundant cytoplasm are *large lymphocytes.* There are normally 1.5–4.0 × 10^9 lymphocytes per litre of blood. They are involved in *immunity and can be subdivided into *B-lymphocytes*, which produce antibodies, and *T-lymphocytes*, which are involved in graft rejection, etc. —**lymphocytic** *adj.*

淋巴細胞　白細胞的一種類型，也存在於淋巴結、脾、胸腺、腸壁和骨髓內。羅曼諾夫斯基染色可見淋巴細胞有緻密的胞核、清亮淺藍色的胞漿。胞漿少的淋巴細胞爲小淋巴細胞，胞漿豐富的爲大淋巴細胞。正常每升血液含有1.5～4.0×10^9個淋巴細胞。淋巴細胞參與免疫反應，可區分爲B淋巴細胞（能製造抗體）和T淋巴細胞（與移植物的排斥有關）等。

lymphocytopenia *n. see* lymphopenia.

淋巴細胞減少

lymphocytosis *n.* an increase in the number of *lymphocytes in the blood. Lymphocytosis may occur in a wide

淋巴細胞增多　血中淋巴細胞數增加，可發生於多種疾病時，如慢性淋巴細

variety of diseases, including chronic lymphocytic *leukaemia and infections due to viruses.

胞性白血病和病毒性感染。

lymphoedema *n.* an accumulation of lymph in the tissues, producing swelling. It may be due to a congenital abnormality of the lymphatic vessels or result from obstruction of the lymphatic vessels by a tumour, parasites, inflammation, or injury. The legs are most often affected. Treatment consists of elastic support, by stockings or bandages, and diuretic drugs. A variety of surgical procedures have been devised but with little success.

淋巴水腫 淋巴在組織內蓄積，引起腫脹。可由淋巴管先天性異常引起，也可爲腫瘤、寄生蟲、炎症或外傷阻塞淋巴管的結果。下肢最常受累。治療包括用彈性支持物如繃帶、長統襪以及使用利尿藥。曾設計了各種外科治療方法但收效甚微。

lymphogranuloma venereum a venereal disease that is caused by a virus and is most common in tropical regions. An initial lesion on the genitals is followed by swelling and inflammation of the lymph nodes in the groin; the lymph vessels in the genital region may become blocked, causing thickening of the skin of that area. Early treatment with sulphonamides or tetracyclines is usually effective.

病毒性淋巴肉芽腫 一種病毒引起的性病，最常見於熱帶地區。開始先有生殖器的損害，然後腹股溝部淋巴結腫大發炎，生殖器局部的淋巴管可被阻塞而引起該部位皮膚增厚。早期用磺胺類或四環素通常有效。

lymphography *n.* the technique of injecting *radio-opaque material into the lymphatic system in a particular region of the body so that X-ray photographs may be taken of the lymph vessels and nodes. Lymphography can indicate the presence of tumours in the lymphatic system.

淋巴造影術 將不透放射線的物質注入身體特定部位的淋巴系統內以拍攝淋巴結和淋巴管X線照片的技術。此法可證實淋巴系統內腫瘤的存在。

lymphoid tissue a tissue responsible for the production of lymphocytes and antibodies. It occurs as discrete organs, in the form of the lymph nodes, tonsils, thymus, and spleen, and also as diffuse groups of cells not separated from surrounding tissue.

淋巴組織 負責生成淋巴細胞和抗體的組織。可以形成獨立的器官，如淋巴結、扁桃腺、胸腺、脾；也可以細胞集聚的形式存在於各種組織中。

lymphoma *n.* any malignant tumour of lymph nodes, excluding Hodgkin's disease. There is a broad spectrum of malignancy, with prognosis ranging from a few months to many years. The patient usually shows evidence of mul-

淋巴瘤 除何傑金氏病以外的所有淋巴結惡性腫瘤。其惡性程度很不一致，患者存活期限爲數月到許多年。病人通常有多發性淋巴結腫大，並可有

tiple enlarged lymph nodes and may have constitutional symptoms such as weight loss, fever, and sweating. Disease is usually widespread, but in some cases is confined to a single area, such as the tonsil. Treatment is with drugs such as chlorambucil or combinations of cyclophosphamide, vincristine and prednisone, sometimes with the addition of doxorubicin and/or bleomycin; response to these drugs is often dramatic. Localized disease may be treated with radiotherapy followed by drugs.

體重減輕、發熱、出汗等全身症狀。疾病常廣泛蔓延，但有些病例僅某一局部受累，如扁桃體。治療藥物包括苯丁酸氮芥或氮芥與環磷醯胺、長春新鹼、强的松聯合使用，有時還可加用阿黴素和／或爭光黴素。對這些藥物的反應常十分顯著。局限性淋巴瘤可用放射治療後加藥物治療。

lymphopenia (lymphocytopenia) *n.* a decrease in the number of *lymphocytes in the blood, which may occur in a wide variety of diseases.

淋巴細胞減少 血內淋巴細胞數量減少，可發生於多種疾病。

lymphopoiesis *n.* the process of the production of *lymphocytes, which occurs in the *bone marrow as well as in the lymph nodes, spleen, thymus gland, and gut wall. The precursor cell from which lymphocytes are derived has not yet been identified.

淋巴細胞生成 發生在骨髓、脾、胸腺和腸壁內的淋巴細胞生成過程。分化爲淋巴細胞，前體細胞迄今尙未確定。

lymphorrhagia *n.* the escape of the lymph from lymphatic vessels that have been injured.

淋巴溢 淋巴從受損淋巴管內逸出。

lymphosarcoma *n.* an old term for certain types of *lymphoma. On the whole these tend to be the types with a better prognosis, and some may not need treatment for months or years after the patient has first been examined.

淋巴肉瘤 某種類型淋巴瘤的舊稱。總體來說，此類腫瘤預後較好，有的在病人初次查出腫瘤後數月甚至數年未予治療也無礙。

lymphuria *n.* the presence in the urine of lymph.

淋巴尿 尿中出現淋巴。

lynoestrenol *n.* a synthetic female sex hormone (*see* progestogen) used mainly in *oral contraceptives, together with an oestrogen. It is also used to treat menstrual disorders.

炔雌烯醇 一種合成的女性激素。主要與雌激素一起用作口服避孕藥。也用於治療月經紊亂。

lys- (lysi-, lyso-) *prefix denoting* lysis: dissolution.

〔前綴〕 **溶解**

lysergic acid diethylamide (LSD) a *psychedelic drug that is also a *hallucinogen. It has been used to aid treatment of psychological disorders. Side-effects include digestive upsets, dizziness, tingling, anxiety, sweating, dilated pupils, muscle incoordination and tremor. Alterations in sight, hearing and other senses occur, psychotic effects, depression, and confusion are common, and tolerance to the drug develops rapidly. Because of these toxic effects, LSD is used only to treat severe cases.

麥角醯二乙胺　一種引起幻覺的藥物，也是一種致幻原。一直用於精神障礙的輔助治療。副作用有：消化道不適、頭暈、麻刺感、焦慮、出汗、瞳孔擴大、共濟失調和震顫。可發生視覺、聽覺或其他感覺異常。精神症狀、抑鬱和精神錯亂常見。迅速發生耐藥性。由於有這些毒性作用，此藥只用於治療嚴重病例。

lysin *n.* a protein component in the blood that is capable of bringing about the destruction (lysis) of whole cells. Names are given to varieties of lysin with different targets; for example, *haemolysin* attacks red blood cells; *leucolysin* white cells; and a *bacteriolysin* bacterial cells.

溶素　血中的一種蛋白質成份，能破壞（溶解）完整的細胞。根據溶解的靶細胞的不同而命名爲不同的溶素，例如溶血素攻擊紅細胞，白細胞溶素破壞白細胞，溶菌素則能溶解細菌細胞。

lysine *n.* an *essential amino acid. *See also* amino acid.

賴氨酸　一種必需氨基酸。

lysis *n.* the destruction of cells through damage or rupture of the plasma membrane, allowing escape of the cell contents. *See also* autolysis, lysozyme.

溶解　藉損傷或破裂細胞膜而破壞細胞，結果造成細胞內容物外溢。

-lysis *suffix denoting* **1.** lysis; dissolution. **2.** remission of symptoms.

〔後綴〕　①**溶解**　②**症狀緩解**

lysogenic *adj.* producing *lysis.

致溶的　引起溶解的。

lysogeny *n.* an interaction between a *bacteriophage and its host in which a latent form of the phage (*prophage*) exists within the bacterial cell, which is not destroyed. Under certain conditions (e.g. irradiation of the bacterium) the phage can develop into an active form, which reproduces itself and eventually destroys the bacterial cell.

噬菌體生成　噬菌體與其宿主之間的一種相互作用過程。此時在細菌細胞內生成一種不活動型噬菌體，而細菌不被破壞。此種噬菌體在一定條件下（如用射線照射細菌）可變爲活動型，不斷增殖並最終破壞細菌細胞。

lysosome *n.* a particle in the cytoplasm of cells that contains enzymes responsible for breaking down sub-

溶酶體　細胞漿內的一種顆粒，內含一些分解細胞內物質的酶，外包一單層

stances in the cell and is bounded by a single membrane. Lysosomes are especially abundant in liver and kidney cells. Foreign particles (e.g. bacteria) taken into the cell are broken down by the enzymes of the lysosomes. When the cell dies, these enzymes are released to break down the cell's components.

膜。溶酶體在肝、腎細胞內特別豐富。異物（如細菌）被攝入細胞後，爲溶酶體的酶所分解。細胞死亡時這些酶被釋出，將細胞成分分解。

lysozyme *n.* an enzyme found in tears and egg white. It catalyses the destruction of the cell walls of certain bacteria. Bacterial cells that are attacked by lysozyme are said to have been *lysed*.

溶菌酶 眼淚和蛋清內的一種酶，能催化某些細菌的細胞壁分解。細菌被溶菌酶破壞的過程稱爲溶菌。

M

M

maceration *n.* **1.** the softening of a solid by leaving it immersed in a liquid. **2.** (in obstetrics) the natural breakdown of a dead fetus within the womb.

浸漬（浸軟） ①把固體浸泡在液體中使其軟化。②（產科）死胎在子宮內自然變形。

macr- (macro-) *prefix denoting* large size. Example: *macrencephaly* (abnormally enlarged brain).

〔前綴〕 **巨，大** 例如：巨腦（腦的異常增大）。

macrocephaly (megalocephaly) *n.* abnormal largeness of the head in relation to the rest of the body. *Compare* microcephaly.

巨頭 頭部異常增大與身體其它部位不成比例。

macrocheilia *n.* hypertrophy of the lips: a congenital condition in which the lips are abnormally large. *Compare* microcheilia.

巨唇 唇肥大：先天性唇異常增大。

macrocyte (megalocyte) *n.* an abnormally large red blood cell (*erythrocyte). *See also* macrocytosis. —**macrocytic** *adj.*

巨紅細胞 異常的大紅細胞。

macrocytosis *n.* the presence of abnormally large red cells (*macrocytes*) in the blood. Macrocytosis is a feature of certain anaemias (*macrocytic anaemias*), including those due to defic-

巨紅細胞症 血中存有異常的大紅細胞。巨紅細胞症是某些貧血（巨紅細胞性貧血），包括維生素 B_{12} 或葉酸缺乏性貧血和

iency of vitamin B_{12} or folic acid, and also of anaemias in which there is an increase in the rate of red cell production.

紅細胞生成速度過快的貧血的一個特徵。

macrodactyly *n.* abnormally large size of one or more of the fingers or toes.

巨指（趾） 一個成多個異常增大的指（趾）。

macrodontia *n.* a condition in which the teeth are unusually large.

巨牙 牙齒異常增大的現象。

macrogamete *n.* the nonmotile female sex cell of the malarial parasite (*Plasmodium*) and other single-celled animals (*see* Protozoa). The macrogamete is similar to the ovum of higher animal groups and larger than the male sex cell (*see* microgamete).

大配子 瘧疾寄生物（瘧原蟲）和其它單細胞動物的無運動的雌性細胞。大配子類似於高等動物的卵並且大於雄性細胞。

macrogametocyte *n.* a cell that undergoes meiosis to form mature female sex cells (macrogametes) of the malarial parasite (*Plasmodium*). Macrogametocytes are found in the blood of man but must be ingested by a mosquito before developing into macrogametes.

大配子體 瘧疾寄生物（瘧原蟲）經過減數分裂而形成成熟雌性細胞（大配子）的一種細胞。大配子體出現在人血中，但是必須通過蚊蟲消化道才能發育成大配子。

macrogenitosoma *n.* excessive bodily growth with marked enlargement of the genitalia. *Macrogenitosoma praecox* is a variant occurring in early childhood.

巨生殖器巨體 身體過度生長並伴有明顯增大的生殖器。早發性巨生殖器巨體是發生在幼年的變異。

macroglia *n.* one of the two basic classes of *glia (the non-nervous cells of the central nervous system), divided into *astrocytes and *oligodendrocytes. *Compare* microglia.

大神經膠質 兩種基本神經膠質中的一種（中樞神經系統的非神經細胞），分爲星形〔膠質〕細胞和少突神經膠質細胞。

macroglobulin (immunoglobulin M) *n.* a protein of the globulin series that is present in the blood and functions as an antibody, forming an effective first-line defence against bacteria in the bloodstream. *See also* immunoglobulin.

巨球蛋白（免疫球蛋白M） 血中具有抗體功能的球蛋白系中的一種蛋白，形成血流中抵禦細菌的第一道防線。

macroglobulinaemia *n.* the presence in the blood of an abnormal form of immunoglobulin-M (*see* macroglobulin), produced by a tumour of the lymphocytes.

巨球蛋白血症 血中出現由淋巴細胞瘤生成的異常的免疫球蛋白M。

macroglossia *n.* an abnormally large tongue. It may be due to a congenital defect, such as thyroid deficiency (cretinism); to infiltration of the tongue with *amyloid or a tumour; or to obstruction of the lymph vessels.

巨舌 異常大的舌。病因可爲先天性缺陷，如甲狀腺功能低下（克汀病），也可爲舌澱粉樣變或舌腫瘤的浸潤以及淋巴管阻塞。

macrognathia *n.* marked overgrowth of one jaw relative to the growth of the other.

巨頜 一側頜明顯地過度生長，與另一側不成比例。

macromastia *n.* abnormally large size of the breasts.

巨乳房 乳房異常增大。

macromelia *n.* abnormally large size of the arms or legs. *Compare* micromelia.

巨肢 上、下肢異常增大。

macronormoblast *n.* an abnormal form of any of the cells (*normoblasts) that form a series of precursors of red blood cells. Macronormoblasts are unusually large but have normal nuclei (*compare* megaloblast); they are seen in certain anaemias in which red cell production is impaired.

巨幼紅細胞 構成紅細胞前體系列的某種細胞（幼紅細胞）發生異常。巨幼紅細胞雖異常增大但胞核正常，可見於某些紅細胞生成障礙性貧血。

macrophage (clasmocyte) *n.* a large scavenger cell (a *phagocyte) present in connective tissue and many major organs and tissues, including the bone marrow, spleen, *lymph nodes, liver (*see* Kuppfer's cells), and the central nervous system (*see* microglia). They are closely related to *monocytes. *Fixed macrophages* (*histiocytes*) are stationary within connective tissue; *free macrophages* wander between cells and aggregate at focal sites of infection, where they remove bacteria or other foreign bodies from blood or tissues. *See also* reticuloendothelial system.

巨噬細胞 存在於結締組織和骨髓、脾、淋巴結、肝和中樞神經系統等許多主要器官和組織中的大游走細胞（清除細胞）。它們與單核細胞密切相關。固定的巨噬細胞（組織細胞）靜止地存在於結締組織內，游離的巨噬細胞游走於細胞間並聚集於感染竈內，以清除血液或組織中的細菌或異物。

macropolycyte *n.* an abnormal form of *neutrophil (a type of white blood cell) the nucleus of which has an excessively large number of lobes. Macropolycytes are seen in vitamin B_{12} or folic acid deficiency.

大多核白細胞 核葉過多的異常中性白細胞（一種白細胞）。大多核白細胞見於維生素B_{12}或葉酸缺乏時。

macropsia *n.* a condition in which objects appear larger than they really

視物顯大症 視物大於客觀物體。病因常爲黃斑受

are. It is usually due to disease of the retina affecting the *macula but may also occur in spasm of *accommodation and in some brain disorders.

損的視網膜疾病，但也可爲（眼）調節痙攣和一些腦疾病。

macroscopic *adj.* visible to the naked eye. *Compare* microscopic.

目視的 肉眼可見的。

macula *n.* (*pl.* **maculae**) **1.** a small anatomical area that is distinguishable from the surrounding tissue. The *macula lutea* is the yellow spot on the retina at the back of the eye, which surrounds the greatest concentration of cones (*see* fovea). Maculae occur in the saccule and utricle of the inner ear (see illustration). Tilting of the head causes the otoliths to bend the hair cells, which send impulses to the brain via the vestibular nerve. *See also* labyrinth. **2.** *see* macule.

斑 區別於周圍組織的一個小的解剖學部位。黃斑是位於眼後視網膜上的黃點，該處是視錐細胞最爲密集的地方。聽斑見於內耳的小囊和橢圓囊內（見圖）。頭的傾斜可引起耳石所致的毛細胞彎曲，後者可將神經衝動經過前庭神經傳送到腦。

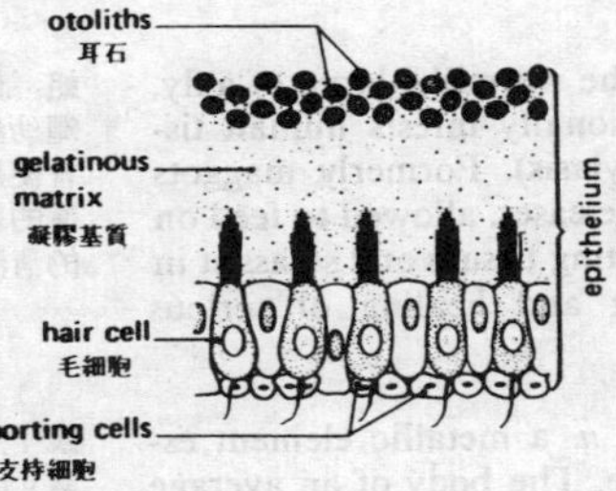

A macula of the inner ear
內耳的斑

macule (macula) *n.* a spot, discoloration, or thickening of the skin that forms a distinct area from the surrounding normal surface. *Compare* papule.

斑〔點〕 明顯不同於周圍正常皮膚表面的斑點、變色或增厚。

maculopapular *adj.* describing a rash that consists of both *macules and *papules.

斑丘疹的 由斑〔點〕和丘疹構成的皮疹。

madarosis *n.* **1.** a congenital deficiency of the eyelashes and eyebrows, which are sometimes absent altogether. **2.** a

睫毛脫落 ①睫毛或眼眉缺失的先天性疾病。有時二者均缺失。 ②慢性潰

deficiency of the eyelashes alone, caused by chronic ulcerative *blepharitis.

瘍性眼瞼炎所致的單純眼睫毛缺失。

Madura foot an infection of the tissues and bones of the foot producing chronic inflammation (mycetoma), occurring in the tropics. It is caused by various filamentous fungi (e.g. *Madurella*) and certain bacteria of the genera *Nocardia* and *Streptomyces*. Medical name: **maduromycosis**.

足分支菌病 脚骨和其它組織的眞菌感染造成的慢性炎症（足分支菌病），見於熱帶。病因爲各種絲狀眞菌（如：馬杜拉分支菌屬）及諾卡氏菌屬和鏈黴菌屬的某些黴菌。

Madurella *n.* a genus of widely distributed fungi. The species *M. grisea* and *M. mycetomi* cause the tropical infection *Madura foot.

馬杜拉分支菌屬 廣泛分佈的眞菌屬。灰色馬杜拉氏菌和足腫分支馬杜拉氏菌造成熱帶的感染——足分支菌病。

maduromycosis *n. see* Madura foot.

足分枝菌病

magenta *n. see* fuchsin.

品紅

maggot *n.* the wormlike larva of a fly, which occasionally infests human tissues (*see* myiasis). Formerly maggots were, in some cases, allowed to feed on dead and rotting tissues and so assist in the cleaning and healing of serious wounds.

蛆 偶然感染人組織的蒼蠅幼蟲。以前，某些病症曾使用蛆來吞食死亡和腐爛的組織以幫助重創傷口的清潔和修復。

magnesium *n.* a metallic element essential to life. The body of an average adult contains about 25 g of magnesium, concentrated mostly in the bones. Magnesium is necessary for the proper functioning of muscle and nervous tissue. It is required as a *cofactor for approximately 90 enzymes. A good source of magnesium is green leafy vegetables.

鎂 生命所必需的金屬元素。健康成人體內大約含25g 鎂，大多數集中於骨內。鎂是維持肌肉和神經組織正常功能所必需的。它是大約 90 種酶的輔因子。綠葉蔬菜是鎂的豐富來源。

magnesium carbonate a weak *antacid used to relieve indigestion and also pain due to stomach and duodenal ulcers; it is also used as a mild laxative. It is usually given with other compounds in mixtures, powders, and tablets.

碳酸鎂 治療消化不良和胃十二指腸潰瘍病的弱抗酸製劑。它也可作爲溫和的緩瀉劑。它通常與其它化合物一起被製成合劑、粉劑和片劑來使用。

magnesium hydroxide a magnesium salt with effects and uses similar to those of *magnesium carbonate. Trade name: **Milk of Magnesia**.

氫氧化鎂 一種類似於碳酸鎂的效果和用途的鎂鹽。商品名：鎂乳。

magnesium sulphate a magnesium salt given in mixtures or enemas to treat constipation (*see* laxative). It is also administered by injection to treat magnesium deficiency.

硫酸鎂 用以治療便秘的鎂鹽合劑或灌腸劑。硫酸鎂注射劑也可用於治療鎂缺乏。

magnesium trisilicate a compound of magnesium with antacid and absorbent properties, used in the treatment of peptic ulcers and other digestive disorders.

三硅酸鎂 具有抗酸和吸收特性的鎂化合物，用於治療消化性潰瘍和其它消化功能紊亂。

mal *n.* illness or disease. *See also* grand mal, petit mal.

病 疾病。

mal- *prefix denoting* disease, disorder, or abnormality.

〔前綴〕 **壞，惡，不良，疾病，紊亂，異常**

malabsorption *n.* a state in which absorption of one or more substances by the small intestine is reduced. It commonly affects fat (causing *steatorrhoea), vitamins (such as B_{12}, folic acid, vitamin D, and vitamin K), *electrolytes (such as calcium, potassium), iron, and amino acids. Symptoms (depending on the substances involved) include weight loss, diarrhoea, anaemia, swelling (oedema), and vitamin deficiencies. The commonest causes are *coeliac disease, *pancreatitis, *cystic fibrosis, *stagnant-loop syndrome, or surgical removal of a length of small intestine.

吸收障礙 小腸內一種或多種物質吸收減少。脂肪（引起脂肪痢）、維生素（如：B_{12}、葉酸、維生素D和維生素K）、電解質（如：鈣、鉀）、鐵和氨基酸的吸收常受影響。根據受影響的不同物質，可有體重減輕、腹瀉、貧血、腫脹（水腫）和維生素缺乏的症狀。常見病因爲麥膠過敏性腹瀉、胰腺炎、腸襻鬱滯綜合徵，或外科小腸部分切除。

malacia *n.* abnormal softening of a part, organ, or tissue, such as bone (*see* osteomalacia).

軟化 身體某部位、器官或組織如骨的異常軟化。

-malacia *suffix denoting* abnormal softening of a tissue. Example: *keratomalacia* (of the cornea).

〔後綴〕 **軟化** 指某組織的異常軟化。如：角膜軟化。

malaise *n.* a general feeling of being unwell. The feeling may be accompanied by identifiable physical discomfort and may indicate the presence of disease.

不適 一種全身的不適感。此不適感可伴有明確的身體某部的不適，並可表示存有某種疾病。

malar bone *see* zygomatic bone. **顴骨**

malaria (ague, marsh fever, periodic fever, paludism) *n.* an infectious disease due to the presence of parasitic protozoa of the genus **Plasmodium* (*P. falciparum*, *P. malariae*, *P. ovale*, or *P. vivax*) within the red blood cells. The disease is transmitted by the *Anopheles* mosquito and is confined mainly to tropical and subtropical areas.

瘧〔疾〕（瘧狀熱，沼澤熱，周期熱） 紅細胞內的瘧原蟲屬（惡性瘧原蟲，三日瘧原蟲，卵形瘧原蟲或間日瘧原蟲）的寄生原蟲所致的感染性疾病。此病經按蚊傳播，主要發生在熱帶和亞熱帶地區。

Parasites in the blood of an infected person are taken into the stomach of the mosquito as it feeds. Here they multiply and then invade the salivary glands. When the mosquito bites an individual, parasites are injected into the bloodstream and migrate to the liver and other organs, where they multiply. After an incubation period varying from 12 days (*P. falciparum*) to 10 months (some varieties of *P. vivax*), parasites return to the bloodstream and invade the red blood cells. Rapid multiplication of the parasites results in destruction of the red cells and the release of more parasites capable of infecting other red cells. This causes a short bout of shivering, fever, and sweating, and the loss of healthy red cells results in anaemia. When the next batch of parasites is released symptoms reappear. The interval between fever attacks varies in different types of malaria: in *quartan malaria* (or *fever*), caused by *P. malariae*, it is three days; in *tertian malaria* (*P. ovale* or *P. vivax*) two days; and in *malignant tertian* (or *quotidian*) *malaria* (*P. falciparum*) – the most severe kind – from a few hours to two days (*see also* blackwater fever). Preventative and curative treatment relies on such drugs as *chloroquine, *mepacrine, and *proguanil.

當蚊子叮咬已感染的人時，人血中的寄生物被帶入蚊子的胃內，在蚊子體內寄生繁殖並侵入唾液腺。當這種蚊子叮咬另一人時，寄生物進入血流而移居到肝臟和其它器官，並在那裏繁殖。經過12天（惡性瘧原蟲）到10個月（某些間日瘧原蟲的變種）的孵化期，寄生物回到血流並侵入紅細胞。寄生物的快速繁殖導致紅細胞的破壞，並釋放更多能感染其它紅細胞的寄生物。由此可引起短暫的寒顫、發熱、出汗和正常紅細胞減少所致的貧血。當下一批寄生物被釋放時，這些症狀重複出現。不同類型的瘧疾有不同的發熱間隔。由三日瘧原蟲引起的三日瘧（或熱），間隔期是三天；由卵形瘧原蟲或間日瘧原蟲引起的間日瘧，間隔期是二天；由惡性瘧原蟲引起的惡性瘧（或日發瘧）是最嚴重的類型，間隔期爲數小時到2天。有效的防治藥物爲氯喹、阿的平和氯胍。

Malassezia *n.* a genus of fungi producing superficial infections of the skin. The species *M. furfur* is the causative organism of a form of ringworm.

馬拉色氏黴菌屬 造成皮膚表面感染的眞菌屬。糠秕馬拉色氏黴菌種是一種癬菌病的病原生物體。

malformation *n.* any variation from the normal physical structure, due either to congenital or developmental defects or to disease or injury.

畸形 因先天或發育上的缺陷以及疾病或損傷所致的正常人體結構的變異。

malignant *adj.* **1.** describing a tumour that invades and destroys the tissue in which it originates and can spread to other sites in the body via the bloodstream and lymphatic system. If untreated such tumours cause progressive deterioration and death. *See* cancer. **2.** describing any disorder that becomes progressively worse if untreated. *Compare* benign.

惡性的 ①發生在身體某部的腫瘤能侵入和破壞其原發組織，並可經血流和淋巴系統傳播到其它部位的那種特性。如未經治療，這種腫瘤可進行性惡化並致死亡。 ②未經治療可進行性惡化的任何病症。

malingering *n.* pretending to be ill, usually in order to avoid work or gain attention. It may be a sign of mental disorder (*see* Munchhausen's syndrome).

裝病（詐病） 爲了引起別人注意或逃避工作而假裝有病。它可爲精神病的一種徵象。

malleolus *n.* either of the two protuberances on each side of the ankle: the *lateral malleolus* at the lower end of the *fibula or the *medial malleolus* at the lower end of the *tibia.

踝 踝關節兩邊的突起。外踝在腓骨的下端，而內踝在脛骨的下端。

malleus *n.* a hammer-shaped bone in the middle *ear that articulates with the incus and is attached to the eardrum. *See* ossicle.

錘骨 位於中耳的連接砧骨並附着在鼓膜上的錘形骨。

Mallory's triple stain a histological stain consisting of water-soluble aniline blue or methyl blue, orange G, and oxalic acid. Before the stain is applied the tissue is mordanted, then treated with acid fuchsin and phosphomolybdic acid. Nuclei stain red, muscle red to orange, nervous tissue lilac, collagen dark blue, and mucus and connective tissue become blue.

馬洛里氏三重染劑 由水溶苯胺藍或甲基藍、橙黃G和草酸構成的一種組織學染劑。使用染劑前，先用媒染劑處理組織，然後用酸品紅和磷鉬酸處理。核被染成紅色，肌肉由紅到橙黃色，神經組織爲淡紫色，膠原組織爲深藍色，黏液和結締組織則變爲藍色。

malnutrition *n.* the condition caused by an improper balance between what an individual eats and what he requires to maintain health. This can result from eating too little (*subnutrition* or *starvation*) but may also imply dietary excess or an incorrect balance of basic food-

營養不良 人體攝入的食物與健康所需的營養不平衡所致的疾病。病因可爲飲食過少（營養不足或飢餓），但也可爲飲食過度或像蛋白質、脂肪和碳水化合物等基本食物攝入不

stuffs such as protein, fat, and carbohydrate. A deficiency (or excess) of one or more minerals, vitamins, or other essential ingredients may arise from *malabsorption of digested food or metabolic malfunction of one or more parts of the body as well as from an unbalanced diet.

平衡。身體某個或多個部位代謝機能障礙，或已消化的食物吸收障礙，以及不平衡飲食可造成一種或多種礦物質、維生素或其它基本成分的缺少（或過多）。

malocclusion *n.* the condition in which the upper and lower teeth are abnormally related.

錯𬌗 上下齒相對關係異常的狀態。

Malpighian body the part of a *nephron comprising the blood capillaries of the glomerulus and its surrounding Bowman's capsule.

馬爾皮基氏小體 由腎小球的毛細血管和它周圍的鮑曼氏囊組成的腎單位的一部分。

Malpighian layer the stratum germinativum: one of the layers of the *epidermis.

馬爾皮基氏層 表皮生發層。爲多層表皮中的一層。

malposition *n.* abnormal location of any part of the body.

錯位 身體任一部分的位置異常。

malpractice *n.* professional misconduct: treatment falling short of the standards of skill and care that can reasonably be expected from a qualified medical practitioner.

醫療差錯 醫務工作中的失誤。因達不到合格的醫務人員所應有的技術標準和疏忽大意所造成的醫療處置失當。

malpresentation *n.* arrival of the fetus at the opening from the womb other than in the normal head-first position (*see* presentation). Malpresentation is likely to make birth difficult and may necessitate delivery by *Caesarean section.

先露異常 胎兒到達子宮口時不同於正常頭先露的位置。先露異常易引起難產並有可能要做剖腹產。

malt *n.* a mixture of carbohydrates, predominantly maltose, produced by the breakdown of starch contained in barley or wheat grains. The cereal grain is allowed to germinate and the malt is extracted with hot water. Malt is used for brewing and distilling; it has been used as a source of nutrients in wasting diseases.

麥芽浸液 由大麥或小麥粒中的澱粉分解產生的以麥芽糖爲主的碳水化合物的混合液。先使麥粒生芽，再用熱水浸出麥芽汁，用於釀造和蒸餾。在消耗性疾病中可用作營養物的一種來源。

Malta fever *see* brucellosis.

馬耳他熱

maltase *n.* an enzyme, present in saliva and pancreatic juice, that converts maltose into glucose during digestion.

麥芽糖酶 唾液和胰液中的能將麥芽糖轉化爲葡萄糖的消化酶。

maltose *n.* a sugar consisting of two molecules of glucose. Maltose is formed from the digestion of starch and glycogen and is found in germinating cereal seeds.

麥芽糖 由葡萄糖的兩分子構成的一種糖。麥芽糖在澱粉和糖原的消化時形成，並且存在於生芽的穀種中。

malunion *n.* deformity of a bone resulting from *union of a fracture in which the bone ends are poorly aligned. Arthritis of adjoining joints may develop as a complication later. *Osteotomy may be needed to correct the deformity and prevent the complication.

〔骨〕連接不正 骨折癒合斷端對接不良所致的骨畸形。鄰近關節的關節炎可能成爲繼發合併症。截骨術可矯正畸形和預防併發症。

mamilla *n. see* nipple.

乳頭

mamillary bodies two paired rounded swellings in the floor of the *hypothalamus, immediately behind the pituitary gland.

乳頭小體 直接位於垂體腺後下丘腦底的兩對圓形隆起。

mamma *n. see* breast.

乳房

mammary gland the milk-producing gland of female mammals. *See* breast.

乳腺 雌性哺乳動物的生乳腺。

mammography *n.* the making of X-ray or infra-red ray photographs of the breast: used for the early detection of abnormal growths. *See also* radiography, thermography.

乳房X線照像術 乳房X線或紅外線照像，用於早期發現異常腫物。

mammoplasty *n.* plastic surgery of the breasts, in order to alter their shape or increase or decrease their size. In the case of sagging breasts skin and glandular tissue are removed and the remaining breast tissue is fixed in the normal position. When the breasts are too small, a *prosthesis may be inserted to improve the contour.

乳房成形術 改變乳房外形和增大或減小乳房的整形外科手術。對乳房下垂的病人，可去除胸部的皮膚和腺體組織，然後將剩餘的乳房組織固定在正常的位置上。當乳房過小時，可植入假體以改善外形。

mammothermography *n.* the technique of examining the breasts for the presence of tumours or other abnormalities by *thermography.

乳房溫度記錄法 用溫度記錄法來檢查乳房腫瘤或其它異常的技術。

M-AMSA (amsacrine) *n.* a *cytotoxic drug undergoing evaluation in the treatment of malignant disease. Side-effects include marrow suppression.

胺苯吖啶 經臨床證實的有效的治療惡性病的細胞毒性藥。副作用有骨髓抑制。

mancinism *n.* the condition of being left-handed.

左利　善用左手。

mandelic acid a drug that prevents bacterial growth and was formerly used to treat infections of the urinary system (it has now largely been replaced by antibiotics). Mandelic acid is administered by mouth.

杏仁酸　預防細菌生長的藥物，曾用於治療泌尿系感染（現在大都已被抗生素取代）。杏仁酸爲口服藥。

mandible *n.* the lower jawbone. It consists of a horseshoe-shaped *body*, the upper surface of which bears the lower teeth (*see* alveolus (def. 2)), and two vertical parts (*rami*). Each ramus divides into a *condyle* and a *coronoid process. The condyle articulates with the temporal bone of the cranium to form the *temporomandibular joint* (a hinge joint). *See also* maxilla, skull. —**mandibular** *adj.*

下頜骨　包括馬蹄形的骨體（其上面支持着下齒）和兩個垂直的部分（支）。每一個支分成一個髁和一個冠狀突。髁與顱的顳骨相連形成顳下頜關節（屈戌關節）。

manganese *n.* a greyish metallic element, the oxide of which, when inhaled by miners in under-ventilated mines, causes brain damage and symptoms very similar to those of *parkinsonism.

錳　淺灰色的金屬元素。在通風不良的井下，礦工吸入錳的氧化物後，可引起腦損傷，並出現類似於帕金森氏綜合徵的症狀。

mania *n.* a state of mind characterized by excessive cheerfulness and increased activity. The mood is euphoric and changes rapidly to irritability. Thought and speech are rapid to the point of incoherence and the connections between ideas may be impossible to follow. Behaviour is overactive, extravagant, overbearing, and sometimes violent. Judgment is impaired, and therefore the sufferer may damage his own interests. There may be grandiose delusions. Treatment is usually with drugs such as lithium or phenothiazines. Hospital admission is frequently necessary. Lithium can also be taken to prevent relapses. *See* manic-depressive psychosis. —**manic** *adj.*

躁狂　以過度歡欣和極其活躍爲特徵的精神狀態。病人情緒欣快並且很易激動。病人可有快速的不連貫的思維和語言，不可能把病人的想法互相聯繫起來。行爲過度活躍、放肆、專橫，有時是狂暴的。判斷力受損，因此患者可做出傷害自身的事。可有誇大妄想。通常可用鋰或吩噻嗪類藥物治療。常需住院。鋰亦用於預防復發。

-mania *suffix denoting* obsession, compulsion, or exaggerated feeling for. Example: *pyromania* (for starting fires).

〔後綴〕　狂，癖　指强迫觀念、强迫行爲或誇大的感覺。例如：放火狂。

manic-depressive psychosis a severe mental illness causing repeated episodes of *depression, *mania, or both. These episodes can be precipitated by upsetting events but are out of proportion to these causes. Sometimes chronic depression or chronic mania can result. There is a genetically inherited predisposition to the illness. Treatment is with *phenothiazine drugs for mania and with *antidepressant drugs or *electroconvulsive therapy for depression. *Lithium can prevent or reduce the frequency and severity of attacks, and the sufferer is usually well in the intervals between them.

躁狂抑鬱性精神病 躁狂、抑鬱或二者反復發作所致的一種嚴重精神病。這些發作可因心緒煩亂而突然發生，但病因與病情不成比例。有時可致慢性抑鬱或慢性躁狂。有遺傳素質的人易患此病。可用吩噻嗪類藥物治療躁狂，用抗抑鬱藥或電驚厥療法治療抑鬱。鋰可預防或減少發作的頻度並減輕其程度。在發作間期，患者通常情況良好。

manikin *n. see* homunculus.

人體模型

manipulation *n.* the use of the hands to produce a desired movement or therapeutic effect in part of the body. Physiotherapists and osteopaths use manipulation to restore normal working to stiff joints.

推拿術 用手在身體某部進行有目的的運動，發揮治療作用。理療和整骨師用推拿術恢復僵直關節的正常功能。

mannitol *n.* a *diuretic administered by injection to supplement other diuretics in the treatment of fluid retention (oedema), to treat some kidney disorders, and to relieve pressure in brain injuries. Headache, chest pain, and dry mouth may occur following injection.

甘露醇 一種利尿藥。在治療液體滯留（水腫）時，通過注射給藥來加强其它利尿藥作用，用以治療某些腎臟病和緩解腦損傷後的顱內壓。注射後可有頭痛、胸痛和口乾的症狀。

mannomustine *n.* a drug that prevents the growth of cancer cells and is used in the treatment of some types of leukaemia and other cancers. It is administered by injection or by mouth and often causes nausea and vomiting. Trade name: **Degranol**.

甘露醇氮芥 可預防癌細胞的生長並可治療不同類型的白血病和其它癌症的藥物。注射或口服。常引起噁心或嘔吐。

Mann-Whitney U test *see* significance.

曼-惠（特尼）二氏U檢驗 非參數性檢驗。

manometer *n.* a device for measuring pressure in a gas. A manometer often consists of a U-tube containing mercury, water, or other liquid, open at one end and exposed to the gas under pressure at the other end. The pressure can be read directly from a graduated scale. *See also* sphygmomanometer.

測壓計 測量氣體中壓力的器械。測壓計常爲一U形管，含有水銀、水或其它液體，開口於一端，而另一端與受壓氣體相接觸，從刻度上可直接讀出壓力。

manpower committee (in Britain) a special committee established regionally (*Regional Manpower Committee*) and centrally (*Central Manpower Committee*) by the Department of Health and Social Security to advise on medical staffing by specialty and to consider the relative numbers of consultants and training grades of doctors in the National Health Service.

人力委員會（英國） 由保健和社會保障部建立的地區性（地區人力委員會）和中央性（中央衛生人力委員會）的特殊委員會。它對國民保健服務制中各專業醫務人員的設置提出建議，並考慮醫師的相對數量及醫生的培訓級別。

Manpower Services Commission *see* Employment Service Division.

人力服務委員會

Mantoux test *see* tuberculin.

芒圖氏試驗

manubrium *n.* (*pl.* **manubria**) **1.** the upper section of the breastbone (*see* sternum). It articulates with the clavicles and the first costal cartilage; the second costal cartilage articulates at the junction between the manubrium and body of the sternum. **2.** the handle-like part of the *malleus (an ear ossicle), attached to the eardrum. —**manubrial** *adj.*

柄 ①胸骨上部。它連接鎖骨和第一肋軟骨，第二肋軟骨連接在胸骨柄和胸骨體的接合處。②附着在鼓膜上的錘骨（一個耳小骨）的柄部。

MAO *see* monoamine oxidase.

單胺氧化酶

MAO inhibitor a drug that prevents the activity of the enzyme *monoamine oxidase (MAO) in brain tissue and therefore affects mood. MAO inhibitors include *iproniazid, isocarboxacid, *phenelzine, and *tranylcypromine. They are *antidepressants, whose use is now restricted because of the severity of their side-effects. These include interactions with other drugs (e.g. ephedrine, amphetamine) and foods containing *tyramine (e.g. cheese) to produce a sudden increase in blood pressure.

單胺氧化酶抑制劑 阻抑單胺氧化酶在腦組織中的活性並因此影響情緒的藥物。單胺氧化酶抑制劑包括異煙醯異丙肼、馬普蘭、苯乙肼和苯環丙胺。這些都是抗抑鬱藥，因其有與其它藥物（如：麻黃鹼，苯異丙胺）和含有酪胺的食物（如：乳酪）相互作用，而使血壓突然升高的嚴重副作用，現在已限制使用。

maple syrup urine disease an inborn defect of amino acid metabolism causing an excess of valine, leucine, isoleucine, and alloisoleucine in the urine, which has an odour like maple syrup. Untreated it leads to mental retardation and death in infancy.

楓糖尿症 氨基酸代謝的先天性缺陷所致的尿中纈氨酸、亮氨酸、異亮氨酸和別異亮氨酸過多，使尿具有楓糖的氣味。不經治療可致精神發育遲緩和嬰兒死亡。

maprotiline *n.* a drug used to treat all types of depression, including that associated with anxiety (*see* antidepressant). It is administered by mouth and may cause drowsiness, dizziness, and tremor. Trade name: **Ludiomil**.

麥普替林 治療包括與焦慮有關的各類抑鬱症的藥物。口服。可引起瞌睡、頭暈和震顫。

marasmus *n.* severe wasting in infants, when body weight is below 75% of that expected for age. The infant looks 'old', pallid, apathetic, lacks skin fat, and has subnormal temperature. The condition may be due to *malabsorption, wrong feeding, metabolic disorders, repeated vomiting, diarrhoea, severe disease of the heart, lungs, kidneys, or urinary tract, or chronic bacterial or parasitic disease (especially in tropical climates). Maternal rejection of an infant may cause marasmus through undereating. Acute infection may precipitate death. Treatment depends on the underlying cause, but initially very gentle nursing and the provision of nourishment and fluids by gradual steps is appropriate for all.

兒童消瘦 體重低於其年齡標準體重75%的嬰兒嚴重消耗性疾病。患兒顯得“老”，蒼白，淡漠，缺少皮下脂肪，體溫低於正常。病因可爲吸收不良，餵養不當，代謝紊亂，反復嘔吐、腹瀉，嚴重的心、肺、腎或泌尿道疾病及慢性的細菌或寄生蟲病（特別是在熱帶）。嬰兒母親拒絕餵食可致攝入過少造成的消瘦。急性感染可致突然死亡。治療取決於基本的病因，但最初非常耐心的護理和逐步供給營養和體液，適用於所有病例。

marble-bone disease *see* osteopetrosis.

骨硬化病

Marburg disease (green monkey disease) a virus disease of vervet (green) monkeys transmitted to man by contact (usually in laboratories) with blood or tissues from an infected animal. Symptoms include fever, malaise, severe headache, vomiting, diarrhoea and bleeding from mucous membranes in the mouth and elsewhere. Treatment with antiserum and measures to reduce the bleeding are sometimes effective.

馬伯格病（綠猴病） 通過接觸（通常在實驗室內）已感染動物的血液或組織，由綠猴傳染給人的一種病毒性疾病。可有發熱、不適、嚴重頭痛、嘔吐、腹瀉和口或其它地方黏膜出血的症狀。有時抗血清療法和減少出血的措施是有效的。

Marfan's syndrome an inherited disorder of connective tissue characterized by excessive height, abnormally long and slender fingers and toes (*arachnodactyly*), heart defects, and partial dislocation of the lenses of the eyes.

馬凡氏綜合征 以身體過高，指、趾異常的長而細，心臟缺陷和眼晶狀體部分脫位爲特徵的遺傳性結締組織疾病。

marihuana *n.* *see* cannabis.

大麻葉

marrow *n.* *see* bone marrow.

骨髓

marsupialization *n.* an operative technique for curing a cyst. The cyst is opened, its contents removed, and the edges then stitched to the skin incision. The wound is kept open until it has healed by *granulation.

造袋術 治療囊腫的手術方法。切開囊腫，清除內容物，然後把囊腫邊緣與皮膚切口縫合起來。開放傷口直到肉芽組織生出，傷口愈口。

Marzine *n. see* cyclizine.

賽克利嗪

masculinization *n.* development of excess body and facial hair, deepening of the voice, and increase in muscle bulk (secondary male sexual characteristics) in a female due to a hormone disorder or to hormone therapy. *See also* virilism, virilization.

男性化 因激素紊亂或激素療法所致的女性體毛和鬍鬚過度發育，嗓音低沉，肌肉發達（男性第二特徵）。

masochism *n.* sexual pleasure derived from the experience of pain. The word is sometimes used loosely for all forms of behaviour that lead to pain or humiliation. *See* perversion. **—masochist** *n.* **—masochistic** *adj.*

受虐狂 因疼痛而獲得的性快感。此詞有時可泛指各種造成疼痛或羞辱的行爲。

massage *n.* manipulation of the soft tissues of the body with the hands. Massage is used to improve circulation, reduce oedema where present, prevent *adhesions in tissues after injury, reduce muscular spasm, and improve the tone of muscles. *See also* effleurage, petrissage, tapotement.

按摩法 用手操作的身體軟組織推拿術。推拿術用於改善循環，減少存在的水腫，預防損傷後的組織黏連，減少肌肉痙攣，如改善肌肉的緊張度。

masseter *n.* a thick muscle in the cheek extending from the zygomatic arch to the outer corner of the mandible. It is important for mastication and acts by closing the jaws.

咬肌 從顴骨弓到下頜骨外角的頰部厚肌肉。它的作用是關閉上下頜，在咀嚼中起重要作用。

mast- (masto-) *prefix denoting* the breast.

〔前綴〕 **乳房**

mastalgia *n.* pain in the breast.

乳腺痛 乳房疼痛。

mastatrophy (mastatrophia) *n.* reduction in size (atrophy) of the breasts.

乳腺萎縮 乳腺的體積減少。

mast cell a large cell in *connective tissue with many coarse cytoplasmic granules. These granules contain the chemicals *heparin, *histamine, and *serotonin, which are released during inflammation and allergic responses.

肥大細胞 結締組織中帶有許多粗細胞質顆粒的大細胞。在炎症和過敏反應時，這些含有肝素、組胺和血清素類化學物質的顆粒被釋放。

mastectomy *n.* surgical removal of a breast. If the operation is to combat cancer a *radical mastectomy* is performed: as well as the breast itself, the lymph nodes in the nearest armpit and the muscles linking the upper part of the chest with the shoulder are also removed, in case the cancer has spread to them.

乳房切除術 外科切除乳房。如果手術治療乳腺癌，就應做乳房根治術。除了切除乳房以外，還應切除已被癌症侵犯的附近腋窩上的淋巴結，以及連接上胸部和肩的肌肉。

mastication *n.* the process of chewing food.

咀嚼 咀嚼食物的過程。

mastitis *n.* inflammation of the breast, usually caused by bacterial infection through damaged nipples. It most often occurs as acute *puerperal mastitis*, which develops during the period of breast-feeding, about a month after childbirth, and sometimes involves the discharge of pus. Chronic *cystic mastitis* has a different cause and does not involve inflammation. The breast feels lumpy due to the presence of cysts, and the condition is thought to be caused by hormone imbalance.

乳腺炎 經受損乳頭的細菌感染所致的乳腺炎。常見的是發生在產後一個月的餵乳期的急性產後乳腺炎。有時流膿。慢性囊性乳腺炎的病因不同，並不伴有炎症。因有囊腫，乳房可凹凸不平，此病可爲激素不平衡所致。

mastoid *n.* the *mastoid process of the temporal bone. *See also* mastoiditis.

乳突

mastoidectomy *n.* an operation to remove some or all of the air cells in the bone behind the ear (the *mastoid process of the temporal bone) when they have become infected (*see* mastoiditis).

乳突切除術 部分或全部切除耳後骨內（顳骨的乳狀突）受感染的含氣腔的手術。

mastoiditis *n.* inflammation of the *mastoid process behind the ear and of the air space (*mastoid antrum*) connecting it to the cavity of the middle ear. It is usually caused by bacterial infection that spreads from the middle ear (*see* otitis (media)). Usually the infection responds to antibiotics, but surgery (*see* mastoidectomy) may be required in severe cases.

乳突炎 耳後乳突以及連接乳突至中耳腔的氣腔（乳突竇）的炎症。病因常爲中耳的細菌感染。通常用抗生素治療有效。重症者可行外科手術。

mastoidotomy *n.* surgical incision of the mastoid bone, usually done to treat infection (*see* mastoidectomy).

乳突鑿開術 外科切開乳突骨，常用於治療感染。

mastoid process a nipple-shaped process on the *temporal bone that extends downward and forward behind the ear canal and is the point of attachment of several neck muscles. It contains many air spaces (*mastoid cells*), which communicate with the cavity of the middle ear via an air-filled channel, the *mastoid antrum*. This provides a possible route for the spread of infection from the middle ear (*see* mastoiditis).

乳突 顳骨上的乳頭狀突，在耳道後向前下方延伸，爲數個頸肌的附着點。它含有許多氣腔（乳突房），經過充滿氣體的管道（乳突竇）與中耳腔相通。這就爲中耳感染的傳播提供了可能的途徑。

mastoplasia (mazoplasia) *n.* increase in the size of the breasts because of multiplication and growth (*hyperplasia) of normal mammary gland cells.

乳房組織增生 因正常的乳腺細胞增殖和生長（增生）所致的乳房體積的增大。

mastoptosis *n.* sagging of the breasts.

乳房下垂

masturbation *n.* physical stimulation of the male or female external genital organs in order to produce sexual pleasure, which may result in orgasm.

手淫 物理刺激男子或女子的外生殖器，以誘發性快感，可達到性慾高潮。

matched pair study *see* case control study.

配對研究

materia medica the study of drugs used in medicine, including *pharmacognosy, *pharmacy, *pharmacology, and therapeutics.

藥物學 醫療用藥的研究。包括生藥學、藥物學、藥理學和治療學。

maternal mortality rate the number of deaths due to complications of pregnancy, childbirth, and the puerperium expressed as a proportion of all births (i.e. including *stillbirths). Formerly the rate was expressed per 1000 births but with the low levels currently reported it is customary to use a base of a 100,000 births. Concern with maternal mortality resulted in Britain in a special confidential enquiry being held into every such death to try and pinpoint the possible shortfall in resources or care.

母親死亡率 妊娠、分娩、產褥期的併發症造成的死亡數目對所有出生數目（即包括死產）的比例。以前是以每 1000 出生次數來表示，但是根據近期報告，母親死亡率很低，故習慣以每 100000 次出生爲基數來表示。隨着對母親死亡率的關注，在英國對這類死亡病例中的每一個人進行了特殊的調查，以努力找出可能存在的對病人關心照顧不够和所需物品供給不足的問題。

matrix *n.* the substance of a tissue or organ in which more specialized structures are embedded; for example, the ground substance of connective tissue.

基質 某一組織或器官中包埋着形態特化的結構的均質性物質。例如：結締組織的基質。

matrix band a flexible strip that is placed round a tooth to restore a wall, thus simplifying insertion of a dental filling.

基層帶 放在牙周圍形成一個壁的柔性帶，以便於插入牙充填物。

maturation *n.* the process of attaining full development. The term is applied particularly to the development of mature germ cells (ova and sperm).

成熟 達到充分發育的過程。特指成熟的胚芽細胞（卵子和精子）的發育。

maxilla *n.* (*pl.* **maxillae** or **maxillas**) loosely, the upper jaw, which bears the upper teeth. Strictly, the maxilla is one of a pair of bones that partly form the upper jaw, the outer walls of the maxillary sinus, and the floor of the orbit. *See also* mandible, skull. —**maxillary** *adj.*

上頜骨 一般指支承上齒的整個上頜。嚴格地說，上頜骨爲形成上頜的一對骨中的一塊骨，它形成上頜竇外壁和眼眶底的一部。

maxillary sinus (maxillary antrum) *see* paranasal sinuses.

上頜竇

maxillofacial *adj.* describing or relating to the region of the face, jaws, and related structures.

頜面的 指面部、頜部及其有關結構的（例如：頜面外科手術）。

maxwell *n.* a unit of magnetic flux equal to a flux of 1 gauss per square centimetre.

麥克斯韋 相當於每平方厘米1高斯通量的磁通量單位。

mazindol *n.* a drug that reduces the appetite and is used in the treatment of obesity. It is administered by mouth and may cause constipation, dry mouth, and insomnia. Trade name: **Teronac**.

氯苯咪吲哚 可減少食慾的治療肥胖症的藥物。口服。副作用可有便秘、口乾和失眠。

McBurney's point the point on the abdomen that overlies the anatomical position of the appendix and is the site of maximum tenderness in acute appendicitis. It lies one-third of the way along a line drawn from the anterior superior iliac spine (the projecting part of the hipbone) to the umbilicus.

麥克伯尼氏點 相應於闌尾解剖部位腹壁上的點。它是急性闌尾炎的最痛的觸痛點。位於髂前上棘（髖骨的突出部分）到臍連線的外三分之一處。

meals on wheels *see* social services.

運送上門飲食

mean (arithmetic mean) *n.* the average of a group of observations calculated by adding their values and dividing by the number in the group. When one or more observations are substan-

均值（算術平均值） 將觀測組中的各觀測值相加，除以組中的觀測次數，計算出的平均數。當一個以上的觀測值與其它

tially different from the rest, which can influence the arithmetic mean unduly, it is preferable to use the *geometric mean* (a similar calculation based on the logarithmic values of the observations) or – more commonly – the *median* (the middle observation of the series arranged in ascending order). A further method of obtaining an average value of a group is to identify the *mode* – the observation (or group of observations when these occur as a continuous quantitative *variable) that occurs most often in the series.

觀測值相差懸殊，它可過度影響算術平均數時，可使用幾何均數（一種基於觀測對數值的類似計算），更常用的是中位數（按遞增順序排列的數列的中部觀測值）。獲得某組均值的另一個方法是識別衆數——即在數列中最常出現的一個觀測值（如觀測值爲連續的變量，則爲一組觀測值）。

measles *n.* a highly infectious virus disease that tends to appear in epidemics every 2–3 years and mainly affects children. After an incubation period of 8–15 days, symptoms resembling those of a cold develop accompanied by a high fever. Small red spots with white centres (*Koplik's spots*) may appear on the inside of the cheeks. On the third to fifth day a blotchy slightly elevated pink rash develops, first behind the ears then on the face and elsewhere; it lasts 3–5 days. The patient is infectious throughout this period. In most cases the symptoms soon subside but patients are susceptible to pneumonia and middle ear infections. Complete recovery may take 2–4 weeks. Vaccination against measles provides effective immunity. Medical names: **rubeola, morbilli**.

麻疹 主要影響兒童的趨向於每2～3年流行一次的高度感染的病毒性疾病。8～15天的潛伏期後，與感冒類似的症狀加重並伴有高燒。頰內出現中心發白的小紅點（科潑力克氏斑）。在第3～5天，首先在耳後，然後在臉及其它部位出現粉紅色的斑丘疹，可持續3～5天。在這個期間，病人是有傳染性的。在大多數病例中，症狀很快消失，但病人易患肺炎和中耳炎。完全恢復需2～4周。麻疹疫苗接種可起有效的免疫作用。

meat- (meato-) *prefix denoting* a meatus. Example: *meatotomy* (incision into the urethral meatus).

〔前綴〕 **道（口）** 管道的開口。例如：尿道口切開術（切開尿道口）。

meatus *n.* (in anatomy) a passage or opening. The *external auditory meatus* is the passage leading from the pinna of the outer *ear to the eardrum. A *nasal meatus* is one of three groovelike parts of the nasal cavity beneath each of the nasal conchae. The *urethral meatus* is the external opening of the urethra.

道 （解剖學）道或口。外耳道是從外耳的耳廓到鼓室的通道。鼻道是在每一個鼻甲下鼻腔的三個溝樣部分之一。尿道口是尿道的外口。

mecamylamine *n.* a drug used to lower high blood pressure. It is administered by mouth and may cause dizziness, blurred vision, digestive upsets, and dry mouth. Trade name: **Inversine**.

美加明 一種降壓藥。口服。服後可有頭暈，視物不清，消化不良和口乾的現象。

mechanoreceptor *n.* a group of cells that respond to mechanical distortion, such as that caused by stretching or compressing a tissue, by generating a nerve impulse in a sensory nerve (*see* receptor). Touch receptors, *proprioceptors, and the receptors for hearing and balance all belong to this class.

機械感受器 通過在感覺神經中產生神經衝動，對牽拉、壓擠所致的機械變形起反應的一組細胞。其中包括觸覺感受器、本體感受器和聽覺及平衡感受器。

mechanotherapy *n.* the use of mechanical equipment during physiotherapy to produce regularly repeated movements in part of the body. This is done to improve the functioning of muscles and joints.

機械療法 在理療中，利用器械的物理作用，在身體某部位產生有規律的反復運動。此法用於改善肌肉和關節的功能。

Meckel's cartilage a cartilaginous bar in the fetus around which the *mandible develops. Part of Meckel's cartilage develops into the malleus (an ear ossicle) in the adult.

美克爾氏軟骨 下頷骨在其周圍發育的胎兒棒狀軟骨。成人後，部分美克爾氏軟骨發育成錘骨（一種耳骨）。

Meckel's diverticulum *see* diverticulum.

美克爾氏憩室

meclozine *n.* an *antihistamine drug used mainly to prevent and treat nausea and vomiting, particularly in travel sickness, and also to relieve allergic reactions. It is administered by mouth.

敏克靜 主要用於預防和治療噁心和嘔吐，特別是暈動病的抗組胺藥。此藥也可治療變態反應。口服。

meconism *n.* poisoning from the effects of eating or smoking *opium or the products derived from it, especially *morphine.

阿片中毒 吃或吸阿片或其製品，特別是嗎啡所致的中毒。

meconium *n.* the first stools of a newborn baby, which are sticky and dark green and composed of cellular debris, mucus, and bile pigments. The presence of meconium in the amniotic fluid during labour indicates fetal distress. *See also* (meconium) ileus.

胎糞 由細胞碎屑、黏液和膽汁色素組成的黏稠的暗綠色的新生兒初便。在分娩時羊水中存有胎糞，表明胎兒呼吸窘迫。

media (tunica media) *n.* **1.** the middle layer of the wall of a *vein or *artery. It

①**血管中膜** 靜脈或動脈壁的中層。它是由彈力纖

is the thickest of the three layers, being composed of elastic fibres and smooth muscle fibres in alternating layers. **2.** the middle layer of various other organs or parts.

維和平滑肌纖維交替組成的三層壁組織中最厚的一層。 ②**中層** 各種其它器官或部位的中層。

medial *adj.* relating to or situated in the central region of an organ, tissue, or the body.

中部的 位於某器官、組織或身體的中部或與之有關的。

median *adj.* **1.** (in anatomy) situated in or towards the plane that divides the body into right and left halves. **2.** (in statistics) *see* mean.

①**正中的** 解剖學用語。把身體分成左右兩半的平面上的。 ②**中位數** 統計學用語。

mediastinitis *n.* inflammation of the midline partition of the chest cavity (mediastinum), usually complicating a rupture of the oesophagus (gullet).

縱隔炎 胸腔中線隔膜（縱隔）的炎症，通常合併食道破裂。

mediastinum *n.* the space in the thorax (chest cavity) between the two pleural sacs. The mediastinum contains the heart, aorta, trachea, oesophagus, and thymus gland and is divided into anterior, middle, posterior, and superior regions.

縱隔 胸（胸腔）中兩個胸膜囊之間的間隙。縱隔含有心臟、主動脉、氣管、食道和胸腺，並且被分成前、中、後和上部。

medical *adj.* **1.** of or relating to medicine, the diagnosis, treatment and prevention of disease. **2.** of or relating to conditions that require the attention of a physician rather than a surgeon. For example, a *medical ward* accommodates patients with such conditions.

①**醫學的** 與疾病的診斷、治療和預防有關的，與醫藥有關的。 ②**內科的** 屬於內科醫生管的病或與其有關的，不屬外科醫生工作範圍的。如：內科病房收住患內科病的病人。

medical certificate a certificate stating a doctor's diagnosis of a patient's medical condition, disability, or fitness to work.

診斷書 表明病人醫療情況、傷殘程度和工作能力的醫生證明書。

medical committee 1. (in a hospital) a group of doctors of consultant grade (some or all of the consultants on the hospital staff) who give medical viewpoints on affairs concerned with overall policies on patient care, resource allocation, and the running of the hospital. Representatives of other hospital professions (nursing, administration, planning, and junior doctors) are usually in

醫學委員會 ①（在醫院裏）對有關病人醫療護理、物資分配和醫院管理等事項的總政策從專業觀點提出意見的經治醫師級組織（醫院內的部分或全體經治醫師）。醫院其它方面的代表（護士、管理人員、計劃人員和低年醫生）通常出席此委員會會

attendance. It is generally subdivided into specialist subgroups known colloquially as the *Cogwheel divisions*, representing the broad divisions of hospital practice (medical, surgical, paediatric, etc.). Usually the chairmen of each Cogwheel division form an executive committee for day-to-day decisions that are ratified at less frequent (quarterly) meetings of the medical committee. **2.** (local) (in Britain) a group of representatives of the general practitioners under contract with a single *Family Practitioner Committee. The members act as spokesmen for the local practitioners, by whom they are elected. Similar arrangements and responsibilities apply for the *local dental committee*, *local pharmaceutical committee*, and the *local optical committee*. **3.** (in Britain) a group of representative specialists and general practitioners who serve as medical advisors and spokesmen to a District or Regional Health Authority (*District Medical Committee* or *Regional Medical Committee*). *See also* National Health Service.

議。委員會一般分成若干專家小組，俗稱"嵌齒輪部門"，代表着醫院各科室部門（內科、外科、兒科等）。通常每個嵌齒輪部門的主席組成決定日常事務的執委會，而這種決定要在醫學委員會會議上通過（醫學委員會開會較少，每季度一次）。②地方醫學委員會（英國的）是全科醫師的代表組織，與"開業醫生管理委員會"簽定獨立的合同。由地方開業醫生選舉出可做爲他們的代言人的代表組成。"地方牙科委員會"、"地方藥學委員會"、"地方眼科委員會"按類似的辦法產生和負有類似的責任。 ③（在英國）由專科醫師和全科醫師代表組成的一個團體。他們充當地區保健局和地段保健局（地區醫學委員會和地段醫學委員會）的醫學顧問和發言人。

medical jurisprudence the study or practice of the legal aspects of medicine. *See* forensic medicine.

法醫學 醫學法律方面的研究或實踐。

Medical Officer of Health formerly, the chief health executive of local government. *See* community physician.

主管保健醫師 以前，地方政府的主要保健行政官員。

medical social worker a person with some medical training, employed to assist patients with domestic problems that may arise through illness.

醫學社會工作人員 受過一些醫學教育，幫助病人處理因疾病所致的家庭問題的工作人員。

medicated *adj.* containing a medicinal drug: applied to lotions, soaps, sweets, etc.

加藥的 洗劑、肥皂、甜食等物品中含有起醫療作用的藥物。

medication *n.* **1.** a substance administered by mouth, applied to the body, or introduced into the body for the purpose of treatment. Medicated dressings are applied to wounds to prevent infection and allow normal healing. *See also*

①**藥物** 爲了治療疾病，通過口服、外用或注入人體的一種物質。外敷藥用於預防傷口感染，使其恢復正常。 ②**藥物療法** 使用藥物治療病人。

premedication. **2.** treatment of a patient using drugs.

medicine *n.* **1.** the science or practice of the diagnosis, treatment, and prevention of disease. **2.** the science or practice of nonsurgical methods of treating disease. **3.** any drug or preparation used for the treatment or prevention of disease, particularly a preparation that is taken by mouth.

①**醫學** 疾病的診斷、治療和預防的科學或實踐。②**內科學** 用非手術方法治療疾病的科學或實踐。③**藥物** 用於預防或治療疾病的任一藥物或製劑，特別是口服製劑。

medicochirurgical *adj.* of or describing matters that are related to both medicine and surgery. A medicochirurgical disorder is one that calls for treatment by both a physician and a surgeon.

內外科的 與內科和外科都有關的或屬於內、外兩科的。內外科疾病是由內科和外科醫生共同治療的疾病。

Mediterranean fever 1. *see* brucellosis. **2.** *see* polyserositis.

地中海熱

medium *n.* **1.** any substance, usually a broth, agar, or gelatin, used for the *culture of microorganisms or tissue cells. An *assay medium* is used to determine the concentration of a growth factor or chemical by measuring the amount of growth it produces in a particular microorganism; all other nutrients are present in amounts adequate for growth. **2.** *see* contrast medium.

培養基 ①用於微生物或組織細胞培養的物質，通常爲肉湯、瓊脂或明膠。鑑定培養基通過測定特殊微生物在培養基中的生長量，來測定生長因素和化學物質的濃度；培養基中所有其它營養物質的量足以供生長之需要。②見對照培養基。

medroxyprogesterone *n.* a synthetic female sex hormone (*see* progestogen) used to treat menstrual disorders, including amenorrhoea, to prevent miscarriage, and (in combination with an oestrogen) in *oral contraceptives. It is administered by mouth or injection. Trade name: **Provera.**

甲孕酮 人工合成的雌性激素。用於治療包括閉經的月經紊亂，預防流產並（與雌激素合用）作爲口服避孕藥。口服或注射。

medulla *n.* **1.** the inner region of any organ or tissue when it is distinguishable from the outer region (the cortex), particularly the inner part of the kidney, adrenal glands, or lymph nodes. **2.** *see* medulla oblongata. **3.** the *myelin layer of certain nerve fibres. **—medullary** *adj.*

髓 ①某些器官或組織的內部結構，以區別於外部結構（皮質），特別是腎、腎上腺或淋巴結的內部結構。②見延髓。③某些神經纖維的髓鞘層。

medulla oblongata (myelencephalon) the extension within the skull of the upper end of the spinal cord, forming the lowest part of the *brainstem. Besides forming the major pathway for nerve impulses entering and leaving the skull, the medulla contains centres that are responsible for the regulation of the heart and blood vessels, respiration, salivation, and swallowing. *Cranial nerves VI–XII leave the brain in this region.

延髓（末腦） 形成腦幹最下部的脊索上端在顱內的延伸部分。除了形成神經衝動進、出顱內的主要通路外，延髓內有負責調節心臟和血管、呼吸、唾液分泌和吞咽的中樞。第6～12顱神經在此離腦。

medullated (myelinated) nerve fibre any nerve fibre that has a sheath of *myelin surrounding and insulating its axon.

有髓〔鞘〕神經纖維 由髓鞘包繞並隔離其軸索的神經纖維。

medulloblastoma *n.* a *cerebral tumour that occurs during childhood. It is derived from cells that have the apparent potential to mature into neurones. The medulloblastoma usually develops adjacent to the fourth ventricle. It causes an unsteady gait and shaky limb movements. Obstruction to the flow of cerebrospinal fluid causes *hydrocephalus. The tumour is sensitive to radiotherapy.

成神經管細胞瘤 兒童腦瘤。它是由有明顯的發育成熟爲神經元傾向的細胞衍變而來。成神經管細胞瘤通常在第四腦室附近生長。它可致步態不穩和震顫性四肢運動。腦脊液流動的梗阻可引起腦積水。腫瘤對放射治療敏感。

mefenamic acid an *analgesic that also reduces inflammation and fever and is used to treat headache, toothache, rheumatic pain, and similar conditions. It is administered by mouth; side-effects include digestive upsets, drowsiness, and skin rashes. Trade name: **Ponstan**.

甲滅酸 用於治療頭痛，牙痛，風濕痛及類似情況並可消炎和退燒的一種止痛藥。口服。副作用有消化不良，瞌睡和皮疹。

mega- *prefix denoting* **1.** large size, or abnormal enlargement or distention. Example: *megacaecum* (of the caecum). **2.** a million. Example: *megavolt* (a million volts).

〔前綴〕 **①巨** 指大的物體或異常增大或膨脹。例如：巨盲腸。 **②一百萬**。例如：兆伏（一百萬伏特）。

megacolon *n.* dilatation, and sometimes lengthening, of the colon. It is caused by obstruction of the colon, *Hirschsprung's disease, or longstanding constipation, or it may occur as a complication of ulcerative *colitis (*toxic megacolon*).

巨結腸 擴張並有時延長的結腸。病因爲結腸梗阻、赫希施普龍氏病、長期便秘，或可以潰瘍性腸炎（毒性巨結腸）併發症的形式出現。

megakaryoblast *n.* a cell that gives rise to the platelet-forming cell *megakaryocyte, found in the blood-forming tissue of the bone marrow. It is derived from a *haemopoietic stem cell and matures via an intermediate stage (*promegakaryocyte*) into a megakaryocyte.

成巨核細胞 骨髓造血組織中生成巨核細胞的一種細胞（巨核細胞是形成血小板的細胞）。它由造血幹細胞衍變而來，並且經過中間階段（幼巨核細胞）發育成熟爲巨核細胞。

megakaryocyte *n.* a cell in the bone marrow that produces *platelets. It is large (35–160 μm in diameter), with an irregularly lobed nucleus, and with *Romanowsky stains its abundant cytoplasm appears pale blue with fine reddish granules. *See also* thrombopoiesis.

巨核細胞 骨髓中生成血小板的細胞。爲大型細胞（直徑爲 35 ~ 160 微米），帶有一個不規則的葉狀核，羅曼諾夫斯基氏染色時，其豐富的胞漿呈淡藍色並帶有細小的微紅的顆粒。

megal- (megalo-) *prefix denoting* abnormal enlargement. Example: ***megalomelia*** (of limbs).

〔前綴〕 **巨** 異常增大。例如：巨肢。

megaloblast *n.* an abnormal form of any of the cells that are precursors of red blood cells (*see* erythroblast). Megaloblasts are unusually large and their nuclei fail to mature in the normal way; they are seen in the bone marrow in certain anaemias (*megaloblastic anaemias*) due to deficiency of vitamin B_{12} or folic acid. —**megaloblastic** *adj.*

幼巨紅細胞 任何一種紅細胞前體細胞的異常形態。幼巨紅細胞異常增大，並且胞核不能以正常形式發育成熟。此細胞見於維生素B_{12}或葉酸缺乏性貧血病人的骨髓中。

megalocephaly *n.* **1.** *see* macrocephaly. **2.** overgrowth and distortion of skull bones (*see* leontiasis).

①巨頭 ②顱骨過度生長變形

megalocyte *n. see* macrocyte.

巨紅細胞

megalomania *n.* delusions of grandeur, such as being God, royalty, etc. It may be a feature of a schizophrenic or manic illness or of cerebral syphilis.

誇大狂 把自己想像爲上帝、皇親等偉大人物的妄想。此乃精神分裂症或躁狂性病以及腦梅毒的一個特徵。

-megaly *suffix denoting* abnormal enlargement. Example: *splenomegaly* (of spleen).

〔後綴〕 **大，巨** 異常增大。例如：脾大。

megaureter *n.* gross dilatation of the *ureter. This occurs above the site of a long-standing obstruction in the ureter, which blocks the free flow of urine from the kidney. A common cause of mega-

巨輸尿管 輸尿管的極度擴張。發生在輸尿管長期阻滯的部位之上，由此阻礙了來自腎臟的尿液的自由流動。

ureter is reflux of urine from the bladder into the ureters (*see* vesicoureteric reflux), but some of the most striking examples are found in so-called *idiopathic megaureter*. In this condition, which may affect one or both ureters, there is a segment of normal ureter of varying length at the extreme lower end of the bladder, above which the ureter is enormously dilated. Both reflux and idiopathic megaureter progress to urinary infection and/or renal impairment. Treatment is by corrective surgery.

巨輸尿管常見病因是尿液從膀胱反流到輸尿管，但一些最典型的病例見於所謂的原發性巨輸尿管。在這種情況下，疾病可發生在一側或雙側輸尿管，在連接膀胱的下端輸尿管可有一段不同長度的正常輸尿管，此段之上的輸尿管明顯擴大。雙側的反流和原發性巨輸尿管可發展成泌尿系感染和/或腎臟損傷。治療此病的方法是施行矯正手術。

megestrol *n.* a synthetic female sex hormone (*see* progestogen) that is used in combination with an oestrogen in *oral contraceptives.

甲地羥孕酮 人工合成的雌性激素，與雌激素合用，作為口服避孕藥。

meibomian cyst *n. see* chalazion.

邁博姆氏囊腫

meibomian glands (tarsal glands) small sebaceous glands that lie under the conjunctiva of the eyelids.

邁博姆氏腺（瞼板腺） 位於眼瞼結膜下的小皮脂腺。

meiosis (reduction division) *n.* a type of cell division that produces four daughter cells, each having half the number of chromosomes of the original cell. It occurs before the formation of sperm and ova and the normal (*diploid) number of chromosomes is restored after fertilization. Meiosis also produces genetic variation in the daughter cells, brought about by the process of *crossing over. Meiosis consists of two successive divisions, each divided into four stages (*see* prophase, metaphase, anaphase, telophase). (See illustration.) *Compare* mitosis. —**meiotic** *adj.*

減數分裂 一種細胞分裂（增殖）的方式。由一個細胞生成四個子細胞，而每個子細胞含有原始細胞半數染色體。它發生在精子和卵子形成之前，受精後染色體數量恢復正常（二倍體）。減數分裂也可產生由交換過程所致的子細胞的遺傳變異。減數分裂由兩次連續的分裂組成，每次分成四個階段（見圖）。

Meissner's plexus (submucous plexus) a fine network of parasympathetic nerve fibres in the wall of the alimentary canal, supplying the muscles and mucous membrane.

麥斯納氏叢（黏膜下叢） 位於消化道壁內，分佈於肌肉和黏膜的一個小副交感神經纖維網。

melaena *n.* black tarry faeces due to the presence of partly digested blood from higher up the digestive tract.

黑糞症 上消化道出血；部分經消化的血液所致的黑色柏油樣便。至少500

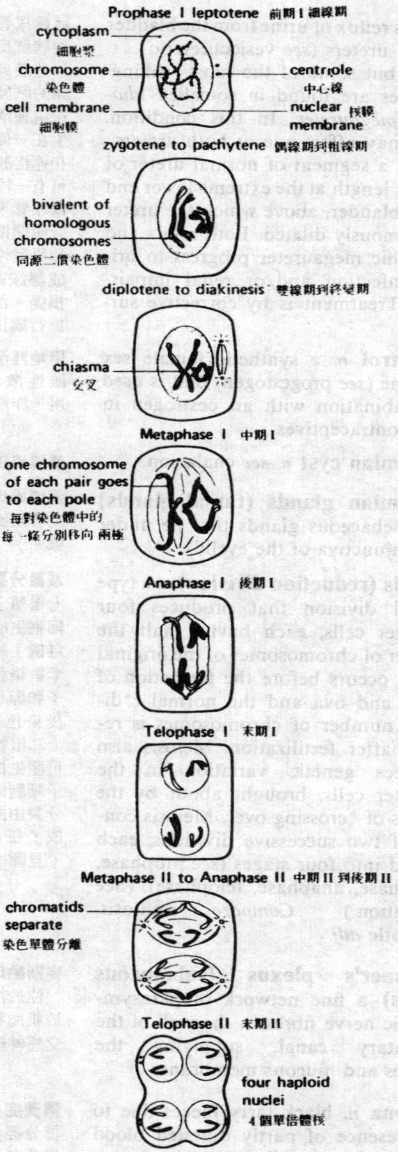

Stages in meiosis
減數分裂各期

Melaena is not apparent unless at least 500 ml of blood has entered the gut. It often occurs after vomiting blood (*see* haematemesis) and the causes are the same.

毫升血進入腸道才會出現黑糞症。此症常發生在嘔血後，其病因同上。

melan- (melano-) *prefix denoting* **1.** black coloration. **2.** melanin. Example: *melanaemia* (presence in the blood).

〔前綴〕 ①**黑色** ②**黑色素** 例如：黑血症（血中有黑色素）。

melancholia *n. see* depression, involutional melancholia.

憂鬱症

melanin *n.* a dark-brown to black pigment occurring in the hair, the skin, and in the iris and choroid layer of the eyes. Melanin is contained within special cells (*chromatophores*); in the skin these are found in the *dermis. Production of melanin in the skin is increased by the action of sunlight (producing tanning), which protects the underlying skin layers from the sun's radiation.

黑〔色〕素 頭髮、皮膚和眼的虹膜和脉絡膜層中深棕到黑色的色素。特殊細胞（色素細胞）內含有黑色素，存在於皮膚的眞皮層內。日光的照射使皮膚內黑色素生成增加（曬黑），由此來保護皮膚下層組織不受日光照射。

melanism (melanosis) *n.* an unusually pronounced darkening of body tissues caused by excessive production of the pigment *melanin. For example, melanism may affect the hair, the skin (after sunburn, during pregnancy, or in *Addison's disease), or the eye.

黑變病（黑色素沉着病） 因黑色素生成過多所致的身體組織異常明顯變暗。例如：黑變病可發生在頭髮、皮膚（日曬，妊娠，或患有阿狄森氏病）或眼睛。

melanocyte (melanophore) *n.* a cell within the epidermis of skin that produces the dark brown pigment *melanin.

黑素細胞 皮膚表皮中可產生暗棕色黑色素的一種細胞。

melanocyte-stimulating hormone (MSH) a hormone synthesized and released by the pituitary gland. In amphibians MSH brings about colour changes in the skin but its physiological role in man is uncertain.

促黑素細胞激素 一種由垂體腺合成並釋放的激素。在兩棲動物中，促黑素細胞激素可改變皮膚的顏色，但它在人體中的生理學作用還不能肯定。

melanoderma *n.* an abnormal increase in the skin pigment (*melanin).

黑皮病 皮膚色素（黑色素）異常增加。

melanoma *n.* a highly malignant tumour of melanin-forming cells, the *melanocytes. Such tumours usually occur in the skin but are also found in the eye and the mucous membranes. They may contain melanin (*melanotic*

黑素瘤 黑色素生成細胞（即黑素細胞）的高度惡性腫瘤。這種腫瘤通常發生在皮膚，但也可見於眼和黏膜。腫瘤可含有黑色

melanomas) or be free of pigment (*amelanotic melanomas*). Spread of this cancer to other parts of the body, especially to the lymph nodes and liver, is common. In these cases melanin or its precursors (*melanogens*) may be excreted in the urine and the whole of the skin may be deeply pigmented.

素（黑變病性黑素瘤）或沒有色素（無黑色素性黑素瘤）。這種癌通常擴散到身體的其它部位，特別是淋巴結和肝臟。在這些病例中，黑色素或它的前體（黑素原）可在尿中被排泄並且整個皮膚可被色素染成深色。

melanonychia *n.* blackening of the nails with the pigment *melanin.

黑甲 帶有黑色素的變黑的指甲。

melanophore *n. see* melanocyte.

黑素細胞

melanoplakia *n.* pigmented areas of *melanin in the mucous membrane lining the inside of the cheeks.

〔口〕黏膜黑斑 頰內黏膜的黑色素沉着部位。

melanosis *n.* **1.** *see* melanism. **2.** a disorder in the body's production of the pigment melanin. **3.** *cachexia associated with the spread of the skin cancer *melanoma. —**melanotic** *adj.*

①**黑變病** ②體內黑色素生成疾病。 ③與黑素瘤的擴散有關的惡病質。

melanuria *n.* the presence of dark pigment in the urine. This may be caused by the presence of melanin or its precursors, in some cases of *melanoma; it may alternatively be caused by metabolic disease, such as *porphyria.

黑尿 尿中有黑色素，在一些黑素瘤的病例中，病因可爲存有黑色素或其前體。黑尿的病因有時也可爲代謝性疾病，例如：卟啉症。

melasma *n. see* chloasma.

黑斑病

melioidosis *n.* a disease of wild rodents caused by the bacterium *Pseudomonas pseudomallei.* It can be transmitted to man, possibly by rat fleas, causing pneumonia, multiple abscesses, and septicaemia. It is often fatal.

類鼻疽 由類鼻疽假單胞菌引起的野生嚙齒動物的疾病。本病可由鼠蚤傳播給人，引起肺炎、多發性膿腫和敗血病。它常常是致命的。

melomelus *n.* a fetus with one or more pairs of supernumery limbs.

贅肢畸胎 有一或有多對額外肢體的胎兒。

melphalan *n.* a drug used to treat various types of cancer, including malignant melanoma, tumours of the breast and ovaries, and Hodgkin's disease. It is administered by mouth or injection. Side-effects include digestive upsets, mouth ulcers, and temporary hair loss. Trade name: **Alkeran**.

左旋溶肉瘤素 治療惡性黑素瘤、乳房和卵巢瘤及何傑金氏病等各種癌病的藥物。口服或注射。副作用有消化不良，口腔潰瘍和暫時脫髮。

membrane *n.* **1.** a thin layer of tissue surrounding the whole or part of an

膜 ①部分或全部地圍繞着某器官、或組織內腔、

organ or tissue lining a cavity, or separating adjacent structures or cavities. *See also* basement membrane, mucous membrane, serous membrane. **2.** the lipoprotein envelope surrounding a cell (*plasma* or *cell membrane*). —**membranous** *adj.*

或區分毗鄰結構、或腔室的一薄層組織。 ②包裹着細胞的脂蛋白被膜（原漿或細胞膜）。

membrane bone a bone that develops in connective tissue by direct *ossification, without cartilage being formed first. The bones of the face and skull are membrane bones.

膜骨 最初沒有軟骨形式，在結締組織中直接骨化而成的一種骨。面骨和顱骨屬於膜骨。

membranous labyrinth *see* labyrinth.

膜迷路

men- (meno-) *prefix denoting* menstruation.

〔前綴〕 **月經**

menarche *n.* the start of the menstrual periods. This may happen at any age between about 10 and 17 years.

月經初潮 月經期的開始。月經可在10到17歲的時期內開始。

mendelism *n.* the theory of inheritance based on *Mendel's laws.

孟德爾氏遺傳學說 基於孟德爾氏定律的遺傳理論。

Mendel's laws rules of inheritance based on the breeding experiments of Gregor Mendel, which showed that the inheritance of characteristics is controlled by particles now known as *genes. In modern terms they are as follows. (1) Each body (somatic) cell of an individual carries two factors (genes) for every characteristic and each gamete carries only one. It is now known that the genes are arranged on chromosomes, which are present in pairs in somatic cells and separate during gamete formation by the process of *meiosis. (2) Each pair of factors segregates independently of all other pairs at meiosis, so that the gametes show all possible combinations of factors. This law applies only to genes on different chromosomes; those on the same chromosome are affected by *linkage. *See also* dominant, recessive.

孟德爾氏定律 基於喬治·孟德爾繁殖實驗的遺傳規律，表明遺傳特性是由現稱爲基因的顆粒控制的。現代術語表示如下：①生物體的每個體細胞中每種遺傳特性都有兩個基因，而每個配子中僅有一個基因。現已知基因均排列在染色體上，在體細胞內染色體是成對的。在形成配子時通過減數分裂的過程而分離。 ②在減數分裂時，每對基因獨立於其它基因而分離，以致配子可有各種各樣的基因組合。此定律僅適用於不同染色體上的基因。在同一個染色體上，它們受連鎖的影響。

menidrosis (menhidrosis) *n.* the production of sweat, sometimes containing

出汗倒經 有時汗中含血以代替正常月經。

blood, instead of the normal menstrual flow.

Ménière's disease (Ménière's syndrome) a disease affecting the inner ear in which deafness is associated with buzzing in the ears (tinnitus) and vertigo; its cause is not known. Typically, the attacks of vertigo are sudden and explosive and associated with pallor, nausea, and vomiting. Between attacks there may be months without symptoms, but as the disease progresses the deafness becomes more marked. Neither medical nor surgical treatment is uniformly successful.

梅尼埃爾氏病（梅尼埃爾氏綜合徵） 病因不明的內耳疾病，其症狀爲耳聾伴有耳內嘈雜聲（耳鳴）和眩暈。典型者，眩暈的發作是突然的和暴發性的，並可有蒼白、噁心和嘔吐。在幾次發作之間，可有數月無症狀，但是當病症發展時，耳聾可更加明顯。內外科治療均無效。

mening- (meningo-) *prefix denoting* the meninges.

〔前綴〕 **腦膜** 指腦〔脊〕膜。

meninges *pl. n.* (*sing.* **meninx**) the three connective tissue membranes that line the skull and vertebral canal and enclose the brain and spinal cord (see illustration). The outermost layer – the *dura mater (pachymeninx) – is inelastic, tough, and thicker than the middle layer (the *arachnoid mater) and the

腦〔脊〕膜 排列在顱骨和椎管內並包圍腦和脊髓的三個結締組織膜（見圖）。最外層爲硬腦〔脊〕膜，無彈性，比較硬，並且厚於中層（蛛網膜）和最內層（軟腦膜）。兩層內膜統稱爲柔腦〔脊〕膜。

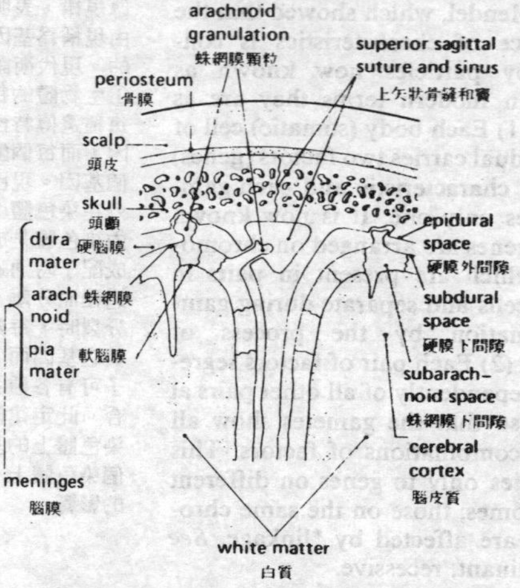

Section through the skull and brain to show meninges
腦和顱骨切面以示腦脊膜

innermost layer (the *pia mater). The inner two membranes are together called the *leptomeninges*; between them circulates the *cerebrospinal fluid.

腦脊液在這兩層膜之間循環流動。

meningioma *n.* a tumour arising from the fibrous coverings of the brain and spinal cord (*meninges). It is usually slow-growing and produces symptoms by pressure on the underlying nervous tissue. In the brain the tumour is a cause of focal *epilepsy and gradually progressive neurological disability. In the spinal cord it causes paraplegia and the *Brown-Séquard syndrome. Some meningiomas (known as *meningeal sarcomas*) are malignant and invade neighbouring tissues. Treatment of the majority of cases is by surgical removal if the tumour is accessible. The more malignant varieties may also require additional radiotherapy. Some patients have been known to have symptoms for as long as 30 years before the tumour has been discovered.

腦〔脊〕膜瘤 在覆蓋腦和脊髓的纖維組織（腦脊膜）上生成的腫瘤。通常生長緩慢並因壓迫下面的神經組織而產生症狀。在腦中，腫瘤是病竈性癲癇和漸近性神經功能喪失的病因。在脊髓，它可引起截癱和布朗-塞卡爾氏綜合徵。一些腦脊膜瘤（稱爲腦脊膜肉瘤）是惡性的，並可侵犯鄰近的組織。大多數病例的治療方法是手術切除。惡性度更高的病變還可進行放射治療。在膜瘤被發現前，一些病人已有長達30年的症狀。

meningism *n.* stiffness of the neck mimicking that found in meningitis. It is most common in childhood and is usually a symptom of chest infection or inflammation in the upper respiratory tract. Examination of the *cerebrospinal fluid reveals no abnormalities.

假性腦〔脊〕膜炎 酷似腦膜炎的頸部僵硬。最常見於兒童，並且通常是胸部感染或上呼吸道炎症的一種症狀。腦脊液檢查未見異常。

meningitis *n.* an inflammation of the *meninges due to infection by viruses or by the bacteria responsible for pneumonia, syphilis, or tuberculosis. Meningitis causes an intense headache, fever, loss of appetite, intolerance to light and sound, rigidity of muscles, especially those in the neck (*see also* Kernig's sign), and in severe cases convulsions, vomiting, and delirium leading to death. Bacterial meningitis can be effectively treated with antibiotics or sulphonamides. Viral meningitis does not respond to drugs; prolonged bed rest, darkness, and quiet is the only treatment. *See also* cerebrospinal fever, leptomeningitis, pachymeningitis.

腦〔脊〕膜炎 由肺炎或梅毒病原體或結核菌和病毒感染所致的腦〔脊〕膜的炎症。腦〔脊〕膜炎可引起劇烈頭痛，發燒，食慾喪失，不能耐受光和聲，肌肉特別是頸部肌肉强直（克尼格氏徵）。重症者，可發生驚厥、嘔吐和譫妄而死亡。抗生素或磺胺藥可有效地治療細菌性腦膜炎。藥物治療病毒性腦膜炎效果不好。唯一的治療方法是長期臥床休息，避免光和聲的刺激。

meningocele *n. see* neural tube defects.
腦〔脊〕膜膨出

meningococcaemia *n.* the presence of meningococci (bacteria of the species *Neisseria meningitidis*) in the bloodstream. *See* meningitis.
腦膜炎雙球菌血症 血流中有腦膜炎雙球菌（腦膜炎雙球菌種的細菌）。

meningococcus *n.* (*pl.* **meningococci**) one of the bacteria causing meningitis: **Neisseria meningitidis*. —**meningococcal** *adj.*
腦膜炎雙球菌 引起腦膜炎的一種細菌：腦膜炎雙球菌。

meningoencephalitis *n.* inflammation of the brain and its membranous coverings (the meninges) caused by infection, as with the mumps virus or *Brucella* (the bacterium causing brucellosis). *Brucellosis may also involve the spinal cord, producing *myelitis with paralysis of both legs, sometimes called *meningomyelitis*.
腦膜腦炎 流行性腮腺炎病毒或布魯氏〔桿〕菌屬（引起布魯氏〔桿〕菌病的細菌）感染引起的腦和腦膜（腦脊膜）的炎症。布魯氏〔桿〕菌病也可累及脊髓，引起伴有雙下肢麻痹的脊髓炎，有時稱爲脊髓脊膜炎。

meningoencephalocele *n. see* neural tube defects.
腦腦膜膨出

meningomyelitis *n. see* meningoencephalitis.
脊髓脊膜炎

meningomyelocele *n. see* neural tube defects.
脊髓脊膜膨出

meningovascular *adj.* relating to or affecting the meninges covering the brain and spinal cord and the blood vessels that penetrate them to supply the underlying neural tissues. The term is usually used to describe secondary syphilitic infection of the nervous system.
腦脊膜血管的 與覆蓋腦和脊髓的腦脊膜以及穿過腦脊膜供養下面神經組織的血管有關的或可影響它們的。此詞常用於神經組織的繼發性梅毒感染。

meninx *n.* the thin layer of mesoderm that surrounds the brain of the embryo. It gives rise to most of the skull and the membranes that surround the brain. *See also* chondrocranium.
原腦〔脊〕膜 圍繞胚腦的薄的中胚層組織。它形成顱和腦周圍膜的最大部分。

meniscectomy *n.* surgical removal of a cartilage (meniscus) in the knee. This is carried out when the meniscus has been torn or is diseased, to relieve pain and 'locking' of the knee joint.
半月板切除術 外科切除膝內的一塊軟骨（半月板）。當半月板撕裂或有病變時可行此術以止痛和"固定"膝關節。

meniscus *n.* (in anatomy) a crescent-shaped structure, such as the fibrocartilaginous disc that divides the cavity of a synovial joint.

半月板 （解剖學）半月形結構，如：分開滑膜關節腔的纖維軟骨盤。

menopause (climacteric) *n.* the time in a woman's life when the ovaries cease to produce an egg cell every four weeks and therefore menstruation ceases and the woman is no longer able to bear children. The menopause can occur at any age between the middle thirties and the late fifties. Menstruation may decrease gradually in successive periods or the intervals between periods may lengthen; alternatively there may be a sudden and complete stoppage of the monthly periods. At the time of the menopause there is a change in the balance of sex hormones in the body, which sometimes leads to hot flushes, palpitations, and dryness of the mucous membrane lining the vagina. Some women may also experience emotional disturbances. **—menopausal** *adj.*

絕經（更年期） 婦女到一定的年齡，卵巢每四周生成一個卵細胞的功能消失，並因此月經停止而不能再生育的時期。絕經可發生在35到近60歲的時期內。在連續的月經期內月經逐步減少或每次月經之間的間期延長，月經也可完全突然停止。在絕經期，體內性激素平衡發生變化，以致有時可出現發熱、潮紅、心悸和陰道內黏膜乾燥。有些婦女也可有情緒紊亂。

menorrhagia (epimenorrhagia) *n.* abnormally heavy bleeding at menstruation, which may or may not be associated with abnormally long periods. Menorrhagia may be associated with high blood pressure, hormonal disturbances, inflammation or tumours (e.g. fibroids) in the pelvic cavity, anaemia, sugar diabetes, kidney disease, and many other conditions.

月經過多（月經過頻過多） 與月經期延長有關或無關的月經期異常的大量出血。月經過多可與高血壓、激素紊亂、骨盆腔內的炎症或腫瘤（如：纖維瘤）、貧血、糖尿病、腎疾病和許多其它情況有關。

menses *n.* the blood and other materials discharged from the womb at menstruation.

月經 月經期從子宮中排出的血和其他物質。

menstrual cycle the periodic sequence of events in sexually mature nonpregnant women by which an egg cell (ovum) is released from the ovary at four-weekly intervals until the change of life (*see* menopause). The stages of the menstrual cycle are shown in the diagram. An ovum develops within a *Graafian follicle in the ovary. When

月經周期 性成熟非妊娠婦女在每四周的間期裏從卵巢內釋放一個卵細胞的周期性、連續性的生理活動，直到生理機能有所改變（絕經）。月經周期的階段如圖所示。卵子在卵巢的格雷夫氏卵泡內發育。暫時的內分泌腺黃體

mature, it bursts from the follicle and travels along the Fallopian tube to the womb. A temporary endocrine gland – the corpus luteum – develops in the ruptured follicle and secretes the hormone *progesterone, which causes the lining of the womb to become thicker and richly supplied with blood in preparation for pregnancy. If the ovum is not fertilized the cycle continues: the corpus luteum shrinks and the womb lining is shed at *menstruation. If fertilization does take place the fertilized ovum becomes attached to the womb lining and the corpus luteum continues to secrete progesterone, i.e. pregnancy begins.

在破裂的卵泡內發育並分泌黃體酮。黃體酮可使子宮內膜增厚，並提供豐富的血流爲妊娠做好準備。如果卵子未受精，月經周期繼續進行：黃體萎縮並且子宮內壁在月經期脫落。如果確已受精，受精卵附着在子宮內壁而且黃體繼續分泌黃體酮，這就是妊娠開始。

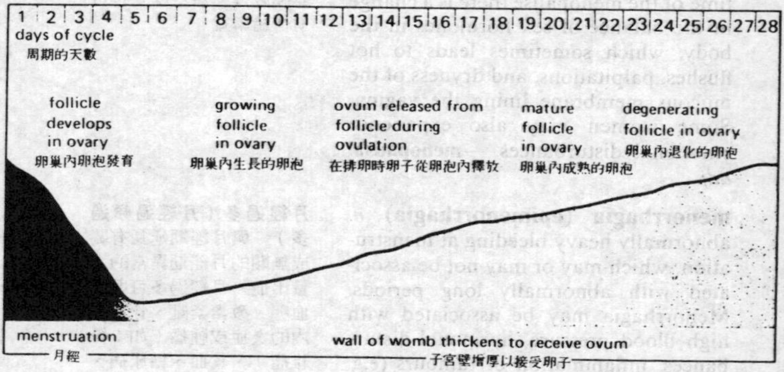

The menstrual cycle
月經周期

menstruation (catamenia) *n.* the discharge of blood and fragments of womb lining from the vagina at intervals of about one month in women of child-bearing age (*see* menarche, menopause). Menstruation is that stage of the *menstrual cycle during which the womb lining, which is thickened in readiness to receive a fertilized egg cell (ovum), is cast off if fertilization does not occur within a limited period of time. The normal duration of discharge varies from three to seven days. In

月經 生育年齡的婦女以一個月爲間期，從陰道內排出子宮內的血和內膜碎片。在月經周期內子宮內膜增厚，以準備接受受精卵細胞（卵子）。如在一定的時間內未受精，子宮內膜脫落，即爲月經。正常月經排出期是3～7天。而不排卵性月經，月經排出時不伴有卵巢內卵細胞的釋放。代償性月經（異位月經）是由其它處黏膜

anovular menstruation, discharge takes place without previous release of an egg cell from the ovary. *Vicarious menstruation* is bleeding from a mucous membrane other than the womb lining when normal menstruation is due. *See also* amenorrhoea, dysmenorrhoea, epimenorrhoea, hypomenorrhoea, menorrhagia, oligomenorrhoea.

出血，而不是像正常月經那樣由子宮內膜出血。

mental[1] *adj.* relating to or affecting the mind.

精神的 與精神有關或影響精神的。

mental[2] *adj.* relating to the chin.

頦的 與頦有關的。

mental age a measure of an individual's level of intellectual functioning; for example, someone described as having a mental age of 6 years would be functioning at the level of an average 6-year-old child. This measure has largely been replaced by a comparison of the functioning of persons of the same age group (*see* intelligence quotient, intelligence test).

智力年齡 對一個人智能水平的測量。如：稱某些人爲6歲智力年齡，即代表他們有平均6歲兒童的智力水平。同年齡組人的智能對比現已基本取代了這種測量。

mental deficiency *see* subnormality.

智力低下

Mental Health Acts the Acts of Parliament governing the care of the mentally disordered. The Mental Health Act 1959 provided the framework for England and Wales; similar Acts in 1960 and 1961 provided for Scotland and Northern Ireland. They abolished the old system of certification and established a legal framework for voluntary treatment of the mentally ill on the same basis as other patients. The Act also provides for *compulsory admission when the mentally disordered put themselves or other people into danger. It also enjoined local authorities to provide for the community treatment of mental disorder. The Mental Health (Amendment) Act of 1982 made further provisions for the protection of the civil rights of patients, the restriction of grounds for detention and compulsory treatment, and for a com-

精神病保健條例 關於精神病人醫療的國會條例。1959年的精神病保健條例爲英格蘭和威爾士規定了保健的基本原則；1960和1961年的相似的條例爲蘇格蘭和北愛爾蘭規定了保健的基本原則。他們廢除了舊的檢定制度，健立了在與其它病人一樣的基礎上自願進行精神病治療的法律原則。當精神病人使自己或他人處境危險時，條例也有强制病人進行治療的內容。條例也責成地方當局對精神病人進行羣體治療。1982年的精神病保健條例（修正案）爲保護病人的公民權，限制禁閉病人和進行强迫性治療，並由一個委員會來管理精神病醫療工作的不同

mission to regulate aspects of the practice of psychiatry (*see* Mental Health Act Commission).

方面，作出了進一步的規定。

Mental Health Act Commission a regulating body set up by the Mental Health (Amendment) Act of 1982. Its members comprise some 90 psychiatrists, nurses, lawyers, members of other clinical professions, and lay people. They have the responsibilities of regularly visiting psychiatric hospitals (yearly for ordinary hospitals; more frequently for *special hospitals), reviewing psychiatric care, giving second opinions on the need for certain psychiatric treatments, and acting as a forum for the discussion of psychiatric issues.

精神病保健條例委員會 根據1982年精神病保健條例（修正案）建立的管理機構。它的成員是由90個精神病醫生、護士、律師、其它臨床專業人員和非專業人員組成。他們負責定期查訪精神病醫院（按年查訪普通醫院，經常查訪專科醫院），檢查精神病醫療情況，對所需的某些精神病治療工作提出參考意見，並且此委員會可作爲討論精神病問題的場合。

mental illness a disorder of one or more of the functions of the mind (such as emotion, perception, memory, or thought), which causes suffering to the patient or others. If the sole problem is that the individual's behaviour as a whole is out of line with society's expectations, then the term 'illness' is not appropriate.
Mental illness should be distinguished from *subnormality, in which an individual has a general failure of development of the normal intellectual capacities. It is broadly divided into *psychosis, in which the capacity for appreciating reality is lost, and *neurosis, in which insight is retained.

精神病 可使病人或其他人遭受痛苦的一種或多種腦功能（如情緒，知覺，記憶或思維）障礙。如果唯一的問題是個人的整個行爲超出了社會預期的範圍，那末用"病"這個名詞就不適當。精神病應與正常智能發育低下所致的低正常智力水平相區別。精神病被廣義地分爲喪失了認識現實能力的精神病和保留有自知力的神經官能症。

mental impairment the presence of seriously antisocial or irresponsible behaviour in a person with mental *subnormality.

精神損傷 精神不正常的人有嚴重的反社會和不負責任的行爲。

mental welfare officer (in Britain) an employee of a local authority with special training in and responsibility for people with mental illness. He obtains court orders for *compulsory admission where necessary and provides surveillance and support for those being

精神病福利官員 （在英國）地方當局的受過特殊訓練的並負責精神病人的僱員。他獲有在必要時進行强迫收容的法庭證明，並監督和資助那些在家中治療或包括出院病人在內

treated at home or in designated hostel accommodation, including those discharged from hospital. *See also* aftercare.

在指定的具有專門設備的處所進行治療的病人。

mento- *prefix denoting* the chin.

〔前綴〕 **頦** 頦骨。

mentum *n.* the chin.

頦

mepacrine *n.* a drug used to treat various infections and infestations, particularly malaria, giardiasis, and taeniasis. It is administered by mouth. Digestive upsets and headache may occur and the skin often turns yellow. Trade names: **Atebrin**, **Quinacrine**.

阿的平 用於治療各種感染和傳染病，特別是瘧疾、梨形鞭毛蟲病和絛蟲病的藥物。口服。可有消化不良和頭痛，並且皮膚常有黃染。

mephenesin *n.* a *muscle-relaxant drug used to relieve muscular spasm and abnormal movements in such diseases as parkinsonism, chorea, and athetosis. It is administered by mouth or injection. Side-effects usually include digestive upsets. Trade name: **Myanesin**.

甲苯丙醇 用於解除在帕金森氏綜合徵、舞蹈病和手足徐動症中的肌肉痙攣和異常運動的一種肌肉鬆弛藥。口服或注射。常見副作用爲消化不良。

meprobamate *n.* a mild *tranquillizer used to relieve anxiety and nervous tension. It is administered by mouth or injection; side-effects include digestive upsets, headache, and drowsiness. Trade names: **Equanil**, **Mepavlon**, **Miltown**.

氨甲丙二酯 解除焦慮和神經緊張的一種輕型安定藥。口服或注射。副作用有消化不良、頭痛和瞌睡。商品名：安寧，眠爾通。

mepyramine *n.* an *antihistamine drug administered by mouth or injection to treat allergies and sensitivity reactions and applied as a cream to treat skin allergies and itching. Drowsiness is a common side-effect and digestive upsets may occur. Trade name: **Anthisan**.

甲氧苄二胺 通過口服或法射治療變態反應和過敏反應的一種抗組胺藥，此藥還可製成乳膏，以治療皮膚變態反應和癢症。副作用常爲瞌睡，也可有消化不良。商品名：馬來酸新安替根。

meralgia paraesthetica painful tingling and numbness felt over the outer surface of the thigh when the lateral cutaneous nerve is trapped as it passes through the fibrous and muscular tissues of the thigh.

感覺異常性股痛 當股外側皮神經在通過股的纖維性和肌性組織時受到牽扯的情況下，股的外表面可有刺痛感和麻木感。

mercaptopurine *n.* a drug that prevents the growth of cancer cells and is administered by mouth, chiefly in the

巯嘌呤 一種防止癌細胞生長的口服藥，主要用於治療某些類型的白血病

treatment of some types of leukaemia (*see* antimetabolite). It commonly reduces the numbers of white blood cells; mouth ulcers and digestive upsets may also occur. Trade name: **Puri-Nethol**.

（見抗代謝產物）。它常可引起白細胞減少，也可引起口腔潰瘍和消化不良。商品名：樂疾寧。

mercurialism (hydrargyria) *n.* mercury poisoning. Metallic mercury is absorbed through the skin and alimentary canal, and its vapour is taken in through the lungs. Acute poisoning causes vomiting, severe abdominal pains, bloody diarrhoea, and kidney damage, with failure to produce urine. Treatment is with *dimercaprol. Chronic poisoning causes mouth ulceration, loose teeth, loss of appetite, and intestinal and renal disturbances, with anaemia and nervous irritability. Treatment is removing the patient from further exposure.

汞中毒（水銀中毒） 金屬汞是通過皮膚和消化道被吸收的，而它的蒸汽是通過肺被吸入的。急性中毒引起嘔吐、嚴重腹痛、血性腹瀉和腎臟損害，並可伴有尿生成障礙。治療可用二巰〔基〕丙醇。慢性中毒可引起口腔潰瘍，牙齒鬆動，食慾喪失和腸道及腎功能紊亂，並可伴有貧血和神經過敏。治療方法是讓病人不再接觸汞。

mercury *n.* a silvery metallic element that is liquid at room temperature. Its toxicity has caused a decline in the use of its compounds in medicine during this century, but mercurial compounds in the form of ointments were formerly used in the treatment of syphilis. The main uses of mercury salts today are in antiseptics, fungicides, and antiparasitic agents. Symbol: Hg. *See also* mercurialism.

汞 在室溫下爲液體的銀色金屬元素。本世紀以來，因其毒性汞化合物在醫藥中的應用已減少，過去汞化合物的藥膏製品用於治療梅毒。目前，汞鹽主要用於防腐劑、殺眞菌劑和抗寄生物劑中。符號：Hg。

merocrine (eccrine) *adj.* describing a type of *secretion in which the glandular cells remain intact during the process of secretion.

部分分泌的（外分泌的） 在分泌過程中，腺細胞保持完整的一種分泌。

merozoite *n.* a stage in the life cycle of the malaria parasite (**Plasmodium*). Many merozoites are formed during the asexual division of the schizont (*see* schizogony). The released merozoites may invade new red blood cells or new liver cells, and continue the asexual phase with the production of yet more merozoites, effectively spreading the infection. Alternatively, merozoites in-

裂殖子 瘧疾寄生物（瘧原蟲）的生活周期的一個階段。許多裂殖子是在裂殖體的無性分裂期形成的。釋放的裂殖子可侵入新的紅細胞或肝細胞，繼續進行無性繁殖，並產生更多的裂殖子，有效地傳播感染。或者，裂殖子侵入紅細胞後，開始進行有

vade red blood cells and begin the sexual cycle with the formation of male and female sex cells (*see* microgametocyte, macrogametocyte).

性繁殖，並形成雄性和雌性性細胞。

mes- (meso-) *prefix denoting* middle or medial.

〔前綴〕 **中間的，中層的**

mesaortitis *n.* inflammation of the middle layer (media) of the wall of the aorta, generally the result of late syphilis. Aneurysm formation may result. The infection can be eradicated with penicillin.

主動脈中層炎 一般爲晚期梅毒所致的主動脈壁中層的炎症。可形成動脈瘤。青黴素可根治此感染。

mesarteritis *n.* inflammation of the middle layer (media) of an artery, which is often combined with inflammation in all layers of the artery wall. It is seen in syphilis, polyarteritis, temporal arteritis, and Buerger's disease.

動脈中層炎 通常合併有動脈壁各層炎症的動脈中層的炎症。此病見於梅毒、多關節炎，顳動脈炎和伯格氏病。

mescaline *n.* an alkaloid present in *mescal buttons* (the dried tops of the Mexican cactus *Lophophora williamsii*) that produces inebriation and vivid colourful hallucinations when ingested.

仙人球毒鹼 威廉斯仙人球花（墨西哥仙人掌屬威廉斯仙人球的乾燥頂部）中的一種鹼。攝入體內時，此鹼能使人產生酒醉狀和鮮明多彩的幻覺。

mesencephalon *n. see* midbrain.

中腦

mesenchyme *n.* the undifferentiated tissue of the early embryo that forms almost entirely from *mesoderm. It is loosely organized and the individual cells migrate to different parts of the body where they form most of the skeletal and connective tissue, the blood and blood system, and the visceral (smooth) muscles.

間〔充〕質 幾乎完全來自中胚層的早期胚胎的未分化組織。它的組織疏鬆，其個別的細胞移行到身體的不同部位，而在各該部位形成骨骼和結締組織、血液和血液系統以及內臟（平滑）肌肉的絕大部分。

mesentery *n.* a double layer of *peritoneum attaching the stomach, small intestine, pancreas, spleen, and other abdominal organs to the posterior wall of the abdomen. It contains blood and lymph vessels and nerves supplying these organs. —**mesenteric** *adj.*

腸繫膜 把胃、小腸、胰、脾和其它腹部器官附着到腹後壁上的一雙層腹膜。它含有供養這些器官的血液、淋巴管和神經。

mesial *adj.* **1.** medial. **2.** relating to or situated in the *median line or plane. **3.** designating the surface of a tooth towards the midline of the jaw.

正中的 ①中間的。②位於中線或正中面的，與中線或正中面有關的。③指朝向頜中線的牙面。

mesiodens *n.* an extra tooth that may occur in the midline of the palate, between the central incisors, and may interfere with their eruption.

額外牙 在腭中線上多生出的一個牙。位於中切牙之間，可對切牙的萌生（長出）造成障礙。

mesmerism *n.* *hypnosis based on the ideas of the 18th-century physician Franz Mesmer, sometimes employing magnets and a variety of other equipment.

催眠術 以18世紀內科醫生弗朗茲·梅斯梅爾的觀點爲基礎的催眠術。有時使用磁鐵和其它各種設備。

mesna *n.* a drug administered intravenously by injection or infusion to prevent the toxic effect of *ifosfamide and *cyclophosphamide on the bladder. It binds with the toxic metabolite acrolein in the urine.

巰乙磺酸鈉 由靜脉注射或輸注的預防異環磷醯胺和環磷醯胺對膀胱的毒性作用的藥物。它與尿中的毒性代謝產物丙烯醛相結合。

mesoappendix *n.* the *mesentery of the appendix.

闌尾繫膜 闌尾的腸繫膜。

mesocolon *n.* the fold of peritoneum by which the colon is fixed to the posterior abdominal wall. Usually only the *transverse* and *sigmoid mesocolons* persist in the adult, attached to the transverse and sigmoid colon, respectively.

結腸繫膜 使結腸固定於腹後壁的腹膜皺襞。成人通常僅有橫結腸和乙狀結腸繫膜，分別附着在橫結腸和乙狀結腸上。

mesoderm *n.* the middle *germ layer of the early embryo. It gives rise to cartilage, muscle, bone, blood, kidneys, gonads and their ducts, and connective tissue. It separates into two layers – an outer *somatic* and an inner *splanchnic mesoderm*, separated by a cavity (*coelom*) that becomes the body cavity. The dorsal somatic mesoderm becomes segmented into a number of *somites. *See also* mesenchyme. —**mesodermal** *adj.*

中胚層 早期胚胎的中胚芽層。它生長成軟骨、肌肉、骨、血、腎臟、性腺及其管道，以及結締組織。它分成二層：即體中胚層和內臟中胚層，二者之間以腔分隔，後來轉變成體腔。背側的體中胚層分成若干個體節。

mesometrium *n.* the broad ligament of the uterus (womb): a sheet of connective tissue that carries blood vessels to the uterus (womb) and attaches it to the abdominal wall.

子宮繫膜 子宮的闊韌帶。攜帶血管到子宮，並將子宮附着在腹壁的結締組織帶。

mesomorphic *adj.* describing a *body type that has a well developed skeletal and muscular structure and a sturdy upright posture. —**mesomorph** *n.* —**mesomorphy** *n.*

中型身材的 指那種骨骼和肌肉結構發育良好並具有强健筆直姿態的體型。

mesonephros (Wolffian body) *n.* the second area of kidney tissue to develop in the embryo. Its excretory function only lasts for a very brief period before it degenerates. However, parts of it become incorporated into the male reproductive structures. Its duct – the *mesonephric* (or *Wolffian*) *duct* – persists in males as the epididymis and vas deferens, which conduct sperm from the testis. —**mesonephric** *adj.*

中腎（午非氏體） 胚胎內第二個腎組織發育區。它僅維持極其短期的排泄功能，後來退化。但是，它的部分組織併入男性生殖結構。它的管道——中腎（或午非氏）管——在男性中存留，成爲從睾丸中引導精液的附睾和輸精管。

mesophilic *adj.* describing organisms, especially bacteria, that grow best at temperatures of about 25–45°C. *Compare* psychrophilic, thermophilic.

適溫的 描述在大約25～45℃的溫度下生長得最好的生物體，特別是細菌。

mesosalpinx *n.* a fold of peritoneum that surrounds the Fallopian tubes. It is the upper part of the broad ligament, which surrounds the womb.

輸卵管繫膜 圍繞着輸卵管的腹膜皺襞。它是圍繞着子宮的闊韌帶的上部。

mesosome *n.* a structure occurring in some bacterial cells, formed by infolding of the cell membrane. Mesosomes are associated with the DNA and play a part in cell division.

間體 因細胞膜內折而形成的一些細菌細胞的結構。間體與DNA有關，而且在細胞分裂中起作用。

mesotendon *n.* the delicate connective tissue membrane that surrounds a tendon.

腱繫膜 腱周圍的柔弱的結締組織膜。

mesothelioma *n.* a tumour of the epithelium making up the pleura, peritoneum, or pericardium. The occurrence of pleural mesothelioma has a strong association with exposure to asbestos dust (*see* asbestosis), and workers in the asbestos industry who develop such tumours are entitled to industrial compensation. In other cases, however, there is no history of asbestos exposure. Some tumours can be surgically removed but most are inoperable; for these cases chemotherapy with *doxorubicin may be tried.

間皮瘤 構成胸膜、腹膜或心包的上皮的腫瘤。胸膜間皮瘤的發生與接觸石棉粉塵有很大關係（見石棉沉着病），石棉工業中患此腫瘤的工人有權享受企業補助。但是，在另外一些病例中，無石棉接觸史。外科手術可切除某些腫瘤，但大多數腫瘤無法切除，對這些病例可試用阿黴素化學療法。

mesothelium *n.* the single layer of cells that lines *serous membranes. It is derived from embryonic mesoderm. *Compare* epithelium.

間皮 覆在漿膜表面的單層細胞。它是由胚胎的中胚層衍變而來的。

mesovarium *n.* the *mesentery of the ovaries.

卵巢繫膜 卵巢的繫膜。

messenger RNA a type of RNA that carries the information of the *genetic code of the DNA from the cell nucleus to the ribosomes, where the code is translated into protein. *See* transcription, translation.

信使RNA 核糖核酸（RNA）的一種。能把脫氧核糖核酸（DNA）的遺傳密碼信息從細胞核携帶到核糖體。在核糖體內密碼被轉譯成蛋白質。

mestranol *n.* a synthetic female sex hormone that is one of the most commonly used oestrogens in *oral contraceptive pills.

炔雌醇甲醚 一種合成的雌性性激素。它是口服避孕藥片中最常用的雌激素之一。

met- (meta-) *prefix denoting* **1.** distal to; beyond; behind. **2.** change; transformation.

〔前綴〕 ①**遠側的，超出，後面** ②**改變，轉變**

metabolism *n.* **1.** the sum of all the chemical and physical changes that take place within the body and enable its continued growth and functioning. Metabolism involves the breakdown of complex organic constituents of the body with the liberation of energy, which is required for other processes (*see* catabolism) and the building up of complex substances, which form the material of the tissues and organs, from simple ones (*see* anabolism). *See also* basal metabolism. **2.** the sum of the biochemical changes undergone by a particular constituent of the body; for example, protein metabolism. **—metabolic** *adj.*

〔新陳〕代謝 ①體內發生的能使身體繼續生長和維持功能的所有化學和物理變化的總和。新陳代謝包括身體複雜有機成分的分解，伴有爲其它過程所需的能量釋放，和從簡單物質合成複雜物質，以構成組織和器官的成分。 ②身體的某特殊成分經歷的生物化學變化的總和，如蛋白質代謝。

metabolite *n.* a substance that takes part in the process of *metabolism. Metabolites are either produced during metabolism or are constituents of food taken into the body.

代謝物 參與代謝過程的某種物質。代謝產物既可是代謝過程中產生的物質，又可是攝入體內的食物成分。

metacarpal **1.** *adj.* relating to the bones of the hand (*metacarpus). **2.** *n.* any of the bones forming the metacarpus.

①**掌的** 與手骨（掌）有關的。 ②**掌骨** 構成掌的一塊骨頭。

metacarpus *n.* the five bones of the hand that connect the *carpus (wrist) to the *phalanges (digits).

掌 把腕連接到指（趾）骨的5個手骨。

metacentric *n.* a chromosome in which the centromere is at or near the centre of the chromosome. —**metacentric** *adj.*

中間着絲粒的〔染色體〕 着絲粒位於或接近染色體中心的〔一種染色體〕。

metacercaria *n.* (*pl.* **metacercariae**) a mature form of the *cercaria larva of a fluke. Liver fluke metacercariae are enveloped by thin cysts and develop on various kinds of vegetation.

後囊蚴 吸蟲尾蚴的成熟形式。肝吸蟲後囊蚴被一薄層囊包繞並在各種植物上發育。

metachromasia (metachromatism) *n.* **1.** the property of a dye of staining certain tissues or cells a colour that is different from that of the stain itself. **2.** the variation in colour produced in certain tissue elements that are stained with the same dye. **3.** abnormal coloration of a tissue produced by a particular stain. —**metachromatic** *adj.*

異染性(變色反應性) ①使被染的某些組織或細胞的顏色不同於染劑本身顏色的染劑特性。 ②同樣的染劑可使某些組織成份產生不同的顏色。 ③某特殊染劑使某組織染色異常。

Metagonimus *n.* a genus of small flukes, usually less than 3 mm in length, common as parasites of dogs and cats in the Far East, N. Siberia, and the Balkan States. Adult flukes of *M. yokogawai* occasionally infect the duodenum of man if undercooked fish (the intermediate host) is eaten. They may cause inflammation and some ulceration of the intestinal lining, which produces a mild diarrhoea. Flukes can be easily removed with tetrachlorethylene.

後殖吸蟲屬 一類小型吸蟲，通常小於3mm，常爲遠東、西伯利亞北部和巴爾幹半島地區狗和貓的寄生物。如果吃了生魚(中間宿主)，橫川後殖吸蟲的成蟲會偶然感染人的十二指腸。它們可引起腸黏膜的炎症和潰瘍，造成輕度腹瀉。四氯乙烯可有效地驅除吸蟲。

metamorphopsia *n.* a condition in which objects appear distorted. It is usually due to a disorder of the retina affecting the *macula (the most sensitive part).

視物變形症 所視物體變形的病症。病因常爲影響黃斑(最敏感部位)的視網膜疾病。

metamyelocyte *n.* an immature *granulocyte (a type of white blood cell), having a kidney-shaped nucleus (*compare* myelocyte) and cytoplasm containing neutrophil, eosinophil, or basophil granules. It is normally found in the blood-forming tissue of the bone marrow but may appear in the blood in a wide variety of diseases, including acute infections. *See also* granulopoiesis.

晚幼粒細胞 一種未成熟的粒細胞(白細胞的一種)。具有腎形核(與中幼粒細胞相比)，並且胞漿內含有嗜中性、嗜酸性或嗜鹼性顆粒。它可正常地出現在骨髓的造血組織內，但也可出現在包括急性感染的許多不同病人的血中。

metanephros *n.* the excretory organ of the fetus, which develops into the kidney and is formed from the rear portion of the *nephrogenic cord. It does not become functional until birth, since urea is transferred across the placenta to the mother.

後腎 發育成腎臟的並由生腎索後部形成的胎兒的排泄器官。出生前，因尿素經過胎盤被轉移到母體，後腎無功能。

metaphase *n.* the second stage of *mitosis and of each division of *meiosis, in which the chromosomes line up at the centre of the *spindle, with their centromeres attached to the spindle fibres.

中期 有絲分裂的第二階段和減數分裂每次分裂的第二階段。此時，隨着它們的着絲粒附着在紡錘體纖維上，染色體排列在紡錘體的中心。

metaphysis *n.* the growing portion of a long bone that lies between the *epiphyses (the ends) and the *diaphysis (the shaft).

幹骺端 位於骨骺（骨端）和骨幹（骨體）之間的長骨的生長部分。

metaplasia *n.* an abnormal change in the nature of a tissue. For instance, columnar epithelium lining the bronchi may be converted to squamous epithelium (*squamous metaplasia*): this may be an early sign of malignant change. *Myeloid metaplasia* is the development of bone marrow elements, normally found only within the marrow cavities of the bones, in organs such as the spleen and liver. This may occur after bone marrow failure.

〔組織〕轉化（化生） 某組織特性的異常變化。如：枝氣管內的柱狀上皮轉化爲鱗狀上皮（鱗狀組織化生），這可作爲惡性變的早期徵象。骨髓組織轉化是骨髓成分的發育，正常情況下僅見於骨髓腔及脾和肝這類器官中。脾和肝內的骨髓組織轉化可發生在骨髓衰竭後。

metastasis *n.* the distant spread of malignant tumour from its site of origin. This occurs by three main routes: (1) through the bloodstream; (2) through the lymphatic system; (3) across body cavities, e.g. through the peritoneum. Highly malignant tumours have a greater potential for metastasis. Individual tumours may spread by one or all of the above routes, although *carcinoma is said classically to metastasize via the lymphatics and *sarcoma via the bloodstream. —**metastatic** *adj.*

轉移 惡性腫瘤從它的原發灶擴散到較遠的部位。轉移有三個途徑：①通過血流；②通過淋巴系統；③穿過體腔，如：通過腹膜。高度惡性的腫瘤轉移的可能性較大。雖然癌症一般被認爲是通過淋巴管擴散，肉瘤是通過血流擴散，但個別腫瘤可通過上述一個或所有途徑擴散。

metastasize *vb.* (of a malignant tumour) to spread by *metastasis.

轉移 （惡性腫瘤）經轉移擴散。

metatarsal 1. *adj.* relating to the bones of the foot (*metatarsus). **2.** *n.* any of the bones forming the metatarsus.

蹠的 ①與脚骨（蹠）有關的。 ②形成蹠的任一骨頭。

metatarsalgia *n.* aching pain in the metatarsal bones of the foot. Repeated injury and deformities of the foot are common causes, and corrective footwear may be prescribed.

蹠〔骨〕痛 脚蹠骨的鈍痛。常見病因爲脚的反覆損傷的畸形，矯形鞋也可爲病因。

metatarsus *n.* the five bones of the foot that connect the *tarsus (ankle) to the *phalanges (toes).

蹠 連接跗骨和趾骨的5個脚骨。

metathalamus *n.* a part of the *thalamus consisting of two nuclei through which impulses pass from the eyes and ears to be distributed to the cerebral cortex.

丘腦後部 由兩個核組成的部分丘腦。眼和耳的衝動可通過丘腦後部被傳導到腦皮層。

metencephalon *n.* part of the hindbrain, formed by the pons and the cerebellum and continuous below with the medulla oblongata. *See* brain.

後腦 菱腦的一部分。由腦橋和小腦構成，向下與延腦相連續。

meteorism *n. see* tympanites.

鼓脹

-meter *suffix denoting* an instrument for measuring. Example: *perimeter* (instrument for measuring the field of vision).

〔後綴〕 **計，表，量器** 指測量儀器，例如：視野計（測量視野的儀器）。

metformin *n.* a drug that reduces blood sugar levels and is used to treat *diabetes. It is administered by mouth and may cause loss of appetite and minor digestive upsets. Trade name: **Glucophage**.

二甲雙胍 降血糖和治療糖尿病的藥。口服。可引起食慾喪失和輕度消化不良。

methadone *n.* a potent narcotic *analgesic drug administered by mouth or injection to relieve severe pain and as a linctus to suppress coughs. It is also used to treat heroin addiction. Digestive upsets, drowsiness, and dizziness may occur, and prolonged use may lead to dependence. Trade name: **Physopeptone**.

美沙酮 用於解除劇痛和用作止咳舐膏劑，經口服或注射的强麻醉鎮痛藥。也可用於治療海洛因成癮。服後可有消化不良、瞌睡和頭暈，長期服用可產生依賴性。

methaemalbumin *n.* a chemical complex of the pigment portion of haemoglobin (*haem*) with the plasma protein *albumin. It is formed in the blood in

正鐵白蛋白 血紅蛋白的色素部分（血紅素）與血漿中的蛋白質（白蛋白）結合而成的化學複合體。

anaemias in which red blood cells are destroyed and free haemoglobin is released into the plasma. In such conditions methaemalbumin can be detected in both the blood and urine.

它在紅細胞被破壞並且游離血紅蛋白被釋放到血漿中的貧血病人血中形成。在這種情況下，血和尿中可發現正鐵白蛋白。

methaemoglobin *n.* a substance formed when the iron atoms of the blood pigment *haemoglobin have been oxidized from the ferrous to the ferric form (*compare* oxyhaemoglobin). Methaemoglobin cannot bind molecular oxygen and therefore cannot transport oxygen round the body. The presence of methaemoglobin in the blood (*methaemoglobinaemia*) may result from ingestion of oxidizing drugs or from an inherited abnormality of the haemoglobin molecule. Symptoms are fatigue, headache, dizziness and *cyanosis.

正鐵血紅蛋白 當血色素（血紅蛋白）的鐵原子從亞鐵被氧化爲高鐵時形成的一種物質。正鐵血紅蛋白不能與氧分子結合，因此不能携帶氧供給全身。血中的正鐵血紅蛋白（正鐵血紅蛋白血症）可因攝入氧化藥物和血紅蛋白分子遺傳異常所引起。症狀爲疲勞、頭痛、頭暈和紫紺。

methandienone *n.* a synthetic male sex hormone with *anabolic properties, used to build up tissues in wasting diseases, such as osteoporosis, and during convalescence. Methandienone is administered by mouth; side-effects are uncommon, but nausea, menstrual abnormalities, and fluid retention may occur. Trade name: **Dianabol**.

去氫甲睾酮 一種合成的男性性激素。用於消耗性疾病中，如在骨質疏鬆〔症〕和恢復期，具有促進組織合成代謝的作用。口服。副作用不常見，但可發生噁心、月經異常和液體滯留。商品名：大力補。

methandriol *n.* a synthetic male sex hormone (*see* androgen) with the same actions and uses as *methandienone. Side-effects may include symptoms of virilization in women, such as growth of body hair and voice changes.

甲雄烯二醇 具有與去氫甲睾酮相同作用和用途的合成男性性激素（見雄激素）。副作用包括婦女的男性化症狀，如體毛生長和嗓音變化等。

methanol *n. see* methyl alcohol.

甲醇

methapyrilene *n.* an *antihistamine used to relieve *hay fever and other allergic reactions. It is administered by mouth and may cause drowsiness.

噻吡二胺 治療枯草熱和其它變態反應的一種抗組胺藥。口服。可引起瞌睡。

methaqualone *n.* a hypnotic and *sedative drug used to treat insomnia. It is administered by mouth; side-effects include headache, drowsiness, and digestive upsets. Trade name: **Revonal**.

安眠酮 治療失眠的催眠和鎮靜藥。口服。副作用有頭痛、瞌睡和消化不良。

methenamine *n. see* hexamine.

烏洛托品

methenolone *n.* a synthetic male sex hormone with body-building actions (*see* anabolic). It is administered by mouth or injection and may cause symptoms of virilization in women, such as growth of body hair and voice changes.

1-甲雄烯醇酮 具有蛋白合成作用的合成男性性激素（見雄激素）。口服或注射。可引起婦女的體毛生長和嗓音變化等男性化症狀。

methimazole *n.* a drug that reduces thyroid activity, used to treat *thyrotoxicosis and to prepare patients for surgical removal of the thyroid gland. It is administered by mouth or injection; side-effects include rashes, digestive upsets, and headache.

甲巰基咪唑 治療甲狀腺毒症和爲甲狀腺外科切除病人作手術前準備的一種降低甲狀腺活性的藥物。口服或注射。副作用有皮疹、消化不良和頭痛。

methionine *n.* a sulphur-containing *essential amino acid. *See also* amino acid.

蛋氨酸 含硫必需氨基酸。

methixene *n.* a drug with effects similar to those of *atropine, used to control the tremors and other symptoms in parkinsonism and to relieve spasm of smooth muscle in digestive disorders. It is administered by mouth; side-effects can include dry mouth, disturbed vision, flushing, and dizziness. Trade name: **Tremonil**.

甲哌噻吨 控制帕金森氏綜合徵中的震顫和其它症狀，並可解除消化道疾病中平滑肌痙攣的、類似於阿托品作用的藥物。口服。副作用有口乾、視力障礙、潮紅和眩暈。

methoin *n.* an *anticonvulsant drug used to prevent or reduce the severity of grand mal fits in *epilepsy. It is administered by mouth; common side-effects are drowsiness, dizziness, and nausea. Trade name: **Mesontoin**.

3-甲基苯乙妥因 預防或減輕癲癇大發作嚴重程度的一種抗驚厥藥。口服。常見副作用爲瞌睡、頭暈和噁心。

methoserpidine *n.* a drug that lowers the blood pressure. It is administered by mouth; common side-effects include lethargy, drowsiness, and digestive upsets. Trade name: **Decaserpyl**.

異利血平 降血壓藥。口服。常見副作用爲昏睡、嗜眠和消化不良。

methotrexate *n.* a drug that interferes with cell growth and is used to treat various types of cancer, including leukaemia (*see* antimetabolite). It is administered by mouth or injection; common side-effects include mouth sores, digestive upsets, skin rashes, and hair loss.

甲氨蝶呤 治療包括白血病的各種癌症的干擾細胞生長藥（見抗代謝產物）。口服或注射。常見副作用有口腔潰瘍、消化不良、皮疹和脫髮。

methotrimeprazine *n.* a tranquillizing, sedative, and analgesic drug used to treat anxiety, tension, and agitation and to relieve moderate or severe pain. It is administered by mouth or injection; common side-effects are drowsiness and weakness. Trade name: **Veractil**.

甲氧異丁嗪 治療焦慮、緊張和激動並解除中、重度疼痛的安定、鎮靜和止痛藥。口服或注射。常見副作用爲瞌睡和虛弱。

methoxamine *n.* a *sympathomimetic drug that causes blood vessels to constrict and thus raises blood pressure. It is administered by injection to maintain the blood pressure during surgical operations. High doses may cause headache and vomiting. Trade name: **Vasoxine**.

甲氧胺 使血管收縮，進而使血壓升高的擬交感神經藥。注射給藥以維持外科手術中的血壓。大劑量可引起頭痛和嘔吐。商品名：美連克新命。

methoxyphenamine *n.* a *sympathomimetic drug used to treat asthma and other allergic conditions, such as rhinitis, and added to cough mixtures. It is administered by mouth and may cause nausea, dizziness, and dry mouth. Trade name: **Orthoxine**.

喘咳寧 治療氣喘和其它變應性疾病和鼻炎的擬交感神經藥。此藥還可加入咳嗽合劑中。口服。可引起噁心，頭暈和口乾。商品名：奧索克新。

methyl alcohol (methanol) wood alcohol: an alcohol that is oxidized in the body much more slowly than ethyl alcohol and forms poisonous products. As little as 10 ml of pure methyl alcohol can produce permanent blindness, and 100 ml is likely to be fatal. The breakdown product formaldehyde is responsible for damage to the eyes; it is itself converted to formic acid, which causes acidosis and death from respiratory failure. *See also* methylated spirits.

甲醇（木醇） 在體內比乙醇氧化慢得多並形成毒性產物的一種醇。僅10毫升純甲醇就可致永久性失明，100毫升就可致命。裂解產物甲醛造成眼的損害，甲醛又自行轉變成甲酸，甲酸可引起酸中毒和呼吸衰竭而死亡。

methylamphetamine *n.* a drug with actions and side-effects similar to those of *amphetamine. It is administered by mouth to treat narcolepsy and parkinsonism and some depressive states, and to reduce appetite. It is also administered by injection in psychiatry, to restore the blood pressure in surgical procedures, and to treat drug overdosage. Its use is restricted to hospitals.

去氧麻黃鹼 作用和副作用類似於苯丙胺的一種藥。口服。治療發作性睡眠、帕金森氏綜合徵和某些抑鬱狀態，並可降低食慾。對精神病人可注射給藥。可恢復外科操作中的血壓，並可治療藥物過量。此藥僅可在醫院內使用。

methylated spirits a mixture consisting mainly of ethyl alcohol with *methyl alcohol and petroleum hydrocar-

甲基化酯劑 主要由乙醇及甲醇和石油烴組成的混合製劑。添加吡啶使酯劑

bons. The addition of pyridine gives it an objectionable smell, and the dye methyl violet is added to make it recognizable as unfit to drink. It is used as a solvent, cleaning fluid, and fuel.

具有難聞的氣味，另外加入甲紫染劑使其易於識別爲不能飲用的物品。它可用作溶劑、清潔液和燃料。

methylcellulose *n.* a compound that absorbs water and is used as a bulk *laxative to treat constipation, to control diarrhoea, and in patients with a *colostomy. It is administered by mouth and usually has no side-effects. Trade names: **Celevac**, **Cellucon**, **Cologel**.

甲基纖維素 一種吸水性化合物，它是治療便秘、控制腹瀉、並用於結腸造口術病人的容積性輕瀉劑。口服。通常無副作用。

methyldopa *n.* a drug that reduces blood pressure (*see* sympatholytic). It is administered by mouth or injection, and drowsiness commonly occurs during the first days of treatment. Trade names: **Aldomet**, **Dopamet**, **Hydromet**, **Medomet**.

甲基多巴 一種降壓藥。口服或注射。在治療的最初幾天常有瞌睡。商品名：愛道美。

methylene blue a blue antiseptic dye that has been used to treat infections of the urinary system, methaemoglobinaemia, and in a test for kidney function. It is also used to stain bacterial cells for microscopic examination.

亞甲藍 已用於治療泌尿系感染、高鐵血紅蛋白血〔症〕和試驗腎功能的一種藍色防腐染劑。也可用於顯微鏡檢查時細菌細胞的染色。

methylergometrine *n.* a drug that stimulates contractions of the womb. It is used in childbirth to control bleeding following delivery and to help the womb return to normal. It is administered by mouth or injection and may cause headache and vertigo.

甲基麥角新鹼 刺激子宮收縮藥。用於控制分娩時胎兒娩出後的出血，並可幫助子宮恢復正常。口服或注射。可引起頭痛和眩暈。

methyl green a basic dye used for colouring the stainable part of the cell nucleus (chromatin) and – with pyronin – for the differential staining of RNA and DNA, which give a red and a green colour respectively.

甲〔基〕綠 一種鹼性染劑。用於對細胞核可染部分（染色質）進行染色；與派若寧合用，可作RNA和DNA的鑑別染色，分別顯示出紅色和綠色。

methylphenidate *n.* a *sympathomimetic drug that also stimulates the central nervous system. It is used to improve mental activity in convalescence and some depressive states and to overcome lethargy associated with drug treatment. It is administered by mouth

苯哌啶醋酸甲酯 一種擬交感神經藥，也可興奮中樞神經系統。此藥用於改善和提高病後恢復期和某些抑鬱狀態病人的精神活動，並克服與藥物治療有關的嗜眠。口服或注射。

or injection; side-effects such as nervousness and insomnia may occur. Trade name: **Ritalin**.

副作用可有神經過敏和失眠。商品名：鹽酸哌醋甲酯。

methyl salicylate oil of wintergreen: a liquid with *counterirritant and *analgesic properties, applied to the skin to relieve pain in lumbago, sciatica, and rheumatic conditions.

水楊酸甲酯 即冬綠油，具有抗刺激和止痛作用的液體，用於皮膚以解除腰痛、坐骨神經痛和風濕症疼痛。

methyltestosterone *n.* a synthetic male sex hormone (*see* androgen) administered by mouth to treat sexual underdevelopment in men. It is also used to suppress lactation, to treat menstrual and menopausal disorders, and to treat breast cancer in women. Side-effects are those of *testosterone.

甲基睾〔丸〕酮 一種人工合成的男性性激素（見雄激素）。口服。用於治療男性性發育不全。也可用於抑制泌乳、治療月經和絕經時的疾病，並可治療女性乳腺癌。副作用與睾丸素的副作用相同。

methylthiouracil *n.* a drug that inhibits thyroid activity, used to treat overactivity of the thyroid gland (*see* thyrotoxicosis). It is administered by mouth; side-effects may include rashes, digestive upsets, and headache.

甲硫氧嘧啶 一種能抑制甲狀腺活動的藥物。用於治療甲狀腺機能亢進。口服。副作用有皮疹、消化不良和頭痛。

methyl violet (gentian violet) a dye used mainly for staining Protozoa.

甲〔基〕紫（龍膽紫） 主要用於染原生動物的染劑。

methyprylone *n.* a hypnotic and *sedative drug used to treat insomnia and to relieve anxiety and tension. It is administered by mouth; side-effects such as headache and drowsiness may occur. Trade name: **Noludar**.

甲乙哌啶酮 治療失眠和解除焦慮及緊張的催眠和鎮靜藥。口服。副作用可有頭痛和瞌睡。商品名：腦了達。

methysergide *n.* a drug used to prevent severe migraine attacks and to control diarrhoea associated with tumours in the digestive system. It is administered by mouth; common side-effects are digestive upsets, dizziness, and drowsiness. Trade name: **Deseril**.

二甲麥角新鹼 預防嚴重偏頭痛發作和控制與消化系統腫瘤有關的腸瀉的藥物。口服。常見副作用有消化不良、眩暈和瞌睡。

metoclopramide *n.* a drug that speeds up digestion. It is used to treat nausea, vomiting, indigestion, heartburn, and flatulence. It is administered by mouth or injection; high doses may cause drowsiness and muscle spasms. Trade names: **Maxolon, Primperan**.

滅吐靈 助消化藥。治療噁心，嘔吐、消化不良、燒心和〔腸胃〕氣脹。口服或注射。大劑量可引起瞌睡和肌肉痙攣。商品名：胃復安。

metolazone *n.* a *diuretic used to treat fluid retention (oedema) and high blood pressure. It is administered by mouth; side-effects include headache, loss of appetite, and digestive upsets, and blood potassium levels may be reduced. Trade name: **Zoroxolyn**.

甲苯喹唑酮 治療液體瀦留（水腫）和高血壓的利尿劑。口服。副作用有頭痛、食慾喪失、消化不良和低血鉀。

metoprolol *n.* a drug that controls the activity of the heart (*see* beta blocker) and is used to treat high blood pressure and angina. It is administered by mouth; the commonest side-effects are tiredness and digestive upsets. Trade names: **Betaloc**, **Lopressor**.

甲氧乙心安 控制心臟活動並治療高血壓和心絞痛的藥物。口服。最常見副作用爲疲乏和消化不良。商品名：美多心安。

metr- (metro-) *prefix denoting* the womb.

〔前綴〕 **子宮**

metralgia *n.* pain in the womb.

子宮痛 子宮內的疼痛。

metre *n.* the *SI unit of length that is equal to 39.37 inches. It is formally defined as the length of the path travelled by light in vacuum during a time interval of 1/299,792,458 of a second. Symbol: m.

米 相當於39.37英寸的長度國際單位。它被正式地規定爲1/299,792,458秒的間隔內，光在眞空中傳播路線的長度。符號：M。

metritis *n.* inflammation of the womb. *See also* endometritis, myometritis.

子宮炎 子宮的炎症。

metrocolpocele *n.* protrusion of the womb into the vagina, which consequently becomes displaced downwards.

子宮陰道膨出 子宮脫入陰道，結果形成子宮向下移位。

metronidazole *n.* a drug used to treat infections of the urinary, genital, and digestive systems, such as trichomoniasis, amoebiasis, and giardiasis, and acute ulcerative gingivitis. It is administered by mouth or in suppositories; side-effects are rare but may include digestive upsets, drowsiness, and headache. Trade name: **Flagyl**.

四硝噻唑 治療毛滴蟲病、阿米巴病和梨形鞭毛蟲病等泌尿、生殖和消化系感染，以及急性潰瘍性牙齦炎的藥物。口服或製成栓劑。偶見副作用，但可有消化不良、瞌睡和頭痛。商品名：滅滴靈。

metropathia haemorrhagica (essential uterine haemorrhage) abnormal loss of blood in the womb, resulting from disease. The lining membrane of the womb usually thickens and there may be fluid-filled sacs in the ovary.

機能性子宮出血（自發性子宮出血） 由疾病所致的子宮異常失血。子宮內膜常變厚，並且卵巢內可有充滿液體的囊。

metroptosis (uterine prolapse) *n.* the downward displacement of the womb. The neck (cervix) of the womb sometimes protrudes from the vaginal opening. The womb usually drops under the influence of gravity because the supporting tissues are weak or damaged, especially in women who have given birth. A surgical operation may be required in order to correct the condition. *Compare* metrocolpocele.

子宮脫垂（子宮脫出） 子宮向下移位。有時子宮頸從陰道口脫出。特別是生育後的婦女因子宮支持組織薄弱或受損，在重力的影響下子宮常下降。可行外科手術矯正此情況。

metrorrhagia *n.* bleeding from the womb when menstruation is not due. Metrorrhagia may indicate the presence of cancer of the cervix (neck of the womb) or some other disease of the womb.

子宮出血 月經期以外的子宮出血。子宮出血可代表存有宮頸癌或子宮的其它疾病。

metrostaxis *n.* a slight but incessant loss of blood from the womb.

子宮滲血 子宮輕微的和持續的出血。

-metry *suffix denoting* measuring or measurement.

〔後綴〕 **測量**

mianserin *n.* a drug used to relieve moderate or severe depression and anxiety. It is administered by mouth; side-effects are usually milder than with other potent antidepressants, the commonest being drowsiness. Trade name: **Bolvidon**.

甲苯吡草 用於解除中、重度抑鬱和焦慮的藥。口服。副作用較其它强效抗抑鬱藥輕，最常見爲瞌睡。

micelle *n.* one of the microscopic particles into which the products of fat digestion (i.e. fatty acids and monoglycerides), present in the gut, are dispersed by the action of *bile salts. Fatty material in this finely dispersed form is more easily absorbed by the small intestine.

微膠粒 在膽汁鹽的作用下，腸道內的脂肪消化產物（如：脂肪酸和單酸甘油酯）分散成的一種微粒。這種小的分散形式的脂肪物質更易被小腸吸收。

micr- (micro-) *prefix denoting* **1.** small size. **2.** one millionth part.

〔前綴〕 ①**小** ②**微** 百萬分之一。

microaerophilic *adj.* describing microorganisms that grow best at very low oxygen concentrations (i.e. below the atmospheric level).

微需氧的 描述在氧濃度極低時（如：低於大氣水平）生長得最好的微生物。

microaneurysm *n.* a minute localized swelling of a capillary wall, which is found in the retina of patients with

微動脉瘤 糖尿病性視網膜病病人視網膜內毛細血管壁上的局限性小腫物，

diabetic *retinopathy. It is recognized as a small red dot when the interior of the eye is examined with an *ophthalmoscope.

當用眼底鏡檢查眼內時，所看到的微動脈瘤爲一小紅點。

microangiopathy *n.* damage to the walls of the smallest blood vessels. It may result from a variety of diseases, including diabetes mellitus, collagen diseases, infections, and cancer. Common manifestations of microangiopathy are kidney failure, haemolysis (damage to red blood cells), and purpura (bleeding into the skin). The treatment is that of the underlying cause.

微血管病 最小血管壁的損傷。病因可爲包括糖尿病、膠原病、感染和癌症的不同疾病。微血管病常見表現形式是腎衰竭、溶血（紅細胞受損）和紫癜（皮下出血）。治療時應治原發病。

microbe *n. see* microorganism.

微生物

microbiology *n.* the science of *microorganisms. Microbiology in relation to medicine is concerned mainly with the isolation and identification of the microorganisms that cause disease. —**microbiological** *adj.* —**microbiologist** *n.*

微生物學 研究微生物的科學。與醫學有關的微生物學主要是研討致病微生物的分離和鑑定等。

microblepharon (microblepharism) *n.* the condition of having abnormally small eyelids.

小〔眼〕瞼 眼瞼小於正常。

microcephaly *n.* abnormal smallness of the head in relation to the size of the rest of the body: a congenital condition in which the brain is not fully developed. *Compare* macrocephaly.

小頭 頭異常小，與身體其它部位不成比例。是一種先天性腦發育不全。

microcheilia *n.* abnormally small size of the lips. *Compare* macrocheilia.

小唇 唇小於正常。

Micrococcus *n.* a genus of spherical Gram-positive bacteria occurring in colonies. They are saprophytes or parasites. The species *M. tetragenus* (formerly *Gaffkya tetragena*) is normally a harmless parasite in man but it can become pathogenic, causing arthritis, endocarditis, meningitis, or abscesses in tissues. It occurs in groups of four.

細球菌屬 結腸內革蘭氏陽性球菌屬。爲腐物寄生物或寄生物。其中的一種四聯細球菌（以前稱爲四聯球菌）是人體中正常的無害寄生物，但它可變成致病菌，引起關節炎、心內膜炎、腦〔脊〕膜炎或組織膿腫。它以四個一組的形式存在。

microcyte *n.* an abnormally small red blood cell (*erythrocyte). *See also* microcytosis. —**microcytic** *adj.*

小紅細胞 一種異常的小型紅細胞。

microcytosis *n.* the presence of abnormally small red cells (*microcytes*) in the blood. Microcytosis is a feature of certain anaemias (*microcytic anaemias*), including iron-deficiency anaemias, certain *haemoglobinopathies, anaemias associated with chronic infections, etc.

小紅細胞症 血中存有異常的小型紅細胞。小紅細胞症是缺鐵性貧血、某種血紅蛋白病和與慢性感染有關的貧血等一類貧血（小紅細胞性貧血）的一個特徵。

microdactyly *n.* abnormal smallness or shortness of the fingers.

細指（趾） 異常小和短的手指或足趾。

microdissection *n.* the process of dissecting minute structures under the microscope. Miniature surgical instruments, such as knives made of glass, are manipulated by means of geared connections that reduce the relatively coarse movements of the operator's fingers into microscopic movements. Using this technique it is possible to dissect the nuclei of cells and even to separate individual chromosomes. *See also* microsurgery.

顯微解剖 在顯微鏡下解剖細微結構的過程。微型外科儀器，如：玻璃刀是通過把術者手指相對粗大的動作轉變爲細微動作的傳動裝置來進行的。使用這種技術可解剖細胞核，甚至分離單個染色體。

microdontia *n.* a condition in which the teeth are unusually small.

小牙 牙齒小於正常。

microelectrode *n.* an extremely fine wire used as an electrode to measure the electrical activity in small areas of tissue. Microelectrodes can be used for recording the electrical changes that occur in the membranes of cells, such as those of nerve and muscle.

微電極 用極微細的電線作電極，以測量小範圍組織內電活動的裝置。微電極可用於記錄發生在細胞膜，如神經和肌肉細胞膜上的電變化。

microfilaria *n.* (*pl.* **microfilariae**) the motile embryo of certain nematodes (*see* filaria). The slender microfilariae, 150–300 μm in length, are commonly found in the circulating blood or lymph of patients suffering an infection with any of the filarial worms, e.g. *Wuchereria.* They mature into larvae, which are infective, within the body of a bloodsucking insect, such as a mosquito.

微絲蚴 某些線蟲的可活動的胚胎。細微絲蚴長150～300微米，常見於任何一種絲蟲（如：吳策線蟲屬）感染的病人血循環或淋巴中。在吸血昆蟲（如蚊子）體內成熟爲幼蟲，具有傳染性。

microgamete *n.* the motile flagellate male sex cell of the malarial parasite (*Plasmodium*) and other single-celled animals (*see* Protozoa). The microgamete is similar to the sperm cell of higher animal groups and smaller than the female sex cell (*see* macrogamete).

小配子 瘧疾寄生物（瘧原蟲屬）和其它單細胞動物（見原生動物）能活動的有鞭毛的雄性性細胞。小配子類似於較高級動物的精子細胞，並且小於雌性性細胞。

microgametocyte *n.* a cell that undergoes meiosis to form 6–8 mature male sex cells (microgametes) of the malarial parasite (**Plasmodium*). Microgametocytes are found in the blood of man but must be ingested by a mosquito before developing into microgametes.

小配子體 瘧疾寄生物（瘧原蟲屬）的一種細胞，減數分裂後形成6～8個成熟雄性性細胞（小配子）。小配子體見於人血中，但是在發育成小配子之前必須被蚊子攝入。

microglia *n.* one of the two basic classes of *glia (the non-nervous cells of the central nervous system), having a mainly scavenging function (*see* macrophage). *Compare* macroglia.

小神經膠質〔細胞〕 兩種基本神經膠質中的一種（中樞神經系統的非神經細胞），主要具有清除功能。

microglossia *n.* abnormally small size of the tongue.

小舌 舌小於正常。

micrognathia *n.* a condition in which one jaw is unusually small.

小頜 頜小於正常。

microgram *n.* one millionth of a gram. Symbol: μg.

微克 百萬分之一克。符號：μg。

micrograph (photomicrograph) *n.* a photograph of an object viewed through a microscope. An *electron micrograph* is photographed through an electron microscope; a *light micrograph* through a light microscope.

顯微照片 通過顯微鏡拍攝某物體的照片。電子顯微照片是通過電子顯微鏡拍攝的，光學顯微照片是通過光學顯微鏡拍攝的。

microgyria *n.* a developmental disorder of the brain in which the folds (convolutions) in its surface are small and its surface layer (cortex) is structurally abnormal. It is associated with mental and physical retardation.

小腦廻 腦表面褶（腦廻）小並且腦皮層（皮質）結構異常的腦發育障礙。它與智力和體力發育遲緩有關。

microhaematocrit *n.* a measurement of the proportion of red blood cells in a volume of circulating blood. It is determined by taking a sample of the patient's blood in a fine tube and spinning it in a centrifuge until settling is complete. *See* packed cell volume.

微紅細胞壓積 一定容量的循環血液中紅細胞所佔比例的測量值。方法是採取病人的血樣品放入一小管內，並將小管置於離心機內，使其旋轉直到完全沉澱。

micromanipulation *n.* the manipulation of extremely small structures under the microscope, as in *microdissection, or *microsurgery.

顯微操作 顯微鏡下，在極小結構上進行的操作，象顯微解剖或顯微外科。

micromastia (micromazia) *n.* the condition of having abnormally small breasts.

小乳房 乳房小於正常。

micromelia *n.* abnormally small size of the arms or legs. *Compare* macromelia.

小肢 上、下肢小於正常。

micrometer *n.* an instrument for making extremely fine measurements of thickness or length, often relying upon the movement of a screw thread and the principle of the *vernier.

測微計 常靠螺紋的運動和微調的原理進行厚度和長度的精細測量的儀器。

micrometre *n.* one millionth of a metre (10^{-6} m). Symbol: μm.

微米 百萬分之一米。符號：μm。

microorganism (microbe) *n.* any organism too small to be visible to the naked eye. Microorganisms include *bacteria, some *fungi, *mycoplasmas, *protozoa, *rickettsiae, and *viruses.

微生物 肉眼看不到的任何小生物〔體〕。微生物包括細菌、某些眞菌、支原體、原生動物、立克次氏體和病毒。

microphotograph *n.* **1.** a photograph reduced to microscopic proportions. **2.** (loosely) a *photomicrograph.

①**縮微照片** 縮小到顯微鏡下才能看清的照片。
②**顯微照片**

micropipette *n.* an extremely fine tube from which minute volumes of liquid can be delivered. It can also be used to draw up minute quantities of liquid for examination. Using a micropipette it is possible to add or take away material from individual cells under the microscope.

微量吸管 用於釋出小量液體的極小管。它也用於吸取檢查用的小量液體。使用微量吸管可以在顯微鏡下添加或取出個別細胞中的物質。

micropsia *n.* a condition in which objects appear smaller than they really are. It is usually due to disease of the retina affecting the *macula but may occur in paralysis of *accommodation and in some brain disorders.

視物顯小症 所視物體小於正常的現象。病因常爲影響黃斑的視網膜病，但也可發生在調節痲痹和某些腦疾病中。

microscope *n.* an instrument for producing a greatly magnified image of an object, which may be so small as to be invisible to the naked eye. *Light* or *optical microscopes* use light as a radia-

顯微鏡 可使肉眼看不到的小物體產生極大的放大圖像的儀器。光學顯微鏡用光作爲觀察樣品的射綫源並且用一套鏡頭，通常

tion source for viewing the specimen and combinations of lenses to magnify the image, usually an *objective and an *eyepiece. *See also* electron microscope, operating microscope, ultramicroscope. —**microscopical** *adj.* —**microscopy** *n.*

爲一個〔接〕物鏡和一個〔接〕目鏡來放大圖像。

microscopic *adj.* **1.** too small to be seen clearly without the use of a microscope. **2.** of, relating to, or using a microscope.

①**顯微鏡的** 小到必須用顯微鏡才能看清的。 ②**顯微鏡下的** 與顯微鏡有關的，或借助於顯微鏡的。

microsome *n.* a small particle consisting of a piece of *endoplasmic reticulum with ribosomes attached. Microsomes are formed when homogenized cells are centrifuged. —**microsomal** *adj.*

微粒體 由附着有核糖體的小塊內質網組成的小顆粒。勻化細胞離心時可形成微粒體。

microsonation *n.* the use of ultrasound waves generated inside the body from an extremely small source, such as the tip of a needle or a bubble within the tissues. This technique is used to obtain a picture of the fine structure of the neighbouring tissues. It is a specialized form of *ultrasonography.

微超聲檢查法 從體內的極小聲源（如插入組織內的針尖和氣囊）產生的超聲波的技術。此技術用於獲得鄰近組織微細結構的圖像。它是超聲波檢查法的特殊形式。

Microsporum *n.* a genus of fungi causing *ringworm of the skin, hair, and nails. The species *M. audouini* causes ringworm of the scalp (tinea capitis).

小孢子菌屬 引起皮膚、毛髮和指甲癬病的眞菌屬。其中的一種奧杜安氏小孢子菌可引起頭皮癬（頭癬）。

microsurgery *n.* the branch of surgery in which extremely intricate operations are performed through highly refined *operating microscopes using miniaturized precision instruments (forceps, scissors, needles, etc.). The technique enables surgery of previously inaccessible parts of the eye, inner ear, spinal cord, and brain (e.g. for the removal of tumours and repair of cerebral aneurysms), as well as the reattachment of amputated fingers (necessitating the suturing of minute nerves and blood vessels) and the reversal of vasectomies.

顯微外科 通過精密度極高的手術顯微鏡，使用微型精密器械（鑷子、剪子、針等），進行極其複雜手術的一種外科。此技術使外科手術可以在以前不易操作的眼、內耳、脊髓和腦（如：切除腫瘤和修補腦動脈瘤）的部位進行，並可進行斷指再植術（必須進行小神經和小血管的縫合）和輸精管切斷術後的再接通。

microtome *n.* an instrument for cutting extremely thin slices of material that can be examined under a micro-

切片機 把材料切成能在顯微鏡下檢查的極薄片的器械。被檢材料通常植於

scope. The material is usually embedded in a suitable medium, such as paraffin wax. A common type of microtome is a steel knife.

適當包埋料中，如：石蠟。常見類型是鋼刀。

microvillus *n.* (*pl.* **microvilli**) one of a number of microscopic hairlike structures (about 5 μm long) projecting from the surface of epithelial cells (*see* epithelium). They serve to increase the surface area of the cell and are seen on absorptive and secretory cells. In some regions (particularly the intestinal tract) microvilli form a dense covering on the free surface of the cells: this is called a *brush border*.

微絨毛 顯微鏡下若干突起於上皮細胞表面的毛髮樣結構（大約5微米長）之一。它們可增加細胞的表面積，並見於吸收和分泌細胞上。在某些部位（特別是腸道），微絨毛形成覆蓋在細胞游離面上的一致密層，稱爲刷狀緣。

microwave therapy a form of *diathermy using electromagnetic waves of extremely short wavelength. In modern apparatus the electric currents induced in the tissues have frequencies of up to 25,000 million cycles per second.

微波療法 用極短波長的電磁波進行的一種透熱法。在先進的儀器中，組織中的感應電流達到250億周/秒的頻率。

micturition *n. see* urination.

排尿

midbrain (mesencephalon) *n.* the small portion of the *brainstem, excluding the pons and the medulla, that joins the hindbrain to the forebrain.

中腦 不包括腦橋和延髓的，連接菱腦與前腦的小部分腦幹。

middle ear (tympanic cavity) the part of the *ear that consists of an air-filled space within the petrous part of the temporal bone. It is lined with mucous membrane and is connected to the pharynx by the *Eustachian tube and to the outer ear by the eardrum (*tympanic membrane). Within the middle ear are three bones – the auditory *ossicles – which transmit sound vibrations from the outer ear to the inner ear (*see* labyrinth).

中耳（鼓室腔） 由顳骨岩部內含氣腔構成的部分耳結構。其表面覆有黏膜，通過咽鼓管與咽相連，通過鼓膜與外耳相連。中耳內有三塊聽小骨，能把聲波從外耳傳到內耳。

midgut *n.* the middle portion of the embryonic gut, which gives rise to most of the small intestine and part of the large intestine. Early in development it is connected with the *yolk sac outside the embryo via the *umbilicus.

中腸 發育成大部分小腸和部分大腸的胚腸的中部。在發育早期，它經過臍部與胚胎外面的卵黃囊相連。

midwifery *n.* the profession of providing assistance and medical care to women undergoing labour and childbirth. *See also* domiciliary midwife, obstetrics. —**midwife** *n.*

助產學 對分娩和臨產的婦女提供幫助和醫療服務的專業。

migraine *n.* a recurrent throbbing headache that characteristically affects one side of the head. There is sometimes forewarning of an attack (an *aura*) consisting of flickering bright lights or blurring of vision, which clears up as the headache develops. It is often accompanied by prostration and vomiting.

偏頭痛 以影響到一側頭爲特點的復發性、搏動性頭痛。有時可有發作先兆，爲閃耀性亮光或視力模糊，頭痛出現後消失。頭痛常伴有虛脫和嘔吐。

miliaria *n. see* prickly heat.

粟疹，痱子，汗疹

miliary *adj.* describing or characterized by very small nodules or lesions, resembling millet seed.

粟粒性的 形容象小米粒樣的極小結節或病竈。

miliary tuberculosis acute generalized *tuberculosis characterized by lesions in affected organs, which resemble millet seeds.

粟粒性結核 以受累器官內小米粒樣病竈爲特徵的急性全身性結核。

milium *n.* (*pl.* **milia**) a white nodule in the skin, particularly on the face. Up to 4 mm in diameter, milia are round masses of *keratin occurring just beneath the outer layer (epidermis) of the skin.

粟粒疹 皮膚內，特別是臉上的白結節。粟粒疹是直徑約爲4毫米的，緊靠皮膚外層（表皮）之下的角蛋白團塊。

milk *n.* the liquid food secreted by female mammals from the mammary gland. It is the sole source of food for the young of most mammals at the start of life. Milk is a complete food in that it has most of the nutrients necessary for life: protein, carbohydrate, fat, minerals, and vitamins. The composition of milk varies very much from mammal to mammal. Cows' milk contains nearly all the essential nutrients but is comparatively deficient in vitamins C and D. Human milk contains more sugar (lactose) and less protein than cows' milk.

奶 由雌性哺乳動物乳腺分泌的液體食物。它是大多數幼小哺乳動物生命初期的唯一食物來源。奶中含有大多數生命必需營養物質：蛋白質、碳水化合物、脂肪、礦物質和維生素，是一種營養全面的食物。不同哺乳動物的奶成分可有很大的變化。牛奶含有幾乎所有的基本營養，但是相對缺少維生素C和D。和牛奶相比，人奶含糖較多，含蛋白質較少。

milk leg *see* white leg.

股白腫

milk teeth *Colloquial.* the deciduous teeth of young children. *See* dentition.

乳牙 幼兒的暫牙，俗稱。

milli- *prefix denoting* one thousandth part.

〔前綴〕 **毫** 千分之一。

milliampere *n.* one thousandth of an ampere (10^{-3} A). Symbol: mA.

毫安〔培〕 千分之一安〔培〕。符號：mA。

milligram *n.* one thousandth of a gram. Symbol: mg.

毫克 千分之一克。符號：mg。

millilitre *n.* one thousandth of a litre. Symbol: ml. *See* litre.

毫升 千分之一升。符號：ml。

millimetre *n.* one thousandth of a metre (10^{-3} m). Symbol: mm.

毫米 千分之一米。符號：mm。

Miltown *n. see* meprobamate.

眠爾通

MIND the National Association for Mental Health. It is a voluntary association, registered as a charity, that promotes the welfare of those with *mental illness through advice, education, campaigning, and the provision of resources.

國家精神衛生協會 志願參加的，以慈善團體的形式出現的協會，它通過諮詢、教育、開展活動和供應物資來促進精神病病人的福利事業。

mineralocorticoid *n. see* corticosteroid.

鹽〔腎上腺〕皮質素類

minim *n.* a unit of volume used in pharmacy, equivalent to one sixtieth part of a fluid *drachm.

量滴 同於藥學調劑的容量單位。相當於一液量打蘭六十分之一。

Minamata disease a form of mercury poisoning (from ingesting methyl mercury in contaminated fish) that caused 43 deaths in the Japanese coastal town of Minimata during 1953–56. The source of mercury was traced to an effluent containing mercuric sulphate from a local PVC factory. Symptoms include numbness, difficulty in controlling the limbs, and impaired speech and hearing.

水俣病 1953～1956年，日本沿海水俣市發生的使43人死亡的汞中毒事例（因攝入被甲基汞污染的魚）。當地聚氯乙烯工廠含硫酸汞的流出物被查證爲汞的來源。症狀包括麻木、四肢失控、言語和聽力受損。

mio- *prefix denoting* **1.** reduction or diminution. **2.** rudimentary.

〔前綴〕 ①**減少，縮小** ②**原基的，退化的**（殘遺痕迹）

miosis (myosis) *n.* constriction of the pupil. This occurs normally in bright light, but persistent miosis is most

縮瞳 瞳孔收縮。在光綫明亮時，瞳孔收縮是正常的，但持續性瞳孔收縮最

commonly due to drug therapy for glaucoma. *See also* miotic. *Compare* mydriasis.

常因青光眼藥物治療引起。

miotic *n.* a drug that causes the pupil of the eye to contract. Miotics, such as *physostigmine and *pilocarpine, are used to counteract the dilation of the pupil caused by drugs such as ephedrine and phenylephrine and to reduce the pressure in the eye in the treatment of glaucoma.

縮瞳藥 使眼瞳孔收縮的藥物。縮瞳藥，如：毒扁豆鹼和毛果芸香鹼，用於對抗麻黃鹼和脫羥腎上腺素類藥引起的瞳孔擴張；在青光眼治療中用於降低眼壓。

miracidium *n.* (*pl.* **miracidia**) the first-stage larva of a parasitic *fluke. Miracidia hatch from eggs released into water with the host's excreta. They have *cilia and swim about until they reach a snail. The miracidia then bore into the snail's soft tissues and there continue their development as *sporocysts.

毛蚴 寄生性吸蟲的初期幼蟲。毛蚴從隨着宿主的排泄物釋放到水中的卵內孵出。它們有纖毛，能游動，當接觸到小螺時，毛蚴鑽入小螺的軟組織，在那裏繼續發育成包蚴。

miscarriage *n. see* abortion.

流產

miso- *prefix denoting* hatred. Example: *misopedia* (of children).

〔前綴〕 **厭** 指憎恨，如：厭子女症。

missed case a person suffering from an infection in whom the symptoms and signs are so minimal that either there is no request for medical assistance or the doctor fails to make the diagnosis. The patient usually has partial immunity to the disease, but since the infecting organisms (pathogens) are of normal virulence, nonimmune contacts can be affected with the full manifestations of the illness. The period of infectivity is confined to the shortened duration of the illness (in contrast to a *carrier, in whom the pathogen is present without necessarily causing any ill effect). Alternatively the subject has had the disease but retains some of the pathogens (e.g. in the throat or bowel) and so acts as a continuing reservoir of infection.

漏診病例 傳染病人的症狀和體徵極其輕微，以致病人沒有就醫要求，或者醫生未能做出診斷。通常此類病人對疾病有部分免疫力。但因病原體具有正常毒力，若接觸未免疫者則可產生疾病的全部表現。傳染期僅限於疾病的較短時間內（與帶菌者有所不同，帶菌者體內雖有致病菌，但不產生任何病狀）。然而，部分免疫病人患本病後可保留某些病原體（如：在喉或腸內），做爲延續的感染竈。

Misuse of Drugs Act (1971) (in the UK) an Act of Parliament restricting the use of dangerous drugs. These controlled drugs include the natural

濫用藥物條例（1971）（英國）限制使用危險藥物的國會條例。被管制的藥物包括天然阿片製劑及

*opiates and their synthetic substitutes, many stimulants (including amphetamine, cocaine, and pemoline), hallucinogens such as LSD and cannabis, and the sedative methaqualone. The Act specifies certain requirements for writing prescriptions for these drugs.

其人工合成替代物，許多興奮劑（包括苯異丙胺、可卡因、苯異妥英），致幻劑如麥角醯二乙胺、大麻和安眠酮鎮靜劑。條例規定了開這些藥物處方的某些條件和要求。

mite *n.* a free-living or parasitic arthropod belonging to a group (Acarina) that also includes the *ticks. Most mites are small, averaging 1 mm or less in length. A mite has no antennae or wings, and its body is not divided into a distinct head, thorax, and abdomen. Medically important mites include the many species causing dermatitis (e.g. *Dermatophagoides*) and the harvest mite (*see* Trombicula), which transmits scrub typhus.

蟎　一種自由生存或寄生性的節肢動物。屬於蟎目（包括蜱和蟎）。大多數蟎是小的，平均長度爲1毫米以下。蟎沒有觸角和翼，而且它的身體不能明顯地分爲頭、胸和腹。在醫學上有重要意義的蟎包括許多可致皮炎的蟎種（如：表皮蟎屬）和可傳播恙蟲病的恙蟎（沙虱）。

mithramycin *n.* an *antibiotic that prevents the growth of cancer cells. It is used mainly to treat cancer of the testis and is administered by injection. Common side-effects are digestive upsets and mouth ulcers and, more seriously, nosebleeds and vomiting of blood.

光輝黴素　預防癌細胞生長的抗生素。它主要用於治療睾丸癌。注射。常見副作用是消化不良和口腔潰瘍，更爲嚴重的是鼻出血和嘔吐。

mitobronitol *n.* a drug that prevents growth of cancer cells, used to treat leukaemia. It is administered by mouth; common side-effects are digestive upsets, hair loss, skin disorders, menstrual abnormalities, and reduction in the numbers of normal blood cells. Trade name: **Myelobromol**.

二溴甘露醇　治療白血病的預防癌細胞生長藥。口服。常見副作用爲消化不良、脫髮、皮膚疾患、月經異常和正常血細胞數量減少。

mitochondrion (chondriosome) *n.* (*pl.* **mitochondria**) a structure, occurring in varying numbers in the cytoplasm of every cell, that is the site of the cell's energy production. Mitochondria contain *ATP and the enzymes involved in the cell's metabolic activities; each is bounded by a double membrane, the inner being folded inwards to form projections (*cristae*). —**mitochondrial** *adj.*

線粒體　每個細胞的胞漿內都存在的一種結構，其數量有多有少，爲細胞能量生成的部位。線粒體含有ATP和參與細胞代謝活動的酶；每一線粒體都被一種雙層膜包裹，內層膜向裏折疊，形成突起。

mitogen *n.* any substance that can cause cells to begin division (*mitosis).

促細胞分裂劑　任何可引起細胞分裂（有絲分裂）的物質。

mitomycin C an antibiotic that inhibits the growth of cancer cells. It causes severe marrow suppression but is of use in the treatment of stomach and breast cancers.

絲裂黴素C 抑制癌細胞生長的抗生素。它可致嚴重的骨髓抑制，但仍用於治療胃癌和乳腺癌。

mitosis *n.* a type of cell division in which a single cell produces two genetically identical daughter cells. It is the way in which new body cells are produced for both growth and repair. Division of the nucleus (*karyokinesis*) takes place in four stages (*see* prophase, metaphase, anaphase, telophase) and is followed by division of the cytoplasm (*cytokinesis*) to form two daughter cells (see illustration). *Compare* meiosis. —**mitotic** *adj.*

有絲分裂 一個單細胞生成兩個基因相同的子細胞的一種細胞分裂型式。爲了生長和修復，有絲分裂是新體細胞生成的途徑。核分裂（間接核分裂）分四個階段，最後細胞漿分裂，形成兩個子細胞。（見圖）

mitral incompetence failure of the *mitral valve to close, allowing a reflux of blood from the left ventricle of the heart to the left atrium. It most often results from scarring of the mitral valve by rheumatic fever, but it can also develop as a complication of myocardial infarction or cardiomyopathies. It may occur as a congenital defect. Its manifestations include breathlessness, atrial *fibrillation, embolism, enlargement of the left ventricle, and a systolic *murmur. Mild cases are symptomless and require no treatment, but in severe cases the affected valve should be replaced with an artificial one (*mitral prosthesis*).

二尖瓣關閉不全 心臟二尖瓣不能關閉，使血液從左心室反流到左心房。最常見的病因是風濕熱所致的二尖瓣瘢痕形成，但它也可是心肌梗塞或心肌病的併發病。它可是先天性缺陷。其表現包括氣短、心房纖顫、栓塞、左心室擴大和收縮期雜音。輕症者無症狀並且無需治療；但重症者，應用人工瓣膜代替受累瓣膜。

mitral stenosis narrowing of the opening of the mitral valve: a result of chronic scarring that follows rheumatic fever. It may be seen alone or combined with *mitral incompetence. The symptoms are similar to those of mitral incompetence except that the patient has a diastolic *murmur. Mild cases need no treatment, but severe cases are treated surgically by reopening the stenosis (*mitral valvotomy*) or by inserting an artificial valve (*mitral prosthesis*).

二尖瓣狹窄 二尖瓣開口狹窄。病因爲風濕熱後的慢性瘢痕形成。它可單獨存在，也可與二尖瓣關閉不全同時存在。除了病人有舒張期雜音外，症狀與二尖瓣關閉不全類似。輕者無需治療，但重者須經外科治療，切開狹窄（二尖瓣瓣膜切開術）或植入人工瓣膜（二尖瓣修復術）。

mitral valve (bicuspid valve) a valve in the heart consisting of two flaps

二尖瓣 附着在左心房和左心室之間的房室口壁上

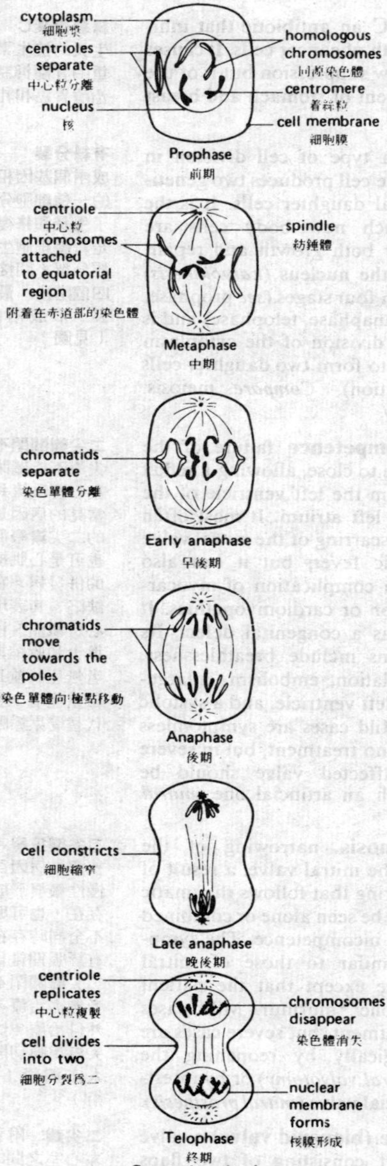

cytoplasm
細胞漿
centrioles
separate
中心粒分離
nucleus
核
homologous
chromosomes
同原染色體
centromere
着絲粒
cell membrane
細胞膜
Prophase
前期
centriole
中心粒
chromosomes
attached
to equatorial
region
附着在赤道部的染色體
spindle
紡錘體
Metaphase
中期
chromatids
separate
染色單體分離
Early anaphase
早後期
chromatids
move
towards the
poles
染色單體向極點移動
Anaphase
後期
cell constricts
細胞縮窄
Late anaphase
晚後期
centriole
replicates
中心粒複製
cell divides
into two
細胞分裂爲二
chromosomes
disappear
染色體消失
nuclear
membrane
forms
核膜形成
Telophase
終期

Stages in mitosis

有絲分裂各期

(cusps) attached to the walls at the opening between the left atrium and left ventricle. It allows blood to pass from the atrium to the ventricle, but prevents any backward flow.

的兩片心臟瓣膜。它允許血液通過心房到心室，但阻止任何反流。

mittelschmerz *n.* pain in the lower abdomen experienced about midway between successive menstrual periods, i.e. when the egg cell is being released from the ovary. *See also* menstrual cycle.

經間痛　在兩次月經周期之間，即當卵巢排卵時，發生的下腹痛。

mixed connective tissue disease a disease with features in common with systemic *lupus erythematosus, *polymyositis, and *scleroderma.

混合性結締組織病　與系統性紅斑狼瘡、多肌炎和硬皮病的特徵相同的一種疾病。

ml *abbrev. for* millilitre. *See* litre.

毫升

MLD minimal lethal dose: the smallest quantity of a toxic compound that is recorded as having caused death. *See also* LD_{50}.

最小致死量　經記錄的某毒性化合物的最小致死量。

mmHg a unit of pressure equal to 1 millimetre of mercury. 1 mmHg = 133.3224 pascals.

毫米汞柱　相當於1毫米汞的壓力單位。1毫米汞柱=133.3224帕斯卡。

modality *n.* **1.** a form of sensation, such as smell, hearing, tasting, or detecting temperature. Differences in modality are not due to differences in the structure of the nerves concerned, but to differences in the working of the sensory receptors and the areas of brain that receive the messages. **2.** one form of therapy as opposed to another, such as the modality of physiotherapy contrasted with that of radiotherapy.

①**感覺道（感覺種型）**感覺的一種類型，例如：嗅、聽、味或溫度覺。感覺道的差別不是有關神經結構的差別所致，而是感覺感受器的工作和接受信息的腦部位的差別所致。②**治療模式**　與另一種療法完全不同的治療方式，如物理療法與放射療法截然不同。

mode *n. see* mean.

衆數

modelling *n.* a technique used in *behaviour modification, whereby an individual learns a behaviour by observing someone else doing it. Together with *prompting, it is useful for introducing new behaviours to the individual.

模擬法　通過觀察其他人的行爲來向別人學習和改進自身行爲的方法。在別人的指點下，應用此方法對於個人學習新行爲是有用的。

modiolus *n.* the conical central pillar of the *cochlea in the inner ear.

蝸軸　內耳蝸的圓錐形中心柱。

Mogadon *n. see* nitrazepam.
硝基安定

molar *n.* in the permanent *dentition, the sixth, seventh, or eighth tooth from the midline on each side in each jaw (*see also* wisdom tooth). In the deciduous dentition, molars are the fourth and fifth teeth from the midline on each side in each jaw.
磨牙 在恒牙列的上下頜每一邊從中線數起的第6、第7或第8顆牙。在乳牙列的上下頜每一邊從中線數起的第4和第5顆牙。

molarity *n.* the strength of a solution, expressed as the weight of dissolved substance in grams per litre divided by its molecular weight, i.e. the number of moles per litre. Molarity is indicated as 0.1 M, 1 M, 2 M, etc.
容積克分子濃度 每升中以克爲單位的溶質的重量除以溶質的分子量所得出的某溶液的濃度，即每升中的克分子數。容積克分子濃度以0.1M、1M、2M等來表示。

molar solution a solution in which the number of grams of dissolved substance per litre equals its molecular weight, i.e. a solution of molarity 1 M.
容積克分子溶液 每升中溶質的克數等於其分子量的溶液，即容積克分子濃度爲1M的溶液。

mole[1] *n.* the *SI unit of amount of substance, equal to the amount of substance that contains as many elementary units as there are atoms in 0.012 kilograms of carbon-12. The elementary units, which must be specified, may be atoms, molecules, ions, electrons, etc., or a specified group of such entities. One mole of a compound has a mass equal to its molecular weight expressed in grams. Symbol: mol.
摩爾 物質的量的國際單位，1摩爾的物質中含有的基本單位的數量等於0.012千克的碳-12所含有的原子數。必須詳細說明基本單位可以是原子、分子、離子、電子等，或其特定的組合。某化合物1摩爾的質量相當於以克表示的此化合物分子量。符號：mol。

mole[2] *n.* an area of pigment, usually brown, in the skin. Some moles are flat; others are raised and occasionally have hairs growing from them. Certain types of mole can become malignant.
痣 皮內的色素區，常爲棕色。有些痣是平的，有的是凸起的並且偶見生出毛髮。某些類型的痣可變爲惡性。

molecular biology the study of the molecules that are associated with living organisms, especially proteins and nucleic acids.
分子生物學 研究與活的生物體——特別是與蛋白和核酸有關的——分子的學科。

molluscum *n.* any of several skin diseases typified by the development of soft rounded tumours. Commonly, the term is used for ***molluscum contagiosum***, a virus disease that produces small rounded pearl-like swellings with cra-
軟疣 以發生軟圓形腫物爲特徵的幾種皮膚病之一。通常指接觸傳染性軟疣，這是一種病毒性疾病，形成小圓形珠樣腫物，其中心凹陷，內含碎

ters containing broken-down matter. The condition is chronic and treatment is by removal with a *curette, *electrocautery, or by instilling carbolic acid locally. *See also* keratoacanthoma (molluscum sebaceum).

屑狀物質。慢性病程。治療方法是用刮器、電烙器去除軟疣或局部滴注石炭酸。

mon- (mono-) *prefix denoting* one, single, or alone.

〔前綴〕 單（一） 指一個，單一或單獨。

mongolism *n. see* Down's syndrome.

先天愚型

Monilia *n.* the former name of the genus of fungi now known as **Candida*.

念珠菌屬 念珠菌屬眞菌的舊名。現已改稱。

moniliasis *n. see* candidiasis.

念珠菌病

monoamine oxidase (MAO) an enzyme that catalyses the oxidation of a large variety of monoamines, including adrenaline, noradrenaline, and serotonin. Monoamine oxidase is found in most tissues, particularly the liver and nervous system. Drugs that act as inhibitors of this enzyme are widely used in the treatment of depression (*see* MAO inhibitor).

單胺氧化酶 催化包括腎上腺素、去甲腎上腺素和血清素的許多不同種類單胺氧化的酶。單胺氧化酶可見於許多不同組織。特別是肝和神經系統。單胺氧化酶抑制劑類的藥物廣泛用於治療抑鬱。

monoarthritis *n. see* arthritis.

單關節炎

monoblast *n.* the earliest identifiable cell that gives rise to a *monocyte. It is probably identical with the *myeloblast and matures via an intermediate stage (*promonocyte*). It is normally found in the blood-forming tissue of the *bone marrow but may appear in the blood in certain diseases, most notably in acute monoblastic *leukaemia.

成單核細胞 可生成單核細胞的最早可識別的細胞，它可能與原始粒細胞完全相同，並經過中間階段（幼單核細胞）而成熟。它可正常地出現在骨髓的造血組織，但也可見於患某種疾病的病人血中，最典型的見於急性成單核細胞性白血病中。

monochromat *n.* a person who is completely colour-blind. There are two types. The *rod monochromat* appears to have totally defective *cones: he has very poor visual acuity as well as the inability to discriminate colours. The *cone monochromat* has normal visual acuity: his cones appear to respond normally to light but to be completely unable to discriminate colours. It is possible in this case that the defect does not lie in the cones themselves but in

全色盲者 完全性色盲的病人。有兩種類型。視桿細胞性全色盲者表現出完全性視錐細胞缺陷；病人視敏度極差，並且不能辨認顏色。視錐細胞性全色盲者有正常的視敏度；病人視錐細胞對光反應正常，但完全不能辨認顏色。在這些病例中，並非視錐細胞本身的缺陷，而是從視錐細胞傳到腦的神

the integration of the nerve impulses as they pass from the cones to the brain. Both types of colour blindness are probably inherited.

經衝動整合缺陷。兩種色盲可能都是遺傳性的。

monoclonal antibody an antibody produced artificially from a cell *clone and therefore consisting of a single type of immunoglobulin. Monoclonal antibodies are produced by fusing antibody-forming lymphocytes from mouse spleen with mouse myeloma cells. The resulting hybrid cells multiply rapidly (like cancer cells) and produce the same antibody as their parent lymphocytes.

單克隆抗體 從一個細胞克隆人工產生的抗體，因此只有單一類型的免疫球蛋白。單克隆抗體是把鼠脾中生成抗體的淋巴細胞與鼠骨髓瘤細胞融合而產生的。所產生的雜種細胞繁殖很快（象癌細胞），並且生成與其親本的淋巴細胞相同的抗體。

monocular *adj.* relating to or used by one eye only. *Compare* binocular.

單眼的 僅用一只眼或與一只眼有關的。

monocyte *n.* a variety of white blood cell, 16–20 μm in diameter, with a kidney-shaped nucleus and greyish-blue cytoplasm (when treated with *Romanowsky stains). Its function is the ingestion of foreign particles, such as bacteria and tissue debris. There are normally 0.2–0.8 $\times$ 10^9 monocytes per litre of blood. —**monocytic** *adj.*

單核細胞 一種帶有腎形核和灰藍色胞漿的、直徑爲16～20微米的白細胞（在用羅曼諾夫斯基氏染劑處理後）。它的功能是吞食異物顆粒，如細菌和組織碎屑。正常時每升血中有0.2～0.8×10^9單核細胞。

monocytosis *n.* an increase in the number of *monocytes in the blood. Monocytosis occurs in a variety of diseases, including certain leukaemias (*monocytic leukaemias*) and infections due to some bacteria and protozoa.

單核細胞增多〔症〕 血中單核細胞數量增多。單核細胞增多〔症〕發生在包括某些白血病（單核細胞性白血病）和由某些細菌和原生動物所致感染造成的疾病中。

monodactylism *n.* the congenital absence of all but one digit on each hand and foot.

單指（趾）〔畸形〕 先天性指（趾）缺失，每只手和脚上只生有一個指（趾）。

monoiodotyrosine *n.* an iodine-containing substance produced in the thyroid gland from which the *thyroid hormones are derived.

單碘酪氨酸 甲狀腺中產生的含碘物質。由此物質衍生出甲狀腺素。

monomania *n.* the state in which a particular delusion or set of delusions is present in an otherwise normally functioning person. *See also* paranoia.

單狂 一個人只有一種特殊的（或一組）妄想狀態，其它功能均正常。

mononeuritis *n.* disease affecting a single peripheral nerve. Entrapment of the nerve or interference with its blood supply are the commonest causes. *Mononeuritis multiplex* is the separate involvement of two or more nerves. *Compare* polyneuropathy.

單神經炎 只影響一根周圍神經的病症。最常見的病因是神經黏連或供血障礙。多神經炎是兩根或數根神經分別受到影響。

mononucleosis *n.* the condition in which the blood contains an abnormally high number of mononuclear leucocytes (*monocytes). *See* glandular fever (infectious mononucleosis).

單核細胞增多〔症〕 血中含有異常大量的單核白細胞（單核細胞）。

monophobia *n.* an extreme fear of being alone.

獨居恐怖 對單獨生活極其恐怖的感覺。

monophyletic *adj.* describing a number of individuals, species, etc., that have evolved from a single ancestral group. *Compare* polyphyletic.

一元的 描述多數個體、物種等等由某單一祖系進化而來的。

monoplegia *n.* paralysis of one limb. —**monoplegic** *adj.*

單癱 一個肢體的癱瘓。

monoploid *adj. see* haploid.

單倍體

monorchism *n.* absence of one testis. This is usually due to failure of one testicle to descend into the scrotum before birth. The term is sometimes used for the condition in which one testicle has been removed surgically or destroyed by injury or disease. If the single testis is normal, no adverse effects result from the absence of the other.

單睾丸 一側睾丸缺失。常因出生前一側睾丸不能下降到陰囊內所致。此術語有時也用於外科切除單側睾丸或單側睾丸因損傷或疾病而受到破壞。如果一側睾丸是正常的，另一側睾丸的缺失就不會產生不良的作用。

monosaccharide *n.* a simple sugar having the general formula $(CH_2O)_n$. Monosaccharides may have between three and nine carbon atoms, but the most common number is five or six. Monosaccharides are classified according to the number of carbon atoms they possess. Thus *trioses* have three carbon atoms, *tetroses* four, *pentoses* five, and *hexoses* six. The most abundant monosaccharide is glucose (a hexose).

單糖 具有共同分子式（CH_2O）^{n}的簡單的糖。單糖可有3～9個碳原子，但最常見的是5或6個。單糖根據它們所擁有的碳原子數來分類：丙糖有3個碳原子，丁糖有4個碳原子，戊糖有5個碳原子，己糖有6個碳原子。存在最多的單糖是葡萄糖（一種己糖）。

monosomy *n.* a condition in which there is one chromosome missing from the normal (*diploid) set. *Compare* trisomy. —**monosomic** *adj.*

單體性 一套正常的染色體組（二倍體）缺失一條染色體。

monozygotic twins *see* twins. **單卵性雙胎**

mons *n.* (in anatomy) a rounded eminence. The *mons pubis* is the mound of fatty tissue lying over the pubic symphysis. **阜** （解剖學）圓形隆起。陰阜是在耻骨聯合上方的脂肪組織隆起（小丘）。

Moraxella *n.* a genus of short rodlike Gram-negative aerobic bacteria, usually occurring in pairs. They exist as parasites in many warm-blooded animals. The species *M. lacunata* causes conjunctivitis. **摩拉克氏菌屬** 短桿狀革蘭氏陰性需氧菌屬，常成對出現。在多種溫血動物體內作爲寄生菌存在。結膜炎摩拉克氏菌可引起結膜炎。

morbid *adj.* diseased or abnormal; pathological. **病的** 疾病的或異常的，病理學的。

morbidity *n.* the state of being diseased. The *morbidity rate* is the number of cases of a disease found to occur in a stated number of the population, usually given as cases per 100,000 or per million. Annual figures for morbidity rate give the incidence of the disease, which is the number of new cases reported in the year. *See also* incidence rate, prevalence rate. **患病** 患有疾病的狀態。患病率是在規定的人口數中所發現的某病病例數，通常以每十萬人口或百萬人口中的患病人數表示。年度患病率的數字可表示該病的發病率，發病率就是一年中所報告的新病例數。

morbilli *n. see* measles. **麻疹**

morbilliform *adj.* describing a skin rash resembling that of measles. **麻疹樣的** 描述一種與麻疹相像的皮疹。

morbus *n.* disease. The term is usually used as part of the medical name of a specific disease. **[疾]病** 此術語通常作爲某特殊疾病的醫學名稱的一部分。

mordant *n.* (in microscopy) a substance, such as alum or phenol, used to fix a *stain in a tissue. **媒染劑** （顯微鏡檢）用於固定組織染劑的一種物質，如明礬或石炭酸。

moribund *adj.* dying. **瀕死的** 臨終的。

morning sickness nausea and vomiting during early pregnancy. In some women the symptoms disappear if a small amount of food is eaten before rising in the morning. *Compare* hyperemesis. Medical name: **nausea gravidarum**. **孕婦噁心** 妊娠早期的噁心和嘔吐。有些婦女如果早晨起床前小量進食，症狀可消失。醫學術語：妊娠期噁心。

moron *n. Obsolete.* a person afflicted by a mild degree of mental subnormality. *See* feeblemindedness. **痴愚者** （廢用詞）精神輕度異常的人。

morphine *n.* a potent analgesic and *narcotic drug used mainly to relieve severe and persistent pain. It is administered by mouth or injection; common side-effects are loss of appetite, nausea, constipation, and confusion. Morphine causes feelings of euphoria; *tolerance develops rapidly and *dependence may occur.

嗎啡 主要用於解除重度和持續性疼痛的强鎮痛和麻醉藥。口服或注射。常見副作用是食慾喪失、噁心、便秘和精神錯亂。嗎啡可引起欣快感，很快産生耐受性並且可産生賴藥性。

morpho- *prefix denoting* form or structure.

〔前綴〕 **形態** 指形狀或結構。

morphoea *n.* a localized form of *scleroderma in which the skin and sometimes the underlying tissues are replaced with connective tissue, forming areas or bands of infiltrating tissue. These bands may follow the course of nerves. The sweat glands and hair follicles disappear in the affected area.

硬斑病 硬皮病的一種局部表現：皮膚（有時包括皮下組織）被結締組織取代，形成浸潤組織區或帶，這些浸潤帶可沿着神經走行分佈。受此病影響的部位、汗腺和毛囊可消失。

morphogenesis *n.* the development of form and structure of the body and its parts.

形態發生 身體及其各部的形態和結構的發育。

morphology *n. see* anatomy.

形態學

-morphous *suffix denoting* form or structure (of a specified kind).

〔後綴〕 **形態** 指（某特殊類型）的形態或結構。

Morquio-Brailsford disease *see* chondrodysplasia.

莫爾基奥-布雷斯福德二氏病

mortality (mortality rate) *n.* the incidence of death in the population in a given period. The ***annual mortality rate*** is the number of registered deaths in a year, multiplied by 1000 and divided by the population at the middle of the year. *See also* infant mortality rate, maternal mortality rate.

死亡率 在一定時期內的人口中死亡的發生率。年死亡率是一年中已登記的死亡數乘1000然後除以年中人口數得出的。

mortification *n. see* necrosis.

壞疽

morula *n.* an early stage of embryonic development formed by *cleavage of the fertilized ovum. It consists of a solid ball of cells and is an intermediate stage between the zygote and *blastocyst.

桑葚胚 由受精卵的卵裂形成的胚胎發育的早期階段。它由一個固體的細胞球組成，並且是合子和胚泡之間的中間階段。

mosaicism *n.* a condition in which the cells of an individual do not all contain

鑲嵌性 一個人細胞內含有的染色體不都是完全相

identical chromosomes; there may be two or more genetically different populations of cells. Often one of the cell populations is normal and the other carries a chromosome defect such as *Down's syndrome or *Turner's syndrome. In affected individuals the chromosome defect is usually not fully expressed. —**mosaic** *adj.*

同的狀態。可有兩個或更多的具有不同遺傳特性的細胞樣羣。此種細胞樣羣之一往往是正常的，而其它的帶有染色體缺陷，如唐斯綜合徵或特納綜合徵。有此種現象的人，染色體缺陷往往不能充分顯示出來。

mosquito *n.* a small winged bloodsucking insect belonging to a large group – the *Diptera (two-winged flies). Its mouthparts are formed into a long proboscis for piercing the skin and sucking blood. Female mosquitoes transmit the parasites responsible for several major infectious diseases, such as *malaria. *See* Anopheles, Aëdes, Culex.

蚊 屬於雙翅目的一種有翼的小吸血昆蟲。它的口器形成一個長喙以刺入皮膚和吸血。雌蚊傳播的寄生蟲可引起幾種主要傳染病（如瘧疾）。

motile *adj.* being able to move spontaneously, without external aid: usually applied to a *microorganism or a cell (e.g. a sperm cell).

能動的 無外力幫助時，可自行移動的，常指微生物或細胞（如：精子）。

motion sickness *see* travel sickness.

暈動〔病〕

motor cortex the region of the *cerebral cortex that is responsible for initiating nerve impulses that bring about voluntary activity in the muscles of the body. It is possible to map out the cortex to show which of its areas is responsible for which particular part of the body. The motor cortex of the left cerebral hemisphere is responsible for muscular activity in the right side of the body.

運動皮層 負責產生神經衝動以引起身體肌肉隨意活動的腦皮質部位。能夠描繪出負責身體某特殊部位運動的具體腦皮質區域。左半腦的運動皮層負責右半邊的肌肉活動。

motor nerve one of the nerves that carry impulses outwards from the central nervous system to bring about activity in a muscle or gland. *Compare* sensory nerve.

運動神經 將衝動從神經中樞傳出而引起某肌肉或腺體活動的一種神經。

motor neurone one of the units (*neurones) that goes to make up the nerve pathway between the brain and an effector organ, such as a skeletal muscle. An *upper motor neurone* has a cell body in the brain and an axon that

運動神經元 組成腦和效應器（如骨骼肌）之間神經通路的單位（神經元）之一。上運動神經元在腦內有一個細胞體和一個延伸到脊髓的軸索，在脊髓

extends into the spinal cord, where it ends in synapses. It is thus entirely within the central nervous system. A *lower motor neurone*, on the other hand, has a cell body in the spinal cord or brainstem and an axon that extends outwards in a cranial or spinal motor nerve to reach an effector.

內終止在突觸處。因此，上運動神經元完全位於中樞神經系統內。另一方面，下運動神經元在脊髓或腦幹內有一個細胞體和一個在顱和脊髓運動神經內延伸出來到達某效應器的軸索。

motor neurone disease a progressive degenerative disease of the motor system occurring in middle age and causing muscle weakness and wasting. It primarily affects the cells of the anterior horn of the spinal cord, the motor nuclei in the brainstem, and the corticospinal fibres. There are three clinically distinct forms: *amyotrophic lateral sclerosis* (*ALS*), *progressive muscular atrophy*, and *progressive bulbar palsy*.

運動神經元病 運動神經系統的一種進行性變性病。見於中年人，可致肌無力和萎縮。它主要影響脊髓的前角細胞、腦幹中的運動核和皮質脊髓纖維。臨床上有三種明顯不同的類型：肌萎縮性〔脊髓〕側索硬化，進行性肌萎縮和進行性延髓麻痹。

mould *n.* any multicellular filamentous fungus that commonly forms a rough furry coating on decaying matter.

黴菌 任何多細胞絲狀黴菌。此菌在腐爛物質上常形成粗毛皮樣包被。

moulding *n.* the changing of the shape of an infant's head during labour, brought about by the pressures to which it is subjected when passing through the birth passage.

兒頭變形 分娩時嬰兒頭形的改變。它是由胎兒通過產道時所承受的壓力所致。

mountain sickness *see* altitude sickness.

高山病

mouthwash *n.* an aqueous solution with antiseptic, astringent, or deodorizing properties used for daily rinsing of the mouth and teeth. Mouthwashes are used to prevent dental *caries (*see also* chlorhexidine) and to treat mild throat infections.

漱口藥 具有防腐、收斂或除臭特性的水溶液。用於每天漱洗口腔和牙齒。漱口藥可預防齲齒和治療輕度咽喉感染。

moxibustion *n.* a form of treatment favoured in Japan, in which cones of sunflower pith or down from the leaves of the plant *Artemisia moxa* are stuck to the skin and ignited. The heat produced by the smouldering cones acts as a counterirritant and is reputed to cure a variety of disorders.

灸術 在日本受人們喜愛的一種治療方法。此療法把向日葵髓或艾葉的茸毛製成的灸炷貼於皮膚上點燃。冒烟的灸炷產生的熱能起一種抗刺激作用並被認爲可治療多種疾病。

MSH *see* melanocyte-stimulating hormone.

促黑素細胞激素

mucilage *n.* (in pharmacy) a thick aqueous solution of a gum used as a lubricant in skin preparations (*see also* glycerin), for the production of pills, and for the suspension of insoluble substances. The most important mucilages are of acacia, tragacanth, and starch.

膠漿 （藥學）濃稠的樹膠水溶液。用作皮膚藥制劑中的潤滑液，亦用於藥片的生產和作爲不溶物質的〔混〕懸液。最重要的膠漿是阿拉伯膠、西黃蓍和澱粉。

mucin *n.* the principal constituent of *mucus. Mucin is a *glycoprotein.

黏蛋白 黏液的主要成分。黏蛋白是一種糖蛋白。

muco- *prefix denoting* **1.** mucus. **2.** mucous membrane.

〔前綴〕 **①黏液②黏膜**

mucocele *n.* a space or organ distended with mucus. For example, it may occur in the gall bladder when the exit duct becomes obstructed so that the mucus secretions are retained and dilate the cavity of the organ. A mucocele in the soft tissues arising from a salivary gland occurs when the duct is blocked or ruptured.

黏液囊腫 因含黏液而腫脹的間隙或器官。當排出管梗阻造成黏液分泌物滯留和管腔擴張時，黏液囊腫可發生在膽囊內。唾液腺的軟組織內的黏液囊腫發生在管道阻塞或破裂時。

mucolytic *n.* an agent, such as carbocysteine or tyloxapol, that dissolves or breaks down mucus. Mucolytics are used to treat chest conditions involving excessive or thickened mucus secretions.

黏液溶解劑 溶解或分解黏液的藥劑。如：羥甲半胱氨酸四丁酚醛。黏液溶解劑用於治療肺部疾病時黏液分泌物過多或黏稠。

mucopolysaccharide *n.* one of a group of complex carbohydrates functioning mainly as structural components in connective tissue. Mucopolysaccharide molecules are usually built up of two repeating sugar units, one of which is an amino sugar. An example of a mucopolysaccharide is *chondroitin, occurring in cartilage.

黏多糖〔類〕 主要是結締組織構成成分的一組複雜糖類之一。黏多糖〔類〕分子通常由重複連接起來的二糖單位組成，其中之一是一種氨基糖。例如，存在於軟骨中的軟骨素，就是一種黏多糖。

mucoprotein *n.* one of a group of proteins found in the *globulin fraction of blood plasma. Mucoproteins are globulins combined with a carbohydrate group (an amino sugar). They are similar to *glycoproteins but contain a greater proportion of carbohydrate.

黏蛋白 含於血漿球蛋白部分之中的一種蛋白。黏蛋白是球蛋白與糖類（一種氨基糖）的結合物，它們與糖蛋白相似，但含糖的比例較大。

mucopurulent *adj.* containing mucus and pus. *See* mucopus.

黏液膿性的 含有黏液和膿的。

mucopus *n.* a mixture of *mucus and *pus.

黏液性膿　黏液和膿的混合物。

Mucor *n.* a genus of mould fungi commonly seen on dead and decaying organic matter. They can be pathogenic in man, causing infections of the skin and respiratory system.

毛黴菌屬　常見於死亡和腐爛有機物上的黴菌屬。它們對人有致病作用，可引起皮膚和呼吸系感染。

mucormycosis *n.* a disease caused by a fungus of the genus *Mucor*, affecting the external ear, skin, and respiratory passages.

毛黴菌病　由毛黴菌屬的黴菌引起的疾病，可影響外耳、皮膚和呼吸道。

mucosa *n. see* mucous membrane. **—mucosal** *adj.*

黏膜

mucous membrane (mucosa) the moist membrane lining many tubular structures and cavities, including the nasal sinuses, respiratory tract, gastrointestinal tract, biliary, and pancreatic systems. The surface of the mouth is lined by mucous membrane, the nature of which varies according to its site. The mucous membrane consists of a surface layer of *epithelium, which contains glands secreting *mucus, with underlying layers of connective tissue (lamina propria) and muscularis mucosae, which forms the inner boundary of the mucous membrane.

黏膜　位於許多管狀結構和腔室內面的濕潤膜。包括鼻竇、呼吸道、胃腸道、膽和胰系統。口腔表面覆有黏膜，黏膜的性質因其部位不同而各異。黏膜由含有分泌黏液的腺體上皮表層，及其下面的結締組織（黏膜固有層）以及形成黏膜內界面的黏膜肌層組成。

mucoviscidosis *n. see* cystic fibrosis.

〔胰管〕黏膜物阻塞症

mucus *n.* a viscous fluid secreted by *mucous membranes in many parts of the body, including the mouth, bronchial passages, and gut. Mucus acts as a protective barrier over the surfaces of the membranes, as a lubricant, and as a carrier of enzymes. It consists chiefly of *glycoproteins, particularly *mucin*, which are responsible for its viscosity. **—mucous** *adj.*

黏液　由身體許多部位（包括口腔、支氣管和腸道）的黏膜所分泌的黏性液體。黏液可作爲黏膜表面的保護層，作爲一種潤滑劑，而且還可作爲酶的載體。它主要由糖蛋白，特別是由決定其黏〔滞〕度的黏蛋白組成。

Müllerian duct *see* paramesonephric duct.

苗勒氏管

multi- *prefix denoting* many; several.

〔前綴〕　**多，多數**

multifactorial *adj.* describing a condition that is believed to have resulted from the interaction of genetic factors,

多因子的　描述據信是由遺傳因子（常爲多基因）與環境因素相互作用所致

usually *polygenes, with an environmental factor or factors. Many disorders, e.g. spina bifida and anencephaly, are thought to be multifactorial.

的疾病。現認爲許多疾病，如脊柱裂和無腦〔畸形〕屬多遺傳因子的範圍。

multifocal lenses lenses in which the power (*see* dioptre) of the lower part gradually increases towards the lower edge. There is no dividing line on the lens as there is between the upper and lower segments of *bifocal lenses. The wearer can see clearly at any distance by lowering or raising his eyes to look through an appropriate part of the lens.

多焦點鏡片 眼鏡下部放大倍數逐漸增加的鏡片。與雙焦點鏡片不同，在其上、下段之間，沒有明顯的分界綫。戴鏡者通過調整眼的高度從鏡片的適當部位，就能看清不同距離的物體。

multigravida *n.* a woman who has been pregnant at least twice.

經孕婦 至少妊娠過兩次的婦女。

multipara *n.* a woman who has given birth to a live child after each of at least two pregnancies.

經產婦 至少妊娠過兩次並且每次妊娠後都曾生出活嬰的婦女。

multiple sclerosis (disseminated sclerosis) a chronic disease of the nervous system affecting young and middle-aged adults. The *myelin sheaths surrounding nerves in the brain and spinal cord are damaged, which affects the function of the nerves involved. The course of the illness is characterized by recurrent relapses followed by remissions. The disease affects different parts of the brain and spinal cord, resulting in typically scattered symptoms. These include unsteady gait and shaky movements of the limbs (ataxia), rapid involuntary movements of the eyes (*nystagmus), defects in speech pronunciation (dysarthria), spastic weakness, and *retrobulbar neuritis. The underlying cause of the nerve damage remains unknown but evidence points to the patient's abnormal response to a viral infection.

多發性硬化 發生於青年和中年人神經系統的慢性病。腦和脊髓內神經周圍的髓鞘被破壞，因而影響了鞘內神經的功能。病程是以復發和緩解相交替爲特徵的。病變侵及腦和脊髓的不同部位，引起典型的散在多病竈症狀。這些症狀包括：步態不穩，四肢震顫性運動（共濟失調），眼的快速不隨意運動（眼球震顫），發音缺陷（構音障礙），肌力減退和球後視神經炎。神經損害的眞正原因仍不清楚，但可見病人對病毒性感染有異常反應的迹象。

multivariate analysis *see* correlation.

多變量分析

mummification *n.* **1.** the conversion of dead tissue into a hard shrunken mass, chiefly by dehydration. **2.** (in dentistry)

①乾屍化 死亡組織轉變爲硬縮團塊，主要因脫水所致。 **②乾髓法** （牙

the application of a fixative to the dental pulp to prevent its decomposition.

科）應用固定液使失活的牙髓乾燥預防其腐敗分解。

mumps *n.* a common virus infection mainly affecting children between the ages of five and 15. Symptoms appear 2–3 weeks after exposure: fever, headache, and vomiting may precede a typical swelling of the *parotid salivary glands. The gland on one side of the face often swells up days before the other but sometimes only one side is affected. The symptoms usually vanish within three days, the patient remaining infectious until the swelling has completely disappeared, but the infection may spread to other salivary glands and to the pancreas, brain, and testicles. In adult men, mumps can cause sterility. Most people acquire immunity through a childhood infection. Medical name: **infectious parotitis**.

流行性腮腺炎 主要發生於5～15歲兒童的常見病毒感染。接觸病毒後2～3周出現病狀：發熱、頭痛和嘔吐，然後出現典型的腮腺腫脹。常是單側腮腺先腫起，數天後另一側才腫起，但有時僅影響單側腺體。症狀通常在三天內消失，腫脹完全消失以前病人具有傳染性，而且感染可傳播到其它涎腺及胰、腦和睾丸。成年男性流行性腮腺炎可致不育。大多數人通過兒童時感染而獲得免疫力。醫學術語：傳染性腮腺炎。

Munchhausen's syndrome a mental disorder in which the patient persistently tries to obtain hospital treatment for an illness that is nonexistent: an extreme form of malingering. The disease may be described in vivid detail, and in some cases injury may be deliberately self-inflicted in an attempt to give the appearance of authenticity to the claims being made.

曼丘森氏綜合徵 一種精神病。在沒有病的情況下病人頑固地堅持要求得到醫治：一種極端的裝病形式。病人可逼眞而又詳細地描述病情，並且在某些病例中爲了證實他們所說的病情而給人以眞實的印象，可有故意傷害自身的情況發生。

murmur (bruit) *n.* a noise, heard with the aid of a stethoscope, that is generated by turbulent blood flow within the heart or blood vessels. Turbulent flow is produced by damaged valves, *septal defects, narrowed arteries, or arteriovenous communications. Heart murmurs can also be heard in normal individuals, especially those who have hyperactive circulation, and frequently in normal children (*innocent murmurs*). Murmurs are classified as *systolic* or *diastolic* (heard in ventricular *systole or *diastole respectively); *continuous mur-*

雜音 借助於聽診器聽到的，由心臟或血管內血液渦流產生的噪聲。渦流是由瓣膜損傷、間隔缺損、動脈狹窄或動靜脈分流造成的。心臟雜音也可見於正常人，特別循環過度活躍的人，並常見於正常兒童（良性雜音）。雜音可分爲收縮〔期〕的或舒張〔期〕的（分別在心室收縮期或舒張期聽到）；連續性雜音可在整個收縮和舒張期聽到。

murs are heard throughout systole and diastole.

muscae volitantes *pl. n.* black spots seen floating before the eyes usually due to the presence of opaque specks in the vitreous humour.

飛蠅幻視 眼前可見漂浮的黑點，通常是玻璃體中存有不透明微粒所致。

muscle *n.* a tissue whose cells have the ability to contract, producing movement or force (see illustration). Muscles possess mechanisms for converting energy derived from chemical reactions into mechanical energy. The major functions of muscles are to produce movements of the body, to maintain the position of the body against the force of gravity, to produce movements of structures inside the body, and to alter pressures or tensions of structures in the body. There are three types of muscle: *striated muscle, attached to the skeleton; *smooth muscle, which is found in such tissues as the stomach, gut, and blood vessels; and *cardiac muscle, which forms the walls of the heart.

肌肉 其細胞能收縮，產生運動或力量的一種組織（見圖）。肌肉具有把化學反應所產生的能量轉變爲機械能的機制。肌肉的主要功能是產生身體的運動、保持在重力作用下身體的姿勢、產生體內結構運動，並且改變體內結構的壓力和張力，肌肉有三種類型：附着在骨骼上的橫紋肌；胃、腸道和血管內的平滑肌；構成心臟壁的心肌。

muscle relaxant an agent that reduces tension in muscles. Drugs such as *chlormezanone, *diazepam, and *mephensin are used to relieve skeletal muscular spasms in various spastic conditions, parkinsonism, and tetanus. Other drugs, e.g. *gallamine, *suxame-

肌肉鬆弛劑 減少肌肉緊張度的藥物。如氯甲噻酮、安定和甲酚甘油醚用於解除在各種痙攣性疾病、帕金森氏綜合徵和破傷風中的骨骼肌痙攣。其它藥物，如：三碘季銨

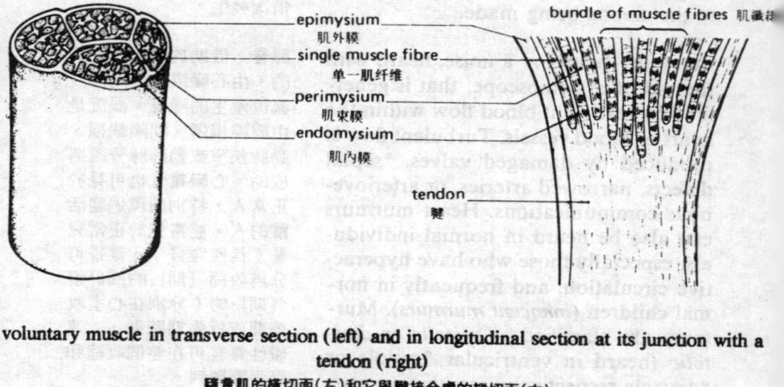

A voluntary muscle in transverse section (left) and in longitudinal section at its junction with a tendon (right)

隨意肌的橫切面（左）和它與腱接合處的縱切面（右）

thonium, and *tubocurarine, paralyse voluntary muscles and are used in addition to anaesthetics to relax the muscles during surgical operations.

酚、琥珀醯膽鹼和筒箭毒鹼可使隨意肌麻痹，在外科手術中與麻醉劑同時使用，可使肌肉鬆弛。

muscle spindle a specialized receptor, sensitive to stretch, that is embedded between and parallel to the fibres of striated muscles. These receptors are important for coordinated muscular movement. *See also* stretch receptor.

肌梭 對牽張敏感的特殊受體，它包埋在橫紋肌纖維之間並與之平行。這些受體在協調肌肉運動中起重要作用。

muscular dystrophy any one of a group of muscle diseases in which there is a recognizable pattern of inheritance. They are marked by weakness and wasting of selected muscles: the affected muscle fibres degenerate and are replaced by fatty tissue. The muscular dystrophies are classified according to the patient's age at onset, distribution of the weakness, the progression of the disease, and the mode of inheritance. Confirmation of the diagnosis is based upon *electromyography and muscle biopsy.

The most common form is *Duchenne dystrophy*, which is inherited as a sex-linked recessive character and is nearly always restricted to boys. It usually begins before the age of four, with selective weakness and wasting of the muscles of the pelvic girdle and back. The child has a waddling gait and *lordosis of the lumbar spine. The calf muscles – and later the shoulders and upper limbs – often become firm and bulky. Although the disease cannot be cured, physiotherapy and orthopaedic measures can relieve the disability. *See also* dystrophia myotonica.

肌營養不良 一種具有遺傳特徵的肌肉病變。它們以選擇性肌無力和萎縮爲特點：受累的肌纖維退化並由脂肪組織取代。肌營養不良的分類是以病人的發病年齡、肌無力的分佈範圍、疾病的進展和遺傳方式爲基礎的。最後確診是根據肌〔動〕電〔流〕描記法和肌肉活組織檢查作出的。

最常見的類型是杜興氏肌營養不良，它是以性連鎖隱性遺傳爲特徵，並且幾乎總是局限於男孩。它通常在4歲前開始發病，伴有選擇性骨盆帶和腰部肌無力和萎縮。兒童可有鴨步〔態〕和腰部的脊柱前凸。小腿肌肉，繼而兩肩和上肢肌肉，常變硬和增大。雖然此病無法治癒，但物理療法和矯形的方法可減輕傷殘。

muscularis *n.* a muscular layer of the wall of a hollow organ (such as the stomach) or a tubular structure (such as the intestine or ureter). The *muscularis mucosae* is the muscular layer of a mucous membrane complex, especially that of the stomach or intestine.

肌層 空腔臟器（如胃）或管狀器官（如腸道或輸尿管）的壁內肌層。黏膜肌層是黏膜肌層複合體，特別是在胃或腸道。

muscular rheumatism any aching pain in the muscles and joints. Commonly the symptoms are due to *fibrositis; wear and tear of the joints (*osteoarthritis); or to inflammation of the muscles associated with abnormal immune reactions (*polymyalgia rheumatica).

肌風濕病 肌肉和關節內的酸痛。此症的病因常爲纖維織炎，關節的磨損和撕裂（骨關節炎），或與異常免疫反應有關的肌肉炎症（風濕性多肌痛）。

musculo- *prefix denoting* muscle.

〔前綴〕 **肌**

musculocutaneous nerve a nerve of the *brachial plexus that supplies some muscles of the arm and the skin of the lateral part of the forearm.

肌皮神經 臂叢的一根神經。支配臂部的某些肌肉和前臂側部的皮膚。

mushroom *n.* the aerial fruiting (spore-producing) body of various fungi. Edible mushrooms include the field and cultivated mushrooms (*Agaricus campestris* and *A. bisporus*), the chanterelle (*Cantherellus cibarius*), and the parasol (*Lepiota procera*). However, great care must be taken in identifying edible fungi. Many species are poisonous, especially the death cap and panther cap (*see* Amanita).

蕈 各種眞菌的氣生子實體（孢子生成）。食用蕈包括野生的和栽培的（如：蘑菇、香菇、草菇、木耳）。在鑑定食用眞菌時，必須十分小心。許多種眞菌是有毒的，特別是毒傘和斑毒蕈（豹紋毒傘）。

mustine (nitrogen mustard) *n.* a drug used to treat various types of cancer, including Hodgkin's disease and some types of leukaemia. It is administered by injection; common side-effects include nausea and vomiting, and the drug may damage the bone marrow, causing serious blood disorders.

氮芥（恩比興） 治療各類癌症包括何傑金氏病和某些白血病的藥物。注射給藥，常見副作用包括噁心和嘔吐。此藥可使骨髓受損，引起嚴重的血液病。

mutagen *n.* an external agent that, when applied to cells or organisms, can increase the rate of *mutation. Mutagens usually only increase the number of mutants formed and do not cause mutations not found under natural conditions. Several kinds of radiation, many chemicals, and some viruses can act as mutagens. *Compare* antimutagen.

誘變劑 用於細胞或機體時，能增加突變率的一種外加物質。誘變劑通常僅增加突變體形成的數量，但不能引起在自然條件下發生不了的突變。數種射綫，許多化學制劑，和某些病毒可起誘變劑的作用。

mutant *n.* **1.** an individual in which a mutation has occurred, especially when

①**突變體** 發生突變的個體。尤指突變效果可見

the effect of the mutation is visible. **2.** a characteristic showing the effects of a mutation. —**mutant** *adj.*

者。②**突變性** 具有突變性能的特徵。

mutation *n.* a change in the genetic material (*DNA) of a cell, or the change this causes in a characteristic of the individual, which is not caused by normal genetic processes. In a *point* (or *gene*) *mutation* there is a change in a single gene; in a *chromosome mutation* there is a change in the structure or number of the chromosomes. All mutations are rare events and may occur spontaneously or be caused by external agents (*mutagens). If a mutation occurs in developing sex cells (gametes) it may be inherited. Mutations in any other cells (*somatic mutations*) are not inherited.

突變 正常遺傳過程中不會發生的某細胞遺傳物質（DNA）的變化，或由這種變化引起的生物體特性的改變。在某點（或基因）突變中，存在着單基因變化；在某染色體突變中，存在着染色體結構和數量上的變化。所有突變均屬罕見，往往是自動發生或由外部作用物（誘變劑）誘發。如果在發育的性細胞（配子）內發生突變，突變是遺傳性的。在任何其它細胞內的突變（體細胞突變）不屬於遺傳性突變。

mutism *n.* inability or refusal to speak; dumbness. Innate speechlessness most commonly occurs in those who have been totally deaf since birth (*deaf-mutism*). Inability to speak may result from brain damage (*see* aphasia). It may also be caused by depression or psychological trauma, in which case the patient either does not speak at all or speaks only to particular persons or in particular situations. This latter condition is called *elective mutism*.
Treatment of mutism due to psychological causes is increasingly by behavioural means, such as *prompting: people that the patient does not address are slowly introduced into the situation where the patient does speak. This may be done either alone or in combination with more traditional psychotherapy. —**mute** *adj.*, *n.*

啞症 不能講話或拒絕講話；瘖啞。先天性啞最常發生在出生後完全性失聽的人中（聾啞症）。不能講話可因腦損害造成。此症也可因抑鬱或心理創傷所致；在這些病例中病人可表現爲完全不講話或僅對某些人或在某殊特場合講話。後者被稱爲選擇性啞症。
心理因素所致啞症的治療愈來愈多地採用行爲療法，如激勵：病人如對某些人不講話，可把這些人慢慢引入病人能够講話的場合中去。可單獨用此療法或與更常用的心理療法結合應用。

mutualism *n.* the intimate but not necessarily obligatory association between two different species of organism in which there is mutual aid and benefit. *Compare* symbiosis.

共生 不同的兩種生物之間共同生存、互助互利的密切而非必需的關係。

my- (myo-) *prefix denoting* muscle.

〔前綴〕**肌**

myalgia *n.* pain in the muscles.

肌痛 肌肉的疼痛。

myasthenia gravis a chronic disease marked by abnormal fatiguability and weakness of selected muscles, which is relieved by rest or *anticholinesterase drugs. The degree of fatigue is so extreme that these muscles are temporarily paralysed. Other symptoms include drooping of the upper eyelid (ptosis), double vision, and *dysarthria. The cause is uncertain, but appears to be associated with impaired ability of the neurotransmitter acetylcholine to induce muscular contraction. It chiefly affects adolescents and young adults (usually women) and adults over 40. Drug treatment and surgical removal of the thymus lessen the severity of the symptoms.

重症肌無力 以選擇性肌肉的異常疲勞和無力爲特徵的一種慢性病。休息或抗膽鹼酯酶藥可治療此症。這些肌肉的疲勞度極高，以致造成暫時性癱瘓。其它症狀包括上瞼下垂、複視和構音障礙。病因不明，但似乎與神經遞質乙醯膽鹼誘導肌肉收縮的能力受損有關。它主要發生於青春期少年、青年（常爲婦女）和40歲以上的成人。藥物治療和外科切除胸腺可減輕症狀。

myc- (myco-, mycet(o)-) *prefix denoting* a fungus.

〔前綴〕 **黴菌，眞菌**

mycelium *n.* (*pl.* **mycelia**) the tangled mass of fine branching threads that make up the feeding and growing part of a *fungus.

菌絲體 構成眞菌攝取營養和生長發育部分的細小分支纏結狀團塊。

mycetoma *n.* a chronic inflammation of tissues caused by a fungus. *See* Madura foot.

足分支菌病 眞菌引起的組織的慢性炎症。

Mycobacterium *n.* a genus of rodlike Gram-positive aerobic bacteria that can form filamentous branching structures. Some species are pathogenic to animals and man: *M. leprae* (*Hansen's bacillus*) causes *leprosy; *M. tuberculosis* (*Koch's bacillus*) causes *tuberculosis. *M. bovis* causes tuberculosis in cattle but can also infect the lungs, joints, and intestines of man.

分支桿菌屬 可形成絲狀分支結構的桿狀革蘭氏陽性需氧菌屬。其中某些菌種對人和動物有致病性。痲風分支桿菌可引起痲風；結核分支桿菌可引起結核。牛〔型〕結核分支桿菌可引起牛的結核，但也可感染人的肺、關節和腸道。

mycology *n.* the science of fungi. *See also* microbiology. —**mycologist** *n.*

眞菌學 研究眞菌的科學。

mycoplasma *n.* one of a group of minute nonmotile microorganisms that lack a rigid cell wall and hence display a variety of forms. They are regarded by some authorities as primitive bac-

支原菌屬 一種小的無運動的微生物。它們缺少堅硬的細胞壁因此形成一個特殊種類。某些權威認爲它們是最初的細菌。此類

teria. The group includes some species that cause severe respiratory disease in cattle, sheep, and goats; one of these, *Mycoplasma pneumoniae*, causes a pneumonia-like disease in man. The group also includes the *pleuropneumonia-like organisms* (*PPLO*).

菌中包括某些可引起牛、羊和山羊嚴重呼吸道疾病的菌種；其中肺炎支原體屬可引起人的肺炎樣病。此類菌中也包括類胸膜肺炎菌。

mycosis *n.* any disease caused by a fungus, including actinomycosis, aspergillosis, cryptococcosis, rhinosporidiosis, ringworm, and sporotrichosis.

眞菌病 眞菌引起的任何疾病。其中包括放線菌病、曲菌病、隱球菌病、鼻孢子蟲病、癬菌病和孢子絲菌病。

mycosis fungoides a disease that is a variety of *reticulosis usually confined to the skin. Chronic irritating eruptions occur, resembling eczema or psoriasis. Purplish tumours develop and then ulcerate. The disease is fatal, though partial remission may be effected with anti-cancer drugs.

蕈樣眞菌病 常局限於皮膚的一種網狀細胞增多病。可有與濕疹或銀屑病相像的慢性刺激性疹。可生成略帶紫色的腫瘤，然後成爲潰瘍。此病是致命的，儘管應用抗癌藥後可有部分緩解。

Mycota *n. see* undecenoic acid.

眞菌 門

mydriasis *n.* widening of the pupil, which occurs normally in dim light. The commonest cause of prolonged mydriasis is drug therapy (*see* mydriatic) or injury to the eye. *See also* cycloplegia. *Compare* miosis.

瞳孔開大 正常情況下，在光線暗淡時瞳孔開大。瞳孔開大時間延長的最常見原因是藥物治療或眼的損傷。

mydriatic *n.* a drug that causes the pupil of the eye to dilate. Examples are *atropine, *cyclopentolate, and *phenylephrine. Mydriatics are used to aid examination of the eye and to treat some eye inflammations such as iritis and cyclitis.

散瞳藥 擴張眼瞳孔的藥。如阿托品、環戊醇胺酯和苯福林。散瞳藥用於幫助檢查眼睛和治療某些眼炎，如虹膜炎和睫狀體炎。

myectomy *n.* a surgical operation to remove part of a muscle.

肌〔部分〕切除術 切除部分肌肉的外科手術

myel- (myelo-) *prefix denoting* **1.** the spinal cord. **2.** bone marrow. **3.** myelin.

〔前綴〕髓 ①脊髓。②骨髓。③髓鞘脂。

myelencephalon *n. see* medulla oblongata.

末腦

myelin *n.* a complex material formed of protein and *phospholipid that is laid down as a sheath around the *axons of certain neurones, known as *myelinated* (or *medullated*) *nerve fibres*. The material is produced and laid down in concentric layers by *Schwann cells at regular intervals along the nerve fibre (see illustrations). Myelinated nerves conduct impulses more rapidly than nonmyelinated nerves.

髓鞘質 蛋白和磷脂形成的一種複合物。它圍繞着某些神經元的軸突形成一種鞘，稱爲有髓〔鞘〕的神經纖維。在神經纖維上每隔一定距離，由許旺氏細胞生成髓鞘質並圍繞成同心層狀（見圖）。有髓鞘的神經傳導衝動快於無髓鞘的神經。

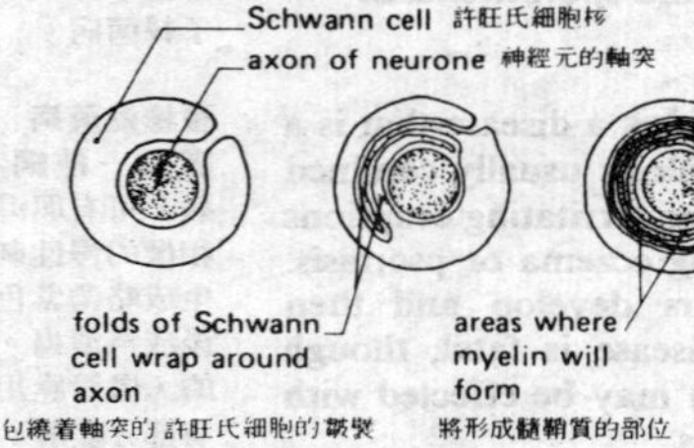

Formation of a myelin sheath by a Schwann cell
許旺氏細胞形成髓鞘質的過程

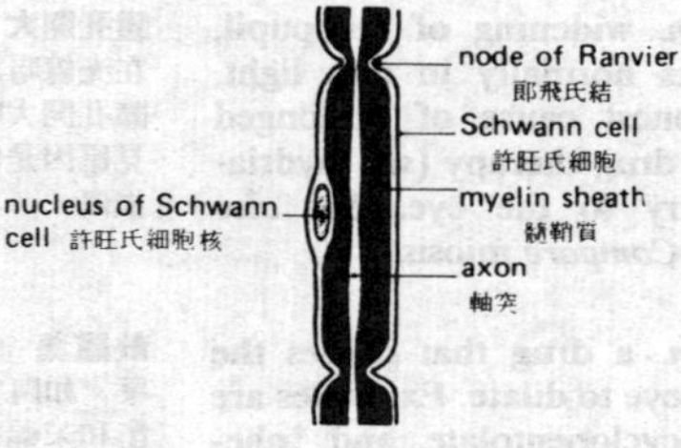

Longitudinal section through a myelinated nerve fibre
髓鞘神經纖維的縱切面

myelination *n.* the process in which *myelin is laid down as an insulating layer around the axons of certain nerves. Myelination of nerve tracts in the central nervous system is completed by the second year of life.

髓鞘形成 髓鞘質在神經軸突的周圍形成絕緣層的過程。中樞神經系統中神經束的髓鞘形成是在出生的第二年完成的。

myelitis *n.* **1.** an inflammatory disease of the spinal cord. The most usual kind (*transverse myelitis*) most often occurs during the development of multiple

①**脊髓炎** 脊髓的炎症。最常見類型（橫貫性脊髓炎）最常發生在多發性硬化的發展過程中；但有時

sclerosis, but it is sometimes a manifestation of *encephalomyelitis, when it can occur as an isolated attack. The inflammation spreads more or less completely across the tissue of the spinal cord, resulting in a loss of its normal function to transmit nerve impulses up and down. It is as though the spinal cord had been severed: paralysis and numbness affects the legs and trunk below the level of the diseased tissue. **2.** inflammation of the bone marrow. *See* osteomyelitis.

可爲腦脊髓炎的一種表現，此時可單獨出現脊髓症狀。炎症幾乎橫貫脊髓組織，以致脊髓喪失正常的向上和向下傳導神經衝動的功能。好象脊髓被切斷一樣，患病組織水平以下的腿和軀幹可發生癱瘓和痲木。②**骨髓炎**

myeloblast *n.* the earliest identifiable cell that gives rise to a *granulocyte, having a large nucleus and scanty cytoplasm. It is normally found in the blood-forming tissue of the bone marrow, but may appear in the blood in a variety of diseases, most notably in acute myeloblastic *leukaemia. *See also* granulopoiesis. —**myeloblastic** *adj.*

原粒細胞 生成粒細胞的最早可鑑別的細胞。它有一個大核和稀疏的細胞漿。正常情況下，見於骨髓造血組織，但也可見於患某種疾病的病人血中，最典型的見於急性原粒細胞性白血病。

myelocele *n. see* neural tube defects.

脊髓突出

myelocyte *n.* an immature form of *granulocyte having a round nucleus (*compare* metamyelocyte) and neutrophil, eosinophil, or basophil granules in its cytoplasm (*compare* promyelocyte). It is normally found in the blood-forming tissue of the bone marrow, but may appear in the blood in a variety of diseases, including infections, infiltrations of the bone marrow, and certain leukaemias. *See also* granulopoiesis.

中幼粒細胞 粒細胞的未成熟形式。其胞漿中有一個圓形核和嗜中性、嗜酸性或嗜中性顆粒。正常情況下，見於骨髓的造血組織，但也可出現在患某種疾病（包括感染、骨髓浸潤和某種白血病）病人的血中。

myelofibrosis *n.* a chronic but progressive disease characterized by *fibrosis of the bone marrow, which leads to anaemia and the presence of immature red and white blood cells in the circulation. Other features include enlargement of the spleen and the presence of blood-forming (myeloid) tissue in abnormal sites, such as the spleen and liver. Its cause is unknown.

骨髓纖維變性 以骨髓的纖維化爲特徵的慢性進行性疾病。它可致貧血和在血循環中出現未成熟的紅細胞和白細胞。其它特徵包括：脾大，在異常部位（如脾和肝）出現造血組織（髓樣組織）。病因不清。

myelography *n.* a specialized method of X-ray examination to demonstrate the spinal canal that involves injection

脊髓〔X線〕造影術 顯示脊髓的X線檢查的特殊方法。此法將不透X線的造

of a radio-opaque contrast medium into the subarachnoid space. The X-rays obtained are called *myelograms*. It is of importance in the recognition of tumours of the spinal cord and other conditions compressing the cord or the nerve roots.

影劑注射到蛛網膜下腔。用此法拍攝的X線照片稱爲"脊髓X線〔造影〕照片"。此方法對於識別脊髓腫瘤和其它壓迫脊髓或神經根的病變是很重要的。

myeloid *adj.* **1.** like, derived from, or relating to bone marrow. **2.** resembling a *myelocyte. **3.** relating to the spinal cord.

①**骨髓樣的** 類似或來自骨髓的，與骨髓有關的。②**中幼粒細胞樣的** 與中幼粒細胞相似的。③**脊髓的** 與脊髓有關的。

myeloid leukaemia a variety of *leukaemia in which the type of blood cell that proliferates abnormally originates in the blood-forming (myeloid) tissue of the bone marrow. Myeloid leukaemias may be acute or chronic and may involve any one of the cells produced by the marrow.

粒細胞性白血病 異常增生的血細胞來源於骨髓造血組織的一種白血病。粒細胞性白血病可爲急性或慢性，並可累及任何由骨髓生成的細胞。

myeloid tissue a tissue in the *bone marrow in which the various classes of blood cells are produced. *See also* haemopoiesis.

骨髓造血組織 骨髓中生成各類血細胞的組織。

myeloma (multiple myeloma, myelomatosis) *n.* a malignant disease of the bone marrow, characterized by two or more of the following criteria: (1) the presence of an excess of abnormal malignant plasma cells in the bone marrow; (2) typical deposits in the bones on X-ray, giving the appearance of holes; (3) the presence in the serum of an abnormal gamma globulin, usually IgG (an immunoglobulin; *see* paraprotein). *Bence-Jones protein may also be found in the serum or urine. The patient may complain of tiredness due to anaemia and of bone pain and may develop pathological fractures. Treatment is usually with such drugs as melphalan or cyclophosphamide, with local radiotherapy to particular areas of pain. Radiotherapy of the whole body is also used in the primary treatment of myeloma. *See also* plasmacytoma.

骨髓瘤（多發性骨髓瘤，骨髓瘤病） 以下列兩種或數種病情爲特徵的骨髓惡性病；①骨髓中存有過多的異常惡性漿細胞；②X線片上可見骨中有典型沉積物，使病變部位呈多孔樣外觀；③血清中存有異常丙種球蛋白，常爲IgG（一種免疫球蛋白）。本斯·瓊斯氏蛋白也可出現在血清或尿中。病人可有因貧血所致的疲勞和骨痛的主訴，並可發展爲病理性骨折。治療常用左旋溶肉瘤素或環磷醯胺等藥，並配合疼痛特殊部位的局部放射治療。全身的放射療法也可作爲骨髓瘤的初期治療。

myelomalacia *n.* softening of the tissues of the spinal cord, most often caused by an impaired blood supply.

脊髓軟化 脊髓組織的軟化。常因血供受損引起。

myelomatosis *n. see* myeloma.

骨髓瘤病

myelomeningocele *n. see* neural tube defects.

脊髓脊膜突出

myenteric reflex a reflex action of the intestine in which a physical stimulus causes the intestine to contract above and relax below the point of stimulation.

腸〔肌〕反射 腸道的反射活動。物理刺激引起刺激部位以上的腸道收縮和刺激部位以下的腸道鬆弛。

myenteron *n.* the muscular layer of the *intestine, consisting of a layer of circular muscle inside a layer of longitudinal muscle. These muscles are used in *peristalsis. —**myenteric** *adj.*

腸肌層 腸的肌層。由內部的環狀肌層和外部的縱肌層組成。這些肌肉在腸蠕動中起作用。

myiasis *n.* an infestation of a living organ or tissue by maggots. The flies normally breed in decaying animal and vegetable matter; myiasis therefore generally occurs only in regions of poor hygiene, and in most cases the infestations are accidental. Various genera may infect man. **Gasterophilus*, **Hypoderma*, **Dermatobia*, and *Cordylobia* affect the skin; *Fannia* invades the alimentary canal and the urinary system; **Phormia* and **Wohlfahrtia* infest open wounds and ulcers; **Oestrus* attacks the eyes; and *Cochliomyia* invades the nasal passages. Treatment of external myiases involves the destruction and removal of maggots followed by the application of antibiotics to wounds and lesions.

蠅蛆病 蛆在活的器官或組織內的寄生。正常情況下，蠅在腐爛的動物和植物中繁殖。因此，蠅蛆病一般僅發生在衛生條件差的地區，大部是偶然感染的。某些蠅屬可感染人。胃蠅屬、皮蠅屬和瘤蠅屬侵襲皮膚；廁蠅屬侵犯消化道和泌尿系；黑花蠅和污蠅屬感染開放的傷口和潰瘍；狂蠅屬侵犯眼睛；錐蠅屬侵犯鼻道。外蠅蛆病的治療包括對傷口和損害部位應用抗生素來殺滅蛆蟲。

mylohyoid *n.* a muscle in the floor of the mouth, attached at one end to the mandible and at the other to the hyoid bone.

下頜舌骨肌 口底的肌肉。此肌的一端附着在下頜骨，另一端附着在舌骨。

myo- *prefix. see* my-.

〔前綴〕 **肌**

myoblast *n.* a cell that develops into a muscle fibre. —**myoblastic** *adj.*

成肌細胞 發展成肌纖維的一種細胞。

myocardial infarction death of a segment of heart muscle, which follows interruption of its blood supply (*see*

心肌梗塞 某一部分心肌在其血供中斷後壞死。心肌梗塞通常局限於左心

coronary thrombosis). Myocardial infarction is usually confined to the left ventricle. The patient experiences a 'heart attack': sudden severe chest pain, which may spread to the arms and throat. The main danger is that of ventricular *fibrillation, which accounts for most of the fatalities. Other *arrhythmias are also frequent; *ectopic beats in the ventricle are especially important as they predispose to ventricular fibrillation. Other complications include heart failure, rupture of the heart, phlebothrombosis, pulmonary embolism, pericarditis, shock, mitral incompetence, and perforation of the septum between the ventricles.

室。病人感到"心臟病突然發作"：突然覺得嚴重胸痛，可傳播到手臂和咽喉。主要危險是心室纖顫，它最易使病人致命。其它心律失常也常發生；心室異位搏動是預示心室纖顫的極重要徵兆。其它併發症包括心衰、心臟破裂、靜脈血栓形成、肺栓塞、心包炎、休克、二尖瓣關閉不全、室間隔穿孔。

The best results from the management of patients with myocardial infarction follow mobile and hospital-based coronary care with facilities for the early detection, prevention, and treatment of arrhythmias and *cardiac arrest. Most survivors of myocardial infarction are able to return to a full and active life, including those who have been successfully resuscitated from cardiac arrest.

隨着急救車的使用和醫院內冠心病監護病房的開展，心肌梗塞病人的管理工作取得了極好的效果，在這種監護醫療中使用了能早期診查、預防和治療心肌梗塞和心搏停止的設備。心肌梗塞的大多數存活者能恢復正常生活，其中包括那些心搏停止後復甦成功的病人。

myocarditis *n.* acute or chronic inflammation of the heart muscle. It may be seen alone or as part of pancarditis (*see* endomyocarditis).

心肌炎 心肌的急性或慢性炎症。它可單獨發病或作爲全心炎的一部分。

myocardium *n.* the middle of the three layers forming the wall of the heart (*see also* endocardium, epicardium). It is composed of *cardiac muscle and forms the greater part of the heart wall, being thicker in the ventricles than in the atria. —**myocardial** *adj.*

心肌〔層〕 構成心臟壁三層組織的中層。它是由心肌組成的並且構成大部分心臟壁。心室的心肌厚於心房。

myoclonus *n.* a sudden spasm of the muscles typically lifting and flexing the arms. Occasional *myoclonic jerks* occur between fits in patients with idiopathic *epilepsy, and myoclonus is a major feature of some progressive neurological illnesses with extensive degeneration of brain cells. —**myoclonic** *adj.*

肌陣攣 肌肉的突然痙攣，多見於手臂。偶然情況下，肌陣攣發生在原發性癲癇病人的兩次發作之間，並且肌陣攣是帶有廣泛腦細胞變性的某些進行性神經性疾病的一個主要特徵。

myocyte *n.* a muscle cell.

肌細胞

myodynia *n.* pain in the muscles.

肌痛 肌肉的疼痛。

myoepithelium *n.* a tissue consisting of cells of epithelial origin having a contractile cytoplasm. Myoepithelial cells play an important role in encouraging the secretion of substances into ducts.

肌上皮 起源於上皮組織細胞的並具有收縮性細胞漿的組織。肌上皮細胞在促進分泌物進入管道中起重要作用。

myofibril *n.* one of numerous contractile filaments found within the cytoplasm of *striated muscle cells. When viewed under a microscope myofibrils show alternating bands of high and low refractive index, which give striated muscle its characteristic appearance.

肌原纖維 橫紋肌細胞的胞漿內發現的有收縮性能的絲狀結構之一。在顯微鏡下觀察時，肌原纖維顯示出高和低折射標誌的交替帶，它可表現出橫紋肌的特性。

myogenic *adj.* originating in muscle: applied to the inherent rhythmicity of contraction of some muscles (e.g. cardiac muscle), which does not depend on neural influences.

肌〔源〕性的 肌肉內起源的：指某些肌肉（如：心肌）收縮的固有節律，此節律不受神經影響的支配。

myoglobin *n.* an iron-containing pigment, resembling *haemoglobin, found in muscle cells. It acts as an oxygen reservoir within the muscle fibres.

肌紅蛋白 肌細胞中存在的、與血紅蛋白相似的一種含鐵色素。它在肌纖維內起着貯存氧的作用。

myoglobinuria *n.* the presence in the urine of the pigment myoglobin.

肌紅蛋白尿 尿中存有肌紅蛋白色素。

myogram *n.* a recording of the activity of a muscle. *See* electromyography.

肌動〔描記〕圖 肌肉活動的記錄。

myograph *n.* an instrument for recording the activity of muscular tissues. *See* electromyography.

肌動描記器 記錄肌組織活動的儀器。

myokymia *n.* prominent quivering of a few muscle fibres, not associated with any other abnormal features. It is a benign condition. *See also* fasciculation.

肌纖維顫搐 少數肌纖維的明顯的顫動。沒有任何其它異常特徵。它是一種良性徵象。

myology *n.* the study of the structure, function, and diseases of the muscles.

肌學 研究肌肉的結構、功能和疾病的學科。

myoma *n.* a benign tumour of muscle. It may originate in smooth muscle (*see* leiomyoma) or in striated muscle (*see* rhabdomyoma).

肌瘤 肌肉的良性瘤。它可發生在平滑肌或橫紋肌肉。

myomectomy *n.* an operation in which benign tumours (fibromyomas or fibroids) are removed from the muscular wall of the womb. It is performed instead of hysterectomy when the patient wishes for further pregnancies.

肌瘤切除術 切除子宮肌壁的良性腫瘤（纖維肌瘤或纖維瘤）的手術。當病人希望保留生育能力時，可行此術以代替子宮切除術。

myometritis *n.* inflammation of the muscular wall (myometrium) of the womb.

子宮肌〔層〕炎 子宮壁肌肉組織（子宮肌層）的炎症。

myometrium *n.* the muscular tissue of the uterus (womb), which surrounds the *endometrium. It is composed of smooth muscle that undergoes small regular spontaneous contractions. The frequency and amplitude of these contractions alter in response to the hormones *oestrogen, *progesterone, and *oxytocin, which are present at particular stages of the menstrual cycle and pregnancy.

子宮肌層 圍繞着子宮內膜的子宮肌組織。它由平滑肌組成，可進行小的規律性的自主收縮。這些收縮的頻率和幅度在雌激素、孕酮和催產素類激素的作用下有所改變。這些激素出現在月經周期和妊娠的特殊階段。

myoneural junction *see* neuromuscular junction.

肌神經接點

myopathy *n.* any disease of the muscles. The myopathies are usually subdivided into those that are inherited (*see* muscular dystrophy) and those that are acquired. The acquired myopathies include *polymyositis and muscular diseases complicating endocrine disorders or carcinoma. All are typified by weakness and wasting of the muscles in the upper parts of the arms and legs.

肌病 肌肉的任一疾病。肌病通常分爲遺傳性的和獲得性的。獲得性肌病包括多肌炎和合併有內分泌病或癌症的肌病。所有肌病都是以臂和腿上部肌肉的無力和萎縮爲特徵的。

myopia (short-sightedness) *n.* the condition in which parallel light rays are brought to a focus in front of the retina (see illustration). Objects further than six metres from the eye are blurred and cannot be made sharp by *accommodation. The condition is corrected by wearing spectacles with concave lenses. *Compare* emmetropia, hypermetropia. —**myopic** *adj.*

近視 平行光線的焦點投射到視網膜前方（見圖）。某物體離眼的距離大於6米時就變得模糊不清並且不能因調節而變得清楚起來。配戴凹透鏡可矯正近視眼。

myoplasm *n.* *see* sarcoplasm.

肌漿

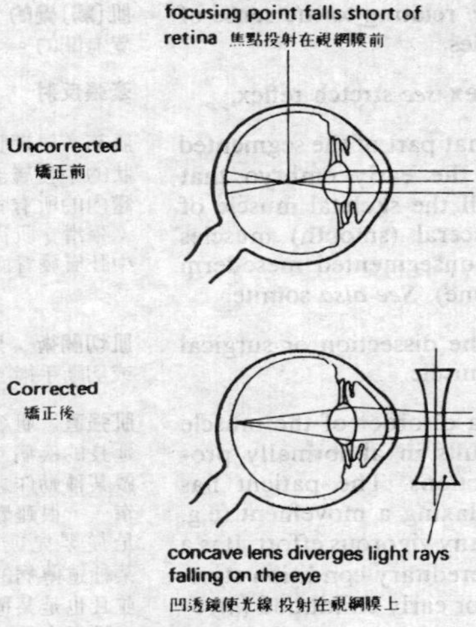

Myopia (short-sightedness)
近視

myoplasty *n.* the plastic surgery of muscle, in which part of a muscle is partly detached and used to repair tissue defects or deformities in the vicinity of the muscle.

肌整形術 肌肉的整形外科手術。此術分離部分肌肉並用以修補肌肉附近組織的缺陷或畸形。

myosarcoma *n.* a malignant tumour of muscle. *See also* leiomyosarcoma, rhabdomyosarcoma.

肌肉瘤 肌肉的惡性瘤。

myosin *n.* the most abundant protein in muscle fibrils, having the important properties of elasticity and contractility. With actin, it comprises the principal contractile element of muscles. *See* striated muscle.

肌球蛋白（肌凝蛋白） 肌原纖維中最豐富的蛋白質。它的重要特徵爲具有彈性和收縮性。它與肌動蛋白（肌纖蛋白）一道，構成肌肉的基本收縮成分。

myosis *n. see* miosis.

瞳孔縮小

myositis *n.* any of a group of muscle diseases in which inflammation and degenerative changes occur. *Polymyositis is the most commonly occurring example, but myositis may be found in relation to systemic *collagen disorders and a minority are caused by bacterial or parasitic infections.

肌炎 發生炎症和變性變化的一類肌病。多肌炎是最常見的病例，但現已發現肌炎與系統性膠原病有關，並且少數病例是由細菌性或寄生蟲性感染引起的。

myotactic *adj.* relating to the sense of touch in muscles.

肌〔觸〕覺的 與肌肉的觸覺有關的。

myotatic reflex *see* stretch reflex.

牽張反射

myotome *n.* that part of the segmented mesoderm in the early embryo that gives rise to all the skeletal muscle of the body. Visceral (smooth) muscles develop from unsegmented mesoderm (*see* mesenchyme). *See also* somite.

肌節 早期胚胎中呈節段狀的中胚層部分，它生成體內的所有骨骼肌。內臟（平滑）肌從未分節段的中胚層發育而來。

myotomy *n.* the dissection or surgical division of a muscle.

肌切開術 某肌肉的剖割或切斷手術。

myotonia *n.* a disorder of the muscle fibres that results in abnormally prolonged contractions. The patient has difficulty in relaxing a movement (e.g. his grip) after any vigorous effort. It is a feature of a hereditary condition starting in infancy or early childhood (*myotonia congenita*) and of a form of muscular dystrophy (*dystrophia myotonica).

肌强直 肌纖維收縮異常延長的疾病。病人在用力做某種動作之後（如：握拳），很難鬆弛下來，它是從嬰兒或幼兒時開始某種遺傳病的一個特徵，並且也是某種肌營養不良（肌强直性營養不良）的一個特徵。

myotonic *adj.* relating to muscle tone.

肌緊張的 與肌緊張有關的。

myotonus *n.* **1.** a tonic muscular spasm. **2.** muscle tone.

①**肌强直** 强直性肌肉痙攣。②**肌緊張**

myringa *n.* the eardrum (*see* tympanic membrane).

鼓膜

myringitis *n.* inflammation of the eardrum. *See* otitis (media).

鼓膜炎

myringoplasty (tympanoplasty) *n.* surgical reconstruction of an eardrum damaged by infection (*otitis media) or injury.

鼓膜成形術 對因感染（中耳炎）或損傷而受到破壞的鼓膜進行重建的外科手術。

myringotomy (tympanotomy) *n.* incision of the eardrum to create an artificial opening, which relieves pressure and allows drainage of fluid from an inflamed middle ear (*otitis media).

鼓膜切開術 在鼓膜上形成人工開口的手術。此術可減輕患有炎症的中耳（中耳炎）內的壓力並可引流其中的液體。

myx- (myxo-) *prefix denoting* mucus.

〔前綴〕 **黏液**

myxoedema *n.* **1.** a dry firm waxy swelling of the skin and subcutaneous tissues found in patients with underac-

黏液〔性〕水腫 ①甲狀腺機能低下的病人皮膚和皮下組織的乾蠟樣腫脹。②

tive thyroid glands (*see* hypothyroidism). **2.** the clinical syndrome due to hypothyroidism in adult life, including coarsening of the skin, intolerance to cold, weight gain, and mental dullness. The symptoms are abolished with thyroxine treatment.

因成人發生的甲狀腺功能減退所致的臨床綜合徵，包括皮膚變粗、怕冷、體重增加、精神遲鈍。用甲狀腺素治療時症狀消失。

myxofibroma *n.* a benign tumour of fibrous tissue that contains myxomatous elements (*see* myxoma) or has undergone mucoid degeneration.

黏液纖維瘤 纖維組織的良性瘤，此瘤含有黏液組織成分或已發生了黏液性變。

myxoma *n.* a benign gelatinous tumour of connective tissue. *Atrial myxoma* is a tumour of the heart, usually of the left side, arising from the septum dividing the two upper chambers. Symptoms may include fever, lassitude, joint pains, and sudden loss of consciousness due to obstruction of the bloodflow. The tumour may be wrongly diagnosed as stenosis of the mitral valve as it can produce a similar murmur. Treatment is by surgical removal. —**myxomatous** *adj.*

黏液瘤 結締組織的良性膠狀瘤，心房黏液瘤是心臟的腫瘤，常發生在左側，起源於心房間隔。症狀有發燒、倦怠、關節痛和因血流梗阻所致的突然意識喪失。因本病能產生與二尖瓣狹窄類似的雜音，故可誤診爲二尖瓣狹窄。治療：外科切除。

myxosarcoma *n.* a *sarcoma containing mucoid material. It is doubtful whether this represents a true entity and it may be simply a variant of other sarcomas, such as a *liposarcoma or a *fibrosarcoma.

黏液肉瘤 含有黏液樣物質的肉瘤。本病係一獨立的肉瘤抑或其它肉瘤（如脂肉瘤或纖維肉瘤）的變種，尚有疑問。

myxovirus *n.* one of a group of RNA-containing viruses that includes those causing influenza in animals and man. The related *paramyxoviruses* include the *respiratory syncytial virus (RSV) and the agents causing measles, mumps, and parainfluenza.

黏液病毒 脫氧核糖核酸（RNA）病毒屬中的一種。其中包括引起動物和人流感的病毒。有關的副黏病毒包括呼吸道合胞病毒（RSV）和引起麻疹、流行性腮腺炎和副流感的病毒。

N

N

nabothian follicle (nabothian cyst, nabothian gland) one of a number of cysts on the neck (cervix) of the womb, near its opening to the vagina. The sacs,

納博特氏濾泡（納博特氏囊腫，納博特氏腺） 子宮頸接近開口處的囊腫。因感染而受損的子宮頸部

which contain a thick liquid, form when the ducts of the glands in the cervix are blocked by a new growth of surface cells (epithelium) over an area damaged through infection.

表層細胞（上皮）的新生物，堵塞了頸部腺體的導管時，形成含有黏稠液體的囊腫。

NAD (nicotinamide adenine dinucleotide) a *coenzyme that acts as a hydrogen acceptor in oxidation-reduction reactions, particularly in the *electron transport chain in cellular respiration. NAD and the closely related coenzyme *NADP* (*nicotinamide adenine dinucleotide phosphate*) are derived from nicotinic acid; they are reduced to *NADH* and *NADPH*, respectively.

二磷酸吡啶核苷酸 在氧化還原反應中作爲氫受體的輔酶。特別是在細胞呼吸的電子轉移鏈上起作用。二磷酸吡啶核苷酸和與其密切相關的輔酶三磷酸吡啶核苷酸是煙酸衍生而來的；它們分別還原爲NADH和NADPH。

NADP (nicotinamide adenine dinucleotide phosphate) *see* NAD.

三磷酸吡啶核苷酸

Naegleria *n.* a genus of *amoebae that normally live in damp soil or mud. *Naegleria* species can, however, live as parasites in man and are believed to have caused some rare, but fatal, infections of the brain.

納格里屬阿米巴 正常情況下生活在潮濕土壤或泥土中的阿米巴屬。但是，納格里屬阿米巴某些種可作爲人的寄生物存在，據信它可引起某些罕見的，但是致命的腦部感染。

naevus *n.* (*pl.* **naevi**) a birthmark: a clearly defined malformation of the skin, present at birth. There are many different types of naevi. Some are composed of small blood vessels (*see* haemangioma). These blood-vessel birthmarks include the *strawberry mark*, which usually disappears in early life, and the *port-wine stain*, which does not disappear and is best left untreated. Another kind of naevus is the *mole.

痣 一種胎記：出生時就有的，界限明顯的皮膚病變。有許多不同類型的痣。某些痣是由小血管組成的。這些血管胎記包括通常在生命早期消失的莓狀痣，和不自動消失的並且最好不加以治療的葡萄酒樣色素斑。另一種痣是胎塊。

Naga sore *see* tropical ulcer.

納加氏潰瘍

nail *n.* a horny structure, composed of keratin, formed from the epidermis on the dorsal surface of each finger and toe (see illustration). The exposed part of the nail is the *body*, behind which is the *root*. The whitish crescent-shaped area at the base of the body is called the *lunula*. Growth of the nail occurs at the end of the nail root by division of the germinative layer of the underlying

甲 每個手指和脚趾背面表皮中形成的，由角蛋白構成的角質結構（見圖）。甲的暴露部位是甲體，甲體的後面是甲根。在甲體基底部的帶白色的新月形區域稱爲弧影。甲的生長發生在甲根的末端，通過甲下表皮生發層（它形成甲床的一部分）

*epidermis (which forms part of the *matrix*). The growing nail slides forward over the *nail bed*. The fold of skin that lies above the root is the *nail fold*; folds of skin on either side of the nail are the *nail walls*. The epidermis of the nail fold that lies next to the nail root is called the *eponychium* (forming the 'cuticle' at the base of the nail). Anatomical name: **unguis**.

的細胞分裂向外生長。生長着的甲在甲床上向前移動，位於甲根上的皮膚〔皺〕襞是甲褶，在甲兩側的皮膚皺襞是甲壁。緊挨着甲根的甲褶的表皮稱爲〔指〕甲上皮（形成在甲基底部的“護膜”）。

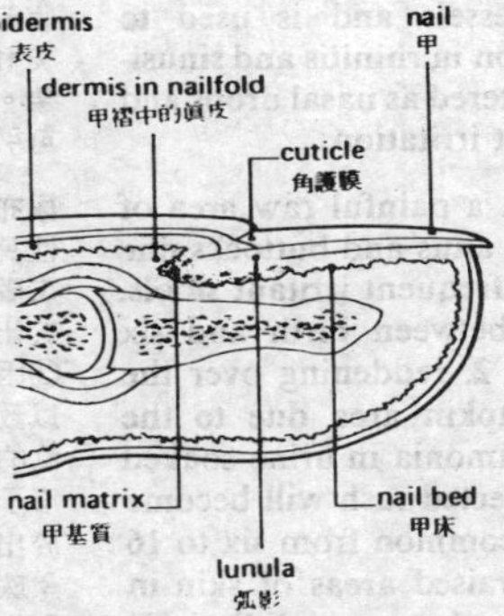

Longitudinal section through the fingertip and nail
指尖和甲的縱切面

nalidixic acid a drug active against various bacteria and used to treat infections of the urinary and digestive systems. It is administered by mouth; common side-effects are nausea, vomiting, and skin reactions. Trade name: **Negram**.

萘啶酸 有效地抗各種細菌並用於治療泌尿系和消化系感染的藥物。口服。常見副作用爲噁心、嘔吐、皮膚反應。

nalorphine *n.* a drug that reduces the effects of morphine and similar narcotic drugs and is used to stimulate breathing and restore consciousness after an overdose of these drugs. It is administered by injection and, given alone, may depress breathing and cause drowsiness or restlessness. Trade name: **Lethidrone**.

烯丙嗎啡 減輕嗎啡和類似麻醉藥作用的藥物。它用於嗎啡類藥物服用過量後刺激呼吸和恢復知覺。注射給藥。單獨用藥可抑制呼吸並引起瞌睡或煩躁。

nandrolone *n.* a synthetic male sex hormone with effects and uses similar to those of *methandienone. It is administered by injection and high doses

諾龍 效果和用途類似於去氫甲睪酮的人工合成男性性激素。注射給藥。大劑量可引起婦女男性化的

may cause signs of *virilization in women. Trade name: **Durabolin**.

症狀。商品名：苯丙酸諾龍。

nano- *prefix denoting* **1.** extremely small size. **2.** one thousand-millionth part (10^{-9}).

〔前綴〕 ①**矮，小** 指極小的物體。 ②**纖，毫微** 10億分之一。

nanometre *n.* one thousand-millionth of a metre (10^{-9} m). One nanometre is equal to 10 angstrom. Symbol: nm.

毫微米 10億分之一米。一毫微米相當於10個埃。符號：nm。

naphazoline *n.* a drug that constricts small blood vessels and is used to relieve congestion in rhinitis and sinusitis. It is administered as nasal drops and may cause slight irritation.

鹽酸萘甲唑啉 使小血管收縮的藥物。用於解除鼻炎和鼻竇炎中的充血現象。製備成滴鼻劑使用，可引起輕度的刺激。

napkin rash 1. a painful raw area of skin around the anus and buttocks due to contact with frequent irritant stools. It is common between birth and six months of age. **2.** reddening over the genitals and napkin area due to the formation of ammonia in urine-soaked napkins. A neglected rash will become ulcerated. It is common from six to 16 months. **3.** red raised areas of skin in the napkin region due to candidiasis. It has some resemblance to *psoriasis, hence its alternative name *napkin psoriasis*.

尿布疹 ①因常接觸刺激性糞便，肛門周圍和臀部皮膚的痛性紅腫。它常見於出生後和6個月之間。②因尿布中的尿形成氨，以致生殖器和尿布覆蓋部位的皮膚變紅。被忽略的疹子將變成潰瘍。它常見於出生後6～16個月。③念珠菌病所致的尿布區域內皮膚的紅腫處。它與銀屑有某些類似的地方，因此它的另一個名稱爲尿布銀屑病。

naprapathy *n.* a system of medicine based on the belief that a great many diseases are attributable to displacement of ligaments, tendons, and other connective tissues and that cure can be brought about only by manipulation to correct these displacements.

推拿療法 一種醫療體系。它基於相信很多疾病是韌帶、肌腱、以及其他結締組織移位造成的，治療方法僅爲通過推拿來矯正這些移位。

naproxen *n.* an analgesic drug that also reduces inflammation and fever. It is used to treat rheumatoid arthritis, ankylosing spondylitis, and gout. It is administered by mouth; side-effects may include digestive upsets and rashes. Trade name: **Naprosyn**.

甲氧萘丙酸 一種鎮痛藥。也有消炎和解熱作用。用於治療風濕性關節炎、强直性脊椎炎、痛風。口服。副作用可有消化不良和發疹。商品名：萘普生。

narcissism *n.* excessive self-regard, with or without some rational basis. In Freudian terms it is a state in which the *ego has taken itself as a love object. Some degree of narcissism is present in

自戀，戀己癖 具備或不具備某些合理原因的過度自我欣賞。在弗洛伊德的術語中，這是自我把自己做爲性愛對象的一種狀

most individuals, but when it is shown to an extreme degree it may be a symptom of schizophrenia, personality disorder, and other conditions. —**narcissistic** *adj.*

態。某種程度的自戀存在於大多數人中，但是當它發展到極其嚴重的程度時，可爲精神分裂症、人格障礙和其他疾病的一種症狀。

narco- *prefix denoting* narcosis; stupor.

〔前綴〕 **麻醉，木僵**

narcolepsy *n.* an extreme tendency to fall asleep in quiet surroundings or when engaged in monotonous activities. The patient can be woken easily and is immediately alert. It is often associated with *cataplexy, and when falling asleep the patient may experience auditory hallucinations or transient attacks of muscular paralysis. —**narcoleptic** *adj.*, *n.*

發作性睡眠 在安靜的環境中或從事單調活動時極易進入睡眠狀態的傾向。病人很易被喚醒，並且可馬上活躍起來。發作性睡眠常與猝倒有關。當熟睡時，病人可有幻聽或短暫發作的肌肉麻痹。

narcosis *n.* a state of diminished consciousness or complete unconsciousness caused by the use of *narcotic drugs, which have a depressant action on the nervous system. The body's normal reactions to stimuli are diminished and the body may become sedated or completely anaesthetized.

麻醉 使用對神經系統有抑制作用的麻醉藥引起的意識朦朧或完全喪失的狀態。麻醉後，身體對刺激的正常反應減弱，並且身體可進入鎮靜狀態或完全麻醉狀態。

narcotic *n.* a drug that induces stupor and insensibility and relieves pain. The term is used particularly for *morphine and other derivatives of opium (*see* opiate) but is also applied to other drugs that depress brain function (e.g. general anaesthetics and hypnotics). In legal terms a narcotic is any addictive drug subject to illegal use. Narcotics (i.e. morphine and morphine-like drugs) have been largely replaced as sleeping drugs because of their ability to cause *dependence and tolerance; they are still used for relief of severe pain (*see* analgesic).

麻醉藥 誘導昏睡、木僵、麻木並可解除疼痛的藥物。麻醉藥特別是指嗎啡和阿片的其它衍化物，但它也指其它抑制腦功能的藥物（例如：全身麻醉藥和安眠藥）。在法律的條文中，麻醉藥是指非法使用的成癮藥。麻醉藥（例如：嗎啡或嗎啡樣藥）大部分已被安眠藥取代，因爲它們能產生賴藥性和耐藥性。麻醉藥仍用於解除重度疼痛。

nares *pl. n.* (*sing.* **naris**) openings of the nose. The two *external* (or *anterior*) *nares* are the nostrils, leading from the nasal cavity to the outside. The two *internal* (or *posterior*) *nares* (*choanae*) are the openings leading from the nasal cavity into the pharynx.

鼻孔 鼻子的開口。兩個外鼻孔（鼻前孔）是鼻腔與外界相通的孔竅。兩個內鼻孔（鼻後孔）是從鼻腔向咽喉的開口。

nasal bone either of a pair of narrow oblong bones that together form the bridge and root of the nose. *See* skull.

鼻骨 共同形成鼻梁和鼻根的一對狹窄長方形骨。

nasal cavity the space inside the nose that lies between the floor of the cranium and the roof of the mouth. It is divided into two halves by a septum: each half communicates with the outside via the nostrils and with the nasopharynx through the posterior nares.

鼻腔 位於口頂和顱底之間的鼻內腔隙，它由中隔分成兩半：每一半經過鼻孔與外界相通，並經過鼻後孔與鼻咽相通。

nasal concha (turbinate bone) any of three thin scroll-like bones that form the sides of the *nasal cavity. The *superior* and *middle nasal conchae* are part of the *ethmoid bone; the *inferior nasal conchae* are a separate pair of bones of the face. *See* skull.

鼻甲 形成鼻腔側壁的三個薄的卷形骨。上鼻甲和中鼻甲是篩骨的一部分；下鼻甲是一對獨立的面骨。

nasion *n.* the point on the bridge of the nose at the centre of the suture between the nasal and frontal bones.

鼻根點 在鼻骨和額骨之間縫中央的、鼻梁上的點。

naso- *prefix denoting* the nose.

〔前綴〕 **鼻**

nasolacrimal *adj.* relating to the nose and the lacrimal (tear-producing) apparatus.

鼻淚的 與鼻和淚器（產生眼淚的器官）有關的。

nasolacrimal duct the duct that passes through the hole (*nasolacrimal canal*) in the palatine bone of the skull. It drains the tears away from the *lacrimal apparatus into the inferior meatus of the nose.

鼻淚管 通過顱的顎骨內孔（鼻淚道）的管。它把淚從淚器中排到鼻的下鼻道內。

nasopharynx (rhinopharynx) *n.* the part of the *pharynx that lies above the soft palate.

鼻咽 軟顎上的咽部分。

nates *pl. n.* the buttocks. —**natal** *adj.*

臀部

National Assistance Act (1945) an Act of Parliament providing for the needs of those who, through age, infirmity, or lack of qualifying contributions, are ineligible for benefit under the terms of the National Insurance Act. Cash payments (*supplementary benefit*) may be made from exchequer funds providing the applicants qualify

國家援助條例（1945）爲那些因年老、疾病、或未作出過一定貢獻的人的需求制定的議會條例。這些不符合享受國家保險條例救濟金的條件。對於在家庭經濟情況調查中符合條件的申請人，可以從國庫基金中支付現金（補充

in a means test. Under the terms of Part III of the Act local authorities are required to provide accommodation for those in need of care and attention that is not otherwise available to them (*Part III accommodation*). Such accommodation has replaced the workhouse, but the associated stigma – and dislike of the means test – deter many who are eligible from applying for help to which they are entitled.

救濟金）。條例第三部分中規定，地方當局要為那些無人照料而需要得到照管和關心的人提供膳宿（第三部分膳宿），這種膳宿條件已代替了濟貧院，但隨之而來的壞名聲，以及對家庭經濟情況調查的厭惡，使許多够條件的人不願申請他們有權得到的幫助。

national census *see* Office of Population Censuses and Surveys.

國家人口普查

National Health Service (in Britain) a comprehensive service offering therapeutic and preventive medical and surgical care, including the prescription and dispensing of medicines, spectacles, and medical and dental appliances. Exchequer funds pay for the services of doctors, nurses, and other professionals and meet a substantial part of the cost of the medicines and appliances. Legislation enacted in 1946 was implemented in 1948 and the services were subjected to substantial reorganization in 1974 and again in 1982. In England overall responsibility is vested in the Secretary of State for Health and Social Security assisted by a comprehensive department (*see* Department of Health and Social Security). Administration is based on a system of delegation downwards and accountability upwards through a hierarchy of 15 regions, each subdivided into a number of districts. In general, *Regional Health Authorities* (*RHA*), whose members are all appointed by the Secretary of State, are responsible for overall planning and monitoring and for allocating funds to the *District Health Authorities* (*DHA*). DHA, whose chairmen are appointed by the Secretary of State and the majority of their members by the RHA, are responsible for local planning, some of which may be delegated to districts. Each tier has a team of officers consisting of a medical officer (*see* community

國民保健服務制（在英國）國家對全民提供內、外各科預防和治療等綜合服務的制度。服務項目包括處方和配藥、眼鏡、以及醫療和牙科用品等。醫生、護士和其它專業人員的工作報酬以及醫藥用品的主要費用由國庫資金中支付。1946年制定的法規於1948年貫徹執行，並且在1974和1982年進行了兩次重大的改革。在英格蘭，保健和社會保障國務大臣在一個綜合性部門的協助下負有全面的責任。行政管理體制是基於自上而下的委派制和自下而上的等級負責制。共分成15個地區，每個地區又分成若干地段，實行分級管理。一般來說，所有地區保健局（RHA）的成員是由國務大臣任命的，這些成員負責全面的計劃和監督，並負責分配資金到地段保健局（DHA）。地段保健局（DHA）局長是由國務大臣任命的，而且他們的大多數成員是由地區保健局（RHA）任命的。地段保健局（DHA）負責局部地段的計劃，其某些成員可被委派到地段去。每一層次都有一個由醫師、行政人

physician), administrator, treasurer, and *nursing officer. The team has executive powers, and decisions are made on the basis of consensus with ultimate accountability to the appropriate authority.

員、財務人員和護師組成的幹部班子。這個班子有行政權力，在作出決定時必須符合於他們向有關當局所負的基本責任。

Health authorities are expected to provide all the normal health services from their own resources except the salaries and fees for general practitioners, pharmacists, opticians, and dentists, which come from a separate fund through the *Family Practitioner Committee. Some of the special resources for patients with rarer complaints are shared on a regional or supraregional basis. Wherever possible, districts have common boundaries with local authorities in order to try and ensure liaison with the Social Service Department, which provides many important services to support the sick and aged (*see* social services). However, many districts include part of more than one local authority since the division tends to be made on the basis of the catchment area of a district general hospital. Executive power is vested in the *District Management Team* (*DMT*), which has equivalent composition to the District Team of Officers with the addition of a general practitioner and a hospital consultant.

各保健局應從他們自己的資金中支付所有正常的保健服務費用，但不包括全科醫師、藥師、眼鏡師和牙醫師的薪金和酬金，這些經費通過開業醫師管理委員會由單獨的基金開支。某些罕見病病人的特殊費用由地區及其以上的機構共同分擔。只要有可能，地段保健局就應儘量與地方有關當局共同合作，以便努力取得和確保與社會服務部門的聯繫，此部門設有資助病人和老年人的許多重要服務項目。但是，許多地段內都包括一個以上的地方當局管界，因爲地段的劃分往往是以地段全科醫院爲中心的，其服務面積不限於一個地方當局管轄。地段管理班子具有行政權力，它的成員構成與地段幹部班子相同，只是增加一名全科醫師和一名醫院經治醫師。

Different arrangements apply in Northern Ireland and Wales, where the appropriate Secretary of State is responsible and the regional tier is omitted. In Scotland (for which there is a separate Act) the Secretary of State is also responsible and there is an intermediate tier by which districts are grouped into areas (*see* Chief Administrative Medical Officer).

在北愛爾蘭和威爾士有不同的管理方法，在那裏由相應的國務大臣負責此項工作，並且不劃分地區的等級。在蘇格蘭（那裏有一個獨立的條例）國務大臣也負責此項工作，並且有一個中層機構把若干地段劃歸幾個行政區。

natriuresis *n.* the excretion of sodium in the urine: a normal phenomenon.

尿鈉排泄 尿中的鈉的排泄，一種正常現象。

natriuretic *n.* an agent that promotes the excretion of sodium salts in the urine. Most *diuretics are natriuretics.

〔促〕尿鈉排泄藥 促使尿中鈉鹽排泄的藥物。大多數利尿劑是〔促〕尿鈉排泄藥。

naturopathy *n.* a system of medicine that relies upon the use of only 'natural' substances for the treatment of disease, rather than drugs. Herbs, food grown without artificial fertilizers and prepared without the use of preservatives or colouring material, pure water, sunlight, and fresh air are all employed in an effort to rid the body of 'unnatural' substances, which are said to be at the root of most illnesses.

自然醫術 不用藥物而僅靠用"自然"物質治病的醫學體系。草藥、非人工肥料培植和未經防腐及着色劑製備的食物、純水、陽光和新鮮空氣都用於去除體內的非自然物質。據說這些物質是大多數疾病的根源。

nausea *n.* the feeling that one is about to vomit, as experienced in seasickness and in morning sickness of early pregnancy. Actual vomiting often occurs subsequently.

噁心 一種想嘔吐的感覺。就像暈船和早孕反應中的感覺一樣。劇烈嘔吐常隨後發生。

navel *n.* see umbilicus.

臍

navicular bone a boat-shaped bone of the ankle (*see* tarsus) that articulates with the three cuneiform bones in front and with the talus behind.

舟骨 踝部的船形骨。它與前面的三個楔骨和後面的距骨相關節。

nearthrosis *n. see* pseudarthrosis.

人造關節

nebula *n.* a faint opacity of the cornea that remains after an ulcer has healed.

角膜雲翳 潰瘍痊癒後角膜上存留的輕度混濁。

nebulizer *n.* an instrument used for applying a liquid in the form of a fine spray.

噴霧器 把液體變成細小的霧滴的器械。

Necator *n.* a genus of *hookworms that live in the small intestine. The human hookworm, *N. americanus*, occurs in tropical Africa, Central and South America, India, and the Pacific Islands. The worm possesses two pairs of sharp cutting plates inside its mouth cavity, which enable it to feed on the blood and tissues of the gut wall. *Compare* Ancylostoma.

板口線蟲屬 生活在小腸內的鈎蟲屬。人類鈎蟲——美洲板口線蟲，見於熱帶非洲、中美洲、南美洲、印度以及太平洋諸島。此蟲的口腔內有兩對銳利的切板，它使此類蟲屬能夠吸食腸壁的血液和組織。

necatoriasis *n.* an infestation of the small intestine by the parasitic hookworm *Necator americanus*. *See also* hookworm disease.

板口線蟲病 寄生鈎蟲——美洲板口線蟲在小腸寄生所致的病。

necro- *prefix denoting* death or dissolution.

〔前綴〕 **壞死** 死亡或溶解。

necrobiosis *n.* a gradual process by which cells lose their function and die. *Necrobiosis lipoidica* is patchy degeneration of the skin causing areas of white scarring and thinning. It is most commonly seen in diabetics but is found occasionally in nondiabetics.

漸進性壞死 細胞喪失其功能並死亡的漸進性過程。脂性漸進性壞死是皮膚斑樣變性所致的局部白色瘢痕並變薄。最常出現於糖尿病中，但也偶見於非糖尿病時。

necrology *n.* the study of the phenomena of death, involving determination of the moment of death and the different changes that occur in the tissues of the body after death.

死亡學 對死亡現象進行的研究。其中包括確定死亡時間和死後體內組織發生的不同變化。

necromania *n.* morbid desire for a dead body or bodies. This may be necrophilism, but the attraction is sometimes not sexual. A bereaved person, for instance, who is not grieving normally, may occasionally treasure the body of a loved one.

戀屍狂 對某個或某些死屍的病態愛好。有時是對異性屍體的戀屍癖，但有時不是由於性的吸引。如：一個居喪的人異常悲痛，可偶然地珍藏他所熱愛的人的屍體。

necrophilism (necrophilia) *n.* sexual attraction to corpses. *See also* perversion. —**necrophile** *n.*

戀屍癖（佯屍癖） 對屍體產生的性吸引。

necropsy *n. see* autopsy.

屍體解剖

necrosis (mortification) *n.* the death of some or all of the cells in an organ or tissue, caused by disease, physical or chemical injury, or interference with the blood supply (*see* gangrene). *Caseous necrosis* occurs in pulmonary tuberculosis, the lung tissue becoming soft, dry, and cheeselike.

壞死（壞疽） 某器官或組織中部分或所有細胞死亡。可爲疾病、物理或化學損傷、血供應障礙所致。乾酪樣壞死發生在肺結核中，肺組織變軟、變乾，呈乾酪樣。

necrospermia *n.* the presence of either dead or motionless spermatozoa in the semen. *See* infertility.

死精症 精液中存有死亡或無運動能力的精子。

necrotomy *n.* **1.** the removal of a dead piece of bone (*see* sequestrum). **2.** dissection of a dead body.

①**死骨切除** 去除死骨塊。 ②**屍體解剖**

needle *n.* a slender sharp-pointed instrument used for a variety of purposes. Needles used for sewing up tissue during surgical operation are of various designs, for specific operations, and are equipped with an eye for threading suture material. Hollow needles are used to inject substances into the body (in hypodermic syringes), to obtain

針 具有多種用途的細而尖銳的器械。外科手術中用於縫合組織的針有不同類型。特殊手術中使用的針具有穿縫線的針眼。空針用於向體內注射物質（在皮下注射器中），獲取組織標本，或從某腔室中抽出液體。

specimens of tissue (*see* biopsy), or to withdraw fluid from a cavity (*see* aspiration). *See also* stop needle.

needling *n.* a form of *capsulotomy in which a sharp needle is used to make a hole in the capsule surrounding the lens of the eye.

針刺術 囊切開術的一種。用一個尖針在眼晶狀體周圍囊上穿一個洞。

negativism *n.* behaviour that is the opposite of that suggested by others. In *active negativism* the individual does the opposite of what he is asked (for example, he screws his eyes up when asked to open them). This is uncommon in adult life and is usually associated with other features of *catatonia. In *passive negativism* the person fails to cooperate (for example, he does not eat). This occurs in *schizophrenia and *depression.

違拗症 與其他人的意見相反的行爲。在主動違拗症中，病人做與別人的要求相反的事情（如：當要求他睜開眼時，他緊閉眼睛）。這在成人中是不常見的，常與緊張症的其它特徵伴發。在被動違拗症中，病人不合作（如不吃飯）。這可發生在精神分裂症和抑鬱症中。

Neisseria *n.* a genus of spherical Gram-negative aerobic nonmotile bacteria characteristically grouped in pairs. They are parasites of animals, and some species are normal inhabitants of the respiratory tract of man. The species *N. gonorrhoeae* (the *gonococcus*) causes *gonorrhoea. Gonococci are found within pus cells of urethral and vaginal discharge; they can be cultured only on serum or blood agar. *N. meningitidis* (the *meningococcus*) causes *cerebrospinal fever and *meningitis. Meningococci are found within pus cells of infected cerebrospinal fluid and blood or in the nasal passages of carriers. They too can only be cultured on serum or blood agar.

奈瑟氏菌屬 革蘭氏陰性、需氧、非運動球菌屬。特徵爲成對聚集在一起。它們是動物的寄生菌，並且某些菌種正常地存在於人的呼吸道。淋病奈瑟氏菌可引起淋病。淋〔病雙〕球菌可見於尿道和陰道排出物的膿細胞內，僅能在血清或血瓊脂平板上培養。腦膜炎奈瑟氏菌（腦膜炎雙球菌）可引起腦脊髓熱和腦〔脊〕膜炎。腦膜炎球菌可見於已感染的脊液和血液的膿細胞內，或見於帶菌者的鼻道內。也僅能在血清或血瓊脂平板上培養。

nematode (roundworm) *n.* any one of a large group of worms having an unsegmented cylindrical body, tapering at both ends. This distinguishes nematodes from other *helminths. Nematodes occur either as free-living forms in the sea, fresh water, and soil or as parasites of plants, animals, and man. *Hookworms and *pinworms infest the alimentary canal. *Filariae are found in the lymphatic tissues. The *guinea

線蟲 具有圓筒形不分段的蟲體，並且兩端逐漸變細的一大類寄生蟲。這可使該蟲區別於其它蠕蟲。線蟲有些是在海水、淡水和土壤中自由生存，有些是植物、動物和人的寄生蟲。鈎蟲和蟯蟲寄生在消化道。線蟲見於淋巴組織中。天竺蠕蟲和盤尾屬常侵入結締組織。某些線蟲

worm and *Onchocerca affect connective tissue. Some nematodes (e.g. pinworms) are transmitted from host to host by the ingestion of eggs; others (e.g. *Wuchereria) by the bite of a bloodsucking insect.

（如：蟯蟲）從宿生到宿主的傳播是攝入蟲卵所致；其它的線蟲（如：吳策線蟲屬）的傳播是由吸血昆蟲的叮咬引起。

Nembutal *n. see* pentobarbitone.

戊巴比妥鈉

neo- *prefix denoting* new or newly formed.

〔前綴〕 **新**

neocerebellum *n.* the middle lobe of the *cerebellum, excluding the pyramid and uvula. In evolutionary terms it is the newest part, occurring only in mammals.

新小腦 不包括蚓錐體和蚓垂的小腦中葉。在種系發育過程中，它是最新的部分，僅見於哺乳動物中。

neologism *n.* (in psychiatry) the invention of words to which meanings are attached. It is common in childhood, but when it occurs in an adult it may be a symptom of a psychotic illness, such as *schizophrenia. It should be distinguished from *paraphasia, in which new meanings are attached to ordinary words.

新語症 （精神病學）具有一定意義的詞滙的發明。此症常見於兒童，但當本症在成人中發生時，可爲精神病（如：精神分裂症）的一種症狀。它應與言語錯亂區別，在言語錯亂中普通的詞滙附加有新的意義。

neomycin *n.* an antibiotic used to treat infections caused by a wide range of bacteria, mainly those affecting the skin and eyes. It is usually applied in creams or drops with other antibiotics, but can also be given by mouth.

新黴素 一種抗生素。用於治療多種細菌（主要爲侵犯皮膚和眼睛的細菌）引起的感染。通常將新黴素與其它抗生素一起製備成乳膏或滴劑使用。但也可口服。

neonatal death rate *see* infant mortality rate.

新生兒〔期〕死亡率

neonate *n.* an infant at any time during the first four weeks of life. The word is particularly applied to infants just born or in the first week of life. —**neonatal** *adj.*

新生兒 出生後四周內的嬰兒。尤指剛出生或出生後一周內的嬰兒。

neopallium *n.* an enlargement of the wall of each cerebral hemisphere. In evolutionary terms it is the newest part of the cerebrum, formed by the development of new pathways for sight and hearing in mammals.

新大腦皮質 每個大腦半球壁的增大部分。在種系發育過程中，它是大腦的最新部分，在哺乳動物由於視覺和聽覺新路徑的發育而形成。

neoplasm *n.* a new and abnormal growth: any *benign or *malignant tumour.

新生物 新的和異常的生長物：任何良性或惡性腫瘤。

neostigmine *n.* a *parasympathomimetic drug that acts by inhibiting the enzyme cholinesterase (*see also* anticholinesterase). It is used mainly to diagnose and treat *myasthenia gravis and as an antidote to some *muscle-relaxant drugs, such as tubocurarine. It is also used to treat some intestinal disorders and glaucoma. Neostigmine is administered by mouth, injection, or in eye-drops; side-effects include digestive upsets and increased saliva flow. Trade name: **Prostigmin**.

新斯的明 可抑制膽鹼酯酶的擬副交感神經藥。主要用於診斷和治療重症肌無力，並作爲某些肌肉鬆弛劑（如：筒箭毒鹼）的解毒劑。也可用於治療某些腸道疾病和青光眼。新斯的明可口服、注射、或作爲滴服劑。副作用包括消化不良和唾液增加。

nephr- (nephro-) *prefix denoting* the kidney(s).

〔前綴〕 **腎**

nephralgia *n.* pain in the kidney. The pain is felt in the loin and can be caused by a variety of kidney complaints.

腎痛 腎臟的疼痛。腰部感到的疼痛，可由多種腎病引起。

nephrectomy *n.* surgical removal of a kidney. When performed for cancer of the kidney, the entire organ is removed together with its surrounding fat and the adjacent adrenal gland (*radical nephrectomy*). Removal of either the upper or lower pole of the kidney is termed *partial nephrectomy*.

腎切除術 外科切除腎臟的手術。當切除腎癌時，需切除整個腎臟以及它周圍的脂肪和鄰近的腎上腺。切除腎上極或下極的手術稱爲腎部分切除術。

nephritis (Bright's disease) *n.* inflammation of the kidney. Nephritis is a nonspecific term used to describe a condition resulting from a variety of causes. *See* glomerulonephritis.

腎炎 腎臟的炎症。腎炎不是一個專門的術語，它用於形容多種不同病因所致的疾病。

nephroblastoma (Wilms' tumour) *n.* a malignant tumour of the kidney found in children (*see* cancer). It is rare over the age of eight years and the most obvious symptom is an abdominal swelling. Treatment is by *nephrectomy followed by radiotherapy and *cytotoxic drugs. Considerable improvement in the results of treatment has occurred in recent years since the use of cytotoxic drugs as a routine.

腎胚細胞瘤（維爾姆斯氏瘤） 兒童的腎惡性瘤。8歲以上少見，其最明顯的症狀是腹部腫塊。治療爲腎切除術，進而使用放射治療和細胞毒性藥物。近年來，因常規使用細胞毒性藥物，治療效果有明顯的改善。

nephrocalcinosis *n.* the presence of calcium deposits in the kidneys. This can be caused by excess calcium in the blood, as caused by overactivity of the

腎鈣質沉着 腎中存有鈣的沉積物。病因可爲甲狀旁腺機能亢進所致的血鈣過多，或可爲腎組織的潛

parathyroid glands, or it may result from an underlying abnormality of the kidney. The cause of nephrocalcinosis must be detected by full biochemical, radiological, and urological investigation so that appropriate treatment can be undertaken.

在異常。腎鈣質沉着須經全面的生物化學、放射學和泌尿科的檢查，找出病因後才能進行適當的治療。

nephrogenic cord either of the paired ridges of tissue that run along the dorsal surface of the abdominal cavity of the embryo. Parts of it develop into the kidney, ovary, or testis and their associated ducts. Intermediate stages of these developments are the *pronephros, *mesonephros, and *metanephros.

生腎索 沿着胚胎腹腔背側排列的成對的組織嵴。部分生腎索發育成腎、卵巢或睾丸及有關的管道。生腎索發育的中間階段爲前腎、中腎和後腎。

nephrolithiasis *n.* the presence of stones in the kidney (*see* calculus). Such stones can cause pain and blood in the urine, but they may produce no symptoms. Full investigation is undertaken to determine the underlying cause of stone formation. When stones are associated with urinary obstruction and infection they usually require surgical removal (*see* nephrolithotomy, pyelolithotomy).

腎石病 腎中存有結石。此種結石可引起尿痛和血尿，但是它們也可不引起任何症狀。爲了確定結石形成的根本原因，須進行全面的檢查。當結石與泌尿系梗阻或感染有關時，常須手術去除。

nephrolithotomy *n.* the surgical removal of a stone from the kidney by an incision into the kidney substance. It is normally performed in combination with an incision into the renal pelvis (*see* pyelolithotomy). *See also* percutaneous nephrolithotomy.

腎石切除術 經腎實質切口進行的腎結石外科切除術。正常情況下，此術常與腎盂切開同時進行。

nephrology *n.* the branch of medicine concerned with the study, investigation, and management of diseases of the kidney. *See also* urology. —**nephrologist** *n.*

腎病學 與腎病的研究、調查和處理有關的醫學分支。

nephron *n.* the active unit of excretion in the kidney (see illustration). Blood, supplied by branches of the renal artery, is filtered through a knot of capillaries (*glomerulus*) into the cup-shaped *Bowman's capsule* so that water, nitrogenous waste, and many other substances (excluding colloids) pass

腎單位 腎臟中具有排泄功能的單位（見圖）。由腎動脈分支供應的血液，通過毛細血管球（腎小球）濾入杯狀的鮑曼氏囊內，以使水、含氮代謝物和許多其它物質（不包括膠體）進入腎小管。在腎

into the *renal tubule*. Here most of the substances are reabsorbed back into the blood, the remaining fluid (*urine) passing into the collecting duct, which drains into the *ureter.

小管中，大多數物質被重吸收回血液中，剩下的液體（尿）進入收集管，此管可將尿液排入輸尿管。

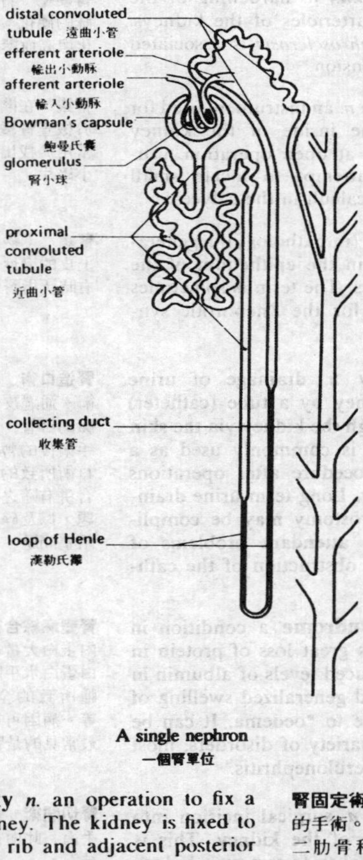

A single nephron
一個腎單位

nephropexy *n.* an operation to fix a mobile kidney. The kidney is fixed to the twelfth rib and adjacent posterior abdominal wall to prevent descent of the kidney on standing (*see* nephroptosis).

腎固定術 固定活動性腎的手術。將腎固定在第十二肋骨和鄰近的後腹壁上，以防站立時腎下垂。

nephroptosis *n.* abnormal descent of a kidney into the pelvis on standing, which may occur if it is excessively mobile (for example, in thin women). If

腎下垂 站立時腎臟異常下降到骨盆。它可發生在腎臟活動度過大時（例如瘦弱婦女）。如腎下垂件

this is accompanied by pain and obstruction to free drainage of urine by the kidney, *nephropexy may be advised.

有疼痛和腎臟排尿障礙，可行腎固定術。

nephrosclerosis *n.* hardening of the arteries and arterioles of the kidneys. *Arteriolar nephrosclerosis* is associated with *hypertension.

腎硬化 腎動脈和腎小動脉的硬化。小動脉性腎硬化與高血壓有關。

nephroscope *n.* an instrument used for examining the inside of the kidney (*nephroscopy*) at open operation, usually in an attempt to locate small fragments of calculi in the calyces.

腎鏡 在開放性手術中用於檢查腎臟內部的器械。常用於找出腎盞內的結石小碎片。

nephrosis *n.* (in pathology) degenerative changes in the epithelium of the kidney tubules. The term is sometimes used loosely for the *nephrotic syndrome.

腎病 （病理學）腎小管上皮的變性性改變。此詞有時泛指腎變病綜合徵。

nephrostomy *n.* drainage of urine from the kidney by a tube (catheter) passing through the kidney via the skin surface. This is commonly used as a temporary procedure after operations on the kidney. Long-term urine drainage by nephrostomy may be complicated by the attendant problems of infection and obstruction of the catheter by debris.

腎造口術 腎臟尿液引流術。通過皮膚置入穿入腎臟的導管。它常作爲腎臟手術後的暫時措施。腎造口術所致的長期尿引流可合併有隨之而來的感染問題，以及碎屑造成的導管阻塞問題。

nephrotic syndrome a condition in which there is great loss of protein in the urine, reduced levels of albumin in the blood, and generalized swelling of the tissues due to *oedema. It can be caused by a variety of disorders, most usually *glomerulonephritis.

腎變病綜合徵 表現爲體內蛋白大量經尿排出、血白蛋白水平降低、以及水腫所致的全身組織腫脹等。病因可爲多種疾病，最常見的是腎小球腎炎。

nephrotomy *n.* surgical incision into the substance of the kidney. This is usually undertaken to remove a kidney stone (*see* nephrolithotomy).

腎切開術 切開腎實質的手術。此術常用於去除腎結石。

nephroureterectomy (ureteronephrectomy) *n.* surgical removal of a kidney together with its ureter. This operation is performed of cancer of the kidney pelvis or ureter. It is also under-

腎輸尿管切除術（輸尿管腎切除術） 切除腎及輸尿管的手術。腎盂或輸尿管癌時行此手術。當腎臟被膀胱輸尿管反流破壞

taken when the kidney has been destroyed by *vesicoureteric reflux, to prevent subsequent continuing reflux into the stump of the ureter that would occur if the kidney alone were removed.

時，也可行此手術，以防單獨切除腎臟後隨之而來的尿液連續反流進入輸尿管殘端。

nerve *n.* a bundle of conducting *nerve fibres (see illustration) that transmit impulses from the brain or spinal cord to the muscles and glands (*motor nerves*) or inwards from the sense organs to the brain and spinal cord (*sensory nerves*). Most large nerves are *mixed nerves*, containing both motor and sensory nerve fibres running to and from a particular region of the body.

神經 傳導神經纖維束（見圖）。可將衝動從腦或脊髓傳導到肌肉和腺體（運動神經），或從感覺器官傳導到腦和脊髓（感覺神經）。大多數大神經是混合神經，含有向身體某部位走行的運動神經和來自此部位的感覺神經。

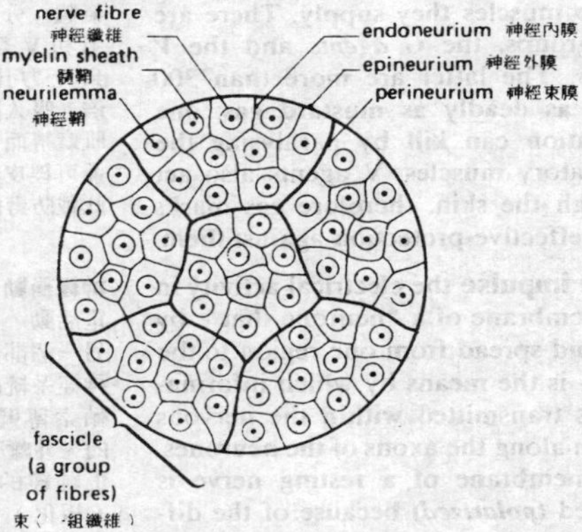

Transverse section through a nerve
神經的橫切面

nerve block a method of producing *anaesthesia in part of the body by blocking the passage of pain impulses in the sensory nerves supplying it. A local anaesthetic, such as lignocaine, is injected into the tissues in the region of a nerve. In this way anaesthesia can be localized, so that minor operations can be performed without the necessity of giving a general anaesthetic.

神經傳導阻滯 通過阻滯感覺神經中痛覺衝動的傳導路，在身體某部位進行麻醉的方法。局部麻醉是將麻醉藥（利多卡因）注射到某神經支配部位的組織內。用此方法，可局限麻醉部位，不須全身麻醉，即可做小手術。

nerve cell *see* neurone.

神經細胞

nerve ending the final part (terminal) of one of the branches of a nerve fibre,

神經末梢 神經纖維分支的終末部分。某種神經元

where a *neurone makes contact either with another neurone at a synapse or with a muscle or gland cell at a neuromuscular or neuroglandular junction.

的神經末梢與另一種神經元相接觸，形成突觸；或與某肌細胞或腺細胞相接觸，形成神經肌肉接頭或神經腺體接頭。

nerve fibre the long fine process that extends from the cell body of a *neurone and carries nerve impulses. Bundles of nerve fibres running together form a *nerve. Each fibre has a sheath, which in medullated nerve fibres is a relatively thick layer containing the fatty insulating material *myelin.

神經纖維 從神經元的細胞體延伸出來並攜帶神經衝動的長細突。走行一致的神經纖維束形成某神經。每個纖維有一個鞘，在有髓鞘的神經纖維中，鞘是較厚的一層，含有脂性絕緣物質——髓磷脂。

nerve gas any gas that disrupts the normal functioning of nerves and thus of the muscles they supply. There are two groups, the *G agents* and the *V agents*. The latter are more than 300 times as deadly as mustard gas: one inhalation can kill by paralysing the respiratory muscles. V agents also act through the skin, therefore gas masks are ineffective protection against them.

神經性毒氣 破壞神經及所支配肌肉的正常功能的氣體。分爲兩類，G 類毒氣和 V 類毒氣。後者的致死力比芥子氣大 300 倍。吸入此氣後可因呼吸肌麻痺而死亡。V 類毒氣還可經皮膚發揮作用，因此戴防毒面具無效。

nerve impulse the electrical activity in the membrane of a *neurone that – by its rapid spread from one region to the next – is the means by which information is transmitted within the nervous system along the axons of the neurones. The membrane of a resting nerve is charged (*polarized*) because of the different concentrations of ions inside and outside the cell. When a nerve impulse is triggered, a wave of *depolarization spreads, and ions flow across the membrane (*see* action potential). Until the nerve has undergone *repolarization no further nerve impulses can pass.

神經衝動 神經元膜內的電活動，它從一個部位到另一個部位迅速傳播，在神經系統內沿着神經元的軸索傳遞信息。因細胞內、外離子濃度不同，靜止神經的膜是帶電荷的（極化）。當一個神經衝動產生時，膜發生去極化，如波狀沿軸索傳播，並且離子透過神經元膜。在神經復極化以前，下一個神經衝動不能通過。

nervous system the vast network of cells specialized to carry information (in the form of *nerve impulses) to and from all parts of the body in order to bring about bodily activity. The brain and spinal cord together form the *central nervous system; the remaining nervous tissue is known as the *peripheral nervous system and includes the

神經系統 專門攜帶信息到身體各部，並攜帶來自身體各部的信息（以神經衝動的形式）以支配身體活動的巨大細胞網絡。腦和脊髓一起形成了中樞神經系統；其餘的神經組織稱爲末梢神經系統並包括自主神經系統。自主神經

*autonomic nervous system, which is itself divided into the sympathetic and parasympathetic nervous systems. The basic functional unit of the nervous system is the *neurone (nerve cell).

系統本身分爲交感神經和副交感神經系統。神經系統的基本功能單位是神經元（神經細胞）。

nettle rash an allergic skin reaction causing blisters and wheals, resembling those caused by nettle stings. *See* urticaria.

蕁麻疹 形成水疱和風團的一種過敏性皮膚反應。類似蕁麻螫刺引起的皮膚反應。

neur- (neuro-) *prefix denoting* nerves or the nervous system.

〔前綴〕**神經**

neural arch *see* vertebra.

神經弓

neural crest the two bands of ectodermal tissue that flank the *neural plate of the early embryo. Cells of the neural crest migrate throughout the embryo and develop into sensory nerve cells and peripheral nerve cells of the autonomic nervous system.

神經嵴 發生於早期胚胎神經板兩側的外胚層組織帶（兩條）。神經嵴的細胞在整個胚胎中移行，並發育成感覺神經細胞和自主神經系統的末梢神經細胞。

neuralgia *n.* a severe burning or stabbing pain often following the course of a nerve. *Postherpetic neuralgia* is an intense debilitating pain felt at the site of a previous attack of shingles. In *trigeminal neuralgia* (*tic douloureux*) there are brief paroxysms of searing pain felt in the distribution of one or more branches of the *trigeminal nerve in the face. The facial pain of *migrainous neuralgia* lasts for 30–60 minutes and occurs at roughly the same time on successive days.

神經痛 常沿着某神經走行發生的嚴重的灼痛或刺痛。帶狀疱疹〔後〕神經痛是在以前發生帶狀疱疹部位的强烈的使人衰憊的疼痛。三叉神經痛可表現爲在面部一個或數個三叉神經分支分佈區有短暫的、陣發性的燒灼樣疼痛。偏頭痛性神經痛的臉部疼痛可持續 30～60 分鐘，並可在連續數天內發生在大致相同的時間裏。

neural plate the strip of ectoderm lying along the central axis of the early embryo that forms the *neural tube and subsequently the central nervous system.

神經板 沿着早期胚胎的中軸排列的外胚層帶。它形成神經管，並進一步形成中樞神經系統。

neural spine the spinous process situated on the neural arch of a *vertebra.

椎骨棘突 位於椎骨神經弓上的棘突。

neural tube the embryological structure from which the brain and spinal cord develop. It is a hollow tube of ectodermal tissue formed when two edges of a groove in a plate of primitive

神經管 發育成腦和脊髓的胚胎結構。它是外胚層組織的一個空管，在原始神經組織盤中一個溝的兩邊融合在一起時形成。正

neural tissue (*neural plate*) come together and fuse. Failure of normal fusion results in a number of congenital defects (*see* neural tube defects).

常融合失敗可導致若干先天缺陷。

neural tube defects a group of congenital abnormalities caused by failure of the *neural tube to close. In *spina bifida the bony arches of the spine, which protect the spinal cord and its coverings (the meninges), fail to close. More severe defects of fusion of these bones result in increasingly serious neurological conditions. A *meningocele* is the protrusion of the meninges through the gap in the spine, the skin covering being vestigial. There is a constant risk of damage to the meninges, with resulting infection. Urgent surgical treatment to protect the meninges is required. In a *meningomyelocele* (*myelomeningocele*, *myelocele*) the spinal cord and the nerve roots are exposed, often adhering to the fine membrane that overlies them. There is a constant risk of infection and this condition is accompanied by paralysis and numbness of the legs and urinary incontinence. *Hydrocephalus and the *Arnold-Chiari malformation are usually present. A failure of fusion at the cranial end of the neural tube (*cranium bifidum*) gives rise to comparable disorders. The bone defect is most often in the occipital region of the skull but it may occur in the frontal or basal regions. A protrusion of the meninges alone is called a *cranial meningocele*. The terms *meningoencephalocele*, *encephalocele*, and *cephalocele* are used to indicate the protrusion of brain tissue through the skull defect. This is accompanied by severe mental and physical disorders.

神經管缺陷 因神經管閉合不良所致的一組先天異常性疾病。脊柱裂是保護脊髓和脊膜的脊柱骨弓閉合不良。這些骨的更嚴重的融合缺陷導致進行性的嚴重的神經性疾病，脊膜突出是脊膜從脊柱間隙突出來，上有殘留皮膚覆蓋。常有脊膜損傷的危險，並伴有繼發性感染。需進行緊急外科治療，以保護脊膜。脊髓脊膜突出（脊髓突出）時，脊髓和神經根暴露，常與覆蓋其上的薄膜黏連。常存有感染的危險，並伴有下肢癱瘓、麻木、尿失禁。常併發腦積水和阿-希二氏畸形。神經管顱末端融合不良可造成類似的病情。骨缺陷最常發生在顱的枕部，但也可發生在額部或顱底部。單純腦膜突出稱爲顱腦脊膜突出。腦腦膜突出、腦突出和腦膨出等術語均指腦組織通過顱骨缺陷向外突出。此種情況可伴有嚴重的精神和軀體上的疾病。

neurapraxia *n.* temporary loss of nerve function resulting in tingling, numbness, and weakness. It is usually caused by compression of the nerve and there is no structural damage involved. Complete recovery occurs.

神經失用症 神經功能的暫時性喪失引起的麻刺感、麻木、無力。病因常爲神經壓迫，並沒有結構上的損害。可完全恢復。

neurasthenia *n.* a set of psychological and physical symptoms, including fatigue, irritability, headache, dizziness, anxiety, and intolerance of noise. It can be caused by organic damage, such as a head injury, or it can be due to neurosis. —**neurasthenic** *adj.*, *n.*

神經衰弱 一組精神上和軀體上的症狀，包括疲勞、過敏、頭痛、頭暈、焦躁和不能耐受噪音。病因可爲器質性損害（如頭部損傷），亦可爲神經官能症。

neurectasis *n.* the surgical procedure for stretching a peripheral nerve.

神經牽伸術 牽伸周圍神經的外科手術。

neurectomy *n.* the surgical removal of the whole or part of a nerve.

神經切除術 切除整根或部分神經的手術。

neurilemma (neurolemma) *n.* the sheath of the *axon of a nerve fibre. The neurilemma of a medullated fibre contains *myelin laid down by Schwann cells. —**neurilemmal** *adj.*

神經鞘 神經纖維軸索的鞘。有髓〔鞘〕纖維的神經鞘含有許旺氏細胞產生的髓鞘脂。

neurilemmoma *n. see* neurofibroma.

神經鞘瘤

neurinoma *n. see* neurofibroma.

神經鞘瘤

neuritis *n.* a disease of the peripheral nerves showing the pathological changes of inflammation. The term is also used in a less precise sense as an alternative to *neuropathy. *See also* retrobulbar neuritis.

神經炎 具有炎症性病理變化的周圍神經病變。神經炎也不準確地用作神經病的代名詞。

neuroanatomy *n.* the study of the structure of the nervous system, from the gross anatomy of the brain down to the microscopic details of neurones.

神經解剖學 研究神經系統結構的學科。包括從腦的肉眼解剖到神經元的顯微鏡下細微結構。

neurobiotaxis *n.* the predisposition of a nerve cell to move towards the source of its stimuli during development.

神經細胞趨生物性 神經細胞在胚胎發育過程中具有的向刺激方向移動的傾向。

neuroblast *n.* any of the nerve cells of the embryo that give rise to functional nerve cells (neurones).

成神經細胞 生成功能性神經細胞（神經元）的胚胎神經細胞。

neuroblastoma *n.* a malignant tumour composed of embryonic nerve cells. It may originate in any part of the sympathetic nervous system, most commonly in the medulla of the adrenal gland, and secondary growths are often widespread in other organs and in bones.

成神經細胞瘤 由胚胎神經細胞構成的惡性瘤。它可起源於交感神經系統的任一部位，最常見於腎上腺髓質。繼發性膜瘤常廣泛分佈在其它器官或骨中。

neurocranium *n.* the part of the skull that encloses the brain.

腦顱 包容腦的部份顱骨。

neurodermatitis (neurodermatosis) *n.* a skin disease in which localized areas itch persistently and, because of constant scratching, become thickened (*see* lichenification). Women suffer more than men and the cause is uncertain, though psychological factors probably play a part. Common sites are the back of the neck, forearm, upper inner thighs, inner side of knees, and outer side of ankle.

神經性皮炎（神經性皮膚病） 局部皮膚持續瘙癢，並因經常抓搔而變厚的一種皮膚病。女性患者多於男性，儘管心理因素可能起一定的作用，但病因仍未確定。常見發病部位是頸後、前臂、股內上側、膝內側和踝外側。

neuroendocrine system the system of dual control of certain activities of the body by means of both nerves and circulating hormones. The functioning of the autonomic nervous system is particularly closely linked to that of the pituitary and adrenal glands. *See* neurohormone, neurosecretion.

神經內分泌系統 由神經和循環於體內的激素對身體某些活動進行雙重控制的系統。自主神經系統的功能與垂體和腎上腺的功能有特別緊密的聯繫。

neuroepithelioma *n.* a malignant tumour of the retina of the eye. It is a form of *glioma and commonly spreads into the brain.

神經上皮瘤 眼視網膜的惡性腫瘤。它是神經膠質瘤的一種形式，並常擴散到腦內。

neuroepithelium *n.* a type of epithelium associated with organs of special sense. It contains sensory nerve endings and is found in the retina, the membranous labyrinth of the inner ear, the mucous membrane lining the nasal cavity, and the taste buds. —**neuroepithelial** *adj.*

神經上皮 與特殊感覺器官有關的一種上皮。它含有感覺神經末梢，並存在於視網膜、內耳的膜迷路、鼻腔內的黏膜和味蕾內。

neurofibril *n.* one of the microscopic threads of cytoplasm found in the cell body of a *neurone and also in the *axoplasm of peripheral nerves.

神經原纖維 顯微鏡下神經細胞的胞漿細絲。見於神經元的細胞體內，也見於周圍神經的軸漿中。

neurofibroma (neurilemmoma, neurinoma, neuroma, Schwannoma) *n.* a benign tumour growing from the fibrous coverings of a peripheral nerve: it is usually symptomless. When it develops from the sheath of a nerve root, it causes pain and may compress the spinal cord.

神經纖維瘤（神經鞘瘤，神經瘤） 從周圍神經的纖維膜上生長出的良性瘤。通常無症狀。當它生在神經根的鞘上時，可引起疼痛並可壓迫脊髓。

neurofibromatosis (von Recklinghausen's disease) *n.* a congenital disease, typified by numerous benign

神經纖維瘤病（雷克林霍會氏病） 以從神經的纖維膜上生長出許多良性瘤

tumours growing from the fibrous coverings of nerves (*see* neurofibroma). Tumours may occur in the spinal canal, where they may press on the spinal cord. The tumours can be felt beneath the skin along the course of the nerves; they sometimes become malignant, giving rise to *neurofibrosarcomas*. Pigmented patches on the skin (*café au lait spots*) are commonly found. This condition is often associated with the adrenal tumour *phaeochromocytoma.

爲特徵的先天性疾病。發生在脊髓中央管的腫瘤可壓迫脊髓。沿着神經的走行，可觸摸到皮下的腫瘤。有時它們可變成惡性的，生成神經纖維肉瘤。皮膚上常出現色素斑。此病常與腎上腺腫瘤——嗜鉻細胞瘤共存。

neurogenesis *n.* the growth and development of nerve cells.

神經發生 神經細胞的生長和發育。

neurogenic *adj.* **1.** caused by disease or dysfunction of the nervous system. **2.** arising in nervous tissue. **3.** caused by nerve stimulation.

神經發生的 ①由神經系統疾病或功能障礙引起的。②起源於神經組織的。③由神經刺激引起的。

neuroglia *n. see* glia.

神經膠質

neurohormone *n.* a hormone that is produced within specialized nerve cells and is secreted from the nerve endings into the circulation. Examples are the hormones oxytocin and vasopressin, produced within the nerve cells of the hypothalamus and released into the circulation in the posterior pituitary gland, and noradrenaline, released from *chromaffin tissue in the adrenal medulla.

神經激素 在特殊的神經細胞內產生的並且從神經末梢分泌到循環中的激素。例如催產素和加壓素是在丘腦下部的神經細胞內產生的，並且從垂體腺釋放進入循環；去甲腎上腺素從腎上腺髓質的嗜鉻組織釋放。

neurohumour *n.* a *neurohormone or a *neurotransmitter.

神經體液 神經激素或神經遞質。

neurohypophysis *n.* the posterior lobe of the *pituitary gland.

垂體神經部 垂體腺的後葉。

neurolemma *n. see* neurilemma.

神經鞘

neurology *n.* the study of the structure, functioning, and diseases of the nervous system (including the brain, spinal cord, and all the peripheral nerves). —**neurological** *adj.* —**neurologist** *n.*

神經病學 研究神經系統（包括腦、脊髓和所有周圍神經）的結構、功能和疾病的學科。

neuroma *n. see* neurofibroma.

神經瘤

neuromuscular junction (myoneural junction) the meeting point of a

神經肌肉接頭（肌神經接點） 神經纖維與其所支

nerve fibre and the muscle fibre that it supplies. Between the enlarged end of the nerve fibre (*motor end-plate*) and the membrane of the muscle is a gap across which a *neurotransmitter must diffuse from the nerve to trigger contraction of the muscle.

配的肌纖維的接〔合〕點。在神經纖維末梢膨大處（運動終板）和肌膜之間有一個間隙，神經遞質必須穿過此間隙，從神經彌散到肌肉，才能引起肌肉收縮。

neuromyelitis optica (Devic's disease) a condition that is closely related to multiple sclerosis. Typically there is a transverse *myelitis, producing paralysis and numbness of the legs and trunk below the inflamed spinal cord, and *retrobulbar (optic) neuritis affecting both optic nerves. The attacks of myelitis and optic neuritis may coincide or they may be separated by days or weeks. Recovery from the initial attack is often incomplete, but relapses appear to be less common than in conventional multiple sclerosis.

視神經脊髓炎（德維克氏病） 與多發性硬化密切相關的一種疾病。典型表現爲橫貫性脊髓炎，產生脊髓炎症部位以下的腿和軀幹的癱瘓和麻木以及影響雙側視神經的球後（視）神經炎。脊髓炎和視神經炎可同時發病，亦可相隔數天或數周分別出現。本病初次發病後的恢復常常是不完全的，但其復發似比常見的多發性硬化少見。

neurone (nerve cell) *n.* one of the basic functional units of the nervous system: a cell specialized to transmit electrical *nerve impulses and so carry information from one part of the body to another (see illustration). Each neurone has an enlarged portion, the *cell body* (*perikaryon*), containing the nucleus; from the body extend several processes (*dendrites*) through which impulses enter from their branches. A longer process, the nerve fibre (*see* axon), extends outwards and carries impulses away from the cell body. This is normally unbranched except at the *nerve ending. The point of contact of one neurone with another is known as a *synapse.

神經元（神經細胞） 神經系統的基本功能單位。是一種特化的細胞，它專門傳遞神經電衝動，將身體某一部位的信息帶到另一部位（見圖）。每個神經元有一個增大的部分，即細胞體（核周體），含有核；從細胞體延伸出幾個短突（樹突），通過這些樹突的分支傳入衝動。一個延伸較長的突（軸索），即神經纖維，傳導衝動離開細胞體。神經纖維正常情況下不分支，除非在神經末梢。某神經元與另一神經元的接觸點稱爲突觸。

neuronophagia *n.* the process whereby damaged or degenerating nerve cells finally disintegrate and are removed by scavenger cells (*phagocytes).

噬神經細胞作用 受損或變性的神經細胞最後裂解並被吞噬細胞清除的過程。

neuronoplasty *n.* reconstructive surgery for damaged or severed peripheral nerves.

神經整形術 受損或切斷的周圍神經的重建術。

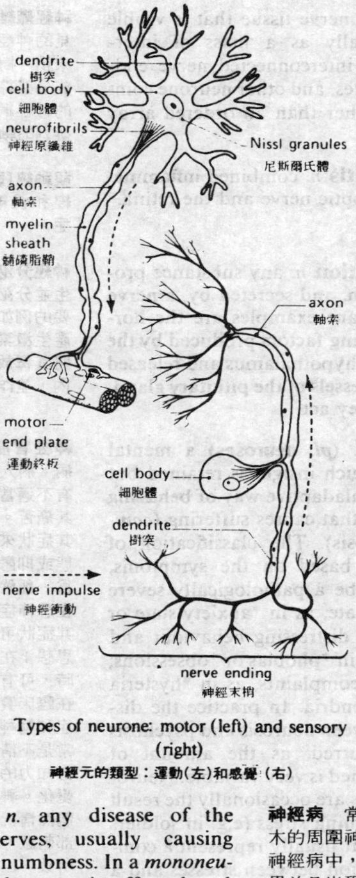

Types of neurone: motor (left) and sensory (right)
神經元的類型：運動(左)和感覺(右)

neuropathy *n.* any disease of the peripheral nerves, usually causing weakness and numbness. In a *mononeuropathy* a single nerve is affected and the extent of the symptoms depends upon the distribution of that nerve. In a *polyneuropathy* many or all of the nerves are involved and the symptoms are most profound at the extremities of the limbs.

神經病 常引起無力和麻木的周圍神經病。在單一神經病中，僅單獨神經受累並且出現症狀的範圍與神經分布的區域一致。在多神經病中，許多或所有的神經受累並且在肢體末端的症狀最嚴重。

neurophysiology *n.* the study of the complex chemical and physical changes that are associated with the activity of the nervous system.

神經生理學 研究與神經系統活動有關的複雜的化學和物理變化的學科。

neuropil *n.* nerve tissue that is visible microscopically as a mass of interwoven and interconnected nerve endings, dendrites, and other neurone components, rather than an ordered array of axons.

神經纖維網 顯微鏡下可見的神經組織。它是神經末梢、樹突和其它神經元成分錯綜交織和互相聯系的神經網，而不是按順序排列的軸索。

neuroretinitis *n.* combined inflammation of the optic nerve and the retina.

視神經〔視〕網膜炎 視神經和視網膜同時患有炎症。

neurosecretion *n.* any substance produced within, and secreted by, a nerve cell. Important examples are the hormone-releasing factors produced by the cells of the *hypothalamus and released into blood vessels of the pituitary gland, on which they act.

神經分泌 由神經細胞產生並分泌的任何物質，重要的例如：丘腦下部細胞產生激素釋放因子，然後將其釋放到垂體腺的血管內，並作用於垂體腺。

neurosis *n.* (*pl.* **neuroses**) a mental illness in which insight is retained but there is a maladaptive way of behaving or thinking that causes suffering (*compare* psychosis). The classification of neuroses is based on the symptoms, which may be a pathologically severe emotional state, as in *anxiety state or *depression; distressing behaviour and thoughts, as in *phobias or *obsessions; or physical complaints, as in *hysteria or *hypochondria. In practice the distinction between neurosis and psychosis is often blurred, as the amount of insight retained is very variable. Neurotic symptoms are occasionally the result of overwhelming stress (e.g. in soldiers in battle), but usually represent a complex interaction between stresses and a vulnerable personality.
Treatment for neurosis can include chemotherapy (often with *tranquillizers), *psychotherapy, or *behaviour therapy. The little evidence there is favours the use of behavioural techniques, such as *desensitization and *flooding. —**neurotic** *adj.*

神經官能症 一種精神病。病人自知力保留，但有不適當的行爲或思想使其痛苦。神經官能症根據其症狀來分類。在焦慮狀態或抑鬱症時，其症狀可爲一種嚴重病態的情感；在恐怖症或强迫觀念時，其症狀可爲困窘的行爲和思想；在癔病或疑病〔症〕時，可有軀體上的症狀。在臨床實踐中，神經官能症和精神病之間的區別常常是不清楚的，因爲保持自知力的多少可有很大的變化。神經官能症的症狀偶然情況下是由極强的外部刺激（士兵在戰鬪中）所致，但通常是由外部刺激和脆弱個性之間複雜的相互作用造成的。
神經官能症的治療包括化學療法（常用安定藥）、心理療法或行爲療法。採用行爲療法，如脫敏〔感作用〕和以恐治恐法，只在極少數病例有效。

neurosurgery *n.* the surgical or operative treatment of diseases of the brain and spinal cord. This includes the

神經外科學 外科或手術治療腦和脊髓疾病的學科。其中包括處理頭部損

management of head injuries, the relief of raised intracranial pressure and compression of the spinal cord, the eradication of infection, the control of intracranial haemorrhage, and the diagnosis and treatment of tumours. The development of neurosurgery has been supported by advances in anaesthetics, radiology, and antiseptics.

傷、解除升高的顱內壓和脊髓的壓力、根除感染、控制顱內出血、診斷及治療腫瘤。神經外科學的發展是以麻醉學、放射學和消毒滅菌方法的進展爲基礎的。

neurosyphilis *n.* *syphilis affecting the nervous system.

神經梅毒 侵犯神經系統的梅毒。

neuroticism *n.* a dimension of personality derived from questionnaires and psychological tests. People with high scores in neuroticism are anxious and intense and more prone to develop neurosis.

神經過敏性 從調查表和心理試驗中測得的一種人格的量度。在神經過敏性調查測驗中，分數較高的人表現爲焦慮和緊張並且更易於發展成神經官能症。

neurotomy *n.* the surgical procedure of severing a nerve.

神經切斷術 切斷神經的外科手術。

neurotoxic *adj.* poisonous or harmful to nerve cells.

神經中毒的 對神經細胞有毒或有害的。

neurotransmitter *n.* a chemical substance released from nerve endings to transmit impulses across *synapses to other nerves and across the minute gaps between the nerves and the muscles or glands that they supply. Outside the central nervous system the chief neurotransmitter is *acetylcholine; *noradrenaline is released by nerve endings of the sympathetic system. In the central nervous system, besides acetylcholine and noradrenaline, *dopamine, *serotonin, *gamma-aminobutyric acid and several other substances are thought to act as transmitters.

神經遞質 由神經末梢釋放的化學物質。此種物質可傳遞衝動穿過突觸到其它神經，也可使衝動穿過神經和所支配的肌肉或神經和所支配的腺體之間的小空隙。在中樞神經系統之外，主要的神經遞質是由交感系統神經末梢釋放的乙醯膽鹼、去甲腎上腺素。在中樞神經系統內，除了乙醯膽鹼和去甲腎上腺素，現認爲多巴胺、5-羥色胺，γ-氨基丁酸和幾種其它物質也起遞質的作用。

neurotrophic *adj.* relating to the growth and nutrition of neural tissue in the body.

神經營養的 與體內神經組織的生成和營養有關的。

neurotropic *adj.* growing towards or having an affinity for neural tissue. The term may be applied to viruses, chemicals, or toxins.

親神經的 朝向神經組織生長或與神經組織有親和力的。此詞適用於病毒、化學物質或毒素。

neutropenia *n.* a decrease in the number of *neutrophils in the blood. Neutropenia may occur in a wide variety of diseases, including certain hereditary defects, aplastic *anaemias, tumours of the bone marrow, *agranulocytosis, and acute leukaemias. It results in an increased susceptibility to infections.

中性白細胞減少〔症〕 血中中性白細胞數量減少。中性白細胞減少〔症〕可發生在許多不同的疾病中，其中包括某些遺傳缺陷、再生障礙性貧血、骨髓腫瘤、粒細胞缺乏症和急性白血病。此症使人易於感染。

neutrophil (polymorph) *n.* a variety of *granulocyte (a type of white blood cell) distinguished by a lobed nucleus and the presence in its cytoplasm of fine granules that stain purple with *Romanowsky stains. It is capable of ingesting and killing bacteria and provides an important defence against infection. There are normally 2.0–7.5 × 10^9 neutrophils per litre of blood.

中性粒細胞（多形核白細胞） 一種粒細胞（血中的一種細胞）。特徵爲有分葉核和在其胞漿中存有小的顆粒，羅曼諾夫斯基染劑可將這些顆粒染成紫色。中性粒細胞能夠消化和殺死細菌並起重要的防禦感染的作用。正常情況下每升血中有2.0～7.5×10^9個中性粒細胞。

newton *n.* the *SI unit of force, equal to the force required to impart to 1 kilogram an acceleration of 1 metre per second per second. Symbol: N.

牛頓 力的國際單位。使1千克物體產生1米/平方秒加速度的力。符號：N。

nexus *n.* (in anatomy) a connection or link.

連結 （解剖學）連接或結合。

niacin *n. see* nicotinic acid.

煙酸

nialamide *n.* a drug with effects similar to *phenelzine, used to treat all types of depression. It is administered by mouth; headache, nausea, dizziness, and giddiness are common side-effects. Trade name: **Niamid**.

煙肼醯胺 與苯乙肼的作用類似的藥物。用於治療各類抑鬱症。口服。常見副作用有頭痛、噁心、頭暈和眩暈。商品名：尼亞醯胺。

niche *n.* (in anatomy) a recess or depression in a smooth surface.

龕 （解剖學）在平滑的表面上的隱窩或凹陷。

nicotinamide *n.* a B vitamin: the amide of *nicotinic acid.

煙醯胺 B族維生素的一種：煙酸的醯胺。

nicotinamide adenine dinucleotide *see* NAD.

二磷酸吡啶核苷酸

nicotine *n.* a poisonous alkaloid derived from *tobacco, responsible for the dependence of regular smokers on cigarettes. In small doses nicotine has a stimulating effect on the autonomic

煙鹼 煙草中所含的一種毒性生物鹼。可造成吸煙成癮者對煙草的依賴性。小量煙鹼對自主神經系統有刺激作用，可使吸煙成

nervous system, causing in regular smokers such effects as raised blood pressure and pulse rate and impaired appetite. Large doses cause paralysis of the autonomic ganglia.

癮者血壓升高、脉率增快和食慾不良。大量煙鹼可使自主神經節痲痹。

nicotinic acid (niacin) a B vitamin. Nicotinic acid is a derivative of pyridine and is interchangeable with its amide, *nicotinamide*. Both forms of the vitamin are equally active. Nicotinamide is a component of the coenzymes *NAD (nicotinamide adenine dinucleotide) and NADP, its phosphate. Nicotinic acid is required in the diet but can also be formed in small amounts in the body from the essential amino acid tryptophan. A deficiency of the vitamin leads to *pellagra. Good sources of nicotinic acid are meat, yeast extracts, and some cereals. Nicotinic acid is present in some cereals (e.g. maize) in a bound unavailable form. The adult recommended intake is 18 mg equivalent per day (1 mg equivalent is equal to 1 mg of available nicotinic acid or 60 mg tryptophan).

煙酸　B族維生素的一種。煙酸是吡啶的衍化物並且可與它的醯胺——煙醯胺互相轉換。這兩種形式的維生素具有同樣的活性。煙醯胺是輔酶 NAD（二磷酸吡啶核苷酸）和它的磷酸鹽 NADP 的一種成分。飲食中需有煙酸，但也可在體內從必需氨基酸——色氨酸中小量形成。缺乏此種維生素可引起糙皮病。煙酸的極好來源是肉、酵母浸出物和某些穀類。有些穀類（如玉米）中的煙酸是以結合的形式存在，無法利用。成人攝入量應爲每日18毫克當量（1毫克當量相當於1毫克可利用的煙酸或60毫克色氨酸）。

nicotinyl *n.* a drug that dilates blood vessels. It is similar to *nicotinic acid and is used to treat disorders due to poor circulation, such as chilblains and Raynaud's disease. It is administered by mouth; side-effects are rare, but temporary flushing of the face may occur. Trade name: **Ronicol**.

煙醇　擴張血管藥。與煙酸類似並用於治療因循環不良所致的疾病，如凍瘡和雷諾氏病。口服。副作用少見，但可發生暫時性臉潮紅。商品名：酒石酸煙醇。

nictitation *n.* exaggerated and frequent blinking or winking of the eyes.

瞬眼（眨眼）　過度用力的和頻繁的瞬眼和眨眼。

nidation *n. see* implantation.

着床

nidus *n.* a place in which bacteria have settled and multiplied because of particularly suitable conditions: a focus of infection.

病竈　因有特別適合的條件細菌易於生活和繁殖的地方：感染竈。

nifuratel *n.* a drug active against various microorganisms, used mainly to treat fungus infections of the genital and urinary systems (such as candidia-

呋喃䓬唑酮　抗各種微生物的藥。主要用於治療生殖泌尿系的眞菌感染（如陰道的念珠菌病）。口服

sis of the vagina). It is administered by mouth and in pessaries; side-effects are rare, but some digestive discomfort may occur. Trade name: **Magmilor**.

和製成陰道栓〔劑〕。副作用少見，但可有些消化不良。商品名：硝呋噻酮。

night blindness the inability to see in dim light or at night. It is due to a disorder of the cells in the retina that are responsible for vision in dim light (*see* rod), and can result from dietary deficiency of *vitamin A. If the vitamin deficiency is allowed to continue night blindness may progress to *xerophthalmia and *keratomalacia. Medical name: **nyctalopia**. *Compare* day blindness.

夜盲　在暗光下或在夜間看不清東西。夜盲爲負責暗光視力的視網膜細胞疾病所致，也可因飲食中維生素A缺乏造成。如果繼續缺少維生素A，夜盲可發展成乾眼病和角膜軟化。

night sweat copious sweating during sleep. Night sweats may be an early indication of tuberculosis or other disease.

盜汗　睡覺時大量出汗。盜汗可爲結核病或其它疾病的早期徵候。

night terror the condition in which a child (usually aged 2–4 years), soon after falling asleep, starts screaming and appears terrified. The child cannot be comforted because he remains mentally inaccessible; the attack ceases when he wakes up fully and is never remembered. Attacks sometimes follow a stressful experience.

夜驚　兒童（常爲2～4歲）入睡後不久，開始尖叫並有驚恐表現的一種病象。因小兒的心靈難以捉摸，不能使之安靜下來。當兒童完全清醒後，發作停止並且兒童本人從不記得此事。有時在精神高度緊張後可有此種現象。

Nile blue an oxazine chloride, used for staining lipids and lipid pigments. *Nile blue A* (*Nile blue sulphate*), which stains fatty acids, changes from blue to purplish at pH 10–11.

尼羅藍　噁嗪氯化物。用於對脂類和脂色素進行染色，尼羅藍A（硫酸尼羅藍）可對脂肪酸進行染色，在 pH 10～11 時從藍色變成略呈紫色。

ninhydrin reaction a histochemical test for proteins, in which ninhydrin (triketohydrindene hydrate) is boiled with the test solution and gives a blue colour in the presence of amino acids and proteins.

〔水合〕茚三酮反應　蛋白的組織化學試驗：將〔水合〕茚三酮加入試驗溶液中煮沸，若有蛋白質和氨基酸存在，則呈藍色。

nipple (mamilla, papilla) *n.* the protuberance at the centre of the *breast. In females the milk ducts open at the nipple.

乳頭　乳房中央的隆起。在雌性動物中，乳腺管在乳頭處開口。

niridazole *n.* an anthelmintic drug used particularly in the treatment of schistosomiasis. It is administered by mouth and side-effects may include agitation and confusion, abdominal discomfort, digestive upsets, and headache. Niridazole should not be used in patients with impaired liver function.

硝噻達唑 一種抗蠕蟲藥。特別用於治療血吸蟲病。口服。副作用可有激動不安、精神混亂、腹部不適、消化不良和頭痛。硝噻達唑禁用於肝功能受損的病人。

Nissl granules collections of dark-staining material, containing RNA, seen in the cell bodies of neurones on microscopic examination.

尼斯爾氏體 含有RNA的深染物質團塊。在顯微鏡檢查時見於神經元的細胞體內。

nit *n.* the egg of a *louse. The eggs of head lice are firmly cemented to the hair, usually at the back of the head; those of body lice are fixed to the clothing. Nits, 0.8 × 0.3 mm, are visible as light white specks.

蟣 蝨卵。頭蝨的卵牢固地黏附在頭髮上，常在頭的後面；體蝨的卵黏附在衣服上。蟣之大小爲0.8×0.3毫米，肉眼可見一微白小粒。

nitrazepam *n.* a *hypnotic drug administered by mouth to treat insomnia and sleep disturbances. It is often preferred to other hypnotics since side-effects are not severe, though morning drowsiness sometimes occurs. Trade names: **Mogadon, Remnos**.

硝基安定 口服安眠藥。用於治療失眠〔症〕和睡眠障礙。因其沒有嚴重的副作用，只是有時早晨略感倦睡，故常選用此種安眠藥。

nitric acid a strong corrosive mineral acid, HNO_3, the concentrated form of which is capable of producing severe burns of the skin. Swallowing the acid leads to intense burning pain and ulceration of the mouth and throat. Treatment is by immediate administration of alkaline solutions, followed by milk or olive oil.

硝酸 一種强腐蝕性無機酸，HNO_3。濃硝酸能造成嚴重的皮膚燒傷。吞服此酸可引起强烈的燒灼性痛以及口腔和咽喉的潰瘍。治療爲立即口服鹼性溶液，然後服用牛奶或〔洋〕橄欖油。

nitrofurantoin *n.* a drug used to treat bacterial infections of the urinary system. It is administered by mouth and may cause nausea, vomiting, and skin rashes. Trade names: **Berkfurin, Furadantin, Furan, Macrodantin**.

硝基呋喃妥英 治療泌尿系細菌感染的藥物。口服。可引起噁心、嘔吐和皮疹。商品名：呋喃咀啶。

nitrogen *n.* a gaseous element and a major constituent of air (79 per cent). Nitrogen is an essential constituent of proteins and nucleic acids and is obtained by man in the form of protein-containing foods (atmospheric nitrogen

氮 一種氣體元素，空氣的主要成分（79%）。氮是蛋白質和核酸的基本成分，人通過攝入含蛋白食物來獲取（大氣氮不能被直接利用）。氮的代謝產

cannot be utilized directly). Nitrogenous waste is excreted as *urea. Symbol: N.

物以尿素的形式被排出。符號：N。

nitrogen mustard *see* mustine.

氮芥

nitroglycerin *n. see* glyceryl trinitrate.

硝酸甘油

nitrous oxide a colourless gas used as an *anaesthetic with good *analgesic properties. It is administered by inhalation, in conjunction with oxygen, and is used as a vehicle for potent anaesthetic vapours, such as halothane. A mixture of oxygen and nitrous oxide provides effective analgesia for some dental procedures and in childbirth; such a state is known as *relative analgesia. Nitrous oxide was formerly referred to as *laughing gas* because of its tendency to excite the patient when used alone.

氧化亞氮　無色氣體，具有良好止痛作用的痲醉劑。它的用法是與氧一起吸入體內，也可用作强痲醉劑（如：氟烷）蒸氣的載體。氧和氧化亞氮的混合劑在某些口腔手術和分娩時可起有效的鎮痛作用。以前氧化亞氮被稱爲笑氣，因爲當單獨使用時它有使病人興奮的趨向。

nm *abbrev. for* nanometre.

〔縮寫〕**毫微米**

NMR *see* nuclear magnetic resonance.

核磁共振

Nocardia *n.* a genus of rodlike or filamentous Gram-positive nonmotile bacteria found in the soil. As cultures age, filaments form branches, but these soon break up into rodlike or spherical cells. Three or more spores may form in each cell; these germinate to form filaments. Some species are pathogenic: *N. asteroides* causes *nocardiosis and *N. madurae* is associated with the disease *Madura foot.

諾卡氏菌屬　存在於土壤中的桿狀或絲狀革蘭氏陽性無運動菌屬。經過一段培養時間，菌絲形成分支，但這些分支不久分裂成桿狀或球狀細胞。在每個細胞內可形成三個或更多的孢子；孢子芽生成菌絲。某種菌種具有致病性：星形諾卡氏菌可引起諾卡氏〔放線〕菌病，杜拉諾卡氏菌與足分支菌病有關。

nocardiosis *n.* a disease caused by bacteria of the genus *Nocardia*, primarily affecting the lungs, skin, and brain, resulting in the formation of abscesses. Treatment involves antibiotics and sulphonamides.

諾卡氏放線菌病　諾卡氏菌屬的細菌引起的疾病。主要影響肺、皮膚和腦，形成膿腫。治療包括使用抗生素和磺胺類藥。

noci- *prefix denoting* pain or injury.

〔前綴〕**傷害，疼痛**

nociceptive *adj.* describing nerve fibres, endings, or pathways that are concerned with the condition of pain.

感受傷害的　與疼痛有關的神經纖維、末梢或通路的形容詞。

noct- (nocti-) *prefix denoting* night.

〔前綴〕**夜間**

noctambulation *n. see* somnambulism.

夢行〔症〕

nocturia *n.* the passage of urine at night. In the absence of a high fluid intake, sleep is not normally interrupted by the need to pass urine. Nocturia usually occurs in elderly men with enlarged prostate glands, and is a common reason for patients to request *prostatectomy.

夜尿症 夜間排尿。在正常情況下，如果沒有大量攝入液體，不會因需排尿而使睡眠中斷。夜尿症常發生在前列腺肥大的老年人，是病人需做前列腺切除術的常見原因。

node *n.* a small swelling or knot of tissue. *See* atrioventricular node, sinoatrial node.

結 組織的小腫物或結節。

node of Ranvier one of the gaps that occur at regular intervals in the *myelin sheath of medullated nerve fibres, between adjacent *Schwann cells.

郎飛氏結 有髓鞘神經纖維的髓磷脂鞘每隔一段距離出現的一個間隙。位於相鄰的許旺氏細胞之間。

nodule *n.* a small swelling or aggregation of cells.

小結 小的腫物或細胞的集團。

noma *n.* a gangrenous infection of the mouth that spreads to involve the face. It is rare in civilized communities and is usually found in debilitated or malnourished individuals. Noma is a severe form of *ulcerative gingivitis.

走馬疳 口腔的壞疽性感染擴散到面部，此病在文明社會裏是罕見的，常見於衰弱或營養不良的人。走馬疳是潰瘍性齦炎的嚴重表現形式。

nondisjunction *n.* a condition in which pairs of homologous chromosomes fail to separate during meiosis or a chromosome fails to divide at *anaphase of mitosis or meiosis. It results in a cell with an abnormal number of chromosomes (*see* monosomy, trisomy).

不分開現象 在減數分裂時成對的同源染色體不能分離，或在有絲分裂的後期染色體不能分離。這種現象造成細胞的染色體數目異常。

nonigravida *n.* a woman who has been pregnant nine times.

第九次孕婦 妊娠過九次的婦女。

nonipara *n.* a woman who has been pregnant at least nine times and has given birth to an infant capable of survival after each of nine pregnancies.

孕$_9$ 至少妊娠過九次的婦女，並且在這九次妊娠的每一次後均生出活嬰。

nonsecretor *n.* a person in whose body fluids it is not possible to detect soluble forms of the A, B, or O agglutinogens that determine blood group. *Compare* secretor.

非分泌者 其分泌物中不能查出可溶性的ABO血型凝集原的人。

noradrenaline (norepinephrine) *n.* a hormone, closely related to *adrenaline and with similar actions, secreted by the medulla of the *adrenal gland and also released as a *neurotransmitter by sympathetic nerve endings. Among its many actions are constriction of small blood vessels leading to an increase in blood pressure, increased blood flow through the coronary arteries and a slowing of the heart rate, increase in the rate and depth of breathing, and relaxation of the smooth muscle in intestinal walls.

去甲腎上腺素 與腎上腺素密切相關並具有類似作用的一種激素。此種激素由腎上腺髓質分泌，也是一種由交感神經末梢釋放的神經遞質。它的許多作用包括小血管收縮造成的血壓升高、冠狀動脈血流增加、心率減慢、呼吸頻率和深度增加，腸壁平滑肌鬆弛。

norepinephrine *n. see* noradrenaline.

去甲腎上腺素

norethandrolone *n.* a synthetic male sex hormone with body-building action. It has the same effects and uses as *methandienone and is administered by mouth or injection.

乙諾酮 具有蛋白合成作用的人工合成男性激素，它有與去氧甲睾酮相同的作用和用途。口服或注射給藥。

norethisterone *n.* a synthetic female sex hormone (*see* progestogen) administered by mouth to treat menstrual disorders, including amenorrhoea. It is also used in oral contraceptives, often in combination with an oestrogen.

炔諾酮 人工合成的雌性激素。口服治療月經紊亂，包括經閉。它也常以與雌激素結合的形式用於口服避孕藥中。

norma *n.* a view of the skull from one of several positions, from which it can be described or measured. For example the *norma lateralis* is a side view of the skull; the *norma verticalis* is the view of the top of the skull.

顱外觀 從幾種不同的位置來觀察顱骨，以描述或測量顱骨。如：側面觀是對顱骨側面進行的觀察；垂直面觀是對顱骨頂部進行的觀察。

normalization *n.* (in psychiatry) the process of making the living conditions of people with mental *subnormality as similar as possible to those of people who are not handicapped. This includes moves to living outside institutions and encouragement to cope with work, pay, social life, and civil rights.

正常化 （精神病學）盡可能使精神異常人的生活條件近似於精神正常人生活條件的過程。其中包括移居到醫院外去，鼓勵他們工作、賺錢、參加社會生活、行使公民權。

normo- *prefix denoting* normality.

〔前綴〕 **正常**

normoblast *n.* a nucleated cell that forms part of the series giving rise to the red blood cells and is normally found in the blood-forming tissue of the bone marrow. Normoblasts pass through

幼紅細胞 生成紅細胞過程中某個階段的有核細胞。正常時存在於骨髓的造血組織中。幼紅細胞經過三個成熟階段：早期

three stages of maturation: *early* (or *basophilic*), *intermediate* (or *polychromatic*), and *late* (or *orthochromatic*) forms. *See also* erythroblast, erythropoiesis.

（或嗜鹼染色的）、中期（或多色的）、晚期（或正染的）。

normocyte *n.* a red blood cell of normal size. A *normocytic anaemia* is one characterized by the presence of such cells. —**normocytic** *adj.*

正常紅細胞 正常大小的紅細胞。正常紅細胞性貧血是以正常紅細胞的存在爲特徵的貧血。

normotensive *adj.* describing the state in which the arterial blood pressure is within the normal range. *Compare* hypertension, hypotension.

血壓正常的 描述動脉血壓在正常範圍內的狀況。

nortriptyline *n.* a tricyclic *antidepressant drug used to relieve all types of depression. It is administered by mouth; side-effects may include dry mouth and drowsiness. Trade names: **Allegron, Aventyl.**

去甲替林 用於解除各類抑鬱〔症〕的三環抗抑鬱藥。口服。副作用可有口乾和頭暈。商品名：去甲阿米替林。

nose *n.* the organ of olfaction, which also acts as an air passage that warms, moistens, and filters the air on its way to the lungs. The *external nose* is a triangular projection in the front of the face that is composed of cartilage and covered with skin. It leads to the *nasal cavity* (*internal nose*), which is lined with mucous membrane containing olfactory cells and is divided into two chambers (*fossae*) by the *nasal septum*. The lateral wall of each chamber is formed by the three scroll-shaped *nasal conchae, below each of which is a groovelike passage (*meatus*). The *paranasal sinuses open into these meatuses.

鼻 嗅覺器官。也是在空氣流向肺時溫暖、濕潤和濾過空氣的氣道。外鼻是臉部的三角形突起，由軟骨構成，其上面覆以皮膚。它與鼻腔（內鼻）相通，鼻腔被含有嗅覺細胞的黏膜覆蓋，由鼻中隔分成左右兩腔，其側壁是由三個卷形鼻甲構成，在每個鼻甲下是一個溝樣的鼻道。鼻旁竇開口於這些鼻道。

nosebleed *n.* bleeding from the nose, which may be caused by physical injury or may be associated with fever, high blood pressure, or blood disorders. The blood often comes from a vessel just inside the nostril, in which case the flow may be stopped by applying pressure on the side of the nose. Otherwise gauze packing may be effective in controlling the loss of blood. Medical name: **epistaxis.**

鼻出血 鼻中出血。病因可爲物理損傷，也可與發燒、高血壓或血液病有關。血液常來自鼻孔淺部的血管，在這種情況下，壓鼻側翼即可止血。否則，用紗布填塞可有效地止血。醫學術詞：鼻衄。

noso- *prefix denoting* disease. 〔前綴〕 **疾病**

nosocomial infection an infection originating in a hospital. It may develop in a hospitalized patient without having been present or incubating at the time of admission, or it may be acquired in hospital but only appears after discharge. The term also includes infections developing among hospital staff.

醫院內感染 在醫院中發生的感染。此感染可發生在入院時沒有得病或處在潛伏期的住院病人，也可在住院期間得病但在出院後才表現出來。此術語也包括在醫院工作人員中發生的感染。

nosology *n.* the naming and classification of diseases.

疾病分類學 對疾病的命名和分類。

Nosopsyllus *n.* a genus of fleas. The common rat flea of temperate regions, *N. fasciatus*, will, in the absence of rats, bite man and may therefore transmit plague or murine typhus from an infected rat population. The rat flea is also an intermediate host for the larval stage of two tapeworms, **Hymenolepis diminuta* and *H. nana*.

病蚤屬 蚤之一屬。溫帶地區常見的一種鼠蚤具帶病蚤，在無鼠時可咬人，因而從感染的鼠羣傳播鼠疫或鼠斑疹傷寒。鼠蚤也是兩種絛蟲——縮小膜殼絛蟲和短膜殼絛蟲的幼蟲期的中間宿主。

nostrils *n. see* nares.

鼻孔

notch *n.* (in anatomy) an indentation, especially one in a bone.

切迹 （解剖學）一種缺痕，特指骨中的切迹。

notifiable disease a disease that must be reported to the health authorities in order that speedy control and preventive action may be undertaken if necessary. In Great Britain such diseases must be notified to the Proper Officer for the control of communicable diseases (formerly to the Medical Officer of Health). They include cholera, diphtheria, dysentery, food poisoning, infective jaundice, malaria, measles, poliomyelitis, smallpox, tuberculosis, typhoid, and whooping cough. The list varies for different countries, being largely dependent on the endemic communicable diseases and the diseases that may be imported.

法定傳染病 必須報告保健當局以便在必要時迅速採取控制和預防措施的疾病。在英國，為了控制傳染病，必須將此種病報告給有關官員（以前是報告主管保健官員）。這種病包括霍亂、白喉、痢疾、食物中毒、傳染性黃疸、瘧疾、痲疹、脊髓灰質炎、天花、結核、傷寒、百日咳。不同的國家可有不同的病種，主要取決於地方性傳染病和由外傳入的疾病。

notochord *n.* a strip of mesodermal tissue that develops along the dorsal surface of the early embryo, beneath the *neural tube. It becomes almost

脊索 沿着早期胚胎的背側面發育的中胚層組織帶，位於神經管之下。因脊椎的發育，它變得幾乎

entirely obliterated by the development of the vertebrae, persisting only as part of the intervertebral discs.

完全閉合，僅留做椎間盤的一部分。

novobiocin *n.* an antibiotic administered by mouth or injection to treat certain infections resistant to other antibiotics. Side-effects, including digestive upsets and rashes, occur frequently and for this reason other antibiotics are usually preferred.

新生黴素　一種抗生素。口服或注射給藥。用於治療對其它抗生素有抗藥性的某些感染。常發生副作用，包括消化不良和出疹等，因此常選用其它抗生素。

nucha *n.* the nape of the neck. **—nuchal** *adj.*

項　頸後部。

nucle- (nucleo-) *prefix denoting* a cell nucleus.

〔前綴〕**核**　指細胞核。

nuclear magnetic resonance (NMR) a technique of chemical analysis that has recently been applied to the diagnosis of brain abnormalities, vascular disease, and cancer. Based on the absorption of specific radio frequencies by atomic nuclei, it enables the imaging of parts of the body in any plane and is without known risk to the patient.

核磁共振(NMR)　一種化學分析技術。最近用診斷腦異常、血管病和癌症。此技術根據原子核吸收特殊頻率的輻射的原理，能使身體各部位的任何平面顯像，並且目前還未發現它有害於人體。

nuclease *n.* an enzyme that catalyses the breakdown of nucleic acids by cleaving the bonds between adjacent nucleotides. Examples are *ribonuclease*, which acts on RNA, and *deoxyribonuclease*, which acts on DNA.

核酸酶　通過鄰近核苷酸之間的鍵裂解來催化核酸分解的一種酶。例如：作用於RNA的核糖核酸酶，作用於DNA的脫氧核糖核酸酶。

nucleic acid either of two organic acids, *DNA or *RNA, present in the nucleus and in some cases the cytoplasm of all living cells. Their main functions are in heredity and protein synthesis.

核酸　存在於一切活細胞的核中並且在某些情況下存在於胞漿中的兩種有機酸DNA或RNA。它們主要是在遺傳和蛋白合成中起作用。

nucleolus *n.* (*pl.* **nucleoli**) a dense spherical structure within the cell *nucleus that disappears during cell division. The nucleolus contains *RNA for the synthesis of *ribosomes and plays an important part in RNA and protein synthesis.

核仁　細胞核內的緻密球形結構。可在細胞分裂中消失。核仁中含有核糖體合成用的RNA並且在RNA和蛋白合成中起重要作用。

nucleoplasm (karyoplasm) *n.* the protoplasm making up the nucleus of a cell.

核質（核漿）　組成細胞核的原生質（原漿）。

nucleoprotein *n.* a compound that occurs in cells and consists of nucleic acid and protein tightly bound together. *Ribosomes are nucleoproteins containing RNA; *chromosomes are nucleoproteins containing DNA.

核蛋白 由緊密結合在一起的核酸和蛋白組成的細胞內化合物。核糖體是含有RNA的核蛋白；染色體是含有DNA的核蛋白。

nucleoside *n.* a compound consisting of a nitrogen-containing base (a *purine or *pyrimidine) linked to a sugar. Examples are *adenosine, *guanosine, *cytidine, *thymidine, and *uracil. *See also* nucleotide.

核苷 由含氮鹼（嘌呤或嘧啶）連接在糖上組成的化合物。如：腺苷、鳥苷、胞核嘧啶、胸腺核苷、和尿嘧啶。

nucleotide *n.* a compound consisting of a nitrogen-containing base (a *purine or *pyrimidine) linked to a sugar and a phosphate group. Nucleic acids (DNA and RNA) are long chains of linked nucleotides (*polynucleotide* chains), which in DNA contain the purine bases adenine and guanine and the pyrimidines thymine and cytosine; in RNA, thymine is replaced by uracil.

核苷酸 由含氮鹼（嘌呤或嘧啶）連接糖和磷酸基組成的化合物。核酸（DNA和RNA）是核苷酸連接成的長鏈（多核苷酸鏈），在DNA中的核苷酸含有嘌呤鹼（腺嘌呤和鳥嘌呤）和嘧啶鹼（胸腺嘧啶和胞嘧啶）；在RNA中，胸腺嘧啶由尿嘧啶取代。

nucleus *n.* **1.** the part of a *cell that contains the genetic material, *DNA. The DNA, which is combined with protein, is normally dispersed throughout the nucleus as *chromatin. During cell division the chromatin becomes visible as *chromosomes. The nucleus also contains *RNA, most of which is located in the *nucleolus. The nucleus is separated from the cytoplasm by a double membrane, the *nuclear envelope*. **2.** an anatomically and functionally distinct mass of nerve cells within the brain or spinal cord.

核 ①細胞中含有遺傳物質DAN的那一部分。與蛋白質結合的DNA正常時作爲染色質瀰散於整個核內。在細胞分裂期間，染色質變爲可見的染色體。核內也含有RNA，大多數RNA位於核仁內。一雙層膜——核膜將細胞核與細胞漿分隔。②腦或脊髓內的神經細胞集團，各具解剖上的和功能上的明顯區別。

nuclide *n.* an artificially produced isotope that emits radioactive waves and may be used in radiotherapy for the treatment of tumours. *See* caesium-137, cobalt, yttrium-90.

〔原子〕核素 人工製造的同位素。它可散發放射波並可用於腫瘤的放射治療。

nuisance *n.* any noxious substance, accumulating in refuse or as dust or effluent, that is deemed by British law to be injurious to health or offensive. It

有害物 蓄積在廢棄物中的或作爲灰塵或廢水排出的任何有毒害的物質。被英國法律認爲損害健康或

can also include dwellings, work premises, or animals.
侵擾居民的有害物也包括住宅、工作場所或動物。

null hypothesis *see* significance.
無效假說

nullipara *n.* a woman who has never given birth to an infant capable of survival.
未產婦 從未生過活嬰的婦女。

nurse *n.* a person trained and experienced in medical matters and entrusted with the care of the sick and the carrying out of medical and surgical routines under the supervision of a doctor. In Britain student nurses must receive a specified period of training in a hospital approved by the General Nursing Council and pass an examination before qualifying for the State Roll of Assistant Nurses (*State Enrolled Nurse*) or State Register of Nurses (*State Registered Nurse*). *See also* domiciliary midwife, health visitor, home nurse, nursing officer, school nurse.
護士 在醫務方面經過培訓和有一定經驗，負責看護病人並在醫生指導下進行內、外科常規工作的人。在英國，護士生必須在全國護士理事會承認的醫院內接受一定時期的培訓，並通過考試合格，然後才能取得國家錄用助理護士和國家注册護士資格。

nursing officer a higher grade of nurse concerned with administration and management in either tier of the British *National Health Service (*Regional* or *District Nursing Officer*). There are in addition the grades of *Principal Nursing Officer*, who has responsibility for part of the nursing organization within a hospital or in community nursing, and *Senior Nursing Officer*, who is responsible for a group of nurses caring for a designated specialty (e.g. surgical).
護師 英國國民保健服務制中的兩級（地區級與地段級）負責行政管理工作的高級護士職稱。此外還有二個職稱：①主任護師，負責某醫院內或社區內的部分護理組織工作；②高級護師，負責某一指定專科（如：外科）的護士小組的工作。

nutation *n.* the act of nodding the head.
點頭 點頭的動作。

nutrient *n.* a substance that must be consumed as part of the diet to provide a source of energy, material for growth, or substances to regulate growth or energy production. Nutrients include carbohydrates, fats, proteins, minerals, and vitamins.
營養素 作爲膳食的成分必須攝取的物質，以提供能量和生長物質的來源，或調節生長和產能的物質。營養素包括碳水化合物、脂肪、蛋白、礦物質和維生素。

nutrition *n.* the study of food in relation to the physiological processes
營養 研究食物及其被身體吸收後的各種生理過程

that depend on its absorption by the body (growth, energy production, repair of body tissues, etc.). The science of nutrition includes the study of diets and deficiency diseases.

（生長、產生能量、身體組織修復等）相互關係。營養學包括對食物和營養缺乏病進行的研究。

nux vomica the seed of the tree *Strychnos nux-vomica*, which contains the poisonous alkaloid *strychnine.

馬錢子 馬錢樹的種子。它含有毒性生物鹼士的寧。

nyct- (nycto-) *prefix denoting* night or darkness.

〔前綴〕 **夜** 指夜晚或黑暗。

nyctalopia *n. see* night blindness.

夜盲〔症〕

nyctophilia *n.* an intense preference for the darkness and an avoidance of activity in daylight hours. This is sometimes a form of social *phobia.

嗜夜癖 極其偏愛黑暗並且躲避開白天進行活動。有時這是社會恐怖〔症〕的一種表現形式。

nyctophobia *n.* extreme fear of the dark. It is common in children and not unusual in normal adults.

黑夜恐怖 對黑暗極其恐懼。它常見於兒童並且在正常成人中也並不少見。

nyctophonia *n.* speaking in the night but not in the daytime: a form of elective *mutism.

白晝失音 晚上講話但白天不講：選擇性啞症的一種。

nymph *n.* **1.** an immature stage in the life history of certain insects, such as grasshoppers and *reduviid bugs. On emerging from the eggs, nymphs resemble the adult insects except that they are smaller, do not have fully developed wings, and are not sexually mature. **2.** the late larval stage of a tick.

若蟲 ①某些昆蟲，如蚱蜢和獵蝽生活史上的未成熟階段。從卵中孵化出來以後，若蟲與成蟲形態類似，只是略小些，翼未完全發育，性未成熟。 ②蜱的幼蟲晚期。

nympho- *prefix denoting* **1.** the labia minora. **2.** female sexuality.

〔前綴〕 **①小陰唇 ②女子性慾**

nymphomania *n.* an extreme degree of sexual promiscuity in a woman. *Compare* satyriasis. —**nymphomaniac** *adj., n.*

慕男狂 女性的極度的性亂交。

nystagmus *n.* rapid involuntary movements of the eyes that may be from side to side, up and down, or rotatory. Nystagmus may be congenital and associated with poor sight; it also occurs in disorders of the part of the brain responsible for eye movements and their coordination and in disorders of the organ of balance in the ear or the

眼球震顫 眼的快速不隨意運動。眼球可向兩側震顫、上下震顫或旋轉式運動。眼球震顫可爲先天性的，並且同時還有視力不良；也可發生在支配眼運動及其協調功能的腦部疾病中，以及耳內平衡器官或其相關腦部的疾病中。

associated parts of the brain. *Optokinetic nystagmus* occurs in normal people when they try to look at a succession of objects moving quickly across their line of sight. Jerking movements sometimes occur in normal people when tired, on exaggerated movement of the eyes. These are called *nystagmoid jerks* and they do not imply disease.

正常人當力圖看淸眼前快速掠過的一系列物體時，可發生視動性眼球震顫。有時正常人因眼球運動過度而疲勞時，也可出現震顫性運動。這叫做眼球震顫樣反射。並不表示有病。

nystatin *n.* an antibiotic active against fungi. It is applied as a cream for skin infections, by mouth for intestinal infections, as pessaries or suppositories for vaginal or anal infections, or as eye-drops for eye infections. Side-effects include mild digestive upsets. Trade name: **Nystan**.

制黴菌素　抗眞菌（黴素）的抗生素。它被製備成膏劑治療皮膚感染，口服治療腸道感染，以子宮托或栓劑的形式治療陰道或肛門感染，或作爲滴眼劑治療眼部感染。副作用爲輕度消化不良。

O

O

oat cell a cell type of carcinoma of the bronchus. Oat cells are small round or oval cells with darkly staining nuclei and scanty indistinct cytoplasm. Oat-cell carcinoma is usually related to smoking and accounts for about one quarter of bronchial carcinomas.

燕麥細胞　支氣管癌細胞的一種類型。燕麥細胞是具有濃染細胞核和小量模糊不清細胞漿的小圓形細胞。燕麥細胞癌常與吸煙有關，約佔支氣管癌的四分之一。

obesity *n.* the condition in which excess fat has accumulated in the body, mostly in the subcutaneous tissues. Obesity is usually considered to be present when a person is 20% above the recommended weight for his/her height and build. The accumulation of fat is caused by the consumption of more food than is required for producing enough energy for daily activities. Obesity is the most common nutritional disorder of recent years. —**obese** *adj.*

肥胖　體內脂肪過度沉積的狀態。主要見於皮下組織。目前一般認爲當一個人的體重超過標準體重的20%時即爲肥胖。脂肪沉積的原因是由於進食產生的熱量多於日常活動所消耗的熱量。肥胖是近年最常見的營養性疾病。

obex *n.* the curved lower margin of the fourth *ventricle of the brain, between the medulla oblongata and the cerebellum.

閂　第四腦室的曲線狀下緣。位於延髓與小腦之間。

objective *n.* (in microscopy) the arrangement of lenses in a light microscope that is nearest to the object under examination and furthest from the *eyepiece. In many microscopes interchangeable objectives with different powers of magnification are provided.

物鏡 光學顯微鏡鏡片。距離受檢標本最近，距離目鏡最遠。多數顯微鏡都配備有不同放大倍數的可交替使用的物鏡。

obligate *adj.* describing an organism that is restricted to one particular way of life; for example, an *obligate parasite* cannot exist without a host. *Compare* facultative.

專性的 描述生存受某種條件限制的生物體的形容詞。如專性寄生蟲就是一種沒有宿主就不能生存的寄生蟲。

observer error *see* validity.

觀察者誤差

obsession *n.* a recurrent thought, feeling, or action that is unpleasant and provokes anxiety but cannot be got rid of. Although an obsession dominates the person, he (or she) realizes its senselessness and struggles to expel it. The obsession may be a vivid image, a thought, a fear (for example, of contamination), or an impulse (for example, to wash the hands repetitively). It is a feature of obsessional neurosis and sometimes of depression and of organic states, such as encephalitis. It can be treated with behaviour therapy and also with psychotherapy and tranquillizers. *See also* anankastic. —**obsessional** *adj.*

强迫觀念 反復出現的違背自己意願的想法、感覺或行動。患者爲之感到焦慮，但是無法擺脫。雖然受這種强迫觀念的支配，但患者仍能認識到它是無意義的，而且想努力解脫。强迫觀念可能是一種鮮明的意象、想法和恐懼（例如：不潔恐懼），或者是一種衝動（例如：反復洗手）。它是强迫性神經症的特有表現，有時也出現於抑鬱症和器質性疾病，如腦炎。可以用行爲療法、心理療法及抗焦慮藥治療。

obstetrics *n.* the branch of medical science concerned with the care of women during pregnancy, childbirth, and the period of about six weeks following the birth, when the reproductive organs are recovering. *Compare* gynaecology. —**obstetrical** *adj.* —**obstetrician** *n.*

產科學 醫學的分支之一。包括妊娠期、分娩期和分娩後大約六周期間的產褥期的治療護理工作，直到其生殖器官恢復正常。

obstipation *n. Chiefly US.* severe or complete constipation.

頑固性便秘 嚴重的或難治性便秘。

obstructive lung disease *see* bronchospasm.

阻塞性肺疾患

obtund *vb.* to blunt or deaden sensitivity; for example, by the application of a local anaesthetic, which reduces or causes complete loss of sensation in nearby nerves.

使遲鈍 使感覺變得遲鈍或麻木。例如：局部應用麻醉藥使該部位神經感覺減弱或完全喪失。

obturator *n.* **1.** *see* obturator muscle. **2.** a wire or rod within a cannula or hollow needle for piercing tissues or fitting aspirating needles. **3.** a removable form of denture that both closes a defect in the palate and also bears artificial teeth for cosmetic purposes. The defect may be congenital, as in a cleft palate, or result from the removal of a tumour.

①**閉孔肌** ②**充填物** 置於套管中的充填物，或中質的或軟質的金屬針芯。③**腭裂充填體** 既可以充填腭裂又帶有美容性的義齒的一種口腔科可摘托牙。這種腭裂可能是先天性的，或者是由於手術摘除腫瘤後形成的。

obturator foramen a large opening in the *hip bone, below and slightly in front of the acetabulum. *See also* pelvis.

閉孔 髖骨上的一個大孔。位於髖臼下前方。

obturator muscle either of two muscles that cover the outer surface of the anterior wall of the pelvis (the *obturator externus* and *obturator internus*) and are responsible for lateral rotation of the thigh and movements of the hip.

閉孔肌 覆蓋於骨盆前壁外表面的兩塊肌肉（閉孔內肌與閉孔外肌）。功能：股骨的外展和髖骨的運動。

obtusion *n.* the weakening or blunting of normal sensations. This may be associated with disease.

感覺遲鈍 正常感覺減弱或遲鈍。可能由疾病引起。

occipital bone a saucer-shaped bone of the *skull that forms the back and part of the base of the cranium. At the base of the occipital are two *occipital condyles*: rounded surfaces that articulate with the first (atlas) vertebra of the backbone. Between the condyles is the *foramen magnum*, the cavity through which the spinal cord passes.

枕骨 位於顱後、顱底部分的淺碟形顱骨。在枕骨的底部有兩個枕骨髁，其圓形的表面與脊柱第一頸椎（環椎）成關節。在這兩髁之間是枕骨大孔，脊髓由此通過。

occiput *n.* the back of the head. —**occipital** *adj.*

枕部 頭顱的後部。

occlusal *adj.* (in dental anatomy) denoting or relating to the biting surface of a premolar or molar tooth.

𬌗面的 在口腔解剖學中指前磨牙或磨牙的咬合面。

occlusal rim the occlusal extension of a denture base to allow the recording of jaw relations in the construction of *dentures.

𬌗堤 製作托牙時用以記錄頜關係的基托上的延長部分。

occlusion *n.* **1.** the closing or obstruction of a hollow organ or part. **2.** (in dentistry) the relation of the upper and

①**閉塞** 空腔臟器或其部分的閉塞。 ②**𬌗** 口腔學中指上、下牙齒接觸時

lower teeth when they are in contact. Maximum contact between the teeth is known as *centric occlusion*. *See also* malocclusion.

的關係。牙齒間最大限度的接觸稱正中牙合。

occult *adj.* not apparent to the naked eye; not easily determined or detected. For example *occult blood* is blood present in such small quantities, for example in the faeces, that it can only be detected microscopically or by chemical testing.

潛隱性 肉眼觀察不明顯的、不易察覺或不易確定的。

occupational disease any one of various specific diseases to which workers in certain occupations are particularly prone. *Industrial diseases*, associated with a particular industry or group of industries, fall within this category. Examples of such diseases include the various forms of *pneumoconiosis, which affect the lungs of workers continually exposed to dusty atmospheres; decompression sickness in divers; poisoning from toxic metals in factory and other workers; and infectious diseases contracted from animals by farm workers. *See also* prescribed disease, sickness benefit.

職業病 從事某種職業的工人易罹患的疾病。與某種特殊工業或某類工業有關的工業病即屬此類。這類疾病包括：由於長期暴露在滿是灰塵的空氣中，工人肺臟受損害的各種類型的塵肺；潛水員的減壓病；工廠有害物質引起的工人的中毒；由於牲畜感染引起的牧場工人的傳染病。

occupational mortality rates and causes of death in relation to different jobs, occupational and socioeconomic groups, or *social class. Because some occupations have older incumbents than others (e.g. judges) allowance for age bias is made by comparing either *standardized mortality ratios* for those aged 15–64 years or related but less familiar indices, such as *comparative mortality figure* or *proportional mortality ratio*.

職業死亡率 與不同工作、職業和社會經濟團體，或社會階級有關的死亡原因與死亡率。某種職業隨着年齡的增長，責任亦愈加重大（如法官），他們領取較其它職業優厚的年資津貼的根據，就是從該職業的死亡率與15～64歲的標準死亡率的比較中得來的，有時也使用較罕用的比較死亡率或死亡率比等指標。

occupational therapy the treatment of physical and psychiatric conditions by encouraging patients to undertake specific selected activities that will help them to reach their maximum level of function and independence in all aspects of daily life. These activities are

職業療法 鼓勵軀體疾病患者與精神病患者從事規定活動的療法。這樣可以儘可能發揮出他們在日常生活中的活動能力和獨立能力。這些活動是根據患者個人的需要事先計劃好

designed to make the best use of the patient's capabilities and are based on individual requirements. They range from woodwork, metalwork, and printing to pottery and other artistic activities, household management, social skills (for psychiatric patients), and leisure activities (for geriatric patients). Occupational therapy also includes assessment for mechanical aids and adaptations in the home.

的，使之最大限度地發揮患者的潛在能力。他們從事木製品、金屬製品和陶器的製做、印刷及其它美術工作、家務工作，學習社交技能（用於精神病患者）和度閒（用於老年患者）。職業療法也包括對機械性醫療輔助裝置和療養所的適應過程。

ochronosis *n.* the presence of brown-black pigment in the skin, cartilage, and other tissues due to the abnormal accumulation of homogentisic acid that occurs in the metabolic disease *alcaptonuria.

褐黃病 由於代謝性疾病尿黑酸尿症時尿黑酸的異常蓄積，引起的皮膚、軟骨和其他組織深褐色色素沉着。

oct- (octa-, octi-, octo-) *prefix denoting* eight.

〔前綴〕 **八**

octigravida *n.* a woman who has been pregnant eight times.

孕₈ 第八次妊娠的婦女。

octipara *n.* a woman who has been pregnant at least eight times and has given birth to an infant capable of survival after each of eight pregnancies.

產₈ 至少有八次妊娠，並分娩過八個活嬰的婦女。

ocular *adj.* of or concerned with the eye or vision.

眼的 與眼睛和視覺有關的。

oculist *n.* a North American term for an *ophthalmologist.

眼科醫師 在北美此詞指眼科學家。

oculo- *prefix denoting* the eye(s).

〔前綴〕 **眼**

oculogyric *adj.* causing or concerned with movements of the eye.

眼動的 與眼球運動有關的。

oculomotor *adj.* concerned with eye movements.

眼球運動的 與眼球運動有關的。

oculomotor nerve the third *cranial nerve (III), which is composed of motor fibres distributed to muscles in and around the eye. Fibres of the parasympathetic system are responsible for altering the size of the pupil and the lens of the eye. Fibres outside the eye run to the upper eyelid and to muscles that turn the eyeball in different directions.

動眼神經 第III對腦神經。由運動性神經纖維組成，分佈於眼內肌和眼外肌。副交感系統的纖維調節瞳孔大小和眼晶狀體形狀。眼外纖維是分佈於眼瞼及使眼球向不同方向轉動的肌肉（眼肌）。

oculonasal *adj.* concerned with the eye and nose.

眼鼻的

odont- (odonto-) *prefix denoting* a tooth. Example: *odontalgia* (toothache).

〔前綴〕 **牙** 例如：牙痛。

odontoblast *n.* a cell that forms dentine. Odontoblasts line the pulp and have small processes that extend into the dentine.

成牙質細胞 形成牙本質的細胞。成牙質細胞覆蓋牙髓並有小突起進入牙本質。

odontoid process a toothlike process from the upper surface of the axis vertebra. *See* cervical vertebrae.

齒突 樞椎上表面的牙齒樣突起。

odontology *n.* the study of the teeth.

牙科學

odontome *n.* an abnormal mass of calcified dental tissue.

牙瘤 鈣化的牙質組織生成的一種異常團塊。

-odynia *suffix denoting* pain in (a specified part).

〔後綴〕 **痛**

odynophagia *n.* a sensation of pain behind the sternum as food or fluid is swallowed; particularly, the burning sensation experienced by patients with reflux *oesophagitis when hot, spicy, or alcoholic liquid is swallowed.

吞咽痛 吞咽食物或飲料時胸骨後的疼痛感覺。尤指逆流性食管炎患者在吞咽熱的、辛辣的和含酒精的飲料時感到的燒灼感。

oedema *n.* excessive accumulation of fluid in the body tissues: popularly known as *dropsy*. The resultant swelling may be local, as with an injury or inflammation, or more general, as in heart or kidney failure. In generalized oedema there may be collections of fluid within the chest cavity (*pleural effusions*), abdomen (*see* ascites), or within the air spaces of the lung (*pulmonary oedema*). It may result from heart or kidney failure, cirrhosis of the liver, acute nephritis, the nephrotic syndrome, starvation, allergy, or drugs (e.g. phenylbutazone or cortisone derivatives). In such cases the kidneys can usually be stimulated to get rid of the excess fluid by the administration of *diuretic drugs. *Subcutaneous oedema* commonly occurs in the legs and ankles due to the influence of gravity and (in women) before menstruation; the swelling subsides with rest and elevation of the legs. —**oedematous** *adj.*

水腫 人體組織內液體的過多瀦留。俗稱浮腫。水腫的發生可以是局部的，如局部外傷或炎症引起的，或者是較大範圍的，如心、腎功能衰竭引起的。全身性水腫時可發生胸腔積液、腹腔積液或肺水腫。水腫可以由心、腎功能衰竭、肝硬變、急性腎炎、腎病綜合徵、長期饑餓、變態反應或藥物（保泰松或可的松類等）引起。這時可以投予作用於腎臟的利尿藥促使過多的液體排出體外。受重力影響和婦女月經前發生的皮下水腫多位於下肢和踝關節部位，在休息和抬高下肢時可消退。

Oedipus complex repressed sexual feelings of a child for its opposite-sexed parent, combined with rivalry towards the same-sexed parent: a normal stage of development, first described by Freud. The end of the Oedipus complex in children is marked by a loss of sexual feelings towards the opposite-sexed parent and an increase in identification with the same-sexed parent. Arrest of development at the Oedipal stage is said to be responsible for sexual deviations and other neurotic behaviour.

伊迪帕斯情綜 子女對異性父母產生的一種被壓抑的性戀心理。與此同時還伴有對同性父母的敵視。此現象首先由弗洛依德描述。他認爲這是兒童心理發育過程中的一個正常的階段。在此階段結束時，對異性父母的性戀心理消失，對同性父母的感情亦趨正常。如果心理發育停止於伊迪帕斯階段，就會發生性心理變態以及其它種種神經異常的行爲。

oesophag- (oesophago-) *prefix denoting* the oesophagus. Example: *oesophagectomy* (surgical removal of).

〔前綴〕 **食管** 例如：食管切除術。

oesophageal ulcer *see* peptic ulcer, oesophagitis.

食管潰瘍

oesophagitis *n.* inflammation of the oesophagus (gullet). Frequent regurgitation of acid and peptic juices from the stomach causes *reflux oesophagitis*, the commonest form, which may be associated with a hiatus *hernia. The main symptoms are heartburn, regurgitation of bitter fluid, and sometimes difficulty in swallowing; complications include bleeding, narrowing (*stricture) of the oesophageal canal, and ulceration. It is treated by antacid medicines, weight reduction, and avoidance of bending; in severe cases surgery may be required. *Corrosive oesophagitis* is caused by the ingestion of caustic acid or alkali. It is often severe and may lead to perforation of the oesophagus or to extensive stricture formation. Treatment includes avoidance of food and administration of antibiotics and corticosteroids; later dilatation of the stricture may be needed. *Infective oesophagitis* is most commonly due to a fungus (*Candida*) infection in debilitated patients, especially those being treated with antibiotics, corticosteroids, and immunosuppressive drugs, but is occasionally due

食管炎 食管的炎症。頻繁的胃酸和消化液的逆流性食管炎，常見於食管裂孔疝。主要症狀有胃灼熱、反酸並且時常有吞咽困難。併發症包括食管出血、狹窄和潰瘍形成。治療應用抗酸藥，控制飲食和避免身體彎曲。嚴重病例需要手術治療。腐蝕性食管炎是由於吞飲苛性酸或鹼造成的。通常很嚴重，可以導致食管穿孔或形成廣泛的狹窄。治療包括禁食、應用抗生素和皮質類固醇；最後需要施行食管擴張術以解除狹窄。感染性食管炎常見於有眞菌感染的虛弱患者，尤其多見於用抗生素、皮質類固醇和免疫抑制性藥物治療時。偶爾可見由病毒（巨大細胞病毒或疱疹病毒）引起者。

to viruses (such as cytomegalovirus or herpes virus).

oesophagocele *n.* protrusion of the lining (mucosa) of the oesophagus (gullet) through a tear in its muscular wall.

食管膨出 通過食管壁肌肉裂口穿出的食管黏膜突起物。

oesophagoscope *n.* an illuminated optical instrument used to inspect the interior of the oesophagus (gullet), dilate its canal (in cases of stricture), obtain material for biopsy, or remove a foreign body. It may be a rigid metal tube or a flexible fibreoptic instrument (*see* gastroscope). —**oesophagoscopy** *n.*

食管鏡 一種有照明裝置的光學器械。用於食管內腔檢查、擴張食管（在狹窄病例）、採取活組織檢查標本或取除異物。食管鏡可以是硬性的金屬管，也可以是柔性的光學纖維器械。

Oesophagostomum *n.* a genus of parasitic nematodes occurring in Brazil, Africa, and Indonesia. It is a rare intestinal parasite of man, producing symptoms of dysentery in cases of heavy infection. The worms may also invade the tissues of the gut wall, giving rise to abscesses. The worms can be eliminated with *tetrachloroethylene.

結節線蟲屬 一屬寄生性線蟲，存在於巴西、非洲和印度尼西亞。是一類罕見的人體腸內寄生蟲。嚴重感染病例可引起痢疾症狀。該類寄生蟲也可以侵襲腸壁組織引起膿腫。治療：用四氯乙烯驅蟲。

oesophagostomy *n.* a surgical operation in which the oesophagus (gullet) is opened onto the neck. It is usually performed after operations on the throat as a temporary measure to allow feeding.

食管造口術 將食管在頸部造口的外科手術。通常在咽部手術後做爲餵飼的一種暫時措施。

oesophagotomy *n.* surgical opening of the oesophagus (gullet) in order to inspect its interior or to remove or insert something.

食管切開術 將食管切開的手術。目的是探查食管內腔，取除異物或插入器械。

oesophagus *n.* the gullet: a muscular tube, about 23 cm long, that extends from the pharynx to the stomach. It is lined with mucous membrane, whose secretions lubricate food as it passes from the mouth to the stomach. Waves of *peristalsis assist the passage of food.

食管 位於咽與胃之間大約23cm長的肌肉管。在食物從口腔通過食管抵達胃的過程中，內層黏膜分泌潤滑食物的黏液。食管蠕動波幫助食物通過。

oestradiol *n.* the major female sex hormone produced by the ovary. *See* oestrogen.

雌二醇 卵巢合成的重要雌激素。

oestriol *n.* one of the female sex hormones produced by the ovary. *See* oestrogen.

雌三醇 卵巢合成的雌激素之一。

oestrogen *n.* one of a group of steroid hormones (including oestriol, oestrone, and oestradiol) that control female sexual development, promoting the growth and function of the female sex organs (*see* menstrual cycle) and female secondary sexual characteristics (such as breast development). Oestrogens are synthesized mainly by the ovary; small amounts are also produced by the adrenal cortex, testes, and placenta. In men excessive production of oestrogen gives rise to *feminization.
Naturally occurring and synthetic oestrogens, given by mouth or injection, are used to treat *amenorrhoea, menopausal disorders, androgen-dependent cancers (e.g. cancer of the prostate), and to inhibit lactation. Synthetic oestrogens are a major constituent of *oral contraceptives. Side-effects of oestrogen therapy may include nausea and vomiting, headache and dizziness, irregular vaginal bleeding, fluid and salt retention, and feminization in men. Oestrogens should not be used in patients with a history of cancer of the breast, womb, or genital tract. —**oestrogenic** *adj.*

雌激素 固醇類激素之一（包括雌三醇、雌酮和雌二醇）。決定女性的成熟，促進女性性器官的功能及女性第二性徵的生長發育（例如乳房的發育）。雌激素主要在卵巢合成。腎上腺皮質、睾丸和胎盤也產生少量雌激素。男子雌激素合成過多會引起女性化。天然的和人工合成的雌激素經口服或注射用於治療經閉、女性更年期障礙、雄激素依賴性癌（前列腺癌等）及抑制泌乳。人工合成的雌激素是口服避孕藥的重要組成成份。雌激素治療的副作用包括噁心、嘔吐、頭痛、眩暈、不規則性陰道出血、水鹽瀦留和男子女性化。雌激素不能用於有乳腺癌、子宮癌或生殖道癌病史的患者。

oestrone *n.* one of the female sex hormones produced by the ovary. *See* oestrogen.

雌酮 卵巢合成的雌激素之一。

Oestrus *n.* a genus of widely distributed nonbloodsucking flies, occurring wherever sheep and goats are raised. The parasitic larvae of *O. ovis*, the sheep nostril fly, may occasionally and accidentally infect man. By means of large mouth hooks, it attaches itself to the conjunctiva of the eye, causing a painful *myiasis that may result in loss of sight. This is an occupational disease of shepherds. Larvae can be removed with forceps following anaesthesia.

狂蠅屬 廣泛分佈的不吸血的飛蠅屬。存在於飼養有綿羊和山羊的地方。寄生在綿羊鼻腔內壁的羊狂蠅幼蟲可以偶然傳染人，以其巨大的口鈎黏附在人眼結膜上，引起疼痛，可以引起失明。蠅蛆病是牧羊人的一種職業病。治療：麻醉後用鑷子自眼內取出幼蟲。

Office of Population Censuses and Surveys (in Britain) a department of central government responsible for the compilation and publication of statistics relating to national and local population and the demographic patterns of births, marriages, and deaths (including the medical cause of death). It organizes a *national census* at ten-yearly intervals based n the actual presence of individuals in a house or institution on a designated night as distinct from their official address.

人口局 （英國）負責收集、滙編、出版全國與各地區人口統計學資料的中央政府部門。統計內容包括出生率、成婚率與死亡率（包括對死亡病因的統計）。每隔10年進行一次全國性調查。全國在統一規定的午夜根據正式戶口所在地（家庭戶口或機關戶口）對實際的人口情況進行全面普查。

ohm *n.* the *SI unit of electrical resistance, equal to the resistance between two points on a conductor when a constant potential difference of 1 volt applied between these points produces a current of 1 ampere. Symbol: Ω.

歐姆 電阻的國際單位制單位。一歐姆相當於某一導體兩點之間用一伏特電壓能產生一安培電流時的電阻强度。符號：Ω。

-oid *suffix denoting* like; resembling. Example: *pemphigoid* (condition resembling pemphigus).

〔後綴〕 **樣，像，類似** 例如：類天疱瘡樣（形狀像天疱瘡）。

ointment *n.* a greasy material, usually containing a medicament, applied to the skin or mucous membranes.

軟膏 油質物質。一般指塗於皮膚或黏膜上的含有藥物成分的軟膏制劑。

oleandomycin *n.* an antibiotic used to treat infections caused by a wide range of bacteria. It is administered by mouth or injection and is usually without side-effects.

夾竹桃黴素 治療細菌感染的廣譜抗生素。口服或注射給藥。通常無副作用。

olecranon process the large process of the *ulna that projects behind the elbow joint.

鷹嘴 位於肘關節後面的尺骨的大的突起部分。

oleic acid *see* fatty acid.

油酸

oleo- *prefix denoting* oil.

〔前綴〕 **油**

oleothorax *n.* the procedure of introducing a light oil into the *pleural cavity so that the lung is allowed to collapse. This was sometimes formerly undertaken to allow healing in a lung damaged by tuberculosis.

人工油胸療法 把輕油輸入胸膜腔引起肺萎縮的治療方法。以前曾用於治療肺結核。

oleum *n.* (in pharmacy) an oil.

油

olfaction *n.* **1.** the sense of smell. **2.** the process of smelling. Sensory cells in the

①嗅覺 ②嗅功能 鼻腔粘膜中的感覺細胞接受在

mucous membrane that lines the nasal cavity are stimulated by the presence of chemical particles dissolved in the mucus. *See* nose. —**olfactory** *adj.*

粘膜中溶解的化學微粒刺激的能力。

olfactory nerve the first *cranial nerve (I): the special sensory nerve of smell. Fibres of the nerve run upwards from smell receptors in the nasal mucosa high in the roof of the nose, through minute holes in the skull, join to form the olfactory tract, and pass back to reach the brain.

嗅神經　第1對腦神經。專司嗅覺的感覺神經。神經纖維從鼻頂部黏膜的嗅覺感受器向上通過顱骨的小孔與嗅束連接，再向後行以達大腦。

olig- (oligo-) *prefix denoting* **1.** few. **2.** a deficiency.

〔前綴〕①少　②缺少

oligaemia *n. see* hypovolaemia.

血量減少

oligoarthritis *n. see* arthritis.

少關節炎

oligodactylism *n.* the congenital absence of some of the fingers and toes.

少指（趾）畸形　先天性指和趾的部分缺失。

oligodendrocyte *n.* one of the cells of the *glia, responsible for producing the *myelin sheaths of the neurones of the central nervous system and therefore equivalent to the *Schwann cells of the peripheral nerves.

少突神經膠質細胞　一種神經膠質細胞。有產生中樞神經系統經元的髓鞘的功能，因此相當於周圍神經的許旺氏細胞。

oligodendroglioma *n.* a tumour of the central nervous system derived from a type of *glia (the supporting tissue) rather than from the nerve cells themselves. *See also* glioma.

少突神經膠質細胞瘤　中樞神經系統的腫瘤。產生於神經膠質（一種支持組織）而非來自神經細胞本身的一種腫瘤。

oligodipsia *n.* a condition in which thirst is diminished or absent.

渴感過弱　口渴的感覺減弱或缺乏。

oligodontia *n.* the congenital absence of some of the teeth.

少牙畸形　先天性部分牙齒缺少。

oligohydramnios *n.* a condition in which the amount of amniotic fluid bathing a fetus during pregnancy is abnormally small. The developing infant may consequently be vulnerable, for example if the mother falls.

羊水過少　妊娠期間浸泡胎兒的羊水量過少。胎兒易受損傷。如母親跌倒時，胎兒亦可能受傷。

oligomenorrhoea *n.* sparse or infrequent menstruation.

月經過少　月經稀少或偶然出現。

oligophrenia *n. Obsolete.* mental *subnormality.

智力發育不全　智力低下的舊稱。

oligospermia *n.* the presence of less than the normal number of spermatozoa in the semen. Normal semen produced on ejaculation usually contains more than 60 million sperm/ml, of which about 80% are motile and morphologically normal. In oligospermia, the sperm usually have poor motility and often include many bizarre and immature forms. Treatment is directed to any underlying cause (such as *varicocele). *See also* infertility.

精子減少 精液中的精子比正常數量少。射精時產生的每毫升正常精液一般包含6千萬個精子以上，其中大約80%形態正常，具有活動能力。精子減少時，精子通常缺乏活動能力並且有很多異常的和未成熟的類型。病因治療（例如精索靜脈曲張）。

oliguria *n.* the production of an abnormally small volume of urine. This may be a result of copious sweating associated with intense physical activity and/or hot weather. It can also be due to kidney disease, retention of water in the tissues (*see* oedema), loss of blood, diarrhoea, or poisoning.

少尿 尿量減少。通常是體力勞動和/或天氣炎熱時大量出汗的結果。亦見於腎臟疾患、水瀦留、失血、腹瀉或中毒時。

olive *n.* a smooth oval swelling in the upper part of the medulla oblongata on each side. It contains a mass of nerve cells, mainly grey matter (*olivary nucleus*). —**olivary** *adj.*

橄欖體 位於延髓上部兩旁的光滑卵圓形隆起。主要是由神經細胞團塊組成的灰質（橄欖核）。

-ology *suffix. see* -logy.

〔後綴〕 **學**

om- (omo-) *prefix denoting* the shoulder.

〔前綴〕 **肩**

-oma *suffix denoting* a tumour. Examples: *hepatoma* (of the liver); *lymphoma* (of the lymph nodes).

〔後綴〕 **瘤** 例如：肝細胞瘤，淋巴（組織）瘤（淋巴結的）。

omentectomy *n.* the removal of all or part of the omentum (the fold of peritoneum between the stomach and other abdominal organs).

網膜切除術 網膜（胃和其它腹腔臟器之間的腹膜褶）全部或部分切除。

omentopexy *n.* an operation in which the *omentum is attached to some other tissue, usually the abdominal wall (in order to improve blood flow through the liver) or the heart (to increase the blood supply to the heart).

網膜固定術 使網膜附着於其它組織，特別是腹壁（爲了改善肝臟的血流）或心臟（以增加心臟的血流供應）的手術。

omentum (epiploon) *n.* a double layer of *peritoneum attached to the stomach and linking it with other abdominal

網膜 將其它膜腔臟器（例如：肝臟、脾臟及小腸）附着於胃的雙重腹膜

organs, such as the liver, spleen, and intestine. The *great omentum* is a highly folded portion of the omentum, rich in fatty tissue, that covers the intestines in an apron-like fashion. It acts as a heat insulator and prevents friction between abdominal organs. The *lesser omentum* links the stomach with the liver. —**omental** *adj.*

層。大網膜是高度反折的網膜的一部分，脂肪組織豐富，呈裙狀覆蓋於小腸，起隔熱和防止腹腔臟器之間互相摩擦的作用。小網膜位於胃和肝臟之間。

Ommaya reservoir a device inserted into the ventricles of the brain to enable the repeated injection of drugs into the cerebrospinal fluid. It is used, for example, in the treatment of malignant meningitis, particularly in children with leukaemia.

御厩氏貯器 插入腦室能够向腦脊液中反復注射藥物的一種器械。用於諸如嚴重腦膜炎的治療，尤其是患有白血病的兒童。

omphal- (omphalo-) *prefix denoting* the navel or umbilical cord.

〔前綴〕 **臍，臍帶**

omphalitis *n.* inflammation of the navel, especially in newborn infants.

臍炎 臍部的炎症。尤其指新生兒。

omphalocele *n.* an umbilical *hernia.

臍突出 臍部發生的疝。

omphalus *n. see* umbilicus.

臍

Onchocerca *n.* a genus of parasitic worms (*see* filaria) occurring in central Africa and central America. The adult worms are found in fibrous nodules within the connective tissues beneath the skin and their presence causes disease (*see* onchocerciasis). Various species of black fly, in which *Onchocerca* undergoes part of its development, transmit the infective larvae to man.

盤尾絲蟲屬 分佈於中非和中美的寄生蟲屬。成蟲存在於皮下發生病變的結締組織的纖維性結節中。寄生於各種黑蠅體內的盤尾絲蟲屬寄生蟲經過一定的發育階段，通過這些黑蠅可以把有傳染性的幼蟲傳染給人。

onchocerciasis *n.* a tropical disease of the skin and underlying connective tissue caused by the parasitic worm *Onchocerca volvulus.* Fibrous nodular tumours grow around the adult worms in the skin; these may take several months to appear, and if secondary bacterial infection occurs they may degenerate into abscesses. The skin also becomes inflamed and itches. The migration of the larvae into the eye can cause total or partial blindness – the *river blindness* of Africa. Onchocerciasis

盤尾絲蟲病 熱帶疾病。由寄生蟲盤尾絲蟲引起的皮膚和皮下結締組織疾病。堅韌的結節瘤圍繞着皮膚中的成蟲生長，經過數月後形成明顯的隆起。如果合併細菌感染，可繼發膿腫、皮膚發炎、發癢。幼蟲移行入眼睛中可以引起全盲或不全盲，即非洲的河源性盲。盤尾絲蟲病多發於中非和中美。應用蘇拉明和乙胺嗪治

occurs in Central Africa and Central America. The drugs *suramin and *diethylcarbamazine are used in treatment; if possible, the nodules are removed as and when they appear.

療；如果條件允許，當結節出現時可以進行手術切除。

onco- *prefix denoting* **1.** a tumour. **2.** volume.

〔前綴〕 ①瘤 ②體積

oncogene *n.* a gene in viruses and mammalian cells that can cause cancer. It probably produces proteins regulating cell division that, under certain conditions, become uncontrolled.

致癌基因 病毒和哺乳動物細胞中存在的能够引起癌症的基因。據稱此基因可產生控制細胞分裂的蛋白，一旦失控，細胞便無限分裂。

oncogenesis *n.* the development of a new abnormal growth (a benign or malignant tumour).

瘤形成 一種異常的新生物（良性或惡性腫瘤）的生成。

oncogenic *adj.* describing a substance, organism, or environment that is known to be a causal factor in the production of a tumour. Some animal viruses are known to be oncogenic; others are suspected of being so in man, including some papovaviruses, adenoviruses, and herpesviruses. *See also* carcinogen.

致腫瘤的 描述具有產生腫瘤的因素的物質、生物或環境的形容詞。已知有些動物的病毒是致腫瘤的；人體內的某些病毒也可能是致腫瘤的。包括部分乳多泡病毒、腺病毒和疱疹病毒。

oncology *n.* the study and practice of treating tumours.

腫瘤學 研究與治療腫瘤的學科。

oncolysis *n.* the destruction of tumours and tumour cells. This may occur spontaneously or, more usually, in response to treatment with drugs or radiotherapy.

癌細胞溶解 腫瘤和腫瘤細胞的溶解過程。可以是自發的；但是更多的情況是應用藥物療法或放射療法的結果。

oncometer *n.* an instrument for measuring the volume of blood circulating in one of the limbs. *See* plethysmography.

器官體積測量器 測量肢體血液循環量的儀器。

oncosphere (hexacanth) *n.* the six-hooked larva of a *tapeworm. If ingested by a suitable intermediate host, such as a pig or an ox, the larva will use its hooks to penetrate the wall of the intestine. The larva subsequently migrates to the muscles, where it develops into a *cysticercus.

六鈎蚴 具有六個口鈎的絛蟲幼蟲。如果被適當的中間宿主嚥下，例如豬或牛，幼蟲將用其口鈎刺入腸壁。接着幼蟲移行至腸壁的肌肉，在這裏發育成爲囊尾蚴。

oncotic *adj.* **1.** characterized by a tumour or swelling. **2.** relating to an increase in volume or pressure.

①腫瘤的 ②腫塊的 ③膨出的 體積或壓力增加的。

oncotic pressure a pressure represented by the pressure difference that exists between the osmotic pressure of blood and that of the lymph or tissue fluid. Oncotic pressure is important for regulating the flow of water between blood and tissue fluid. *See also* osmosis.

膨脹壓 血液與淋巴液或組織液之間的滲透壓不同而產生的壓力。膨脹壓的主要作用調節血液和組織液之間的液體流動。

oneir- (oneiro-) *prefix denoting* dreams or dreaming.

〔前綴〕 **夢**

oneirism *n.* day-dreaming. Obviously this is a normal phenomenon, but in excess it may impair the ability to cope with life. This is a feature of *schizoid and *asthenic personalities.

夢樣狀態 白日夢或耽於幻想。任人皆知這是一種正常現象，但是超過界限將影響日常生活能力。這是精神分裂型人格和無力型人格的特徵。

onomatomania *n.* the repeated intrusion of a specific word or a name into a person's thoughts: a form of *obsession.

强迫性名詞追思 强迫觀念的一種類型。患者反復想到某一特殊名稱或單詞而困擾不能自拔。

onomatopoiesis *n.* inventing words that reflect the sound made by the object or event to be described. It is one of the principles that guide some schizophrenics in the production of *neologisms.

詞語創新 模仿被描述事物發出的聲音來創造新語。是精神分裂症病人在創造新語時所遵循的一條原則。

ontogeny *n.* the history of the development of an individual from the fertilized egg to maturity.

個體發生 從受精卵到成熟個體的發育過程。

onych- (onycho-) *prefix denoting* the nail(s).

〔前綴〕 **甲**

onychauxis *n.* thickening or overgrowth of the nails.

甲肥厚 指〔趾〕甲增厚或增生。

onychia *n.* inflammation of the matrix of the *nail, which results in loss of the nail.

甲床炎 指〔趾〕甲床的炎症。可以引起指〔趾〕甲的脫落。

onychogryphosis *n.* gross thickening and hardening of the nail, which becomes elongated and deformed. The cause is unknown.

甲彎曲 指〔趾〕甲的明顯增厚變硬、延長變形。病因不明。

onycholysis *n.* separation or loosening of part or all of a nail from its bed, often due to a poor blood supply. The condition may occur in *psoriasis and in fungus infection of the skin and nail bed.

甲脫離 指〔趾〕甲部分或全部從指〔趾〕甲床分離或脫落。常因供血不足引起。可能與銀屑病及皮膚和指〔趾〕甲床的眞菌感染有關。

onychomadesis *n.* loss of the nails.

甲缺失 指〔趾〕甲的脫落。

onychomycosis *n.* fungus infection of the nails, usually caused by **Epidermophyton* or **Candida*. The nails become white, opaque, thickened, and brittle. *See also* ringworm.

甲癬 指〔趾〕甲的眞菌感染。常因表皮癬菌屬或念珠菌屬感染引起。指〔趾〕甲呈白色，無光澤，質硬，脆。

onychosis *n.* any disease or deformity of the nails.

甲病 指〔趾〕甲疾病或畸形的總稱。

O'nyong nyong fever (joint-breaker fever) an East African disease caused by an *arbovirus and transmitted to man by mosquitoes of the genus **Anopheles*. The disease is similar to *dengue and symptoms include rigor, severe headache, an irritating rash, fever, and pains in the joints. The patient is given drugs to relieve the pain and fever.

奧紐紐熱（關節裂痛熱） 蚊媒病毒感染。東非一種經按蚊屬按蚊傳播的疾病。這種病與登革熱相似，症狀包括寒戰、劇烈頭痛、搔癢性皮疹、發熱和關節痛。服藥後患者可以解除疼痛和發熱。

oo- *prefix denoting* an egg; ovum.

〔前綴〕 ①卵 ②卵巢

oocyesis (ovariocyesis) *n.* the development of an embryo in the ovary: ovarian pregnancy. *See also* ectopic pregnancy.

卵巢妊娠 胚胎在卵巢內發育。

oocyst *n.* a spherical structure, 50–60 μm in diameter, that develops from the zygote (*see* ookinete) of the malarial parasite (*Plasmodium*) on the outer wall of the mosquito's stomach. The oocyst steadily grows in size and its contents divide repeatedly to form *sporozoites, which are released into the body cavity of the mosquito when the oocyst bursts.

卵囊 直徑爲50～60μm的球形組織。存在於蚊胃的外側壁，由瘧原蟲的受精卵發育形成。卵囊逐漸長大，不斷分裂形成子孢子，當卵囊脹破時，形成的子孢子進入蚊的體腔。

oocyte *n.* a cell in the ovary that undergoes *meiosis to form an ovum. *Primary oocytes* develop from *oogonia in the fetal ovary as they enter the early

卵母細胞 經過減數分裂形成卵子的卵巢細胞。在胚胎期卵巢中，卵原細胞在減數分裂早期時開始形

stages of meiosis. Only a fraction of the primary oocytes survive until puberty, and even fewer will be ovulated. At ovulation the first meiotic division is completed and a *secondary oocyte* and a *polar body* are formed. Fertilization stimulates the completion of the second meiotic division, which produces a second polar body and an ovum.

成初級卵母細胞。初級卵母細胞只有一小部分能存活到青春期，其中能形成成熟卵子的就爲數更少。排卵時第一次減數分裂已經完成，並且形成了次級卵母細胞和極體。受精促進第二次減數分裂的完成，產生二極體和成熟卵子。

oogenesis *n.* the process by which mature ova (egg cells) are produced in the ovary (see illustration). Primordial germ cells multiply to form *oogonia, which start their first meiotic division to become *oocytes in the fetus. This division is not completed until each oocyte is ovulated. The second division is only completed on fertilization. Each meiotic division is unequal, so that one large ovum is produced with a much smaller polar body.

卵〔子〕發生 卵巢成熟卵細胞產生的過程（見圖）原始胚細胞增殖形成卵原細胞。卵原細胞在胚胎期開始第一次減數分裂轉變成卵母細胞。這種分裂一直持續到每個卵母細胞排卵時。第二次細胞分裂在受精時才能完成。每次減數分裂都不是相等的，產生一個有很小的極體和一個大的卵子。

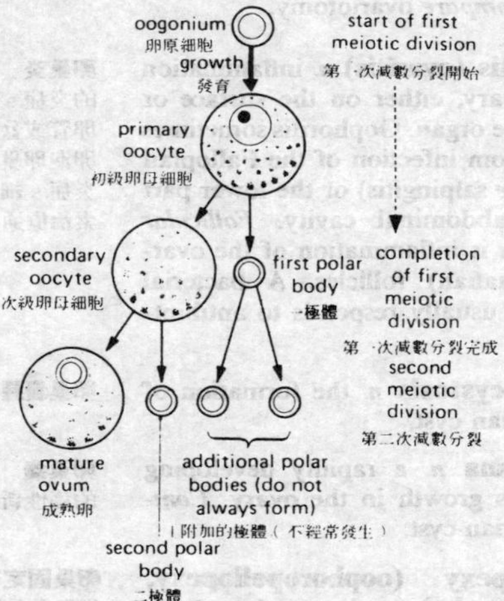

Oogenesis
卵子發生

oogonium *n.* (*pl.* **oogonia**) a cell produced at an early stage in the formation of an ovum (egg cell). Primordial germ cells that have migrated to the embry-

卵原細胞 卵細胞發育早期出現的一種細胞。移行到胚胎卵巢的原始胚細胞增殖形成大量小卵原細

onic ovary multiply to form numerous small oogonia. After the fifth month of pregnancy they enter the early stages of the first meiotic division to form *oocytes. *See also* oogenesis.

胞。妊娠五個月以後，進入第一次減數分裂早期，形成卵母細胞。

ookinete *n.* the motile elongated *zygote of the malarial parasite (**Plasmodium*), formed after fertilization of the *macrogamete. The ookinete bores through the lining of the mosquito's stomach and attaches itself to the outer wall, where it later forms an *oocyst.

動合子 能活動的細長瘧原蟲合子。形成於巨配子受精之後。動合子穿過蚊的胃壁粘膜附着在外側壁，然後形成卵囊。

oophor- (oophoro-) *prefix denoting* the ovary.

〔前綴〕**卵巢**

oophoralgia (ovarialgia, ovaralgia) *n.* pain in the ovary.

卵巢痛

oophorectomy (ovariectomy) *n.* surgical removal of an ovary, performed, for example, when the ovary contains tumours or cysts or is otherwise diseased. *Compare* ovariotomy.

卵巢切除術 卵巢發生腫瘤、囊腫或其它病變時，進行卵巢外科切除的手術。

oophoritis (ovaritis) *n.* inflammation of an ovary, either on the surface or within the organ. Oophoritis sometimes results from infection of the Fallopian tubes (*see* salpingitis) or the lower part of the abdominal cavity. *Follicular oophoritis* is inflammation of the ovarian (Graafian) follicles. A bacterial infection usually responds to antibiotics.

卵巢炎 卵巢表面或內部的炎症。卵巢炎經常由輸卵管或盆腔的感染引起。卵泡卵巢炎是卵巢卵泡的炎症。細菌性感染用抗生素治療通常有效。

oophorocystosis *n.* the formation of an *ovarian cyst.

卵巢囊腫形成

oophoroma *n.* a rapidly developing cancerous growth in the ovary. *Compare* ovarian cyst.

卵巢瘤 卵巢的生長迅速的癌性新生物。

oophoropexy (oophoropeliopexy, oophorrhaphy) *n.* the stitching of a displaced ovary to the wall of the pelvic cavity.

卵巢固定術 將移位的卵巢與骨盆壁縫合起來的手術。

operant *adj.* describing a unit of behaviour that is defined by its effect on the environment. *See* conditioning.

操作的 對環境產生影響的行爲因素。

operating microscope a binocular microscope used in surgery, e.g. in operations to remove a blood clot from an artery (*see* endarterectomy). The field of operation is illuminated through the objective lens by a light source within the microscope (see illustration). Many models incorporate a beam splitter and a second set of eyepieces, to enable the surgeon's assistant to view the operation.

手術顯微鏡 外科用雙筒（雙目鏡）顯微鏡。例如在行動脉血栓手術時使用的顯微鏡。通過帶有光源的顯微鏡使手術視野變得清晰。很多型號都裝配有分光鏡和附加目鏡，可以使外科醫生的助手也能觀察到手術。

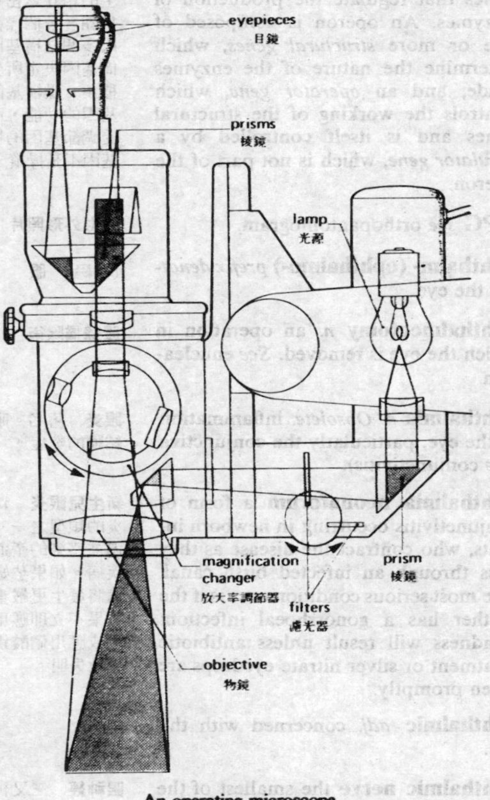

An operating microscope
手術顯微鏡

operculum *n.* (*pl.* **opercula**) **1.** a plug of mucus that blocks the cervical canal of

①**栓** 阻塞妊娠婦女子宮頸管的黏液栓。 ②**滋養**

the womb in a pregnant woman. **2.** (in embryology) a plug of fibrin and blood cells that develops over the site at which a developing fertilized ovum has become embedded in the wall of the womb. **3.** (in neurology) one of the folded and overlapping regions of cerebral cortex that conceal the *insula on each side of the brain.

層蓋 （胚胎學）着床處出現的使受精卵能够植入子宮壁的纖維素和血細胞的栓子。 ③**島蓋** （神經解剖學）位於腦兩側掩蓋腦島的大腦皮質褶叠區。

operon *n.* a group of closely linked genes that regulate the production of enzymes. An operon is composed of one or more *structural genes*, which determine the nature of the enzymes made, and an *operator gene*, which controls the working of the structural genes and is itself controlled by a ***regulator gene***, which is not part of the operon.

操縱子 一組能控制酶產生的相互緊密相連的基因集團。一個操縱子由一個或多個結構基因構成。結構基因決定所生成的酶的種類。操縱基因控制結構基因的功能，而它本身又受調節基因的控制。調節基因不是操縱子的部分。

OPG *see* orthopantomogram.

正影外形照片

ophthalm- (ophthalmo-) *prefix denoting* the eye.

〔前綴〕 **眼**

ophthalmectomy *n.* an operation in which the eye is removed. *See* enucleation.

眼球摘除術

ophthalmia *n. Obsolete.* inflammation of the eye, particularly the conjunctiva (*see* conjunctivitis).

眼炎 舊名。眼的，尤指結膜的炎症。

ophthalmia neonatorum a form of conjunctivitis occurring in newborn infants, who contract the disease as they pass through an infected birth canal. The most serious condition occurs if the mother has a gonorrhoeal infection: blindness will result unless antibiotic treatment or silver nitrate eyedrops are given promptly.

新生兒眼炎 新生兒結膜炎的類型之一。新生兒通過被感染的產道時感染的疾病。如果孕婦感染有淋病將發生更嚴重的後果，如果不立即應用抗生素治療或應用硝酸銀滴眼液將導致失明。

ophthalmic *adj.* concerned with the eye.

眼的

ophthalmic nerve the smallest of the three branches of the *trigeminal nerve. It supplies sensory fibres to the eyeball, conjunctiva, and lacrimal gland, to a small region of the nasal mucous mem-

眼神經 三叉神經三個分支中最小的一支。有感覺纖維分布於眼球、結膜、淚腺、鼻黏膜的一小部分以及鼻、額和頭的皮膚。

brane, and to the skin of the nose, brows, and scalp.

ophthalmitis *n.* inflammation of the eye. *See* conjunctivitis, uveitis.

眼炎

ophthalmodynamometry *n.* measurement of the blood pressure in the vessels of the retina of the eye. A small instrument is pressed against the eye until the vessels are seen (through an *ophthalmoscope) to collapse. The pressure recorded by the instrument reflects the pressure within the vessels of the retina. In certain disorders of the blood circulation to the eye, the pressure in the vessels is reduced and the vessels can be made to collapse by a pressure that is lower than normal.

視網膜血壓檢查法 測量視網膜血壓的方法。用一個小型壓力計用力靠在眼球上，直到觀察到（通過眼底鏡）血管萎陷。此時儀器上的壓力即視網膜血管的壓力。有某種眼部血液循環機能失調時，視網膜血壓下降，使用比正常低的壓力就能使其靜脈萎陷。

ophthalmologist *n.* a doctor who specializes in the diagnosis and treatment of eye diseases.

眼科學家 專門從事眼科疾病的診斷和治療工作的醫生。

ophthalmology *n.* the branch of medicine that is devoted to the study and treatment of eye diseases. —**ophthalmological** *adj.*

眼科學 專門進行眼科疾病治療和研究的醫學分支。

ophthalmometer *n. see* keratometer.

檢眼計（眼屈光計）

ophthalmoplegia *n.* paralysis of the muscles of the eye. *Internal ophthalmoplegia* affects the muscles inside the eye: the iris (which controls the size of the pupil) and the ciliary muscle (which is responsible for *accommodation). *External ophthalmoplegia* affects the muscles that move the eye.

眼肌麻痹 眼部肌肉的麻痹。眼內肌麻痹影響眼內肌肉：虹膜肌（調節瞳孔大小）和睫狀肌（調節晶體厚度）。眼外肌麻痹影響眼球運動肌肉。

ophthalmorrhexis *n.* rupture of the eyeball. This is usually due to a severe blow to the eye.

眼球破裂 眼球的破裂傷。經常由眼受到猛擊引起。

ophthalmoscope *n.* an instrument for examining the interior of the eye (see illustration). There are two types. The *direct ophthalmoscope* enables a fine beam of light to be directed into the eye and at the same time allows the exam-

檢眼鏡（眼底鏡） 檢查眼底的器械（見圖）。有兩種類型。直接檢眼鏡用細小的光束直接照射到眼底，檢查者可以觀察到光束到達眼底的地方。檢查

iner to see the spot where the beam falls inside the eye. Examiner and subject are very close together. In the *indirect ophthalmoscope* an image of the inside of the eye is formed between the subject and the examiner; it is this image that the examiner sees. The examiner and subject are almost at arm's length apart. —**ophthalmoscopy** *n.*

者和受檢查距離非常近。間接檢眼鏡眼底像形成於檢查者與受檢者之間，檢查者見到的就是這個像。檢查者與受檢者之間大約離開一臂長的距離。

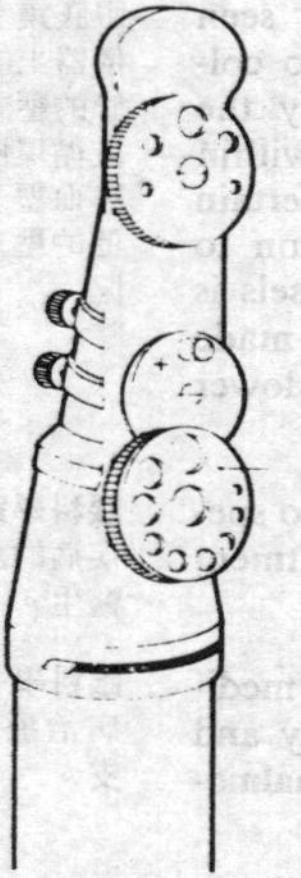

An ophthalmoscope
檢眼鏡

ophthalmotomy *n.* the operation of making an incision in the eyeball.

眼球切開術

ophthalmotonometer (tonometer) *n.* a small instrument for measuring the pressure inside the eye. There are two types, both applied to the cornea after a drop of local anaesthetic has been put in the eye. The *indentation* (*Schiotz*) *tonometer* uses a small plunger that indents the cornea by an amount corresponding to the softness (determined by pressure) of the eye. The *applanation tonometer* measures the pressure required to flatten a constant area of the cornea. A high pressure is required when the pressure inside the eye is increased, and vice versa.

眼壓計 測量眼內部壓力的小型儀器。有兩種類型，不論哪一種類型都要在角膜滴加局麻藥後才能放置到眼球上。凹壓式眼壓計使用硬度不同的（取決於眼壓）壓迫器在角膜上壓出凹痕。平壓式眼壓計則是將角膜某部分壓平。眼壓增高時，施壓要大；眼壓減低時，施壓要小。

-opia *suffix denoting* a defect of the eye or of vision. Example: *asthenopia* (eyestrain).

〔後綴〕 **視力不足** 例如：視力疲勞（眼疲勞）。

opiate *n.* one of a group of drugs derived from opium, including *apomorphine, *codeine, *morphine, and *papaverine. Opiates depress the central nervous system: they relieve pain, suppress coughing, and stimulate vomiting. The most important opiate – morphine – and its synthetic derivative heroin are *narcotics, producing feelings of euphoria before inducing stupor. They are only used for severe pain since they cause *dependence.

阿片制劑 從阿片中提取的一組藥劑。包括阿朴嗎啡、可卡因、嗎啡和罌粟。阿片制劑抑制中樞神經系統：鎮痛、止咳和引起嘔吐。最主要的阿片制劑——嗎啡和其合成衍生物海洛因是麻醉藥，在引起昏睡以前產生欣快感。因能夠引起賴藥性，故僅用於劇烈疼痛。

opisth- (opistho-) *prefix denoting* **1.** dorsal; posterior. **2.** backwards.

〔前綴〕 **①背的，後面的 ②向後的**

opisthorchiasis *n.* a condition caused by the presence of the parasitic fluke **Opisthorchis* in the bile ducts. The infection is acquired through eating raw or undercooked fish that contains the larval stage of the parasite. Heavy infections can lead to considerable damage of the tissues of the bile duct and liver, progressing in advanced cases to *cirrhosis. Symptoms may include loss of weight, abdominal pain, indigestion, and sometimes diarrhoea. The disease, occurring in E Europe and the Far East, is treated with *chloroquine.

後睾吸蟲病 寄生於膽管內的後睾吸蟲屬吸蟲引起的疾病。感染是由於進食生的或半熟的含有幼蟲的魚引起。嚴重感染能導致肝和膽管組織的大量損害，發展爲肝硬化。症狀包括：消瘦、腹痛和消化不良，有時可以引起腹瀉。該病存在於東歐和遠東地區。應用氯喹治療。

Opisthorchis *n.* a genus of parasitic flukes occurring in E Europe and parts of SE Asia. *O. felineus* is normally a parasite of fish-eating mammals but accidental infections of man have occurred. The adult flukes, which live in the bile ducts, can cause *opisthorchiasis.

後睾吸蟲屬 分佈於東歐和東南亞部分地區的寄生蟲屬。貓後睾吸蟲一般是食魚哺乳動物的寄生蟲，但可以偶爾傳染於人。成蟲寄生在膽管內，引起後睾吸蟲病。

opisthotonos *n.* the position of the body in which the head, neck, and spine are arched backwards. It is assumed involuntarily by patients with tetanus and strychnine poisoning.

角弓反張 頭、頸和脊柱向後彎成弓形的體位。是破傷風和士的寧（番木鱉鹼）中毒病人的一種强迫體位。

opium *n.* an extract from the poppy *Papaver somniferum*, which has analgesic and narcotic action due to its content of *morphine. It has the same uses and side-effects as morphine and prolonged use may lead to *dependence. *See also* opiate.

阿片 罌粟屬植物白花罌粟的提取物。由於含嗎啡，所以具有止痛和痲醉作用。與嗎啡具有相同的作用和副作用，長期使用可產生賴藥性。

opponens *n.* one of a group of muscles in the hand that bring the digits opposite to other digits. For example, the *opponens pollicis* is the principal muscle causing opposition of the thumb.

對掌肌 手部肌羣之一。可使手指對向其它各指運動。例如：拇指對掌肌是使拇指對向運動時的主要肌肉。

opposition *n.* (in anatomy) the position of the thumb in relation to the other fingers when it is moved towards the palm of the hand.

對向 （解剖學）拇指向掌面運動時與其它手指的位置關係。

-opsia *suffix denoting* a condition of vision. Example: *erythropsia* (red vision).

〔後綴〕 **視** 例如：紅視。

opsonic index a numerical measurement of the power of a person's serum to attack invading bacteria and prepare them for destruction by *phagocytes. It is measured by dividing the average number of bacteria in the blood per phagocyte in the presence of immune serum by the corresponding number in the presence of normal serum. A vaccine increases the opsonic index.

調理指數 測定病人血清使入侵細菌變得易被白細胞吞噬的能力的數字指標。即：病人血清平均每一個白細胞吞噬的細菌數，與正常人的血清平均每一個白細胞吞噬的細菌數之比，疫苗接種能使調理指數增加。

opsonin *n.* a serum component that attaches itself to invading bacteria and apparently makes them more attractive to *phagocytes and thus more likely to be engulfed and destroyed.

調理素 血漿的組成成分。調理素與入侵細菌結合，使這些細菌更容易吸引吞噬細胞，從而更容易被吞噬和破壞。

opsonization *n.* the process by which opsonins render bacteria more attractive to *phagocytes by attaching themselves to their outer surfaces and changing their physical and chemical composition.

調理素作用 調理素結合在細菌的外表面，改變細菌的物理和化學構成，使細菌更能吸引吞噬細胞的過程。

opt- (opto-) *prefix denoting* vision or the eye.

〔前綴〕 **眼，視力**

optic *adj.* concerned with the eye or vision.

視力的，眼的

optical activity the property possessed by some substances of rotating the plane of polarization of polarized light. A compound that rotates the plane to the left is described as *laevorotatory* (or l-); one that rotates the plane to the right is described as *dextrorotatory* (or d-).

旋光性 某些物質具有的能使偏振光的偏振面發生旋轉的性質。旋光面向左的化合物稱作左旋體；旋光面向右的稱作右旋體。

optical committee (local) *see* medical committee (local).

眼科委員會（地區的）

optic atrophy degeneration of the optic nerve. It may be secondary to disease within the eye or it may follow damage to the nerve itself resulting from injury or inflammation.

視神經萎縮 視神經的退化、變性。可以繼發於眼的疾病，也可以繼發於神經本身的損傷或感染。

optic chiasma (optic commissure) the X-shaped structure formed by the two optic nerves, which pass backwards from the eyeballs to meet in the midline beneath the brain, near the pituitary gland (see illustration). Nerve fibres from the nasal side of the retina of each eye cross over to join fibres from the lateral side of the retina of the opposite eye. The optic tracts resulting from the junction pass backwards to the occipital lobes.

視交叉 由兩束視神經組成的X形結構。由眼球向後走行，交叉於腦的中下方垂體附近。起始於視網膜鼻側的神經纖維與對側眼起始於視網膜顳側的纖維相結合。視束是指從結合點向眼球後到枕葉的部分。

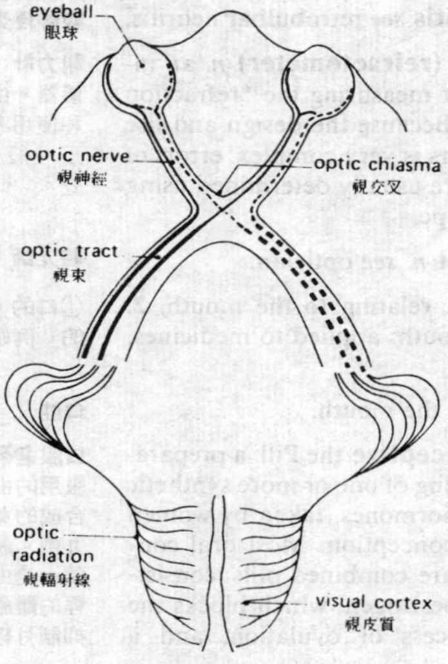

The optic chiasma
視交叉

optic cup either of the paired cup-shaped outgrowths of the embryonic brain that form the retina and iris of the eyes.

視杯 胚胎時腦的一對杯狀突起。形成視網膜和虹膜。

optic disc (optic papilla) the start of the optic nerve, where nerve fibres from the rods and cones leave the eyeball. *See* blind spot.

視神經乳頭 視神經的起點。即神經纖維從視網膜的視桿細胞和視錐細胞離開眼球的地方。

optic foramen the groove in the top of the *orbit that contains the optic nerve and the ophthalmic artery.

視神經管 位於眶頂部的溝。容納視神經和眼動脉。

optician *n.* a person who either makes and fits glasses (*dispensing optician*) or who both tests people for glasses and also makes and fits them (*ophthalmic optician* or *optometrist*).

眼鏡師 製作和配眼鏡（配鏡師），或者是既負責驗光（驗光師）又負責製作和配眼鏡的人。

optic nerve the second *cranial nerve (II), which is responsible for vision. Each nerve contains about one million fibres that receive information from the rod and cone cells of the retina. It passes into the skull behind the eyeball to reach the *optic chiasma, after which the visual pathway continues to the cortex of the occipital lobe of the brain on each side.

視神經 第II對腦神經。爲視覺神經。每束視神經都約含百萬條神經纖維，接受來自視網膜的視桿細胞和視錐細胞的信息。由眼球進入顱內到達視交叉，然後到達腦兩側的枕葉皮質。

optic neuritis *see* retrobulbar neuritis.

視神經炎

optometer (refractometer) *n.* an instrument for measuring the *refraction of the eye. Because the design and use of optometers is very complex, errors of refraction are usually determined using a *retinoscope.

視力計 檢查眼屈光度的儀器。由於視力計的設計和使用非常複雜，屈光不正一般使用視網膜鏡檢查。

optometrist *n. see* optician.

驗光師

oral *adj.* **1.** relating to the mouth. **2.** taken by mouth: applied to medicines, etc.

①口的，口腔的 ②口服的 例如口服藥等。

oral cavity the mouth.

口腔

oral contraceptive the Pill: a preparation, consisting of one or more synthetic female sex hormones, taken by women to prevent conception. Most oral contraceptives are combined pills, consisting of an *oestrogen, which blocks the normal process of ovulation, and a

口服避孕藥 婦女避孕時服用的由一種或多種人工合成的女性性激素組成的丸劑。最常見的口服避孕藥，是由抑制正常排卵過程的雌激素和作用於垂體抑制月經周期正常調節的

*progestogen, which acts on the pituitary gland to block the normal control of the menstrual cycle. Progestogens also alter the lining of the womb and the viscosity of mucus in its outlet, the cervix, so that conception is less likely should ovulation occur. These pills are taken every day for three weeks and then stopped for a week, during which time menstruation occurs. Side-effects may include headache, weight gain, nausea, skin changes, and depression. There is also a small risk that blood clots may form in the veins, especially those of the legs (which may lead to *pulmonary embolism), or that prolonged use of hormonal contraceptives may reduce fertility. The unwanted pregnancy rate is less than 1 per 100 woman-years.

Other hormonal contraceptives include *minipills*, which rely on a progestogen alone, and injections of progestogen, which need be given only every three months. The unwanted pregnancy rate is slightly higher with these preparations: 1–2 per 100 woman-years.

孕激素組成的複合丸劑。孕激素還可以改變子宮內膜和子宮頸黏液稠度，從而減少排卵期妊娠的可能性。這些丸劑每天服用，持續三個星期，停藥一個星期，停藥期出現月經。副作用包括頭痛、體重增加、噁心、皮膚變化和精神抑鬱。而少見的病例可能形成靜脈血栓，尤其是股靜脈的血栓，可以導致肺栓塞。長期應用激素類避孕藥能使生育能力降低。避孕失敗率低於1%（婦女-年）。其它激素類避孕藥包括只含有孕激素的小型丸劑和每三個月只需應用一次的孕激素注射劑。其避孕失敗率稍高：1～2%(婦女-年)。

oral rehabilitation the procedure of rebuilding a dentition that has been mutilated as a result of disease, wear, or trauma.

口腔康復　牙齒由於疾病、磨損或外傷引起殘缺後的恢復過程。

Orbenin *n. see* cloxacillin sodium.

氯唑青黴素

orbicularis *n.* either of two circular muscles of the face. The *orbicularis oris*, around the mouth, closes and compresses the lips. The *orbicularis oculi*, around each orbit, is responsible for closing the eye.

輪匝肌　面部的環形肌肉。口輪匝肌在口唇周圍，功能是閉合口唇。眼輪匝肌在雙眼的周圍，功能是閉合眼睛。

orbit *n.* the cavity in the skull that contains the eye. It is formed from parts of the frontal, sphenoid, zygomatic, lacrimal, ethmoid, palatine, and maxillary bones. —**orbital** *adj.*

眶　容納眼球的顱骨陷窩。由額骨、蝶骨、顴骨、淚骨、篩骨、腭骨和上頜骨組成。

orbitotomy *n.* a surgical incision into the bony orbit containing the eye.

眶切開術　切開容納眼球的骨性眶的外科手術。

orchi- (orchido-, orchio-) *prefix denoting* the testis or testicle. Example: *orchioplasty* (plastic surgery of).

〔前綴〕 **睪丸** 例如：睪丸成形術。

orchidalgia *n.* pain in the testicle. The pain may not be due to a primary condition of the testicle itself: it may be caused by a hernia in the groin, the presence of a stone in the lower ureter, or the presence of a *varicocele.

睪丸痛 睪丸的疼痛。其疼痛可能不是主要由睪丸本身引起；而是由於腹股溝疝、輸尿管下部結石，或者精索靜脈曲張引起。

orchidectomy *n.* surgical removal of a testis, usually to treat such diseases as *seminoma (a malignant tumour of the testis). Removal of both testes (*castration) causes sterility.

睪丸切除術 切除睪丸的外科手術。一般是在睪丸出現像精原細胞瘤（睪丸的惡性腫瘤）這樣的疾病時進行。切除雙側睪丸（閹割）引起不育。

orchidopexy *n.* the operation of mobilizing an undescended testis in the groin and fixing it in the scrotum. The operation should be performed well before puberty to allow the testis every chance of normal development (*see* cryptorchidism).

睪丸固定術 將腹股溝內隱睪固定到陰囊內的手術。手術必須在青春期前進行，睪丸才能正常發育。

orchidotomy *n.* an incision into the testis, usually done to obtain *biopsy material for histological examination, particularly in men with few or no sperm in their semen (*see* azoospermia, oligospermia).

睪丸切開術 睪丸切開的手術。一般用於組織學檢查以獲得活組織檢查標本，尤其是對於精液中缺少或完全沒有精子的病人。

orchitis *n.* inflammation of the testis. This causes pain, redness, and swelling of the scrotum, and may be associated with inflammation of the epididymis (*epididymo-orchitis*). The condition may affect one or both testes; it is usually caused by infection spreading down the vas deferens but can develop in mumps. Mumps orchitis affecting both testes may result in sterility. Treatment of epididymo-orchitis is by local support and administration of analgesics and antibiotics; mumps orchitis often responds to *corticosteroids.

睪丸炎 睪丸的炎症。引起陰囊的紅腫和疼痛，並且可合併附睪炎，可爲一側或雙側，感染一般是由輸精管下行性蔓延引起，但也可合併於腮腺炎。腮腺炎性睪丸炎累及雙側睪丸，可以導致不育。附睪炎的治療包括局部支托，給予鎮痛和抗生素；腮腺炎性睪丸炎應用皮質類固醇常有效。

orciprenaline *n.* a drug used to relieve bronchitis and asthma. It has the same

間羥異丙腎上腺素 治療氣管炎和哮喘的藥物。與

actions and side-effects as *isoprenaline. Trade name: **Alupent**.

異丙腎上腺素有相同的療效和副作用。商品名：（硫酸）異丙喘寧。

orf *n.* a virus infection of sheep and goats that can be transmitted to man, causing a mild skin eruption on the fingers, hands, and forearms.

羊痘疱 綿羊和山羊的病毒性傳染病。可以傳染於人。引起手指、手和前臂的輕度皮疹。

organ *n.* a part of the body, composed of more than one tissue, that forms a structural unit responsible for a particular function (or functions). Examples are the heart, lungs, and liver.

器官 身體的一部份。由幾種組織組成，形成一個結構單位，具有特殊的功能。例如：心臟、肺和肝臟。

organelle *n.* a structure within a cell that is specialized for a particular function. Examples of organelles are the nucleus, endoplasmic reticulum, Golgi apparatus, lysosomes, and mitochondria.

細胞器 具有特殊功能的細胞內結構。例如：細胞核、內質網、高爾基氏器、溶酶體和線粒體。

organic *adj.* **1.** relating to any or all of the organs of the body. **2.** describing chemical compounds containing carbon, found in all living systems.

①**器官的** 與人體器官之一或全部有關的。 ②**有機的** 生物界中存在的含碳化合物的。

organic disorder a disorder associated with changes in the structure of an organ or tissue. *Compare* functional disorder.

器質性疾病 組織或器官發生結構改變的疾病。

organism *n.* any living thing, which may consist of a single cell (*see* microorganism) or a group of differentiated but interdependent cells.

生物體 有生命的機體，可以由單細胞組成，也可以由分化的但是相互依賴的細胞羣組成。

organo- *prefix denoting* organ or organic. Examples: *organogenesis* (formation of); *organopathy* (disease of).

〔前綴〕 **器官** 例如：器官發生，器官病。

organ of Corti (spiral organ) the sense organ of the *cochlea of the inner ear, which converts sound signals into nerve impulses that are transmitted to the brain via the cochlear nerve.

柯替氏器（螺旋器） 內耳耳蝸的聽覺器官。把聲音信號轉換成神經衝動通過耳蝸神經傳入大腦。

organ of Jacobson (vomeronasal organ) a small blind sac in the wall of the nasal cavity. In man it never develops properly and has no function, but in lower animals (e.g. snakes) it is one of the major organs of olfaction.

雅各布遜氏器（犁鼻器） 鼻腔壁的小盲囊。在人體發育不良，沒有功能，但在低等動物（例如蛇）則是嗅覺的重要器官之一。

organotrophic *adj. see* heterotrophic. **器官營養的**

orgasm *n.* the climax of sexual excitement, which – in men – occurs simultaneously with *ejaculation. In women its occurrence is much more variable, being dependent upon a number of physiological and psychological factors.

性慾高潮 性興奮的高峯。男性在性慾高潮的同時射精。女性性高潮的發生相當不穩定，取決於多種生理的和精神的因素。

oriental sore (Baghdad boil, Delhi boil, Aleppo boil) a skin disease, occurring in tropical and subtropical Africa and Asia, caused by the parasitic protozoan *Leishmania tropica* (*see* leishmaniasis). The disease commonly affects children and takes the form of a slow-healing open sore or ulcer, which sometimes becomes secondarily infected with bacteria. Antibiotics are administered to combat the infection.

東方瘡 發生在熱帶亞熱帶的非洲和亞洲的一種皮膚病。由寄生蟲熱帶利甚曼原蟲屬原蟲引起。這種疾病一般感染小兒，引起難以癒合的瘡腫和潰瘍。有時可以發生由細菌引起的繼發性感染。給予抗生素抗感染。

orientation *n.* (in psychology) awareness of oneself in time, space, and place. Orientation may be disturbed in such conditions as organic brain disease, toxic drug states, and concussion.

定向 （精神病學）時間、空間、地點的自我意識。器質性腦病、藥物中毒階段和腦震盪時定向能力將會受到影響。

origin *n.* (in anatomy) **1.** the point of attachment of a muscle that remains relatively fixed during contraction of the muscle. *Compare* insertion. **2.** the point at which a nerve or blood vessel branches from a main nerve or blood vessel.

起端 （解剖學）①肌肉收縮過程中保持相對固定的肌肉附着點。 ②神經幹或血管幹的分支處。

ornithine *n.* an *amino acid produced in the liver as a by-product during the conversion of ammonia to *urea.

鳥尿酸 肝臟合成的氨基酸之一。係氨合成尿素的過程中的產物。

Ornithodoros (Ornithodorus) *n.* a genus of soft *ticks, a number of species of which are important in various parts of the world in the transmission of *relapsing fever.

鈍緣蜱屬 軟蜱中的一屬。有很多種類在世界各地回歸熱的傳播上十分重要。

ornithosis *n.* an infectious disease of birds, primarily pigeons, due to a virus-like organism of the genus *Chlamydia*; it can be transmitted to man and causes symptoms resembling those of pneumonia. *Compare* parrot disease.

鳥疫 鳥類的一種傳染性疾病。最初發生在鴿子，由衣原體屬的病毒樣生物引起。這種病能傳染於人，並引起類似肺炎的症狀。

oro- *prefix denoting* the mouth. 〔前綴〕 **口**

oro-antral fistula a connection between the mouth and the maxillary sinus (antrum) as a sequel to tooth extraction. It may resolve or require surgical closure.

口腔上頜竇瘻 拔牙後出現的口腔和上頜竇之間的瘻道。可以自然癒合或需要外科縫合。

oropharynx *n.* the part of the *pharynx that lies between the soft palate and the hyoid bone (which is situated near the upper portion of the epiglottis).

口咽 位於軟腭和舌骨之間的咽部（會厭上部附近）。

Oroya fever *see* bartonellosis.

奧羅亞熱

orphenadrine *n.* a drug that relieves spasm in muscle, used to treat all types of parkinsonism. It is administered by mouth or injection; side-effects may include dry mouth, sight disturbances, and difficulty in urination. Trade name: **Disipal**.

鄰甲苯海拉明 肌鬆藥，治療各型帕金森氏病。口服或注射。副作用有口乾、視力模糊及排尿障礙。

ortho- *prefix denoting* **1.** straight. Example: *orthograde* (having straight posture). **2.** normal. Example: *orthocrasia* (normal reaction to drugs).

〔前綴〕①**直的** 例如：直體步行的（採取直立的姿勢）。 ②**正常的** 例如：正常反應性（對藥物的正常反應）。

orthochromatic *adj.* describing or relating to a tissue specimen that stains normally.

正染的 着色正常的組織標本的。

orthodiagraph *n.* an X-ray photograph designed to give an undistorted picture of part of the body so that accurate measurements may be made from it.

正影描記器 能描繪出身體某一部位的正常形像，因而能够進行準確測量的X線描記器。

orthodontic appliance an appliance used to move teeth as part of orthodontic treatment. A *fixed appliance* is fitted to the teeth and used to perform complex tooth movements; it is used by dentists with specialist training. A *removable appliance* is a dental plate with appropriate retainers and springs to perform simple tooth movements; it is removed from the mouth for cleaning by the patient.

正牙器 牙列正畸治療時用於移動牙齒的裝置。固定正牙器在牙齒上，可以進行複雜的牙齒運動；由受過專門訓練的牙科醫生使用。活動正牙器是帶有與齒槽外形相吻合的固位體和彈簧的托牙板，可以進行簡單的牙齒運動；患者可以把它從口腔中取出來進行清洗。

orthodontics *n.* the branch of dentistry concerned with the growth and development of the dentition and the

正畸學 與牙齒生長發育和牙齒不齊的治療有關的牙科學分支。

treatment of irregularities. *See* orthodontic appliance. —**orthodontic** *adj.*

orthopaedics *n.* the science or practice of correcting deformities caused by disease of or damage to the bones and joints of the skeleton. This specialized branch of medicine may require the use of surgery, manipulation, traction, or special apparatus. —**orthopaedic** *adj.*

矯形學 矯正由於疾病或骨和關節損傷引起的畸形的學科。是醫學領域的一個專門學科，需要使用手術、推拿、牽引，或者特殊裝置等。

orthopantomogram (OPG) *n.* a special form of tomogram (*see* tomography) that provides a picture of all the teeth of both jaws on one film.

正位全頜斷層照片 X線斷層攝影的特殊類型。在一張照片上提供上下頜的全部牙齒像。

orthophoria *n.* the condition of complete balance between the movements of the two eyes, such that perfect alignment is maintained even when one eye is covered. This theoretically normal state is in fact rarely seen, since most people have a slight tendency to squint (*see* heterophoria).

正視 兩眼球的運動完全平衡的狀態。當一雙眼睛被遮住時兩眼視線仍完全保持平行。事實上理論上的正視十分少見。大多數人具有輕度斜視的傾向。

orthopnoea *n.* breathlessness that prevents the patient from lying down, so that he has to sleep propped up in bed or sitting in a chair. —**orthopnoeic** *adj.*

端坐呼吸 病人因呼吸困難而不能平卧的狀態。他們只能用手支撐在床上或坐在椅子上睡眠。

orthoptics *n.* the practice of using nonsurgical methods, particularly eye exercises, to treat abnormalities of vision and of coordination of eye movements (most commonly strabismus (squint) and amblyopia). Orthoptics also includes the detection and measurement of the degree of such abnormalities. —**orthoptist** *n.*

視軸矯正法 使用非手術方法，主要是用眼球運動操治療視力和眼球運動調節（尤其是斜視和弱視）異常的方法。視軸矯正法也包括各種異常度數的檢測和測量。

orthoptoscope *n. see* amblyoscope.

視軸矯正器

orthostatic *adj.* relating to the upright position of the body: used when describing this posture or a condition caused by it. *Orthostatic hypotension*, for example, is low blood pressure found in some patients when they stand upright.

直立的 描述身體的直立姿勢。或這種姿勢引起的後果的形容詞。例如：直立性低血壓就是某些病人當他們站立的時候發生血壓下降。

os¹ *n.* (*pl.* **ossa**) a bone.

骨

os² *n.* (*pl.* **ora**) the mouth or a mouth-like part.

口 口或口樣結構。

osche- (oscheo-) *prefix denoting* the scrotum. Example: *oscheocele* (a scrotal hernia).

〔前綴〕 **陰囊** 例如：陰囊疝。

oscilloscope *n.* a cathode-ray tube designed to display electronically a wave form corresponding to the electrical data fed into it. Oscilloscopes are used to provide a continuous record of many different measurements, such as the activity of the heart and brain. *See* electrocardiography, electroencephalography.

示波器 用電子學方法顯示相當於電測數據的波形的陰極射線管。示波器用於提供大量不同檢測的連續記錄。尤其是對於心臟和腦的活動。

osculum *n.* (in anatomy) a small aperture.

小口 （解剖學）小孔。

-osis *suffix denoting* **1.** a diseased condition. Examples: *nephrosis* (of the kidney); *leptospirosis* (caused by *Leptospira* species). **2.** any condition. Example: *narcosis* (of stupor). **3.** an increase or excess. Example: *leucocytosis* (of leucocytes).

〔後綴〕 ①**病態** 例如：腎病，鉤端螺旋體病（由鉤端螺旋體屬寄生引起）。 ②**狀態** 例如：麻醉狀態（意識喪失）。 ③**增加** 例如：白細胞增多。

osm- (osmo-) *prefix denoting* **1.** smell or odour. **2.** osmosis or osmotic pressure.

〔前綴〕 ①**嗅覺，氣味** ②**滲透，滲透壓**

osmic acid *see* osmium tetroxide.

鋨酸

osmiophilic *adj.* describing a tissue that stains readily with osmium tetroxide.

嗜鋨的 易染四氧化鋨的組織的。

osmium tetroxide (osmic acid) a colourless or faintly yellowish compound used to stain fats or as a *fixative in the preparation of tissues for microscopical study. Osmium tetroxide evaporates readily, the vapour having a toxic action on the eyes, skin, and respiratory tract.

四氧化鋨（鋨酸） 無色或淺黃色化合物。用於組織標本的脂肪着色或固定，以便在顯微鏡下觀察。四氧化鋨易揮發，其揮發物對眼睛、皮膚和呼吸道有毒性作用。

osmole *n.* a unit of osmotic pressure equal to the molecular weight of a solute in grams divided by the number of ions or other particles into which it dissociates in solution.

滲克分子 滲透壓單位。相當於用溶質的克分子量除以溶液中離解的離子或其他粒子的數量。

osmoreceptor *n.* a group of cells in the *hypothalamus that monitor blood concentration. Should this increase abnormally, as in dehydration, the osmo-

滲透壓感受器 位於丘腦下部控制血液濃度的細胞羣。如果血液濃度異常增高，例如在脫水時，滲透

receptors send nerve impulses to the hypothalamus, which then increases the rate of release of *vasopressin from the posterior pituitary gland. Loss of water from the body in the urine is thus restricted until the blood concentration returns to normal.

壓感受器向丘腦下部輸送神經衝動，增加垂體後葉加壓素釋放。這樣，體內水份通過尿的排泄受到限制，直到血液濃度恢復正常。

osmosis *n.* the passage of a solvent from a less concentrated to a more concentrated solution through a *semipermeable membrane. This tends to equalize the concentrations of the two solutions. In living organisms the solvent is water and cell membranes function as semipermeable membranes, and the process of osmosis plays an important role in controlling the distribution of water. The *osmotic pressure* of a solution is the pressure by which water is drawn into it through the semipermeable membrane; the more concentrated the solution (i.e. the more solute molecules it contains), the greater its osmotic pressure. **—osmotic** *adj.*

滲透〔作用〕 溶劑通過半透膜從低濃度溶液移向高濃度溶液的過程。最後趨向於兩種溶液濃度的平衡。有生命的生物界，溶劑是水，細胞膜的功能類似半透膜，而且滲透壓在控制體內水份平衡方面起着重要作用。溶液的滲透壓是使水通過半透膜移向該溶液的壓力。高濃度溶液（例如含有大量溶質分子等），其滲透壓也高。

osseous *adj.* bony: applied to the bony parts of the inner ear (cochlea, semicircular canals, labyrinth).

骨的 骨性的。如內耳（耳蝸、半規管、迷路）的骨性部分。

ossicle *n.* a small bone. The *auditory ossicles* are three small bones (the incus, malleus, and stapes) in the middle *ear. They transmit sound from the outer ear to the labyrinth (inner ear).

小骨 小的骨頭。聽小骨是位於中耳的三塊小骨（鐙骨、錘骨和砧骨）。聽小骨把來自外耳的聲音傳向迷路（內耳）。

ossification (osteogenesis) *n.* the formation of *bone, which takes place in three stages by the action of special cells (osteoblasts). A meshwork of collagen fibres is deposited in connective tissue, followed by the production of a cementing polysaccharide. Finally the cement is impregnated with minute crystals of calcium salts. The osteoblasts become enclosed within the matrix as *osteocytes* (*bone cells*). In *intracartilaginous* (or *endochondral*) *ossification* the bone replaces cartilage. This process starts to occur soon after the end of the second month of embryonic life. *Intramembranous ossification*

骨化 骨的形成過程。在特殊細胞（成骨細胞）的作用下分三個階段完成。首先在結締組織中形成膠原纖維網絡，接着產生起黏固作用的黏多糖，最後在黏多糖內充滿細小的鈣鹽結晶。成骨細胞被基質包圍，成爲骨細胞。軟骨骨化是指軟骨組織被骨組織所代替。這個過程在胚胎第二個月末立即開始。膜內骨化是指膜成骨（顱骨）的形成過程。此過程開始於胚胎早期，在出生時仍未完成。

is the formation of a *membrane bone (e.g. a bone of the skull). This starts in the early embryo and is not complete at birth (*see* fontanelle).

ost- (oste-, osteo-) *prefix denoting* bone. Examples: *ostalgia* (pain in); *osteocarcinoma* (carcinoma of); *osteonecrosis* (death of); *osteoplasty* (plastic surgery of).

〔前綴〕 **骨** 例如：骨痛，骨癌，骨壞死，骨成形術。

ostectomy *n.* the surgical removal of a bone or a piece of bone. *See also* osteotomy.

骨切除術 切除骨或者一段骨頭的手術。

osteitis *n.* inflammation of bone, due to infection, damage, or metabolic disorder. *Osteitis fibrosa cystica* refers to the characteristic cystic changes that occur in bones during long-standing *hyperparathyroidism. *See also* Paget's disease (of bone) (osteitis deformans).

骨炎 感染、損傷或代謝紊亂引起的骨的炎症。囊狀纖維性骨炎是長期患甲狀旁腺機能亢進時骨的特殊的囊腫性變。

osteo- *prefix. see* ost-.

〔前綴〕 **骨**

osteoarthritis (osteoarthrosis) *n.* a disease of joint cartilage, associated with secondary changes in the underlying bone, which may ultimately cause pain and impair the function of the affected joint (usually the hip, knee, and thumb joints). The condition may result from overuse and is most common in those past middle life; it may also complicate many other diseases involving joints, such as *rheumatoid arthritis (*secondary osteoarthritis*). Osteoarthritis is recognized on X-ray by narrowing of the joint space (due to loss of cartilage) and the presence of *osteophytes and irregularity at the bone margins. Treatment consists of aspirin and other analgesics, reduction of pressure across the joint (by weight loss and the use of a walking stick in osteoarthritis of the hip), and corrective and prosthetic surgery.

骨關節炎 關節軟骨的疾病。合併所屬骨的繼發性改變，最後可以引起關節的疼痛和功能障礙（一般是髖關節、膝關節和拇指關節）。可由關節活動過度引起，尤其是中年人。這種病還可以合併許多其他關節疾病，尤其是風濕樣關節炎（繼發性骨關節炎）。骨關節炎的診斷可以根據X線照片上出現關節間隙狹窄（由於軟骨缺損）、骨贅及骨緣參差不齊。治療：給予阿司匹林和其他鎮痛藥，減輕關節負荷（髖關節炎時，減輕體重與使用拐杖）以及行整復手術。

osteoarthropathy *n.* any disease of the bone and cartilage adjoining a joint. *Hypertrophic osteoarthropathy* is characterized by the formation of new bony

骨關節性疾病 關節端的骨和軟骨疾病的總稱。肥大性骨關節病特徵是新骨組織的形成。患肺膿腫、

tissue and occurs as a complication of chronic diseases of the chest, including pulmonary abscess, mesothelioma, and lung cancer.
間皮瘤和肺癌等慢性呼吸系統疾病時可併發本病。

osteoarthrosis *n. see* osteoarthritis.
骨關節病 骨關節炎。

osteoarthrotomy *n.* surgical excision of the bone adjoining a joint.
骨關節端切除術 骨關節端的外科切除手術。

osteoblast *n.* a cell, originating in the mesoderm of the embryo, that is responsible for the formation of *bone. *See also* ossification.
成骨細胞 來源於胚胎中胚層的細胞。功能是骨的形成。

osteochondritis *n.* inflammation of a bone associated with pain: the deposition of abnormal bony tissue seen on X-ray (*see* osteosclerosis). The cause is not known and the condition is frequently self-limiting, though permanent deformity of the affected bone may result. Treatment is with analgesics. *See also* Köhler's disease, Legg-Calvé-Perthes disease.
This condition was formerly known as *osteochondrosis.*
骨軟骨炎 合併疼痛的骨炎症。X線照片上可見異常骨組織的沉積。病因不明。這種病的病程通常是自限的，但可留下骨組織永久性畸形。治療應用鎮痛藥。這種病從前稱爲骨軟骨病。

osteochondritis dissecans release of a small fragment (or fragments) of bone and cartilage into a joint, most frequently the knee, with resulting pain, swelling, and limitation of movement. If the condition persists, or relapses frequently, *arthrotomy, followed by extraction of the bone fragments, may be required.
分離性骨軟骨炎 關節腔中有骨和軟骨的碎片游離。多發生於膝關節，引起疼痛、腫脹和活動受限。如果這種病長期不癒或者經常復發，通過關節切開術摘除骨片則是必要的。

osteochondroma *n.* (*pl.* **osteochondromata**) a bone tumour composed of cartilage-forming cells. It appears as a painless mass, usually at the end of a long bone, and is most common between the ages of 10 and 25. As a small proportion of these tumours become malignant if untreated, they are excised.
骨軟骨瘤 類軟骨細胞形成的骨腫瘤。一般在長骨端出現無痛性團塊，多發年齡爲10～25歲。如果不進行治療，其中少數骨軟骨瘤發生惡變，就要進行手術切除。

osteochondrosis *n. see* osteochondritis.
骨軟骨病

osteoclasia (osteoclasis) *n.* **1.** the deliberate breaking of a malformed or
①**折骨術** 折斷畸形的或連接不正的骨，以矯正畸

malunited bone, carried out by a surgeon to correct deformity. Also called: **osteoclasty**. **2.** dissolution of bone through disease (*see* osteolysis).

形的外科手術。 ②**骨質溶解** 疾病導致的骨的溶解。

osteoclasis *n.* **1.** remodelling of bone by *osteoclasts, during growth or the healing of a fracture. **2.** *see* osteoclasia.

①**骨重建** 骨在生長或骨折痊癒後由於破骨細胞的作用發生的骨組織的重新排列。 ②**折骨術** ③**骨質溶解**

osteoclast *n.* **1.** a large multinucleate cell that resorbs calcified bone. Osteoclasts are only found when bone is being resorbed and may be seen in small depressions on the bone surface. **2.** a device for fracturing bone for therapeutic purposes.

①**破骨細胞** 重新吸收已鈣化的骨的大多核細胞。破骨細胞僅在骨質被吸收時出現，在骨表面表現爲細小的凹陷。 ②**折骨器** 爲了治療目的而折斷骨的器械。

osteoclastoma *n.* a rare tumour of bone, caused by proliferation of *osteoclast cells.

破骨細胞瘤 罕見的骨腫瘤。由破骨細胞的異常增生引起。

osteocyte *n.* a bone cell: an *osteoblast that has ceased activity and has become embedded in the bone matrix.

骨細胞 停止活動並且包埋在骨基質中的成骨細胞。

osteodystrophy *n.* any generalized bone disease resulting from a metabolic disorder. *Renal osteodystrophy* is the characteristic change in bones occurring in chronic kidney failure.

骨營養不良 代謝紊亂引起的全身性骨疾患的總稱。腎病性骨營養不良是在慢性腎衰時骨骼發生的特殊變化。

osteogenesis *n. see* ossification.

骨發生

osteogenesis imperfecta (fragilitas ossium) a congenital disorder in which the bones are unusually brittle and fragile. No treatment is available, but the tendency to fracture sometimes diminishes at adolescence.

成骨不全 骨骼的先天性疾病。骨質異常脆弱。治療無效，但是到了青春期骨折經常有減少的趨勢。

osteology *n.* the study of the structure and function of bones and related structures.

骨骼學 研究骨骼及與之有關的部分的功能和結構的學科。

osteolysis (osteoclasia) *n.* dissolution of bone through disease, commonly by infection or loss of the blood supply (ischaemia) to the bone. In *acro-osteolysis* the terminal bones of the fingers or toes are affected: a common

骨質溶解 疾病引起的骨的溶解。一般由感染或骨骼供血不足引起。肢骨質溶解影響指或趾的末端骨。某些侵犯血管的疾病（包括雷諾氏病）、硬皮

feature of some disorders involving blood vessels (including *Raynaud's disease), *scleroderma, and systemic *lupus erythematosus.

病和全身性紅斑狼瘡等皆可出現此種現象。

osteoma *n.* a benign bone tumour. A *cancellous osteoma* (*exostosis*) is an outgrowth from the end of a long bone, usually rising to a point. A *compact osteoma* (*ivory tumour*) is usually harmless but may rarely compress surrounding structures, as within the skull. An *osteoid osteoma* is an overgrowth of bone-forming cells, usually causing pain in the middle of a long bone. Compact and osteoid osteomas are treated by surgical excision.

骨瘤 艮性骨腫瘤。鬆質骨瘤是長骨端的突起物，常是尖形的。密質骨瘤經常是艮性的，偶可壓迫周圍組織，如顱骨瘤。骨樣骨瘤是成骨細胞過度增生的結果。經常引起長骨中間部位的疼痛。密質骨瘤和骨樣骨瘤需要手術切除治療。

osteomalacia *n.* softening of the bones caused by a deficiency of *vitamin D, either from a poor diet or lack of sunshine or both. It is the adult counterpart of *rickets. Vitamin D is necessary for the uptake of calcium from food; the deficiency therefore leads to progressive decalcification of bony tissues, often causing bone pain. The condition may become irreversible if treatment with vitamin D is not given. Osteomalacia is most common in the Middle and Far East, particularly in women of child-bearing age in whom calcium is lost from the skeleton during pregnancy.

骨軟化 維生素D缺乏引起的骨骼軟化。由於食物中缺乏維生素D或陽光照射不足，或者兩者同時存在。本病是成人的佝僂病。維生素D是從食物中攝取鈣所必需的物質：缺乏時導致進行性骨組織脫鈣，經常引起骨痛。如果不用維生素D進行治療，這種狀態將成爲不可逆的。骨軟化多見於中東、遠東，尤其是妊娠期骨骼中鈣減少的生育年齡的婦女。

osteomyelitis *n.* inflammation of the bone marrow due to infection. This is a hazard following compound fractures and must be rigorously guarded against whenever the marrow is exposed during bone or joint surgery. It may also be caused by blood-borne microorganisms. In *acute osteomyelitis*, most common in children, there is severe pain, swelling, and redness at the site, often in the shaft of a long bone, accompanied by general illness and high fever. *Chronic osteomyelitis* may follow the acute form or develop insidiously; tuberculosis and syphilis are occasional causes. Both forms are treated by anti-

骨髓炎 感染引起的骨髓炎症。本病是哆開性骨折的嚴重的併發症，在骨或關節手術時對暴露在外的骨髓必須嚴加保護。本病亦可由血源性感染引起。急性骨髓炎多發生於兒童，病變部位有劇痛、紅腫，多發生於長骨幹部，伴有全身症狀與高熱。慢性骨髓炎可由急性型轉變而來，或潛隱發生。結核與梅毒是可能的病因。兩種類型的治療都應用大劑量抗生素，某些病例則需要外科引流。不及時治療

biotics in high dosage, and in some cases drainage by surgery may be necessary. Delay in eradicating the infection may lead to bone shortening and deformity.

感染，可以導致骨的短縮和畸形。

osteopathy *n.* a system of healing based on the theory that most diseases are caused by displacement of bones from their correct positions. Treatment, by manipulation and massage, provides relief for many disorders of bones and joints. **—osteopath** *n.* **—osteopathic** *adj.*

整骨療法 有一種理論認爲，大多數疾病都是由於骨的位置不正產生的，根據這種理論產生了整骨療法。治療：應用手法推拿。此法可爲許多骨關節疾病解除痛苦。

osteopetrosis (Albers-Schönberg disease, marble-bone disease) *n.* a congenital abnormality in which bones become abnormally dense and brittle and tend to fracture. Affected bones appear unusually opaque to X-rays. *See also* osteosclerosis.

骨硬化病（阿爾伯斯-尙堡氏病，骨石化病）骨質異常緻密、脆弱，容易發生骨折的先天性病變。病變骨X線透過性異常減弱。

osteophyte *n.* a projection of bone, usually shaped like a rose thorn, that occurs at sites of cartilage degeneration or destruction near joints and intervertebral discs. Osteophyte formation is an X-ray sign of *osteoarthritis but is not a cause of symptoms in itself.

骨贅 骨的突起物。呈玫瑰刺狀，一般發生於軟骨變性部位或者關節和椎間盤破壞區附近。骨贅形成是骨關節炎的X線徵，但並非產生症狀的原因。

osteoporosis *n.* loss of bony tissue, resulting in bones that are brittle and liable to fracture. Infection, injury, and *synovitis can cause localized osteoporosis of adjacent bone. Generalized osteoporosis is common in the elderly, and in women often follows the menopause. It is also a feature of *Cushing's disease and prolonged steroid therapy. The condition may be prevented by oestrogen therapy in the menopause (this use of oestrogens is controversial).

骨質疏鬆〔症〕 骨組織缺乏。導致骨骼脆弱，容易發生骨折。感染、外傷和滑膜炎都能引起鄰近骨局部骨質疏鬆。全身性骨質疏鬆常見於老年人和絕經後的婦女。庫興氏病和長期應用皮質醇治療也可引起本病。在絕經期可以用雌激素（此法尙有爭議）預防發病。

osteosarcoma *n.* a malignant bone tumour. It is usually seen in children and adolescents but can occur in adults of all ages, often in association with *Paget's disease of bone. Osteosarcomas can also occur in soft tissue in elderly patients. In children the usual site for the tumour is the leg, particu-

骨肉瘤 惡性骨腫瘤。多見於兒童和青少年，也可發生於任何年齡的成年人，經常合併骨的變形性骨炎（佩季氏病）。骨肉瘤也能發生於老年病人的軟組織。兒童腫瘤的多發部位是腿，尤其是股骨。

larly the femur. Secondary growths (metastases) are common, most frequently in the lungs (though other sites, such as the liver, may also be involved). The symptoms are usually pain and swelling at the site of the tumour and there is often a history of preceding trauma, although it is doubtful whether this contributes to the cause. Treatment of disease localized to the primary site is by amputation of the limb. Many centres also give postoperative drug therapy in an attempt to kill any residual microscopic tumour that might have already spread. Drugs used include doxorubicin, vincristine, cyclophosphamide, and methotrexate.

轉移常見，肺部轉移最多（也可轉移到其他部位，如肝臟）。臨床症狀：常有腫瘤部位的疼痛和腫脹，病前常有外傷史，不過外傷是否爲病因尚未確定。治療：尚未轉移者用截肢術。許多醫院術後再用藥物療法以消滅任何可能轉移了的殘留的微小腫瘤。藥物包括阿黴素、長春新鹼、環磷醯胺和甲氨蝶呤。

osteosclerosis *n.* an abnormal increase in the density of bone, as a result of poor blood supply, chronic infection, or tumour. The affected bone is more opaque to X-rays than normal bone. *See also* osteopetrosis.

骨硬化 骨質密度的異常增加。係供血不足、慢性感染或者腫瘤引起。病變骨組織的X線透過性比正常骨組織弱得多。

osteotome *n.* a surgical chisel designed to cut bone (see illustration).

骨鑿 鑿骨用的外科鑿子（見圖）。

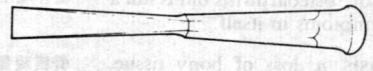

An osteotome
骨鑿

osteotomy *n.* a surgical operation to cut a bone into two parts, followed by realignment of the ends to allow healing. The operation is performed to reduce pain and disability in an arthritic joint, for cases in which conservative treatment has failed. Osteotomy of the jaws is performed to improve severe discrepancies in jaw relation.

切骨術 將骨切成兩部分，再將斷端重新結合以達到治療目的的外科手術。這種手術用於保守治療無效的關節炎患者，可減輕疼痛和恢復功能。頜切骨術用於改善頜關節的嚴重錯位。

ostium *n.* (*pl.* **ostia**) (in anatomy) an opening. The *ostium abdominale* is the opening of the Fallopian tube into the abdominal cavity.

口（解剖學）開口。腹腔口是輸卵管的腹腔內開口。

-ostomy *suffix. see* -stomy.

〔後綴〕**造口術，造瘻術，吻合術**

ot- (oto-) *prefix denoting* the ear. Example: *ototomy* (surgical incision of).

〔前綴〕**耳** 例如：耳切開術。

otalgia *n.* pain in the ear. Apart from local causes it may be due to a lesion of the geniculate ganglion of the facial nerve (*geniculate otalgia*) or to *herpes zoster affecting the facial nerve (Ramsay Hunt syndrome).

耳痛 耳的疼痛。除了局部原因以外，可能由面神經膝狀神經節的損害（膝狀神經節耳痛）或者是帶狀疱疹累及面神經所引起。

otic *adj.* relating to the ear.

耳的

otic capsule the cup-shaped cartilage in the head of an embryo that later develops into the bony *labyrinth of the ear.

耳囊 胚胎期頭部的杯狀軟骨。以後發展成爲耳的骨迷路。

otitis *n.* inflammation of the ear. *Otitis externa* is inflammation of the canal between the eardrum and the external opening of the ear (the external auditory meatus) and is often found in swimmers (*swimmer's ear*). *Otitis media* is inflammation, usually due to viral or bacterial infection, of the middle ear (the chamber lying behind the eardrum and containing the three bony ossicles that conduct sound to the inner ear). Symptoms include severe pain and a high fever; unless treated (with antibiotics), it may lead to conductive *deafness. *Secretory otitis media* (glue ear) is a chronic accumulation of fluid in the tympanic cavity, causing deafness (*see* grommet). *Otitis interna* (*labyrinthitis*) is inflammation of the inner ear, causing the sudden onset of vomiting, vertigo, and loss of balance.

耳炎 耳的炎症。外耳炎是鼓室與耳的外界開口之間的耳道（外耳道）的炎症，常見於游泳者（游泳者耳）。中耳炎經常是由病毒或細菌的感染引起的。中耳是位於鼓膜內方的腔室，有三塊向內耳傳達聲音的聽小骨。症狀包括：劇痛和高熱，如果不應用抗生素治療將導致傳導性耳聾。分泌性中耳炎（膠耳）是鼓室腔內液體的慢性蓄積，也能引起耳聾。內耳炎（迷路炎）是內耳的炎症，可引起突發性嘔吐、眩暈和身體平衡失調。

otoconium *n. see* otolith.

耳石

otocyst *n.* a small cavity in the mesoderm of the head of an embryo that later develops into the membranous *labyrinth of the ear.

聽囊 胚胎時位於頭部的中胚層的小腔。以後發展成爲耳的膜迷路。

otolaryngology *n.* the study of diseases of the ears and larynx.

耳喉科學 研究耳和喉科疾病的學科。

otolith (otoconium) *n.* one of the small particles of calcium carbonate associated with a macula in the *saccule or *utricle of the inner ear.

耳石 存在於內耳球囊或橢圓囊斑上的碳酸鈣微粒。

otology *n.* the study of diseases of the ear. **耳科學** 研究耳疾病的學科。

-otomy *suffix. see* -tomy. 〔後綴〕 **切開術**

otomycosis *n.* a fungus infection of the ear, causing irritation and inflammation of the canal between the eardrum and the external opening of the ear (external auditory meatus). It is one of the causes of *otitis externa. **耳眞菌病** 耳的眞菌感染。引起外耳道的感染和刺激症狀。是外耳炎的原因之一。

otoplasty *n.* surgical repair or reconstruction of the ears after injury or in the correction of a congenital defect (such as 'bat ears'). **耳成形術** 耳外傷後或者矯正先天性缺陷的外科修復或再建手術。

otorhinolaryngology *n.* the study of ear, nose, and throat diseases (i.e. ENT disorders). **耳鼻喉科學** 研究耳、鼻和咽喉疾病的學科。

otorrhagia *n.* bleeding from the ear. **耳出血**

otorrhoea *n.* any discharge from the ear, commonly a purulent discharge in chronic middle ear infection (*otitis media). **耳液溢** 耳有液體外溢的病變。一般指慢性中耳炎的膿性液溢。

otosclerosis *n.* a hereditary disorder causing deafness in adult life. An overgrowth of the bone of the inner ear leads to the third ear ossicle (the stapes) becoming fixed to the fenestra ovalis, which separates the middle and inner ears, so that sounds cannot be conducted to the inner ear. *Deafness is progressive and may become very severe, but surgical treatment is highly effective (*see* fenestration, stapedectomy). **耳硬化症** 引起成人耳聾的遺傳性疾病。由內耳骨生長出的突起物使第三塊聽小骨（鐙骨）固定在前庭窗上，把中耳和內耳隔開，這樣聲音就不能傳達到內耳。耳聾可以發展。而且可以變得非常嚴重，但是外科治療是非常有效的。

otoscope *n. see* auriscope. **耳鏡**

ouabain *n.* a drug that stimulates the heart and is used to treat heart failure and other heart conditions. It is administered by mouth or injection and has the same actions and side-effects as *digitalis. **苦毒毛旋花子甙** 治療心衰和其它心臟疾病的强心藥。口服或注射給藥，其作用和副作用與洋地黃相同。

outbreeding *n.* the production of offspring by parents who are not closely related. *Compare* inbreeding. **遠系繁殖** 由沒有明顯血緣關係的父母生育後代。

outer ear the pinna and the external auditory meatus of the *ear.

外耳 耳廓和外耳道的總稱。

out-patient *n.* a patient who receives treatment at a hospital, either at a single attendance or at a series of attendances, but is not admitted to a bed in a hospital ward. Large hospitals have *clinics at which out-patients with various complaints can be given specialist treatment. *Compare* in-patient.

門診病人 到醫院就醫的病人。可能是一次就診，也可能多次複診，但不住院。大醫院都設有門診部對各種病人進行專科治療。

oval window *see* fenestra (ovalis).

卵圓窗

ovari- (ovario-) *prefix denoting* the ovary.

〔前綴〕 **卵巢**

ovarian cyst a fluid-filled sac, one or more of which may develop in the ovary. Although most ovarian cysts are not malignant, they may reach a very large size or become twisted on their stalks, producing pain and vomiting. In such cases the cysts are usually surgically removed.

卵巢囊腫 卵巢單發或多發的充滿液體的囊腫。雖然多數卵巢囊腫不惡變，但是可以達到非常大的程度，或者形成蒂扭轉，引起疼痛和嘔吐。這樣的囊腫一般採取手術切除治療。

ovariectomy *n. see* oophorectomy.

卵巢切除術

ovariocele *n.* hernia of an ovary.

卵巢突出 卵巢的疝。

ovariocyesis *n. see* oocyesis.

卵巢妊娠

ovariotomy *n.* **1.** incision into or surgical removal of an ovary. **2.** surgical removal of a tumour of the ovary.

①**卵巢切開術，卵巢切除術** 卵巢的切開或切除手術。 ②**卵巢腫瘤切除術** 卵巢腫瘤的外科切除手術。

ovaritis *n. see* oophoritis.

卵巢炎

ovary *n.* the main female reproductive organ, which produces ova (egg cells) and steroid hormones in a regular cycle (*see* menstrual cycle) in response to hormones (*gonadotrophins) from the anterior pituitary gland. There are two ovaries, situated in the lower abdomen, one on each side of the womb (*see* reproductive system). Each ovary contains numerous *follicles*, within which the ova develop (see illustration), but only a small proportion of them reach maturity (*see* Graafian follicle, oogene-

卵巢 主要的雌性生殖器官。在垂體前葉激素（促性腺激素）的影響下周期地排卵和分泌固醇類激素。兩個卵巢位於下腹部子宮的兩側。每個卵巢都有大量的卵泡，卵子就在其中發育（見圖），但是達到成熟的卵子的比例極小。卵泡分泌雌激素和少量的雄激素。排卵後在破裂的卵泡部位形成的黃體分泌孕酮。雌激素和孕酮

sis). The follicles secrete *oestrogen and small amounts of androgen. After ovulation a *corpus luteum forms at the site of the ruptured follicle and secretes progesterone. Oestrogen and progesterone regulate the changes in the womb throughout the menstrual cycle and pregnancy. —**ovarian** *adj.*

在月經周期和妊娠期間調節子宮內變化。

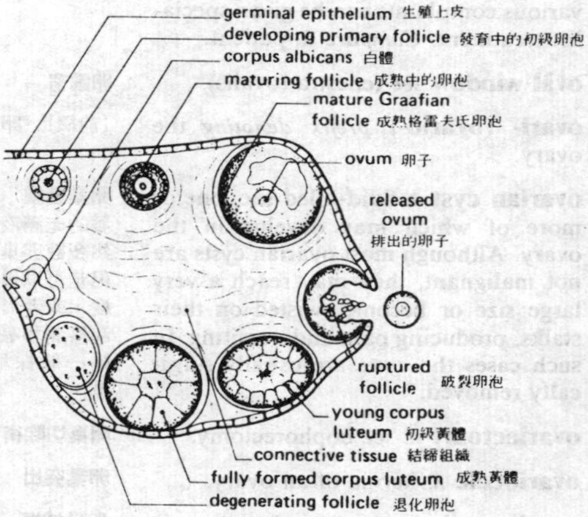

Section of the ovary showing ova in various stages of maturation
各種成熟階段的卵子的卵巢斷面圖

overbite *n.* the vertical overlap of the upper incisor teeth over the lower ones.

覆聆 上切牙與下切牙的垂直重疊。

overcompensation *n.* (in psychology) the situation in which a person tries to overcome a disability by making greater efforts than are required. This may result in the person becoming extremely efficient in what he (or she) is trying to achieve; alternatively, excessive overcompensation may be harmful to the person.

過度補償 （心理學）做出比實際需要更大的努力以克服能力缺陷的心理狀態。雖然這可以使人在工作中效果卓著，過份的過度補償却可以給人帶來危害。

overjet *n.* the horizontal overlap of the upper incisor teeth in front of the lower ones.

覆蓋 上切牙與下切牙前後的水平重疊。

overt *adj.* plainly to be seen or detected: applied to diseases with observa-

明顯的 容易察覺和容易發現的。描述那些有顯著

ble signs and symptoms, as opposed to those whose presence may not be suspected for years despite the fact that they cause insidious damage. An infectious disease becomes overt only at the end of an incubation period.

症狀和體徵的疾病。與此相反，另外一些疾病儘管引起隱性損害，却長期不能被發現。傳染病只有潛伏期末期才變得明顯起來。

ovi- (ovo-) *prefix denoting* an egg; ovum.

〔前綴〕 **卵，蛋**

oviduct *n. see* Fallopian tube.

輸卵管

ovulation *n.* the process by which an ovum is released from a mature *Graafian follicle. The fluid-filled follicle distends the surface of the ovary until a thin spot breaks down and the ovum floats out surrounded by a cluster of follicle cells (the cumulus oophoricus) and starts to travel down the Fallopian tube to the womb. Ovulation is stimulated by the secretion of *luteinizing hormone by the anterior pituitary gland.

排卵 卵子從成熟格雷夫氏卵胞釋放的過程。充滿液體的卵泡使卵巢表面膨脹，直到在一薄弱的部位破裂，被卵泡細胞團（卵丘）包埋着的卵子浮游出來，沿着輸卵管到達子宮。垂體前葉的促黃體激素的分泌促進排卵。

ovum (egg cell, vitellus) *n.* the mature female sex cell (*see* gamete). The term is often applied to the secondary *oocyte although this is technically incorrect. The final stage of meiosis occurs only when the oocyte has been activated by fertilization.

卵子 成熟的雌性性細胞。這個名詞經常用於次級卵母細胞，但這在專業上是錯誤的。只有在受精後次級卵母細胞被激活才開始進入減數分裂的後期。

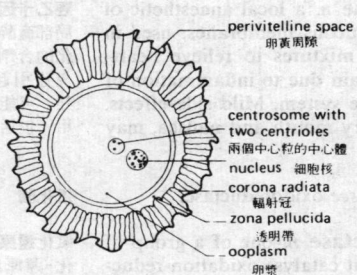

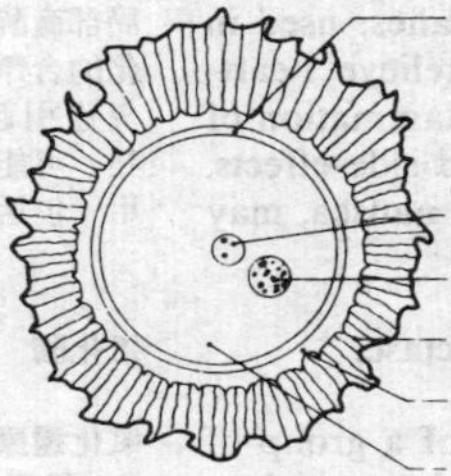

A mature ovum (magnification about x 600)
成熟卵子（放大約 600 倍）

oxacillin *n.* an antibiotic used to treat infections caused by a wide variety of bacteria. It is administered by mouth or injection; side-effects include allergic reactions and digestive upsets.

苯甲異噁唑青黴素 治療細菌感染的廣譜抗生素。口服或注射給藥。副作用包括過敏反應和消化道不適。

oxalic acid an extremely poisonous acid, $C_2H_2O_4$. It is a component of some bleaching powders and is found in many plants, including sorrel and the leaves of rhubarb. Oxalic acid is a powerful local irritant; when swallowed it produces burning sensations in the mouth and throat, vomiting of blood, breathing difficulties, and circulatory collapse. Treatment is with calcium lactate or other calcium salts, lime water, or milk.

草酸 劇毒性酸，$C_2H_2O_4$。是某些漂白粉的成分，也存在於許多植物中，包括酸模和大黃的葉。草酸是一種强烈的局部刺激藥，吞服後產生口咽部的灼熱的感覺、嘔血、呼吸困難以及循環性虛脱。治療應用乳酸鈣或其它鈣鹽、石灰水或奶液。

oxalosis *n.* an inborn defect of metabolism causing deposition of oxalate in the kidneys and elsewhere and eventually leading to renal failure.

草酸血症 草酸在腎臟和身體的其它部位蓄積的先天性代謝障礙。可以導致腎衰。

oxaluria *n.* the presence in the urine of oxalic acid or oxalates, especially calcium oxalate. Excessive amounts of oxalates are excreted in *oxalosis.

草酸尿 尿中出現草酸或草酸鹽，尤其是草酸鈣。草酸血症時尿中出現大量的草酸鹽。

oxazepam *n.* a tranquillizing drug used to relieve anxiety and tension and for the treatment of alcoholism. It is administered by mouth and commonly causes drowsiness. Trade name: **Serenid**. *See also* tranquillizer.

去甲羥基安定 安定藥。用於減輕焦慮和緊張，治療酒精中毒。口服。常引起嗜眠。商品名：舒寧。

oxethazaine *n.* a local anaesthetic of skin and mucous membranes, used in indigestion mixtures to relieve heartburn and pain due to inflammation of the digestive system. Mild side-effects, including dry mouth and nausea, may occur.

羥乙卡因 皮膚和黏膜的局部麻醉藥。用於不易消化的合劑以減輕消化系統炎症引起的疼痛和胃灼熱。可能出現輕微的副作用，包括口乾和噁心。

oxidase *n. see* oxidoreductase.

氧化酶

oxidoreductase *n.* one of a group of enzymes that catalyse oxidation-reduction reactions. This class includes the enzymes formerly known either as *dehydrogenases* or as *oxidases*.

氧化還原酶 一組催化氧化-還原反應的酶。這類酶包括過去稱爲脱氫酶或氧化酶等類的酶。

oximeter *n.* an instrument for measuring the proportion of oxygenated haemoglobin (oxyhaemoglobin) in the blood.

血氧計 檢測血液中載氧血紅蛋白（氧合血紅蛋白）的儀器。

oxolinic acid an antibacterial drug used to treat infections of the urinary system. It is administered by mouth; side-effects may include digestive upsets and disturbances of vision. Trade name: **Prodoxol**.

噁喹酸 治療泌尿系統感染的抗生素。口服。副作用包括消化系統不適和視覺障礙。

oxprenolol *n.* a drug that controls the activity of the heart (*see* beta blocker), used to treat angina, high blood pressure, and abnormal heart rhythm. It is administered by mouth or injection; side-effects may include dizziness, drowsiness, headache, and digestive upsets. Trade name: **Trasicor**.

烯丙氧心安 調節心臟功能的藥物。用於治療心絞痛、高血壓和心律失常。口服或注射。副作用包括頭暈、嗜睡、頭痛和消化道不適。商品名：心得安。

oxycephaly (turricephaly) *n.* a deformity of the bones of the skull giving the head a pointed appearance. —**oxycephalic** *adj.*

尖頭〔畸形〕 頭呈尖狀的顱骨畸形。

oxygen *n.* an odourless colourless gas that makes up one-fifth of the atmosphere. Oxygen is essential to most forms of life in that it combines chemically with glucose (or some other fuel) to provide energy for metabolic processes. In man oxygen is absorbed into the blood from air breathed into the lungs. Oxygen is administered therapeutically in various conditions in which the tissues are unable to obtain an adequate supply through the lungs (*see* oxygenator, (oxygen) tent). Symbol: O.

氧 無色、無味的氣體。佔空氣的五分之一。氧是大多數以氧化葡萄糖（或某些其它能源）作爲代謝過程中能源的生命的基礎。人體中的氧是通過呼吸空氣進入肺而被血液吸收的。在各種通過肺吸收的氧不能滿足組織需要的疾病中，吸氧有治療作用。

oxygenator *n.* a machine that oxygenates blood outside the body. It is used together with pumps to maintain the patient's circulation while he is undergoing open heart surgery (*see* heart-lung machine) or to improve the circulation of a patient with heart or lung disorders that lower the amount of blood oxygen.

氧合器 體外血液充氧的器械。與泵一起使用以維持心臟外科手術病人的血液循環，或者改善血氧含量低的心、肺疾病患者的循環。

oxygen deficit a physiological condition that exists in cells during periods of temporary oxygen shortage. During periods of violent exertion the body requires extra energy, which is obtained

缺氧 暫時性氧缺乏期間細胞的生理狀態。過勞期間，身體需要額外的能量，在氧缺乏的情況下，以葡萄糖分解來獲得能

by the breakdown of glucose in the absence of oxygen, after the available oxygen has been used up. The breakdown products are acidic and cause muscle pain. The oxygen required to get rid of the breakdown products (called the oxygen deficit) must be made available after the exertion stops.

量。分解產物是酸性的，可引起肌肉疼痛。消除分解產物所需要的氧（稱爲氧債）必須在勞動停止後才能償還。

oxygen tent *see* tent.

氧幕

oxyhaemoglobin *n.* the bright-red substance formed when the pigment *haemoglobin in red blood cells combines reversibly with oxygen. Oxyhaemoglobin is the form in which oxygen is transported from the lungs to the tissues, where the oxygen is released. *Compare* methaemoglobin.

氧合血紅蛋白 紅細胞的血紅蛋白與氧可逆性結合時形成的鮮紅物質。氧以氧合血紅蛋白的形式從肺被輸送並釋放到組織中。

oxymesterone *n.* a synthetic male sex hormone with body-building action. It has the same action and uses as *methandienone.

羥甲睾酮 人工合成的雄性性激素。具有促進身體合成代謝的功能。作用與去氫甲基睾丸素相同，用途也類似。

oxyntic cells (parietal cells) cells of the *gastric glands that secrete hydrochloric acid in the fundic region of the stomach.

泌酸細胞（壁細胞） 胃腺細胞。位於胃的基底部，分泌鹽酸。

oxypertine *n.* a major *tranquillizer used to treat anxiety and tension in mental illnesses such as schizophrenia. It is administered by mouth and commonly causes drowsiness, dizziness, and restlessness, especially in high doses. Trade name: **Integrin**.

氧苯哌吲哚 重要的安定藥。用於治療像精神分裂症這樣的精神病引起的焦慮和緊張。口服。經常引起頭暈、嗜眠和坐立不安，尤其是在大劑量服用時。商品名：奥潑定。

oxyphenbutazone *n.* an *analgesic that also reduces inflammation and fever. It is used mainly to relieve pain in rheumatoid arthritis, gout, and similar conditions. It is administered by mouth or in suppositories; common side-effects include nausea, rashes, dizziness, and mouth ulcers. Trade name: **Tanderil**.

羥基保泰松 解熱、抗炎、鎮痛藥。主要用於治療類風濕性關節炎、痛風和類似疾病引起的疼痛。口服或應用栓劑。經常出現的副作用包括噁心、蕁疹、頭暈和口腔潰瘍。

oxyphencyclimine *n.* a drug with actions similar to *atropine. Since it

羥苯環嘧 作用類似阿托品的藥物。由於其吸收過

slows down the digestive processes, it is used to treat stomach and duodenal ulcers and other digestive disorders. It is administered by mouth; side-effects include dry mouth, thirst, and disturbances of vision. Trade name: **Daricon**.

程緩慢，被用於治療胃和十二指腸潰瘍以及其它消化系統疾病。口服。副作用包括口乾、口渴和視覺障礙。

oxytetracycline *n.* an *antibiotic used to treat infections caused by a wide variety of bacteria. It is administered by mouth or injection or applied to the skin in a cream; side-effects are those of the other *tetracyclines. Trade names: **Abbocin, Berkmycen, Clinimycin, Galenomycin, Imperacin, Oxydon, Oxymycin, Stecsolin, Terramycin, Unimycin.**

氧四環素　治療細菌感染的廣譜抗生素。口服或注射，也可以用其乳膏劑塗於皮膚。副作用與其它四環素類藥物相同。商品名：土黴素。

oxytocia *n.* labour and childbirth of exceptionally short duration.

分娩急速　在特別短的時間內的分娩。

oxytocic *n.* a drug that induces or accelerates labour by stimulating the muscles of the womb to contract. *See also* oxytocin.

催產藥　使子宮平滑肌收縮，導致或促進分娩的藥物。

oxytocin *n.* a hormone, released by the pituitary gland, that causes increased contraction of the womb during labour and stimulates the ejection of milk from the breasts. Oxytocin may be given by mouth or injection to assist labour.

〔後葉〕催產素　垂體釋放的一種激素。在分娩期間增加子宮的收縮力，並且刺激乳房的奶液分泌。人工合成的催產素可以口服或注射以幫助分娩。

oxyuriasis *n. see* enterobiasis.

蟯蟲病

Oxyuris *n. see* pinworm.

尖尾線蟲屬

ozaena *n.* a disorder of the nose in which the bones forming the sides of the nasal cavity become atrophied, with the production of an offensive discharge and crusts.

臭鼻〔症〕　鼻腔兩翼骨性部分萎縮，產生刺激性分泌物並結痂的鼻疾病。

ozone *n.* a poisonous gas containing three oxygen atoms per molecule. Ozone is a very powerful oxidizing agent and is formed when oxygen or air is subjected to electric discharge. Ozone is found in the atmosphere at very high altitudes and is responsible for destroying a large proportion of the sun's ultraviolet radiation. Without this absorption by ozone the earth would be

臭氧　每分子含有三個氧原子的刺激性氣體。臭氧是極强的氧化劑，在氧或空氣發生放電現象時形成。臭氧存在於大氣層的高層，對自然光中紫外線輻射具有很大的破壞作用。沒有臭氧的這種吸收作用，地球將遭受致命量的紫外線輻射。

subjected to a lethal amount of ultraviolet radiation.

P

P

Pacchionian body *see* arachnoid villus. **蛛網膜粒**

pacemaker *n.* **1.** a device used to produce and maintain a normal heart rate in patients who have *heart block. The unit consists of a battery that stimulates the heart through an insulated electrode wire attached to the surface of the ventricle (*epicardial pacemaker*) or lying in contact with the lining of the heart (*endocardial pacemaker*). A pacemaker may be used as a temporary measure with an external battery or it may be permanent, when the whole apparatus is surgically implanted under the skin. Some pacemakers stimulate the heart at a fixed rate; others sense when the natural heart rate falls below a predetermined value and then stimulate the heart (*demand pacemaker*). **2.** the part of the heart that regulates the rate at which it beats: the *sinoatrial node.

①**起搏器**　心臟傳導阻滯病人用於心臟起搏和維持正常心律的裝置。該裝置由一電池組成，通過絕緣電極線與心外膜相連（心外膜起搏器）或與心內膜相連（心內膜起搏器）以刺激心臟。起搏器與外接電池相連，可作爲臨時起搏措施；用手術將整個起搏器植入皮下，也可作爲持久起搏措施。有的起搏器是以固定頻率刺激心臟；有的起搏器是在心臟自發頻率低於預定值時才起作用（按需心臟起搏器）。②**起搏點**　心臟中調節心律的部位，稱作竇房結。

pachy- *prefix denoting* **1.** thickening of a part or parts. **2.** the dura mater. 〔前綴〕 ①**部分增厚** ②**硬腦〔脊〕膜**

pachydactyly *n.* abnormal enlargement of the fingers and toes, occurring either as a congenital abnormality or as part of an acquired disease (such as *acromegaly).

指（趾）肥大　手指或脚趾異常增大。可以是先天性的疾病，也可以是後天性疾病的一種表現（如肢端巨大症）。

pachydermia *n.* any abnormal thickening of the skin. **皮肥厚**　皮膚異常增厚。

pachyglossia *n.* abnormal thickness of the tongue. **舌肥厚**　舌異常增厚。

pachymeningitis *n.* inflammation of the dura mater, one of the membranes (meninges) covering the brain and spinal cord (*see* meningitis).

硬腦（脊）膜炎　覆蓋於腦和脊髓的硬腦脊膜層發生的炎症。

pachymeninx *n.* the *dura mater, outermost of the three meninges.

硬腦（脊）膜 三層腦膜的最外一層。

pachyonychia *n.* thickening of the nails. Rarely, this may occur as an inherited disease.

甲肥厚 指（趾）甲的增厚。是一種少見病。可見於遺傳性疾病。

pachysomia *n.* thickening of parts of the body, which occurs in certain diseases.

軀體肥厚 身體某部分增厚。見於某些疾病。

pachytene *n.* the third stage of the first prophase of *meiosis, in which *crossing over begins.

粗線期 減數分裂前期第一期的第三階段。該期染色體開始交換。

Pacinian corpuscles sensory receptors for touch in the skin, consisting of sensory nerve endings surrounded by capsules of membrane in 'onion-skin' layers. They are especially sensitive to changes in pressure and so detect vibration particularly well.

環層小體 皮內觸覺感受器。由許多呈同心層排列（洋葱皮樣）的被囊包繞，中央爲感覺神經末梢。它們對壓力變化，尤其是震動覺特别敏感。

pack *n.* a pad of folded moistened material, such as cotton-wool, applied to the body or inserted into a cavity.

敷料 用潮濕的脫脂棉等摺叠成墊。用以包敷體表或塡塞腔洞。

packed cell volume (haematocrit) the volume of the red cells (erythrocytes) in blood, expressed as a fraction of the total volume of the blood. The packed cell volume is determined by centrifuging blood in a tube and measuring the height of the red-cell column as a fraction of the total.

紅細胞壓積 紅細胞在血液中的容積。用紅細胞在血液整個容積中所佔百分比來表示。紅細胞壓積是將試管中血液離心沉澱，測量紅細胞柱的高度，並算出它佔總血量的百分比數。

pad *n.* cotton-wool, foam rubber, or other material used to protect a part of the body from friction, bruising, or other unwanted contact.

墊 用脫脂棉、泡沫塑料或其他材料製做的墊子。用來保獲身體某部分，以防受到磨擦、挫傷或其他不必要的接觸。

paed- (paedo-) *prefix denoting* children.

〔前綴〕 **兒童**

paederasty *n.* *sodomy with a boy or a young man.

鷄奸兒童 對男性兒童或青少年的一種違反道德的性變態行爲。

paediatrics *n.* the general medicine of childhood. Handling the sick child requires a special approach at every age from birth (or premature birth) to adolescence and also a proper under-

兒科學 兒科學專業的總稱。處理從出生（或早產）至青春期的各階段兒童疾病需要不同的特殊方法，對父母情況也需有適

standing of parents. It also requires detailed knowledge of genetics, obstetrics, psychological development, management of handicaps at home and in school, and effects of social conditions on child health. The preventive measures associated with all these aspects of paediatrics are the concern of *community physicians (child health) of area health authorities or community paediatricians (hospital-based *consultants). *See also* child health clinic. —**paediatrician** *n.*

當的了解。兒科醫生還必須具備遺傳學、產科學、生理發育、家庭和學校對殘疾兒童的護理，以及社會環境對兒童健康的影響等方面的詳盡的知識。有關以上各方面的預防措施，則是地方保健局的公共保健醫師與醫院的兒科保健醫師所關心的內容。

paedodontics *n.* the branch of dentistry concerned with the care and treatment of children's teeth.

兒童牙科學 牙科的一個分支學科。專門研究兒童期牙齒保健與牙病治療。

paedophilia *n.* sexual attraction to children (of either sex). Sexual activity with any children under the age of 16 is illegal in the UK. The condition is usually caused by psychological and social factors, which affect the development of sexuality. Paedophiles may seek treatment because of society's disapproval: *behaviour therapy can be used, or the sexual drive can be reduced by drug treatment. —**paedophile** *n.* —**paedophilic** *adj.*

戀童癖 對男性或女性兒童產生的性戀。在英國與任何不滿16歲兒童發生性行爲都是非法的。這種異常性行爲常由於心理因素和社會因素所引起。這種疾病影響性生理的正常發育。患者由於受到社會非難，要求治療。可用行爲療法或藥物治療來抑制性衝動。

Paget's disease 1. a chronic disease of bones, occurring in the elderly and most frequently affecting the skull, backbone, pelvis, and long bones. Affected bones become thickened and their structure disorganized: X-rays reveal patchy *sclerosis. Severe continuous pain may result, which is relieved by a prolonged course of *thyrocalcitonin injections. Medical name: **osteitis deformans**. **2.** an inflammatory condition of the nipple, resembling eczema in appearance, associated with underlying cancer of the milk ducts of the breast. *See also* breast cancer.

①**變形性骨炎** 骨的一種慢性疾病。見於老年人，最常侵襲的部位是頭顱、脊柱、骨盆及長骨。受侵部位的骨組織變厚，其結構遭到破壞。X線可見斑片狀硬化。該病可引起持續性的劇痛，長期注射降血鈣素可減輕。 ②**乳頭乳暈炎性癌變** 乳頭的一種炎症。外觀與濕疹相似，併發於潛伏的乳腺癌。

paint *n.* (in pharmacy) a liquid preparation that is applied to the skin or mucous membranes. Paints usually

塗劑 藥物的一種劑型。塗於皮膚或黏膜的一種液體製劑。塗劑中常含有消

contain antiseptics, astringents, caustics, or analgesics.
毒劑、收斂劑、腐蝕劑或鎮痛藥等。

palaeo- *prefix denoting* **1.** ancient. **2.** primitive.
〔前綴〕 **①老，古，舊 ②原始的，初級的**

palaeocerebellum *n.* the anterior lobe of the cerebellum. In evolutionary terms it is one of the earliest parts of the hindbrain to develop in mammals.
舊小腦 小腦前葉。在進化過程中，哺乳動物的小腦前葉是後腦（菱腦）最早生長發育部位之一。

palaeopathology *n.* the study of the diseases of man and other animals in prehistoric times, from examination of their bones or other remains. By examining the bones of specimens of Neanderthal man it has been discovered that spinal arthritis was a disease that existed at least 50,000 years ago.
古生物病理學 用檢查古人或古獸遺骨或遺跡的方法來研究史前期人與其他動物疾病的學科。通過對尼安德特爾人骨標本檢查，人們發現脊柱關節炎是一種至少在五萬年以前就已存在的疾病。

palaeostriatum *n. see* pallidum.
舊紋狀體

palaeothalamus *n.* the anterior and central part of the *thalamus, older in evolutionary terms than the lateral part, the neothalamus, which is well developed in apes and man.
舊丘腦 丘腦前部與中央部。在進化過程中，它們比丘腦側部（新丘腦）生成較早。新丘腦在人類與猿類發育良好。

palate *n.* the roof of the mouth, which separates the mouth from the nasal cavity and consists of two portions. The *hard palate*, at the front of the mouth, is formed by processes of the maxillae and palatine bones and is covered by mucous membrane. The *soft palate*, further back, is a movable fold of mucous membrane that tapers at the back of the mouth to form a fleshy hanging flap of tissue – the *uvula*.
腭 口腔頂部。它將口腔與鼻腔隔開。腭由硬腭與軟腭兩部分組成。硬腭位於口腔前部，由上頜骨突和腭骨構成，並被黏膜覆蓋。軟腭在口腔後部深處，是塊可移動的黏膜皺襞。該皺襞在口腔底部逐漸變窄，形成一條懸垂的肉質瓣組織——懸雍垂。

palatine bone either of a pair of approximately L-shaped bones of the face that contribute to the hard *palate, the nasal cavity, and the orbits. *See* skull.
腭骨 面部一對近似"L"形的骨。它構成硬腭、鼻腔與眼眶的一部分。

palato- *prefix denoting* **1.** the palate. **2.** the palatine bone.
〔前綴〕 **①腭 ②腭骨**

palatoplasty *n.* plastic surgery of the roof of the mouth, usually to correct cleft palate or other defects present at birth.
腭成形術 口腔頂部成形手術。通常用以矯正腭裂或其他在出生時就出現的缺損。

palatorrhaphy *n. see* staphylorrhaphy.
腭裂縫合術

pali- (palin-) *prefix denoting* repetition or recurrence.

〔前綴〕 **重複，復發**

palilalia *n.* a disorder of speech in which a word spoken by the individual is rapidly and involuntarily repeated. It is seen, with other tics, in the *Gilles de la Tourette syndrome. It is also encountered when encephalitis or other processes damage the *extrapyramidal system of the brain.

言語重複 一種語言障礙。患者講話時，吐字速度快，並且不自主地重複。圖雷特氏綜合徵的病人可有此症狀，並伴有其他抽搐症狀。腦炎或其他病變引起腦錐體外系受損的病人也可出現此症狀。

palindromic *adj.* relapsing: describing diseases or symptoms that recur or get worse.

復發的，再發的，回歸的 用以描述疾病或症狀的復發或惡化。

palingraphia *n.* writing in which the words and letters are reversed so that they appear as mirror images. Adoption of this as a consistent style is usually a matter of voluntary choice or is *hysterical; very occasionally it follows brain damage. Mirror-image reversals of single letters are common in children learning to write and in older children whose language abilities are impaired.

倒寫症 寫出的單詞和字母是顛倒的，呈鏡像樣。採用這一固定寫法，通常是故意的或是歇斯底里性的；腦損傷的病人偶爾也可有此現象。初學書寫的兒童或患言語障礙的大齡兒童反寫個別字母也是常見的。

paliphrasia *n.* repetition of phrases while speaking: a form of *stammering or a kind of *tic.

短語重複 講話時反復重複某一短語，並伴有口吃或抽搐。

palliative *n.* a medicine that gives temporary relief from the symptoms of a disease but does not actually cure the disease. Palliatives are often used in the treatment of such diseases as cancer.

姑息劑 使病人暫時緩解症狀，但實際上並不能治癒疾病的藥物。姑息劑常用以對付諸如癌症一類的疾病。

pallidectomy *n.* a neurosurgical operation to destroy or modify the effects of the globus pallidus (*see* basal ganglia). This operation was used for the relief of *parkinsonism and other conditions in which involuntary movements are prominent.

蒼白球切開術 一種破壞或改變蒼白球作用的神經外科手術。該手術用以緩解帕金森氏綜合徵及其他以不自主運動症狀爲主的疾病的症狀。

pallidum (palaeostriatum) *n.* one of the dense collections of grey matter, deep in each cerebral hemisphere, that go to make up the *basal ganglia.

蒼白球 大腦灰質密集匯合的一部分。位於每側大腦半球深部，構成腦基底神經節。

pallium *n.* the outer wall of the cerebral hemisphere as it appears in the

大腦蒼白質 哺乳動物腦進化的早期階段的大腦半

early stages of evolution of the mammalian brain. In the modern brain it corresponds to the *cerebral cortex.

球外壁。相當於現代動物的大腦皮質。

pallor *n.* abnormal paleness of the skin, due to reduced blood flow or lack of normal pigments. Pallor may be associated with an indoor mode of life; it may also indicate shock, anaemia, cancer, or other diseases.

蒼白 由於血流量減少或正常色素缺少所引起的皮膚異常發白。蒼白可能與缺乏戶外活動有關，也可能是休克、貧血、癌症或其他疾病的一種表現。

palmitic acid *see* fatty acid.

軟脂酸

palpation *n.* the process of examining part of the body by careful feeling with the hands and fingertips. Using palpation it is possible, in many cases, to distinguish between swellings that are solid and those that are cystic (*see* fluctuation). Palpation is also used to discover the presence of a fetus in the womb (*see* ballottement).

觸診 用手與指尖仔細觸摸來檢查人體某部位的方法。觸診可用以鑑別多種疾病的實性腫物與囊性腫物，也可用以檢查宮內的胎兒。

palpebral *adj.* relating to the eyelid (palpebra).

瞼的 與眼瞼有關的。

palpitation *n.* an awareness of the heart beat. This is normal with fear, emotion, or exertion. It may also be a symptom of neurosis, arrhythmias, heart disease, and overactivity of the circulation (as in thyrotoxicosis).

心悸 心臟跳動的感覺。人在恐懼、激動或用力過度時感覺到心跳是正常的。心悸也能是神經質、心律不齊、心臟病，以及血循環過速的（像甲狀腺毒症的）症狀。

palsy *n.* paralysis. This archaic word is retained in compound terms, such as *Bell's palsy, *cerebral palsy, and *Todd's palsy.

麻痹 這是保留在複合詞中使用的舊詞，像面神經麻痹，大腦性麻痹和托德氏麻痹等。

paludism *n. see* malaria.

瘧疾

pan- (pant(o)-) *prefix denoting* all; every: hence (in medicine) affecting all parts of an organ or the body; generalized.

〔前綴〕 **全部，廣泛** 在醫學方面指影響全身的或整個器官的；普遍性的。

panacea *n.* a medicine said to be a cure for all diseases and disorders, no matter what their nature. Unfortunately panaceas do not exist, despite the claims of many patent medicine manufacturers.

萬應藥 據説是一種能治癒各種疾病的藥物，不管是何種疑難病症。儘管許多專賣藥的製造商聲稱生產出了此藥，但遺憾的是萬應藥根本不存在。

Panadol *n. see* paracetamol.

醋氨酚

pancarditis *n. see* endomyocarditis.

全心炎

pancreas *n.* a compound gland, about 15 cm long, that lies behind the stomach. One end lies in the curve of the duodenum; the other end touches the spleen. It is composed of clusters (*acini*) of cells that secrete *pancreatic juice. This contains a number of enzymes concerned in digestion. The juice drains into small ducts that open into the *pancreatic duct*. This unites with the common *bile duct and the secretions pass into the duodenum. Interspersed among the acini are the *islets of Langerhans – isolated groups of cells that secrete the hormones *insulin and *glucagon into the bloodstream.

胰腺 一種位於胃後長約 15 cm 的複合腺，其一端在十二指腸彎曲部，另一端與脾相接。胰腺由分泌胰液的細胞團（腺泡）組成。胰液含有多種消化酶。胰液排入通向胰管的小導管。胰管與總膽管匯合，其分泌液流入十二指腸。腺泡中分佈有胰島（郎格罕氏島——孤立的細胞團），它們向血液中分泌胰島素和高血糖素等激素。

pancreas divisum a congenital abnormality in which the pancreas develops in two parts draining separately into the duodenum, the small ventral pancreas through the main ampulla and the larger dorsal pancreas through an accessory papilla. In rare instances this is associated with recurrent abdominal pain, probably due to inadequate drainage of the dorsal pancreas. Diagnosis is made by *ERCP.

胰腺分離 一種先天畸形。在胰腺發育過程中，形成了兩個胰腺，各個胰腺的胰管都分別開口於十二指腸。小的腹胰以主胰管開口於壺腹部，較大的背胰以副胰管開口於乳頭。少數病人可伴有反覆發作性腹痛，這很可能是由於背胰引流異常所致。用內窺鏡逆行性胰膽管造影術可作出診斷。

pancreatectomy *n.* surgical removal of the pancreas. *Total pancreatectomy* (*Whipple's operation*) involves the entire gland and part of the duodenum. In *subtotal pancreatectomy* most of the gland is removed, usually leaving a small part close to the duodenum. In *partial pancreatectomy* only a portion of the gland is removed. The operations are performed for tumours in the gland or because of chronic or relapsing *pancreatitis. After total or subtotal pancreatectomy it is necessary to administer pancreatic enzymes with food to aid its digestion and insulin injections to replace that normally secreted by the gland.

胰腺切除術 切除胰腺的手術。胰腺全切術（惠普爾氏手術）是指切除全部胰腺及部分十二指腸。胰腺次全切術指切除大部分胰腺，通常留下靠近十二指腸的小部分。胰腺部分切除術，指僅切除一部分胰腺。胰腺腫瘤、慢性或反復發作性胰腺炎患者均適宜做胰腺切除手術。在做胰腺全切手術或次全切手術後，病人有必要在進食的同時服用胰酶以助消化，並注射胰島素以代替胰腺的正常分泌。

pancreatic juice the digestive juice secreted by the *pancreas. Its pro-

胰液 胰腺分泌的消化液。十二指腸受到來自胃

duction is stimulated by hormones secreted by the duodenum, which in turn is stimulated by contact with food from the stomach. If the duodenum produces the hormone *secretin the pancreatic juice contains a large amount of sodium bicarbonate, which neutralizes the acidity of the stomach contents. Another hormone (*see* cholecystokinin-pancreozymin) causes the production of a juice rich in digestive enzymes, including trypsinogen and chymotrypsinogen (which are converted to *trypsin and *chymotrypsin in the duodenum), *amylase, *lipase, and *maltase.

中食物接觸刺激隨之分泌激素，該激素又刺激胰腺分泌消化液。如果十二指腸分泌了腸促胰液素，胰液就會含有大量可中和胃酸的碳酸氫鈉。另一種激素可促使生成一種富含多種消化酶的消化液，該消化液的消化酶包括胰蛋白酶原、胰凝乳蛋白酶原（在十二指腸內分別轉化爲胰蛋白酶和胰凝乳蛋白酶）、澱粉酶、脂酶和麥芽糖酶等。

pancreatin *n.* an extract obtained from the *pancreas, containing the pancreatic enzymes. Pancreatin is administered for conditions in which pancreatic secretion is deficient; for example, in pancreatitis.

胰酶　從胰腺中提取的一種含有胰酶的物質。胰酶用於胰腺分泌物不足的病人，例如，胰腺炎患者。

pancreatitis *n.* inflammation of the pancreas. *Acute pancreatitis* is a sudden illness in which the patient experiences severe pain in upper abdomen and back, with shock; its cause is uncertain. It may be mistaken for a perforated peptic ulcer but differs from this condition in that the level of the enzyme *amylase in the blood is raised. The main complication is formation of a *pseudocyst. Treatment consists of intravenous feeding (no food or drink should be given by mouth), and *anticholinergic drugs. *Relapsing pancreatitis*, in which the above symptoms are recurrent and less severe, may be associated with gallstones or alcoholism; prevention is by removal of gallstones and avoidance of alcohol and fat. *Chronic pancreatitis* may produce symptoms similar to relapsing pancreatitis or may be painless; it leads to pancreatic failure causing *malabsorption and *diabetes mellitus. The pancreas often becomes calcified, producing visible shadowing on X-rays. The

胰腺炎　胰腺的炎症。急性胰腺炎是一種突發性疾病，發病時病人感覺到上腹部和背部劇痛，可併發休克。病因不明。該病易誤診爲消化性潰瘍穿孔，但急性胰腺炎病人血中澱粉酶常升高。主要併發症是形成假性囊腫。治療：靜脉輸注營養液（不得經口腔進食和給水）和給予抗膽鹼藥。復發性胰腺炎病人的上述症狀是反覆發作性的，但程度較輕，也可能併發膽石症或酒精中毒，預防措施是摘除膽石、禁酒與限制脂肪類食物。慢性胰腺炎病人的症狀可能與復發性胰腺炎相類似，或可能無疼痛症狀。該病可導致胰腺衰竭，引起營養吸收障礙和糖尿病。做X線檢查時，可見胰腺鈣化陰影。治療：伴有吸收障礙的病人，在低脂飲食的同時，

malabsorption is treated by a low-fat diet with pancreatic enzyme supplements, and the diabetes with insulin.

給予胰酶，糖尿病人給予胰島素製劑。

pancreatogram *n.* a radiographic image of the pancreatic ducts obtained by injecting a contrast medium into them by direct puncture under *ultrasound guidance, at the time of laparotomy or by *ERCP.

胰腺圖 施行剖腹術或內窺鏡逆行性胰膽管造影術時，在超聲波指導下，直接給胰腺穿刺注射造影劑所取得的胰管X線圖像。

pancreatotomy *n.* surgical opening of the duct of the pancreas in order to inspect the duct, to join the duct to the intestine, or to inject contrast material in order to obtain X-ray pictures of the duct system.

胰切開術 爲了檢查胰管或使胰管與腸相吻合，或者爲了拍攝胰管系統X線圖像注射造影劑而施行的胰管切開手術。

pancreozymin *n. see* cholecystokinin-pancreozymin.

促胰酶素

pancytopenia *n.* a simultaneous decrease in the numbers of red cells (*anaemia), white cells (*neutropenia), and platelets (*thrombocytopenia) in the blood. It occurs in a variety of disorders, including aplastic *anaemias, *hypersplenism, and tumours of the bone marrow.

全血細胞减少 血液中紅細胞（貧血）、白細胞（中性白細胞减少症）、血小板（血小板减少症）的數量同時减少。見於再生障礙性貧血、脾功能亢進、骨髓瘤等各種疾病。

pandemic *n.* an *epidemic so widely spread that vast numbers of people in different countries are affected. The Black Death, the epidemic plague that ravaged Europe in the fourteenth century and killed over one third of the population, was a classical pandemic. —**pandemic** *adj.*

大流行病 一種流行廣泛，使得不同國家的絕大多數人遭受傳染的流行病。十四世紀歐洲流行黑死病（鼠疫），，造成三分之一以上的人口死亡，是歷史上有名的一次瘟疫大流行。

panhysterectomy *n.* the surgical removal of the entire womb, including its neck (cervix). *See* hysterectomy.

全子宮切除術 包括宮頸在內的整個子宮切除手術。

panhysterocolpectomy *n.* surgical removal of the entire womb and the vagina.

全子宮陰道切除術 切除整個子宮和陰道的手術。

panhystero-oophorectomy *n.* surgical removal of the entire womb and of one or both ovaries.

全子宮卵巢切除術 切除全部子宮並摘除一側或雙側卵巢的手術。

panhysterosalpingo-oophorectomy *n.* surgical removal of the entire womb, the ovaries, and the *Fallopian tubes.

全子宮輸卵管卵巢切除術 切除全部子宮、卵巢和輸卵管的手術。

panmixis *n.* random mating within a population, i.e. when there is no selection of partners on religious, racial, social, or other grounds.

隨機交配 羣體中隨意婚配，也就是說選擇配偶不受宗教、種族、社會地位或其他因素的影響。

panniculitis *n.* inflammation of the layer of fat beneath the skin (*panniculus adiposus*), leading to multiple tender nodules in the thighs, trunk, and breasts. When there are other features, including fever and enlargement of the liver and spleen, the condition is known as the *Weber-Christian disease*.

脂膜炎 皮下脂肪層（脂膜）的炎症。可使大腿、軀幹、乳房等部位生長出許多觸痛性結節。當伴有其他症狀（包括發燒與肝腫大）時，人們稱之爲韋-克二氏病（結節性非化膿性脂膜炎）。

panniculus *n.* a membranous sheet of tissue. For example, the *panniculus adiposus* is the fatty layer of tissue underlying the skin.

膜 薄膜樣組織層。例如，脂膜爲皮下脂肪層組織。

pannus *n.* invasion of the outer layers of the cornea of the eye by tissue containing many blood vessels, which grows in from the conjunctiva. It is seen as a response to inflammation of the cornea or conjunctiva, particularly in *trachoma.

血管翳，角膜翳 眼角膜外層受到從結膜生長出來的，含有許多血管的組織的侵襲。人們認爲角膜翳是角膜或結膜的一種炎症反應，多見於沙眼。

panophthalmitis *n.* inflammation involving the whole of the interior of the eye.

全眼球炎 整個眼睛內部的炎症。

Panstrongylus *n.* a genus of large bloodsucking bugs (*see* reduviid). *P. megistus* is important in transmitting *Chagas' disease to man in Brazil.

錐蝽屬 一種大型的吸血昆蟲屬（見獵蝽）。在巴西，大錐蝽是傳播恰加斯氏病的主要媒介。

pant- (panto-) *prefix. see* pan-.

〔前綴〕 **全，總，泛**

pantothenic acid a B vitamin that is a constituent of *coenzyme A. It plays an important role in the transfer of acetyl groups in the body. Pantothenic acid is widely distributed in food and a deficiency is therefore unlikely to occur.

泛酸 構成輔酶A的維生素B類中的一種。它在人體中對乙醯基的轉移起着重要的作用。泛酸在食物中分佈廣泛，因此在人體中不大可能缺乏。

pantropic *adj.* describing a virus that can invade and affect many different tissues of the body, for example the nerves, skin, or liver, without showing a special affinity for any one of them.

泛向的 用來描述能夠侵入和感染人體許多不同組織，例如，神經、皮膚或肝臟等的病毒。它對任何一種組織並不表現出特殊的親和力。

papain *n.* a preparation that contains one or more protein-digesting enzymes.

番木瓜酶 從番木瓜果中提取的，含有一種或多種

It is obtained from the pawpaw fruit and is used as a digestant.

蛋白消化酶的製劑。用作消化劑。

Papanicolaou test (Pap test) a test to detect cancer of the neck (cervix) or lining (endometrium) of the womb. A specimen of tissue taken from the womb is stained and examined under the microscope for the presence of abnormal cells.

帕帕尼科拉烏氏試驗 檢查子宮頸癌或子宮內膜癌的一種試驗。從子宮內取組織標本，經染色後，再在顯微鏡下檢查異常細胞。

papaverine *n.* an alkaloid, derived from opium, that relaxes smooth muscle. It is administered by mouth or injection to treat muscle spasm in such conditions as colic and in sprays for the relief of asthma. It may cause abnormal heart rate.

罌粟鹼 從阿片中提取出來的一種生物鹼。具有鬆弛平滑肌的作用。口服或注射。可治療肌痙攣，如絞痛；通過噴霧給藥可緩解哮喘。罌粟鹼可能引起心律失常。

papilla *n.* (*pl.* **papillae**) any small nipple-shaped protuberance. Several different kinds of papillae occur on the *tongue, in association with the taste buds. The *optic papilla* is an alternative name for the *optic disc.

乳頭 小乳頭狀隆凸。舌上生長有含有味蕾的幾種不同的乳頭。視神經乳頭是視神經盤的別稱。

papillitis *n.* inflammation of the first part of the optic nerve (the optic disc or optic papilla), i.e. where the nerve leaves the eyeball.

視神經乳頭炎 視神經自眼球發出的開始部分（視神經盤或視神經乳頭）的炎症。

papilloedema *n.* swelling of the first part of the optic nerve (the optic disc or optic papilla).

視神經乳頭水腫 視神經自眼球發出的開始部分（視神經盤或視神經乳頭）的腫脹。

papilloma *n.* a benign growth on the surface of skin or mucous membrane (for example, in the womb). Papillomas, which develop from the *epidermis, are usually in the form of a conical, flattish, or stalked protuberance, 2–5 mm in diameter. *Warts are a type of papilloma.

乳頭狀瘤 生長在皮膚表面或黏膜（如子宮內）上的良性腫瘤。從表皮生長出來的乳頭狀瘤，通常呈圓錐形，頂稍平，或為帶蒂的隆凸，直徑2～5 mm。疣就是乳頭狀瘤的一種類型。

papillomatosis *n.* a condition in which many *papillomas grow on an area of skin or mucous membrane.

乳頭狀瘤病 在皮膚或黏膜有許多乳頭狀瘤生長的疾病。

papillotomy *n.* the operation of cutting the *ampulla of Vater to widen its outlet in order to improve bile drainage and allow the passage of stones from

十二指腸乳頭切開術 切開十二指腸法特氏壺腹，來擴大其出口，使得膽汁引流通暢，膽石順利通過

the common bile duct. It is usually performed using a diathermy wire through a *duodenoscope following *ERCP.

總膽管的手術。該手術通常在內窺鏡逆行性胰膽管造影後，用一條導熱金屬絲通過十二指腸鏡進行。

papovavirus *n.* one of a group of small DNA-containing viruses producing tumours (usually malignant) in animals (subgroup *polyoma viruses*) and non-malignant tumours in animals and man (subgroup *papilloma viruses*).

乳多泡病毒 脫氧核糖核酸小病毒族的一種。這族病毒通常能引起動物的惡性腫瘤，如多瘤病毒亞族；有些能引起動物和人的良性腫瘤，如乳頭病毒亞族。

Pappataci fever *see* sandfly fever.

白蛉熱

papule *n.* a small superficial raised abnormality or spot on the skin. It usually forms part of a rash, such as appears with chickenpox.

丘疹 生長在皮膚表面的微小隆起。通常是皮疹的一種，如患水痘時出現的皮疹。

papulo- *prefix denoting* a papule or pimple.

〔前綴〕 **丘疹，膿疱**

papulosquamous *adj.* **1.** describing a rash that is both papular and scaly. **2.** denoting a group of skin diseases that have this characteristic, including *pityriaris rosea, seborrhoeic *dermatitis, *lichen planus, and *psoriasis.

丘疹鱗屑性的 ①描述一種既有丘疹特點，又有鱗屑特點的皮疹。②指一組具有丘疹和鱗屑的皮膚病，包括玫瑰糠疹、皮脂溢性皮炎、扁平苔蘚和銀屑病等。

para- *prefix denoting* **1.** beside or near. Example: *paranasal* (near the nasal cavity). **2.** resembling. Example: *paradysentery* (a mild form of dysentery). **3.** abnormal. Example: *paralalia* (abnormal speech).

〔前綴〕 ①**旁，附近** 例如，鼻旁的（鼻腔附近）。 ②**類，副，擬** 例如，副痢疾（一種輕型痢疾）。 ③**異常，倒錯，錯亂** 例如，構音倒錯（一種語言障礙）。

para-aminobenzoic acid a naturally occurring drug used in lotions and creams to prevent sunburn. It was formerly administered by mouth to treat certain infections now treated with antibiotics. High doses may cause nausea, vomiting, itching, and rashes.

對氨苯甲酸 一種天然藥物。洗劑和乳膏用來防曬。從前口服治療某些感染，現在已被抗生素代替。大劑量可引起噁心、嘔吐、瘙癢和皮疹等副作用。

para-aminosalicylic acid (PAS) a drug, chemically related to aspirin, used – in conjunction with isoniazid or streptomycin – to treat various types of tuberculosis. It is administered by mouth and commonly causes nausea, vomiting, diarrhoea, and rashes.

對氨水楊酸 一種抗結核藥。化學結構與阿司匹林相似，和異菸肼鏈黴素併用於治療各種結核病。口服常引起噁心、嘔吐、腹瀉和皮疹等副作用。

paracentesis *n.* tapping: the process of drawing off excess fluid from a part of the body through a hollow needle or *cannula.

穿刺術 穿刺放液法。是一種通過空心針或插管把身體某部位過量液體抽出來的方法。

paracetamol *n.* an *analgesic drug that also reduces fever. It is used to treat mild or moderate pain, such as headache, toothache, and rheumatism. It is administered by mouth and may cause digestive upsets; overdosage causes liver damage. Trade names: **Panadol**, **Panasorb**, **Salzone**.

對乙醯氨基酚 一種具有退燒作用的鎮痛藥。用於解除輕度的或中度的疼痛，如頭痛、牙痛和風濕病。口服可引起消化道的不適，過量用藥能引起肝臟的損害。商品名：撲熱息痛。

paracholia *n. Archaic.* disordered bile secretion.

泌膽障礙 膽汁分泌障礙的舊稱。

Paracoccidioides *n.* a genus of yeast-like fungi causing infection of the skin and mucous membranes. The species *P. brasiliensis* causes a chronic skin disease, South American *blastomycosis.

芽生菌屬 酵母菌樣的眞菌屬。能引起皮膚和黏膜的感染。巴西芽生菌能引起一種慢性皮膚病，即南美芽生菌病。

paracusis *n.* any abnormality of hearing.

聽覺倒錯 任何一種聽覺的異常。

paradidymis *n.* the vestigial remains of part of the embryonic *mesonephros that are found near the testis of the adult. Some of the mesonephric collecting tubules persist as the functional *vasa efferentia but the rest degenerate almost completely. A similar vestigial structure (the *paroophoron*) is found in females.

旁睾 胚胎期中腎的部分殘留物。見於成人睾丸附近。中腎中某些集合管仍起着輸出管的作用，但其餘的幾乎完全退化。人們發現在女性中也有類似結構，即卵巢旁體。

paradoxical breathing breathing movements seen in patients with broken ribs: on inhalation the chest wall moves in instead of out, and vice versa on exhalation.

反常呼吸 見於肋骨骨折患者的一種呼吸運動。病人在吸氣時胸壁向內運動，呼氣時反而向外運動。

paraesthesiae *pl. n.* spontaneously occurring abnormal tingling sensations, sometimes described as *pins and needles*. They are symptoms of partial damage to a peripheral nerve, such as that caused by external pressure on the affected part. *Compare* dysaesthesiae.

感覺異常 自發的異常刺痛感覺。有時描述爲針刺感。這是周圍神經部分受損（患部受到外界壓力）而引起的症狀。

paraffin *n.* one of a series of hydrocarbons derived from petroleum. *Paraffin wax* (*hard paraffin*), a whitish mixture

石蠟 自石油中提煉的一組碳氫化合物中的一種。固體石蠟爲一種固體碳氫

of solid hydrocarbons melting at 45–60°C, is used in medicine mainly as a base for ointments; it is also used for *embedding specimens for microscopical study. *Liquid paraffin* is a mineral oil, which has been used as a laxative.

化合物的微白色混合物，在45°～60℃溫度中熔化，醫學上主要用作藥膏基質；也可用於鏡檢時包埋標本。液體石蠟爲一種礦物油，用作輕瀉劑。

paraffinoma *n.* a type of tumour induced by the presence in the tissues of paraffin wax, formerly used in cosmetic surgery to increase the size of the female breasts.

石蠟瘤 由於存在於人體組織中的固體石蠟而引起的一種腫瘤。從前，整容外科常用石蠟作爲充填物來增大女性乳房的體積。

paraformaldehyde *n.* a white crystalline polymer of formaldehyde, used as a disinfectant fumigant and in the treatment of certain skin disorders.

多聚甲醛 甲醛的白色結晶聚合物。用作消毒的熏劑和用來治療某些皮膚病。

paraganglion *n.* one of the small oval masses of cells found in the walls of the ganglia of the sympathetic nervous system, near the spinal cord. They are *chromaffin cells, like those of the adrenal gland, and may secrete adrenaline.

副神經節 在脊髓附近的交感神經系統神經節的壁內發現的一種小卵圓形的細胞團。該細胞團，與腎上腺的細胞一樣，是嗜鉻細胞，可分泌腎上腺素。

parageusia (parageusis) *n.* abnormality of the sense of taste.

味覺異常

paragonimiasis (endemic haemoptysis) *n.* a tropical disease, occurring principally in the Far East, caused by the presence of the fluke **Paragonimus westermani* in the lungs. The infection is acquired by eating inadequately cooked shellfish, such as crayfish and crabs. Symptoms resemble those of chronic *bronchitis, including the coughing up of blood and difficulty in breathing (dyspnoea). Paragonimiasis is treated with the drugs bithionol and chloroquine.

並殖吸虫病 主要發生於遠東地區的一種熱帶病，由存在於肺中的衛斯特曼氏並殖吸虫引起。該病是由於吃尙未烹調熟的蝲蛄、蟹等甲殼類動物而引起的感染。患者的症狀與慢性支氣管炎相類似，可出現咳血和呼吸困難。常用硫雙二氯酚和氯喹來治療。

Paragonimus *n.* a genus of large tropical parasitic *flukes that are particularly prevalent in the Far East. The adults of *P. westermani* live in the lungs of man, where they cause destruction and bleeding of the tissues (*see* paragonimiasis). However, they may also be found in other organs of the body. Eggs are passed out in the sputum and the

並殖吸蟲屬 主要流行於遠東地區的一種大體形熱帶寄生吸蟲屬。衛斯特曼氏並殖吸蟲的成蟲寄居於人的肺內，破壞肺組織，而引起肺組織出血（見肺吸蟲病）。人們發現它也可以在人體其他器官內寄生。蟲卵隨痰排出。幼蟲

larvae undergo their development in two other hosts, a snail and a crab.
在成長過程中還要經歷螺和蟹兩個宿主。

paragranuloma *n.* an old term for one of the types of *Hodgkin's disease. It is now known as *lymphocyte-predominant Hodgkin's disease* and has the best prognosis of all the types.
類肉芽腫 何傑金氏病的一種類型的舊稱。現稱淋巴細胞為主型何傑金氏病。在所有類型中該型預後最好。

paragraphia *n.* a disorder of writing, involving the omission or transposition of letters or of whole words. The appearance of this in adult life is usually due to damage to the brain. In childhood it usually reflects a developmental delay in learning to write correctly.
書寫倒錯 包括漏字母、漏詞或把字母或詞顛倒換位的書寫障礙。成人出現這種現象，通常是由於大腦損傷所致；兒童則通常是學習書寫方面的智力發育緩慢的表現。

para-influenza viruses a group of large RNA-containing viruses that cause infections of the respiratory tract producing mild influenza-like symptoms. They are included in the paramyxovirus group (*see* myxovirus).
副流感病毒 一組大體形的核糖核酸病毒。該病毒能引起呼吸道的感染。患者出現輕型流感樣的症狀。該病毒屬於副黏液病毒組。

paraldehyde *n.* a *hypnotic and *anticonvulsant drug used to induce sleep in mental patients and to control convulsions in tetanus. It is administered by mouth, injection, or in suppositories; side-effects may include digestive upsets and, in large doses, prolonged unconsciousness. *Tolerance and *dependence may result from prolonged use of the drug.
三聚乙醛 一種有安眠和抗驚厥作用的藥物。用於精神病患者的催眠和控制破傷風病人的抽搐。可通過口服、注射或使用栓劑給藥。副作用有消化不良和（大劑量用藥可致）長時間的意識喪失。長期用藥可產生耐藥性和賴藥性。

paralysis *n.* muscle weakness that varies in its extent, its severity, and the degree of *spasticity or flaccidity according to the nature of the underlying disease and its distribution in the brain, spinal cord, peripheral nerves, or muscles. *See also* diplegia, hemiplegia, paraplegia, poliomyelitis. —**paralytic** *adj.*
麻痹，癱瘓 肌肉無力。根據原發病性質和原發病竈在腦、脊髓、周圍神經或肌肉的分佈情況的不同，其肌無力的影響範圍、嚴重程度、痙攣或鬆弛程度亦有所不同。

paramedian *adj.* situated close to or beside the *median plane.
正中旁的 位於正中矢狀平面的附近或旁邊。

paramedical *adj.* describing or relating to the professions closely linked to the medical profession and working in
關係醫學的（醫務人員） 描述與醫學專業密切相關的專業。該專業人員與

conjunction with them. Such professions require expert knowledge and experience in certain fields, but no medical degree. Paramedical personnel in a hospital include the nurses, radiographers, physiotherapists, and dietitians.

醫學專業人員相互配合，共同工作。關係醫學專業工作人員需要具備某些方面的專門知識和經驗，但並沒有醫學學位。醫院中關係醫學專業工作人員包括護士、放射科技師、理療師和營養師。

paramesonephric duct (Müllerian duct) either of the paired ducts that form adjacent to the *mesonephric ducts in the embryo. In the female these ducts develop into the Fallopian tubes, womb, and part of the vagina. However, in the male they degenerate almost completely.

副中腎管　胚胎期靠近中腎管形成的一對導管。在女性該管發育成輸卵管、子宮和陰道的一部分，而在男性則幾乎全部退化。

parameter *n.* (in medicine) a measurement of some factor, such as blood pressure, pulse rate, or haemoglobin level, that may have a bearing on the condition being investigated.

參數　在醫學上指血壓、脉搏頻率、血紅蛋白的數量指標。該指標對觀察的疾病有着重要的意義。

paramethadione *n.* an *anticonvulsant drug used to prevent or reduce petit mal fits in epilepsy. It is administered by mouth; the commonest side-effects include drowsiness, digestive upsets, and blurred vision. Trade name: **Paradione**.

對甲雙酮　一種抗驚厥藥。用來預防或控制癲癇小發作。口服。最常見副作用包括：倦眠、胃腸不適和視力模糊。商品名：帕朧二酮。

parametric test *see* significance.

參數試驗

parametritis (pelvic cellulitis) *n.* inflammation of the loose connective tissue and smooth muscle around the womb (the parametrium). The condition may be associated with *puerperal fever.

子宮旁（組織）炎　子宮周圍的平滑肌和疏鬆結締組織（子宮旁組織）的炎症。該病可能與產褥熱有關。

parametrium *n.* the layer of connective tissue surrounding the womb.

子宮旁組織　子宮周圍的結締組織層。

paramnesia *n.* a distorted memory, such as *confabulation or *déjà vu.

記憶錯誤　一種記憶障礙。如虛談症或似曾相識症。

paramyoclonus multiplex a benign disorder of the nervous system that is characterized by brief irregular twitch-like contractions of the muscles of the limbs and trunk.

多發性肌陣攣　神經系統的一種良性疾病。其特徵爲軀幹和四肢肌肉短暫的不規則的顫搐樣攣縮。

paramyotonia congenita a rare constitutional disorder in which prolonged contraction of muscle fibres (*see* myotonia) develops when the patient is exposed to cold. This may be due to a disorder of potassium metabolism.

先天性肌强直病 一種罕見的全身性疾病。當病人受到冷刺激時，肌肉纖維收縮時間延長。這可能是鉀代謝障礙所致。

paranasal sinuses the air-filled spaces, lined with mucous membrane, within some of the bones of the skull. They open into the nasal cavity, via the meatuses, and are named according to the bone in which they are situated. They comprise the *frontal sinuses* and the *maxillary sinuses* (one pair of each), the *ethmoid sinuses* (consisting of many spaces inside the ethmoid bone), and the two *sphenoid sinuses*. (See illustration.)

鼻旁竇 一些顱骨內襯有黏膜的充氣腔。它們通過鼻道，開口於鼻腔，並根據其所位於的骨而命名。鼻旁竇包括額竇和上頜竇（各一對）、篩竇（由篩骨內許多腔構成），以及兩個蝶竇（見圖）。

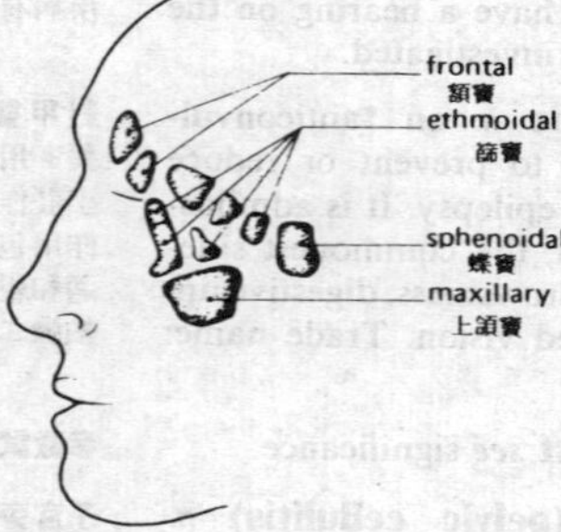

Paranasal sinuses projected to the surface
鼻旁竇表面投影

paranoia *n.* a mental disorder characterized by *delusions organized into a system, without hallucinations or other marked symptoms of mental illness. It is a rare chronic condition; most people with such delusions will in time develop signs of other mental illness.
The same term is sometimes used more loosely for a state of mind in which the individual has a strong belief that he is persecuted by others. His behaviour is therefore suspicious and isolated. This can be a result of *personality disorder

偏執狂 以系統性妄想爲主要特徵，而不伴有幻覺或其他明顯精神病症狀的一種精神性疾病。這是一種罕見的慢性病。伴有妄想的絕大部分患者將來都會出現其他精神病症狀。
上述術語（指偏執狂）有時應用的範圍較廣，像用於具有一種受他人迫害的强烈信念的精神病患者。這種病人行爲常常是多疑的和孤立的，這可能是人

as well as mental illnesses causing *paranoid states.

格障礙的後果，也可能是類偏執狂型精神病的後果。

paranoid *adj.* **1.** describing a mental state characterized by fixed and logically elaborated *delusions. There are many causes, including paranoid *schizophrenia, *manic-depressive psychosis, organic psychoses such as *alcoholism, *paraphrenia, and severe emotional stress. **2.** describing a personality distinguished by such traits as excessive sensitivity to rejection by others, suspiciousness, hostility, and self-importance.

類偏狂 ①描寫一種以固定的和有邏輯的妄想爲特徵的精神狀態。原因很多，包括類偏狂型精神分裂症、躁狂抑鬱型精神病，以及諸如酒精中毒、妄想痴呆等器質性精神病和受到嚴重的感情創傷等。 ②描寫一種對其他人的不友好行爲過度敏感的人格。該人常表現爲多疑、存有敵意、妄自尊大。

paraparesis *n.* weakness of both legs, resulting from disease of the nervous system.

下身輕癱 由神經系統疾病引起的雙腿無力症。

paraphasia *n.* a disorder of language in which unintended syllables, words, or phrases are interpolated in the patient's speech. A severe degree of paraphasia results in speech that is a meaningless jumble of words and sounds, called *jargon aphasia*.

言語錯亂 病人在講話時無意識地增添音節、單詞或短語的一種語言障礙。嚴重言語錯亂的病人，講話中無意識地把詞意和語音弄得雜亂無章。此種疾病稱之爲雜亂性失語。

paraphimosis *n.* retraction and constriction of the foreskin behind the glans penis. This occurs in some patients with *phimosis on erection of the penis: the tight foreskin cannot be drawn back over the glans and becomes painful and swollen. Manual replacement of the foreskin can usually be achieved under local or general anaesthesia, but *circumcision is required to prevent a recurrence.

箝頓包莖 陰莖頭包皮回縮與縮窄。見於有些包莖患者的陰莖勃起時，緊綳的包皮不能從陰莖頭上縮回，並產生疼痛與腫脹。通常在局痲或全痲下，施行包皮的手法復位，但爲了防止復發，需要做包皮環切術。

paraphrenia *n.* a mental disorder characterized by systematic *delusions and prominent *hallucinations but without any other marked symptoms of mental illness. The only loss of contact with reality is in areas affected by the delusions and hallucinations. It is typically seen in the elderly and deaf. Some sufferers, if followed up over a period of years, eventually show other symptoms of *schizophrenia. It is therefore

妄想痴呆 一種以系統性妄想和明顯的幻覺爲特徵，但不伴有任何其他明顯精神病症狀的精神病。與現實關系破壞的只限於受妄想和幻覺影響那部分。該典型症狀見於上了年紀的人和聾人。如果對有些患者隨訪數年，最終會發現他們出現精神分裂症的其他症狀。因此，妄

debatable whether paraphrenia constitutes a separate entity.

想痴呆是不是一種獨立疾病，人們還是有爭議的。

paraplegia *n.* *paralysis of both legs, usually due to disease or injury of the spinal cord. It is often accompanied by loss of sensation below the level of the injury and disturbed bladder function. —**paraplegic** *adj.*, *n.*

截癱 通常由脊髓性疾病或損傷所引起的下肢癱瘓。常伴有脊髓損傷部水平以下的感覺喪失和膀胱功能失調。

paraprotein *n.* an abnormal protein of the *immunoglobulin series. Paraproteins appear in malignant disease of the spleen, bone marrow, liver, etc. Examples of paraproteins are *myeloma globulins, *macroglobulin, and *Bence-Jones protein.

病變蛋白 免疫球蛋白組中的一種異常蛋白。該蛋白的出現表明在脾臟、骨髓、肝臟等有惡性病變。病變蛋白有骨髓瘤球蛋白、巨球蛋白和本瓊氏蛋白。

parapsoriasis *n.* any one of a group of skin diseases (*erythrodermas) that develop slowly and are typified by chronic red scaly patches that resemble psoriasis.

類銀屑病 一組發展緩慢、並以與銀屑病相似的、長期不癒的紅色鱗屑斑為特徵的皮膚病（紅皮病）。

parapsychology *n.* the study of *extrasensory perception, *psychokinesis, and other mental abilities that appear to defy natural law.

通靈學 研究超感知覺、精神能量以及似乎違反自然法則的其他精神能力的學科。

paraquat *n.* the chemical compound dimethyl dipyridilium, widely used as a weed-killer. When swallowed it exerts its most serious effects upon the lungs, the tissues of which it destroys after a few days. Paraquat poisoning is almost invariably fatal.

百草枯 二甲基二吡啶化合物。廣泛使用的一種除草劑。當誤服該除草劑時，對肺影響極大，數日後肺組織受到破壞。百草枯中毒幾乎都難免於死。

parasite *n.* any living thing that lives in (*see* endoparasite) or on (*see* ectoparasite) another living organism (*see* host). The parasite, which may spend all or only part of its existence with the host, obtains food and/or shelter from the host and contributes nothing to its welfare. Some parasites cause irritation and interfere with bodily functions; others destroy host tissues and release toxins into the body, thus injuring health and causing disease. Human parasites include fungi, bacteria, viruses, protozoa, and worms. *See also* commensal, symbiosis. —**parasitic** *adj.*

寄生物 任何寄生於其他生物體內或體表的生物。該寄生物的整個生活周期或僅部分生活周期可以在其宿主體內度過，從宿主體攝取養料和（或）寄生於宿主體，而對宿主並沒有一點好處。有些寄生物能夠刺激宿主機體，並引起功能失調；另外一些寄生物能破壞宿主組織，並釋放毒素，因而損害宿主健康和引起疾病。人體寄生物包括黴菌、細菌、病毒、原蟲、蠕蟲等。

parasiticide *n.* an agent, such as *gamma benzene hexachloride, that destroys parasites (excluding bacteria and fungi). *See also* acaricide, anthelmintic, trypanocide.

殺寄生蟲藥 殺滅寄生蟲（不包括細菌與黴菌）的藥劑。如丙種六六六。

parasitology *n.* the study and science of parasites.

寄生蟲學 研究寄生物的學科。

parasternal *adj.* situated close to the sternum. The *parasternal line* is an imaginary vertical line parallel to and midway between the lateral margin of the sternum and the vertical line through the nipple.

胸骨旁的 位於胸骨旁邊的。胸骨旁線是一條假想的垂直線，它是胸骨外側線和乳線之間的中線。

parasuicide *n.* a self-injuring act (such as an overdose of sleeping tablets) that is not motivated by a genuine wish to die. It differs from attempted *suicide in being common in young people who are distressed but not seriously mentally ill. However, many people who have acted in this way go on to attempt, or even to achieve, suicide. Help in sorting out their difficulties should therefore be given. *See also* Samaritans.

類自殺 一種自我傷害行爲。如服用過量安眠藥片。該行爲並沒有眞想死的念頭。類自殺與青年人因痛苦而企圖自殺是不同的，而青年人受痛苦折磨想死並不是嚴重的精神病。許多人曾有過這種行爲，並不斷產生想死念頭，或甚至已達到自殺目的。對這些人，我們應當給予一些幫助，以便使他們從痛苦中解脫出來。

parasympathetic nervous system one of the two divisions of the *autonomic nervous system, having fibres that leave the central nervous system from the brain and the lower portion of the spinal cord and are distributed to blood vessels, glands, and the majority of internal organs. The system works in balance with the *sympathetic nervous system, the actions of which it frequently opposes.

副交感神統系統 兩部分自主神經系統中的一部分。該神經系統的纖維是從位於腦和脊髓較低部位的中樞發出，並分佈於血管、腺體，以及大多數的內臟器官。副交感神經系統的功能與交感神經系統功能相互平衡，其作用往往是相反的。

parasympatholytic *n.* a drug opposing the effects of the *parasympathetic nervous system. The actions of parasympatholytic drugs are *anticholinergic* (i.e. preventing acetylcholine from acting as a neurotransmitter); they include relaxation of smooth muscle, decreased secretion of saliva, sweat, and digestive juices, and dilation of the pupil of the

抗副交感神經藥 一種與副交感神經系統作用相對抗的藥物。其藥物作用是抗膽鹼能的，也就是作爲一種神經遞質來阻止乙醯膽鹼發揮作用。包括鬆弛平滑肌，減少唾液、汗液和消化液的分泌，以及擴瞳等。阿托品及其類似藥

eye. *Atropine and similar drugs have these effects; they are used in the treatment of peptic ulcers (e.g. *propantheline) and parkinsonism (e.g. *chlorphenoxamine), to relieve spasm of smooth muscle (*see* spasmolytic), and as *mydriatics. Characteristic side-effects include dry mouth, thirst, blurred vision, dry skin, increased heart rate, and difficulty in urination.

物均有這些作用。這類藥用於治療消化性潰瘍（如普魯本辛）和帕金森氏綜合徵（如氯甲苯醇銨）、解除平滑肌痙攣，以及作爲擴瞳藥。其特有的副作用包括：口乾、渴感、視力模糊、皮膚乾燥、心率加快和排尿困難。

parasympathomimetic *n.* a drug that has the effect of stimulating the *parasympathetic nervous system. The actions of parasympathomimetic drugs are *cholinergic* (resembling those of *acetylcholine) and include stimulation of skeletal muscle, *vasodilatation, depression of heart rate, increasing the tension of smooth muscle, increasing secretions (such as saliva), and constricting the pupil of the eye. They are used in the treatment of *myasthenia gravis (*see* anticholinesterase), glaucoma (*see* miotic), and some heart and circulatory conditions (e.g. *carbachol) and to restore intestinal and bladder function after surgery (e.g. bethenecol).

擬副交感神經藥 一種具有興奮副交感神經系統的作用的藥物。該藥物具有膽鹼能的作用（與乙醯膽鹼作用相似），包括興奮骨骼肌、擴張血管、減低心率、增强平滑肌張力、增加分泌（如唾液）、縮小瞳孔等。用以治療重症肌無力、青光眼和某些心血管系統疾病（如卡巴可），以及手術後腸與膀胱功能的恢復。

paratenon *n.* the tissue of a tendon sheath that fills up spaces round the tendon.

腱旁組織 一種充塡於腱周圍間隙的腱鞘組織。

parathion *n.* an organic phosphorus compound, used as a pesticide, that causes poisoning when inhaled, ingested, or absorbed through the skin. Like several other organic phosphorus compounds, it attacks the enzyme *cholinesterase and causes excessive stimulation of the parasympathetic nervous system. The symptoms are headache, sweating, salivation, lacrimation, vomiting, diarrhoea, and muscular spasms. Treatment is by administration of *atropine.

對硫磷 一種用作殺蟲劑的有機磷化合物。當人們吸入、食入或經皮膚吸收時，能引起中毒。該化合物同其他幾種有機磷化合物一樣，均能夠破壞膽鹼脂酶，引起副交感神經系統過度興奮。出現頭痛、出汗、流涎、流淚、嘔吐、腹瀉、肌痙攣等症狀。可用阿托品治療。

parathormone *n. see* parathyroid hormone.

甲狀旁腺激素

parathyroidectomy *n.* surgical removal of the parathyroid glands, usu-

甲狀旁腺切除術 切除甲狀旁腺的外科手術。通常

ally as part of the treatment of *hyperparathyroidism.

作爲治療甲狀旁腺機能亢進的一種手段。

parathyroid glands two pairs of yellowish-brown *endocrine glands that are situated behind, or sometimes embedded within, the *thyroid gland. They are stimulated to produce *parathyroid hormone by a decrease in the amount of calcium in the blood.

甲狀旁腺 位於甲狀腺後或有時包埋於甲狀腺內的兩對淡黃褐色的內分泌腺。當血鈣濃度下降時，能分泌甲狀旁腺激素。

parathyroid hormone (parathormone) a hormone, synthesized and released by the parathyroid glands, that controls the distribution of calcium and phosphate in the body. A high level of the hormone causes transfer of calcium from the bones to the blood; a deficiency lowers blood calcium levels, causing *tetany. This condition may be treated by injections of the hormone. *Compare* thyrocalcitonin.

甲狀旁腺激素 由甲狀旁腺合成和分泌的一種激素。該激素能够調節體內鈣與磷的分佈。激素濃度升高可促使骨鈣轉移到血中；激素不足時，血鈣下降，引起手足搐搦，可注射甲狀旁腺激素治療。

paratyphoid fever an infectious disease caused by the bacterium *Salmonella paratyphi A*, *B*, or *C*. Bacteria are spread in the faeces of patients or carriers, and outbreaks occur as a result of poor sanitation or unhygienic food-handling. After an incubation period of 1–10 days, symptoms, including diarrhoea, mild fever, and a pink rash on the chest, appear and last for about a week. Treatment with chloramphenicol is effective. Vaccination with *TAB provides temporary immunity against paratyphoid A and B.

副傷寒 由甲型、乙型或丙型副傷寒沙門氏菌引起的傳染病。這類細菌通過病人或帶菌者的糞便傳播。該病暴發常由於衛生條件差或吃了不潔淨食物所致。在1～10天的潛伏期後，出現腹瀉、低燒和胸部淡紅色丘疹等症狀，持續一週左右。用氯黴素治療有效。接種副傷寒疫苗可產生預防甲、乙型副傷寒的暫時性的免疫力。

pareidolia *n.* misperception of random stimuli as real things or people, as when faces are vividly seen in the flames of a fire.

幻想性錯覺 病人常把某些非眞實性刺激誤認爲眞人或眞物。例如，從火焰中看到一個逼眞的人面。

parenchyma *n.* the functional part of an organ, as opposed to the supporting tissue (*stroma*).

實質 器官的功能部分。係與支持組織（基質）相對而言。

parenteral *adj.* administered by any way other than through the mouth:

腸胃外的 除經口腔以外的其他任何給藥方法。例

applied, for example, to the introduction of drugs or other agents into the body by injection.

如採用注射方法將藥物或其他物質注入體內。

paresis *n.* muscular weakness caused by disease of the nervous system. It implies a lesser degree of weakness than *paralysis*, although the two words are often used interchangeably.

輕癱 由神經系統疾病引起的肌無力。輕癱與癱瘓兩個詞，雖然常常交替使用，但前者（輕癱）指的肌無力程度較輕一些。

paries *n.* (*pl.* **parietes**) **1.** the enveloping or surrounding part of an organ or other structure. **2.** the wall of a cavity.

壁 ①器官或其他結構的包裹部分或外圍部分。②腔壁。

parietal *adj.* **1.** of or relating to the inner walls of a body cavity, as opposed to the contents: applied particularly to the membranes lining a cavity (*see* peritoneum, pleura). **2.** of or relating to the parietal bone.

①**壁的** 體腔內壁的或與體腔內壁有關的。壁與內容物是相對而言的。特別多用於描述體腔內膜。②**頂骨的** 頂骨的或與頂骨有關的。

parietal bone either of a pair of bones forming the top and sides of the cranium. *See* skull.

頂骨 構成顱頂部和顱雙側部一對骨頭。

parietal cells *see* oxyntic cells.

壁細胞

parietal lobe one of the major divisions of each cerebral hemisphere (*see* cerebrum), lying behind the frontal lobe, above the temporal lobe, and in front of the occipital lobe. It is thus beneath the crown of the skull. It contains the *sensory cortex and *association areas.

頂葉 每側腦半球的一個主要組成部分。位於額葉後部、顳葉上部和枕葉的前方。因此，它緊靠顱冠之下。頂葉有感覺皮層和聯想區。

parity *n.* the condition of a woman with regard to the number of pregnancies she has had that have each resulted in the birth of an infant capable of survival.

經產狀況 有關婦女懷孕並活產次數的情況。

parkinsonism *n.* a disorder of middle-aged and elderly people characterized by tremor, rigidity and a poverty of spontaneous movements. The first and most prominent symptom is tremor, which often affects one hand, spreading first to the leg on the same side and then to the other limbs. It is most pronounced in resting limbs, interfering with such actions as holding a cup. The patient has an expressionless face, an

帕金森氏綜合徵 一種以震顫、肌強直和自發運動缺乏爲主要特徵的中老年疾病。最早出現的和最明顯的症狀是震顫。它常從一隻手發作開始，再傳到同側腿部，然後又傳到其他肢體。在肢體作擱置某物的動作時，震顫症狀最爲明顯，妨礙像拿杯子這樣的動作。患者面部無表

unmodulated voice, and an increasing tendency to stoop (a shuffling run is needed to maintain balance). Parkinsonism is a disease affecting the basal ganglia of the brain for which in many cases no cause can be found. Drug-induced parkinsonism may complicate the use of psychoactive substances, including the phenothiazines, butyrophenones, and metoclopramide. Uncommonly it can be attributed to the late effects of *encephalitis or coal-gas poisoning or to *Wilson's disease. Relief of the symptoms may be obtained with *anticholinergic drugs and *levodopa.

情、發音單調。並且有日益加重的駝背（為了保持平衡，病人跑動時出現一種笨拙的步態）。帕金森氏綜合徵是由於腦基底神經節受侵襲所引起的。許多病例尚無法查明其原因。由於藥物能引起帕金森氏綜合徵，因此，在使用對精神活動有影響的藥物包括吩噻嗪、苯丙甲酮、胃復安等藥時，應特別謹慎。帕金森氏綜合徵有時也偶見於威爾遜氏病、腦炎或煤氣中毒後期的病人。可用抗膽鹼能藥和左旋多巴來減輕症狀。

paromomycin *n.* an antibiotic, active against intestinal bacteria and amoebae used to treat dysentery and gastroenteritis. It is administered by mouth; side-effects include stomach pains, itching, and heartburn.

巴龍黴素　一種具有抗腸道細菌和阿米巴作用的抗生素。用於治療痢疾和胃腸炎。口服。副作用包括：胃痛、瘙癢、胃灼熱等。

paronychia *n.* inflammation and swelling of the skin folds and tissues surrounding a fingernail or toenail. Chronic paronychia is usually caused by the fungus **Candida* or it can occur in psoriasis. Acute paronychia is the result of bacterial infection. *See also* whitlow.

甲溝炎　手指甲或腳趾甲周圍的皮膚皺摺與組織發生的炎症和腫脹。慢性甲溝炎通常由念珠菌引起，或見於銀屑病病人；急性甲溝炎由細菌感染所致。

paroophoron *n.* the vestigial remains of part of the *mesonephric duct in the female, situated next to each ovary. It is associated with a similar structure, the *epoophoron*. Both are without known function.

卵巢旁體　女性中腎管的部分殘遺組織。位於每側卵巢的附近。它與另一種相似的結構——卵巢冠有關。兩者的功能均不明。

parosmia *n.* any disorder of the sense of smell.

嗅覺倒錯　一種嗅覺失常。

parotid gland one of a pair of *salivary glands situated in front of each ear. The openings of the parotid ducts (*Stensen's ducts*) are on the inner sides of the cheeks, opposite the second upper molar teeth.

腮腺　位於每側耳前的一對唾液腺中的任何一個。腮腺管（斯滕森氏管）開口於頰內側，與第二上磨牙相對。

parotitis *n.* inflammation of the parotid salivary glands. *See* mumps (infectious parotitis).

腮腺炎 腮腺發生的炎症。

parous *adj.* having given birth to one or more children.

經產的 分娩過一個或多個嬰兒的。

paroxysm *n.* **1.** a sudden violent attack, especially a spasm or convulsion. **2.** the abrupt worsening of symptoms or recurrence of disease. —**paroxysmal** *adj.*

①**發作** 一種突然而猛烈的發病過程。特別指痙攣或抽搐。 ②**陣發** 症狀突然加重或疾病的反復發作。

parrot disease an infectious disease of parrots and budgerigars due to a virus-like organism of the genus *Chlamydia*; it can be transmitted to man and causes headache, bleeding from the nose, shivering, fever, and complications involving the lungs. Untreated the disease can be fatal, but it responds to tetracyclines or penicillin. Medical name: **psittacosis**. *Compare* ornithosis.

鸚鵡熱 由一種類似病毒的衣原體屬引起鸚鵡和澳洲長尾小鸚鵡的傳染病。它能够傳給人。患者出現頭痛、鼻出血、寒顫、發燒和肺併發症。如不治療可以引起死亡。四環素或青黴素治療有效。

pars *n.* a specific part of an organ or other structure, such as any of parts of the pituitary gland.

部分 器官或其他結構的特殊部分。例如，垂體的任何一部分。

Part III accommodation *see* National Assistance Act.

第三部分膳宿

parthenogenesis *n.* reproduction in which an organism develops from an unfertilized ovum. It is common in plants and occurs in some lower animals (e.g. aphids).

單性生殖 從一個未受精卵生長發育成一個生物的生殖過程。單性生殖常見於植物和某些較低級動物（如蚜蟲類）。

partially sighted register (in Britain) a list of persons who have poor sight but are not technically blind. In general their sight is adequate to permit the performance of tasks for which some vision is essential. *Compare* blind register.

弱視登記表 在英國用的一種具有弱視但並非全盲的視力登記表。一般來講，這些人的視力能够從事一些需要一定視力的工作。

parturition *n.* childbirth. *See* labour.

分娩

parvi- *prefix denoting* small size.

〔前綴〕 **小** 指小體積的。

PAS *see* para-aminosalicylic acid.

對氨水楊酸

pascal *n.* the *SI unit of pressure, equal to 1 newton per square metre. Symbol: Pa.

帕斯卡 國際單位制的壓力單位。1個單位等於每平方米1牛頓。符號爲Pa。

Paschen bodies particles that occur in the cells of skin rashes in patients with *cowpox or *smallpox; they are thought to be the virus particles.

帕興氏小體 在牛痘或天花病人的皮疹細胞中所形成的包涵體。人們認爲該包涵體就是病毒顆粒。

passive movement movement not brought about by a patient's own efforts. Passive movements are induced by manipulation of the joints by a physiotherapist. They are useful in maintaining function when a patient has nerve or muscle disorders that prevent voluntary movement.

被動運動 不靠病人自身力量而靠外力引起的運動。由理療醫師推拿關節引起的運動就屬於被動運動。當病人患有妨礙隨意運動的神經或肌肉性疾病時，被動運動有助於保持功能。

pass pointing (past pointing) failure to touch a chosen target with an outstretched hand when the eyes are closed. It is a sign of imbalance in the function of the labyrinth of the inner ear. The hand moves towards the side of the affected labyrinth.

過指徵 閉上雙眼時，伸出的手摸不准所選擇的目標。這是內耳迷路平衡功能障礙的一個症狀。手常偏向內耳迷路患側。

paste *n.* (in pharmacy) a medicinal preparation of a soft sticky consistency, which is applied externally.

糊劑 藥物劑型。一種外敷的稀薄而黏稠的藥物制劑。

Pasteurella a genus of small rodlike Gram-negative bacteria that are parasites of animals and man. The species *P. pestis* causes *plague in man, and *P. tularensis* causes *tularemia.

巴斯德氏菌屬 一種寄生於動物和人體的小桿狀革蘭氏陰性桿菌屬。鼠疫巴斯德氏菌種能引起人的鼠疫，土拉巴斯德氏菌種能引起土拉菌病。

pasteurization *n.* the treatment of milk by heating it to 65°C for 30 minutes, or to 72°C for 15 minutes, followed by rapid cooling, to kill such bacteria as those of tuberculosis and typhoid.

巴〔斯德〕氏消毒法 把牛奶加熱到65℃維持30分鐘，或加熱到72℃維持15分鐘，再立即冷却的處理法。該消毒法可殺滅結核和傷寒桿菌等。

pastille *n.* a medicinal preparation containing gelatine and glycerine, usually coated with sugar, that is dissolved in the mouth so that the medication is applied to the mouth or throat.

錠劑 通常爲外包糖衣內含明膠和甘油的一種藥物劑型。用於口腔含化，以治療口咽部疾患。

patch test a test to discover which, if any, of a number of possible substances is responsible for a patient's allergy. Small quantities of different allergens are applied either to light scratches on

斑貼試驗 一種檢查某些物質是否能引起病人的過敏反應的試驗。方法是將小量的過敏原放在輕輕劃破的手臂或背部的皮膚

the skin of the arm or back or beneath plaster. In common allergies the offending substance causes a patch of swelling and a typical red flare in the skin in 5 to 15 minutes. A delayed reaction may take 24 to 72 hours to develop.

上，再貼上膠布。呈陽性反應者一般在5～15分鐘內皮膚出現明顯的紅腫斑，反應遲緩者，可在24～72小時內出現以上皮膚反應。

patella *n.* the lens shaped bone that forms the kneecap. It is situated in front of the knee in the tendon of the quadriceps muscle of the thigh. *See also* sesamoid bone.

髕骨 構成膝蓋的扁豆形骨。位於膝前方，與股四頭肌腱相連。

patellar reflex the knee jerk, in which stretching the muscle at the front of the thigh by tapping its tendon below the knee cap causes a *reflex contraction of the muscle, so that the leg kicks. This is a test of the connection between the sensory nerves attached to stretch receptors in the muscle, the spinal cord, and the motor neurones running from the cord to the thigh muscle, all of which are involved in the reflex. Disease or damage may result in absence of the reflex.

膝反射 輕輕叩擊膝蓋下方的肌腱，使大腿前部肌肉緊張，引起肌肉反射性收縮，導致小腿跳動。該反射用以檢查由肌肉牽張感受器發出的感覺神經與脊髓和從脊髓走向大腿肌肉的運動神經之間的相互聯系情況。以上諸環節都與反射有關。任一部位受到損傷或遭到疾病侵襲，均可導致反射消失。

patent ductus arteriosus *see* ductus arteriosus.

動脉導管

path- (patho-) *prefix denoting* disease. Example: *pathophobia* (morbid fear of).

〔前綴〕 **病** 指疾病。例如，疾病恐怖。

pathogen *n.* a microorganism, such as a bacterium, that parasitizes an animal (or plant) or man and produces a disease.

病原體 寄生於動物（或植物）或人，並能引起疾病的微生物。例如細菌。

pathogenic *adj.* capable of causing disease. The term is applied to a parasitic microorganism (especially a bacterium) in relation to its host. —**pathogenicity** *n.*

致病性 能引起疾病的。該術語用於描述寄生物（尤其指細菌）與其宿主間的關係。

pathognomonic *adj.* describing a symptom or sign that is characteristic of or unique to a particular disease. The presence of such a sign or symptom allows positive diagnosis of the disease.

特殊病徵的 描述某種特殊疾病所特有的或僅有的症狀或體徵。一旦出現該症狀或體徵，有助於對該病作出明確的診斷。

pathological *adj.* relating to or arising from disease. For example, a pathological *fracture is one associated with disease of the bone.

病理性 與疾病有關的或由疾病引起的。例如，病理性骨折與骨的疾病有關。

pathology *n.* the study of disease processes with the aim of understanding their nature and causes. This is achieved by observing samples of blood, urine, faeces, and diseased tissue obtained from the living patient or at autopsy, by the use of X-rays, and by many other techniques. (*See* biopsy.) *Clinical pathology* is the application of the knowledge gained to the treatment of patients. —**pathologist** *n.*

病理學 以研究疾病的性質和病因爲目的的一門學科。該學科的知識是通過觀察血液、尿液、糞便標本和由患病活體採取病變組織標本或屍體解剖標本獲得的。也可借助於X射綫和許多其他方法來進行研究。臨床病理學是將獲得的知識具體用於患者的應用學科。

-pathy *suffix denoting* **1.** disease. Example: *nephropathy* (of the kidney). **2.** therapy. Example: *osteopathy* (by manipulation).

〔後綴〕 ①**疾病** 例如腎病。 ②**療法** 例如按骨療法。

pauciarthritis *n. see* arthritis.

少關節炎

pavementation (pavementing) *n.* the sticking of white blood cells to the linings of the finest blood vessels (capillaries) when inflammation occurs.

鋪壁 炎症時白細胞貼附於最細的血管（毛細血管）內壁的現象。

peau d'orange a dimpled appearance of the skin over a breast tumour, resembling the surface of an orange. The skin is thickened and the openings of hair follicles and sweat glands are enlarged.

橘皮現象 覆蓋於乳房腫瘤的皮膚呈點狀陷窩外觀的現象。與橘子皮類似，皮膚變厚，毛囊孔與汗腺擴大。

pecten *n.* **1.** the middle section of the anal canal, below the anal valves (*see* anus). **2.** a sharp ridge on the upper branch of the pubis (part of the hip bone). —**pectineal** *adj.*

①**肛門梳** 肛瓣下方肛管的中間部分。 ②**恥骨梳** 恥骨上枝的銳嵴（髖骨部分）。

pectoral *adj.* relating to the chest.

胸的

pectoral girdle *see* shoulder girdle.

肩胛帶

pectoral muscles the chest muscles (see illustration). The *pectoralis major* is

胸肌 胸部肌肉（見圖）。胸大肌是一塊大的

a large fan-shaped muscle that works over the shoulder joint, drawing the arm forward across the chest and rotating it medially. Beneath it, the *pectoralis minor* depresses the shoulder and draws the scapula down towards the chest.

扇形肌肉，它的功能是支配肩關節，使手臂前伸和向內旋轉；胸大肌下面是胸小肌，它使肩關節下降和肩胛骨內收。

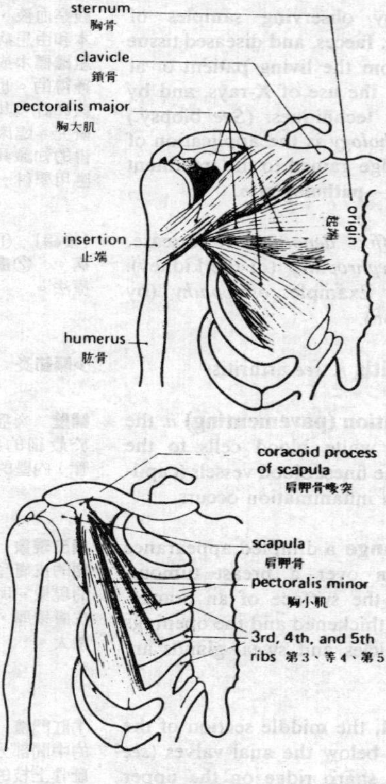

Pectoral muscles
胸肌

pectoriloquy *n.* abnormal transmission of the patient's voice sounds through the chest wall so that they can be clearly heard through a stethoscope. Whispered sounds (*whispering pectoriloquy*) can be heard over the lung of a patient with pneumonia.

胸語音　病人經胸壁非正常傳導的聲音。該種聲音借助聽診器可清晰地聽到。肺炎病人肺部可聽到耳語胸語音（低音胸語音）。

pectus *n.* the chest or breast.

胸

pedicle *n.* **1.** the narrow neck of tissue connecting some tumours to the normal tissue from which they have developed. **2.** (in plastic surgery) a narrow folded tube of skin by means of which a piece of skin used for grafting remains attached to its original site. A pedicle graft is used when the recipient site is unsuited to take an independent skin graft (for example, because of poor blood supply). *See also* **flap**, **skin graft**. **3.** (in anatomy) any slender stemlike process.

蒂 ①某些腫瘤與其賴以生長的正常組織之間相連的狹窄頸樣組織。 ②（在整形外科手術中）由移植皮片摺疊成的狹窄的管狀物，該皮片仍附着於原取皮膚部位。當接受植皮部位（例如，由於供血不足）不宜採用分離的移植皮片時，可採用蒂狀移植皮片。 ③（解剖學）任何細長的莖狀突起。

pediculicide *n.* an agent that kills lice; for example *benzyl benzoate, and *gamma benzene hexachloride.

①滅蝨的 ②滅蝨藥 殺滅蝨子的藥物。例如，苯甲酸苄酯和丙體六六六。

Pediculoides (Pyemotes) *n.* a genus of widely distributed tiny predaceous mites. *P. ventricosus* occasionally attacks man and causes an allergic dermatitis called *grain itch*. This complaint most usually affects those people coming into contact with stored cereal products, such as hay and grain.

蒲蟎屬 廣泛分布的小捕食蟎的一個屬。袋形蝨蟎偶爾可侵襲人體，並引起稱之爲穀癢病的變應性皮炎。該病人常有接觸過貯存的穀類植物（如乾草和穀物）的歷史。

pediculosis *n.* an infestation of the body and/or scalp with lice of the genus **Pediculus*, which causes intense itching; continued scratching by the patient may result in bacterial infection of the skin. Untreated pediculosis of the scalp can lead to a condition in which the hair becomes matted together by the exudate from weeping skin lesions. Body lice are destroyed by dusting the body and clothes with DDT powder; head lice are eliminated with gamma benzene hexachloride

蝨病 由體蝨和/或頭蝨引起的疾病。有奇癢，由於病人不斷抓搔，常可引起皮膚的細菌性感染。未經治療的頭蝨病常由於頭皮患病部位的滲出液，致使頭髮糾結成團。在身體和衣服上撒滴滴涕粉可殺滅體蝨；用丙體六六六可殺滅頭蝨。

Pediculus *n.* a widely distributed genus of lice. There are two varieties of the species affecting man: *P. humanus capitis*, the head louse; and *P. humanus corporis*, the body louse. The presence of these parasites can irritate the skin (*see* pediculosis), and in some parts of the world body lice are involved in

蝨屬 一種廣泛分布的蝨屬。侵襲人體的有頭蝨和體蝨兩種。這類寄生蟲能引起皮膚的炎症，世界上某些地方的體蝨可傳播回歸熱和斑疹傷寒。

transmitting *relapsing fever and *typhus.

pedometer *n.* a small portable device that records the number of paces walked, and thus the approximate distance covered. A pedometer is usually attached to the leg or hung at the belt.

步數計 一種小型的手提式的能記錄行走步數的裝置，因此，也能測出行路的大約距離。步數計通常繫在腿上或懸掛在腰帶上。

peduncle *n.* a narrow process or stalk-like structure, serving as a support or a connection. For example, the *middle cerebellar peduncle* connects the pons and cerebellum.

脚，蒂，莖 起支持或連接作用的狹突或莖狀（蒂狀、柄狀）結構。例如，連接腦橋和小腦的小腦脚。

pellagra *n.* a nutritional disease due to a deficiency of *nicotinic acid (a B vitamin). Pellagra results from the consumption of a diet that is poor in either nicotinic acid or the amino acid tryptophan, from which nicotinic acid can be synthesized in the body. It is common in maize-eating communities. The symptoms of pellagra are scaly dermatitis on exposed surfaces, diarrhoea, and depression.

糙皮病 一種由於缺乏煙酸（一種維生素B）引起的營養性疾病。糙皮病是由於飲食中缺乏煙酸或一種氨基酸（色氨酸）所致。色氨酸在人體中能合成爲煙酸。該病常見以玉米爲主食的地區。糙皮病的症狀有暴露的皮膚患脫屑性皮炎、腹瀉和抑鬱症。

pellicle *n.* a thin layer of skin, membrane, or any other substance.

表膜，表皮 一薄層皮膚、膜或任何其他組織。

pelvic girdle (hip girdle) the bony structure to which the bones of the lower limbs are attached. It consists of the right and left *hip bones.

骨盆帶 與下肢骨相連的骨結構，由左、右髖骨組成。

pelvimetry *n.* the measurement of the four internal diameters of the pelvis (transverse, anteroposterior, left oblique, and right oblique). Pelvimetry helps in determining whether it will be possible for a fetus to be delivered in the normal way. Abnormality of the outlet of the pelvis may be an indication for Caesarean section.

骨盆測量法 測量骨盆四條內徑（橫徑、前後徑、左斜徑和右斜徑）的方法。骨盆測量法有助於判斷或決定胎兒能否正常分娩。骨盆出口不正常可能是剖腹產手術的適應症。

pelvis *n.* (*pl.* **pelves**) **1.** the bony structure formed by the *hip bones, *sacrum, and *coccyx: the bony pelvis (see illustration). The hip bones are fused at the back to the sacrum to form a rigid structure that protects the organs of the

①骨盆 由髖骨、骶骨和尾骨構成的骨質結構（見圖）。骶骨與髖骨合併形成堅硬的結構，以保護下腹部的器官，並與下肢肌肉和骨相連接。 **②下腹**

lower abdomen and provides attachment for the bones and muscles of the lower limbs. **2.** the lower part of the abdomen. **3.** the cavity within the bony pelvis. **4.** any structure shaped like a basin, e.g. the expanded part of the ureter in the kidney (*renal pelvis*). —**pelvic** *adj.*

部 ③骨盆內腔，盆腔 ④任何一種形狀像盆的結構。如輸尿管在腎內的擴大部位（腎盂）。

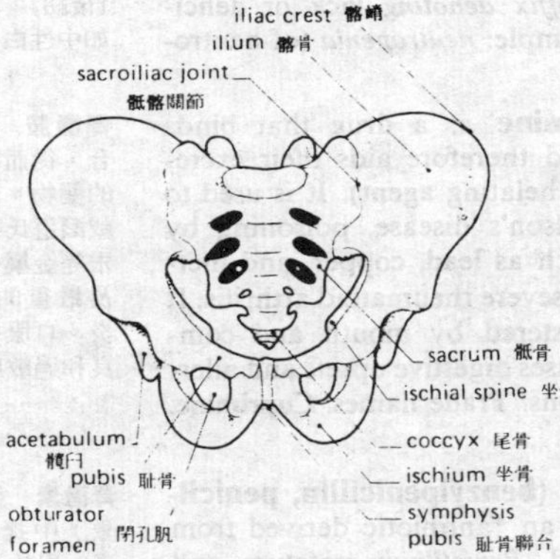

The male pelvis (ventral view)
男性骨盆（前面觀）

pemphigoid *n.* any of a group of skin disorders that resemble pemphigus but are distinct from it. A common type affects the elderly, with large, sometimes bloody, blisters occurring on the trunk and limbs. Attacks may be short or recurrent.

類天疱瘡 一組類似天疱瘡但又與天疱瘡不同的皮膚病。普通型見於老年人，在軀幹與四肢出現大的、有時帶血的大疱。病期可能不長，或者反覆發作。

pemphigus *n.* any of several distinctive skin diseases marked by successive outbreaks of blisters. There are several types; for example, *benign familial pemphigus*, which is a hereditary condition; and *pemphigus vulgaris*, a rare serious disease occurring in middle age and initially affecting the mucous membranes.

天疱瘡 以連續出現大疱爲特徵的一組皮膚病。該病有幾種類型，例如，良性家族天疱瘡（一種遺傳性疾病），尋常天疱瘡（見於中年人的一種以侵犯黏膜爲主的罕見的嚴重疾病）。

penetrance *n.* the frequency with which the characteristic controlled by a gene is seen in the individuals possessing it. Complete penetrance occurs

外顯率 受某個遺傳基因所控制的特徵在含有該基因的個體中的出現率。當已知含有某基因的全部個

when the characteristic is seen in all individuals known to possess the gene. If a percentage of individuals with the gene do not show its effects, penetrance is incomplete. In this way a characteristic in a family may appear to 'skip' a generation.

體均出現某特徵時，就稱爲完全外顯率。如果帶該種基因的個體的百分比不足以顯示出其影響時，就稱之爲不完全外顯率。在這種情況下，某家族中的某一特徵就可能出現隔代遺傳。

-penia *suffix denoting* lack or deficiency. Example: *neutropenia* (of neutrophils).

〔後綴〕 **缺乏，減少** 例如中性白細胞減少症。

penicillamine *n.* a drug that binds metals and therefore aids their excretion (*see* chelating agent). It is used to treat *Wilson's disease, poisoning by metals such as lead, copper, and mercury, and severe rheumatoid arthritis. It is administered by mouth and commonly causes digestive upsets and allergic reactions. Trade names: **Cuprimine**, **Distamine**.

青黴胺 能與金屬相結合，從而有助於金屬排泄的藥物。該藥常用於治療威爾遜氏病，由鉛、銅和汞等金屬引起的中毒，以及嚴重的類風濕性關節炎。口服。常引起消化不良和過敏反應等副作用。

penicillin (benzylpenicillin, penicillin G) *n.* an *antibiotic derived from the mould *Penicillium notatum* and used to treat infections caused by a wide variety of bacteria. It is usually administered by injection, but taken orally is widely used to treat dental abscesses and remains the antibiotic of choice for their treatment. There are few serious side-effects, but some patients are allergic to penicillin and develop such reactions as skin rashes, swelling of the throat, and fever. Trade names: **Crystapen**, **Falapen**, **Icipen**, **Stabillin**.
There are several similar drugs prepared from *P. notatum* (*see* benethamine penicillin, benzathine penicillin) and a number of antibiotics derived from the penicillins (including *ampicillin and *cloxacillin), known as *semi-synthetic penicillins*.

青黴素 從黴菌（特異青黴）中提取的一種抗生素。用於治療由不同細菌引起的感染。通常注射用藥；但在治療牙膿腫時廣泛採取口腔內用藥，至今仍爲治療該種感染的首選藥物。嚴重副作用少見，但某些病人對青黴素有過敏反應，出現如皮疹、咽喉水腫、發燒等反應。
有幾種由特異青黴製取的類似藥物和一些由青黴素衍化而得的抗生素（包括氨苄青黴素和鄰氯青黴素）都稱爲半合成青黴素。

penicillinase *n.* an enzyme-like substance, produced by some bacteria, that is capable of antagonizing the antibacterial action of *penicillin. Purified

青黴素酶 由某些細菌產生的能對抗青黴素抗菌作用的一種酶樣物質。從蠟樣芽胞桿菌株中提純的青

penicillinase, obtained from a strain of **Bacillus cereus*, may be used to treat reactions to penicillin. It is also used in diagnostic tests to isolate microorganisms from the blood of patients receiving penicillin.

黴素酶可用於治療青黴素反應。它也可用於對從接受青黴素治療的病人血液中分離出來的微生物進行診斷檢查。

Penicillium *n.* a genus of mouldlike fungi that commonly grow on decaying fruit, bread, or cheese. The species *P. chrysogenum* is the major natural source of the antibiotic *penicillin. Some species of *Penicillium* are pathogenic to man, causing diseases of the skin and respiratory tract.

青黴屬　一種通常在腐爛的水果、麵包或乳酪上生長的黴菌樣的眞菌屬。產黃青黴是抗生素青黴素的主要自然來源。青黴屬的某些菌種是引起人體皮膚病和呼吸道疾病的致病菌。

penis *n.* the male organ that carries the *urethra, through which urine and semen are discharged (see illustration). Urination can occur in the normal hanging position. Most of the organ is composed of erectile tissue (*see* corpus cavernosum, corpus spongiosum), which becomes filled with blood under conditions of sexual excitement so that the penis is erected. In this position it can act as a sexual organ, capable of entering the vagina and ejaculating semen. *See also* glans, prepuce.

陰莖　帶有尿道的男性器官。尿和精液通過尿道排出（見圖）。在正常懸垂位，可以排尿。該器官主要由勃起組織組成，在性慾衝動時，勃起組織充血，陰莖勃起。在此情況下，它可作爲性器官，進入陰道並射精。

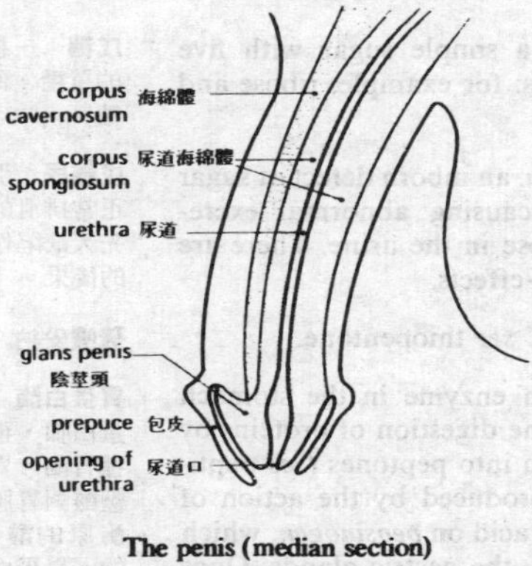

The penis (median section)
陰莖（正中切面）

pent- (penta-) *prefix denoting* five.

〔前綴〕　五

pentaerythritol *n.* a drug that dilates blood vessels and is used in the treat-

季戊四醇　一種用於治療心絞痛與其他心臟病的血

ment of angina and other heart conditions. It is administered by mouth and may cause headache and indigestion. Trade names: **Cardiacap**, **Mycardol**, **Pentral**, **Peritrate**.

管擴張藥。口服。可引起頭痛和消化不良。

pentagastrin *n.* a synthetic hormone that has the same effects as *gastrin in stimulating the secretion of gastric juice from the stomach. It is injected to test for gastric secretion in the diagnosis of digestive disorders. Trade name: **Peptavlon**.

五肽胃泌素 一種能刺激胃分泌消化液，與促胃液素有相同作用的合成激素。在診斷消化障礙時，通過注射，檢查胃液的分泌情況。

pentazocine *n.* a potent *analgesic drug used to relieve moderate or severe pain. It is administered by mouth, injection, or in suppositories; side-effects include dizziness and digestive upsets. Trade name: **Fortral**.

戊唑辛 一種用於緩解中等度或劇烈疼痛的强鎮痛藥。有口服劑、注射劑或栓劑。副作用有頭暈、消化不良。商品名：鎮痛新。

pentobarbitone *n.* a *barbiturate drug used to relieve insomnia and agitation and also as an *anticonvulsant. It is administered by mouth, injection, or in suppositories. Side-effects include rashes, digestive upsets, and lethargy, and prolonged use may lead to *dependence. Trade name: **Nembutal**.

戊巴比妥 一種具有催眠與鎮靜，並且也有抗驚厥作用的巴比妥類藥物。有口服劑、注射劑或栓劑。副作用有皮疹、噁心、暈眩。長期使用可產生賴藥性。

pentose *n.* a simple sugar with five carbon atoms: for example, ribose and xylose.

戊糖 一種帶五個碳原子的單糖。例如，核糖和木糖。

pentosuria *n.* an inborn defect of sugar metabolism causing abnormal excretion of pentose in the urine. There are no serious ill-effects.

戊糖尿 引起尿中戊糖非正常排泄的一種糖代謝的先天缺陷性疾病。無嚴重的後果。

Pentothal *n. see* thiopentone.

硫噴妥鈉

pepsin *n.* an enzyme in the stomach that begins the digestion of proteins by splitting them into peptones (*see* peptidase). It is produced by the action of hydrochloric acid on *pepsinogen*, which is secreted by the gastric glands. Once made, pepsin itself can act on pepsinogen to produce more pepsin.

胃蛋白酶 把蛋白分解爲蛋白腖，再進行消化的一種胃酶。胃蛋白酶是通過鹽酸對胃腺分泌的胃蛋白酶原的酸化作用而生成的。胃蛋白酶一旦生成之後，它本身就能對胃蛋白酶原起催化作用，從而產生更多的胃蛋白酶。

pepsinogen *n. see* pepsin.

胃蛋白酶原

peptic *adj.* **1.** relating to pepsin. **2.** relating to digestion.

①胃蛋白酶的 ②消化的

peptic ulcer a breach in the lining (mucosa) of the digestive tract produced by digestion of the mucosa by pepsin and acid. This may occur when pepsin and acid are present in abnormally high concentrations or when some other mechanism reduces the normal protective mechanisms of the mucosa; bile salts may play a part, especially in stomach ulcers. A peptic ulcer may be found in the oesophagus (*oesophageal ulcer*, associated with reflux *oesophagitis); the stomach (*see* gastric ulcer); duodenum (*see* duodenal ulcer); jejunum (*jejunal ulcer*, usually in the *Zollinger-Ellison syndrome); in a Meckel's *diverticulum; and close to a *gastroenterostomy (*stomal ulcer*, *anastomatic ulcer*, *marginal ulcer*).

消化性潰瘍 由於胃蛋白酶和胃酸對黏膜的消化作用在消化道內壁（黏膜）產生的病損。這可能由於胃蛋白酶與胃酸過濃或某些其他原因減低了黏膜的正常保護作用而引起。膽汁酸鹽對胃潰瘍的形成可能起着一種特殊作用。在食管（與回流性食管炎伴發的食管潰瘍）、胃、十二指腸、空腸（通常在卓-埃二氏綜合徵中的空腸潰瘍）、美克爾憩室和靠近胃腸吻合術的地方（吻合口潰瘍、吻合處潰瘍、邊緣潰瘍）都有可能發現潰瘍。

peptidase *n.* one of a group of digestive enzymes that split proteins in the stomach and intestine into their constituent amino acids. The group is divided into *endopeptidases and *exopeptidases.

肽酶 一組消化酶中的一種。它將胃、腸中的蛋白質分解爲其構成單位氨基酸。該組消化酶分爲肽鏈內斷酶和肽鏈端解酶。

peptide *n.* a molecule consisting of two or more *amino acids linked by bonds between the amino group (-NH) and the carboxyl group (-CO). This bond is known as a *peptide bond*. *See also* polypeptide.

肽 由兩個或多個氨基酸組成的分子結構，在氨基團（－NH）與羧基團（－CO）之間以鏈相連。該腱稱爲肽腱（見多肽）。

peptone *n.* a large protein fragment produced by the action of enzymes on proteins in the first stages of protein digestion.

蛋白腖 大的蛋白質裂解產物。在蛋白消化過程的第一階段，通過酶對蛋白質的消化作用而產生。

peptonuria *n.* the presence in the urine of *peptones, intermediate compounds formed during the digestion of proteins.

腖尿 尿中出現蛋白腖。蛋白腖爲蛋白質消化過程中形成的中間化合物。

perception *n.* (in psychology) the process by which information about the world, received by the senses, is analysed and made meaningful. Abnormalities of perception include *hallucinations, *illusions, and *agnosia.

知覺 （心理學）對通過感覺所接受的關於各種事物的信息進行分析，並賦予意義的加工過程。異常性知覺有幻覺、錯覺及失認症。

percussion *n.* the technique of examining part of the body by tapping it with the fingers or an instrument (*plessor*) and sensing the resultant vibrations. With experience it is possible to detect the presence of abnormal solidification or enlargement in different organs and the presence of fluid, for example in the lungs.

叩診 用手指或器械（叩診槌）輕敲身體某個部位，並感覺其產生的振動的查體技術。有經驗者可以檢查出不同器官的異常實變或腫大和積液（如在肺部）。

percutaneous *adj.* through the skin: often applied to the route of administration of drugs in ointments, etc., which are absorbed through the skin.

經皮膚的 通過皮膚。常爲油膏等製劑的給藥途徑。該製劑通過皮膚吸收。

percutaneous nephrolithotomy a technique of removing stones from the kidney via an endoscope passed into the kidney through a track from the skin surface previously established by the presence of a catheter.

經皮腎結石切除術 一種借助內窺鏡從腎臟切除結石的手術。內窺鏡通過預先從皮膚表面借助導管建立的徑路進入腎臟。

perforation *n.* the creation of a hole in an organ, tissue, or tube. This may occur in the course of a disease (e.g. a *duodenal ulcer, colonic *diverticulitis, or stomach cancer), allowing the contents of the intestine to enter the peritoneal cavity, which causes acute inflammation (*peritonitis) with sudden severe abdominal pain and shock. Treatment is usually by surgical repair of the perforation, but conservative treatment with antibiotics may result in spontaneous healing. Perforation may also be caused accidentally by instruments – for example a gastroscope may perforate the stomach, a curette may perforate the womb – or by injury; for example to the eardrum.

穿孔 在某器官、組織或管道內發生孔洞。這可能發生於某種疾病（如十二指腸潰瘍、結腸憩室炎或胃癌）。如腸內容物進入腹腔，能引起具有突發性腹部劇烈疼痛與休克症狀的急性炎症（腹膜炎）。治療通常採用外科手術修復穿孔處，但用抗生素保守療法也可能自癒。醫療器械也有可能造成事故性穿孔，如胃鏡可造成胃穿孔，刮匙可造成子宮穿孔；外傷也可造成穿孔，如耳鼓室的外傷性穿孔。

perfusion *n.* **1.** the passage of fluid through a tissue, especially the passage of blood through the lung tissue to pick up oxygen from the air in the alveoli, which is brought there by *ventilation, and release carbon dioxide. If ventilation is impaired deoxygenated venous blood is returned to the general circulation. If perfusion is impaired insufficient gas exchange takes place. **2.** the

灌流 ①液體通過組織的過程。特別指血液通過肺組織，從肺泡的空氣中獲取氧的過程。借助於換氣，吸取氧氣釋放出二氧化碳。如果發生換氣障礙，脫氧靜脈血液仍回流入大循環。如果灌流功能受到損傷，空氣就不能進行充分交換。②有意地

deliberate introduction of fluid into a tissue, usually by injection into the blood vessels supplying the tissue.

將液體輸入某組織。通常用注射法向支配該組織的血管輸注液體。

peri- *prefix denoting* near, around, or enclosing. Examples: *pericardial* (around the heart); *peritonsillar* (around a tonsil).

〔前綴〕 **附近，周圍** 例如心包的（心臟周圍），扁桃體周的（扁桃體周圍的）。

periadenitis *n.* inflammation of tissues surrounding a gland.

腺周炎 腺體周圍組織發生的炎症。

perianal haematoma (external haemorrhoid) a small painful swelling beside the anus, occurring after a bout of straining to pass faeces or coughing. Perianal haematomas are caused by the rupture of a small vein in the anus. They often heal spontaneously but occasionally rupture. Rarely this is followed by abscess formation. If severe pain continues, surgical removal can be undertaken. *See also* haemorrhoids.

肛門周圍血腫（外痔） 在排大便困難或陣咳後於肛門附近出現的小的疼痛性的血腫。肛門周圍血腫是由於肛門內小靜脉破裂而引起，常能自癒，偶可破裂。伴發膿腫者很少見。如果劇烈疼痛持續不止，可採用手術切除。

periapical *adj.* around an apex, particularly the apex of a tooth. The term is applied to bone surrounding the apex and to X-ray views of this area.

尖周的 尖端周圍。特指齒根尖。該術語用於描述根尖周圍的骨骼及其X綫所見。

periarteritis nodosa *see* polyarteritis nodosa.

結節性動脉外膜炎

periarthritis *n.* inflammation of tissues around a joint capsule, including tendons and *bursae. *Chronic periarthritis*, which may be spontaneous or follow injury, is a common cause of pain and stiffness of the shoulder; it usually responds to local steroid injections or physiotherapy.

關節周炎 關節囊周圍組織，包括肌腱和滑液囊的炎症。慢性關節周炎，可能是自發的，也可能是外傷引起的，是肩關節疼痛和僵直的常見原因。通常採用局部類固醇注射或物理療法。

pericard- (pericardio-) *prefix denoting* the pericardium.

〔前綴〕 **心包**

pericardectomy *n.* surgical removal of the membranous sac surrounding the heart (pericardium). It is used in the treatment of chronic constrictive pericarditis and chronic pericardial effusion (*see* pericarditis).

心包切除術 切除心臟周圍膜囊（心包）的手術。用於治療慢性縮窄性心包炎和慢性的心包腔積液。

pericardiocentesis *n.* removal of excess fluid from within the sac (pericardium) surrounding the heart by means of needle *aspiration. *See* pericarditis, hydropericardium.

心包穿刺放液術 用針吸出心包腔內的過量的液體。

pericardiolysis *n.* the surgical separation of *adhesions between the heart and surrounding structures within the ribcage (*adherent pericardium*). The operation has now fallen into disuse.

心包鬆解術 在胸腔內將心臟與其周圍結構分離（黏連的心包）的外科手術。這種手術現已不用。

pericardiorrhaphy *n.* the repair of wounds in the membrane surrounding the heart (pericardium), such as those due to injury or surgery.

心包縫合術 修補心包傷口（如由外傷或手術所致）的手術。

pericardiostomy *n.* an operation in which the membranous sac around the heart is opened and the fluid within drained via a tube. It is sometimes used in the treatment of septic pericarditis.

心包造口術 打開心包膜，並用導管引流其中液體的手術。該手術有時用於治療膿毒性心包炎。

pericarditis *n.* acute or chronic inflammation of the membranous sac (pericardium) surrounding the heart. Pericarditis may be seen alone or as part of pancarditis (*see* endomyocarditis). It has numerous causes, including virus infections, uraemia, and cancer. *Acute pericarditis* is characterized by fever, chest pain, and a pericardial friction rub. Fluid may accumulate within the pericardial sac (*pericardial effusion*). Rarely, chronic thickening of the pericardium (*chronic constrictive pericarditis*) develops. This interferes with activity of the heart and has many features in common with *heart failure, including oedema, pleural effusions, ascites, and engorgement of the veins. Constrictive pericarditis most often results from tubercular infection.

The treatment of pericarditis is directed to the cause. Pericardial effusions may be aspirated by a needle inserted through the chest wall. Chronic constrictive pericarditis is treated by surgical removal of the pericardium (*pericardectomy*).

心包炎 心臟周圍膜囊（心包）的急性或慢性炎症。心包炎可單獨存在，或作爲全心炎的一部分出現。該病有許多病因，包括病毒感染、尿毒症和癌症等。急性心包炎以發燒、胸痛和心包摩擦音爲其特徵。心包腔內可能有積液（心包滲出液）。很少情況下，可發展爲慢性縮窄性心包炎。慢性縮窄性心包炎妨礙了心臟的跳動，並且出現與心力衰竭相似的症狀，包括浮腫、胸膜滲出液、腹水和靜脈充血等。縮窄性心包炎多由於結核感染所致。

心包炎針對病因進行治療。心包滲出液可用針經胸壁穿刺進入心包腔抽出。慢性縮窄性心包炎可用心包切除術治療。

pericardium *n.* the membrane surrounding the heart, consisting of two portions. The outer *fibrous pericardium* completely encloses the heart and is attached to the large blood vessels emerging from the heart. The internal *serous pericardium* is a closed sac of *serous membrane: the inner visceral portion (*epicardium*) is closely attached to the muscular heart wall and the outer parietal portion lines the fibrous pericardium. Within the sac is a very small amount of fluid, which prevents friction as the two surfaces slide over one another as the heart beats. —**pericardial** *adj.*

心包 包圍心臟的膜。它由兩部分組成：外層爲心包纖維層，它把心臟完全包圍，並與從心臟發出的大血管相連；內層爲漿膜密閉囊，其內壁（心外膜）與心肌壁緊密相連，其外壁與心包纖維層相連。囊內有很少量液體，當心臟跳動時，可防止心包兩層表面相互摩擦。

pericardotomy *n.* surgical opening or puncture of the membranous sac (pericardium) around the heart. It is required to gain access to the heart in heart surgery and to remove excess fluid from within the pericardium.

心包切開術 切開或針刺心包的外科手術。在做心臟手術時，爲了接近心臟或從心包內排出過量液體時可採用該種手術。

perichondritis *n.* inflammation of cartilage and surrounding soft tissues, usually due to chronic infection. A common site is the external ear.

軟骨膜炎 軟骨及其週圍組織的炎症。通常是由慢性感染所致，外耳是常發部位。

perichondrium *n.* the dense layer of fibrous connective tissue that covers the surface of *cartilage.

軟骨膜 覆蓋於軟骨表面的纖維結締組織的緻密層。

pericolpitis (paracolpitis) *n.* inflammation of the connective tissues around the vagina.

陰道周炎 陰道周圍結締組織發生的炎症。

pericoronitis *n.* inflammation around the crown of a tooth, particularly a partially erupted third molar.

牙冠周炎 牙冠周圍，特指未完全萌出的第三磨牙周圍的炎症。

pericranium *n.* the *periosteum of the skull.

顱骨膜

pericystitis *n.* inflammation in the tissues around the bladder, causing pain in the pelvis, fever, and symptoms of *cystitis. It usually results from infection in the Fallopian tubes or womb, but can occasionally arise from severe infection in a *diverticulum of the bladder itself. Treatment of pericystitis is directed to the underlying cause

膀胱周炎 膀胱周圍組織的炎症。它能引起盆腔部位疼痛、發燒和膀胱炎等症狀。通常由於輸卵管或子宮感染引起，但偶爾由於膀胱憩室本身的嚴重感染引起。膀胱周炎應針對其主要病因進行治療，通常包括抗生素藥物療法。

and usually involves antibiotic therapy. Pericystitis associated with a pelvic abscess clears when the abscess is surgically drained.

伴有盆腔膿腫的膀胱周炎，一旦手術引流膿腫之後，病情就會減輕。

pericyte *n.* a type of cell surrounding the smallest blood vessels (terminal arterioles and venules and capillaries). It is not capable of contraction, and its function is uncertain.

周皮細胞，外膜細胞 包圍着最小血管（末梢動脉、靜脉、毛細血管）的一型細胞。該型細胞不能收縮，其功能尚不清楚。

periderm *n. see* epitrichium.

皮上層

perifolliculitis *n.* inflammation around the hair follicles.

毛囊周炎 毛囊周圍發生的炎症。

perihepatitis *n.* inflammation of the membrane covering the liver. It is usually associated with abnormalities of the liver (including liver abscess, cirrhosis, tuberculosis) or in chronic peritonitis.

肝周炎 肝臟包膜的炎症。常伴有肝臟其他病變（包括肝膿腫、肝硬化、肝結核）或慢性腹膜炎。

perikaryon *n. see* cell body.

核周體

perilymph *n.* the fluid between the bony and membranous *labyrinths of the ear.

外淋巴 位於內耳骨迷路與膜迷路之間的液體。

perimeter *n.* an instrument for mapping the absolute extent of the *visual field (see illustration). The patient looks steadily at a target in the centre of the inner surface of the hemisphere. Ob-

視野計 一種測量視野絕對範圍的儀器（見圖）。病人注視着半球內表面的中心目標，說出他在半球內表面看見的物體。這樣

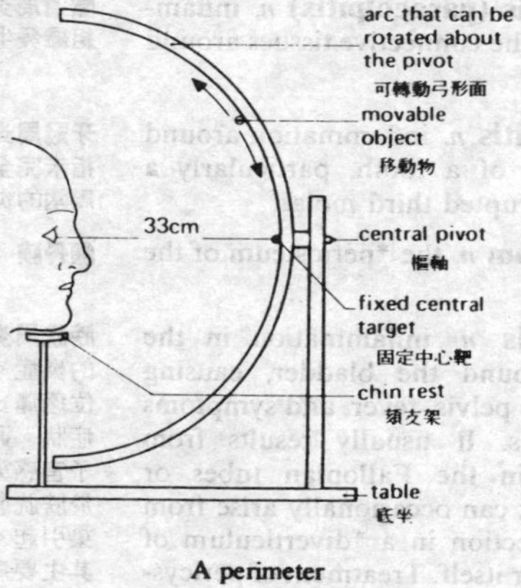

A perimeter
視野計

jects·are presented on this surface and the patient says if he sees them. The edge of the visual field can be defined and any gaps in the field can be detected. There are several types of perimeter. In the *static perimeter* the movable object is replaced by a system of tiny lights, set in a black background, that can be flashed singly or in patterns. If the patient has a field defect he will fail to see the lights that flash in the area of the defect. —**perimetry** *n.*

就能確定其視野邊界並檢查出其視野的任何缺陷。視野計有幾種類型。固定視野計上無移動物體，而在黑色背景上裝一組能單獨閃光或同時構成圖形的小燈泡。如果病人視野的某部位有缺陷，就看不見該視野區域的閃光燈泡。

perimetritis *n.* inflammation of the membrane on the outer surface of the womb. The condition may be associated with *parametritis.

子宮外膜炎 子宮外膜層的炎症。該病可伴發子宮旁組織炎。

perimetrium *n.* the *peritoneum of the womb (uterus).

子宮外膜 子宮的腹膜層。

perimysium *n.* the fibrous sheath that surrounds each bundle of *muscle fibres.

肌束膜 包裹各條肌纖維的纖維鞘。

perinatal *adj.* relating to the period from about three months before to one month after birth.

圍產期的 大約從出生前三個月到出生後一個月這段時期的。

perinatal mortality rate *see* infant mortality rate.

圍產期死亡率

perineoplasty *n.* a tissue-grafting operation to repair the area between the vulva and anus (the perineum).

會陰成形術 修復外陰與肛門之間區域（會陰）的一種組織移植手術。

perineorrhaphy *n.* the stitching of a tear, possibly sustained during childbirth, in the region between the vulva and anus (the perineum). The operation may involve repair of the vaginal wall.

會陰縫合術 縫合在外陰與肛門之間區域（會陰）可能在分娩期間造成的裂傷的手術。該手術可包括陰道壁的修復。

perinephritis *n.* inflammation of the tissues around the kidney. This is usually due to spread of infection from the kidney itself (*see* pyelonephritis, pyonephrosis). The patient has pain in the loins, fever, and fits of shivering. Prompt treatment of the underlying

腎周炎 腎周圍組織的炎症。通常由於腎臟本身感染蔓延引起。病人可有腰痛、發燒和寒顫等症狀。爲了預防膿腫形成，應及時治療腎臟的主要感染。

renal infection is required to prevent progression to an abscess.

perineum *n.* the region of the body between the anus and the urethral opening, including both skin and underlying muscle. In females it is perforated by the vaginal opening. —**perineal** *adj.*

會陰 位於肛門與尿道口之間的區域，包括皮膚和下層肌肉。女性的會陰有陰道開口。

perineurium *n.* the sheath of connective tissue that surrounds individual bundles (fascicles) of nerve fibres within a large *nerve.

神經束膜 在大的神經內包裹各條神經纖維的結締組織鞘。

periodic acid-Schiff (PAS) reaction a test for the presence of glycoproteins, polysaccharides, certain mucopolysaccharides, glycolipids, and certain fatty acids in tissue sections. The tissue is treated with periodic acid, followed by *Schiff's reagent. A positive reaction is the development of a red or magenta coloration.

高碘酸席夫氏反應 一種檢查組織切片中是否含有糖蛋白、多糖、某種黏多糖、糖脂和某種脂肪酸的試驗。該組織切片用高碘酸處理後，再用席夫氏試劑染色。陽性反應呈紅色或品紅色。

periodic fever *see* malaria.

周期熱

periodontal *adj.* denoting or relating to the tissues surrounding the teeth.

牙周的 指牙齒周圍組織的。

periodontal abscess an abscess that arises in the periodontal tissues and is invariably an acute manifestation of periodontal disease.

牙周膿腫 牙周圍組織發生的膿腫，常爲牙周的一種急性炎症。

periodontal disease disease of the tissues that support and attach the teeth – the gums, periodontal membrane, and alveolar bone. It is caused by the metabolism of bacterial *plaque on the surfaces of the teeth adjacent to these tissues. Periodontal disease includes *gingivitis and the more advanced stage of *periodontitis*, which results in the formation of spaces between the gums and the teeth (*periodontal pockets*), the loss of some fibres that attach the tooth to the jaw, and the loss of bone. The disease is widespread and is the most common cause of tooth loss in older people. Poor oral hygiene is a major contributory factor, but the resistance of the patient has some influence.

牙周病 支撑和緊貼牙齒的組織（牙齦、牙周膜和牙槽骨）的疾病。該病是由於受到靠近這些組織的牙齒表面菌斑中的細菌代謝作用而引起。牙周病包括齦炎和牙周炎的後期，此時牙齦與牙齒之間形成空隙（牙周袋），牙齒與頜骨相連的某些纖維骨質皆受損。牙周病廣泛存在，是老年人牙齒脫落最常見的原因。口腔衛生差是主要的致病因素，但與病人抵抗力下降也有一定的關係。

periodontal membrane (periodontal ligament) the ligament around a *tooth, by which it is attached to the bone.

牙周膜（牙周韌帶） 牙齒周圍的韌帶，牙齒通過該韌帶與骨相連。

periodontal pocket a space between the gingival tissues and tooth occurring in periodontitis. *See* periodontal disease.

牙周袋 在牙齦組織與牙齒之間形成的空隙，常由牙周炎引起。

periodontium *n.* the tissues that support and attach the teeth: the gums (*see* gingiva), *periodontal membrane, alveolar bone, and *cementum.

牙周組織 支撐和緊貼牙齒的組織。包括牙齦、牙周膜、牙槽骨和牙骨質。

periodontology *n.* the branch of dentistry concerned with the tissues that support and attach the teeth and the prevention and treatment of *periodontal disease.

牙周病學 牙科學的分支學科。係研究有關支撐和緊貼牙齒的組織，以及防治牙周病的一門學科。

periosteum *n.* a layer of dense connective tissue that covers the surface of a bone except at the articular surfaces. The outer layer of the periosteum is extremely dense and contains a large number of blood vessels. The inner layer is more cellular in appearance and contains osteoblasts and fewer blood vessels. The periosteum provides attachment for muscles, tendons, and ligaments.

骨膜 除關節表面外所有覆蓋骨表面的緻密結締組織層。骨膜外層非常緻密，並含有大量血管；骨膜內層外觀疏鬆，含有成骨細胞和少量血管。肌肉、肌腱和韌帶附着在骨膜上。

periostitis *n.* inflammation of the membrane surrounding a bone (*see* periosteum). *Acute periostitis* results from direct injury to the bone and is associated with a *haematoma, which may later become infected. The uncomplicated condition subsides quickly with rest and anti-inflammatory analgesics. *Chronic periostitis* sometimes follows but is more often due to an inflammatory disease, such as tuberculosis or syphilis, or to a chronic ulcer overlying the bone involved. Chronic periostitis causes thickening of the underlying bone, which is evident on X-ray.

骨膜炎 包裹骨骼的膜層發生的炎症。急性骨膜炎由於直接骨外傷引起，伴有血腫，隨後可能引起感染。如無併發症，進行休息和使用抗炎止痛藥治療，能很快緩解。有時可引起慢性骨膜炎，但慢性骨膜炎的大多數還是由某種特殊炎症疾病引起，如結核、梅毒和患骨上方的慢性潰瘍等。慢性骨膜炎能引起骨膜炎症下方的骨質增厚，這一特徵可在X綫下顯示出來。

peripheral nervous system all parts of the nervous system lying outside the

外周神經系統 除中樞神經系統（大腦與脊髓）以

central nervous system (brain and spinal cord). It includes the *cranial nerves and *spinal nerves and their branches, which link the receptors and effector organs with the brain and spinal cord. *See also* autonomic nervous system.

外的全部神經系統。該系統包括顱神經、脊神經和它們的分支。這些分支將感受器和效應器與大腦和脊髓連接起來。

periphlebitis *n.* inflammation of the tissues around a vein: seen as an extension of *phlebitis.

靜脉周炎 靜脉周圍組織的炎症。是靜脉炎蔓延的結果。

perisalpingitis *n.* inflammation of the membrane on the outer surface of a Fallopian tube.

輸卵管腹膜炎 輸卵管外膜層的炎症。

perisplenitis *n.* inflammation of the external coverings of the spleen.

脾周炎 脾臟外部覆蓋組織的炎症。

peristalsis *n.* a wavelike movement that progresses along some of the hollow tubes of the body. It occurs involuntarily and is characteristic of tubes that possess circular and longitudinal muscles, such as the *intestines. It is induced by distension of the walls of the tube. Immediately behind the distension the circular muscle contracts. In front of the distension the circular muscle relaxes and the longitudinal muscle contracts, which pushes the contents of the tube forward. —**peristaltic** *adj.*

蠕動 沿着身體某些空心管道前進的一種波浪形運動。是具有環狀肌和縱向肌的管道器官（如腸）所特有的一種不隨意運動。它是由於管壁擴張引起的。緊接管壁擴張，其後部的環狀肌收縮。前部的環狀肌鬆弛，而縱向肌收縮，於是便把管道內容物向前推進。

peritendineum *n.* the fibrous covering of a tendon.

腱鞘 覆蓋於肌腱的纖維層。

peritendinitis *n. see* tenosynovitis.

腱鞘炎

peritomy *n.* an eye operation in which an incision of the conjunctiva is made in a complete circle around the cornea. It is performed for the relief of *pannus.

球結膜環狀切開術 在球結膜上沿角膜做一完全性環狀切開的眼科手術。該手術用來緩解角膜翳。

peritoneoscope *n. see* laparoscope.

腹腔鏡

peritoneum *n.* the *serous membrane of the abdominal cavity (see illustration). The *parietal peritoneum* lines the walls of the abdomen, and the *visceral peritoneum* covers the abdominal organs. *See also* mesentery, omentum. —**peritoneal** *adj.*

腹膜 腹腔的漿膜層（見圖）。腹膜壁層內襯於腹壁，而腹膜臟層覆蓋於腹部器官。

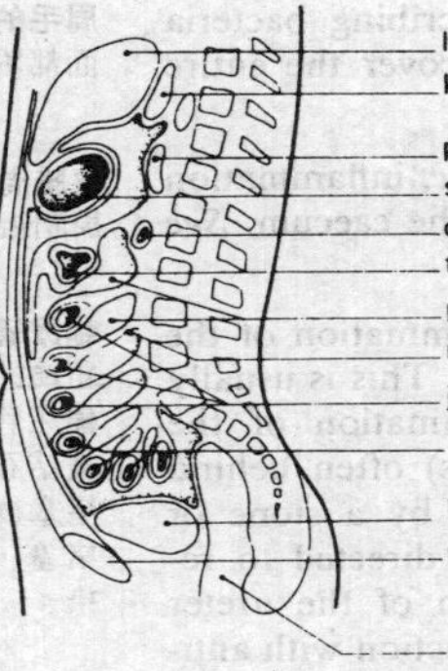

Sagittal section of the abdomen to show arrangement of the peritoneum
表示腹膜分佈的腹腔縱切面圖

peritonitis *n.* inflammation of the *peritoneum. *Primary peritonitis* is caused by bacteria spread via the bloodstream: examples are *pneumococcal peritonitis* and *tuberculous peritonitis.* Symptoms are diffuse abdominal pain and swelling, with fever and weight loss. Fluid may accumulate in the peritoneal cavity (*see* ascites) or the infection may complicate existing ascites. *Secondary peritonitis* is due to perforation or rupture of an abdominal organ (for example, a duodenal ulcer or the vermiform appendix), allowing access of bacteria and irritant digestive juices to the peritoneum. This produces sudden severe abdominal pain, first at the site of rupture but becoming generalized. Shock develops, and the abdominal wall becomes rigid; X-ray examination may reveal gas within the peritoneal cavity. Treatment is usually by surgical repair of the perforation, but in some cases conservative treatment using antibiotics and intravenous fluid may be used. *Subphrenic abscess is a possible complication.

腹膜炎 腹膜的炎症。原發性腹膜炎是由細菌經血液傳播引起，例如肺炎球菌腹膜炎和結核性腹膜炎。症狀爲瀰散性腹部疼痛和腹脹，並伴有發燒和體重減輕。腹腔內可有腹水，可合併其他細菌感染。繼發性腹膜炎是由於腹部器官穿孔或破裂（例如十二指腸潰瘍或闌尾炎）細菌和刺激性消化液進入腹腔所致。這樣就會引起突發性的劇烈腹痛，先在破裂處，繼而遍及全腹部。出現休克、腹壁變硬。X線檢查可發現腹腔內充有氣體。治療：通常用手術修復穿孔，但有些病例也採用抗生素和靜脈輸液等保守療法。

peritonsillar abscess *see* quinsy.

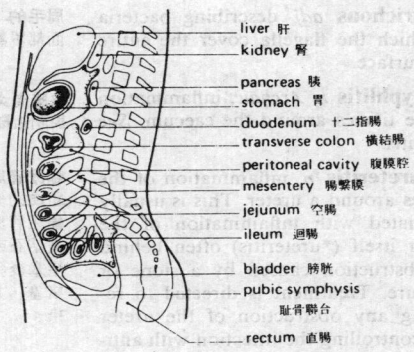

扁桃體周膿腫

peritrichous *adj.* describing bacteria in which the flagella cover the entire cell surface.

周毛的 描述整個細胞表面都覆蓋有鞭毛的細菌。

perityphlitis *n. Archaic.* inflammation of the tissues around the caecum. *See* typhlitis.

盲腸周炎 （舊稱）盲腸周圍組織發生的炎症。

periureteritis *n.* inflammation of the tissues around a ureter. This is usually associated with inflammation of the ureter itself (*ureteritis) often behind an obstruction caused by a stone or stricture. Treatment is directed to relieving any obstruction of the ureter and controlling the infection with antibiotics.

輸尿管周炎 輸尿管周圍組織的炎症。該病通常與輸尿管炎有關，常在尿道被結石或因尿道狹窄引起堵塞後發病。治療：解除堵塞，用抗生素控制感染。

perle *n.* a soft capsule containing medicine.

珠劑 一種內含藥物的軟膠囊。

perleche *n.* dryness and cracking of the corners of the mouth, sometimes with infection. Perleche may be caused by persistent lip licking or by a vitamin-deficient diet.

傳染性口角炎 口角乾裂，有時伴有感染。該病可能由於持續不斷地舔唇，或由於食物中缺乏某種維生素所引起。

pernicious *adj.* describing diseases that are highly dangerous or likely to result in death if untreated. *See also* pernicious anaemia.

惡性的 描述具有極大危險性或若不治療很可能致死的疾病。

pernicious anaemia a form of *anaemia resulting from deficiency of *vitamin B_{12}. This in turn results either from failure to produce the substance (*intrinsic factor) that facilitates absorption of B_{12} from the bowel or from dietary deficiency of the vitamin. Pernicious anaemia is characterized by defective production of red blood cells and the presence of *megaloblasts in the bone marrow. In severe forms the nervous system is affected (*see* subacute combined degeneration of the cord). The condition is treated by injections of vitamin B_{12}.

惡性貧血 一種由缺乏維生素 B_{12} 而引起的貧血。這是由於不能產生促進從腸內吸收維生素 B_{12} 的物質（內因子）或由於飲食中缺乏該種維生素所致。惡性貧血是以紅細胞的生成缺陷和骨髓中出現巨成紅細胞爲其特徵。病情嚴重時，神經系統也受到影響。該病用注射維生素 B_{12} 來治療。

pernio *n. see* chilblain.

凍瘡

perniosis *n.* any one of a group of conditions caused by the effect of persistent cold on individuals whose skin

凍瘡病 皮膚血管特別敏感的人受到持續寒冷刺激時產生的一組疾病。小動

blood vessels are especially sensitive. The small arteries constrict and the capillaries dilate slowing the blood flow. The blood loses all its oxygen and fluid passes from the stagnant capillary blood into the tissues. The affected area becomes blue, swollen, and cold. Perniosis includes such conditions as *chilblains, *acrocyanosis, *erythrocyanosis, and *Raynaud's disease.

脉收縮和毛細血管擴張，從而血流速度減慢。血氧耗盡，液體通過鬱血的毛細血管進入組織。患部發青、腫脹和寒冷。凍瘡病包括諸如凍瘡、手足發紺、紺紅皮病和雷諾氏病等。

pero- *prefix denoting* deformity; defect. Example: *peromelia* (of the limbs).

〔前綴〕 **殘缺，畸形**

peroneal *adj.* relating to or supplying the outer (fibular) side of the leg.

腓骨的，腓側的 小腿外側的。

peroneus *n.* one of the muscles of the leg that arises from the fibula. The *peroneus longus* and *peroneus brevis* are situated at the side of the leg and inserted into the metatarsal bones of the foot. They help to turn the foot outwards.

腓骨肌 起自腓骨的小腿肌肉。腓長肌與腓短肌均位於小腿一側，止於蹠骨，使脚向外旋轉。

peroxidase *n.* an enzyme, found mainly in plants but also present in leucocytes and milk, that catalyses the dehydrogenation (oxidation) of various substances in the presence of hydrogen peroxide (which acts as a hydrogen acceptor, being converted to water in the process).

過氧化物酶 主要存在於植物中，但在白細胞和牛奶中也能發現的一種酶。在存在有過氧化氫的條件下，它能催化各種物質的脫氫作用。過氧化氫作爲氫的受體出現，在該反應過程中轉化爲水。

peroxisome *n.* a small structure within a cell that is similar to a *lysosome but contains different enzymes, some of which may take part in reactions involving hydrogen peroxide.

過氧化物酶體 細胞內的一種小結構，它與溶酶體相似，但含有的酶不同，其中有些酶參與過氧化氫的反應。

perphenazine *n.* a major *tranquillizer used to relieve anxiety, tension, and agitation and to prevent nausea and vomiting. It is administered by mouth or injection; side-effects are similar to those of *chlorpromazine. Trade name: **Fentazin**.

羥哌氯丙嗪 一種用於治療焦慮、緊張和激動，並能預防噁心和嘔吐的重要安定藥。口服或注射。副作用與氯丙嗪相同。商品名：奮乃靜。

perseveration *n.* excessive persistence at a task that prevents the individual from turning his attention to new situations. It is a symptom of organic disease

持續症 不論情況發生任何變化，患者的注意力仍持續地固定於某一事件。這是大腦的器質性病變的

of the brain and sometimes of obsessional neurosis.

症狀，有時爲强迫性神經官能症的症狀。

personality *n.* (in psychology) an enduring disposition to act and feel in particular ways that differentiate one individual from another. These patterns are sometimes conceptualized as different categories (*see* personality disorder) and sometimes as different dimensions (*see* extroversion, neuroticism).

人格 （心理學）個人固定的性格。每個人的性格各不相同，都有其行動和表達感情的特殊方式。不同的人格有時按特殊類型分類，有時按其不同的特徵分類。

personality disorder a deeply ingrained and maladjusted pattern of behaviour, persisting through many years. It is usually manifest by the time the individual is adolescent. The abnormality of behaviour must be sufficiently severe that it causes suffering, either to the patient or to other people (or to both). Some such personalities mature into happier people. Most forms of psychotherapy claim to be of therapeutic value, but the worth of any treatment remains debatable. *See* anankastic, asthenic, hysterical, paranoid, psychopath, schizoid.

人格障礙 持續多年的一種根深蒂固的，適應不良的行爲模式。人格障礙通常在青少年的時期即表現出來。這種行爲異常必須是嚴重的，足能引起患者本人或他人（或兩者）的痛苦。某些人格障礙隨着年齡的增大而逐漸好轉。多種類型的心理療法均宣稱有療效，但任何一種治療效果都有爭議。

perspiration *n.* *sweat or the process of sweating. *Insensible perspiration* is sweat that evaporates immediately from the skin and is therefore not visible; *sensible perspiration* is visible on the skin in the form of drops.

出汗 汗或排汗的過程。不顯汗指汗液從皮膚立即蒸發，因而是看不見的；顯汗是指汗液在皮膚上以汗珠形式出現，因而是可見的。

Perthes' disease *see* Legg-Calvé-Perthes disease.

佩特茲氏病，骨骺骨軟骨病

pertussis *n. see* whooping cough.

百日咳

perversion *n.* any abnormal sexual behaviour. (An equivalent term with less derogatory implications is *deviation*). The abnormality may be in the sexual object (as in *homosexuality and *fetishism) or in the activity engaged in (for example, *sadism and *exhibitionism). The activity is sexually pleasurable.
The definition of what is normal varies with different cultures. Treatment is necessary only when the perversion

性行爲異常 任何一種異常的性行爲。性行爲異常還有一個含有較少貶義的同義詞，即性心理變態。異常性行爲可以指性的對像，如同性戀和戀物癖；或者指所採取的性行爲方式，如施虐狂和露陰癖。以上異常性活動能使病人獲得性滿足。藥物治療的唯一效果是使性慾下降。

causes suffering. Some people may find that *counselling helps them to adjust to their deviation. Others may wish for treatment to change the deviation: *aversion therapy is used, also *conditioning normal sexual fantasies to pleasurable behaviour. The only helpful effect of drugs is to reduce sexual drive generally.

pes *n.* (in anatomy) the foot or a part resembling a foot.

足，脚 解剖學用語。指脚或類似脚的部位。

pes cavus *see* claw-foot.

弓形足

pes planus *see* flat-foot.

扁平足

pessary *n.* **1.** a plastic or metal instrument, often ring-shaped, that fits into the vagina and keeps the womb in position: used to treat *prolapse. **2.** a plug or cylinder of cocoa butter or other soft material containing a drug that is fitted into the vagina for the treatment of gynaecological disorders, e.g. vaginitis. Also called: **vaginal suppository**.

①**子宮托** 一種用於治療子宮脫垂的器具。常將該器具置入陰道內，使子宮保持正常位置。通常由塑料或金屬製成，呈環形。②**陰道栓劑** 用含有藥物的可可豆脂或其他柔軟材料製成的一種栓劑。放入陰道內，用以治療婦科疾病，如陰道炎等。又稱陰道栓劑。

pesticide *n.* a chemical agent used to kill insects or other organisms harmful to crops and other cultivated plants. Some pesticides, such as *parathion and *dieldrin, have caused poisoning in human beings and livestock after accidental exposure.

農藥 用於殺滅昆蟲和對莊稼與其他農作物有害的生物的化學製劑。有些農藥，例如對硫磷和狄氏劑，因意外接觸可引起人畜中毒。

petechia *n.* (*pl.* **petechiae**) a small round flat dark-red spot caused by bleeding into the skin or beneath the mucous membrane. Petechiae occur, for example, in the *purpuras.

瘀斑 一種因皮膚或黏膜下出血引起的平坦的小圓形暗紅色斑。如發生於紫癜病人的瘀斑。

pethidine *n.* a potent *analgesic drug with mild sedative action, used to relieve moderate or severe pain. It is administered by mouth or injection; side-effects may include nausea, dizziness, and dry mouth, and *dependence may occur with prolonged use.

哌替啶 一種用於緩解中度或劇烈疼痛的，並具有弱鎮靜作用的有效鎮痛藥。口服或注射。副作用可有：噁心、頭暈和口乾。用藥期過長可產生賴藥性。

petit mal a form of idiopathic epilepsy in which there are brief spells of uncon-

癲癇小發作 爲特發性癲癇的一種類型。發作時出

sciousness, lasting for a few seconds, during which posture and balance are maintained. The eyes stare blankly and there may be fluttering movements of the lids and momentary twitching of the fingers and mouth. The electroencephalogram characteristically shows bisynchronous wave and spike discharges (3 per second) during the attacks and at other times. Attacks are sometimes provoked by overbreathing or intermittent photic stimulation. As the stream of thought is completely interrupted, children with frequent petit mal may have learning difficulties. Petit mal seldom appears before the age of three or after adolescence.
Drug treatment (with *sodium valproate or *ethosuximide) is usually effective. Petit mal often subsides spontaneously in adult life. It may be accompanied or followed by grand mal.

現暫時性的意識喪失，可持續幾秒，同時姿態保持平衡，兩眼木然凝視，眼瞼顫動、手指與嘴出現瞬息間的抽搐。腦電圖在發作時和在其他時間均顯示以雙同步波和尖峯型放電（每秒3次）爲特徵的異常電波。有時由於呼吸過度或間斷性光刺激而誘發該病發作。兒童有頻繁癲癇小發作者，由於思維的連續性完全中斷，學習可能發生困難。三歲以前或青春期以後，很少有癲癇小發作出現。
通常用藥物（丙戊酸鈉或乙琥胺）治療見效。在成年時期，癲癇小發作常自然消失。癲癇小發作還可伴發或轉變爲癲癇大發作。

Petri dish a flat shallow circular glass or plastic dish with a pillbox-like lid, used to hold solid agar or gelatin media for culturing bacteria.

佩特里細菌培養皿　一種用以培養細菌的淺底圓形帶扁平蓋的玻璃碟或塑料碟。內盛固體瓊脂或明膠培養基。

petrissage *n.* kneading: a form of *massage in which the skin is lifted up, pressed down and squeezed, and pinched and rolled. Alternate squeezing and relaxation of the tissues stimulates the local circulation and may have a pain-relieving effect in muscular disorders.

揉捏法　按摩的一種類型。指在按摩時把皮膚提起、下按、擠壓、捏緊、揉搓。用這種相互交替擠壓和放鬆組織的方法刺激局部的血循環，從而可解除由肌肉病症所引起的疼痛。

petrositis *n.* inflammation of the petrous part of the *temporal bone (which encloses the inner ear), usually due to an extension of *mastoiditis.

顳骨岩部炎　顳骨（內耳位於顳骨中）岩部發生的炎症。通常由乳突炎蔓延引起。

petrous bone *see* temporal bone.

顳骨岩部

-pexy *suffix denoting* surgical fixation. Example: *omentopexy* (of the omentum).

〔後綴〕 **固定術**　指手術固定。例如，網膜固定術。

Peyer's patches oval masses of *lymphoid tissue on the mucous membrane lining the small intestine.

派伊爾氏淋巴集結　內襯於小腸黏膜上面的淋巴組織卵圓形塊。

Peyronie's disease a dense fibrous plaque in the penis, which can be felt in the erectile tissue as an irregular hard lump. The penis curves or angulates at this point on erection and pain often results. The cause is unknown and treatment unsatisfactory. The pain usually subsides spontaneously, but impotence often results.

佩羅尼氏病，纖維性海綿體炎 陰莖內的一種緻密纖維組織斑。可在海綿體（勃起組織）中觸摸到不規則硬塊。在陰莖勃起時，陰莖此處呈弧形或棱形彎曲，並感到疼痛。病因不明，治療效果不滿意。疼痛通常自然消失，但常導致陽萎。

pH a measure of the concentration of hydrogen ions in a solution, and therefore of its acidity or alkalinity. A pH of 7 indicates a neutral solution, a pH below 7 indicates acidity, and a pH in excess of 7 indicates alkalinity.

氫離子指數 測定溶液中的氫離子濃度的指標。以此得知它為酸性或鹼性。氫離子指數是7時為中性，小於7為酸性，大於7為鹼性。

phaco- *prefix. see* phako-.

〔前綴〕 ①**晶狀體** ②**透鏡**

phaeochromocytoma *n.* a small vascular tumour of the inner region (medulla) of the adrenal gland. By its uncontrolled and irregular secretion of the hormones *adrenaline and *noradrenaline, the tumour causes attacks of raised blood pressure, increased heart rate, palpitations, and headache.

嗜鉻細胞瘤 一種腎上腺髓質的小血管瘤。患者由於腎上腺髓質失去控制，不規則地分泌腎上腺素和去甲腎上腺素，從而引起突發性血壓升高、心率加快、心悸和頭痛等症狀。

phag- (phago-) *prefix denoting* **1.** eating. **2.** phagocytes.

〔前綴〕 ①**吞噬** ②**吞噬細胞**

phage *n. see* bacteriophage.

噬菌體

phagedaena *n.* rapidly spreading ulceration with sloughing of dead skin. *See also* bedsore.

崩蝕性潰瘍，蝕瘡 一種帶有壞死性腐肉的，並可迅速蔓延的皮膚潰瘍。

-phagia *suffix denoting* a condition involving eating.

〔後綴〕 **噬** 指與吞食有關的情況或狀態。

phagocyte *n.* a cell that is able to engulf and digest bacteria, protozoa, cells and cell debris, and other small particles. Phagocytes include many white blood cells (*see* leucocyte) and *macrophages, which play a major role in the body's defence mechanism. —**phagocytic** *adj.*

吞噬細胞 一種能夠吞噬和消化細菌、原生動物、細胞、細胞碎片和其他微小顆粒的細胞。吞噬細胞包括各種白細胞和吞噬細胞。它在人體的防禦機能方面起着主要作用。

phagocytosis *n.* the engulfment and digestion of bacteria and other foreign

吞噬作用 指某種細胞（即吞噬細胞）對細菌和

particles by a cell (*see* phagocyte). *Compare* pinocytosis.
其他外來微小顆粒的吞噬和消化過程。

phako- (phaco-) *prefix denoting* the lens of the eye.
〔前綴〕 **晶體** 指眼睛的晶狀體。

phakoemulsification *n.* the process of softening the lens of the eye before removing it in a method of surgery for cataract. A fine probe is inserted into the lens and the emulsification is commonly performed by ultrasonic vibration.
晶體乳化 爲白內障外科手術的一種方法。在眼晶狀體摘除以前，先進行晶體的軟化步驟。把一根細探針插入晶體中，通過超聲波振動來進行乳化。

phalangeal cells rows of supporting cells between the sensory hair cells of the organ of Corti (*see* cochlea).
指細胞 柯替氏器（螺旋器）的感覺毛細胞之間排列成行的支撐細胞。

phalangectomy *n.* surgical removal of one or more of the small bones (phalanges) in the fingers or toes.
指（趾）骨切除術 切除手指或脚趾的一塊或多塊小形骨（指或趾骨）的手術。

phalanges *n.* (*sing.* **phalanx**) the bones of the fingers and toes (digits). The first digit (thumb/big toe) has two phalanges. Each of the remaining digits has three phalanges. —**phalangeal** *adj.*
指（趾）骨 手指和脚趾的骨。第一個手指（拇指）和脚趾（蹞趾）有兩塊指（趾）骨，其他每個指（趾）均有三塊指（趾）骨。

phalangitis *n.* inflammation of a finger or toe, causing swelling and pain. The condition may be caused by infection of the soft tissues, tendon sheaths, bone, or joints or by some rheumatic diseases, such as *psoriatic arthritis. *See also* dactylitis.
指（趾）骨炎 手指或脚趾發生的炎症，常引起腫脹和疼痛。該炎症可能由於軟組織、腱鞘、骨或關節的感染或者因某些風濕性疾病（如銀屑病性關節炎）而引起。

phalanx *n. see* phalanges.
指（趾）骨

phalloplasty *n.* surgical reconstruction or repair of the penis. It is required for congenital deformity of the penis, as in *hypospadias or *epispadias, and sometimes also following injury to the penis with loss of skin.
陰莖成形術 重建或修補陰莖的外科手術。陰莖先天性畸形的病人，如尿道上裂或尿道下裂，和有時陰莖因外傷其皮膚缺損的病人，都有必要做這種手術。

phallus *n.* the embryonic penis, before the urethral duct has reached its final state of development.
初陰 指尿道發育完全之前的胚胎期陰莖。

phanero- *prefix denoting* visible; apparent.
〔前綴〕 **可見的，明顯的**

phaneromania *n.* an excessively strong impulse to touch or rub parts of one's own body.

自體觸摸癖 一種觸摸或摩擦自己身體某些部位的强烈衝動。

phantasy *n. see* fantasy.

幻想

phantom limb the sensation that an arm or leg, or part of an arm or leg, is still attached to the body after it has been amputated. Pain may seem to come from the amputated part. This may arise because of stimulation of the amputation stump, which contains severed nerves that formerly carried messages from the removed portion.

幻肢 病人被截肢後，還認爲被截掉的臂或腿，或者是臂或腿的某部分依然存在的一種幻覺。被截肢的部位似乎感覺到疼痛。這可能由殘端的刺激而引起，殘端含有被切斷的、從前傳遞被截肢體部位信息的神經。

phantom tumour a swelling, in the abdomen or elsewhere, caused by local muscular contraction or the accumulation of gases, that mimics a swelling caused by a tumour or other structural change. The condition is usually associated with emotional disorder, and the 'tumour' may disappear under anaesthesia.

幻想瘤 因局部肌肉收縮或氣體積聚引起腹部或其他部位的腫脹。它酷似由於腫瘤或其他結構發生變化所引起的腫塊，這常與情緒障礙有關，在使用麻醉劑的情况下，所謂腫瘤可能消失。

pharmaceutical *adj.* relating to pharmacy.

藥學的

pharmaceutical committee (local) *see* medical committee (local).

藥學委員會

pharmacist *n.* a person who is qualified by examination and registered and authorized to dispense medicines or to keep open a shop for the sale and dispensing of medicines.

藥劑師 通過考試並注册的有配方與開設藥房資格的人員。

pharmaco- *prefix denoting* drugs. Example: *pharmacophobia* (morbid fear of).

〔前綴〕 **藥物** 例如，藥物恐怖。

pharmacognosy *n.* the knowledge or study of pharmacologically active principles derived from plants.

生藥學 研究植物中的藥效成分的學科。

pharmacology *n.* the science of the properties of drugs and their effects on the body. **—pharmacological** *adj.*

藥理學 研究有關藥物性質和藥物對人體作用的學科。

pharmacomania *n.* an abnormal desire for taking medicines.

藥物癖 想服藥的一種異常慾望。

pharmacopoeia *n.* a book containing a list of the drugs used in medicine, with details of their formulae, methods of preparation, dosages, standards of purity, etc.

藥典 記載醫用藥物及其分子式、制劑方法、劑量、純度標準等的書籍。

pharmacy *n.* **1.** the preparation and dispensing of drugs. **2.** premises registered to dispense medicines and sell poisons.

①**藥劑學** 有關藥物製劑和配方的學科。 ②**藥房** 經登記准許出售一般藥物和麻醉藥的商店。

pharyng- (pharyngo-) *prefix denoting* the pharynx. Example: *pharyngopathy* (disease of).

〔前綴〕 **咽** 例如咽病。

pharyngeal arch (branchial or **visceral arch)** any of the paired segmented ridges of tissue in each side of the throat of the early embryo that correspond to the gill arches of fish. Each arch contains a cartilage, a cranial nerve, and a blood vessel. Between each arch there is a *pharyngeal pouch.

咽弓，鰓弓 胚胎早期咽喉部兩側的成對存在的分節弓狀組織。它相當於魚鰓弓。每側咽弓都含有軟骨、腦神經和血管。咽弓之間有咽囊。

pharyngeal cleft (branchial or **visceral cleft)** any of the paired segmented clefts in each side of the throat of the early embryo that correspond to the gills of fish. Soon after they have formed they close to form the *pharyngeal pouches, except for the first cleft, which persists as the external auditory meatus.

鰓裂 胚胎早期咽喉部兩側成對存在的分節裂縫。相當於魚鰓。它們形成後，除第一對裂縫繼續發育生長為外耳道外，其餘的裂縫很快關閉形成咽囊。

pharyngeal pouch (branchial or **visceral pouch)** any of the paired segmented pouches in the side of the throat of the early embryo. They give rise to the tympanic cavity, the parathyroid glands, the thymus, and probably the thyroid gland.

咽囊 胚胎早期的咽喉兩側成對存在的分節的囊。它們生長發育為中耳鼓室、甲狀旁腺、胸腺或許還有甲狀腺。

pharyngectomy *n.* surgical removal of part of the pharynx.

咽部分切除術 切除部分咽喉的手術。

pharyngismus *n.* spasmodic contraction of the muscles of the pharynx.

咽痙攣 咽喉的肌肉呈痙攣性收縮。

pharyngitis *n.* inflammation of the part of the throat behind the soft palate (pharynx). It produces *sore throat and is usually associated with *tonsillitis.

咽炎 軟腭後的咽喉部位發生的炎症。它能引起咽喉疼痛，並常伴發扁桃體炎。

pharyngocele *n.* a pouch or cyst opening off the pharynx (*see* branchial cyst). **咽突出** 開口於咽喉的囊。

pharyngoplegia *n.* muscular paralysis of the pharynx. **咽肌麻痹** 咽喉部肌肉麻痹。

pharyngoscope *n.* an *endoscope for the examination of the pharynx. **咽鏡** 一種檢查咽喉的內窺鏡。

pharynx *n.* a muscular tube, lined with mucous membrane, that extends from the beginning of the oesophagus (gullet) up to the base of the skull. It is divided into the *nasopharynx, *oropharynx, and *laryngopharynx (see illustration) and it communicates with the posterior *nares, *Eustachian tube, the mouth, larynx, and oesophagus. The pharynx acts as a passageway for food from the mouth to the oesophagus, and as an air passage from the nasal cavity and mouth to the larynx. It also acts as a resonating chamber for the sounds produced in the larynx. —**pharyngeal** *adj.* **咽** 從食道起端開始一直延伸至顱底的內襯黏膜的肌肉性管道，它分爲鼻咽、口咽、喉咽（見圖），並與後鼻孔、咽鼓管、口腔、喉和食管相通。咽是食物從口腔到達食管和空氣從鼻腔與口腔到達喉部的通道。同時也是喉部發出的聲音的共鳴箱。

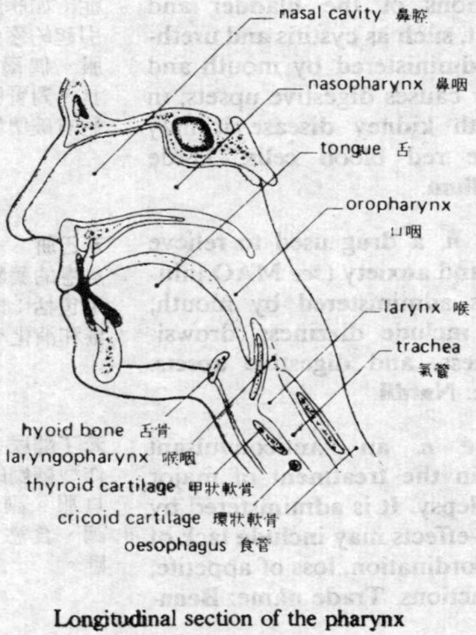

Longitudinal section of the pharynx
咽的縱切面圖

phenacemide *n.* an *anticonvulsant drug used in the treatment of epilepsy. **苯乙醯脲** 一種用於治療癲癇的抗驚厥藥。口服。

It is administered by mouth; side-effects include digestive upsets, fever, and rash. Mental changes and damage to liver, kidneys, and bone marrow may also occur.

副作用包括：消化不良、發燒和皮疹。也可發生精神變化和肝、腎、骨髓的損傷。

phenacetin *n.* an *analgesic drug that also reduces fever, used to relieve mild or moderate pain. It is administered by mouth; side-effects may include sweating and skin rashes. Because prolonged high doses may cause kidney damage, its use in Britain was restricted by law in 1974.

非那西丁　退燒鎮痛藥。用於緩解輕度或中等度疼痛。口服。副作用有出汗和皮疹。大劑量長期用藥，可導致腎臟的損害。英國於1974年頒布法律，該藥在英國使用受到限制。

phenazocine *n.* an *analgesic drug used for rapid relief of moderate or severe pain. It is administered by mouth or injection; side-effects may include digestive upsets and dizziness, and prolonged use may lead to *dependence. Trade name: **Narphen**.

非那唑辛　一種用於緩解中度或劇烈疼痛的速效鎮痛藥。口服或注射。副作用有消化不良和頭暈。長期用藥可產生賴藥性。商品名爲納爾芬。

phenazopyridine *n.* an *analgesic drug used to relieve pain in inflammatory conditions of the bladder and urinary tract, such as cystitis and urethritis. It is administered by mouth and occasionally causes digestive upsets; in patients with kidney disease it may damage the red blood cells. Trade name: **Pyridium**.

鹽酸苯偶氮吡胺　一種用於緩解由於膀胱和尿道炎症（如膀胱炎、尿道炎）引起的疼痛的鎮痛藥。口服。偶爾能引起消化不良。對腎臟病患者的紅細胞有破壞作用。

phenelzine *n.* a drug used to relieve depression and anxiety (*see* MAO inhibitor). It is administered by mouth; side-effects include dizziness, drowsiness, tiredness, and digestive upsets. Trade name: **Nardil**.

苯乙肼　一種治療抑鬱和焦慮的藥物。口服。副作用包括：頭暈、嗜眠、疲倦和消化不良。

pheneturide *n.* an *anticonvulsant drug used in the treatment of major types of epilepsy. It is administered by mouth; side-effects may include lack of muscular coordination, loss of appetite, and skin reactions. Trade name: **Benuride**.

苯丁醯尿　一種治療大發作型癲癇的抗驚厥藥物。口服。副作用有共濟失調、食慾不振和過敏反應。

phenformin *n.* a drug that reduces blood sugar levels and is used to treat *diabetes. It is administered by mouth;

苯乙雙胍　一種治療糖尿病的降血糖藥物。口服。副作用有口中出現金屬味

side-effects include a metallic taste in the mouth and digestive upsets. Trade names: **Dibotin, Dipar, Meltrol**.

和消化不良。商品名：降糖靈。

phenindione *n.* an *anticoagulant drug used to treat thrombosis in the blood vessels of the heart and limbs. It is administered by mouth or injection; side-effects may include skin rashes, fever, and diarrhoea. Trade name: **Dindevan**.

苯茚二酮 一種治療心臟與肢體血管中的血栓的抗凝血藥物。口服或注射。副作用可有皮疹、發燒和腹瀉。

pheniramine *n.* an *antihistamine used to treat allergic reactions such as hay fever and hives. It is administered by mouth or is applied to the skin in an ointment; side-effects may include drowsiness, digestive upsets, and skin reactions. Trade name: **Daneral**.

非尼蠟明 一種治療如枯草熱和蕁麻疹等變態反應性疾病的抗組胺藥物。口服或用其軟膏塗抹皮膚。副作用有瞌睡、消化不良和皮膚過敏反應。商品名：抗感明。

phenmetrazine *n.* a drug that reduces the appetite and was formerly used in the treatment of obesity. It is administered by mouth and its actions and side-effects are similar to those of *amphetamine. Prolonged use and large doses may cause mental depression and *dependence.

苯甲嗎啉 一種從前用於治療肥胖症的食慾抑制藥。口服。其作用和副作用均與苯丙胺相似。長期和大劑量用藥可引起精神抑鬱症和賴藥性。

phenobarbitone *n.* a *barbiturate drug used to treat insomnia and anxiety and as an anticonvulsant in the treatment of epilepsy. It is administered by mouth or injection; side-effects may include drowsiness and skin sensitivity reactions, and dependence may result from continued use.

苯巴比妥，魯米那 一種治療失眠和焦慮的巴比妥類藥，也是一種治療癲癇的抗驚厥藥。口服或注射。副作用有瞌睡和皮膚過敏反應。持續不斷用藥可產生賴藥性。

phenol (carbolic acid) *n.* a strong *disinfectant used for cleansing wounds, treating inflammations of the mouth, throat, and ear, and as a preservative in injections. It is administered as solution, ointments, and lotions and is highly toxic if taken by mouth.

苯酚 一種用於清洗傷口，治療口腔炎、咽喉炎、耳炎的强效力消毒劑。也可用作注射液中的防腐劑。使用的劑型有溶液、軟膏、洗劑。該消毒劑有劇毒，禁忌內服。

phenolphthalein *n.* an irritant *laxative administered by mouth, usually given at night to act the following morning. Side-effects may include stomach cramps.

酚酞 一種口服輕瀉劑。通常夜間給藥，次晨才起作用。副作用可有胃部（痛性）痙攣。

phenolsulphonphthalein *n.* a red dye administered by injection in a test for kidney function.

酚磺酞 在做腎功能試驗時注射用的一種紅色染料。

phenothiazines *n.* a group of chemically related compounds with various pharmacological actions. Some (e.g. *chlorpromazine and *trifluoperazine) are major *tranquillizers; others (e.g. *piperazine) are anthelmintics.

吩噻嗪 一組藥效不同，但化學結構相似的化台物。有些藥物，如氯丙嗪和三氟拉嗪均是主要的安定藥；而另外一些藥物，如哌嗪是驅蟲藥。

phenotype *n.* the observable characteristics of an individual, which result from interaction between the genes he possesses (*genotype) and the environment.

表型 由一個人的固有基因（基因型）和其外在環境因素間相互作用而形成的外顯的特徵。

phenoxybenzamine *n.* a drug that dilates blood vessels (*see* vasodilator). It is used to reduce blood pressure and to treat conditions involving poor circulation, such as Raynaud's disease and chilblains. It is administered by mouth or injection and may cause dizziness and fast heart beat. Trade name: **Dibenyline**.

苯氧苄胺 一種擴張血管藥。用於降低血壓和治療一些血循環不良性疾病，如雷諾氏病和凍瘡。口服或注射。副作用有頭暈和心跳加快。

phenoxymethylpenicillin *n.* an *antibiotic, similar to *penicillin, used to treat infections caused by a wide variety of microorganisms. It is administered by mouth and may cause diarrhoea and allergic reactions.

苯氧甲基青黴素 一種作用和結構與青黴素相似的抗生素。用於治療多種細菌引起的感染。口服。副作用有腹瀉和過敏反應。

phensuximide *n.* an *anticonvulsant drug used to prevent or reduce petit mal fits in epilepsy. It is administered by mouth; side-effects may include dizziness, drowsiness, nausea, and loss of appetite.

苯琥胺 一種預防或治療癲癇小發作的抗驚厥藥物。口服。副作用有頭暈、嗜眠、噁心和食慾不振。

phentermine *n.* a *sympathomimetic drug that suppresses the appetite and is used in the treatment of obesity. It is administered by mouth; side-effects include dry mouth, nausea, and restlessness, and continued use produces *tolerance. Trade names: **Duromine**, **Ionamin**.

苯〔叔〕丁胺 一種抑制食慾的擬交感神經藥。用於治療肥胖症。口服。副作用有口乾、噁心、煩躁不安。連續不斷用藥可產生耐藥性。

phentolamine *n.* a drug that dilates blood vessels (*see* vasodilator) and is

酚胺唑啉 一種擴張血管藥。用於降低嗜鉻細胞瘤

used to reduce blood pressure in *phaeochromocytoma and to treat conditions of poor circulation such as Raynaud's disease and chilblains. It is administered by mouth or injection; side-effects include fast heart beat and digestive upsets. Trade name: **Rogitine**.

患者的血壓和治療一些血液循環不良性疾病，如雷諾氏病和凍瘡。口服或注射。副作用有心跳加快和消化不良。

phenylalanine *n.* an *essential amino acid that is readily converted to tyrosine. Blockade of this metabolic pathway gives rise to *phenylketonuria, which is associated with the excretion of large amounts of phenylalanine and phenylpyruvic acid in the urine and retarded mental development.

苯丙氨酸　一種易於轉化爲酪氨酸的必需氨基酸。這一代謝途徑一旦受到阻礙，便會引起苯丙酮酸尿症，這時尿中含有大量苯丙氨酸和苯丙酮酸，並且影響智力發育。

phenylbutazone *n.* an *analgesic drug that reduces fever and inflammation and is used to relieve pain in rheumatic and related diseases. It is administered by mouth or injection; common side-effects include digestive upsets, rashes, and fluid retention. Trade names: **Butazolidin**, **Butazone**, **Flexazone**.

二苯丁唑酮布他酮　一種具有退燒和消炎作用的鎮痛藥。用於緩解風濕病和有關疾病的疼痛。口服或注射。常見的副作用有消化不良、皮疹和液體瀦留。商品名：保泰松。

phenylephrine *n.* a drug that constricts blood vessels (*see* sympathomimetic). It is given by injection to increase blood pressure, in a nasal spray to relieve nasal congestion, and in eye-drops to dilate the pupils. Irritation may occur when applied. Trade name: **Neophryn**.

脫羥腎上腺素　一種血管收縮藥。通過注射給藥能使血壓上昇；通過鼻腔噴霧能使鼻腔的充血減輕；用作滴眼劑能擴瞳。外用時有刺激作用。商品名：新福林。

phenylketonuria *n.* an inborn defect of protein metabolism causing an excess of the amino acid phenylalanine in the blood, which damages the nervous system and leads to severe mental retardation. Screening of newborn infants by testing a blood sample for phenylalanine (the *Guthrie test*) enables the condition to be detected soon enough for dietary treatment to prevent any brain damage: the baby's diet contains proteins from which phenylalanine has been removed. The gene responsible for phenylketonuria is recessive, so that a child is affected only if both parents are carriers of the defective gene.

苯丙酮酸尿　一種造成血中苯丙氨酸過量的先天性蛋白代謝障礙疾病。苯丙氨酸對神經系統有損害作用，並導致嚴重的智力遲鈍。通過驗血檢查新生兒血液中苯丙氨酸的濃度（加斯里試驗）能很快確診該病。及時採用飲食療法（嬰兒食取不含有苯丙氨酸的蛋白食物）可防止大腦損害。由於苯丙酮酸尿症的致病基因是隱性的，所以只有雙親均是缺陷基因的攜帶者，兒童才會得病。

phenylpropanolamine *n.* a drug with actions similar to those of *ephedrine. It is used to relieve allergic conditions, such as asthma and hay fever, and nasal congestion, and is administered by mouth, injection, or by inhalation. Side-effects may include dizziness, headache, digestive disorders, sweating, and thirst.

苯丙醇胺 一種作用與麻黃鹼相類似的藥物。用於治療如哮喘、枯草熱等過敏性疾病和鼻腔充血。口服、注射或吸入。副作用有頭暈、頭痛、消化不良、出汗和口渴等。

phenylthiocarbamide (PTC) *n.* a substance that tastes bitter to some individuals but is tasteless to others. Response to PTC appears to be controlled by a single pair of genes (*alleles): ability to taste PTC is *dominant to the inability to taste it.

苯硫脲 一些人感到有苦味，但另一些人却並不覺着有苦味的一種物質。人們對苯硫脲的反應似乎是受等位基因的控制。能嘗出苯硫脲苦味的人遠比嚐不出的人多。

phenytoin *n.* an *anticonvulsant drug used to control major (grand mal) and focal fits. It is administered by mouth or injection; the side-effects include gum hypertrophy, hirsutism, and skin rashes. Overdosage causes unsteadiness. Trade name: **Epanutin**.

苯妥英 一種用於控制癲癇大發作和局部發作的抗驚厥藥。口服或注射。副作用有牙齦肥大、多毛〔症〕和皮疹。用藥過量可引起共濟失調與震顫。

phial *n.* a small glass bottle for storing medicines or poisons.

管〔形〕瓶 一種用於貯藏藥物或毒藥的小玻璃瓶。

-philia *suffix denoting* morbid craving or attraction. Example: *nyctophilia* (for darkness).

〔後綴〕 **癖、嗜** 指病態的嗜好。例如，嗜夜癖。

phimosis *n.* narrowing of the opening of the foreskin, which cannot therefore be drawn back over the underlying glans penis. This predisposes to inflammation (*see* balanitis, balanoposthitis), which results in further narrowing. Treatment is by surgical removal of the foreskin (*circumcision).

包莖 包皮開口狹窄。包皮不能從陰莖頭（龜頭）上回縮復位。可誘發炎症，導致進一步狹窄。治療：手術切除包皮（包皮環切術）。

phleb- (phlebo-) *prefix denoting* a vein or veins. Example: *phlebectopia* (abnormal position of).

〔前綴〕 **靜脉** 如靜脉異位。

phlebectomy *n.* the surgical removal of a vein (or part of a vein), sometimes performed for the treatment of varicose veins in the legs (*varicectomy*).

靜脉切除術 切除一根靜脉或部分靜脉的手術。該手術有時用於治療腿部靜脉曲張。

phlebitis *n.* inflammation of the wall of a vein, which is most commonly seen in the legs as a complication of *varicose veins. A segment of vein becomes painful and tender and the surrounding skin feels hot and appears red. Thrombosis (*thrombophlebitis*) commonly develops. Treatment consists of elastic support together with drugs, such as phenylbutazone, to relieve the inflammation and pain. Anticoagulants are not used (*compare* phlebothrombosis). Phlebitis may also complicate sepsis (*see* pylephlebitis) or cancer, especially of the stomach, bronchus, or pancreas. In pancreatic cancer the phlebitis may affect a variety of veins (*thrombophlebitis migrans*).

靜脉炎 靜脉管壁的炎症。通常爲靜脉曲張的併發症，常見於腿部，靜脉的一段產生疼痛、觸痛，其周圍皮膚發熱並呈紅色。患處常易形成血栓（血栓性靜脉炎）。治療：用彈性綳帶包紮，內服保泰松類藥物以消炎鎮痛。不得使用抗凝血藥物。靜脉炎也可以與膿毒血症或癌症併發，尤其是胃癌、支氣管癌或胰腺癌。在胰腺癌時，可引起多發性靜脉炎（游走性血栓性靜脉炎）。

phlebography *n. see* venography.

靜脉造影術

phlebolith *n.* a stone-like structure, usually found incidentally on abdominal X-ray, that results from deposition of calcium in a venous blood clot. It appears as a small round white opacity in the pelvic region. It does not produce symptoms and requires no treatment.

靜脉石 通常在用X線檢查腹部時偶爾發現的一種石狀結構。該結構是由靜脉血管凝塊中鈣沉積物所形成的。它在骨盆部位以一個小圓形的白色不透光斑顯示出來。本病沒有症狀，不需要治療。

phlebosclerosis (venosclerosis) *n.* a rare degenerative condition, of unknown cause, that affects the leg veins of young men. The vein walls become thickened and feel like cords under the skin. It is not related to arteriosclerosis and needs no treatment.

靜脉硬化 一種罕見的、病因不明的、侵襲年輕人腿部靜脉的變性疾病。靜脉管壁增厚，觸摸時皮下像有繩索樣物。它與動脉硬化無關，不需治療。

phlebothrombosis *n.* obstruction of a vein by a blood clot, without preceding inflammation of its wall. It is most common within the deep veins of the calf of the leg (in contrast to thrombophlebitis, which affects superficial leg veins (*see* phlebitis)). Prolonged bed rest, heart failure, pregnancy, injury, and surgery predispose to thrombosis by encouraging sluggish blood flow. Many of these conditions are associated with changes in the clotting factors in

靜脉血栓形成 由於血凝塊而不是由於靜脉炎引起的靜脉堵塞。該病最常見的發生部位是小腿肚的深靜脉（與血栓性靜脉炎的發生部位不同，血栓性靜脉炎主要侵襲腿部表淺靜脉）。長期卧床休息、心衰、妊娠、外傷及手術時血流緩慢，是導致血栓形成的主要原因。多數病例與血液中凝血因素改變有

the blood that increase the tendency to thrombosis; these changes also occur in some women taking oral contraceptives.
The affected leg may become swollen and tender. The main danger is that the clot may become detached and give rise to *pulmonary embolism. Regular leg exercises help to prevent phlebothrombosis, and anticoagulant drugs (such as warfarin and heparin) are used in prevention and treatment. Large clots may be removed surgically in the operation of *thrombectomy* to relieve leg swelling.

關。凝血因素的變化助長了血栓形成的趨勢。有些用口服避孕藥的婦女可發生這種凝血因素的改變。
患腿出現腫脹和觸痛。主要的危險是凝血塊可脫落引起肺栓塞。有規律地進行腿部鍛煉有助於預防靜脈血栓形成；抗凝血藥（如苄丙酮香豆素和肝素等）也可用於預防和治療；大凝血塊可施行血栓切除術以消除腿部腫脹。

Phlebotomus *n. see* sandfly.

白蛉屬

phlebotomy (venesection) *n.* the surgical opening or puncture of a vein in order to remove blood (in the treatment of *polycythaemia) or to infuse fluids, blood, or drugs in the treatment of many conditions. It may also be required for cardiac *catheterization and *angiocardiography.

靜脉切開術，放血術 用於放血（治療紅細胞增多症）或用於輸液、輸血或給藥（治療多種疾病）的切開或穿刺靜脉的手術。做心臟導管插入術與心血管造影術時也可能需要做靜脉切開術。

phlegm *n.* a nonmedical term for *sputum.

黏痰 痰的俗稱。

phlegmon *n. Archaic.* inflammation of connective tissue, leading to ulceration.

蜂窩織炎 舊稱。一種能引起潰瘍的結締組織炎症。

phlycten *n.* a small pinkish-yellow nodule surrounded by a zone of dilated blood vessels that occurs in the conjunctiva or in the cornea. It develops into a small ulcer that heals without trace in the conjunctiva but produces some residual scarring in the cornea. Phlyctens, which are prone to recur, are thought to be due to a type of allergy to the tubercle bacillus.

水疱 一種發生於結膜或角膜的，被血管擴張區域所包圍的橘紅色小結節。它可發展成小潰瘍，癒後在結膜上不留痕跡，但在角膜上殘留有瘢痕。水疱易復發，人們認爲它是一種由結核桿菌引起的變態反應性疾病。

phobia *n.* a pathologically strong *fear of a particular event or thing. Avoiding the feared situation may severely restrict one's life and cause much suffering. The main kinds of phobia are *specific phobias*, (isolated fears of parti-

恐怖症 病人對某種特殊的事物所產生的一種病理性的、强烈的恐懼感。爲了廻避恐懼處境，病人可能嚴格地限制自己的生活範圍，因而十分痛苦。恐

cular things, such as sharp knives); *agoraphobia; *social phobias* of encountering people; and *animal phobias*, as of spiders, rats, or dogs (*see also* preparedness). Treatment is with behaviour therapy, especially *desensitization and *flooding. *Psychotherapy and drug therapy are also useful.

怖症的主要類型有：特殊物體恐怖（只對某種特殊物體，如鋒利的刀剪，產生恐怖），曠野恐怖，社交恐怖和動物恐怖（如對蜘蛛、老鼠或狗等的恐怖）。採用行爲療法（特別是脫敏療法和以恐治恐法）治療。心理療法與藥物療法也有效。

-phobia *suffix denoting* morbid fear or dread.

〔後綴〕 **恐怖** 病態性的恐懼。

phocomelia *n.* congenital absence of the upper arm and/or upper leg, the hands or feet or both being attached to the trunk by a short stump. The condition is extremely rare except as a side-effect of the drug *thalidomide taken during early pregnancy.

短肢畸形 上臂和/或大腿的先天性短缺。手或脚或手脚兩者靠短殘肢與軀幹相連。該病主要由妊娠早期服用酞胺哌啶酮藥所引起，其他原因引起者極少見。

pholcodine *n.* a drug that suppresses coughs and reduces irritation in the respiratory system (*see* antitussive). It is administered by mouth in cough mixtures and sometimes causes nausea and drowsiness.

嗎啉乙嗎啡 一種鎮咳和減輕呼吸系統刺激的藥物。口服。係止咳合劑成份之一。有時會引起噁心、困倦等副作用。

phon *n.* a unit of loudness of sound. The intensity of a sound to be measured is compared by the human ear to a reference tone of 2×10^{-5} pascal sound pressure and 1000 hertz frequency. The intensity of the reference tone is increased until it appears to be equal in loudness to the sound being measured; the loudness of this sound in phons is then equal to the number of decibels by which the reference tone has had to be increased.

叻 音響單位。音響的强度是用人耳對所測音和人耳對2×10^{-5}帕斯卡聲壓與1000赫茲頻率的標準音作比較而測出的。把標準音不斷升高到與所測者相等，標準音升高的分貝數就等於這個音的音響單位〔叻〕數。

phon- (phono-) *prefix denoting* sound or voice.

〔前綴〕 **聲音**

phonasthenia *n.* weakness of the voice, especially when due to fatigue.

發音無力 聲音微弱。特別指由於疲勞所引起的發音微弱。

phonation *n.* the production of vocal sounds, particularly speech.

發音 發出聲音。尤其指語音。

phonocardiogram *n. see* electrocardiophonography. —**phonocardiography** *n.*

心音圖

-phoria *suffix denoting* (in ophthalmology) an abnormal deviation of the eyes or turning of the visual axis. Example: *heterophoria* (tendency to squint).

〔後綴〕 **隱斜視** （眼科學）非正常的眼睛偏斜或視軸转向偏差。

Phormia *n.* a genus of non-bloodsucking flies, commonly known as blowflies. The maggot of *P. regina* normally breeds in decaying meat but it has occasionally been found in suppurating wounds, giving rise to a type of *myiasis.

黑花蠅屬 一種非吸血蠅屬。通稱爲麗蠅。黑花蠅通常在腐肉中生蛆，但蠅蛆在化膿傷口中也可偶爾見到，能引起一種蠅蛆病。

phosgene *n.* a poisonous gas developed during World War I. It is a choking agent, acting on the lungs to produce *oedema, with consequent respiratory and cardiac failure.

光氣 第一次世界大戰期間研製出來的一種窒息性毒氣。它能引起肺水腫，從而導致呼吸困難和心衰。

phosphagen *n.* creatine phosphate (*see* creatine).

磷酸肌酸

phosphataemia *n.* the presence of phosphates in the blood. Sodium, calcium, potassium, and magnesium phosphates are normal constituents.

磷酸鹽血 血中含有磷酸鹽。鈉、鈣、鉀及鎂的磷酸鹽是血液的正常成分。

phosphatase *n.* one of a group of enzymes capable of catalysing the hydrolysis of phosphoric acid esters. An example is glucose-6-phosphatase, which catalyses the hydrolysis of glucose-6-phosphate to glucose and phosphate. Phosphatases are important in the absorption and metabolism of carbohydrates, nucleotides, and phospholipids and are essential in the calcification of bone. *Acid phosphatase* is present in kidney, semen, serum, and the prostate gland. *Alkaline phosphatase* occurs in teeth, developing bone, plasma, kidney, and intestine.

磷酸酯酶 一種能够催化磷酸酯水解的酶，如葡萄糖-6-磷酸酯酶。該酶能催化葡萄糖-6-磷酸水解爲葡萄糖和磷酸鹽。磷酸酯酶在碳水化合物（糖類）、核苷酸和磷脂的吸收與代謝過程中起重要作用，並且在骨鈣化中也是必不可少的。酸性磷酸酯酶存在於腎臟、精液、血清及前列腺中；鹼性磷酸酯酶存在於牙齒、血漿、腎臟、腸和生長發育的骨中。

phosphatidylcholine *n. see* lecithin.

磷脂醯膽鹼，卵磷脂

phosphatidylserine *n.* a cephalin-like phospholipid containing the amino acid serine. It is found in brain tissue. *See also* cephalin.

磷脂醯絲氨酸 一種含有氨基酸絲氨酸的腦磷脂樣磷脂。該物質存在於腦組織中。

phosphaturia (phosphuria) *n.* the presence of an abnormally high concentration of phosphates in the urine, making it cloudy. The condition may be associated with the formation of stones (calculi) in the kidneys or bladder.

磷酸鹽尿 在尿液中含有一種使尿液渾濁的、異常高濃度的磷酸鹽。該病可能與腎臟結石或膀胱結石的形成有關。

phosphocreatine *n.* creatine phosphate (*see* creatine).

磷酸肌酸

phosphofructokinase *n.* an enzyme that catalyses the conversion of fructose-6-phosphate to fructose-1,6-diphosphate. This is an important reaction occurring during the process of *glycolysis.

磷酸果糖激酶 一種能够催化6-磷酸果糖轉化爲1，6-二磷酸果糖的酶。這是在糖原酵解過程中發生的一個重要化學反應。

phospholipid *n.* a *lipid containing a phosphate group as part of the molecule. Phospholipids are constituents of all tissues and organs, especially the brain. They are synthesized in the liver and small intestine and are involved in many of the body's metabolic processes. Examples are *cephalins, *lecithins, plasmalogens, and phosphatidylserine.

磷脂 一種在分子結構中含有磷酸鹽基團的脂類。磷脂是所有組織和器官，特別是大腦的組成成分。它們在肝臟和小腸中合成，並參與體內許多代謝過程。例如腦磷脂、卵磷脂、縮醛磷脂和磷脂醯絲氨酸等皆屬磷脂類。

phosphonecrosis *n.* the destruction of tissues caused by excessive amounts of phosphorus in the system. The tissues likely to suffer in phosphorus poisoning are the liver, kidneys, muscles, bones, and the cardiovascular system.

磷毒性壞死 在某系統中由於磷過量而引起組織的破壞。磷中毒時易受破壞的組織有肝、腎、肌肉、骨和心血管系統。

phosphorus *n.* a nonmetallic element. Phosphorus compounds are major constituents in the tissues of both plants and animals. In man, phosphorus is mostly concentrated in *bone. However, certain phosphorus-containing compounds – for example adenosine triphosphate (*ATP) and *creatine phosphate – play an important part in energy conversions and storage in the body. In a pure state, phosphorus is toxic.

磷 一種非金屬元素。在動物和植物的組織中，磷化合物是主要組成成分。人體中的磷大部分集中在骨內，但某些含磷化合物，如三磷酸腺苷和磷酸肌酸，對於人體能量的轉化和貯存起着重要的作用。單純的磷對人體是有毒的。

phosphorylase *n.* any enzyme that catalyses the combination of an organic molecule (usually glucose) with a phosphate group (phosphorylation). Phos-

磷酸化酶 任何一種能催化有機分子（通常爲葡萄糖）與磷酸鹽基團化合（磷酸化）的酶。磷酸化

phorylase is found in the liver and kidney, where it is involved in the breakdown of glycogen to glucosé-1-phosphate. 酶存在於肝和腎中，該酶在此參與把糖原分解爲1-磷酸葡萄糖的化學反應。

phot- (photo-) *prefix denoting* light. 〔前綴〕 **光**

photalgia *n.* pain in the eye caused by very bright light. **光痛** 由於强光刺激而引起眼痛。

photocoagulation *n.* the destruction of tissue by heat released from the absorption of light shone on it. In eye disorders the technique is used to destroy diseased retinal tissue, occurring, for example, as a complication of diabetes; and to produce scarring between the retina and choroid, thus binding them together, in cases of *detached retina. Several instruments are available for producing the intense light needed; the principle is similar when lasers are used. **光照性凝固法** 利用光照部位光吸收時釋放出的熱能來破壞組織。該項技術用於治療眼科疾病，如用來破壞糖尿病併發症的病變視網膜組織。在視網膜脫離的患者中，可把視網膜和脉絡膜之間燒灼成疤，使兩者黏合在一起。有好幾種可以發出所需强光的儀器，其原理皆與激光相似。

photodermatitis *n.* a condition in which the skin becomes sensitized to a substance (certain antiseptics used in soaps may be a trigger) but only those parts of the skin subsequently exposed to light react by developing *dermatitis. **光照性皮炎** 皮膚對某種物質產生過敏（肥皂中用的某些防腐劑可能是觸發劑），但只有隨後暴露於光的部分皮膚才發生皮炎的一種疾病。

photomicrograph *n.* an enlarged photographic record of an object taken through an optical or electron microscope. *Compare* microphotograph. **顯微照片** 把光學顯微鏡或電子顯微鏡拍攝的物像放大的照片。

photophobia *n.* an abnormal intolerance of light, in which exposure to light produces intense discomfort of the eyes with tight contraction of the eyelids and other reactions aimed at avoiding the light. In most cases the light simply aggravates already existing discomfort from eye disease. Photophobia may be associated with dilation of the pupils as a result of drug administration or with migraine, measles, German measles, or meningitis. **畏光** 一種極端畏懼光綫的症狀。患者一旦暴露於光下時，眼睛感到極不舒服，出現眼瞼緊閉和其他廻避光綫的反應。在大多數病人中，光只能使眼病原有的不適感加重。畏光還可能與因用藥造成的瞳孔擴大、偏頭痛、痲疹、風疹、腦膜炎有關。

photophthalmia *n.* inflammation of the eye due to exposure to light. It is **强光眼炎** 因暴露於强光下引起的眼睛炎症。通常

usually caused by the damaging effect of ultraviolet light on the cornea, for example in snow blindness.

由於角膜受到紫外綫的損害而造成，例如：雪盲。

photopic *adj.* relating to or describing conditions of bright illumination. For example, *photopic vision* is vision in bright light, in which the *cones of the retina are responsible for visual sensation. —**photopia** *n.*

明視的 關於或描述光照明的。例如，明視覺是指在亮光下的視覺，這時視錐細胞對視覺起作用。

photopsia *n.* the sensation of flashes of light caused by irritation of the retina of the eye, usually due to inflammation or slight movements of the retina.

閃光幻覺 由於眼睛視網膜的刺激作用而引起的閃光感覺。通常是由於視網膜炎或視網膜輕微的運動所致。

photoretinitis *n.* damage to the retina of the eye caused by looking at the sun without adequate protection for the eyes. The retina may be burnt by the intense light focused on it; this affects the central part of the visual field, which may be permanently lost (*sun blindness*).

光照性視網膜炎 眼睛在無適當防護的情況下注視太陽產生的視網膜損傷。强光聚焦在視網膜上，可燒損視網膜。如影響到視野中央部位，視力可能永久喪失（日光盲）。

photosensitivity *n.* abnormal and severe reaction of the skin to sunlight. —**photosensitive** *adj.*

光敏感性 皮膚對陽光產生的一種非正常的和嚴重的反應。

photosynthesis *n.* the process whereby green plants and some bacteria manufacture carbohydrates from carbon dioxide and water, using energy absorbed from sunlight by the green pigment chlorophyll. In green plants this complex process may be summarized thus:

$$6CO_2 + 6H_2O \rightarrow C_6H_{12}O_6 + 6O_2$$

光合作用 綠色植物和某些細菌通過光合作用，利用葉綠素從日光中吸收的能量，將二氧化碳和水合成碳水化合物的過程。在綠色植物中，這個複雜程序可以概括爲：$6CO_2 + 6H_2O \rightarrow C_6H_{12}O_6 + 6O_2$

phototaxis *n.* movement of a cell or organism in response to a stimulus of light.

趨光性 在光刺激的影響下細胞和生物的運動。

photuria *n.* the excretion of phosphorescent urine, which glows in the dark, due to the presence of certain phosphorus-containing compounds derived from phosphates.

發光尿 一種磷光尿。該種尿液在黑暗中閃閃發光。這是由於尿中有來自磷酸鹽的某些含磷化合物所致。

phren- (phreno-) *prefix denoting* **1.** the mind or brain. **2.** the diaphragm. **3.** the phrenic nerve.

〔前綴〕 ①**精神或大腦** ②**膈** ③**膈神經**

phrenemphraxis (phreniclasia) *n.* surgical crushing of a portion of the *phrenic nerve. This paralyses the diaphragm on the side operated upon, which is then pushed up by the abdominal contents, so pressing on the lung and partially collapsing it. Deliberate collapsing of the lung was a technique formerly used in the treatment of pulmonary tuberculosis.

膈神經壓軋術 壓軋部分膈神經的手術。手術側的膈發生癱瘓，腹部內容物便把膈往上推，從而壓迫肺臟，使部分肺萎陷。在以前，有意識地使部分肺萎陷是治療肺結核的一種方法。

-phrenia *suffix denoting* a condition of the mind. Example: ***hebephrenia*** (schizophrenia affecting young adults).

〔後綴〕 **精神狀態** 例如：青春型精神分裂症。

phrenic avulsion the surgical removal of a section of the *phrenic nerve, which paralyses the diaphragm. The procedure was used as a means of resting a lung infected with tuberculosis.

膈神經抽出術 切除部分膈神經，使膈肌癱瘓的手術。該手術曾用於使有結核病變的肺活動量減少。

phrenicectomy *n.* surgical division or removal of part of the phrenic nerve. Partial removal of the nerve produces the same results as *phrenemphraxis and division (phrenicotomy); it is done because the nerve sometimes regenerates after the other procedures.

膈神經切除術 切斷或切除部分膈神經的手術。部分膈神經切除術與膈神經壓軋術和膈神經切斷術產生同樣的效果。由於使用其他方法以後，有時膈神經能够再生，所以才用膈神經切除術。

phreniclasia *n. see* phrenemphraxis.

膈神經壓軋術

phrenic nerve the nerve that supplies the muscles of the diaphragm. On each side it arises in the neck from the third, fourth, and fifth cervical spinal roots and passes downwards between the lungs and the heart to reach the diaphragm. Impulses through the nerves from the brain bring about the regular contractions of the diaphragm during breathing.

膈神經 分佈於膈肌的神經。每側神經起自頸內第三、第四和第五頸神經根，並通過兩側肺與心臟之間往下到横膈膜。在呼吸期間，來自腦神經的衝動引起膈有規律的收縮。

phrenology *n.* the study of the bumps on the outside of the skull in order to determine a person's character. It is based on the mistaken theory that the skull becomes modified over the different functional areas of the cortex of the brain.

顱相學 根據顱骨外形的隆起來推斷一個人性格的學科。它認爲覆蓋腦皮質不同的功能區域的顱骨會起變化。這種理論基礎是錯誤的。

phthiriasis *n.* infestation of the crab louse, **Phthirus pubis*, which causes intense itching; continued scratching by the patient may result in bacterial infection of the skin. Phthiriasis can be treated with applications containing gamma benzene hexachloride.

蝨病 由於陰蝨感染人體，引起奇癢的一種疾病。患者不斷地搔癢可以導致皮膚的細菌性感染。本病可用含有丙體六六六的藥物治療。

Phthirus *n.* a widely distributed genus of lice. The crab (or pubic) louse, *P. pubis*, is a common parasite of man that lives permanently attached to the body hair, particularly that of the pubic or perianal regions but also on the eyelashes and the hairs in the armpits. Crab lice are not known to transmit disease but their bites can irritate the skin (*see* phthiriasis). An infestation may be acquired during sexual intercourse or from hairs left on clothing, towels, and lavatory seats.

陰蝨屬 一種廣泛分布的蝨屬。陰蝨是人體的一種普通寄生蟲，它們永久性地寄生於體毛，特別是陰毛或肛周部的體毛，但也可寄生於睫毛和腋毛中。尚無陰蝨能傳染疾病的報導，但它們的叮咬能刺激皮膚。人們通過性交或從留在衣服、毛巾或馬桶上的體毛而傳染。

phthisis *n.* a former name for: **1.** any disease resulting in wasting of tissues; **2.** pulmonary *tuberculosis.

①肺結核 ②消耗性疾病（舊稱）

phycomycosis *n.* a disease caused by parasitic fungi of the genera *Rhizopus*, *Absidia*, and **Mucor*. The disease affects the sinuses, the central nervous system, the lungs, and the skin tissues. The fungi are able to grow within the blood vessels of the lungs and nervous tissue, thus causing blood clots which cut off the blood supply (*see* infarction). Treatment with the antibiotic *amphotericin has proved effective.

藻菌病 由根黴菌屬、犁頭黴菌屬和毛黴菌屬的寄生眞菌引起的一種疾病。常侵襲鼻竇、中樞神經系統、肺和皮膚組織。眞菌能够在肺血管中和神經組織中生長，因而產生血凝塊，阻斷血液的供應（梗塞形成）。已經證明用抗生素二性黴素治療有效。

phylogenesis *n.* the evolutionary history of a species or individual.

系統發育，種系統育 生物種系或個體的發展史。

physi- (physio-) *prefix denoting* **1.** physiology. **2.** physical.

〔前綴〕 **①生理學 ②物理的，軀體的**

physical *adj.* (in medicine) relating to the body rather than to the mind. For example, a *physical sign* is one that a doctor can detect when examining a patient, such as abnormal dilation of the pupils or the absence of a knee-jerk

身體的 指與身體有關的而不是與精神有關的。例如，檢查病人時醫師發現的體徵，像異常的瞳孔散大或膝反射消失等。

reflex (*see also* functional disorder, organic disorder).

physical medicine a medical specialty established by the Royal Society of Medicine in 1931. Initially the members pioneered clinics devoted to the diagnosis and management of rheumatic diseases, but later extended their interests to the *rehabilitation of patients with physical disabilities ranging from asthma and hand injuries to back trouble and poliomyelitis. The term has caused confusion in recent years, with many doctors preferring the description *rheumatology and rehabilitation* for this specialist activity. Since 1972, however, when the Royal College of Physicians approved it, physical medicine has become the generally accepted term. *See also* rheumatology.

軀體醫學 在1931年，由英國皇家醫學會創立的一個醫學專業。最初倡用於臨床的醫生們只用於診斷和治療風濕性疾病，但後來逐漸擴大到軀體傷殘病人的康復，包括哮喘、手外傷、腰背痛、脊髓灰質炎等。

近年來這個術語已引起混亂，許多醫生把這類獨特的專業稱之爲風濕病學和康復醫學。但自1972年以來，經英國皇家內科學院認可軀體醫學這一術語才被普遍採用。

physician *n.* a registered medical practitioner who specializes in the diagnosis and treatment of disease by other than surgical means. In the USA the term is applied to any authorized medical practitioner. *See also* Doctor.

內科醫師 專門從事診斷和治療疾病，但不用外科方法的注册醫師。在美國該術語適用於任何被批准的行醫者。

physiological solution one of a group of solutions used to maintain tissues in a viable state. These solutions contain specific concentrations of substances that are vital for normal tissue function (e.g. sodium, potassium, calcium, chloride, magnesium, bicarbonate, and phosphate ions, glucose, and oxygen). An example of such a solution is *Ringer's solution.

生理鹽水溶液 一組用以維持組織處於生活狀態的溶液。其中含有特定濃度的維持組織正常功能所必需的物質，如鈉、鉀、鈣、氯、鎂、碳酸氫鹽、磷酸鹽離子、葡萄糖和氧等。林格氏溶液就是這類液體。

physiology *n.* the science of the functioning of living organisms and of their component parts. —**physiological** *adj.* —**physiologist** *n.*

生理學 研究生物及其組成部分功能的學科。

physiotherapy *n.* the branch of treatment that employs physical methods to promote healing, including the use of light, infrared and ultraviolet rays, heat, electric current, massage, manipulation, and remedial exercise.

物理治療，理療 採用物理方法促使病人恢復健康的治療學中的一個分支學科。這些物理方法包括使用日光、紅外線、紫外線、熱、電流、按摩、推拿以及醫療體操等。

physo- *prefix denoting* air or gas.

〔前綴〕 **氣，空氣**

physostigmine (eserine) *n.* a *parasympathomimetic drug used mainly to constrict the pupil of the eye and to reduce pressure inside the eye in glaucoma. It is administered by injection, in eye-drops, or in an ointment; side-effects include digestive upsets and salivation.

毒扁豆鹼 主要用於縮瞳和降低青光眼患者眼內壓的一種擬副交感神經藥。注射或配成眼藥水或軟膏使用。副作用有消化不良和流涎。

phyt- (phyto-) *prefix denoting* plants; of plant origin.

〔前綴〕 **植物，植物源的**

phytomenadione *n.* a form of *vitamin K occurring naturally in green plants but usually synthesized for use as an antidote to overdosage with anticoagulant drugs. It promotes the production of prothrombin, essential for the normal coagulation of blood.

維生素K_1 在綠色植物中自然存在的一種維生素K，但通常人工合成。在抗凝血劑過量時用作拮抗劑。它促使正常凝血過程所必需的凝血酶的生成。

phytophotodermatitis *n.* an eruption of large blisters occurring after exposure to light in people who have been in contact with certain plants, such as wild parsnip or cow parsley, to which they are sensitive.

植物性日光照性皮炎 對某些植物（如野生歐洲防風或歐芹等）過敏的人接觸這類植物後再受到日光的照射時出現的大型水疱疹。

phytotoxin *n.* any poisonous substance (toxin) produced by a plant, such as any of the toxins produced by fungi of the genus **Amanita*.

植物毒素 由某種植物產生的有毒物質（毒素）。如捕繩蕈菌屬類眞菌產生的毒素。

pia (pia mater) *n.* the innermost of the three *meninges surrounding the brain and spinal cord. The membrane is closely attached to the surface of the brain and spinal cord, faithfully following each fissure and sulcus. It contains numerous finely branching blood vessels that supply the nerve tissue within. The subarachnoid space separates it from the arachnoid.

軟腦膜 包圍着腦與脊髓的三層腦脊膜中最裏邊的一層。軟腦膜緊貼於腦和脊髓表面，並深入到裂溝的深部。它含有許多分佈到腦內神經組織中去的小血管。蛛網膜下腔把蛛網膜與軟腦膜隔開。

pian *n. see* yaws.

雅司病

pica *n.* the indiscriminate eating of non-nutritious or harmful substances, such as grass, stones, or clothing. It is common in early childhood but may also be found in mentally handicapped

異食癖 不加選擇地吃些無營養或有害的物質（如草、石或衣服之類）的癖好。該病在幼兒期較常見，但在心理缺陷和精神

and psychotic patients. Although thought to be completely nonadaptive, recent evidence suggests that some patients showing pica may have particular mineral deficiencies (such as iron deficiency).

病患者當中也能見到。最近有些材料證明，某些有異食癖表現的病人可能缺乏某種特殊的礦物質（如缺鐵），但未獲一致公認。

Pick's disease a rare cause of dementia in middle-aged people. The damage is mainly in the frontal and temporal lobes of the brain, in contrast with the diffuse degeneration of *Alzheimer's disease.

皮克氏病　一種罕見的中年痴呆病。與阿爾茨海默氏病（早老性痴呆）的彌漫性變性不同，本病的主要損害位於腦的額葉和顳葉內。

pico- *prefix denoting* one million-millionth (10^{-12}).

〔前綴〕 **沙，毫纖，皮可** (10^{-12})

picornavirus *n.* one of a group of small RNA-containing viruses (pico = small; hence pico-RNA-virus). The group includes *Coxsackie viruses, *echoviruses, *polioviruses, and *rhinoviruses.

細小核糖核酸病毒，微小RNA病毒　一組含有核糖核酸的小病毒。該組病毒包括：柯薩奇病毒、人腸道細胞病變孤兒病毒、脊髓灰質炎病毒和鼻病毒。

picric acid (trinitrophenol) a yellow crystalline solid used as a dye and as a tissue *fixative.

三硝基苯酚　一種用作染劑和組織固定劑的黃色結晶固體。

piedra *n.* a fungal disease of the hair in which the hair shafts carry hard masses of black or white fungus. The black fungus, *Piedraia hortai*, is found mainly in the tropics and the white variety, *Trichosporon cutaneum*, in temperate regions.

熱帶毛孢子菌病　一種在毛幹上攜帶有黑色或白色眞菌硬塊的毛發眞菌病。黑色眞菌爲霍塔氏毛孢子菌，主要見於熱帶地區；而白色菌種爲白色毛孢子菌，見於溫帶地區。

pigeon chest forward protrusion of the breastbone resulting in deformity of the chest. The condition is painless and harmless.

鷄胸　胸骨向前突出，導致胸廓變形，該種畸形旣無痛又無害。

pigeon toes an abnormal posture in which the toes are turned inwards. It is often associated with *knock-knee.

鴿趾，內收足　一種脚趾向內收的反常姿勢。常與膝外翻有關。

pigment *n.* a substance giving colour. Physiologically important pigments include the blood pigments (especially *haemoglobin), *bile pigments, and retinal pigment (*see* rhodopsin). The pigment *melanin occurs in the skin and in the iris of the eye. Important plant

色素　着色的物質。在生理上重要的色素包括：血色素（特別是血紅蛋白）、膽色素和視網膜色素。黑色素存在於皮膚中和眼虹膜內。植物的主要色素有葉綠素和類胡蘿蔔素。

pigments include *chlorophyll and the *carotenoids.

pigmentation *n.* coloration produced in the body by the deposition of one pigment, especially in excessive amounts. Pigmentation may be produced by natural pigments, such as bile pigments (as in jaundice) or melanin, or by foreign material, such as lead or arsenic in chronic poisoning.

色素沉着 由於體內某種色素沉積（尤指色素過量）而引起的着色。色素沉着可由體內固有的色素引起，如（在黃疸病人中的）膽色素或黑色素；也可由外來物質引起，如在慢性中毒中的鉛或砷。

piles *n. see* haemorrhoids.

痔

pili (fimbriae) *pl. n.* (*sing.* **pilus, fimbria**) hairlike processes present on the surface of certain bacteria. They are thought to be involved in adhesion of bacteria to other cells and in transfer of DNA during *conjugation.

菌毛 生長於某些細菌表面的毛狀突起。人們認爲該種突起能使細菌與其他細胞粘連在一起，並能在接合生殖期使脫氧核糖核酸轉移。

pill *n.* **1.** a small round ball, sometimes coated with sugar, that contains one or more medicinal substances in solid form. It is taken by mouth. **2. the Pill** *see* oral contraceptive.

①**丸劑** 含有一種或多種藥物的、有時外加糖衣的一種小圓球形的固體藥劑。口服。 ②**口服避孕藥**。

pillar *n.* (in anatomy) an elongated apparently supportive structure. For example, the *pillars of the fauces* are folds of mucous membrane on either side of the opening from the mouth to the pharynx.

弓，柱，脚 在解剖學上指一種明顯延長的支撑結構。例如，舌腭弓就是咽部兩側的黏膜皺襞。

pilo- *prefix denoting* hair. Example: *pilosis* (excessive development of).

〔前綴〕 **毛，髮** 如多毛〔症〕。

pilocarpine *n.* a drug with actions and uses similar to those of *physostigmine. It is administered as eye-drops and may cause digestive upsets and salivation if absorbed into the system.

毛果芸香鹼 一種與毒扁豆鹼作用與用途相似的藥物。配成滴眼藥水使用。如被消化系統吸收，可引起消化不良和流涎。

pilomotor nerves sympathetic nerves that supply muscle fibres in the skin, around the roots of hairs. Activity of the sympathetic nervous system causes the muscles to contract, raising the hairs and giving the 'gooseflesh' effect of fear or cold.

立毛神經，毛髮運動神經 分布於皮膚內毛根周圍的肌纖維的交感神經。當受到恐懼和寒冷的刺激時，交感神經系統興奮引起肌肉收縮，從而使得毛髮竪立，出現鷄皮疙瘩。

pilonidal sinus a short tract leading from an opening in the skin in or near the cleft at the top of the buttocks and

藏毛竇、骶尾竇 由皮膚開口處通向或接近骶裂頂的短的含毛管道。該竇可

containing hairs. The sinus may be recurrently infected, leading to pain and the discharge of pus. Treatment is by surgical opening and cleaning of the sinus.

能反復感染，引起疼痛和流膿。治療：手術切開和清潔竇道。

pilosebaceous *adj.* relating to the hair follicles and their associated sebaceous glands.

毛囊〔腺〕皮脂腺的

pilus *n.* a hair. *See also* pili.

毛，髮

pimel- (pimelo-) *prefix denoting* fat; fatty.

〔前綴〕 ①**脂，脂肪** ②**脂的，脂肪的**

pimozide *n.* a major *tranquillizer used to relieve hallucinations and delusions occurring in schizophrenia. It is administered by mouth; side-effects may include skin rashes, tremors, and abnormal movements. Trade name: **Orap**.

哌迷清 一種用於治療精神分裂症患者出現的幻覺和妄想的強安定藥。口服。副作用可有皮疹、震顫和運動障礙。

pimple *n.* a small inflamed swelling on the skin that contains pus. It may be the result of bacterial infection of a skin pore that has become obstructed with fatty secretions from the sebaceous glands. Pimples occurring in large numbers on the chest, back, and face are usually described as *acne, a common condition of adolescence.

小膿疱 一種含有膿液的小形炎性疱疹。該膿疱可能由於來自皮脂腺的脂肪分泌物阻塞了皮膚毛孔而引起的細菌性感染。患者胸、背、面部出現大量小膿疱時通常稱爲痤瘡，是青春期的一種常見病。

pincement *n.* one of the techniques used in massage, in which pinches of the patient's flesh are taken between finger and thumb and twisted or rolled before release. This is said to improve the tone of the skin, improve circulation, and alleviate underlying pain.

搴按法 按摩用的一種手法。用拇指和手指捏起病人的肌肉，搴揉後再放鬆。據說搴按法可增强皮膚張力、改善血液循環和減輕搴按部位的疼痛。

pineal body (pineal gland) a pea-sized mass of tissue attached by a stalk to the posterior wall of the third ventricle of the brain, deep between the cerebral hemispheres at the back of the skull. It may play a part in initiating the development of the gonads, but this is uncertain; in other mammals it secretes the hormone-like substance *melatonin*. The gland becomes calcified as age

松果體 通過一個蒂附着於頭顱後部兩側大腦半球之間深部的、第三腦室後壁的豆粒大小的一塊組織。該組織可能有促使性腺發育的作用，但尚未肯定。在其他哺乳動物中，松果體分泌激素類物質——褪黑激素。該腺體隨着年齡的增大逐漸鈣

progresses, providing a useful landmark in X-rays of the skull. Anatomical name: **epiphysis**.

化，為頭顱X線檢查提供了有用的界線標記。

pinguecula *n.* a degenerative change in the conjunctiva of the eye, seen most commonly in the elderly and in those who live in hot dry climates. Thickened yellow triangles develop on the conjunctiva at the inner and outer margins of the cornea.

結膜黃斑 常見於老年人和生活在炎熱乾燥地區居民中的眼結膜的變性病變。在角膜內、外緣的結膜上生長有黃色增厚的三角形物。

pink disease a severe illness of children of the teething age, marked by pink cold clammy hands and feet, heavy sweating, raised blood pressure, rapid pulse, photophobia, loss of appetite, and insomnia. It has been suggested that the condition is an allergic reaction to mercury, since it used to occur when teething powders, lotions, and ointments containing mercury were used. Although there is no definite proof of this, the disease has virtually disappeared since all mercury-containing paediatric preparations have been banned. Medical names: **acrodynia, erythroedema, erythromelalgia.**

紅皮水腫性多發性神經病 出牙期兒童的一種嚴重疾病。該病的主要表現為手足發紅冰冷黏濕、多汗、高血壓、脉促、畏光、食慾不振和失眠等。該病往往在使用含汞的牙粉、洗劑和軟膏時發病，因而曾被認為是由汞引起的一種變態反應性疾病。雖然還無確切的證據，但自從含汞兒童日用品一律禁用後，該病基本上已不復存在。醫學術語：肢痛症、紅皮水腫病、紅斑性肢痛病。

pink eye *see* conjunctivitis.

紅眼，急性結膜炎

pinna (auricle) *n.* the flap of skin and cartilage that projects from the head at the exterior opening of the external auditory meatus of the *ear (see illustration). In man the pinna is largely vestigial but it may be partly concerned with detecting the direction of sound sources.

耳廓 從頭部外耳道外開口處向外突起的由皮膚和軟骨構成的瓣狀物（見圖）。人的耳廓大部分退化，但它與辨別聲源方向可能有些關係。

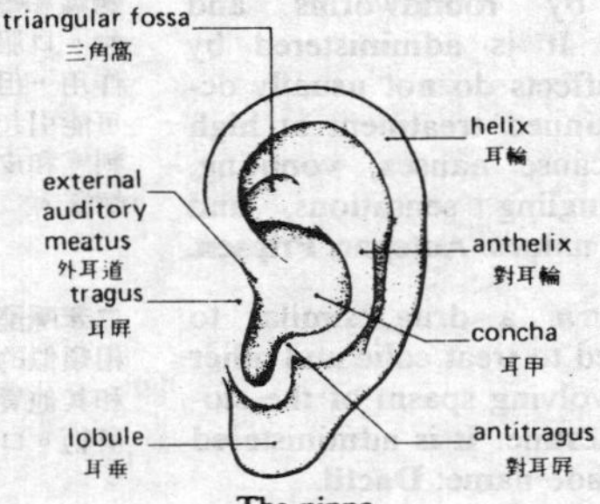

The pinna
耳廓

pinocytosis *n.* the intake of small droplets of fluid by a cell by cytoplasmic engulfment. It occurs in many white blood cells and in certain kidney and liver cells. *Compare* phagocytosis.

吞飲作用 細胞通過胞漿的吞食作用來攝取液體微滴的過程。該現象發生於許多白細胞中和某些腎和肝臟細胞中。

pinta *n.* a skin disease, prevalent in tropical America, that seems to affect only the dark-skinned races. It is caused by the *spirochaete *Treponema carateum*, a microorganism similar to those causing *yaws and *syphilis. The disease is thought to be transmitted either by direct contact between individuals or by flies that carry the infective spirochaetes on their bodies. Symptoms include thickening and eventual loss of pigment of the skin, particularly on the hands, wrists, feet, and ankles. Pinta is rarely disabling or fatal and is treated successfully with *penicillin.

品他病 流行於熱帶美洲的，好像只感染黑色皮膚人種的一種皮膚疾病。該病是由品他病密螺旋體引起，此螺旋體與引起雅司病和梅毒的微生物相似。人們認爲這種病可能由於人與人之間的直接接觸，或者由於攜帶有密螺旋體的蒼蠅傳播而引起。症狀包括皮膚色素沉積而最後消失，在手、腕、足和踝部的皮膚色尤爲顯著。品他病很少有致殘或致死的，並且用青黴素治療效果很好。

pinworm (threadworm) *n.* a parasitic nematode worm of the genus *Enterobius* (*Oxyuris*), which lives in the upper part of the large intestine of man. The threadlike female worm, some 12 mm long, is larger than the male; it emerges from the anus in the evening to deposit its eggs, and later dies. If the eggs are swallowed by man and reach the intestine they develop directly into adult worms. Pinworms cause *enterobiasis, a disease common in children throughout the world.

蟯蟲（線蟲） 棲居於人大腸上部的寄生性蟯蟲屬線蟲。線狀雌蟲長約12mm，比雄蟲體大，夜晚從肛門鑽出來產卵，隨後死亡。蟲卵若被人吞吃進入腸內，就會直接發育爲成蟲。蟯蟲所引起的蟯蟲病是全世界兒童的常見病。

piperazine *n.* a drug used to treat infestations by roundworms and threadworms. It is administered by mouth; side-effects do not usually occur, but continued treatment at high doses may cause nausea, vomiting, headache, tingling sensations, and rashes. Trade names: **Antepar, Pripsen**.

哌嗪 一種用於治療由蛔蟲和蟯蟲引起感染的藥物。口服。通常不發生副作用，但持續大劑量服用可能引起嘔吐、頭痛、麻刺感和皮疹。商品名：驅蛔靈。

piperidolate *n.* a drug, similar to *atropine, used to treat colic and other conditions involving spasm of the stomach and intestine. It is administered by mouth. Trade name: **Dactil**.

二苯哌酯 一種與阿托品相類似的，用於治療絞痛和其他胃腸痙攣性疾病的藥物。口服。

piriform fossae two pear-shaped depressions that lie on either side of the opening to the larynx.

梨狀隱窩 位於喉嚨出口兩側的兩個梨狀凹陷。

pisiform bone the smallest bone of the wrist (*carpus): a pea-shaped bone that articulates with the triquetral bone and, indirectly by cartilage, with the ulna.

豌豆骨 腕骨中最小的一塊豌豆狀的骨頭。它與三角骨相關節，並通過軟骨與尺骨間接相關節。

pit *n.* (in anatomy) a hollow or depression, such as any of the depressions on the surface of an embryo marking the site of future organs.

凹 在解剖學中指凹陷或窩。如在胚胎表面上則代表着將來生長出的器官位置的各種窩。

pithiatism *n.* the treatment of certain disorders by persuading the patient that all is well. Disorders that disappear in these circumstances are regarded as manifestations of psychological disturbance and are classified as hysterical disorders.

說服療法 通過勸說治療無器質性疾病的病人的方法。若經該療法治療後病情好轉，就可以看作是心理性障礙，並且可歸類爲癔病性疾病。

pithing *n.* the laboratory procedure in which a part or the whole of the central nervous system of an experimental animal (such as a frog) is destroyed, usually by inserting a probe through the foramen magnum, in preparation for physiological or pharmacological experiments.

腦脊髓刺毀法 爲進行生理學或藥理學試驗所作的一種實驗室手術。通常是用探針刺透試驗動物（例如青蛙）的枕骨大孔，以破壞其部分或全部中樞神經系統。

pitting *n.* the formation of depressed scars, as occurs on the skin following smallpox or acne. *Pitting oedema* is swelling of the tissues due to excess fluid in which fingertip pressure leaves temporary indentations in the skin.

凹陷，凹痕 下陷的瘢痕。如患天花或痤瘡後在皮膚上留下的凹陷性瘢痕。凹陷性水腫（指壓性水腫）是由於組織內積液過多引起的浮腫，用指尖按壓水腫的皮膚會留有暫時性凹陷。

pituicyte *n.* a type of cell found in the posterior lobe of the pituitary gland, similar in appearance to an *astrocyte, with numerous fine branches that end in contact with the lining membrane of the blood channels in the gland.

垂體〔後葉〕細胞 位於垂體腺後葉的一種細胞。該細胞與星形〔膠質〕細胞的外形相似，有許多細小分支。這些細小分支末梢與腺體血管內壁相接觸。

pituitary gland (hypophysis) the master endocrine gland: a pea-sized body attached beneath the *hypothalamus in a bony cavity at the base of the skull. It has an anterior lobe (*adenohy-*

垂體 最重要的內分泌腺。爲在顱底骨腔內附着於下丘腦下方的一個豌豆大小的腺體。它的前葉（腺性垂體）分泌促甲狀

pophysis), which secretes *thyroid-stimulating hormone, *ACTH (adrenocorticotrophic hormone), *gonadotrophins, *growth hormone, *prolactin, *lipotrophin, and *melanocyte-stimulating hormone. The secretion of all these hormones is regulated by specific *hormone releasing factors*, which are produced in the hypothalamus. The posterior lobe (*neurohypophysis*) secretes *vasopressin and *oxytocin, which are synthesized in the hypothalamus and transported to the pituitary, where they are stored before release.

腺激素、促腎上腺皮質激素、促性腺激素、生長激素、催乳素、促脂解激素和促黑色素細胞激素等。所有這些激素的分泌均受下丘腦產生的專門的激素釋放因子的調節。後葉（神經性垂體）分泌加壓素和催產素。這些分泌物先在下丘腦合成再輸送到垂體貯存。

pityriasis *n.* (originally) any of a group of skin diseases typified by the development of fine branlike scales. The term is now used only with a modifying adjective. For instance, *pityriasis rosea* is a common skin complaint, of unknown cause, in which flat pink oval spots (macules) develop on the trunk and upper parts of the limbs. It occurs mainly in young people in spring and autumn and typically starts with a localized patch of spots that precedes the general eruption by about seven days. *Pityriasis alba* is a very common condition in children and adolescents in which uneven round pale macules appear on the face. This disease may persist until adulthood. *See also* dandruff (pityriasis capitis), liver spot.

糠疹 本詞原來指任何一種以細糠樣皮屑爲特徵的皮膚病，但現在僅與一個限定性形容詞合用。例如，玫瑰糠疹，指一種病因不明的常見皮膚疾病，特點爲在軀幹和肢體上部生長有扁平的卵圓形紅斑。該病主要在春、秋季發病，常見於青年人。特徵是起初出現局限性的斑點，繼而在大約七天後全身出疹。白糠疹是兒童和青年人最常見的皮膚病，特點爲在面部出現隆起的圓形白斑。此病可以一直延續到成年。

pivot joint *see* trochoid joint.

車輪關節，旋轉關節

placebo *n.* a medicine that is ineffective but may help to relieve a condition because the patient has faith in its powers. New drugs are tested against placebos in clinical trials: the drug's effect is compared with the *placebo response*, which occurs even in the absence of any pharmacologically active substance in the placebo.

安慰劑 實際上無效，但由於病人確信有效，而且用後有助於緩解病情的一種藥物。安慰劑在新藥的臨床試驗中作對照用，即將新藥的療效與並無任何藥理作用的安慰劑所產生的“安慰效應”進行比較。

placenta *n.* an organ within the uterus (womb) by means of which the embryo is attached to the wall of the uterus. Its primary function is to provide the

胎盤 在子宮內胚胎藉以附着於子宮壁的器官。它的主要功能是給胚胎提供營養、排除廢物和交換呼

embryo with nourishment, eliminate its wastes, and exchange respiratory gases. This is accomplished by the close proximity of the maternal and fetal blood systems within the placenta. It also functions as a gland, secreting *chorionic gonadotrophin, *progesterone, and oestrogens, which regulate the maintenance of pregnancy. *See also* afterbirth. —**placental** *adj.*

吸氣體。這是通過母體和胎盤內胎兒血液系統的緊密相連來完成的。胎盤也具有腺體的功能，可分泌絨〔毛〕膜促性腺激素、孕酮和雌激素。這些分泌物能够維持妊娠。

placenta praevia the attachment of the placenta to the lower part of the womb (instead of to the upper part, as is normal). As it grows, the placenta may partially or completely cover the outlet from the womb to the vagina. Slight bleeding may occur from about the seventh month of pregnancy, and anaemia may develop. Childbirth may be made difficult because the placenta hinders the movement of the infant through the vagina and delivery by Caesarean section may be necessary.

前置胎盤 附着於子宮下部（正常時則附着於子宮上部）的胎盤。隨着胎兒的生長發育，胎盤可能會部分地或全部地覆蓋於子宮通往陰道的出口。大約從妊娠的第七個月起開始小量出血，並可引起貧血。因爲胎盤妨礙嬰兒通過陰道，可能造成難產而需採用剖腹產手術。

placentography *n.* *radiography of the pregnant womb in order to determine the position of the *placenta. *See also* placenta praevia.

胎盤造影術 爲了確定胎盤位置所採用的妊娠子宮的X線照像術。

placode *n.* any of the thickened areas of ectoderm in the embryo that will develop into nerve ganglia or the special sensory structures of the eye, ear, or nose.

基板 在胚胎中外胚層的任何增厚區域。它將發育成神經節或眼、耳、鼻等特殊感覺結構。

plagiocephaly *n.* any distortion or lack of symmetry in the shape of the head, usually due to irregularity in the closure of the sutures between the bones of the skull.

斜頭〔畸形〕 任何一種變形或不對稱的頭形。這常由於頭顱骨縫的不規則接合所致。

plague *n.* **1.** any epidemic disease with a high death rate. **2.** an acute epidemic disease of rats and other wild rodents caused by the bacterium *Pasteurella pestis*, which is transmitted to man by rat fleas. *Bubonic plague*, the most common form of the disease, has an incubation period of 2–6 days. Headache, fever, weakness, aching limbs, and delirium develop and are followed

①**瘟疫** 任何一種死亡率高的流行性疾病。②**鼠疫** 由鼠疫巴斯德菌引起家鼠和其他野生嚙齒動物的一種急性傳染病。該病可通過鼠蚤傳染給人。腺鼠疫爲最常見的一種。潛伏期2～6天。症狀可有頭痛、發燒、虛弱無力、肢體疼痛、譫妄，隨後繼發

by acute painful swellings of the lymph nodes (*see* bubo). In favourable cases the buboes burst after about a week, releasing pus, and then heal. In other cases bleeding under the skin, producing black patches, can lead to ulcers, which may prove fatal (hence the former name *Black Death*). In the most serious cases bacteria enter the bloodstream (*septicaemic plague*) or lungs (*pneumonic plague*); if untreated, these are nearly always fatal. Treatment with tetracycline, streptomycin, and chloramphenicol is effective; vaccination against the disease provides only partial protection.

淋巴結急性腫痛。輕症病人的淋巴結約持續一周後潰破、流膿、然後痊癒；在其他病人中，皮下出血產生黑斑，最後能引起可致命的潰瘍（舊稱：黑死病，因此而得名）；最嚴重的病人，細菌進入血流（敗血性鼠疫）或肺（肺鼠疫），如不進行治療，這些病人幾乎全部死亡。用四環素、鏈黴素和合黴素治療均有效，預防接種僅起部分作用。

plane *n.* a level or smooth surface, especially any of the hypothetical flat surfaces – orientated in various directions – used to divide the body; for example, the *coronal and *sagittal planes.

平面 平的或光滑的表面。特指在各個方向上用以劃分身體部位的假設的任何平面。例如，冠狀面和矢狀面。

planoconcave *adj.* describing a structure, such as a lens, that is flat on one side and concave on the other.

平凹的 描述一面平而另一面凹的鏡片或類似的結構。

planoconvex *adj.* describing a structure, such as a lens, that is flat on one side and convex on the other.

平凸的 描述一面平而另一面凸的鏡片或類似的結構。

plantar *adj.* relating to the sole of the foot (*planta*). *See also* flexion.

足底的，蹠的 與脚底有關的。

plantar arch the arch in the sole of the foot formed by anastomosing branches of the plantar arteries.

蹠弓，足底弓 在脚底內由足底動脈吻合支形成的弓。

plantar reflex a reflex obtained by drawing a bluntly pointed object along the outer border of the sole of the foot from the heel to the little toe. The normal *flexor response* is a bunching and downward movement of the toes. An upward movement of the great toe is called an *extensor response* (or *Babinski reflex*). In all persons over the age of 18 months this is a sensitive indication of disease in the brain or spinal cord.

蹠反射，足底反射 用鈍尖頭的物體從足跟沿脚底外緣到小趾劃線所引起的一種反射。正常的屈肌反應是脚趾屈曲向下運動。大拇趾向上的運動稱作伸肌反應（或稱巴彬斯奇氏反射）。這一反射是檢查所有年滿18個月的人們患大腦或脊髓性疾病的可靠方法。

plantar wart a wart occurring in the skin on the sole of the foot, usually at the base of the toes. *See* wart.

足蹠疣，蹠疣 生長在足底皮膚中的一種疣。通常位於足趾根部。

plantigrade *adj.* walking on the entire sole of the foot: a habit of man and some animals.

蹠行的 用整個足底（脚掌）行走。係人類和某些哺乳動物的習慣。

plaque *n.* **1.** a layer that forms on the surface of a tooth, principally at its neck, composed of bacteria in an organic matrix. Under certain conditions the plaque may cause *gingivitis, *periodontal disease, or *dental caries. The purpose of oral hygiene is to remove plaque. **2.** a raised circular patch of skin or mucous membrane resulting from local damage, usually due to infection.

①**菌斑，牙斑** 主要在牙頸部的牙齒表面由有機基質中的細菌形成的一層膜。在一定的條件下，菌斑可引起牙齦炎、牙周病或齲齒。口腔衛生的目的就在於清除菌斑。 ②**斑** 通常由於感染、局部受傷而引起皮膚或黏膜的一種隆起的圓形斑。

-plasia *suffix denoting* formation; development. Example: *hyperplasia* (excessive tissue formation).

〔前綴〕 **形成，生長** 例如，增生（組織生長過度）。

plasm- (plasmo-) *prefix denoting* **1.** blood plasma. **2.** protoplasm or cytoplasm.

〔前綴〕 ①**血漿** ②**原生質或細胞質**

plasma (blood plasma) *n.* the straw-coloured fluid in which the blood cells are suspended. It consists of a solution of various inorganic salts of sodium, potassium, calcium, etc., with a high concentration of protein (approximately 70 g/l) and a variety of trace substances.

血漿 懸浮有血細胞的草黃色液體。它由鈉、鉀、鈣等各種無機鹽溶液和高濃度的蛋白質（約70g/1）以及各種微量元素組成。

plasmacytoma *n.* a malignant tumour of plasma cells, very closely allied to *myeloma. It usually occurs as a solitary tumour of bone, but may be multiple. Less frequently it affects soft tissues, usually the upper air passages. All of these tumours may produce the abnormal gamma globulins that are characteristic of myeloma, and they may progress to widespread myeloma. The soft-tissue tumours often respond to radiotherapy and to such drugs as melphalan and cyclophosphamide; the bone tumours are less responsive. Tumours originating in soft tissue may spread to bone, producing an appear-

漿細胞瘤 漿細胞的一種惡性腫瘤。與骨髓瘤同屬一類。它通常是單獨的骨瘤，也可能是多發性的，有時侵犯上呼吸道的軟組織。這些腫瘤均可以產生骨髓瘤所特有的異常丙種球蛋白，並可發展爲擴散性骨髓瘤。用放射療法和苯丙氨酸氮芥與環磷醯胺類藥物療法對軟組織腫瘤通常是有效的；而對骨腫瘤的療效較差。起源於軟組織的腫瘤可能蔓延到骨骼，在用X線檢查時顯示出與骨髓瘤相同的迹像，

ance on X-ray identical to myeloma deposits; these secondary growths often resolve completely after radiological treatment.

這些繼發性腫瘤經放射治療常全部消失。

plasmalogen *n.* a phospholipid, found in brain and muscle, similar in structure to *lecithin and *cephalin.

縮醛磷脂 存在於腦和肌肉中的磷脂，其結構與腦磷脂和卵磷脂相似。

plasmapheresis *n.* a method of removing a quantity of plasma from the blood. Blood is withdrawn from the patient and allowed to settle in a container. The plasma is drawn off the top of the blood, and the blood cells are then transfused back into the patient.

去血漿法 從血液中去掉血漿的方法。從病人身上抽取血漿，並將血靜置於一容器內，從血液頂部吸出血漿，然後，把血細胞輸回給患者。

plasmidotrophoblast (syncytiotrophoblast) *n.* that part of the *trophoblast that loses its cellular structure and becomes a *syncytium. This is the invasive part of the trophoblast, which erodes the maternal tissues and forms the villi of the placenta.

合胞體滋養層 滋養層失去它的細胞結構而成爲合胞體的那部分。這就是滋養層突出的部分，該部分侵入母體組織而形成胎盤絨毛。

plasmin (fibrinolysin) *n.* an enzyme that digests the protein fibrin. Its function is the dissolution of blood clots (*see* fibrinolysis). Plasmin is not normally present in the blood but exists as an inactive precursor, *plasminogen*.

纖維蛋白溶酶 一種消化蛋白纖維的酶。其功能是溶解血凝塊。平時血液中是沒有纖維蛋白溶酶的，但有其非活性的前身物質纖維蛋白溶酶原。

plasminogen *n.* a substance normally present in the blood plasma that may be activated to form *plasmin. *See* fibrinolysis.

纖維蛋白溶酶原 平時血漿中就存在的，可被激活而變成纖維蛋白溶酶的一種物質。

Plasmodium *n.* a genus of protozoans (*see* Sporozoa) that live as parasites within the red blood cells and liver cells of man. The parasite undergoes its asexual development (*see* schizogony) in man and completes the sexual phase of its development (*see* sporogony) in the stomach and digestive glands of a bloodsucking **Anopheles* mosquito. Four species cause *malaria in man: *P. vivax*, *P. ovale*, *P. falciparum*, and *P. malariae*.

瘧原蟲屬 寄生於人體紅細胞和肝細胞中的原蟲屬。該寄生蟲在人體內進行無性生殖，而在吸血按蚊的胃和消化腺中完成其有性生殖期。引起人瘧疾病的四種原蟲爲：間日瘧原蟲、卵形瘧原蟲、惡性瘧原蟲和三日瘧原蟲。

plasmolysis *n.* a process occurring in bacteria and plants in which the protoplasm shrinks away from the rigid cell wall when the cell is placed in a *hypertonic solution. This is due to withdrawal of water from the cell by *osmosis.

胞質皺縮 當細胞和植物細胞被放置於高滲溶液中時，原生質從堅硬的細胞壁脫離並收縮（退縮）的過程。這是由於水通過滲透作用從細胞內逸出所致。

plaster *n.* adhesive tape used in shaped pieces or as a bandage to keep a dressing in place.

膠布 可剪成不同形狀黏貼用的橡皮膏，也可用以固定敷料。

plaster model (in dentistry) an accurate cast of the teeth and jaws made from modified plaster of Paris. A pair of models are used to study the dentition, particularly before treatment. Models are also used to construct dentures, orthodontic appliances, or such restorations as crowns.

石膏模型 （牙科學）用煅石膏加工製成的一種牙齒和頜骨的精確模型。這種成對的模型用於牙列研究，特別在治療以前。模型也可用於鑄造托牙、口腔整畸矯正器或冠修復體。

plaster of Paris a preparation of gypsum (calcium sulphate) that sets hard when water is added. It is used in various modified forms in dentistry to make *plaster models. It is also used in orthopaedics for preparing plaster *casts.

煅石膏 加水時可變硬的一種石膏（硫酸鈣）制劑。牙科學中用以鑄造各種不同形狀的石膏模型。在骨科中也用來製造筒形石膏夾。

plastic lymph a transparent yellowish liquid produced in a wound or other site of inflammation, in which connective tissue cells and blood vessels develop during healing.

成形性淋巴，機化性淋巴 在創傷或其他炎症部位所產生的一種淡黃色的透明液體。當創傷癒合時，結締組織細胞和血管在該液體中生長。

plastic surgery a branch of surgery dealing with the reconstruction of deformed or damaged parts of the body. It also includes the replacement of parts of the body that have been lost. If performed simply to improve appearances plastic surgery is called *cosmetic surgery*, but most plastic surgery involves the treatment and repair of burns or accidents and the correction of congenital defects, such as harelip and cleft palate.

整形外科 專門用於矯正人體畸形部位或修復人體的損傷部位的外科分支學科。它也包括裝配（置換）已喪失的人體部位。單純為改善容貌施行的成形外科手術稱作整容外科，但大部分整形外科是治療和修復燒傷或意外傷害，以及矯正先天性畸形，如兔唇和腭裂。

plastron *n.* the breastbone (*sternum) together with the costal cartilages attached to it.

胸板 胸骨和附着於胸骨的肋軟骨合稱。

-plasty *suffix denoting* plastic surgery. Example: *labioplasty* (of the lips).

〔後綴〕 **成形術，整形術，整復術** 指整形外科手術，例如，唇成形術。

platelet (thrombocyte) *n.* a disc-shaped structure, 1–2 μm in diameter, present in the blood. With *Romanowsky stains platelets appear as fragments of pale-blue cytoplasm with a few red granules. They have several functions, all relating to the arrest of bleeding (*see* blood coagulation). There are normally 150–400 × 10^9 platelets per litre of blood. *See also* thrombopoiesis.

血小板 存在於血液中的盤狀結構，直徑1～2 μm。用羅曼諾夫斯基氏染色劑染色的血小板，呈現出帶幾個紅色顆粒的淺藍色胞漿碎片。它們具有幾種功能，所有這些功能都與止血有關。正常人的每升血液中含有血小板爲150～400×10^9。

platy- *prefix denoting* broad or flat.

〔前綴〕 **闊，扁平**

platyhelminth *n. see* flatworm.

扁蠕虫，扁體動物

platysma *n.* a broad thin sheet of muscle that extends from below the collar bone to the angle of the jaw. It depresses the corner of the mouth.

〔頸〕闊肌 從鎖骨下延伸到頜骨角的一塊寬闊而薄的肌肉。功能：壓口角向下。

pledget *n.* a small wad of dressing material, such as lint, used either to cover a wound or sore or as a plug.

塡蓋料 由敷料材料如絨布製成的一種小的敷料塊或敷料卷，用來覆蓋或塡塞傷口。

-plegia *suffix denoting* paralysis. Example: *hemiplegia* (of one side of the body).

〔後綴〕 **麻痹，癱瘓** 例如，偏癱。

pleio- (pleo-) *prefix denoting* **1.** multiple. **2.** excessive.

〔前綴〕 **①多的 ②過多的**

pleiotropy *n.* a situation in which a single gene is responsible for more than one effect in the *phenotype. The mutation of such a gene will therefore have multiple effects. —**pleiotropic** *adj.*

〔基因〕多效性 單一基因對表型具有多種制約作用。因而突變基因也具有多種作用。

pleocytosis *n.* the presence of an abnormally large number of lymphocytes in the cerebrospinal fluid, which bathes the brain and spinal cord.

腦脊液淋巴細胞增加 指在浸泡腦與脊髓的腦脊髓液體中出現異常大量的淋巴細胞。

pleomastia (polymastia) *n.* multiple breasts or nipples. These are usually symmetrically arranged along a line between the mid point of the collar bone and the pelvis (the nipple line).

多乳房〔畸形〕 多個乳房或乳頭。這些乳頭通常沿着鎖骨中點和骨盆的延線（乳線）對稱地排列。

pleomorphism *n.* the condition in which an individual assumes a number of different forms during its life cycle. The malarial parasite (*Plasmodium*) displays pleomorphism.

多形性 一生物體在它的生活周期中能以多種不同形態出現的現象。瘧原虫就表現爲多形性的。

pleoptics *n.* special techniques practised by orthoptists (*see* orthoptics) for developing normal function of the macula (the most sensitive part of the retina), in people whose macular function has previously been disturbed because of strabismus (squint).

弱視眼操練〔療〕法，增視法 爲了使由於斜視而影響黃斑功能的患者恢復其黃斑（網膜中最敏感的部分）的正常功能，由視軸矯正醫師指導的一種特殊操練方法。

plerocercoid *n.* a larval stage of certain tapeworms, such as **Diphyllobothrium latum*. It differs from the *cysticercus (another larval form) in being solid and in lacking a cyst or bladder.

全尾蚴，裂頭蚴 某些縧蟲（如闊節裂頭縧蟲）的幼蟲期。它與囊尾蚴（另一種幼蟲形式）不同之處就在於實而無囊。

plessimeter (pleximeter) *n.* a small plate of bone, ivory, or other material pressed against the surface of the body and struck with a *plessor in the technique of *percussion.

叩診板 用骨、象牙或其他材料製成的一種小板。叩診時，將叩診板壓在身體表面並用叩診槌敲擊該板。

plessor (plexor) *n.* a small hammer used to investigate nervous reflexes and in the technique of *percussion.

叩診槌 用來檢查神經反射或叩診操作時用的一種小槌。

plethora *n.* any excess of any bodily fluid, especially blood (*see* hyperaemia). —**plethoric** *adj.*

多血〔症〕 體液過多。尤指血液過多。

plethysmography *n.* the process of recording the changes in the volume of a limb caused by alterations in blood pressure. The limb is inserted into a fluid-filled watertight casing (*oncometer*) and the pressure variations in the fluid are recorded.

體積描記法 記錄由於血壓的變化而引起的肢體體積變化的一種技術。將肢體插入一個充滿液體的密封筒（器官體積測量器）內，並記錄液體內壓力的變化。

pleur- (pleuro-) *prefix denoting* **1.** the pleura. **2.** the side of the body.

〔前綴〕 ①**胸膜** ②**身體側面**

pleura *n.* the covering of the lungs (*visceral pleura*) and of the inner surface of the chest wall (*parietal pleura*). (See illustration.) The covering consists of a closed sac of *serous membrane, which has a smooth shiny moist surface due to the secretion of small amounts of fluid. This fluid lubricates the opposing vis-

胸膜 覆蓋於肺（胸膜臟層，肺胸膜）和胸壁內表面（胸膜壁層）的膜（見圖）。它是由一個密封的漿膜囊構成。由於分泌少量液體，胸膜表面是平滑光亮而濕潤的。這種液體對胸膜的臟層與壁層表面

ceral and parietal surfaces so that they can slide painlessly over each other during breathing. —**pleural** *adj.*

起潤滑作用，以致當呼吸時臟、壁層兩個表面相互滑動而不產生疼痛。

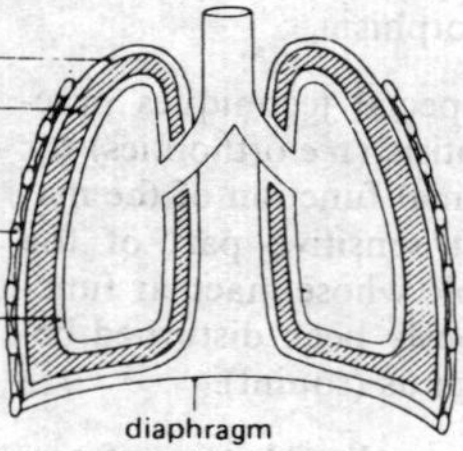

The pleura
胸膜

pleuracentesis *n. see* pleurocentesis.

胸腔穿刺術

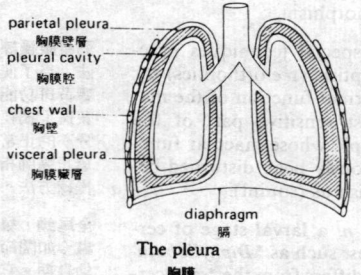

pleural cavity the space between the visceral and parietal *pleura, which is normally very small as the pleural membranes are in close contact. The introduction of fluid (*pleural effusion*) or gas separates the pleural surfaces and increases the volume of the pleural space.

胸膜腔　在胸膜臟層與壁層之間形成的腔隙。正常情況下，因爲兩層胸膜緊密地接觸，所以它們之間的空隙非常狹小。如有液體（胸膜腔積液）或氣體進入，將壁層與臟層表面隔開，可擴大胸膜腔隙的容積。

pleurectomy *n.* surgical removal of part of the *pleura, which is sometimes done to overcome recurrent *pneumothorax or to remove diseased areas of pleura.

胸膜部分切除術　有時爲了防止氣胸復發或爲了除去胸膜患病區域而做的部分胸膜切除的手術。

pleurisy *n.* inflammation of the *pleura, usually due to pneumonia in the underlying lung. The normally shiny and slippery pleural surfaces lose their sheen and become slightly sticky, so that there is pain on deep breathing and a characteristic 'rub' can be heard through a stethoscope. Pleurisy is always associated with some other disease in the lung, chest wall, diaphragm, or abdomen.

胸膜炎　通常由於胸膜所覆蓋的肺部組織發炎引起胸膜的炎症反應。正常時光滑的胸膜表面失去其光澤而變得有些粗糙不平，以致在深呼吸時引起疼痛。用聽診器可聽到一種特有的摩擦音，胸膜炎常與肺部、胸壁、膈或腹部的其他疾病有關。

pleurocele *n.* herniation of the pleura. *See* hernia.

胸膜疝　胸膜突出

pleurocentesis (pleuracentesis, thoracentesis, thoracocentesis) *n.* in-

胸腔穿刺術　爲了抽出胸腔液體、血液、膿液或氣

sertion of a hollow needle into the *pleural cavity through the chest wall in order to withdraw fluid, blood, pus, or air.

體，將空心針經胸壁刺入胸膜腔的手術。

pleurodesis *n.* the artificial production of pleurisy by chemical or mechanical means to obliterate the *pleural cavity, in order to prevent recurrent, usually malignant, pleural effusions.

胸膜固定術 爲了防止（通常爲惡性）胸膜滲液反復發作，用化學或機械方法造成人爲的胸膜炎，以閉鎖胸腔。

pleurodynia *n.* severe paroxysmal pain arising from the muscles between the ribs. It is often thought to be of rheumatic origin.

胸膜痛，胸肌痛 由肋間肌肉產生的劇烈的陣發性疼痛。人們通常認爲是由風濕所致。

pleurolysis (pneumolysis) *n.* surgical stripping of the parietal *pleura from the chest wall to allow the lung to collapse. The procedure was used in the days before effective antituberculous drugs to help tuberculosis to heal.

胸膜鬆解術 從胸壁剝離胸膜壁層引起肺萎陷的手術。在沒有抗結核特效藥物之前，該手術是治療結核病的一種輔助手段。

pleuropneumonia *n.* inflammation involving both the lung and pleura. *See* pleurisy, pneumonia.

胸膜肺炎 發生在胸膜與肺的炎症。

pleuropneumonia-like organisms (PPLO) *n. see* mycoplasma.

類胸膜肺炎微生物

pleurotomy *n.* surgical incision of the pleura. *See* pleurectomy.

胸膜切開術 將胸膜切開的一種手術。

pleurotyphoid *n.* *typhoid fever involving the lungs.

胸膜型傷寒 有肺部感染的傷寒。

pleximeter *n. see* plessimeter.

叩診板

plexor *n. see* plessor.

叩診槌

plexus *n.* a network of nerves or blood vessels. *See* brachial plexus.

叢 神經或血管的一種網狀結構。

plica *n.* a fold of tissue; for example, the *plica sublingualis*, the mucous fold in the floor of the mouth. —**plicate** *adj.*

〔皺〕襞，褶 組織的皺褶。例如，"舌下襞"即口腔底部的黏膜皺襞。

plication *n.* a surgical technique in which the size of a hollow organ is reduced by taking tucks or folds in the walls.

摺疊術 在空心器官的壁上打褶或摺疊，使其體積縮小的一種外科手術。

plombage *n.* **1.** a technique used in surgery for the correction of a *detached retina. A small piece of silicone

充塡術 ①用於治療視網膜脫離的一種外科手術。將一小片硅有機樹脂塑料

plastic is sewn on the outside of the eyeball to produce an indentation over the region where a retinal hole has been found. **2.** the insertion of plastic balls into the pleural cavity to cause collapse of the lung. This was done in the days before effective antituberculous drugs to help tuberculosis to heal.

縫在眼球外，以壓迫形成的視網膜孔的區域。②將塑料球充塡入胸腔引起肺萎陷。該方法是在沒有抗結核特效藥物以前，用於治療結核病的一種輔助手段。

plumbism *n.* lead poisoning. *See* lead[1].

鉛中毒

pluri- *prefix denoting* more than one; several.

〔前綴〕 **多**

pneo- *prefix denoting* breathing; respiration.

〔前綴〕 **呼吸**

pneum- (pneumo-) *prefix denoting* **1.** the presence of air or gas. Example: *pneumocolon* (within the colon). **2.** the lung(s). Example: *pneumogastric* (relating to the lungs and stomach). **3.** respiration.

〔前綴〕 ①**氣** 含有空氣或氣體。例如，結腸積氣。 ②**肺** 例如，肺胃的（與肺和胃有關的）。③**呼吸**

pneumat- (pneumato-) *prefix denoting* **1.** the presence of air or gas. **2.** respiration.

〔前綴〕 ①**氣，氣體** 含有空氣或氣體。 ②**呼吸**

pneumatization *n.* the presence of air-filled cavities in bone, such as the sinuses of the skull.

氣腔形成 骨內形成充滿氣體的腔，如顱骨中的竇。

pneumatocele *n.* herniation of lung tissue. *See* hernia.

肺膨出 肺組織突出。

pneumaturia *n.* the presence in the urine of bubbles of air or other gas, due to the formation of gas by bacteria infecting the urinary tract or to an abnormal connection (fistula) between the urinary tract and bowel.

氣尿 尿中含有由尿道的細菌感染或由尿與腸不正常溝通（瘻管）而產生空氣或其他氣體的氣泡。

pneumo- *prefix. see* pneum-.

〔前綴〕 ①**氣，氣體** ②**肺** ③**呼吸**

pneumocephalus (pneumocele) *n.* the presence of air within the skull, usually resulting from a fracture passing through one of the air sinuses. There may be a leak of cerebrospinal fluid at the site of the fracture, manifested as a watery discharge from the nose. Pneumocephalus can best be detected by plain X-rays of the skull,

顱腔積氣 通常由於顱骨骨折穿透氣竇而在顱內出現氣體。在骨折處可能有腦脊液漏出，表現爲從鼻流出水樣液體。顱腔積氣通過普通X線顱骨照像術很容易發現：顱腔內顯示出氣體和液體之間的水平面。

which show air and a fluid level inside a cavity.

pneumococcus *n.* (*pl.* **pneumococci**) the bacterium associated with pneumonia: **Streptococcus pneumoniae*. —**pneumococcal** *adj.*

肺炎球菌 與肺炎有關的細菌：肺炎鏈球菌。

pneumoconiosis *n.* a lung disease caused by inhaling dust. The dust particles must be less than 0.5 μm in diameter to reach the depths of the lung and there is usually a long period after initial exposure before shadows appear on the chest X-ray and breathlessness develops. In practice industrial exposure to coal dust (*anthracosis*), silica (*see* silicosis), and asbestos (*see* asbestosis) produces most of the cases of pneumoconiosis. In Britain such cases are examined by the Pneumoconiosis Medical Panels, on whose advice statutory compensation for industrial injury is awarded.

肺塵埃沉着病，塵肺 由吸入塵埃所引起的一種肺部疾病。塵埃顆粒的直徑必須小於0.5 μm才能到達肺的深部，而且從開始接觸塵埃到胸部X線檢查顯示出陰影以及出現氣喘症狀通常需經過較長一段時間。實際上，大部分肺塵埃沉着病均是由於接觸煤（炭末沉着病）、硅（矽肺或硅肺）、石棉（石棉沉着病）等工業粉塵所引起的。在英國，這類疾病通過肺塵病醫療保險機構的檢查並提出處理意見，發給患者法定工傷事故賠償金。

Pneumocystis *n.* a genus of protozoans. The species *P. carinii* causes pneumonia in immunosuppressed patients, usually following intensive chemotherapy (*see also* AIDS). The infection is fatal if untreated, but it can be overcome with high doses of *co-trimoxazole.

肺孢子蟲屬 原生動物的一個屬。卡氏肺囊蟲種能引起免疫受抑制病人的肺部炎症。該種免疫力受抑制通常是由於用大劑量化學藥物長期治療所引起的。這種感染如不進行治療可導致死亡，但大劑量複方新諾明可治療該病。

pneumocyte *n.* a type of cell that lines the walls separating the air sacs (*see* alveolus) in the lungs. Type I pneumocytes are flat and inconspicuous. Type II pneumocytes are cuboidal and secrete *surfactant.

肺細胞 覆蓋於肺泡壁上的一類細胞。Ⅰ型肺細胞呈扁平形，很不明顯；Ⅱ型肺細胞呈立方形，能分泌表面活性物質。

pneumoencephalography *n.* a technique used in the X-ray diagnosis of disease within the skull. Air is introduced into the cavities (ventricles) of the brain to displace the cerebrospinal fluid, thus acting as a *contrast me-

氣腦造影術 爲診斷顱內疾病採用的X線照影的一種技術。將氣體注入腦室來取代其中的腦脊液。這些氣體起着造影劑的作用，在X線照片上能顯示

dium. X-ray photographs show the size and disposition of the ventricles and the subarachnoid spaces.

出腦室和蛛網膜下腔的大小及其位置改變。

pneumograph *n.* an instrument used to record the movements made during respiration.

呼吸描記器 用來記錄呼吸運動的一種儀器。

pneumohaemothorax *n. see* haemopneumothorax.

血氣胸

pneumohydrothorax *n. see* hydropneumothorax.

水氣胸

pneumolysis *n. see* pleurolysis.

〔胸膜外〕肺鬆解術

pneumon- (pneumono-) *prefix denoting* the lung(s). Example: *pneumonopexy* (surgical fixation to the chest wall).

〔前綴〕 **肺** 例如，肺固定術。

pneumonectomy *n.* surgical removal of a lung, usually for cancer.

肺切除術 通常由於治療癌症所採用的切除肺的外科手術。

pneumonia *n.* inflammation of the lung caused by bacteria, in which the air sacs (*alveoli) fill up with pus so that air is excluded and the lung becomes solid (*see* consolidation). The symptoms depend on the amount of lung involved and the virulence of the bacteria, but they generally include cough and chest pain, with shadows on the chest X-ray. The most common type is *bronchopneumonia*, which starts around the bronchi and bronchioles. *Lobar pneumonia* affects whole lobes of either or both lungs and is caused by certain strains of *Streptococcus pneumoniae*; *hypostatic pneumonia* develops in dependant parts of the lung in people who are otherwise ill, chilled, or immobilized. The bacteria that cause pneumonia are usually sensitive to *antibiotics, and recovery is usually quick. *Compare* pneumonitis.

肺炎 由細菌引起的肺部炎症。這時肺炎症部位的肺泡內充滿膿液，空氣排出，而發生肺實變。症狀的輕重取決於肺受侵襲部位的大小和細菌的毒力大小，但一般均有咳嗽和胸痛，並在胸部X線檢查時出現陰影。最常見的類型是支氣管肺炎，這種肺炎侵襲支氣管和細支氣管。大葉性肺炎常侵襲一側或兩側肺的整個肺葉，這種肺炎是由肺炎鏈球菌的某些菌株引起的。墜積性肺炎發生於患有其他疾病、受寒或胸腔運動受阻的病人的肺的下部。引起肺炎的細菌常對抗生素敏感，因而通常很快康復。

pneumonitis *n.* inflammation of the lung that is confined to the walls of the air sacs (alveoli) and often caused by viruses or unknown agents. It may be acute and transient or chronic, leading

局限性肺炎 常由病毒引起的或病因不明的，局限於肺泡壁的肺部炎症。該病可以是急性的和短暫的或慢性的，並可導至逐漸

to increasing respiratory disability. It does not respond to antibiotics but corticosteroids may be helpful. *Compare* pneumonia.

加重的呼吸困難。局限性肺炎對抗生素不敏感，但用皮質類固醇治療可能有效。

pneumopericardium *n.* the presence of air within the membranous sac surrounding the heart. *See* hydropneumopericardium.

心包積氣，氣心包 心包腔內積有氣體。

pneumoperitoneum *n.* air or gas in the peritoneal or abdominal cavity, usually due to a perforation of the stomach or bowel. A former treatment of tuberculosis was the deliberate injection of air into the peritoneal cavity to allow the tuberculous lung to be rested (*artificial pneumoperitoneum*).

氣腹 通常由胃或腸穿孔引起的腹膜腔積氣。以前治療結核時曾有意地往腹腔內注入氣體，以便使患結核的肺部得到休息（人工氣腹）。

pneumoradiography *n.* X-ray examination of part of the body using a gas, such as air or carbon dioxide, as a *contrast medium. For example, introduction of air into the ventricles of the brain enables them to be distinguished by X-rays; in their normal (fluid-filled) state they are not sufficiently contrasted with the brain tissue itself.

充氣造影術 使用氣體（如空氣或二氧化碳）作爲造影劑，對身體某部分進行X線檢查的方法。例如，將空氣注入腦室使得它們易通過X線顯影。在正常的腦室中是充滿液體的，與腦組織本身難以區別。

pneumothorax *n.* air in the *pleural cavity. Any breach of the lung surface or chest wall allows air to enter the pleural cavity, causing the lung to collapse. The leak can occur without apparent cause, in otherwise healthy people (*spontaneous pneumothorax*), or result from injuries to the chest (*traumatic pneumothorax*). In *tension pneumothorax* a breach in the lung surface acts as a valve, admitting air into the pleural cavity when the patient breathes in but preventing its escape when he breathes out. This air must be let out by surgical incision.
A former treatment for pulmonary tuberculosis – *artificial pneumothorax* – was the deliberate injection of air into the pleural cavity to collapse the lung and allow the tuberculous areas to heal.

氣胸 胸腔內積氣。肺表面或胸壁的任何裂隙都能使空氣進入胸腔，引起肺萎陷。在其他方面都健康的人無明顯原因發生的氣胸爲自發性氣胸，由於胸部受傷發生的氣胸爲創傷性氣胸。在張力性氣胸中，肺表面的裂隙起着活塞作用，當病人吸氣時，空氣得以進入胸膜腔；當病人呼氣時，則可阻擋空氣逸出。這種積氣必須通過手術切開才能排出。治療肺結核的舊方法（人工氣胸）即有意地將空氣注入胸膜腔，使肺萎陷，而促使患結核的肺部區域得以痊癒。

-pnoea *suffix denoting* a condition of breathing. Example: *dyspnoea* (breathlessness).

〔後綴〕 **呼吸** 例如，呼吸困難。

pock *n.* a small pus-filled eruption on the skin characteristic of *chickenpox and *smallpox rashes. *See also* pustule.

痘疱 水痘和牛痘所特有的，皮膚上的一種充滿膿液的小疱疹。

pocket *n.* (in dentistry) *see* periodontal pocket.

袋 （牙科）

pod- *prefix denoting* the foot.

〔前綴〕 **足，脚**

podagra *n.* gout of the foot, especially the big toe.

〔足〕痛風 脚的痛風病，特指大拇趾的。

podalic version altering the position of a fetus in the womb so that its feet will emerge first at birth. *See also* version.

胎足倒轉術 轉換子宮內胎兒的位置以使在分娩時胎兒的雙脚先露的手術。

-poiesis *suffix denoting* formation; production. Example: *haemopoiesis* (of blood cells).

〔後綴〕 **產生，生、造** 例如，血細胞生成。

poikilo- *prefix denoting* variation; irregularity.

〔前綴〕 **異，變，不規則**

poikilocyte *n.* an abnormally shaped red blood cell (*erythrocyte). Poikilocytes may be classified into a variety of types on the basis of their shape; for example elliptocytes (ellipsoid) and schistocytes (semilunar). *See also* poikilocytosis.

異形紅細胞 形狀異常的紅細胞。異形紅細胞根據其形狀可分爲各種類型。例如橢圓形紅細胞和裂紅細胞（半月形）。

poikilocytosis *n.* the presence of abnormally shaped red cells (*poikilocytes) in the blood. Poikilocytosis is particularly marked in *myelofibrosis but can occur to some extent in almost any blood disease.

異形紅細胞症 血液中出現形狀異常的紅細胞（異形紅細胞）。異形紅細胞症在骨髓纖維變性中特別明顯，但在幾乎所有血液疾病中均能出現某種程度的異形紅細胞。

poikiloderma *n.* a condition in which the skin atrophies and becomes pigmented, giving it a mottled appearance.

皮膚異色病 由皮膚萎縮和色素沉着，而呈現出花斑狀皮膚外觀的一種疾病。

poikilothermic *adj.* cold-blooded: being unable to regulate the body temperature, which fluctuates according to

冷血動物的，變溫動物的 冷血的，不能夠調節體溫的，體溫隨着環境溫度

that of the surroundings. Reptiles and amphibians are cold-blooded. *Compare* homoiothermic. —**poikilothermy** *n.*

的變化而變化的。爬行類與兩棲類皆爲冷血動物。

pointillage *n.* a procedure in massage in which the operator's fingers are pressed, fingertip first, deep into the patient's skin. This is done to manipulate underlying structures and break up adhesions that may have formed following injury.

指尖按摩法 操作者用手指（指尖向下）深深按壓入皮膚的一種按摩方法。這是爲了使推拿的力量施於皮下結構，從而分離受傷後可能形成的黏連。

poison *n.* any substance that irritates, damages, or impairs the activity of the body's tissues. In large enough doses almost any substance acts as a poison, but the term is usually reserved for substances, such as arsenic, cyanide, and strychnine, that are harmful in relatively small amounts.

毒物 任何對人體組織功能有刺激、破壞或損傷作用的物質。幾乎任何物質在足夠大的劑量時都會成爲毒物。但該詞通常僅用於相當小的劑量即有損害作用的物質，如砷、氰化物、士的寧等。

Poisson distribution *see* frequency distribution.

泊松分佈

polar body one of the small cells produced during the formation of an ovum from an *oocyte that does not develop into a functional egg cell.

極體 在卵子形成期，從未發育爲功能卵細胞的卵母細胞中生長出的一種小細胞。

poldine *n.* a drug, similar to *atropine, that inhibits gastric secretion and is used to treat such disorders as gastric and duodenal ulcers. It is administered by mouth; side-effects may include dry mouth, blurred vision, difficulty in urination, and fast heart beat. Trade name: **Nacton.**

波爾定 一種作用與阿托品相似的藥物。該藥具有抑制胃分泌功能的作用，用於治療胃和十二指腸潰瘍等疾病。口服。副作用可有口乾、視力模糊、排尿困難和心跳快。

pole *n.* (in anatomy) the extremity of the axis of the body, an organ, or a cell.

極 在解剖學中指身體、器官或細胞軸的末端。

poli- (polio-) *prefix denoting* the grey matter of the nervous system.

〔前綴〕 **灰質** 指神經系統的灰色物質。

polioencephalitis (viral encephalitis) *n.* a virus infection of the brain, causing particular damage to the *grey matter of the cerebral hemispheres and the brainstem. The infection is usually transmitted to man by the bite of a mosquito or tick. Some forms of this illness are endemic in a particular locality (e.g. Japanese (B) encephalitis); others have occurred as epidemics, e.g.

腦灰質炎 一種對腦半球和腦幹的灰質造成特殊損傷的腦病毒性感染。這種感染通常是由於蚊子或蜱叮咬後傳播給人的。這類疾病中的某些類型是一些特定地區的地方病（如，日本乙型腦炎）；另外一些是流行病，如昏睡性腦炎（昏睡病）。

encephalitis lethargica (sleepy sickness). *See also* encephalitis.

polioencephalomyelitis *n.* any virus infection of the central nervous system affecting the grey matter of the brain and spinal cord. *Rabies is the outstanding example.

腦脊髓灰質炎 一種侵襲腦和脊髓灰質的中樞神經系統的病毒感染。狂犬病就是一個顯著的例子。

poliomyelitis (infantile paralysis, polio) *n.* an infectious virus disease affecting the central nervous system. The virus is excreted in the faeces of an infected person and the disease is therefore most common where sanitation is poor. However, epidemics may occur in more hygienic conditions, where individuals have not acquired immunity to the disease during infancy. Symptoms commence 7–12 days after infection. In most cases paralysis does not occur: in *abortive poliomyelitis* only the throat and intestines are infected and the symptoms are those of a stomach upset or influenza; in *nonparalytic poliomyelitis* these symptoms are accompanied by muscle stiffness, particularly in the neck and back. *Paralytic poliomyelitis* is much less common. The symptoms of the milder forms of the disease are followed by weakness and eventual paralysis of the muscles: in *bulbar poliomyelitis* the muscles of the respiratory system are involved and breathing is affected.

There is no specific treatment, apart from measures to relieve the symptoms: cases of bulbar polio may require the use of a *respirator. Immunization, using the *Sabin vaccine (taken orally) or the *Salk vaccine (injected), is highly effective.

脊髓灰質炎 一種侵襲中樞神經系統的病毒感染性疾病。該病毒隨着受感染病人的糞便排出，因此，在衛生條件差的地區，該病最爲常見。但在嬰兒期對該病未獲得免疫力的人，在衛生條件較好的地區也可以患流行性脊髓灰質炎。在感染後的7～12日內開始出現症狀。在大多數病人中不出現痲痹的症狀。僅在喉與腸部位的感染是頓挫性脊髓灰質炎。其症狀與胃腸疾病或流行性感冒的症狀相同。非痲痹性脊髓灰質炎病人，除有以上症狀以外，還可併發肌强直，特別是頸、背肌肉的强直。痲痹性脊髓灰質炎較少見。該病輕型的症狀是先有肌無力，最後結局是肌痲痹。在延髓型脊髓灰質炎中，呼吸系統的肌肉受累而影響呼吸。

除了採取緩解症狀的措施以外，尚沒有特殊的治療方法。延髓型脊髓灰質炎的患者可能還需使用呼吸器。用薩賓氏疫苗（口服）或索爾克氏疫苗（注射）免疫接種有顯著的效果。

poliosis *n.* premature greying of the hair.

白髮〔症〕 頭髮早白。

poliovirus *n.* one of a small group of RNA-containing viruses causing *poliomyelitis. They are included within the *picornavirus group.

脊髓灰質炎病毒 一小組能引起脊髓灰質炎的核糖核酸病毒中的一種。它們屬於細小核糖核酸病毒組。

pollex *n.* (*pl.* **pollices**) the thumb.
拇指，拇

pollinosis *n.* a more precise term than *hayfever for an allergy due to the pollen of grasses, trees, or shrubs.
花粉病　由草、樹或灌木的花粉引起的一種變態反應性疾病。花粉病一詞比枯草熱一詞更爲確切。

poly- *prefix denoting* **1.** many; multiple. **2.** excessive. **3.** generalized; affecting many parts.
〔前綴〕①多，多數　②過多，過度　③遍及全身的，全身的，多發的

polyarteritis nodosa (periarteritis nodosa) a disease of unknown cause in which there is patchy inflammation of the walls of the arteries. It is one of the *collagen diseases. Common manifestations are arthritis, neuritis, asthma, skin rashes, hypertension, kidney failure, and fever. The inflammation is suppressed by corticosteroid drugs (such as prednisolone).
結節性多動脉炎　多處動脉壁上出現炎症斑塊的一種病因不明的疾病。該病是膠原病的一種。常見的表現有關節炎、神經炎、氣喘、皮疹、高血壓、腎衰和發燒。用皮質類固醇藥如强的松龍可控制炎症。

polyarthritis *n.* rheumatic disease involving several to many joints, either together or in sequence, causing pain, stiffness, swelling, tenderness, and loss of function. *Rheumatoid arthritis is the most common cause.
多關節炎　同時或陸續侵襲幾處至許多處關節的風濕性疾病。該病能引起關節的疼痛、强直、腫脹、觸痛和功能喪失等症狀。類風濕性關節炎爲最常見的病因。

polychromasia (polychromatophilia) *n.* the presence of certain blue red blood cells (*erythrocytes) seen in blood films stained with *Romanowsky stains, as well as the normal pink cells. The cells that appear blue are juvenile erythrocytes (*see* reticulocyte).
多染〔性〕細胞增多　經羅曼諾夫斯基染色劑處理的血片上，除見到正常粉紅色細胞外，還可見到某些帶藍色的紅細胞。帶藍色的細胞是未成熟的紅細胞。

polycoria *n.* a rare congenital abnormality of the eye in which there are one or more holes in the iris in addition to the pupil.
多瞳〔畸形〕，多瞳症　一種罕見的先天性眼睛畸形。該病人的眼睛中除有瞳孔外，在虹膜內還有一個或多個孔。

polycystic disease of the kidneys an inherited disorder, transmitted as an autosomal *dominant, in which the substance of both kidneys is largely replaced by numerous cysts. Symptoms – including *haematuria, urinary tract infection, and hypertension-appear be-
多囊腎　由常染色體顯性等位基因傳遞的一種遺傳性疾病。該遺傳病患者的兩側腎臟實質的大部分被許多囊腫所取代。病人常在20～40歲之間出現血尿、尿道感染和高血壓等

tween the ages of 20 and 40 and are associated with chronic kidney failure.

症狀，還可併發慢性腎功能衰竭。

polycythaemia *n.* an increase in the haemoglobin concentration of the blood. This may be due either to a decrease in the total volume of the plasma (*relative polycythaemia*) or to an increase in the total volume of the red cells (*absolute polycythaemia*). The latter may occur as a primary disease (*see* polycythaemia vera) or as a secondary condition in association with various respiratory or circulatory disorders that cause deficiency of oxygen in the tissues and with certain tumours, such as carcinoma of the kidney.

紅細胞增多症 血液中血紅蛋白濃度增高。這可能是由於血漿總量的減少（相對性的紅細胞增多）或由於紅細胞的總量增加而引起。後者（紅細胞總量增加）即可能是原發性疾病；也可能併發於引起組織缺氧的各種呼吸系或循環系疾病，或併發於某些腫瘤，如腎癌。

polycythaemia vera (erythraemia, Vaquez-Osler disease) a disease in which the number of red cells in the blood is greatly increased (*see also* polycythaemia). There is often also an increase in the numbers of white blood cells and platelets. Symptoms include headache, thromboses, *cyanosis, and *plethora. Polycythaemia vera may be treated by blood-letting, but more severe cases are best treated by radiotherapy. The cause of the disease is not known.

眞性紅細胞增多（紅細胞增多症，瓦-奧二氏病） 血液內紅細胞數大量增加的一種疾病。其中的白細胞和血小板也往往同時增加。症狀包括頭痛、血栓形成、發紺和多血質外觀。眞性紅細胞增多可以通過放血來治療，但較嚴重的病人使用放射療法效果最好。此病病因不明。

polydactylism *n. see* hyperdactylism.

多指（趾）〔畸形〕

polydipsia *n.* abnormally intense thirst, leading to the drinking of large quantities of fluid. This is a symptom typical of diabetes mellitus and diabetes insipidus.

煩渴 能飲用大量液體的異常强烈的口渴現象。煩渴是糖尿病和尿崩症的一個典型的症狀。

polygene *n.* one of a number of genes that together control a single characteristic in an individual. Each polygene has only a slight effect and the expression of a set of polygenes is the result of their combined interaction. Characteristics controlled by polygenes are usually of a quantitative nature, e.g. height. *See also* multifactorial. —**polygenic** *adj.*

多基因 在個體中共同控制單獨一個性狀的數個基因中的一個。每一多基因僅起一點微小的作用，而一套多基因的表現正是它們聯合起來相互作用的結果。多基因所控制的通常是一個數量性狀，例如，高度。

polymastia *n. see* pleomastia.

多乳房

polymer *n.* a substance formed by the linkage of a large number of smaller molecules known as *monomers*. An example of a monomer is glucose, whose molecules link together to form glycogen, a polymer. Polymers may have molecular weights from a few thousands to many millions. Polymers made up of a single type of monomer are known as *homopolymers*; those of two or more monomers as *heteropolymers*.

聚合物，聚合體 由許多個稱作單體的較小分子連接而組成的一種物質。例如，葡萄糖是一個單體，其分子聯接在一起就構成糖原——聚合物。聚合物的分子量可為數千甚至數百萬。由單純一種單體組成的聚合物稱作同型聚合物；由兩種或更多種單體組成的聚合物稱作異型聚合物。

polymorph (polymorphonuclear leucocyte) *n. see* neutrophil.

多形核白細胞

polymorphism *n.* (in genetics) a condition in which a chromosome or a genetic character occurs in more than one form, resulting in the coexistence of more than one morphological type in the same population.

多形〔態〕，多形變態 （遺傳學）一個染色體或一種遺傳特性以多種形式出現，以致在同一羣體中同時出現多種形態特徵。

polymyalgia rheumatica a rheumatic disease causing aching and progressive stiffness of the muscles of the shoulders and hips. The condition is most common in the elderly, rarely occurring before the age of 50. The symptoms respond rapidly and effectively to corticosteroid treatment, which must usually be continued for several years. It is often associated with temporal *arteritis.

風濕性多肌痛 一種能引起肩部和髖部肌肉疼痛和逐漸强直的風濕性疾病。該病最常見於老年人，小於五十歲的人較少見。用皮質類固醇治療，症狀可迅速緩解。但通常必須持續用藥數年。該病常併有顳動脉炎。

polymyositis *n.* a generalized disease of the muscles that may be acute or chronic. It particularly affects the muscles of the shoulder and hip girdles, which are weak and tender to the touch. Microscopic examination of the affected muscles shows diffuse inflammatory changes, and relief of the symptoms is obtained with *corticosteroid drugs. The skin may be reddened and atrophic. *See also* dermatomyositis.

多肌炎 一種急性或慢性的侵襲全身肌肉的疾病。該病特別易侵襲肩胛帶和髖帶，可有無力和觸痛的症狀。患部肌肉在顯微鏡下檢查，可顯示出瀰漫性炎症病變的特徵。皮質類固醇藥物有緩解症狀的作用。皮膚可有發紅和萎縮的現象。

polymyxin B an *antibiotic used to treat infections caused by Gram-negative bacteria, especially **Pseudomonas*. It is usually administered by injection but is also taken by mouth or applied as

多黏菌素B 用於治療由革蘭氏陰性菌，特別是假單胞菌屬引起的感染的一種抗生素。通常注射給藥，但也可以口服，爲治

a solution or ointment for ear and eye infections. The drug may cause mild dizziness. Trade name: **Aerosporin**.

療耳和眼的感染則可配製成溶液或軟膏使用。該藥可以引起輕微的頭暈。

polyneuritis *n.* any disorder involving all the peripheral nerves. The term is often used interchangeably with *polyneuropathy although its specific use implies inflammation of the nerves.

多神經炎 任何侵襲所有周圍神經的疾病。雖然該詞的含義是專指神經炎症，但它往往與多神經病一詞交替使用。

polyneuropathy *n.* any disease involving all of the peripheral nerves. The symptoms first affect the tips of the fingers and toes (i.e. the extremities of the nerve fibres) and subsequently spread towards the trunk. The symptoms are usually roughly symmetrical. *See* neuropathy.

多神經病 任何侵犯全部周圍神經的疾病。症狀先在指尖和趾尖（神經纖維末梢）出現，隨後擴散到軀幹，並且往往大體上對稱。

polynucleotide *n.* a long chain of linked *nucleotides, of which molecules of DNA and RNA are made.

多核苷酸 由核苷酸聯接成的一條長鏈，脫氧核糖核酸和核糖核酸分子即由此鏈構成。

polyopia *n.* the sensation of multiple images of one object. It is sometimes experienced by people with early cataract. *See also* diplopia.

視物顯多症 一物多像感（視一物却產生多個形像的感覺）。白內障病人有時早期可有此症狀。

polyorchidism *n.* a congenital abnormality resulting in more than two testes.

多睾〔畸形〕 長有兩個以上睾丸的先天性畸形。

polyp (polypus) *n.* a growth, usually benign, protruding from a mucous membrane. Polyps are commonly found in the nose and sinuses, giving rise to obstruction, chronic infection, and discharge. They are often present in patients with allergic rhinitis, in whom they may develop in response to long-term antigenic stimulation. Other sites of occurrence include the ear, the stomach, and the bowel. Polyps are usually removed surgically (*see* polypectomy).

息肉 從黏膜突出來的腫瘤，通常爲良性的。息肉常見於鼻腔和鼻竇，可引起阻塞、慢性炎症和溢液等症狀。息肉常見於患有變應性鼻炎的病人，可能由於長期的抗原刺激而產生。易發的其它部位包括耳、胃和腸。息肉通常採用外科手術切除。

polypectomy *n.* the surgical removal of a *polyp. The technique used depends upon the site and size of the polyp, but it is often done by cutting

息肉切除術 切除息肉的外科手術。所採用的手術方法取决於息肉所在部位和其大小。通常使用電烙

across the base using a wire loop (snare) through which is passed a coagulating *diathermy current.

勒除器在息肉根部進行勒除。

polypeptide *n.* a molecule consisting of three or more amino acids linked together by *peptide bonds. *Protein molecules are polypeptides.

多肽 由以肽鏈相連的三個或更多個氨基酸所組成的分子。蛋白分子就屬於多肽。

polyphagia *n.* gluttonous excessive eating.

貪食〔症〕 一種不知飽的暴食症。

polypharmacy *n.* treatment of a patient with more than one type of medicine.

複方藥療法，多味藥療法 讓病人服用多於一種藥劑的治療方法。

polyphyletic *adj.* describing a number of individuals, species, etc., that have evolved from more than one ancestral group. *Compare* monophyletic.

多元的，多系的，多源的 描述從不止於一個祖系演化而來的許多個體或物種。

polyploid *adj.* describing cells, tissues, or individuals in which there are three or more complete sets of chromosomes. *Compare* diploid, haploid. —**polyploidy** *n.*

多倍體的 描述在細胞、組織或個體中有三套或更多套完整的染色體的。

polypoid *adj.* having the appearance of a *polyp.

息肉狀的 具有息肉樣外觀的。

polyposis *n.* a condition in which numerous polyps form in an organ or tissue. *Familial polyposis coli* is a hereditary disease in which multiple polyps develop in the colon at puberty. As these polyps often become malignant, patients are usually advised to undergo total removal of the colon. *Compare* pseudopolyposis.

息肉病 在器官或組織中形成許多息肉的一種疾病。家族性結腸息肉病是一種遺傳性疾病，特點是在青春期結腸內生長出許多息肉。因爲這些息肉常能轉變爲惡性的，所以通常建議病人將結腸全部切除。

polypus *n. see* polyp.

息肉

polyradiculitis (polyradiculopathy) *n.* any disorder of the peripheral nerves (*see* neuropathy) in which the brunt of the disease falls on the nerve roots where they emerge from the spinal cord. An abnormal allergic response in the nerve fibres is thought to be the cause of this condition. The *Guillain-Barré syndrome is an example.

多神經根炎 一種主要侵襲來自脊髓的神經根部位的周圍神經疾病。人們認爲多神經根炎的病因可能是神經纖維的一種過敏反應。格－巴二氏綜合徵（急性感染性多神經炎）就是一個例子。

polyribosome *n. see* polysome.

多核糖體，多核糖核蛋白體

polysaccharide *n.* a *carbohydrate formed from many monosaccharides joined together in long linear or branched chains. Polysaccharides have two important functions: (1) as storage forms of energy; for example *glycogen in animals and man and *starch in plants, and (2) as structural elements; for example *mucopolysaccharides in animals and man and *cellulose in plants.

多糖 由呈長線形的或支鏈形的許多單糖連接在一起構成的一種碳水化合物。多糖具有兩種重要功能：①作爲能量的一種貯存形式，例如人體內與動物體內的糖原，植物中的澱粉。②作爲組織結構的組成成分，例如人體和動物體中的黏多糖，植物中的纖維素。

polyserositis *n.* inflammation of the membranes that line the chest, abdomen, and joints, with accumulation of fluid in the cavities. Commonly the condition is inherited and intermittent and is termed *familial Mediterranean fever*. If complicated by infiltration of major organs by a glycoprotein (*see* amyloidosis) the disease usually proves fatal.

多漿膜炎 內襯於胸、腹腔和關節的膜發生炎症，並伴有腔內積液。該病通常是遺傳性的和間歇性的，並稱爲家族性地中海熱。如果該病還伴有主要器官的糖蛋白浸潤時，往往是致命的。

polysome (polyribosome) *n.* a structure that occurs in the cytoplasm of cells and consists of a group of *ribosomes linked together by *messenger RNA molecules: formed during protein synthesis.

多核糖體，多核糖核蛋白體 存在於細胞質中的，由信使核糖核酸分子連接在一起形成的核糖體的複合結構。它是在蛋白的合成過程中形成的。

polyspermia *n.* **1.** excessive formation of semen. **2.** *see* polyspermy.

①精液過多 ②多精受精，多精入卵

polyspermy (polyspermia) *n.* fertilization of a single ovum by more than one spermatozoon: the development is abnormal and the embryo dies.

多精受精，多精入卵 不止一個精子與單個卵子相接合的受精過程。這種受精卵的發育是不正常的，胚胎不能存活。

polythelia *n.* a congenital excess of nipples (*see* pleomastia).

多乳頭〔畸形〕 一種先天性乳頭過多的畸形。

polyuria *n.* the production of large volumes of urine, which is dilute and of a pale colour. The phenomenon may be due simply to excessive liquid intake or to disease, particularly diabetes mellitus, diabetes insipidus, and kidney disorders.

多尿〔症〕 排出大量呈稀釋狀態的、淡色的尿液。該現象可能是由於單純地飲水過多，也可能由於某種疾病，特別是糖尿病、尿崩症和腎臟疾病所引起。

pompholyx *n.* *eczema of the hands and feet. Because the horny layer of the

汗疱 手與脚上的濕疹。由於這些部位皮膚的表皮

skin in these parts is so thick the vesicles typical of eczema cannot rupture; they therefore persist in the skin, looking like rice grains. There is intense itching until the skin eventually peels. There may be secondary infection due to scratching. Pompholyx is commonest in early adulthood and attacks occur suddenly, lasting up to six weeks. The disease may be recurrent or persist as a chronic condition.

角質層太厚，以致水泡型濕疹的小水泡不能破裂。因此這些小水泡看上去像存留在皮膚內的米粒。直到角質層最終脫落後，奇癢才能消失。由於不斷的搔抓，可以繼發感染。汗疱在成年人的早期最爲常見，突然發病，持續達六周。該病可能反復發病或像慢性病一樣持續存在。

pons *n.* **1.** *see* pons Varolii. **2.** any portion of tissue that joins two parts of an organ.

①**腦橋** ②**橋** 連接一個器官的兩部分的組織部位。

pons Varolii (pons) the part of the *brainstem that links the medulla oblongata and the thalamus, bulging forwards in front of the cerebellum, from which it is separated by the fourth ventricle. It contains numerous nerve tracts between the cerebral cortex and the spinal cord and several nuclei of grey matter. From its front surface the *trigeminal nerves emerge.

腦橋 連接延髓和丘腦的腦幹部分。它在小腦前方向前膨出，被第四腦室與小腦分隔開。腦橋含有大量連接大腦皮質與脊髓的神經束和一些灰質核。三叉神經就從腦橋的前表面發出。

popliteus *n.* a flat triangular muscle at the back of the knee joint, between the femur and tibia, that helps to flex the knee. —**popliteal** *adj.*

膕肌 位於股骨和脛骨之間的，膝關節後的一塊扁平形的三角肌。它能幫助膝關節屈曲。

porcelain *n.* (in dentistry) a ceramic material used to construct tooth-coloured crowns.

瓷，瓷料 在牙科中用於鑄造牙齒本色齒冠的一種陶瓷材料。

pore *n.* a small opening; for example, *sweat pores* are the openings of the sweat glands on the surface of the skin.

孔 一種小的開口。例如，汗孔是皮膚表面汗腺的開口。

porencephaly *n.* an abnormal communication between the lateral *ventricle and the surface of the brain. This is usually a consequence of brain injury or cerebrovascular disease; uncommonly it may be a developmental defect, when it would most likely affect both lateral ventricles.

腦穿通〔畸形〕 在側腦室與腦表面之間形成一個異常通道。該種畸形往往由腦外傷或腦血管疾病所致。兩側腦室穿通畸形可能是一種發育缺陷，但這種情况並不多見。

porocephaliasis *n.* a rare infestation of the nasal cavities, windpipe, lungs, liver, or spleen by the nymphs of the

蛇舌狀蟲病 由寄生性節肢動物蛇舌狀蟲屬（洞頭蟲屬）的若蟲（蛹）引起

parasitic arthropod *Porocephalus. Man becomes infected on consumption of water or uncooked vegetables contaminated with the parasite's eggs. There may be some abdominal pain while the parasite is in the gut but generally there are no symptoms. Porocephaliasis has been occasionally reported in negroes of central Africa.

的鼻腔、氣管、肺、肝或脾臟的一種罕見的感染。人可能由於飲用或進食由寄生蟲卵汚染的生水或生菜而引起感染。當寄生蟲進入腸內時，病人可能有些腹痛的症狀，但一般情況下並沒有任何症狀。蛇舌狀蟲病在中非的黑人中曾經偶爾有過報導。

Porocephalus *n.* a genus of wormlike arthropods occurring mainly in tropical Africa and India. The legless adults are parasites in the lungs of snakes. The eggs, which are ejected with the snake's bronchial secretions, may be accidentally swallowed by man. The larva bores through the gut wall and usually migrates to the liver, where it develops into a nymph (*see* porocephaliasis).

蛇舌狀蟲屬 一種主要生活在熱帶非洲和印度的蠕蟲樣節肢動物屬。這種無腿成蟲寄生於蛇的肺內。隨着蛇支氣管分泌物一同吐出來的蟲卵，可能偶然被人吞嚥下去。幼蟲穿過腸壁，通常遷移到肝臟，在肝臟發育成若蟲（蛹）。

porphin *n.* a complex nitrogen-containing ring structure and parent compound of the *porphyrins.

卟吩 一種含有氮環結構的化合物，是卟啉的母體。

porphobilinogen *n.* a pigment that appears in the urine of individuals with acute *porphyria, causing it to darken if left standing.

卟啉膽色素原 急性卟啉症患者尿液中出現的一種色素。如尿液靜置，顏色可由淺變深。

porphyria *n.* one of a group of rare inherited disorders due to disturbance of the metabolism of the breakdown products (*porphyrins) of the red blood pigment haemoglobin. The defect may be primarily in the liver (*hepatic porphyria*) or in the bone marrow (*erythropoietic porphyria*) or both. The prominent features include the excretion of porphyrins and their derivatives in the urine, which may change colour on standing (*see* porphobilinogen); sensitivity of the skin to sunlight causing chronic inflammation or blistering; inflammation of the nerves (neuritis); mental disturbances; and attacks of abdominal pain.

卟啉症 血紅蛋白分解產物（卟啉）代謝失調所引起的一種罕見的遺傳性疾病。該代謝缺陷最初可能在肝臟（肝卟啉症）或在骨髓（紅細胞生成性卟啉症）或者在肝與骨髓兩者中發生。主要特徵是尿液中有卟啉和其衍生物排出。如尿靜置不動，這些尿中的物質可能變色；皮膚對日光過敏，可引起慢性皮膚炎症或起疱、神經炎、精神失常和腹部疼痛。

porphyrin *n.* one of a number of pigments derived from *porphin, which are widely distributed in living things.

卟啉 從卟吩衍生而來的多種色素中的一種。卟吩廣泛分布於生物之中。所

All porphyrins form chelates with iron, magnesium, zinc, nickel, copper, and cobalt. These chelates are constituents of *haemoglobin, *myoglobin, the *cytochromes, and chlorophyll, and are thus important in many oxidation/reduction reactions in all living organisms. *See also* protoporphyrin IX.

有卟啉都和鐵、錳、鋅、鎳、銅、鈷結合成螯合物。這些螯合物是血紅蛋白、肌紅蛋白、細胞色素和葉綠素的組成成分，因此它們在所有生物的許多氧化與還原反應中起着重要作用。

porphyrinuria *n.* the presence in the urine of breakdown products of the red blood pigment haemoglobin (porphyrins), sometimes causing discoloration. *See* porphyria, porphobilinogen.

卟啉尿 尿中出現紅色的血液色素血紅蛋白的分解產物（卟啉）。有時可使尿變色。

porta *n.* the aperture in an organ through which its associated vessels pass. Such an opening occurs in the liver (*porta hepatis*).

門 在某器官中其有關管道通過的口。如肝門。

portacaval anastomosis (portacaval shunt) 1. a surgical technique in which the hepatic portal vein is joined to the inferior vena cava. Blood draining from the abdominal viscera is thus diverted past the liver. It is used in the treatment of *portal hypertension, since – by lowering the pressure within the veins of the stomach and oesophagus – it prevents serious bleeding into the gastrointestinal tract. **2.** any of the natural communications between the branches of the hepatic portal vein in the liver and the inferior vena cava.

①門腔靜脈〔吻合〕分流術 一種將肝臟門靜脈與下腔靜脈相連接的外科手術。此術可使腹腔內臟回流的血液改道繞過肝臟。該手術用於治療門靜脈高壓，從而降低胃與食管內的靜脈壓，以防止胃腸道嚴重的出血。 **②門腔靜脈分流** 指肝門靜脈支與下腔靜脈之間形成的任何自然通路。

portal *adj.* **1.** relating to the portal vein or system. **2.** relating to a porta.

門的 ①有關門靜脈或門靜脈系統的。②門的。

portal hypertension a state in which the pressure within the hepatic *portal vein is increased, causing enlargement of the spleen, enlargement of veins in the oesophagus (gullet) (which may rupture to cause severe bleeding), and accumulation of fluid in the peritoneal cavity (ascites). The commonest cause is *cirrhosis, but other diseases of the liver or thrombosis of the portal vein will also produce it. Treatment is by *diuretic drugs, but under some circumstances surgery to join the portal vein to the inferior vena cava (bypass-

門靜脈高血壓 肝臟門靜脈血壓增高，引起脾臟腫大、食管靜脈擴張（可發生破裂導致嚴重的出血）和腹腔積液（腹水）。引起門靜脈高血壓最常見的原因是肝硬變，但其他肝臟疾病或門靜脈血栓形成也能引起本病。治療：可使用利尿藥，但在某些情況下需採用肝門靜脈與（繞過肝的）下腔靜脈相吻合的手術。

ing the liver) may be necessary (*see* portacaval anastomosis).

portal system a vein or group of veins that terminates at both ends in a capillary bed. The best known is the *hepatic portal system*, which consists of the *portal vein and its tributaries (see illustration). Blood is drained from the spleen, stomach, pancreas, and small and large intestines into veins that merge to form the portal vein leading to the liver. Here the portal vein branches, ending in many small capillaries called *sinusoids. These permit the passage into the liver cells of nutrients absorbed by blood from the intestines.

門靜脉系統 兩端都與毛細血管相接連的一種靜脉。最典型的是肝門靜脉系統，它由門靜脉及其分支組成（見圖）。脾、胃、胰、小腸和大腸的靜脉血液進入通向肝臟的門靜脉。在此處，門靜脉分支終止於稱爲竇狀隙的許多小毛細血管。血液從腸中吸收的營養通過竇狀隙進入肝細胞。

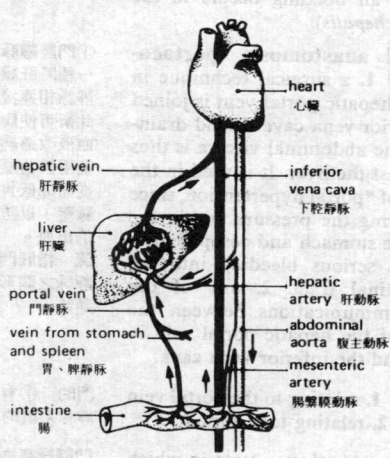

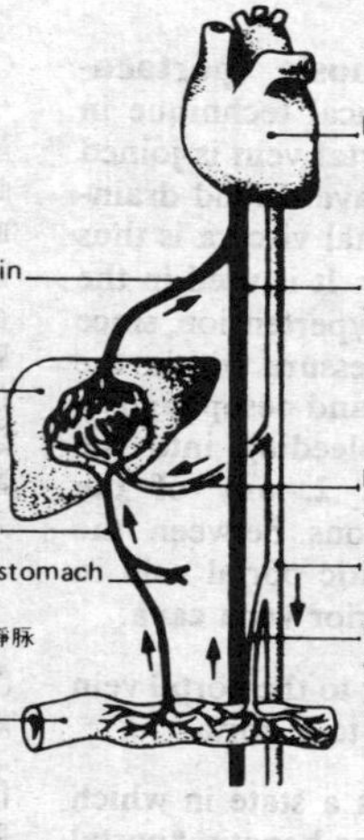

The hepatic portal system
肝門靜脉系統

portal vein a short vein, about 8 cm long, forming part of the hepatic *portal system. It receives many tributaries, including the splenic vein from the spleen and pancreas, the gastric vein from the stomach, the mesenteric vein from the small and large intestines, and the rectal vein from the rectum and anus.

門靜脉 一條長約8cm的短靜脉，爲肝臟門靜脉系統的一個構成部分。它接受許多所屬分支的靜脉血液，包括脾、胰的脾靜脉，來自胃的胃靜脉，來自小腸和大腸的腸繫膜靜脉以及來自直腸和肛門的直腸靜脉。

positron emission tomography (PET) a technique used to evaluate activity of brain tissues by measuring the emission of radioactive particles from molecules of radiation-labelled 2-deoxyglucose. This substance is accepted by brain cells in much the same way as glucose, but it is metabolized very slowly after uptake by functioning neurones. Metabolic activity is reduced in damaged brain tissues and radioactive emissions from these areas is absent or reduced considerably if scanned by tomography equipment designed to detect radiation. The 2-deoxyglucose, usually tagged with radioactive oxygen, is injected into the patient to be examined. PET examinations are employed in the diagnosis and treatment of patients suffering from cerebral palsy and similar types of brain damage. *See also* tomography. *Compare* computerized axial tomography (CAT).

正電子發射計算體層攝影術(PET) 通過測量放射性示蹤分子2-脫氧葡萄糖中放射性粒子的放射性來估價腦組織功能的技術。2-脫氧葡萄糖和葡萄糖同樣，均可被腦細胞吸收。但前者被功能性神經元吸收後，代謝非常緩慢。該物質在受損傷的腦組織中代謝功能減弱，如這時使用為測量放射物質而設計的體層照相掃描時，可看到這些區域的放射物質缺乏或大大減少。2-脫氧葡萄糖通常用放射性氧作示蹤標記，注射入病人體內以備檢查。正電子發射計算體層攝影術用於診斷和治療大腦性麻痹和其他類似的腦損傷患者。

posology *n.* the science of the dosage of medicines.

劑量學 研究藥物劑量的科學。

Possum *n.* a device that enables severely paralysed patients to use typewriters, adding machines, telephones, and a wide variety of other machines. Modern Possums are operated by micro-switches that require only the slightest movement in any limb. The original device worked by blowing and sucking a mouthpiece. The name derives from *Patient-Operated Selector Mechanism* (*POSM*).

殘人用多功能操作器 一種幫助嚴重癱瘓的病人使用打字機、加法器、電話機及其他多種機器的裝置。現代殘人用多功能操作器裝有微型旋鈕，只要任何一個肢體（手或脚）的輕微運動就能操作。最初這種裝置是通過對口罩的吹吸來操作的。"Possum" 一詞是從 "Patient-Operated Selector Mechanism" 的字頭(POSM)縮寫而成。

post- *prefix denoting* **1.** following; after. Example: *postepileptic* (after an epileptic attack). **2.** (in anatomy) behind. Example: *postoral* (behind the mouth).

〔前綴〕 ①**後的** 例如癲癇發作後的。 ②（解剖學）**後方的** 例如口後的。

postcentral *adj.* **1.** situated behind any centre. **2.** situated behind the central fissure of the brain.

中央後的，中樞後的 ①位於任何中央後的。②位於大腦中央溝後的。

postcibal *adj.* occurring after eating.

食後的

posterior *adj.* situated at or near the back of the body or an organ.

後的，後面的 位於或靠近身體或某器官之後的。

postero- *prefix denoting* posterior. Example: *posterolateral* (behind and at the side of).

〔前綴〕 **後部，在後** 指後面的。例如後外側的。

posteroanterior *adj.* from the back to the front. In radiology it denotes a view in the *coronal plane.

後前〔位〕的 從後到前。在放射學中指冠狀平面的視像。

postganglionic *adj.* describing a neurone in a nerve pathway that starts at a ganglion and ends at the muscle or gland that it supplies. In the sympathetic nervous system, postganglionic fibres are *adrenergic, unlike those in the parasympathetic system, which are *cholinergic. *Compare* preganglionic.

〔神經〕節後的 描述某神經徑路中起於神經節止於它所支配的肌肉或腺體的神經元。在交感神經系統中，節後纖維是腎上腺素能神經，副交感神經系統則全屬於膽鹼能神經。

posthetomy *n.* an obsolete term for *circumcision.

包皮環切除術 該詞現已廢用。

posthitis *n.* inflammation of the foreskin. This usually occurs in association with inflammation of the glans penis (*balanitis*; *see* balanoposthitis). Pain, redness, and swelling of the foreskin occurs due to bacterial infection. Treatment is by antibiotic administration, and subsequent *circumcision prevents further attacks.

包皮炎 包皮發生的炎症。通常與龜頭炎併發。該病是由於細菌感染引起，常出現包皮疼痛、紅腫。治療：使用抗生素消炎，癒後採用包皮環切術以防止再發。

posthumous birth 1. delivery of a child by *Caesarean section after the mother's death. **2.** birth of a child after the father's death.

死後生產 ①母親死後，採用剖腹產手術取出嬰兒。 ②父親死後分娩出的嬰兒。

post mortem Latin: after death. *See* autopsy.

死後

postoperative *adj.* following operation: referring to the condition of a patient or to the treatment given at this time.

手術後的 做了手術以後的。指病人的手術後情況或術後這段時間所接受的治療。

postpartum *adj.* relating to the period of a few days immediately after birth.

產後的 有關產後數日內的。

postprandial *adj.* occurring after eating.

食後的 食後發生的。

postural muscles (antigravity muscles) muscles (principally exten-

姿勢肌（抗引力肌） 對抗地心引力，以維持身體

sors) that serve to maintain the upright posture of the body against the force of gravity.

直立姿勢的肌肉（主要指伸肌）。

potassium chloride a salt of potassium used to prevent and treat potassium deficiency, especially during treatment with certain diuretics. It is administered by mouth or injection; some irritation in the digestive system may occur after oral administration. Trade names: **Kalium**, **Kay-Cee-L**, **K-Contin**, **Slow-K**.

氯化鉀 預防和治療鉀缺乏的一種鉀鹽。主要在用某些利尿劑治療時使用。口服或注射。口服後可能對消化系統有某些刺激作用。

potassium hydroxyquinoline a salt of potassium that has antifungal, antibacterial, and deodorant activities. It is applied to the skin in creams or lotions to treat skin infections and occasionally causes skin irritation.

羥喹啉鉀 一種能够抗黴菌、抗細菌和具有除臭作用的鉀鹽。用法：將乳劑或洗液搽於皮膚上，以治療皮膚的感染。偶爾對皮膚可產生刺激作用。

potassium perchlorate a salt of potassium that is used to treat overactivity of the thyroid gland (thyrotoxicosis). It is administered by mouth; side-effects may include digestive upsets and rashes. Trade name: **Peroidin**.

高氯酸鉀 一種治療甲狀腺功能亢進（甲狀腺毒症）的鉀鹽。口服。副作用可有消化不良和皮疹。

potassium permanganate a salt of potassium used for disinfecting and cleansing wounds and as a general skin *antiseptic. It irritates mucous membranes and is poisonous if taken into the body.

高錳酸鉀 一種用作一般皮膚消毒劑的鉀鹽。用於消毒和清洗傷口。該藥有刺激黏膜的作用，如進入體內可引起中毒。

Pott's disease *tuberculosis of the backbone, usually transmitted by infected cows' milk. Untreated, it can lead to a hunchback deformity.

波特氏病，脊柱骨疽 經常由受到感染的乳牛的牛奶傳染的一種脊椎結核。如不治療，能引起駝背。

pouch *n.* (in anatomy) a small sac-like structure, especially occurring as an outgrowth of a larger structure.

囊 在解剖學中指一種小的袋狀結構，特別是在較大的結構上生長的囊。

poultice (fomentation) *n.* a preparation of hot moist material applied to any part of the body to increase local circulation, alleviate pain, or soften the skin to allow matter to be expressed from a boil. Poultices containing kaolin retain heat for a considerable period during use.

泥罨劑，泥敷劑 一種由熱的濕潤的材料配製的敷劑。該敷劑可塗抹於身體任何部位，以促進局部血循環、減輕疼痛或軟化皮膚使膿腫（癤）中的膿液易於擠出。爲了使得熱敷有效期延長，泥罨劑含有保溫的高嶺土。

Poupart's ligament *see* inguinal ligament.

普帕爾氏韌帶

powder *n.* (in pharmacy) a medicinal preparation consisting of a mixture of two or more drugs in the form of fine particles.

散劑，粉劑 （藥劑學用語）一種由兩種或數種藥物混合配成的細小顆粒狀的藥物製劑。

pox *n.* **1.** an infectious disease causing a skin rash. **2.** a rash of pimples that become pus-filled, as in *chickenpox and *smallpox.

痘 ①引起皮疹的傳染病。 ②一種充滿膿液的小膿疱疹，例如水痘和天花。

poxvirus *n.* one of a group of large DNA-containing viruses including those that cause *smallpox (variola) and *cowpox (vaccinia) in man, and pox and tumours in animals.

痘病毒 一組大型脫氧核糖核酸病毒，包括引起人體天花和牛痘的病毒和引起動物痘瘡和腫瘤的病毒。

PPLO *see* mycoplasma.

類胸膜肺炎微生物

practolol *n.* a drug administered by mouth or injection to control abnormal heart rhythm (*see* beta blocker). It has the side-effects of *propranolol and, in addition, more serious side-effects, particularly affecting the eyes and skin, which led to its withdrawal in 1975. Trade name: **Eraldin**.

醋氨心安 一種用於控制異常心律的口服或注射藥物。該藥可有萘心安的副作用和其他更爲嚴重的副作用，還有影響眼睛和皮膚的副作用，因此，於1975年該藥已禁止使用。

pre- *prefix denoting* **1.** before; preceding. Example: *premenstrual* (before menstruation); *prenatal* (before birth). **2.** (in anatomy) in front of; anterior to. Example: *precardiac* (in front of the heart); *prepatellar* (in front of the patella).

〔前綴〕 ①**前** 例如月經前，產前。 ②（解剖學）**前方的** 例如心前區的，髕前的。

pre-agonal *adj.* relating to the phenomena that precede the moment of death. *See also* agonal.

瀕死的 有關死前的現象（症狀和體徵）。

precancerous *adj.* describing a growth that is not yet malignant but that is known to become so if left untreated. *Leukoplakia of the vulva is known to be a precancerous condition. *See also* metaplasia.

癌前期的 指一種雖然不是惡性的，但是如不治療，可以變爲惡性的疾病。已知外陰白斑病就是一種癌前期的疾病。

precipitin *n.* any antibody that combines with its antigen to form a complex that comes out of solution and is seen as a precipitate. The antibody-antigen reaction is specific; the precipitin reaction

沉澱素 由任何抗體與其抗原結合而構成的一種複合物。這種物質在溶液中呈沉澱物析出。抗體-抗原反應是特異性的，因

is therefore a useful means of confirming the identity of an unknown antigen or establishing that a serum contains antibodies to a known disease. This test may be performed in watery solution or in a semisolid medium such as agar gel. *See also* agglutination.

此，沉澱反應對鑑定某種未知抗體方面是一種有效的方法。該試驗可以在水溶液中或在半固體培養基（如瓊脂凝膠）中進行。

precipitinogen *n.* any antigen that is precipitated from solution by a *precipitin.

沉澱原，沉澱素原 使用沉澱素從溶液中沉澱出來的任何抗原。

precision attachment (in dentistry) a special machined joint that holds certain types of partial *dentures in place. The attachment is in two parts, one fixed to the denture and the other fixed to a crown on one of the teeth abutting the denture.

精確附着，槽溝附着 （牙科學）把某種類型的部分托牙固定在適當的位置上的一種經特殊加工的接合體。該接合體一部分固定在托牙上，另一部分固定在橋基牙的牙冠上。

precocity *n.* an acceleration of normal development. The intellectually precocious child has a high IQ and may become isolated from his contemporaries or frustrated at school. Mental illness is less common than in those who develop normally. —**precocious** *adj.*

早熟 一種超正常的發育。智力早熟的兒童智商高，可能和他（她）的同齡人不合羣或在學校受到冷遇。早熟兒童患精神病者比發育正常兒童少見。

precordium *n.* the region of the thorax immediately over the heart. —**precordial** *adj.*

心前區 胸部體表與心臟相應的部位。

precuneus *n.* an area of the inner surface of the cerebral hemisphere on each side, above and in front of the *corpus callosum. *See* cerebrum.

楔前葉 位於每側大腦半球內表面的，胼胝體上部和前部區域。

predisposition *n.* a tendency to be affected by a particular disease or kind of disease. Such a tendency may be hereditary or may arise because of such factors as lack of vitamins, food, or sleep. *See also* diathesis.

誘因 具有易患某種特殊疾病或某類疾病的傾向。該傾向可以遺傳或者由於因缺乏某維生素、食物或睡眠等因素而產生。

prednisolone *n.* a synthetic *corticosteroid used to treat rheumatic diseases and inflammatory and allergic conditions. It is administered by mouth, injected into joints, or applied in creams, lotions, and ointments (for skin conditions). Side-effects are those of *cortisone. Trade names: **Codelcortone,**

潑尼松龍 一種用於治療風濕性的疾病、炎症和變態反應性疾病的合成皮質類固醇。口服或關節內注射或者製成乳劑、洗劑和軟膏劑外用（適用於皮膚病）。副作用同可的松。

Delta-Cortef, Deltacortril, Deltastab, Precortisyl, Prednesol.

prednisone *n.* a synthetic *corticosteroid used to treat rheumatic diseases, severe allergic conditions, inflammatory conditions, and leukaemia. It is administered by mouth and side-effects are those of *cortisone. Trade names: **Deltacortone, Di-Adreson.**

强的松 用於治療風濕性疾病、嚴重的變態反應疾病、炎症和白血病的一種合成皮質類固醇。口服。副作用同可的松。

pre-eclampsia *n.* a condition that affects women at an advanced stage of pregnancy and is marked by high blood pressure, swelling of the ankles, and the presence of protein in the urine. Pre-eclampsia sometimes develops into a much more serious condition involving convulsions (*see* eclampsia). *See also* toxaemia of pregnancy.

子癇前期 婦女妊娠晚期出現的一種病，其特徵爲血壓升高、踝關節腫脹和蛋白尿。子癇前期有時會發展成更爲嚴重的疾病，如驚厥等。

prefrontal lobe the region of the brain at the very front of each cerebral hemisphere (*see* frontal lobe). The functions of the lobe are concerned with emotions, memory, learning, and social behaviour. Nerve tracts in the lobe are cut during the operation of prefrontal *leucotomy.

額前葉 每側大腦半球最前部位。該葉的功能與情感、記憶、學習能力和社交行爲有關。在做腦白質切斷術時，額前葉神經束便被切斷。

preganglionic *adj.* describing fibres in a nerve pathway that end in a ganglion, where they form synapses with *postganglionic fibres that continue the pathway to the effector organ, muscle or gland.

神經節前的 指在神經徑路中終止於神經節的纖維。它們在該神經節中與繼續通向效應器、肌肉或腺體的神經節後纖維構成突觸。

pregnancy *n.* the period during which a woman carries a developing fetus. Pregnancy lasts for approximately 266 days, from *conception until the baby is born, and the fetus normally develops in the womb (*compare* ectopic pregnancy). During pregnancy menstruation is absent, there may be a great increase in appetite, and the breasts increase in size; the woman may also experience *morning sickness. These and other changes are brought about by a hormone (*progesterone) produced at first by the ovary and later by the *placenta. Definite evidence of preg-

妊娠 婦女懷有正在發育的胎兒的時期。胎兒在子宮中正常發育，從受孕直到嬰兒出生，妊娠期持續爲266天。妊娠期月經停止，食慾可能大增，乳房增大，也可以有晨間噁心。這些變化和其他一些變化均是由於最初從卵巢和後期從胎盤分泌的激素（孕酮）所引起的。通過做各種妊娠試驗和聽到胎兒心音即可確診妊娠。

nancy is provided by various *pregnancy tests and by the detection of the heart beat of the fetus. Medical name: **cyesis**. *See also* pseudocyesis (phantom pregnancy). —**pregnant** *adj.*

pregnancy test any of several methods used to demonstrate whether or not a woman is pregnant. A commonly used laboratory test of early pregnancy is based on detection of a hormone, *chorionic gonadotrophin, in the urine. Mixture of a few drops of urine with a test solution containing an antibody that reacts with the hormone gives an almost immediate result. The test becomes positive within a month of conception and false-positive results are very rare. Alternative tests that require a woman to take hormonal drugs should be avoided if the pregnancy is intended, since there is a risk of damage to the developing embryo.

妊娠試驗 任何一種可用於證明婦女是否懷孕的方法。一種常用於妊娠早期的化驗是以檢查尿中是否有絨毛膜促性腺激素爲依據的。用幾滴尿液與含抗體的試劑相混合，這時試劑中的抗體與尿中的激素（抗原）產生反應。這樣幾乎可以立即得出結果。該試驗在妊娠一個月內就呈陽性反應，而假陽性反應結果極罕見。如果懷孕後有意保胎，孕婦應禁用激素藥物等其他檢驗，因爲這樣對發育中的胚胎有損害。

pregnanediol *n.* a steroid that is formed during the metabolism of the female sex hormone *progesterone. It occurs in the urine during pregnancy and certain phases of the menstrual cycle.

孕烷二醇 一種在女性激素——孕酮的代謝過程中形成的固醇類化合物，見於妊娠期和月經周期某些階段的尿中。

pregnenolone *n.* a steroid synthesized in the adrenal glands, ovaries, and testes. Pregnenolone is an important intermediate product in steroid hormone synthesis and can – depending on the pathways followed – be converted to corticosteroids (glucocorticoids or mineralocorticoids), androgens, or oestrogens.

孕烯醇酮 一種在腎上腺、卵巢和睾丸中合成的固醇類化合物。孕烯醇酮在固醇類化合物激素的合成過程中是一種重要的中間產物。按照不同的途徑，孕烯醇酮能轉化爲皮質激素類（糖皮質激素或鹽皮質激素）、雄激素或雌激素。

premature beat *see* ectopic beat.

過早收縮，期外收縮，額外收縮

premature birth birth of a baby before full term. Since the date of conception is often not precisely known, a premature baby is defined as one weighing less than 2500 g (5½ lb) at birth. If such babies are unable to maintain a normal body temperature

早產 嬰兒於足月以前分娩。由於懷孕日期並不是無法確切知道，所以在生產時凡體重不足2500克（5½磅）的嬰兒均規定爲早產兒。如果這些早產兒自己不能維持正常體

they require special care in an incubator.

溫，就需要把他們放入保溫箱中進行特殊護理。

premature ejaculation emission of semen (and consequent loss of erection) during the initial stages of preparation for sexual intercourse, before insertion into the vagina or immediately afterwards.

射精過早，早泄 在準備性交的開始階段，陰莖還未插入陰道或剛插入就發生遺精（隨之發生陽萎）。

premedication *n.* drugs administered to a patient before an operation (usually one in which an anaesthetic is used). Premedication usually comprises injection of a *sedative, to calm the patient down, together with a drug, such as *atropine, to dry up the secretions of the lungs (which might otherwise be inhaled during anaesthesia).

前驅給藥法，術前用藥法 在手術前給病人用藥（通常用麻醉劑）。術前用藥法通常包括：爲使病人安靜下來的鎮靜注射劑和使病人肺分泌物減少的藥物（如阿托品），後者是爲了避免在麻醉時將分泌物吸入。

premenstrual tension a condition of nervousness, irritability, emotional disturbance, headache, and/or depression affecting some women for up to about ten days before menstruation. The condition is associated with the accumulation of salt and water in the tissues. It usually disappears soon after menstruation begins.

經前期緊張 有些婦女在月經前10天左右就開始出現神經過敏、易怒、情緒障礙、頭痛和/或抑鬱等症狀。該病伴有組織水腫（水鹽瀦留）。一旦月經來潮，以上症狀通常立即消失。

premenstruum *n.* the stage of the *menstrual cycle immediately preceding menstruation.

經前期 在月經周期中緊挨來月經前的一段時間。

premolar *n.* either of the two teeth on each side of each jaw behind the canines and in front of the molars in the adult *dentition.

前磨牙，雙尖牙 在成人牙列中位於尖牙後和磨牙前的雙側頜骨上的兩顆牙齒。

premyelocyte *n. see* promyelocyte.

早幼粒細胞，前髓細胞

prenatal diagnosis (antenatal diagnosis) diagnostic procedures carried out on pregnant women in order to discover genetic or other abnormalities in the developing fetus. The investigations involve the use of X-rays, *ultrasound scanning, *thermography, and analysis of amniotic fluid (obtained by *amniocentesis) or of fetal blood (obtained by *fetoscopy). Some of the techniques, including amniocentesis,

產前診斷 爲了發現正在生長發育中的胎兒遺傳方面的以及其他方面的異常情況而對孕婦所進行的檢查。檢查方法包括使用X線檢查、超聲波掃描、體溫記錄法、羊水（通過羊膜穿刺術取得羊水）或胎兒血液（通過胎兒鏡取得胎血）的分析。有些檢查技術，包括羊膜穿刺術，

involve possible risks to the mother and/or fetus and should not be undertaken without good cause. If the results indicate that the child is likely or certain to be born with severe malformation or abnormality, the possibility of abortion is discussed by the doctors involved and the parents.

對母親和/或胎兒可能具有危險性，如沒有充分的理由不要輕易採用。如果檢查結果表明，嬰兒在出生時很可能或肯定有嚴重的畸形或異常，有關醫生和嬰兒父母可商討是否需要墮胎。

prenylamine *n.* a drug that dilates blood vessels (*see* vasodilator). It is administered by mouth to treat angina; side-effects at high doses may include digestive upsets, skin reactions, and drowsiness. Trade name: **Synadrin**.

雙苯丙胺 一種擴張血管藥物。口服用以治療心絞痛。大劑量用藥可引起消化不良、皮膚過敏反應和倦眠等副作用。商品名：心可定。

preoperative *adj.* before operation: referring to the condition of a patient or to treatment, such as sedation, given at this time.

手術前的 做手術以前的。術前這一段時間的病人情况或對病人所作的處理情况。（如讓病人處於鎮靜的狀態）。

preparedness *n.* (in psychology) a quality of some stimuli that makes them much more likely to give rise to a pathological fear. For example, animals or high places are much more likely to become the subject of a *phobia than are plants or clothes. One theory is that individuals are genetically predisposed to *conditioning of fear to objects that have been a biological threat during the evolution of mankind.

恐怖素質 在心理學中指某些刺激所具有的更容易引起病理性恐怖的性質。例如，動物或高處就比植物或衣服更易成爲病理性恐怖的對象。有一種理論認爲：從遺傳學的觀點來看，人對那些在人類進化過程中曾經成爲威脅生命的客體，容易產生恐懼。

prepubertal *adj.* relating to or occurring in the period before puberty.

青春期前的 關於或發生於青春期以前的時期的。

prepuce (foreskin) *n.* the fold of skin that grows over the end (glans) of the penis. On its inner surface modified sebaceous glands (*preputial glands*) secrete a lubricating fluid over the glans. The accumulation of this secretion is known as *smegma. The foreskin is often surgically removed in infancy (*see* circumcision). The fold of skin that surrounds the clitoris is also called the prepuce. —**preputial** *adj.*

包皮 生長並覆蓋於陰莖末端（龜頭）上面的皮褶。在包皮的內表面上有皮脂腺（包皮腺），該皮脂腺（包皮腺）能够分泌一種潤滑液，在龜頭上起潤滑作用。聚集的分泌物稱爲包皮垢。包皮在嬰兒期常採用外科手術切除。陰蒂周圍的皮褶也稱爲包皮。

preputial glands modified sebaceous glands on the inner surface of the *prepuce.

包皮腺 位於包皮內表面的起潤滑作用的皮脂腺。

prepyramidal *adj.* **1.** situated in the middle lobe of the cerebellum, in front of the *pyramid. **2.** describing nerve fibres in tracts that descend from the cerebral cortex to the spinal cord, before the crossing over that occurs at the pyramid of the medulla oblongata.

錐體前的 ①位於錐體前的小腦中葉內的。②指從大腦皮質脊髓的下行束在延髓錐體發生交換（交叉）之前的神經纖維。

presby- (presbyo-) *prefix denoting* old age.

〔前綴〕 **老年**

presbyacusis *n.* the progressive perceptive *deafness that occurs with age.

老年性耳聾 見於老年人的進行性的耳聾。

presbyopia *n.* difficulty in reading at the usual distance (about one foot from the eyes) and in performing other close work, due to the decline with age in the ability of the eye to alter its focus to see close objects clearly. This is caused by gradual loss of elasticity of the lens of the eye which thus becomes progressively less able to increase its curvature in order to focus on near objects.

老視 年老人在看近距離物體時調節眼焦距的能力減弱，因此在通常的距離（離眼睛一英尺左右）閱讀和從事其他近距離工作有困難。這是由於眼球晶狀體的彈性逐漸消失所致。因此，為了聚焦於近距離物體時，要增加晶狀體的曲度，就變得越來越困難。

prescribed disease one of a number of illnesses (currently 48) arising as a result of employment requiring close contact with a hazardous substance or circumstance. Examples include poisoning by such chemicals as mercury or benzene, decompression sickness in divers, and infections such as *anthrax in those handling wool. Some diseases that occur widely in the population may be prescribed in relation to a specific occupation (e.g. deafness in those working with pneumatic drills or tuberculosis in mortuary attendants).

法定性職業病 由於在所從事的職業中不得不（需要）與有害物質或環境密切接觸而引起的一類疾病（現有48種）。如汞、苯等化學物質的中毒、潛水員的減壓病、接觸（加工）羊毛的工人感染的炭疽病等。有些在人羣中廣泛發生的疾病已被認定與某些特殊的職業有關（例如，使用氣鑽的工人所患耳聾病或停屍室工作人員的結核病等）。

prescription *n.* a written direction from a registered medical practitioner to a pharmacist for preparing and dispensing a drug.

處方，藥方 醫師給藥劑師開的關於配製藥物與發藥的書面指示。

presenility *n.* premature ageing of the mind and body, so that a person shows the reduction in mental and physical abilities normally found only in old age. *See also* dementia, progeria. —**presenile** *adj.*

早老 身心早衰。一個人出現的通常只在老年人中才見到的心理和生理功能的減退。

presentation *n.* the part of the infant's body that appears first at the opening from the neck of the womb during childbirth, as perceived on inserting the finger into the vagina. Normally the head appears first (*cephalic presentation*). However, the infant's buttocks (*see* breech presentation), its side (*transverse presentation*), its feet, or the placenta (*see* placenta praevia) may be the first parts to appear. These and other abnormal presentations may cause complications during childbirth, and an attempt may be made to correct them (*see* cephalic version).

先露 在分娩時用手指插入陰道檢查，在宮頸口觸到的最先露出的嬰兒身體部分。正常應該是嬰兒的頭先露出。但是嬰兒的臀部、身體側部（橫位）、脚部或胎盤都可能是先露出的部分。在分娩時，這些不正常的先露均可以導至難產，可採取措施糾正。

pressor *n.* an agent that raises blood pressure. *See* vasoconstrictor.

升壓藥 升高血壓的藥物。

pressure point a point at which an artery lies over a bone on which it may be compressed by finger pressure, to arrest haemorrhage beyond. For example, the femoral artery may be compressed against the pelvic bone in the groin.

壓迫點 動脉跨越骨上的某一點。在該處用手指壓迫動脉，可以阻止遠側的出血。例如：可在腹股溝處將股動脉壓向骨盆。

pressure sore *see* bedsore.

褥瘡

presymptomatic *adj.* describing or relating to a symptom that occurs before the typical symptoms of a disease. *See also* prodromal.

症狀發生前的 指發生在疾病典型症狀之前的。

presystole *n.* the period in the cardiac cycle just preceding systole.

收縮前期 心動周期中在剛開始收縮之前的時期。

prevalence rate a measure of morbidity based on current sickness in a population, estimated either at a particular time (*point prevalence*) or over a stated period (*period prevalence*). It can be expressed either in terms of sick people (persons) or episodes of sickness per 1000 individuals at risk. *Compare* incidence rate.

現患率 測定某特定時刻（時點患病率）或某段時間（時期患病率）內人羣中的現有疾病的患病率。現患率可以每1000受威脅者中的病人數或發病次數表示。

preventive dentistry the branch of dentistry concerned with the prevention of dental disease. It includes dietary

預防牙醫學 牙醫學中關於牙病預防的分支學科。包括飲食諮詢、口腔衛生

counselling, advice on oral hygiene, and the application of *fluoride and *fissure sealants to the teeth.

指導、氟化物和牙裂隙充填劑的應用。

preventive medicine the branch of medicine whose main aim is the prevention of disease. This is a wide field, in which workers tackle problems ranging from the immunization of persons against infectious diseases, such as diphtheria or whooping-cough, to finding methods of eliminating *vectors, such as malaria-carrying mosquitoes.

預防醫學 以預防疾病爲基本目的的醫學分支學科。這是一個廣泛的領域，從抗白喉、百日咳之類傳染病的人體免疫接種到尋找消滅病媒（如攜帶瘧原蟲的蚊子）的方法，都包括在內。

priapism *n.* persistent erection of the penis. It is commonly due to a blood clot in the erectile tissue of the penis and is most often encountered in patients with kidney failure undergoing intermittent *dialysis. Treatment is by early surgical removal of the blood clot and the construction of a venous shunt to permit blood flow from the penis.

陰莖異常勃起 指陰莖持續勃起狀態。一般系由陰莖勃起組織中的血凝塊引起，最常見於因腎衰竭而做周期性透析的患者。治療：及早外科摘除血凝塊，建立靜脈分流以幫助血液回流。

prickle cells cells with cytoplasmic processes that form intercellular bridges. The germinative layer of the *epidermis is sometimes called the prickle cell layer.

棘細胞 以胞漿突起形成細胞間橋的細胞。表皮生發層有時稱爲棘細胞層。

prickly heat (heat rash) an itchy rash of small raised red spots. It occurs usually on the face, neck, back, chest, and thighs. Infants and obese people are susceptible to prickly heat, which is most common in hot moist weather. Medical name: **miliaria**.

汗疹 一種隆起的小紅點狀癢疹。常發生於顏面、頸項、背、胸和大腿皮膚。嬰兒和肥胖者易生汗疹，汗疹最多見於濕熱氣候。

prilocaine *n.* a local *anaesthetic used particularly in ear, nose, and throat surgery and in dentistry. It is applied in a solution to mucous membranes or injected. High doses may cause methaemoglobinaemia and cyanosis. Trade name: **Citanest**.

丙胺卡因 一種局部麻醉藥，主要用於耳鼻喉科手術和牙科。其溶液用於黏膜或注射。大劑量可引起正鐵血紅蛋白血症和紫紺。

primaquine *n.* a drug used to treat malaria. It is administered by mouth, usually in combination with other antimalarial drugs, such as *chloroquine.

伯氨喹 一種抗瘧藥物。口服。通常與其它抗瘧藥（如氯喹）合用。大劑量可引起血液病變（如

High doses may cause blood disorders (such as methaemoglobinaemia or haemolytic anaemia) and digestive upsets. Trade name: **Mysoline**.

正鐵血紅蛋白血症或溶血性貧血）和胃腸紊亂。

primary medical care *see* general practitioner.

初級衛生保健

prime *vb.* (in chemotherapy) to administer small doses of *cyclophosphamide prior to high-dose chemotherapy and/or radiotherapy. This causes proliferation of the primitive bone marrow cells and aids subsequent regeneration of the bone marrow.

基礎投藥 （化學治療）在大劑量化學治療和/或放射治療前給予小劑量環磷醯胺，以引起原始骨髓細胞增殖，促進隨後的骨髓再生。

prime mover *see* agonist.

主動肌

primidone *n.* an *anticonvulsant drug used to treat major (grand mal) epilepsy. It is administered by mouth; common side-effects, which are usually transient, include drowsiness, muscle incoordination, digestive upsets, vertigo, and sight disturbances. Trade name: **Mysoline**.

撲癇酮 一種治療癲癇大發作的抗驚厥藥。口服。常見副作用多爲短暫性，有睏倦、共濟失調、胃腸紊亂、眩暈和輕度視覺障礙等。

primigravida (unigravida) *n.* a woman experiencing her first pregnancy.

初孕婦 初次妊娠的婦女。

primipara (unipara) *n.* a woman who has given birth to one infant capable of survival.

初產婦 初娩過一個活嬰的婦女。

primitive streak the region of the embryo that proliferates rapidly, producing mesoderm cells that spread outwards between the layers of ectoderm and endoderm.

原條 胚的一部分。該部迅速增殖，產生中胚層細胞，在內胚層和外胚層之間向外擴展。

primordial *adj.* (in embryology) describing cells or tissues that are formed in the early stages of embryonic development.

原始的 （胚胎學）指胚發育早期形成的細胞和組織。

pro- *prefix denoting* **1.** before; preceding. **2.** a precursor. **3.** in front of.

〔前綴〕 ①前 ②**前體** ③**在前面**

probability *n. see* significance.

概率，機率

proband *n. see* propositus.

先證者

probang *n.* a long flexible rod with a small sponge, ball, or tuft at the end,

食管-氣管內除鯁器 爲一可彎曲的長桿，末端裝

used to remove obstructions from the larynx or oesophagus (gullet). A probang is also used to apply medication to these structures.

有海綿、球頭或馬鬃、用於解除喉或食管阻塞。還可用以對上述部位進行藥物治療。

probe *n.* a thin rod of pliable metal, such as silver, with a blunt swollen end. The instrument is used for exploring cavities, wounds, *fistulas, or sinus channels.

探針 一種用柔韌金屬（如銀）製成的末端鈍圓的細桿。用於探測腔洞、創口、瘻管或竇道。

probenecid *n.* a drug that reduces the level of uric acid in the blood (*see* uricosuric drug) and is used chiefly in the treatment of gout. It is administered by mouth; mild side-effects, such as digestive upsets, dizziness, and skin rashes, may occur. Trade name: **Benemid**.

羧苯磺胺 降低血中尿酸的藥物。主要用於治療痛風。口服。可有輕度副作用，如胃腸紊亂、頭暈、皮疹。

procainamide *n.* a drug that slows down the activity of the heart and is used to control abnormal heart rhythm. It is administered by mouth or injection; side-effects may include digestive upsets, dizziness, and allergic reactions. Trade name: **Pronestyl**.

普魯卡因醯胺 降低心率的藥物。用於控制心律異常。口服或注射。副作用有：胃腸紊亂、頭暈、皮疹。

procaine *n.* a local *anaesthetic administered by injection for *spinal anaesthesia. It was formerly used in dentistry. Side-effects are uncommon, but allergic reactions may occur. Trade name: **Novutex**.

普魯卡因 局部麻醉藥。注射，用於脊髓麻醉。過去一度用於牙科。副作用少見，可有變應性反應。

procaine penicillin an *antibiotic, consisting of penicillin and procaine, used to treat infections caused by organisms sensitive to penicillin. It is injected into muscle so that the penicillin is released slowly and remains effective for some time. Trade names: **Bicillin, Depocillin**.

普魯卡因青黴素 由青黴素和普魯卡因組成的抗生素。用於治療對青黴素敏感的細菌感染。肌肉注射，因青黴素釋放緩慢，可使藥效維持一段時間。

procarbazine *n.* a drug that inhibits growth of cancer cells by preventing cell division and is used to treat such cancers as Hodgkin's disease. It is administered by mouth; common side-effects include loss of appetite, nausea, vomiting, diarrhoea, and mouth sores. Trade name: **Natulan**.

甲基苄肼 一種藉阻止細胞分裂而抑制癌細胞生長的藥物。多用於治療何傑金病之類的癌瘤。口服。常見副作用爲食慾不振、噁心、嘔吐、腹瀉、口腔潰瘍。

process *n.* (in anatomy) a thin prominence or protuberance; for example, any of the processes of a vertebra.

突 （解剖學）細小的突起或隆突。例如：所有脊椎骨上的突。

prochlorperazine *n.* a major *tranquillizer used to treat schizophrenia and other mental disorders, migraine, vertigo, nausea, and vomiting. It is administered by mouth, injection, or in suppositories; side-effects include drowsiness and dry mouth, and high doses may cause tremors and abnormal muscle movements. Trade name: **Stemetil**.

甲哌氯丙嗪 一種重要的安定藥。用於治療精神分裂症和其它精神障礙、偏頭痛、眩暈、噁心、嘔吐。口服、注射或製成栓劑。副作用：睏倦、口乾，大劑量可引起震顫和異常肌肉活動。

procidentia *n.* the complete downward displacement (*prolapse) of an organ, especially the womb (*uterine procidentia*), which protrudes from the vaginal opening. Uterine procidentia may result from injury to the floor of the pelvic cavity.

脫垂 器官全部下垂移位狀態。例如：子宮脫垂時子宮可自陰道口突出，膀胱脫垂可由盆腔底部損傷引起。

proct- (procto-) *prefix denoting* the anus and/or rectum.

〔前綴〕 ①肛 ②直腸

proctalgia (proctodynia) *n.* pain in the rectum or anus. In *proctalgia fugax* severe pain suddenly affects the rectum and may last for minutes or hours; attacks may be days or months apart. There is no structural disease and the pain is probably due to muscle spasm. Relief is sometimes obtained from a bowel action, inserting a finger into the rectum, or from a hot bath.

肛痛 直腸或肛部疼痛。患痙攣性肛痛時直腸突發劇烈疼痛，持續幾分鐘至幾小時；兩次發作可間隔幾天至幾個月。不能查出器質性病變，疼痛可能出自肌痙攣。排便、用指插入肛門，或者行熱水坐浴，有時可解除疼痛。

proctatresia *n. see* imperforate anus.

肛門閉鎖

proctectasia *n.* enlargement or widening of the rectum, usually due to long-standing constipation (*see* dyschezia).

直腸擴張 直腸擴大或增粗，多為長時間便秘所致。

proctectomy *n.* surgical removal of the rectum. It is usually performed for cancer of the rectum and requires the construction of a permanent opening in the colon (*see* colostomy).

直腸切除術 外科手術切除直腸。通常於直腸癌時施行，同時須於結腸建立一永久性開口。

proctitis *n.* inflammation of the rectum. Symptoms are ineffectual straining to empty the bowels (*tenesmus), diarrhoea, and often bleeding. Proctitis

直腸炎 直腸的炎症。症狀為竭力想解盡大便而總是徒勞（裏急後重），腹瀉，常有便血。直腸炎總

is invariably present in ulcerative *colitis and sometimes in *Crohn's disease, but may occur independently (*idiopathic proctitis*). Rarer causes include damage by irradiation (for example in radiation therapy for cervical cancer) or by *lymphogranuloma venereum.

是與潰瘍性結腸炎伴存有時亦見於節段性回腸炎，但也可獨立存在（特發性直腸炎）。更少見的原因是照射（如用放射線治療子宮頸癌）或性病性淋巴肉芽腫的損害。

proctocele (rectocele) *n.* bulging or pouching of the rectum, usually a forward protrusion of the rectum into the vagina in association with prolapse of the womb.

直腸突出 直腸膨出或鼓凸。通常是向前突入陰道，與子宮脫垂併存。

proctoclysis *n.* an infusion of fluid into the rectum: formerly used to replace fluid but rarely employed now.

直腸滴注法 向直腸內注入液體。過去用於置換體液，現罕用。

proctocolectomy *n.* a surgical operation in which the rectum and colon are removed. In *panproctocolectomy* the whole rectum and colon are removed, necessitating a permanent opening of the ileum (*see* ileostomy). This is usually performed for ulcerative *colitis.

直腸結腸切除術 切除直腸和結腸的外科手術。全直腸結腸切除術是將直腸和結腸全部切除，同時須做廻腸永久開口。此術常於潰瘍性結腸炎時施行。

proctocolitis *n.* inflammation of the rectum and colon, usually due to ulcerative *colitis. *See also* proctitis.

直腸結腸炎 通常由潰瘍性結腸炎所致的直腸和結腸炎症。

proctodeum *n.* the site of the embryonic anus, marked by a depression lined with ectoderm. The membrane separating it from the hindgut breaks down in the third month of gestation. *Compare* stomodeum.

肛道 胚胎期肛門的部位，爲一襯被外胚層的凹窩。將肛道與後腸隔開的膜於妊娠第三個月消失。

proctodynia *n. see* proctalgia.

肛部痛

proctology *n.* the study of disorders of the rectum and anus.

肛腸病學 研究有關直腸和肛門疾病的學科。

proctorrhaphy *n.* a surgical operation to stitch tears of the rectum or anus.

直腸縫合術 縫合直腸或肛門撕裂的外科手術。

proctoscope *n.* an illuminated instrument through which the lower part of the rectum and the anus may be inspected and minor procedures (such as injection therapy for haemorrhoids) carried out. —**proctoscopy** *n.*

直腸鏡 一種用於檢查直腸下部和肛門並可進行簡單操作（如注射藥物治療痔瘡）的帶照明裝置的器械。

proctosigmoiditis *n.* inflammation of the rectum and the sigmoid (lower) colon. *See also* proctocolitis.

直腸乙狀結腸炎 直腸和乙狀結腸（下段結腸）的炎症。

proctotomy *n.* incision into the rectum or anus to relieve *stricture (narrowing) of these canals or to open an imperforate (closed) anus.

直腸切開術 切開直腸或肛門以解除縮窄或者爲肛門閉鎖開口的手術。

procyclidine *n.* a drug, similar in its effects to *atropine, used to reduce muscle tremor and rigidity in parkinsonism. It is administered by mouth or injection; common side-effects include dry mouth, blurred vision, and giddiness. Trade name: **Kemadrin**.

普環啶 一種作用類似阿托品的藥物。用以減輕震顫性麻痹的肌震顫和肌强直。口服或注射。常見副作用爲口乾、視物模糊、眩暈。

prodromal *adj.* relating to the period of time between the appearance of the first symptoms of an infectious disease and the development of a rash or fever. A *prodromal rash* is one preceding the full rash of an infectious disease.

前驅期的 指急性傳染病時從初始症狀出現到出現皮疹或發熱之間那段時間。前驅疹是指傳染病在出現典型皮疹之前出現的疹子。

prodrome *n.* a symptom indicating the onset of a disease.

前驅症狀 疾病初起時的症狀。

proenzyme (zymogen) *n.* the inactive form in which certain enzymes (e.g. digestive enzymes) are originally produced and secreted. The existence of this inactive form prevents the enzyme from breaking down the cells in which it was made. Once the proenzyme has been secreted it is converted to the active form.

前酶（酶原） 某些酶（如消化酶）在剛產生和分泌時的無活性型。這種型的存在使酶不致將製造它的細胞分解破壞。前酶一旦泌出，便轉變爲活性型。

proerythroblast *n.* the earliest recognizable precursor of the red blood cell (erythrocyte). It is found in the bone marrow and has a large nucleus and a cytoplasm that stains deep blue with *Romanowsky stains. *See also* erythroblast, erythropoiesis.

原成紅細胞 紅細胞的最早可辨認的祖細胞。可在骨髓內見到，有一巨大的核，胞漿爲羅曼諾夫斯基染色法染成深藍色。

profunda *adj.* describing blood vessels that are deeply embedded in the tissues they supply.

深的 指深埋於所供應組織內的血管。

progeria *n.* a very rare condition in which all the signs of old age appear and progress in a child, so that 'senility' is reached before puberty.

早老，早衰 一種罕見的狀況：早在兒童期即出現全部老年期徵象，並迅速發展，以致未到青春期即已老態龍鍾。

progesterone *n.* a steroid hormone secreted by the *corpus luteum of the ovary, the placenta, and also (in small amounts) by the adrenal cortex and testes. It is responsible for preparing the inner lining (endometrium) of the womb for pregnancy. If fertilization occurs it maintains the womb throughout pregnancy and prevents the further release of eggs from the ovary. *See also* menstrual cycle.

孕酮 由卵巢黃體、胎盤以及少量由腎上腺皮質和睾丸分泌的一種固醇類激素。功能爲使子宮內膜適應妊娠的需要。一旦受精成功，孕酮在整個妊娠期維持子宮的妊娠狀態並防止卵巢再次排卵。

progestogen *n.* one of a group of naturally occurring or synthetic steroid hormones, including *progesterone, that maintain the normal course of pregnancy. Progestogens are used to treat threatened or habitual abortion, premenstrual tension, *amenorrhoea, and abnormal bleeding from the womb. Because they prevent ovulation, progestogens are a major constituent of *oral contraceptives. Synthetic progestogens may be taken by mouth but the naturally occurring hormone must be given by intramuscular injection.

孕激素 一類天然生成或人工合成的固醇類激素，其中包括維持正常妊娠進程的孕酮。多用於治療先兆流產、習慣性流產、月經前緊張症狀、月經失調子宮異常出血。因有抑制排卵作用，成爲口服避孕藥的主要成分。合成孕激素可口服，天然生成者只能肌肉注射。

proglottis *n.* (*pl.* **proglottids** or **proglottides**) one of the segments of a *tapeworm. Mature segments, situated at the posterior end of the worm, each consist mainly of a branched uterus packed with eggs.

節片 絛蟲的一個體節。成熟的節片位於絛蟲後端，每個節片主要由含卵的分支狀子宮組成。

prognathism *n.* the state of one jaw being markedly larger than the other and therefore in front of it. —**prognathic** *adj.*

凸頜 一頜明顯大於另一頜而呈向前方突出的狀態。

prognosis *n.* an assessment of the future course and outcome of a patient's disease, based on knowledge of the course of the disease in other patients together with the general health, age, and sex of the patient.

預後 對病人所患疾病的未來發展過程和結局的估計。預後是依據他人患該病的過程的知識結合現病人的一般狀況、年齡、性別等而做出的。

proguanil *n.* a drug that kills malaria parasites and is used in the prevention and treatment of malaria. It is administered by mouth and rarely causes side-effects. Trade name: **Paludrine**.

氯胍 殺瘧原蟲藥。用於預防和治療瘧疾。口服，偶有副作用。

proinsulin *n.* a substance produced in the pancreas from which the hormone *insulin is derived.

前胰島素 在胰腺內生成的胰島素前體物質。

projection *n.* (in psychology) the attribution of one's own qualities to other people. In psychoanalytic psychology this is one of the *defence mechanisms; people who cannot tolerate their own feelings (e.g. anger) may cope by imagining that other people have those feelings (e.g. are persecuting).

投射 （心理學）將自己的品質推諉於他人。在精神分析心理學中這是一種防御機制：有的人對於自己的情感（如憤怒）不願承認，却老是想象別人具有這種情感（如正在迫害他）。

projective test a way of measuring aspects of personality, in which the subject is asked to talk freely about ambiguous objects. His responses are then analysed. Examples are the *Rorschach test and the Thematic Apperception Test (in which the subject invents stories about a set of pictures).

投射試驗 一種測試性格諸方面的方法。要求受試者對相互矛盾的事物自由發表意見，然後對他的表現進行分析。屬於這類試驗的有墨迹試驗和主題統覺試驗（令受試者對一組圖畫虛構故事）。

prolactin (lactogenic hormone, luteotrophic hormone, luteotrophin) *n.* a hormone, synthesized and stored in the anterior pituitary gland, that stimulates milk production after childbirth and also stimulates production of *progesterone by the *corpus luteum in the ovary. In both sexes excessive secretion of prolactin gives rise to abnormal production of milk (galactorrhoea).

催乳素，生乳素，促黃體激素 一種在垂體前葉內合成和貯存的激素。在分娩後刺激泌乳，並能刺激卵巢黃體產生孕酮。催乳素分泌過多可使女性和男性發生乳汁異常分泌（乳溢）。

prolapse *n.* downward displacement of an organ or a part from its normal position. This may happen if the supporting tissues are weak. The womb (*see* metroptosis) and rectum are most commonly affected by this condition.

脫垂，下垂 器官或其部分從正常位置下垂移位。可發生於支持組織薄弱的情況下。最常受累的是子宮和直腸。

prolapsed intervertebral disc (PID) a 'slipped disc': protrusion of the pulpy inner material of an *intervertebral disc through the fibrous outer coat, causing pressure on adjoining nerve roots, ligaments, etc. The condition often results from sudden twisting or bending of the backbone. Pressure on a nerve root causes *sciatica, and if severe may damage the nerve's function, leading to abnormalities or loss of sensation, muscle weakness, or loss of tendon reflexes.

椎間盤脫出 椎間盤滑出。盤內部的髓樣物質穿過纖維性外膜向前方突出，造成對鄰近的神經根、韌帶的壓迫。常爲脊柱突然彎扭或屈曲的結果。壓迫神經根引起坐骨神經痛，如壓迫嚴重，可使神經功能受損，導至感覺異常或喪失，肌無力或腱反射消失。治療：睡硬床，徹底休息，手法推

Treatment is by complete bed rest on a firm surface, manipulation, *traction, and analgesics; if these fail, the protruding portion of the disc is surgically removed (*see* laminectomy).

拿，牽引，給鎮靜藥。若上述治療無效，則須外科手術切除椎間盤的前突部分。

proline *n.* an *amino acid found in many proteins.

脯氨酸 多種蛋白質中均含有的一種氨基酸。

promazine *n.* a major *tranquillizer used to relieve agitation, confusion, severe pain, anxiety, nausea, and vomiting and in the treatment of alcoholism and drug withdrawal symptoms. It is administered by mouth or injection; common side-effects are drowsiness and dizziness. Trade name: **Sparine.**

丙嗪 一種重要的安定藥。用以消除激動、精神混亂、嚴重疼痛、焦慮、噁心、嘔吐、並可治療酒精中毒和麻醉藥戒斷綜合徵。口服或注射。常見副作用爲困倦和眩暈。

promegakaryocyte *n.* an immature cell, found in the bone marrow, that develops into a *megakaryocyte.

前巨核細胞 在骨髓中見到的一種不成熟細胞。以後分化爲巨核細胞。

promethazine *n.* a powerful *antihistamine drug used to treat allergic conditions and – because of its sedative action – insomnia. It is also used as an *antitussive in cough mixtures. Promethazine is administered by mouth or injection; side-effects include drowsiness, dizziness, and confusion. Trade name: **Phenergan.**

異丙嗪 一種强有力的抗組胺藥。用於治療變應性疾病。因有鎮靜作用，可治失眠。還可作爲止咳合劑中的鎮咳藥。副作用有困倦、眩暈、精神混亂。商品名：非那根。

prominence *n.* (in anatomy) a projection, such as a projection on a bone.

隆凸 （解剖學）凸起。如骨上的隆凸。

promontory *n.* (in anatomy) a projecting part of an organ or other structure.

岬 （解剖學）器官或其他結構的隆凸部分。

prompting *n.* a technique used in *behaviour modification to elicit a response not previously present. The subject is made to engage passively in the required behaviour by instructions or by being physically put through the movements. The behaviour can then be rewarded (*see* reinforcement). This is followed by *fading*, in which the prompting is gradually withdrawn and the reinforcement maintained.

激勵 在行爲矯正中使用的一種技巧。旨在引出原先不存在的反應。藉助於指導或幫助患者做出某種動作，使他被動地發生所要求的行爲。此時可予以獎勵（强化）。接着進行淡化，即漸漸停止激勵，而强化繼續進行。

promyelocyte (premyelocyte) *n.* one of the series of cells that gives rise to the *granulocytes (a type of white blood

早幼粒細胞 發育爲粒細胞（血液白細胞的一個類型）的細胞系列中的一種

cell). It has abundant cytoplasm that, with *Romanowsky stains, appears blue with reddish granules (*compare* myeloblast, myelocyte). Promyelocytes are normally found in the blood-forming tissue of the bone marrow but may appear in the blood in a variety of diseases. *See also* granulopoiesis.

細胞。胞漿豐富，羅曼諾夫斯基染色染爲藍色，胞核呈微紅色。正常見於骨髓造血組織，但許多疾病中可在血液中出現。

pronation *n.* the act of turning the hand so that the palm faces downwards. In this position the bones of the forearm (radius and ulna) are crossed. *Compare* supination.

旋前 使掌面朝下的手的旋轉動作。前臂在旋前時其尺骨和橈骨的位置相互交換。

pronator *n.* any muscle that causes pronation of the forearm and hand; for example, the *pronator teres*, a two-headed muscle arising from the humerus and ulna, close to the elbow, and inserted into the radius.

旋前肌 使前臂和手旋前的肌肉。例如，旋前圓肌以兩個頭起於肱骨和尺骨，緊貼肘彎，止於橈骨。

prone *adj.* **1.** lying with the face downwards. **2.** (of the forearm) in the position in which the palm of the hand faces downwards (*see* pronation). *Compare* supine.

①**俯卧** 面朝下的。②**旋前** 手掌面朝下的位置。

pronephros *n.* the first kidney tissue that develops in the embryo. It is not functional and soon disappears. *Compare* mesonephros, metanephros.

前腎 胚胎期最初發生的腎組織。無功能，且很快消失。

pronucleus *n.* (*pl.* **pronuclei**) the nucleus of either the ovum or spermatozoon after fertilization but before the fusion of nuclear material. The pronuclei are larger than the normal nucleus and have a diffuse appearance.

原核 受精後核物質融合前卵子或精子的核。原核較通常的核大。

propanidid *n.* an *anaesthetic that is injected to give rapid complete anaesthesia for a short period of time, for use in minor surgical operations. Side-effects may include digestive upsets, abnormal muscle movements, and a fall in blood pressure. Trade name: **Epontol**.

普爾安 一種麻醉藥，注射後迅速產生短暫的完全麻醉。用於外科小手術。副作用有胃腸紊亂、肌肉異常動作、血壓下降。

propantheline *n.* a drug that decreases activity of smooth muscle (*see* parasympatholytic) and is used to treat dis-

丙胺太林 降低平滑肌活動的藥物。用於治療消化系統疾病（如胃十二指腸

orders of the digestive system, including stomach and duodenal ulcers, and enuresis (bed wetting). It is administered by mouth or injection; side-effects include dry mouth and blurred vision. Trade name: **Pro-Banthine**.

潰瘍）和遺尿症（尿床）。口服或注射。副作用有口乾和視物模糊。商品名：普魯本辛。

properdin *n.* a group of substances in blood plasma that, in combination with *complement and magnesium ions, is capable of destroying certain bacteria and viruses. The properdin complex occurs naturally, rather than as the result of previous exposure to microorganisms, and its activity is not directed against any particular species. *Compare* antibody.

備解素 血漿內的一組與補體和鎂離子結合後具有破壞某些細菌和病毒的能力的物質。備解素複合物是天然存在的，並非經微生物預先作用後產生，其作用也不針對任何特定微生物。

Proper Officer *see* community physician.

專務幹事

prophase *n.* the first stage of *mitosis and of each division of *meiosis, in which the chromosomes become visible under the microscope. The first prophase of meiosis takes place in five stages (*see* leptotene, zygotene, pachytene, diplotene, diakinesis).

前期 有絲分裂或每次減數分裂的第一階段。該時染色質在顯微鏡下變爲可見。減數分裂的前期分爲5個階段。

prophylactic *n.* an agent that prevents the development of a condition or disease. An example is *glyceryl trinitrate, which is used to prevent attacks of angina.

預防藥 防止疾病或症狀發生的藥物。例如：硝酸甘油用於預防心絞痛發作。

prophylaxis *n.* any means taken to prevent disease, such as immunization against diphtheria or whooping cough, or *fluoridation to prevent dental decay in children. —**prophylactic** *adj.*

預防 預防疾病的一切手段。如預防白喉和百日咳的免疫接種，預防兒童齲齒的氟化法等。

propositus (proband) *n.* the first individual studied in an investigation of several related patients with an inherited or familial disorder.

先證者 在對一些患某遺傳病或家族性疾病的病人進行調查時第一個被研究的病人。

propranolol *n.* a drug (*see* beta blocker) used to treat abnormal heart rhythm, angina, and high blood pressure and also taken to relieve anxiety. It is administered by mouth or injection; common side-effects include digestive

心得安 一種治療心律失常、心絞痛、高血壓和解除焦慮症的藥物。口服或注射。常見副作用爲胃腸紊亂、失眠、倦怠。

upsets, insomnia, and lassitude. Trade name: **Inderal**.

proprietary name (in pharmacy) the trade name of a drug: the name assigned to it by the firm that manufactured it. For example, Mogadon is the proprietary name for nitrazepam.

藥品專利名 （藥劑學）藥物的商品名。由製造廠家命名。例如：莫加酮是硝基安定的藥品專利名稱。

proprioceptor *n.* a specialized sensory nerve ending (*see* receptor) that monitors internal changes in the body brought about by movement and muscular activity. Proprioceptors located in muscles and tendons transmit information that is used to coordinate muscular activity (*see* stretch receptor, tendon organ). *See also* mechanoreceptor.

本體感受器 一種特化的神經末梢，監測由動作和肌活動引起的體內改變。本體感受器位於肌肉和肌腱內，傳送信息以調整肌活動。

proptometer *n. see* exophthalmometer.

突眼計

proptosis *n.* forward displacement of an organ, especially the eye (*see* exophthalmos).

突出 器官（主要是眼球）前突移位。

propylthiouracil *n.* a drug that reduces thyroid activity and is used to treat *thyrotoxicosis and to prepare patients for surgical removal of the thyroid gland. It is administered by mouth; side-effects may include rashes and digestive upsets.

丙基硫尿嘧啶 降低甲狀腺活性的藥物。用於治療甲狀腺中毒症以及行甲狀腺切除術病人的術前準備。口服。副作用有皮疹和胃腸紊亂。

prorennin *n. see* rennin.

前凝乳酶

prosencephalon *n.* the forebrain.

前腦

prosop- (prosopo-) *prefix denoting* the face. Example: *prosopodynia* (pain in).

〔前綴〕 **面** 例如面痛。

prospective study 1. a forward-looking review of a group of individuals in relation to morbidity. **2.** *see* cohort study.

前瞻性研究 ①對一組個體可能患某種疾病的預見性調查。 ②參見隊列研究。

prostaglandin *n.* one of a group of hormone-like substances present in a wide variety of tissues and body fluids (including the womb, brain, lungs, kidney, and semen). Prostaglandins have many actions, one of which is to cause contraction of the womb: for this reason

前列腺素 廣泛存在於組織和體液（子宮、腦、肺、腎和精液）中的一組激素樣物質。具有多種作用，其中的一種作用是引起子宮收縮，因此一直用於助產和引導流產。

they have been used therapeutically to aid labour and induce abortion.

prostatectomy *n.* surgical removal of the prostate gland. The operation is necessary to relieve retention of urine due to enlargement of the prostate or to cure the symptoms of frequency and poor urinary flow due to the same cause. The operation can be performed through the bladder (*transvesical prostatectomy*) or through the surrounding capsule of the prostate (*retropubic prostatectomy*). In the operation of *transurethral prostatectomy* (*transurethral resection*) the obstructing prostate can be removed through the urethra using a *resectoscope.

前列腺切除術 外科切除前列腺。爲解除前列腺增大所致尿豬留、尿頻、尿流不暢等症狀，須做前列腺切除術。手術可經膀胱（經膀胱前列腺切除術）或經前列腺包囊（恥骨後前列腺切除術）進行。引起阻塞的前列腺還可經尿道用前列腺切除鏡切除。

prostate gland a male accessory sex gland that opens into the urethra just below the bladder and vas deferens (see illustration). During ejaculation it secretes an alkaline fluid that forms part of the *semen. The prostate may become enlarged in elderly men. This obstructs the neck of the bladder, impairing urination. The bladder dilates and the increased pressure is transmitted through the ureters to the kidney nephrons, leading to damage and impaired function of the kidneys. Treatment is by *prostatectomy.

前列腺 單個的男性附屬性腺，在膀胱和輸精管下方開口於尿道（見圖）。射精時前列腺分泌鹼性液體，參與精液的組成。老年人可發生前列腺肥大，阻塞膀胱頸部而影響排尿。膀胱擴張，增高的內壓傳到腎臟的腎單位，使腎受損害，導至腎功能障礙。治療：手術切除前列腺。

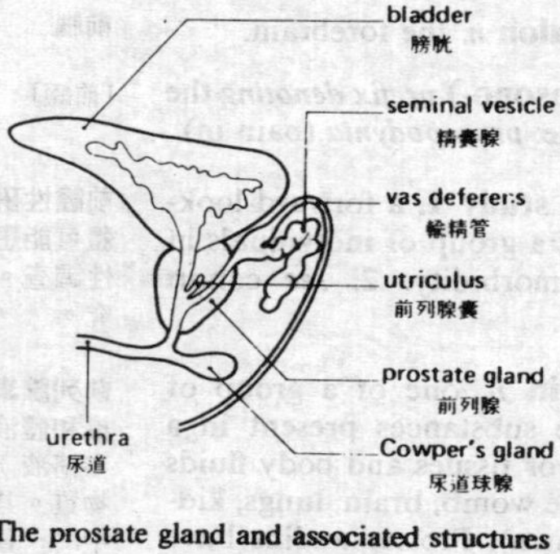

The prostate gland and associated structures (median view)
前列腺及其有關結構（正中斷面觀）

prostatitis *n.* inflammation of the prostate gland. This may be due to bacterial infection and can be either acute or chronic. In acute prostatitis the patient has all the symptoms of a urinary infection, including pain in the perineal area, temperature, and shivering. Treatment is by antibiotic administration. In chronic prostatitis the urinary symptoms are variable; if urinary obstruction develops, transurethral *prostatectomy is indicated.

前列腺炎 前列腺的炎症。可由細菌感染引起，有急性和慢性之分。急性前列腺炎病人具有尿路感染的全部症狀，包括會陰部疼痛、發熱、寒戰。用抗生素治療。慢性前列腺炎有不同的尿路症狀，如發生阻塞，則可行經尿道前列腺切除術。

prostatorrhoea *n.* an abnormal discharge of fluid from the prostate gland. This occurs in some patients with acute *prostatitis, who complain of a profuse discharge from the urethra. The discharge is usually thin and watery and is often sterile on culture. The discharge usually subsides when the underlying prostatitis is controlled.

前列腺液溢 前列腺排液異常。某些急性前列腺炎病人訴說尿道淋漓，排出的液體常呈稀薄水樣，細菌培養常陰性。當其原發前列腺炎得到控制後，排液隨着消失。

prosthesis (*pl.* **prostheses**) *n.* any artificial device that is attached to the body as an aid. Prostheses include dentures, artificial limbs, hearing aids, implanted pacemakers, and many other substitutes for parts of the body that are missing or nonfunctional. —**prosthetic** *adj.*

假體 裝在身體上起輔助作用的人工裝置。假體包括托牙、假肢、助聽器、植入式起搏器，以及其它許多用以替代缺失的或喪失功能的身體部分的置代物。

prosthetic dentistry the branch of dentistry concerned with the provision of dentures.

牙修復學 從事托牙製備的牙科學分支。

protamine *n.* one of a group of simple proteins that can be conjugated with nucleic acids to form nucleoproteins. Protamine can also be combined with *insulin to form *protamine zinc insulin*, which – when injected – is absorbed much more slowly than ordinary insulin and thus reduces the frequency of injections.

精蛋白 一種單純蛋白質，可與核酸結合成核蛋白。精蛋白還可與胰島素結合形成精蛋白鋅胰島素，本品注射後的吸收較普通胰島素慢得多，因而減少了注射次數。

protanopia *n.* a defect in colour vision in which affected persons are insensitive to red light and confuse reds, yellows, and greens. *Compare* deuteranopia, tritanopia.

紅色盲 對紅色光不敏感，不能區別紅、黃、綠色的色覺缺陷。

protease *n. see* proteolytic enzyme.

蛋白酶

protein *n.* one of a group of organic compounds of carbon, hydrogen, oxygen, and nitrogen (sulphur and phosphorus may also be present). The protein molecule is a complex structure made up of one or more chains of *amino acids, which are linked by peptide bonds. Proteins are essential constituents of the body; they form the structural material of muscles, tissues, organs, etc., and are equally important as regulators of function, as enzymes and hormones. Proteins are synthesized in the body from their constituent amino acids, which are obtained from the digestion of protein in the diet. Excess protein, not required by the body, can be converted into glucose and used as an energy source.

蛋白質 一類由碳、氫、氮（還可有硫、磷）組成的有機化合物。蛋白質分子是由一條或多條藉肽鏈連接的氨基酸構成的複雜結構。蛋白質是機體的必需成分，它們形成肌肉、組織、器官等的結構物質，其重要性與功能的調節物——酶和激素等同。蛋白質在體內由其組成成分氨基酸合成，氨基酸則係通過消化食物中的蛋白質獲得。機體不需要的過剩蛋白質轉化爲葡萄糖做爲能源使用。

proteinuria *n.* the presence of protein in the urine. This may indicate the presence of damage to, or disease of, the kidneys. *See also* albuminuria.

蛋白尿 尿中出現蛋白質。表示腎臟損害或腎臟疾病。

proteolysis *n.* the process whereby complex protein molecules, obtained from the diet, are broken down by digestive enzymes in the stomach and small intestine into their constituent amino acids, which are then absorbed into the bloodstream. *See* endopeptidase, exopeptidase. —**proteolytic** *adj.*

蛋白分解 食物中的複雜蛋白質分子在胃和小腸內被消化酶分解爲其組成成分氨基酸的過程。氨基酸被吸收進入血液。

proteolytic enzyme (protease) a digestive enzyme that causes the breakdown of protein. *See* endopeptidase, exopeptidase.

蛋白分解酶（蛋白酶） 分解蛋白質的消化酶。

proteose *n.* a product of the hydrolytic decomposition of protein.

䏡 蛋白的水解產物。

Proteus *n.* a genus of rodlike Gram-negative flagellate highly motile bacteria common in the intestines and in decaying organic material. All species can decompose urea. Some species may cause disease in man: *P. morganii* is associated with acute enteritis in children, and *P. vulgaris* can cause urinary tract infections.

變形桿菌屬 一屬革蘭染色陰性、有鞭毛、活動性强的桿狀菌。通常存在於小腸與腐敗的有機物質中。所有的種均能分解尿素。有些種能引起人體疾病。如摩根變形桿菌與兒童急性小腸炎有關，普通變形桿菌能引起尿路感染。

prothionamide *n.* a drug used in the treatment of tuberculosis. It is administered by mouth, usually together with other antituberculosis drugs; side-effects may include loss of appetite and digestive upsets. Trade name: **Trevintix**.

丙硫異煙胺 一種治療結核病的藥物。口服。通常與其它抗結核藥同用。副作用有食慾喪失和胃腸紊亂。

prothipendyl *n.* a *tranquillizer and *sedative drug used to relieve anxiety, agitation, restlessness, and excitement, to induce sleep, and to prevent nausea and vomiting. It is administered by mouth or injection; common side-effects are dry mouth and abdominal pains. Trade name: **Tolnate**.

丙胺氮嗪 一種安定、鎮靜藥。用於解除焦慮、激動、不安、興奮，引導入眠，並有防噁心、嘔吐的作用。口服或注射。常見副作用爲口乾和腹痛。

prothrombin *n.* a substance, present in blood plasma, that is the inactive precursor from which the enzyme *thrombin is derived during the process of *blood coagulation. *See also* coagulation factors.

前凝血酶 凝血酶的無活性前體。存在於血漿內，在凝血過程中轉化爲凝血酶。

proto- *prefix denoting* **1.** first. **2.** primitive; early. **3.** a precursor.

〔前綴〕 ①**第一** ②**原始，早期** ③**前體**

protodiastole *n.* the short period in the cardiac cycle between the end of systole and the closure of the *aortic valve marking the start of diastole.

舒張前期 心動週期中在收縮結束和主動脈瓣關閉（標示舒張開始）之間的短暫瞬間。

protopathic *adj.* describing the ability to perceive only strong stimuli of pain, heat, etc. *Compare* epicritic.

粗的 指僅能感受强的疼痛、熱的刺激的能力。

protoplasm *n.* the material of which living cells are made, which includes the cytoplasm and nucleus. —**protoplasmic** *adj.*

原生質，原漿 活細胞的構成物質，包括胞漿和胞核。

protoplast *n.* a bacterial or plant cell without its cell wall.

原生質體 失去細胞壁的細菌或植物細胞。

protoporphyrin IX the most common type of *porphyrin found in nature. It is a constituent of haemoglobin, myoglobin, most of the cytochromes, and the commoner chlorophylls.

原卟啉IX 自然界中最常見的卟啉類型。爲血紅蛋白、肌紅蛋白、多數細胞色素以及一般葉綠素的組成成分。

Protozoa *n.* a group of microscopic single-celled animals. Most Protozoa

原生動物門 一類僅能在顯微鏡下觀察到的單細胞

are free-living but some are important disease-causing parasites of man; for example, *Plasmodium, *Leishmania, and *Trypanosoma cause *malaria, *kala-azar, and *sleeping sickness respectively. *See also* amoeba.

動物。多數營獨立生活，但有些爲人類致病的微生物。例如：瘧原蟲屬、利什曼原蟲屬、錐蟲屬，可分別引起瘧疾、利什曼病和昏睡病。

protozoan *n.* a single-celled animal. *See* Protozoa.

原生動物 單細胞動物。

protozoology *n.* the study of single-celled animals (*Protozoa).

原生動物學 研究單細胞動物的科學。

protriptyline *n.* a tricyclic *antidepressant drug used to treat moderate or severe depression, especially in apathetic and withdrawn patients. It is administered by mouth; side-effects include dry mouth, blurred vision, fast heart beat, digestive disturbances, and skin rashes. Trade name: **Concordin**.

普羅替林 一種三環結構的抗憂鬱藥。用於治療中度或重症抑鬱症，特別是表現淡漠和孤僻的病人。口服。副作用有口乾、視物模糊、心動過速、胃腸紊亂、皮疹。

protrusion *n.* (in dentistry) **1.** forward movement of the lower jaw. **2.** a *malocclusion in which some of the teeth are further forward than usual. *Compare* retrusion.

前伸 （牙科學）①下頜向前的運動。②部分牙過分前突的錯牙合。

protuberance *n.* (in anatomy) a rounded projecting part, e.g. the projecting part of the chin (*mental protuberance*).

隆凸 （解剖學）圓形隆起部。如下巴的隆凸部（頦隆凸）。

provitamin *n.* a substance that is not itself a vitamin but can be converted to a vitamin in the body. An example is β-carotene, which can be converted into vitamin A.

前維生素 本身不是維生素然而能在體內轉化爲維生素的物質。例如：β-胡蘿蔔素可轉化爲維生素A。

proximal *adj.* (in anatomy) situated close to the origin or point of attachment or close to the median line of the body. *Compare* distal.

近側的 （解剖學）緊臨起點或附着點的，或者靠近身體正中線的。

prurigo *n.* a chronic itchy skin disease of unknown cause. It usually starts in childhood with small pale pimples arising deep in the skin. Prurigo may occur in association with hay fever or asthma or start in warm weather. Treatment is unsatisfactory and relapses are frequent.

癢疹 一種原因不明的慢性皮膚瘙癢症。通常始於兒童期，表現爲自皮膚深層突起的蒼白丘疹。可與枯草熱或哮喘病同時存在，多在溫暖氣候發作。缺乏有效治療，常復發。

pruritus *n.* itching, caused by local irritation of the skin or sometimes nervous disorders. Severe itching is a symptom of some forms of jaundice. Pruritus of the vulva in women may be due to vaginal infection, in some cases caused by yeast organisms that flourish in diabetes, when the urine contains sugar. Pruritus of the anal region may be due to poor hygiene, haemorrhoids, or the presence of intestinal worms.

瘙癢 局部皮膚刺激引起的癢感。有時發生於神經疾患。嚴重瘙癢可爲某些類型黃疸的症狀。婦女外陰瘙癢可由陰道炎症引起，而在患糖尿病的婦女，因尿含糖致使酵母菌繁殖而引起瘙癢。肛門瘙癢的原因是衛生不良、痔瘡或腸蠕蟲病。

prussic acid *see* hydrocyanic acid.

氫氰酸

psammoma *n.* a tumour containing gritty sandlike particles (*psammoma bodies*). Such tumours may be found in the meninges (the membranes surrounding the brain), the ovary, etc.

沙粒瘤 一種含沙樣顆粒（沙粒瘤小體）的腫瘤。可見於腦膜、卵巢等處。

psellism *n.* a deficiency of articulation of speech, such as *stammering.

口吃 一種言語發音缺陷，如說話結巴。

pseud- (pseudo-) *prefix denoting* superficial resemblance to; false.

〔前綴〕 **表面相似，假的**

pseudarthrosis (nearthrosis) *n.* a 'false' joint, formed around a displaced bone end after dislocation. Congenital hip dislocation may result in a pseudarthrosis.

假關節 脫位後在移位骨端周圍形成的假性連結。先天性髖關節脫位可導至假關節形成。

pseudoagglutination *n.* the misleading appearance of clumping during an antiserum-antigen test as a result of incorrect temperature or acidity of the solutions used.

假凝集 由於溫度或所用溶液酸度不合適在抗血清-抗原試驗中出現的使人誤解的凝塊現象。

pseudocholinesterase *n.* an enzyme found in the blood and other tissues that – like *cholinesterase – breaks down acetylcholine, but much more slowly. Not being localized at nerve endings, it plays little part in the normal breakdown of acetylcholine in synapses and at neuromuscular junctions.

假膽鹼酯酶 血液和其他組織中存在的一種與膽鹼酯酶相似、能分解乙醯膽鹼但速度大爲緩慢的酶。此酶因不存在於神經末梢，故在突觸內或神經肌肉接頭處的乙醯膽鹼分解中不起作用。

pseudocoxalgia *n.* *see* Legg-Calvé-Perthes disease.

假性髖關節痛

pseudocrisis *n.* a false crisis: a sudden but temporary fall of temperature in a patient with fever. The pseudocrisis is followed by a return to the fever.

假驟退 假的熱驟退：發熱病人體溫突然短時間下降，其後又行升高。

pseudocroup *n.* spasmodic contraction of the larynx that is not caused by inflammation of the glottis or associated with coughing. It occurs particularly in children with rickets.

假格魯布 喉的痙攣性收縮，其原因不是聲門炎症，且不伴有咳嗽。主要見於佝僂病患兒。

pseudocryptorchidism *n.* apparent absence of the testes. This is quite common in young boys, who retract their testes into the groin due to involuntary or reflex contraction of the cremasteric muscle of the suspensory cord. The condition is only important in that it needs to be distinguished from true failure of descent of the testes into the scrotum, which requires early surgical treatment (*see* cryptorchidism).

假隱睾 外表缺乏睾丸的形態。較多見於青少年，係由於精索提睾肌不隨意性或反射性收縮使睾丸回縮在腹股溝部。這種狀態僅在需要與眞性睾丸不能降入陰囊相區別時才有意義。後者需早期外科手術。

pseudocyesis (phantom pregnancy) *n.* a condition in which a nonpregnant woman exhibits symptoms of pregnancy, e.g. enlarged abdomen, increased weight, morning sickness, and absence of menstruation. The condition usually has an emotional basis and is determined by hormones secreted by the pituitary gland.

假孕 未孕婦女顯示妊娠徵象（腹部膨隆，體重增加，晨起噁心，無月經）的狀況。通常爲情緒性，係垂體分泌激素所致。

pseudocyst *n.* a fluid-filled space without a proper wall or lining, within an organ. A *pancreatic pseudocyst* may develop in cases of chronic pancreatitis or as a complication of acute pancreatitis. As the pseudocyst, which is filled with enzyme-rich pancreatic juice, slowly expands it may cause episodes of abdominal pain accompanied by a rise in the level of enzymes in the blood. It may be felt by abdominal examination, or may be seen by radiology as it displaces other organs. Treatment is by surgical drainage, usually by the technique of joining the pseudocyst to the stomach (*marsupialization).

假囊腫 器官內的充滿液體而無適當包壁或內膜的腔。胰腺假囊腫可發生於慢性胰腺炎，或者是急性胰腺炎的合併症。當充盈富含酶的胰液的假囊腫慢慢增大時，可引起腹痛伴有血中酶濃度增高。腹部檢查可觸知假囊腫，當它推擠其它器官移位時，可在X線下查見。治療一般爲應用溝通假囊腫和胃的手術進行外科引流。

pseudogout *n.* joint pain and swelling, resembling gout, caused by crystals of

假痛風 由焦磷酸鈣結晶沉着於滑膜和滑囊液內所

calcium pyrophosphate in the synovial membrane and fluid. *See also* chondrocalcinosis.

致的很像痛風的關節腫痛。

pseudohermaphroditism *n.* a congenital abnormality in which the external genitalia of a male or a female resemble those of the opposite sex; for example, a woman would have enlarged labia and clitoris, resembling a scrotum and penis respectively.

假兩性畸形 一種先天性異常，表現爲男性或女性外生殖器與異性相似。例如，女病人的陰唇和陰蒂增大，相應地類似陰囊和陰莖。

pseudohypertrophy *n.* increase in the size of an organ or structure caused by excessive growth of cells that have a packing or supporting role but do not contribute directly to its functioning. The result is usually a decline in the efficiency of the organ although it becomes larger. —**pseudohypertrophic** *adj.*

假性肥大 僅起充塡或支持作用的細胞過度生長所致的器官或結構的體積增大。器官或結構的功能並不能增强，結果往往器官增大而其功能却降低。

pseudohypoparathyroidism *n.* a syndrome of mental retardation, restricted growth, and bony abnormalities due to a genetic defect that causes lack of response to the hormone secreted by the *parathyroid glands. Treatment with calcium and vitamin D can reverse most of the features.

假甲狀旁腺功能減退 一種表現爲智力落後、生長受阻和骨骼異常的綜合徵，係因基因缺陷而對甲狀旁腺分泌的激素缺乏反應所致。用鈣和維生素D治療可使多數症狀好轉。

pseudologia fantastica the telling of elaborate and fictitious stories as if they were true. Often some facts are woven into the tissue of lies. While not necessarily a symptom of illness, it is sometimes a feature of chronic mental illness and of personality disorders, particularly psychopathy.

幻想性謊言癖 繪聲繪色地將編造的故事說得如同眞有其事。經常是將某些事實編織在謊言之中。這雖非一定是疾病的症狀，但有時可爲慢性精神疾病和人格障礙（尤其是精神變態）的表現。

pseudomembrane *n.* a false membrane, consisting of a layer of exudate on the surface of the skin or a mucous membrane. In diphtheria a pseudomembrane forms in the throat.

假膜 皮膚或黏膜表面由一層滲出物構成的假膜。患白喉時喉內可形成假膜。

Pseudomonas *n.* a genus of rodlike motile pigmented Gram-negative bacteria. Most live in soil and decomposing organic matter; they are involved in recycling nitrogen, converting nitrates to ammonia or free nitrogen. The spe-

假單胞菌屬 革蘭染色陰性、有活動能力、含色素的桿狀菌屬。多數生存於土壤內，能分解有機物，參與氮的再循環，將硝酸鹽變爲氨或游離氮。綠膿

cies *P. aeruginosa* is pathogenic to man, occurring in pus from wounds; it is associated with urinary tract infections. *P. pseudomallei* is the causative agent of *melioidosis.

假單胞菌爲人類致病菌，存在於創傷的膿內，與尿路感染有關。類鼻疽桿菌是類鼻疽病的病原菌。

pseudomutuality *n.* a disorder of communication within a family in which a superficial pretence of closeness and reciprocal understanding belies a lack of real feeling. It has been alleged, but not proved, to be a factor in the backgrounds of schizophrenics.

假親密 家庭內部交往的障礙。表面上做作的親熱和相互理解掩飾着實際上的無感情。人們認爲這是精神分裂症的背景因素之一，但此點未能證實。

pseudomyxoma *n.* a mucoid tumour of the peritoneum, often seen in association with *myxomas of the ovary. In *pseudomyxoma peritonei* material from a myxoma, usually in the ovary, is spilled into the peritoneal cavity and continues to be produced within the abdomen, often to massive proportions.

假黏液瘤 腹膜的黏液樣瘤，常與卵巢黏液瘤並存。卵巢黏液瘤內的物質溢出進入腹膜腔，並在腹膜腔內不斷生成，以致常可達到巨大程度。

pseudoneuritis *n.* a condition that resembles *retrobulbar neuritis but is not due to inflammation. The most usual cause is blockage of blood vessels in the optic nerve (*ischaemic optic neuropathy*).

假視神經炎 一種與球後視神經炎相似的非炎性疾病。最常見的原因是視神經內血管阻塞（缺血性視神經病）。

pseudophakos *n.* the state of the eye after the natural lens has been replaced by a plastic lens implanted inside the eye, approximately in the position previously occupied by the natural lens. This is a modern form of surgery for cataract.

假晶狀體 眼內天然晶狀體被植入的塑料晶狀體取代（後者大致佔據天然晶狀體原先的位置）。此係一新型晶狀體手術。

pseudoplegia *n.* paralysis of the limbs not associated with organic abnormalities. *See also* hysterical.

假癱 沒有器質性病變的肢體癱瘓。

pseudopodium *n.* (*pl.* **pseudopodia**) a temporary and constantly changing extension of the body of an amoeba or an amoeboid cell (*see* phagocyte). Pseudopodia engulf bacteria and other particles as food and are responsible for the movements of the cell.

假足，僞足 阿米巴或阿米巴樣細胞胞體的短暫或持續的延伸。假足能吞食細菌或其它顆粒，並使細胞運動。

pseudopolyposis *n.* a condition in which .the bowel lining (mucosa) is covered by elevated or protuberant plaques (*pseudopolyps*) that are not true *polyps but abnormal growth of inflamed mucosa. It is usually found in chronic ulcerative *colitis. The pseudopolyps may be seen with the *sigmoidoscope or *colonoscope (through which they may be sampled for microscopic examination) or by barium enema examination.

假息肉症 腸黏膜表面覆蓋着突起或隆起的斑塊（假息肉）。這些斑塊不是眞正的息肉而是發炎黏膜的異常生長物。通常見於慢性潰瘍性結腸炎。可在乙狀結腸鏡或結腸鏡下（可取樣做顯微鏡檢查）或做鋇劑灌腸檢查發現。

pseudopseudohypoparathyroidism *n.* a condition in which all the symptoms of *pseudohypoparathyroidism are present but the patient's response to parathyroid hormone is normal. It is often found in families affected with pseudohypoparathyroidism.

假性假甲狀旁腺功能減退 具有假甲狀旁腺功能減退的全部症狀但對甲狀旁腺激素反應正常。常見於假甲狀旁腺功能減退病人的家庭成員。

pseudotumour cerebri *see* benign intracranial hypertension.

腦假瘤

psilosis *n. see* sprue.

口炎性腹瀉

psittacosis *n. see* parrot disease.

鸚鵡熱

psoas (psoas major) *n.* a muscle in the groin that acts jointly with the iliacus muscle to flex the hip joint (see illustration). A smaller muscle, *psoas minor*, has the same action but is often absent.

腰肌（腰大肌） 位於腹股溝部的肌肉，與髂肌共同使髖關節屈曲（見圖）。腰小肌的作用相同，但腰小肌常闕如。

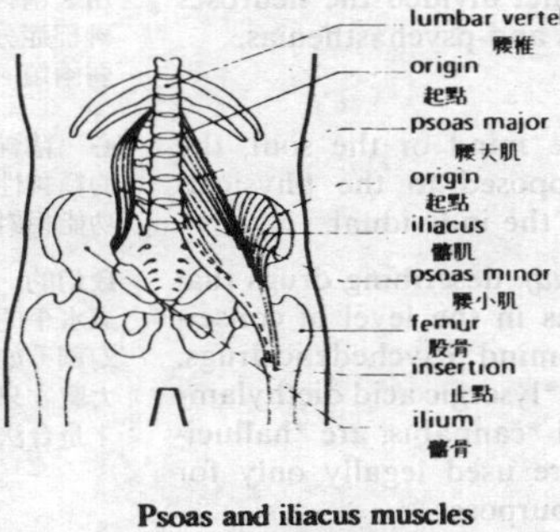

Psoas and iliacus muscles
腰肌與髂肌

psoriasis *n.* a chronic skin disease in which itchy scaly red patches form on

銀屑病 一種慢性皮膚病，其特徵爲在肘、前

the elbows, forearms, knees, legs, scalp, and other parts of the body. Psoriasis is one of the commonest skin diseases in Britain, affecting about 1% of the population, but its cause is not known. The disorder often runs in families and may be brought on by anxiety; it is rare in infants and the elderly, the commonest time of onset being in childhood or adolescence. It sometimes occurs in association with arthritis (*see* psoriatic arthritis). Occasionally the disease may be very severe, affecting much of the skin and causing considerable disability in the patient. There is no known cure and treatment is palliative with lotions or ointments.

臂、膝、小腿、頭皮及身體其它部位皮膚上形成癢性鱗片狀紅色斑。銀屑病是英國最常見的皮膚病，波及大約1%的人口。原因不明。家庭成員常相繼發生而引起焦慮。嬰兒和老人少見，最常在兒童和青少年時期發作，有時可與關節炎並存。偶可十分嚴重，侵犯大部分皮膚，病人明顯喪失勞動能力。尚無有效治療，用洗劑或軟膏可減輕症狀。

psoriatic arthritis arthritis associated with *psoriasis. It occurs in only a small minority of patients with psoriasis but may be painful and disabling. It often affects small joints, such as the terminal joints of the fingers and toes, or the spine (*spondylitis) and sacroiliac joints (*sacroiliitis).

銀屑病性關節炎 伴同銀屑病的關節炎。銀屑病病人患關節炎者極少，有關節痛和喪失勞動能力。通常侵犯小關節（如指、趾的末端關節）脊柱（脊椎炎）或骶髂關節（骶髂關節炎）。

psych- (psycho-) *prefix denoting* **1.** the mind; psyche. **2.** psychology.

〔前綴〕 ①**精神，心理** ②**心理學**

psychasthenia *n.* an obsolete term for a group of neuroses including phobias, anxiety states, and obsessions. The psychiatrist P. Janet divided the neuroses into *hysterias and psychasthenias.

精神衰弱 指包括恐懼症、焦慮狀態、强迫症的一組神經症。此詞已廢用。精神病學家讓奈曾將神經症分爲癔症和精神衰弱兩類。

psyche *n.* the mind or the soul; the mental (as opposed to the physical) functioning of the individual.

心 精神或靈魂。指個體的精神性功能（與軀體性功能相對立）。

psychedelic *adj.* describing drugs that induce changes in the level of consciousness of the mind. Psychedelic drugs, which include *lysergic acid diethylamide (LSD) and *cannabis, are *hallucinogens and are used legally only for experimental purposes.

致幻的 指能引出精神意識水平的改變的藥物。致幻劑（如麥角醯二乙胺、大麻）只有用於實驗目的才是合法的。

psychiatrist *n.* a medically qualified physician who specializes in the study and treatment of mental disorders.

精神病學家 獲得行醫資格的以研究和治療精神障礙爲專長的醫生。

psychiatry *n.* the study of mental disorders and their diagnosis, management, and prevention. —**psychiatric** *adj.*

精神病學 研究精神障礙及其診斷、處理和預防的科學。

psychic *adj.* **1.** of or relating to the *psyche. **2.** relating to parapsychological phenomena. **3.** describing a person who is endowed with extrasensory or psychokinetic powers.

①精神的 ②心靈學的 ③稟賦超感官或精神致動能力者

psychoanalysis *n.* a school of psychology and a method of treating mental disorders based upon the teachings of Sigmund Freud (1856–1939). Psychoanalysis employs the technique of *free association in the course of intensive *psychotherapy in order to bring repressed fears and conflicts to the conscious mind, where they can be dealt with (*see* repression). It stresses the dynamic interplay of unconscious forces and the importance of sexual development in childhood for personality development. —**psychoanalyst** *n.* —**psychoanalytic** *adj.*

精神分析 心理學派之一。一種以弗洛伊德(1856～1939)學說爲依據的精神障礙治療方法。精神分析在積極的心理治療過程中應用自由聯想技術，目的是使被壓抑的恐懼和衝突進入意識領域以便進行治療。精神分析强調下意識力量之間的相互作用以及兒童性發育在人格發育中的重要性。

psychodrama *n.* a form of group psychotherapy in which individuals acquire insight into themselves by acting out situations from their past with other group members. *See* group therapy.

心理劇 一種集體心理治療形式。病人個體通過與集體內其他成員表演他們既往體驗過的情景從而達到洞察自我。

psychogenic *adj.* having an origin in the mind rather than in the body. The term is applied particularly to symptoms and illnesses.

精神性的，心理性的 起源於精神而非驅體的。此詞主要用於描述症狀和疾病。

psychogeriatrics *n.* the branch of psychiatry that deals with the mental disorders of old people. —**psychogeriatric** *adj.*

老年精神病學 探討老年人精神障礙的精神病學分支。

psychokinesis *n.* a supposed ability of some individuals to alter the state of an object by the power of the mind alone, without any physical intervention. *See also* parapsychology.

精神致動 假定在某些人身上賦有的只用精神力量不加任何物理干預就能改變客體狀態的能力。

psychologist *n.* a person who is engaged in the scientific study of the mind. He may work in a university, in industry, in schools, or in a hospital. A

心理學家 從事心理科學研究的工作者。心理學家可在大學、企業、學校或醫院內工作。臨床心理學

clinical psychologist has been trained in aspects of the assessment and treatment of the ill and handicapped. He usually works in a hospital, often as one of a multidisciplinary team. An *educational psychologist* has been trained in aspects of the cognitive and emotional development of children. He usually works in close association with schools and advises on the management of children.

家須具備評定和治療疾病和殘疾的知識，通常在醫院工作，並常作爲多科性醫療隊的一員。教育心理學家則須具備兒童認知和感情發育方面的知識，通常與學校密切聯繫，對兒童的管理提出建議。

psychology *n.* the science concerned with the behaviour of man and animals. Different schools of psychology have used different methods and theories. *Experimental psychology* uses laboratory experiments to study processes such as motivation and learning. *Ethology* investigates animal behaviour by observation in the natural environment. *Introspectionist psychology* used the method of trained subjects describing their own mental states. Other schools include *behaviourism, *gestaltism, and *psychoanalysis. —**psychological** *adj.*

心理學 研究人和動物行爲的科學。不同的心理學派應用不同的理論和方法。實驗心理學應用實驗室方法研究動機和學習這類過程。習性學通過自然環境中的觀察研究動物的行爲。內省主義心理學應用讓受試者描述他們自己的心理狀態的方法。此外還有行爲主義、完形主義和精神分析等學派。

psychometrics *n.* the measurement of individual differences in psychological functions (such as intelligence and personality) by means of standardized tests. —**psychometric** *adj.*

心理測驗 應用標準化手段測定心理功能（如智力和個性）的個體差異。

psychomotor *adj.* relating to muscular and mental activity. The term is applied to disorders in which muscular activities are affected by cerebral disturbance.

精神運動的 指肌肉和精神的活動。此詞用於肌肉活動受大腦障礙影響的疾病。

psychomotor epilepsy *see* epilepsy.

精神運動性癲癇

psychoneurosis *n.* a *neurosis that is manifest in psychological rather than organic symptoms.

精神性神經症 精神症狀比器質性症狀明顯的神經症。

psychopath *n.* a person who behaves in an antisocial way and shows little or no guilt for antisocial acts and little capacity for forming emotional relationships with others. There is some evidence that EEG patterns of psychopaths are abnormal. Psychopaths tend

精神病態者 以反社會方式行動、對其反社會行爲不自覺有罪、並且不能與他人建立感情關係的人。已有一些證據表明，精神病態者的腦電圖類型是異常的。這種病人對治療反

to respond poorly to treatment but many mature as they age. *See also* personality disorder. —**psychopathic** *adj.* —**psychopathy** *n.*

應不佳，但到老年會明顯好轉。

psychopathology *n.* **1.** the study of mental disorders, with the aim of explaining and describing aberrant behaviour. *Compare* psychiatry. **2.** the symptoms, collectively, of a mental disorder. —**psychopathological** *adj.*

精神病理學 ①研究精神障礙，解釋和描述異常行爲的科學。②某種精神障礙的症狀總和。

psychopharmacology *n.* the study of the effects of drugs on mental processes and behaviour, particularly *psychotropic drugs.

精神藥理學 研究藥物（主要是精神治療藥）對心理過程和行爲的影響的科學。

psychophysiology *n.* the branch of psychology that records physiological measurements, such as the electrical resistance of the skin, the heart rate, the size of the pupil, and the electroencephalogram, and relates them to psychological events. —**psychophysiological** *adj.*

心理生理學 生理學的分支，記錄各種生理學測量結果，諸如皮膚電阻抗、心率、瞳孔大小、腦電圖等，並用以與心理學變化相聯繫。

psychosexual development the process by which an individual becomes more mature in his sexual feelings and behaviour. Gender identity, sex-role behaviour, and choice of sexual partner are the three major areas of development. The phrase is sometimes used specifically for a sequence of stages, supposed by psychoanalytic psychologists to be universal, in which oral, anal, phallic, latency, and genital stages successively occur. These stages reflect the parts of the body on which sexual interest is concentrated during childhood development.

性心理發育 個體在其性的情感和行爲方面變得成熟的過程。性確認、性行爲和選擇性伴侶，是發育的三個主要方面。此術語有時專指口、肛、外生殖器、潛伏期和生殖期諸階段依次出現的過程（精神分析派心理學家認爲這種次序是普遍存在的）。這些階段反映了兒童發育過程中性興趣所集中注意的身體部分。

psychosis *n.* a severe mental illness in which the sufferer loses contact with reality. *Delusions and *hallucinations occur and thought processes may be altered. The major varieties are *organic* and *functional*; in the latter no physical cause has been demonstrated. The most important functional psychoses are *schizophrenia and *manic-depressive

精神病 喪失與現實世界接觸能力的嚴重精神障礙。病人有各種幻覺和妄想，思維過程可發生變態。分器質性和功能性兩類。功能性精神病沒有軀體性原因，最重要的有精神分裂症和躁鬱性精神病。還有一些不屬於兩者

psychosis. Psychoses not typical of either of these also occur: *oneiroid psychosis* is characterized by an acute dreamlike confused state; *cycloid psychosis* by a tendency to recur; and *schizoaffective psychosis* by the presence of both schizophrenic and manic-depressive qualities. —**psychotic** *adj.*

的精神病：如夢魘樣精神病以急性夢樣混亂迷惘狀態爲特徵；類循環型精神病有復發傾向；分裂情感性精神病則是精神分裂症與躁鬱症並存。

psychosomatic *adj.* relating to or involving both the mind and body: usually applied to illnesses that are caused by the interaction of mental and physical factors. Certain physical illnesses, including asthma, eczema, and peptic ulcer, are thought to be in part a response to psychological and social stresses. Psychological treatments sometimes have a marked effect, but are usually much less effective than physical treatments for such illnesses.

心身的 與精神和軀體有關或涉及兩者的。通常用於由精神和軀體因素相互影響所致的疾病。某些軀體疾病如哮喘、濕疹和消化性潰瘍，被認爲是某種程度社會心理應激的反映。對於這類疾病，心理治療有時有顯效，但通常療效遠不如軀體治療。

psychosurgery *n.* surgery of the brain to relieve psychological symptoms. The operation most commonly performed is *leucotomy, but *cingulectomy and amygdalectomy are sometimes also used. These are all irreversible treatments and are therefore reserved for the most severe and intractable of symptoms, particularly severe chronic anxiety, depression, and untreatable pain. Side-effects can be severe but are less common with modern selective operations. —**psychosurgical** *adj.*

精神外科學 旨在解除精神症狀的大腦外科手術。最常用的是腦白質切斷術，有時也採用扣帶回切除術和扁桃切除術。此類手術均爲破壞性治療，因而只用於最嚴重和難治的病症，主要爲慢性焦慮症、抑鬱症和頑固性疼痛。副作用可很嚴重，但在施行現代精確選擇性破壞手術後已不多見。

psychotherapy *n.* psychological (as opposed to physical) methods for the treatment of mental disorders and psychological problems. There are many different approaches to psychotherapy, including *psychoanalysis, *client-centred therapy, and *group therapy. These approaches share the views that the relationship between therapist and client is of prime importance, that the goal is to help personal development and self-understanding generally rather than to remove symptoms, and that the therapist does not direct the client's

心理療法 治療精神障礙和心理方面問題的心理學（與軀體的相對立）方法。手段多種多樣，有精神分析、患者中心治療法、集體療法等。這些療法都是基於如下觀點：醫者與患者之間的關係是最重要的，治療的總目標是促進個體的正常發展和全面自我認識，而不局限於消除症狀，醫者讓患者自己去解決所存在的問題。上述療法均已廣泛用於治

decisions. They have all been very widely applied to differing clinical conditions but are of unknown value as treatments of mental illness. *See also* behaviour therapy, counselling. —**psychotherapeutic** *adj.* —**psychotherapist** *n.*

療各種臨床疾病，但作爲精神疾病的療法，其價值尚未肯定。

psychoticism *n.* a dimension of personality derived from psychometric tests, which appears to indicate a degree of emotional coldness and some cognitive impairment.

心理評析法 一種人格的量度法。係從心理測驗得出的結果進行評析。用以指明情緒淡漠和某些認知能力損害的程度。

psychotropic *adj.* describing drugs that affect mood. *Antidepressants, *sedatives, *stimulants, and *tranquillizers are psychotropic.

精神治療藥 影響心境的藥物。抗抑鬱藥、鎮靜藥、興奮藥和安定藥都是精神治療藥。

psychro- *prefix denoting* cold.

〔前綴〕 **冷**

psychrophilic *adj.* describing organisms, especially bacteria, that grow best at temperatures of 0–25°C. *Compare* mesophilic, thermophilic.

嗜冷的 指那些在0～25℃生長最好的有機體（主要是細菌）。

PTC *see* phenylthiocarbamide.

苯硫脲

pterion *n.* the point on the side of the skull at which the sutures between the *parietal, *temporal, and *sphenoid bones meet.

翼點 顱骨上頂骨、顳骨和蝶骨的骨縫匯合點。

pteroylglutamic acid *see* folic acid.

蝶醯穀氨酸

pterygium *n.* a triangular overgrowth of the cornea, usually the inner side, by thickened and degenerative conjunctiva. It is most commonly seen in people from dry hot dusty climates, and only rarely interferes with vision.

翼狀胬肉 角膜（通常爲內側）的三角形贅生物，係來自增厚、變性的結膜。最常見於在乾熱多塵環境中生活的人們。偶可影響視力。

pterygo- *prefix denoting* the pterygoid process of the sphenoid bone. Example: *pterygomaxillary* (of the pterygoid process and the maxilla).

〔前綴〕 **翼** 指蝶骨翼突。例如，翼突上頜的（翼突和上頜骨的）。

pterygoid process either of two large processes of the *sphenoid bone.

翼突 蝶骨兩個大突起之一。

ptomaine *n.* any of various substances produced in decaying foodstuffs and responsible for the unpleasant taste and smell of such foods. These compounds

屍鹼 食物腐敗時產生的各種使該食物具有惡味和惡臭的物質。這類化合物包括腐胺、屍胺、神經

– which include putrescine, cadaverine, and neurine – were formerly thought to be responsible for food poisoning, but although they are often associated with toxic bacteria they themselves are harmless.

鹼，過去曾被認爲是食物中毒的原因；它們雖常與致毒性細菌同時存在，其實本身是無害的。

ptosis *n.* drooping of the upper eyelid, for which there are several causes. It may be due to a disorder of the third cranial nerve (*oculomotor nerve), in which case it is likely to be accompanied by paralysis of eye movements causing double vision and an enlarged pupil. When part of *Horner's syndrome, ptosis is accompanied by a small pupil and an absence of sweating on that side of the face. It may be due to *myasthenia gravis, in which the ptosis increases with fatigue and is part of a more widespread fatiguable weakness. Ptosis may also occur as an isolated congenital feature or as part of a disease of the eye muscles, when it is associated with weak or absent eye movements.

瞼下垂　上眼瞼下垂。有幾種原因。可發生於第Ⅲ對顱神經（動眼神經）障礙時，常伴有眼球運動麻痺，引起複視和一側瞳孔擴大。當做爲霍納綜合徵的一部分時，瞼下垂伴有患側瞳孔縮小和面部汗閉。重症肌無力時可有瞼下垂，下垂程度隨疲勞而增加，成爲全身疲乏無力的一部分。瞼下垂也可是單獨的先天性病症或眼肌病的部分，後者瞼下垂與眼球運動減弱或消失同時存在。

-ptosis *suffix denoting* a lowered position of an organ or part; prolapse. Example: *colpoptosis* (of the vagina).

〔後綴〕 **下垂**　指器官或部分的位置過低；脫垂。例如陰道下垂。

ptyal- (ptyalo-) *prefix denoting* saliva. Example: *ptyalorrhoea* (excessive flow of).

〔前綴〕 **唾液，涎**　例如流涎（唾液大量流出）。

ptyalin *n.* an enzyme (an *amylase) found in saliva.

唾液澱粉酶　一種唾液酶（澱粉酶）。

ptyalism (sialorrhoea) *n.* the excessive production of saliva: a symptom of certain nervous disorders, poisoning (by mercury, mushrooms, or organophosphates), or infection (rabies). *Compare* xerostomia.

唾液分泌過多（流涎）　唾液生成過多。爲某些神經障礙、中毒（汞中毒、毒蕈中毒、有機磷中毒）、感染（狂犬病）的症狀。

ptyalith *n.* a stone (*calculus) in a salivary gland or duct.

涎石　唾液腺或導管中的結石（鈣）。

ptyalography *n. see* sialography.

涎管X線造影術

puberty *n.* the time at which the onset of sexual maturity occurs and the re-

青春期　生殖器官開始發揮功能的性成熟時期。兩

productive organs become functional. This is manifested in both sexes by the appearance of *secondary sexual characteristics (e.g. deepening of the voice in boys; growth of breasts in girls) and in girls by the start of *menstruation. These changes are brought about by an increase in sex hormone activity due to stimulation of the ovaries and testes by pituitary hormones. *See also* androgen, oestrogen. —**pubertal** *adj.*

性的第二性徵顯露（如：男孩嗓音低沉，女孩乳房發育等），女孩開始有月經。這些變化是由於垂體激素刺激卵巢和睾丸，使其分泌性激素的活動增强的結果。

pubes *n.* **1.** the body surface that overlies the pubis, at the front of the pelvis. It is covered with *pubic hair*. **2.** *see* pubis. —**pubic** *adj.*

①**陰阜**　骨盆前面、包蓋恥骨的體表部分。陰阜表面覆有陰毛。　②**恥骨**

pubiotomy *n.* an operation to divide the pubic bone near the symphysis, the front midline where the left and right pubic bones meet. Pubiotomy is performed during childbirth if it is necessary to increase the size of an abnormally small pelvis to allow passage of the child.

恥骨切開術　在恥骨聯合即左右恥骨匯合處前正中附近分離恥骨的手術。此術在分娩中當骨盆過小而需擴大以允許胎兒通過時施行。

pubis *n.* (*pl.* **pubes**) a bone forming the lower and anterior part of each side of the *hip bone (*see also* pelvis). The two pubes meet at the front of the pelvis at the *pubic symphysis*. *See also* pubes.

恥骨　構成一側髖骨的前部和下部的骨。左右恥骨在骨盆前面恥骨聯合處匯合。

Public Health Inspector the former title of the Environmental Health Officer.

公共衛生督察　環境衛生官員的舊稱。

Public Health Laboratory (in Britain) a regional service, with headquarters at Colindale, to assist with the investigation and control of infections. Such laboratories are a separate organization from hospital laboratories, which are under the control of District Health Authorities, but they can be located within a hospital and can contribute to the day-to-day diagnosis of hospital in-patients and out-patients.

公共衛生實驗室　（英國）總部設在科林代爾的地區性機構，協助傳染病的調查和控制工作。這種實驗室與醫院實驗室沒有關係，後者受地段保健局領導。這種實驗室也可設在醫院內，協助醫院的住院和門診患者的日常診斷業務。

pudendum *n.* (*pl.* **pudenda**) the external genital organs, especially those of the female (*see* vulva). —**pudendal** *adj.*

陰部　外生殖器（主要指女性）。

puerpera *n.* a woman who has recently given birth and whose womb has not yet returned to its normal nonpregnant dimensions.

產婦 分娩後子宮尚未恢復到正常未孕時大小的婦女。

puerperal (puerperous) *adj.* relating to childbirth or the period that immediately follows it.

產褥的，產後的 指分娩或緊接分娩後的一段時間。

puerperal fever (childbed fever) blood poisoning (*septicaemia) in a mother shortly after childbirth resulting from infection of the lining of the womb or the vagina, which have been torn or bruised during labour. Increased standards of hygiene in midwifery and the use of such antibiotics as penicillin have reduced the numbers of deaths caused by puerperal fever from the formerly high level almost to nil.

產褥熱 分娩後不久發生的產婦血液中毒症（敗血症），其根源是分娩時子宮或陰道內膜受損或撕裂而致的感染。以前產褥熱死亡率很高，隨着助產衛生標準的提高和青黴素之類抗生素的應用，死亡率已接近零。

puerperalism *n.* illness of a mother or her baby associated with childbirth.

產褥病 與分娩有關的產婦或嬰兒的疾病。

puerperium (childbed) *n.* the period of up to about six weeks after childbirth, during which the size of the womb decreases to normal.

產褥期 分娩後約6周的這段時間，其間子宮縮至正常大小。

Pulex *n.* a genus of widely distributed *fleas. *P. irritans*, the human flea, is a common parasite of man and its bite may give rise to intense irritation and bacterial infection. It is an intermediate host for larvae of the tapeworms **Hymenolepis* and **Dipylidium*, which it can transmit to man, and it may also be involved in the transmission of plague.

蚤屬 一種廣泛分佈的蚤。人蚤爲最常見的人體寄生蟲，咬人後可引起劇癢和細菌感染。爲膜殼絛蟲和複孔絛蟲幼蟲的中間宿主，可將兩者傳給人；還可參與鼠疫的傳播。

pulicide *n.* any chemical agent, for example *DDT or malathion, used for killing fleas.

滅蚤劑 用於殺蚤的化學劑，如滴滴涕、馬拉硫磷。

pulmo- (pulmon(o)-) *prefix denoting* the lung(s).

〔前綴〕 **肺**

pulmonary *adj.* relating to, associated with, or affecting the lungs.

肺的 與肺有關的，伴同肺的，影響肺的。

pulmonary artery the artery that conveys blood from the heart to the lungs for oxygenation: the only artery in the body containing deoxygenated blood. It leaves the right ventricle and passes

肺動脈 將來自心臟的血液輸送到肺進行氧合的動脈，是體內唯一含有脫氧血的動脈。肺動脈離開右心室上行5cm處分爲2

upwards for 5 cm before dividing into two, one branch going to each lung. Within the lungs each pulmonary artery divides into many fine branches, which end in capillaries in the alveolar walls. *See also* pulmonary circulation.

支，分別進入兩肺。在肺內又分爲大量細支，最後止於肺泡壁內的毛細血管。

pulmonary circulation a system of blood vessels effecting transport of blood between the heart and lungs. Deoxygenated blood leaves the right ventricle by the pulmonary artery and is carried to the alveolar capillaries of the lungs. Gaseous exchange occurs, with carbon dioxide leaving the circulation and oxygen entering. The oxygenated blood then passes into small veins leading to the pulmonary veins, which leave the lungs and return blood to the left atrium of the heart. The oxygenated blood can then be pumped around the body via the *systemic circulation.

肺循環　在心與肺之間輸送血液的血管系統。由肺動脈攜帶脫氧血離開右心室，到達肺的肺泡毛細血管，進行氣體交換，二氧化碳離開循環，氧氣進入循環。氧合血經小靜脈入肺靜脉，肺靜脉離開肺而將血液回送到左心房。氧合血遂通過體循環而流向全身。

pulmonary embolism obstruction of the *pulmonary artery or one of its branches by an *embolus, usually a blood clot derived from *phlebothrombosis of the leg veins. Large pulmonary emboli result in acute heart failure or sudden death. Smaller emboli cause death of sections of lung tissue, pleurisy, and haemoptysis (coughing of blood). Minor pulmonary emboli respond to the *anticoagulant drugs heparin and warfarin. Major pulmonary embolism is treated by *embolectomy or by dissolution of the blood clot with an infusion of *streptokinase. Recurrent pulmonary embolism may result in *pulmonary hypertension.

肺栓塞　肺動脉或其一支爲栓子（通常爲來自腿部靜脉血栓性靜脉炎的血凝塊）所阻塞。大的肺栓子導致急性心力衰竭或猝死。較小的栓塞引起肺組織段壞死、胸膜炎和咯血。抗凝血藥肝素和華法令對小的肺栓塞有作用。大的肺栓塞可用栓子切除術或注入鏈激酶溶解血凝塊治療。復發性肺栓塞可引起肺動脉高壓。

pulmonary hypertension a condition in which there is raised blood pressure within the blood vessels supplying the lungs (the pulmonary artery blood pressure is normally much lower than the pressure within the aorta and its branches). Pulmonary hypertension may complicate pulmonary embolism, *septal defects, heart failure, diseases of the mitral valve, and chronic lung

肺動脉高壓　供應肺的血管內血壓升高（肺動脉血壓正常時遠低於主動脉及其分支的血壓）。肺動脉高壓可發生於肺栓塞、間隔缺損、心力衰竭、二尖瓣病和肺慢性疾病。有的找不到任何原因，稱爲原發性肺動脉高壓。病人發生右心室擴大、心力衰

diseases. It may also develop without any known cause (*primary pulmonary hypertension*). The right ventricle enlarges and heart failure, fainting, and chest pain occur. The treatment is that of the cause; drugs used to control *hypertension are ineffective.

竭、昏厥和胸痛。針對原因治療；藥物控制高血壓不能奏效。

pulmonary stenosis congenital narrowing of the outlet of the right ventricle of the heart to the pulmonary artery. The defect may be in the pulmonary valve (*valvular stenosis*) or in the outflow tract of the right ventricle below the valve (*infundibular stenosis*). It may be isolated or combined with other heart defects (e.g. *tetralogy of Fallot). Severe pulmonary stenosis may produce angina pectoris, faintness, and heart failure. The defect is corrected by surgery.

肺動脈狹窄 肺動脈自右心室發出處的先天性縮窄。此缺陷可位於肺動脈瓣（動脈瓣狹窄）或瓣膜下方右心室流出道（動脈圓錐狹窄）。本病可獨立存在也可合併其他心臟缺陷(如法魯四聯症)。重症者可引起心絞痛、昏厥和心力衰竭。須做手術糾正缺陷。

pulmonary tuberculosis *see* tuberculosis.

肺結核

pulmonary vein a vein carrying oxygenated blood from the lung to the left atrium. *See* pulmonary circulation.

肺靜脈 將氧合血從肺輸送到左心房的靜脈。

pulp *n.* **1.** a soft mass of tissue (for example, of the spleen). **2.** the mass of connective tissue in the *pulp cavity*, at the centre of a *tooth. It is surrounded by dentine except where it communicates with the rest of the body at the apex.

髓 ①鬆軟的組織團塊（如脾髓）。②牙中央髓腔內的結締組織。牙髓四周爲牙本質包圍，僅通過根尖孔與身體其它部分相通。

pulpitis *n.* inflammation of the pulp of a tooth: a frequent cause of toothache.

牙髓炎 牙髓的炎症，爲牙痛的常見原因。

pulse *n.* a series of pressure waves within an artery caused by contractions of the left ventricle and corresponding with the heart rate (the number of times the heart beats per minute). It is easily detected on such superficial arteries as the radial artery near the wrist and the carotid artery in the neck. The average adult pulse rate at rest is 60–80 per minute, but exercise, injury, illness, and emotion may produce much faster rates.

脈搏 由左心室收縮產生的與心率（每分鐘的心跳次數）一致的動脈內壓力波系列。在淺表的動脈，如腕部附近的橈動脈和頸部的頸動脈上，很容易測到。成人安靜時的脈搏率爲每分鐘60～80次，鍛煉、受傷、患病和情緒激動時脈搏顯著增快。

pulsus paradoxus a large fall in systolic blood pressure and pulse volume when the patient breathes in. It is seen in constrictive *pericarditis, pericardial effusion, and asthma.

奇脉 病人吸氣時心收縮期血壓和脉搏容量顯著下降的現象。可見於縮窄性心包炎、心包滲液和哮喘。

pulvinar *n.* the expanded posterior end of the *thalamus.

丘腦枕 丘腦膨大的後端。

punch-drunk syndrome a group of symptoms consisting of progressive *dementia, tremor of the hands, and epilepsy. It is a consequence of repeated blows to the head that have been severe enough to cause *concussion.

擊暈綜合徵 由進行性痴獃、手震顫和癲癇組成的一組症狀。爲頭部反復遭受足以引起腦震盪的嚴重打擊的結果。

punctum *n.* (*pl.* **puncta**) (in anatomy) a point or small area, especially the *puncta lacrimalia* – the two openings of the tear ducts in the inner corners of the upper and lower eyelids (*see* lacrimal apparatus).

點 （解剖學）點和小區，主要指淚點，即上下眼瞼內背部的淚管的兩個開口。

puncture 1. *n.* a wound made accidentally or deliberately by a sharp object or instrument. Puncture wounds need careful treatment as a small entry hole in the skin can disguise serious injury in an underlying organ or tissue. Punctures are also performed for diagnostic purposes, in order to withdraw tissue or fluid for examination. *See also* lumbar puncture. **2.** *vb.* to pierce a tissue with a sharp instrument.

刺傷，穿刺 ①用尖銳物體或工具意外或故意地造成的傷口。刺傷須細心治療，因小的皮膚入口可掩蓋深處器官組織的嚴重損傷。穿刺可用於診斷目的，抽出組織或液體做檢查。②用尖銳工具刺穿組織。

pupil *n.* the circular opening in the centre of the *iris, through which light passes into the lens of the eye. —**pupillary** *adj.*

瞳孔 虹膜中央的環狀孔，光線通過瞳孔穿透眼晶狀體。

pupillary reflex (light reflex) the reflex change in the size of the pupil according to the amount of light entering the eye. Bright light reaching the retina stimulates nerves of the *parasympathetic nervous system, which cause the pupil to contract. In dim light the pupil opens, due to stimulation of the *sympathetic nervous system. *See also* iris.

瞳孔反射（光反射） 瞳孔隨進入眼內光線的量而改變大小的反射。强光抵達視網膜，刺激副交感神經系統的神經，引起瞳孔縮小。在弱光下由於交感神經系統的興奮，瞳孔開大。

purgation *n.* the use of drugs to stimulate intestinal activity and clear the bowels. *See* laxative.

催瀉 用藥物刺激腸管活動，清除糞便。

purgative *n. see* laxative.

催瀉藥

purine *n.* a nitrogen-containing compound with a two-ring molecular structure. Examples of purines are adenine and guanine, which form the *nucleotides of nucleic acids, and uric acid, which is the end-product of purine metabolism.

嘌呤 帶雙環分子結構的含氮化合物。嘌呤的代表是腺嘌呤和鳥嘌呤，它們構成核酸的核苷酸。嘌呤代謝的終產物是尿酸。

Purkinje cells nerve cells found in great numbers in the cortex of the cerebellum. The cell body is flask-shaped, with numerous dendrites branching from the neck and extending fanwise among other cells towards the surface and a long axon that runs from the base deep into the cerebellum (see illustration).

浦肯野細胞 大量存在於小腦皮質內的神經細胞。胞體呈細頸燒瓶狀，有衆多樹突枝從頸部發出，並在其它細胞之間呈扇形向皮質表面散開；一條長的軸突從基部伸向小腦深部（見圖）。

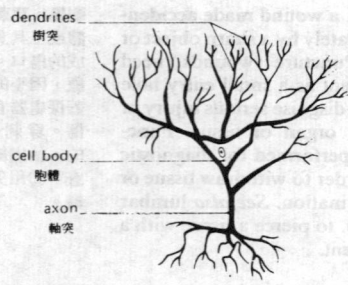

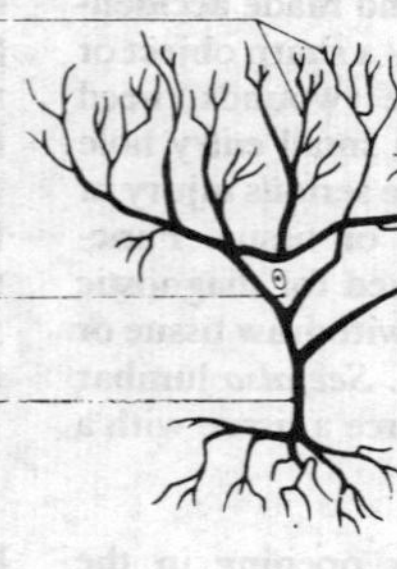

A Purkinje cell
浦肯野細胞

Purkinje fibres *see* atrioventricular bundle.

浦肯野纖維

purpura *n.* a skin rash resulting from bleeding into the skin from small blood vessels (capillaries); the individual purple spots of the rash are called *petechiae*. Purpura may be due either to defects in the capillaries (*nonthrombocytopenic purpura*) or to a deficiency of blood platelets (*thrombocytopenic purpura*). *Acute idiopathic thrombocyto-*

紫癜 皮膚小血管（毛細血管）出血造成的皮疹。單個的紫色皮疹點稱爲瘀點。紫癜的原因可以是毛細血管缺陷（非血小板減少性紫癜）或血小板缺陷（血小板減少性紫癜）。急性特發性血小板性紫癜是一種兒童疾病，患兒體

penic purpura is a disease of children in which antibodies are produced that destroy the patient's platelets. The child usually recovers without treatment. *See also* thrombocytopenia, Schönlein-Henoch purpura.

內產生破壞血小板的抗體。患者一般可自癒。

purulent *adj.* forming, consisting of, or containing pus.

膿性的 生膿的，由膿構成的，含膿的。

pus *n.* a thick yellowish or greenish liquid formed at the site of an established infection. Pus contains dead white blood cells, both living and dead bacteria, and fragments of dead tissue. *See also* mucopus, seropus.

膿 在感染部位生成的稠厚、帶黃色或帶綠色的液體。膿內含有死亡的白細胞、活的或死的細菌以及壞死組織碎片。

pustule *n.* a small pus-containing blister on the skin.

膿疱 皮膚上的含膿小疱。

putamen *n.* a part of the lenticular nucleus (*see* basal ganglia).

殼 豆狀核的一部分。

putrefaction *n.* the process whereby proteins are decomposed by bacteria. This is accompanied by the formation of amines (such as *putrescine* and *cadaverine*) having a strong and very unpleasant smell.

腐敗 細菌分解蛋白質的過程。此過程同時有胺類（如腐胺和屍胺）產生，後者發出强烈惡臭。

putrescine *n.* an amine formed during *putrefaction.

腐胺 腐敗過程中生成的一種胺。

py- (pyo-) *prefix denoting* pus; a purulent condition. Example: *pyoureter* (pus in a ureter).

〔前綴〕 **膿** 例如輸尿管積膿。

pyaemia *n.* blood poisoning by pus-forming bacteria released from an abscess. Widespread formation of abscesses may develop, with fatal results. *Compare* sapraemia, septicaemia, toxaemia.

膿毒血症 化膿菌從膿腫釋出的毒所致的血液中毒症。可發生廣泛分佈的膿腫，導至死亡結局。

pyarthrosis *n.* an infected joint filled with pus. Drainage, combined with antibiotic treatment, is necessary, though the joint may already be severely damaged if diagnosis is late.

關節積膿 關節感染而充滿膿液。如延誤診斷，關節已遭受嚴重損害，則須做切開引流，並用抗生素。

pyel- (pyelo-) *prefix denoting* the pelvis of the kidney. Example: *pyelectasis* (dilation of).

〔前綴〕 **腎盂** 例如腎盂擴張。

pyelitis *n.* inflammation of the pelvis of the kidney (the part of the kidney from which urine drains into the ureter). This is usually caused by a bacterial infection, which may develop in any condition causing obstruction to the flow of urine. The patient experiences pain in the loins, shivering, and a high temperature. Treatment is by the administration of a suitable antibiotic, together with analgesics and a high fluid intake. Any underlying abnormality of the urinary system must be relieved to prevent further attacks.

腎盂炎 腎盂（腎的一部分，尿由此流入輸尿管）的炎症。常爲細菌感染所致，後者可由任何使尿流阻塞的疾病引起。病人有腰痛、寒戰、高熱。治療爲給予適宜的抗生素、鎮痛劑或大量飲水。腎盂以下的尿路系統的任何異常均須解除，以防再發。

pyelocystitis *n.* inflammation of the renal pelvis and urinary bladder (*see* pyelitis, cystitis).

腎盂膀胱炎 腎盂和膀胱的炎症。

pyelogram *n.* *see* intravenous pyelogram, pyelography.

腎盂X線照片

pyelography (urography) *n.* X-ray examination of the kidneys using *radio-opaque contrast material. In *intravenous pyelography* (*excretion urography*) the contrast medium is injected into a vein and is concentrated and excreted by the kidneys (*see* intravenous pyelogram). In *retrograde pyelography*, fine catheters are passed up the ureter to the kidneys at *cystoscopy and contrast material is injected directly into the renal pelvis to allow X-ray examination. The X-ray pictures obtained from these procedures are called *pyelograms*.

腎盂X線造影術 應用造影劑做腎臟X線檢查。做經靜脉腎盂X線造影術（排泄性腎X線造影術）時造影劑注入靜脉內，然後在腎內濃集和排出。逆行性腎盂X線造影術是在膀胱鏡下將細導管向上經輸尿管送抵腎臟，直接向腎盂內注入造影劑，進行X線檢查。由此獲得的X線照片稱爲腎盂X線照片。

pyelolithotomy *n.* surgical removal of a stone from the kidney through an incision made in the pelvis of the kidney. The incision is usually made into the posterior surface of the pelvis (*posterior pyelotomy*) to gain access to the stone, which can then be lifted clear.

腎盂結石切除術 通過腎盂部所做的切口除去腎內結石的手術。切口通常做在腎盂後側表面（後側腎盂切開術），以便接近和除盡結石。

pyelonephritis *n.* bacterial infection of the kidney substance. In *acute pyelonephritis*, the patient has pain in the loins, a high temperature, and shivering fits. Treatment is by the administration of

腎盂腎炎 細菌所致的腎實質炎症。急性腎盂腎炎病人有腰部痛、高熱和寒顫發作。治療用相應的抗生素，同時須做全面泌尿

an appropriate antibiotic, and a full urological investigation is conducted to determine any underlying abnormality and prevent recurrence. In *chronic pyelonephritis*, the kidneys become small and scarred and kidney failure ensues. *Vesicoureteric reflux in childhood is one of the causes.

系統檢查，以發現任何潛在的異常，從而防止再發。在慢性腎盂腎炎，腎臟結疤縮小，最後發生腎衰竭。在兒童膀胱輸尿管尿液返流是腎盂炎發病原因之一。

pyeloplasty *n.* an operation to relieve obstruction at the junction of the pelvis kidney and the ureter. *See* hydronephrosis, Dietl's crisis.

腎盂成形術 解除腎盂和輸尿管接合部阻塞的手術。

pyelotomy *n.* surgical incision into the pelvis of the kidney. This operation is usually undertaken to remove a stone (*see* pyelolithotomy) but is also necessary when surgical drainage of the kidney is required by a catheter or tube.

腎盂切開術 手術切開腎盂。此術常用於除去結石，當用導管進行腎臟外科引流時也是必做的。

Pyemotes *n. see* Pediculoides.

蝨形蟎

pyg- (pygo-) *prefix denoting* the buttocks.

〔前綴〕 **臀**

pykno- *prefix denoting* thickness or density.

〔前綴〕 **濃厚，緻密**

pyknolepsy *n. Obsolete.* a very high frequency of *petit mal attacks.

癲癇小發作 廢用詞。頻度極高的癲癇小發作。

pyknosis *n.* the process in which the cell nucleus is thickened into a dense mass, which occurs when cells die. —**pyknotic** *adj.*

核固縮 細胞核濃縮爲高密度團塊的過程，發生於細胞死亡時。

pyl- (pyle-) *prefix denoting* the portal vein.

〔前綴〕 **門靜脉**

pylephlebitis (portal pyaemia) *n.* septic inflammation and thrombosis of the hepatic portal vein. This is a rare result of the spread of infection within the abdomen (as from appendicitis). The condition causes severe illness, with fever, liver abscesses, and *ascites. Treatment is by antibiotic drugs and surgical drainage of abscesses.

門靜脉炎（門靜脉膿血症） 肝門靜脉的敗血性炎症和血栓形成。爲腹腔內感染（如起源於闌尾炎）蔓延的罕見結果。病情嚴重，伴有發熱、肝膿腫和腹水。治療：使用抗菌藥物和膿腫外科引流。

pylethrombosis *n.* obstruction of the portal vein by a blood clot (*see* thrombosis). It can result from infection of

門靜脉血栓形成 門靜脉被血凝塊阻塞。可起自嬰兒臍部感染、門靜脉炎、

the umbilicus in infants, pylephlebitis, cirrhosis of the liver, and liver tumours. *Portal hypertension is a frequent result.

肝硬化和肝腫瘤。其常見結果爲門靜脉高壓。

pylor- (pyloro-) *prefix denoting* the pylorus. Example: *pyloroduodenal* (of the pylorus and duodenum).

〔前綴〕 **幽門** 例如幽門十二指腸的。

pylorectomy *n.* a surgical operation in which the muscular outlet of the stomach (*pylorus) is removed. *See* antrectomy, pyloroplasty.

幽門切除術 切除胃肌性出口部(幽門)的外科手術。

pyloric stenosis narrowing of the muscular outlet of the stomach (*pylorus). This causes delay in passage of the stomach contents to the duodenum, which leads to repeated vomiting (sometimes of food eaten more than 24 hours earlier), and sometimes visible distension and movement of the stomach. If the condition persists the patient loses weight, becomes dehydrated, and develops *alkalosis. *Congenital hypertrophic pyloric stenosis* occurs in babies about 10 to 14 days old (particularly boys) in which the thickened pyloric muscle can be felt as a nodule. Treatment is by the surgical operation of *pyloromyotomy (Ramstedt's operation). Recovery is usually complete and the condition does not recur. Pyloric stenosis in adults is caused either by a *peptic ulcer close to the pylorus or by a cancerous growth invading and obstructing the pylorus. Treatment is by surgical removal or bypass (*see* gastroenterostomy).

幽門狹窄 胃肌性出口部(幽門)狹窄。可引起胃內容物進入十二指腸延遲，從而導至反復嘔吐(有時可嘔出24小時以前進食的食物)，有時肉眼可見胃部膨隆和胃蠕動。如狹窄狀態持續存在，病人體重下降，脫水，出現鹼中毒。先天性肥大性幽門狹窄見於生後10～14天的嬰兒(男嬰居多)，肥厚的幽門肌觸診像一個結節。治療：做幽門肌切開術(臘姆斯提特手術)常可徹底恢復，不復發。成人幽門狹窄係由近幽門部胃潰瘍或癌生長侵襲並阻塞幽門所致。治療：外科切除或建立旁路。

pyloromyotomy (Ramstedt's operation) *n.* a surgical operation in which the muscle around the outlet of the stomach (pylorus) is divided down to the lining (mucosa) in order to relieve congenital *pyloric stenosis.

幽門肌切開術(臘姆斯提特手術) 將環繞胃出口部(幽門)的肌肉分離直達黏膜下以鬆解先天性幽門狹窄的外科手術。

pyloroplasty *n.* a surgical operation in which the outlet of the stomach (pylorus) is widened by a form of reconstruction. It is done to allow the contents of the stomach to pass more easily into the

幽門成形術 使胃出口部(幽門)擴大的外科重建手術。做此手術目的是使胃內容物易於進入十二指腸，特別是在做迷走神經

duodenum, particularly after *vagotomy to treat peptic ulcers (which would otherwise cause delay in gastric emptying). 切斷術治療消化性潰瘍後（因該手術又可使胃排空延遲）。

pylorospasm *n.* closure of the outlet of the stomach (pylorus) due to muscle spasm, leading to delay in the passage of stomach contents to the duodenum and vomiting. It is usually associated with duodenal or pyloric ulcers. **幽門痙攣** 胃出口（幽門）由於肌痙攣而關閉，導至胃內容物進入十二指腸延遲和發生嘔吐。通常與胃或十二指腸潰瘍同時存在。

pylorus *n.* the lower end of the *stomach, which leads to the duodenum. It terminates at a ring of muscle – the *pyloric sphincter* – which contracts to close the opening by which the stomach communicates with the duodenum. —**pyloric** *adj.* **幽門** 胃的下端，接連十二指腸。幽門末端爲一環形肌（幽門括約肌），此肌收縮時使胃與十二指腸相交通的開口關閉。

pyo- *prefix. see* py-. 〔前綴〕 **膿**

pyocele *n.* a swelling caused by an accumulation of pus in a part of the body. **膿性囊腫** 膿蓄積於身體局部形成的膿脹。

pyocolpos *n.* the presence of pus in the vagina. **陰道積膿** 陰道內有膿。

pyocyanin *n.* an antibiotic substance produced by the bacterium **Pseudomonas aeruginosa* and active principally against Gram-positive bacteria. **綠膿菌素** 綠膿桿菌產生的一種抗菌物質，主要抗革蘭陽性細菌。

pyoderma *n.* any infected skin disease in which pus is produced. **膿皮病** 任何有膿生成的感染性皮膚病。

pyogenic *adj.* causing the formation of pus. Pyogenic bacteria include *Staphylococcus aureus*, *Streptococcus hemolyticus*, and *Neisseria gonorrhoeae*. **生膿的** 引起膿生成的。例如生膿菌，包括金黃色葡萄球菌、溶血性鏈球菌和奈瑟淋球菌。

pyometra *n.* the presence of pus in the womb. **子宮積膿** 子宮內有膿。

pyometritis *n.* inflammation of the womb, with the formation of pus. **膿性子宮炎** 伴有膿生成的子宮炎症。

pyomyositis *n.* bacterial or fungal infection of a muscle resulting in painful inflammation. **膿性肌炎** 細菌或眞菌感染所致的肌肉痛性炎症。

pyonephrosis *n.* obstruction and infection of the kidney resulting in pus formation. A kidney stone is the usual **腎盂積膿** 腎的阻塞和感染導至膿生成。腎結石是阻塞的常見原因，腎因積

cause of the obstruction, and the kidney becomes distended by pus and destroyed by the inflammation, which extends into the kidney substance itself and sometimes into the surrounding tissues (*see* perinephritis). Treatment is urgent *nephrectomy under antibiotic cover.

膿而膨脹，並爲炎症所破壞，炎症向腎實質內擴展，有時可侵入腎周圍組織。治療：在抗生素控制下緊急施行腎切除術。

pyopneumothorax *n.* pus and gas or air in the *pleural cavity. The condition can arise if gas is produced by gas-forming bacteria as part of an *empyema or if air is introduced during attempts to drain the pus from an empyema. Alternatively a *hydropneumothorax may become infected.

膿氣胸 胸膜腔內有膿和氣體（或空氣）。當膿胸中的細菌爲產氣菌，或者從膿胸引流膿時導入了空氣，即可發生膿氣胸。此外，水氣胸也可因感染而變爲膿氣胸。

pyorrhoea *n.* a former name for *periodontal disease.

膿溢 牙周病的舊名。

pyosalpingitis *n.* inflammation of a Fallopian tube, with the formation of pus.

膿性輸卵管炎 伴有膿生成的輸卵管炎症。

pyosalpingo-oophoritis *n.* inflammation of an ovary and Fallopian tube, with the formation of pus.

膿性輸卵管卵巢炎 伴有膿生成的輸卵管和卵巢的炎症。

pyosalpinx *n.* the accumulation of pus in a Fallopian tube.

輸卵管積膿 輸卵管內有膿蓄積。

pyosis *n.* the formation and discharge of pus.

化膿 膿生成和排膿。

pyothorax *n. see* empyema.

膿胸

pyr- (pyro-) *prefix denoting* **1.** fire. **2.** a burning sensation. **3.** fever.

〔前綴〕 ①**炎** ②**燒灼感** ③**發熱**

pyramid *n.* **1.** one of the conical masses that make up the medulla of the *kidney, extending inwards from a base inside the cortex towards the pelvis of the kidney. **2.** one of the elongated bulging areas on the anterior surface of the *medulla oblongata in the brain, extending downwards to the spinal cord. **3.** one of the divisions of the vermis of the *cerebellum in the middle lobe. **4.** a protrusion of the medial wall of the vestibule of the middle ear.

錐體，圓錐 ①構成腎髓質的圓錐形團塊，基底在腎皮質下面，尖頂朝向腎盂。②延髓（向下延續到脊髓）前表面上的長形隆起區域。③小腦中央葉蚓部的一部分。④中耳前庭內側壁上的錐狀隆起。

pyramidal cell a type of neurone found in the *cerebral cortex, with a pyramid-shaped cell body, a branched dendrite extending from the apex towards the brain surface, several dendrites extending horizontally from the base, and an axon running in the white matter of the hemisphere (see illustration).

錐體細胞 存在於大腦皮質中的一類神經元。胞體呈錐體狀，一條樹突枝從尖頂發出，走向大腦表面，另有幾條樹突枝從基底水平向外伸展，一條軸突則在半球的白質內行進（見圖）。

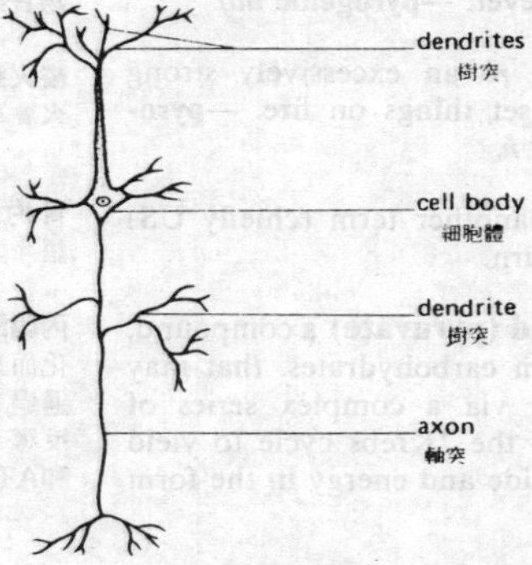

A pyramidal cell
錐體細胞

pyramidal system a collection of nerve tracts within the *pyramid of the medulla oblongata, en route from the cerebral cortex to the spinal cord. Within the pyramid fibres cross from one side of the brain to the opposite of the spinal cord; this is called the *decussation of the pyramids*.

錐體系統 由大腦皮質到脊髓，途經延髓，在延髓錐體內的神經束集合體。兩側的神經纖維在錐體內相互交叉，走向對側脊髓，稱爲錐體交叉。

pyrazinamide *n.* a drug administered by mouth, usually in combination with other drugs, to treat tuberculosis. Side-effects may include digestive upsets, joint pains, gout, fever, and rashes, and high doses may cause liver damage. Trade name: **Zinamide**.

吡嗪醯胺 一種口服藥，常與其它藥合用以治療結核病。副作用爲胃腸紊亂、關節痛、痛風、發熱和皮疹，大劑量可引起肝損害。

pyret- (pyreto-) *prefix denoting* fever.

〔前綴〕 **發熱**

pyrexia *n. see* fever.

發熱

pyridoxal phosphate a derivative of vitamin B_6 that is an important *coenzyme in certain reactions of amino-acid metabolism. *See* transamination.

磷酸吡哆醛 維生素B_6的衍生物。爲氨基酸代謝中某些反應的輔酶。

pyridoxine *n. see* vitamin B_6.

吡哆醇

pyrimidine *n.* a nitrogen-containing compound with a ring molecular structure. The commonest pyrimidines are cytosine, thymine, and uracil, which form the *nucleotides of nucleic acids.

嘧啶　一類帶單環分子結構的含氮化合物。最普通的嘧啶有胞嘧啶、胸腺嘧啶和尿嘧啶，三者參與生成核酸的核苷酸。

pyrogen *n.* any substance or agent producing fever. —**pyrogenic** *adj.*

致熱原　所有引起發熱的物質或因子。

pyromania *n.* an excessively strong impulse to set things on fire. —**pyromaniac** *adj.*, *n.*

縱火癖　十分强烈的想放火燒東西的衝動。

pyrosis *n.* another term (chiefly US) for *heartburn.

胃灼熱　燒心的另一術語。主要在美國使用。

pyruvic acid (pyruvate) a compound, derived from carbohydrates, that may be oxidized via a complex series of reactions in the *Krebs cycle to yield carbon dioxide and energy in the form of ATP.

丙酮酸　由碳水化合物衍化而來的一種化合物，可通過三羧酸循環中一系列反應，氧化生成二氧化碳和ATP形式的能量。

pyuria *n.* the presence of pus in the urine, making it cloudy. This is a sign of bacterial infection in the urinary tract.

膿尿　含膿的混濁尿。爲尿路細菌感染的現象之一。

Q

Q

Q fever an acute infectious disease of cattle, sheep, and goats that is caused by a *rickettsia, *Coxiella burnetti*, and can be transmitted to man primarily through contaminated unpasteurized milk. The disease lasts about two weeks and causes fever, severe headache, and respiratory problems. Treatment with tetracyclines or chloramphenicol is effective. *See also* typhus.

Q熱　一種由伯特納氏立克次體引起的牛、羊和山羊的急性傳染病。主要通過汚染的未經消毒的牛奶傳染給人。此病持續約兩周，可引起發熱、劇烈頭痛和呼吸道症狀。用四環素或氯黴素治療有效。

quadrantanopia *n.* absence or loss of one quarter of the *visual field (i.e. upper nasal (inner), upper temporal

象限盲　四分之一視野區（上鼻側、上顳側、下鼻側或下顳側）缺損或喪

(outer), lower nasal (inner), or lower temporal (outer)). In *homonymous quadrantanopia* the same quarter is lost in the field of vision of each eye.

失。同向性象限盲時，兩眼相同的四分之一視野喪失。

quadrate lobe one of the lobes of the *liver.

肝方葉 肝臟的一葉。

quadratus *n.* any of various four-sided muscles. The *quadratus femoris* is a flat muscle at the head of the femur, responsible for lateral rotation of the thigh.

方肌 四邊形的肌肉，股方肌是股骨頭上的一塊扁平肌肉，司大腿的外旋。

quadri- *prefix denoting* four. Example: *quadrilateral* (having four sides).

〔前綴〕 **四** 例如：四邊形（有四個邊）。

quadriceps *n.* one of the great extensor muscles of the legs. It is situated in the thigh and is subdivided into four distinct portions: the *rectus femoris* (which also flexes the thigh), *vastus lateralis*, *vastus medialis*, and *vastus intermedius* (see illustration).

四頭肌 下肢大的伸肌之一，位於大腿，分爲四個不同部分：股直肌（亦可使大腿彎曲），股外肌，股內肌和股中間肌（見圖）。

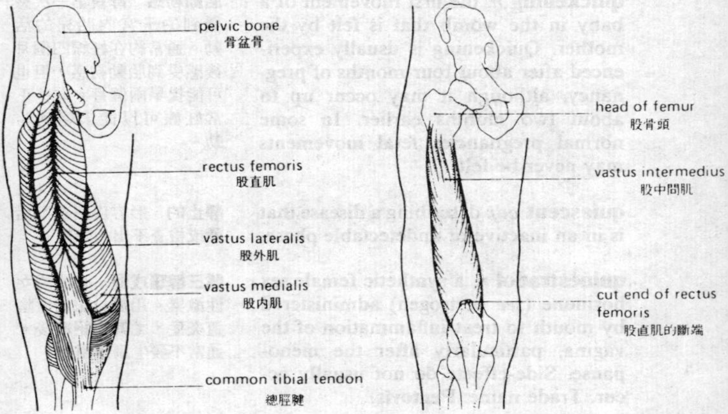

Components of the quadriceps femoris
四頭肌的組成

quadripara *n.* a woman who has been pregnant at least four times and who has given birth to an infant capable of survival after each of four pregnancies.

產$_4$ 至少有四次妊娠的婦女，且每次妊娠皆分娩出一個能存活的嬰兒。

quadriplegia (tetraplegia) *n.* paralysis affecting all four limbs. —**quadriplegic** *adj.*, *n.*

四肢麻痹（四肢癱） 累及四個肢體的麻痹。

quarantine *n.* the period for which a person (or animal) is kept in isolation to prevent the spread of a contagious disease. The original quarantine was a period of 40 days, but different diseases now have different quarantine periods.

檢疫期 爲防止傳染病的播散而將人（或動物）隔離的期限。原定檢疫期爲40天，但現在不同的疾病有不同的檢疫期限。

quartan fever *see* malaria.

三日瘧

Queckenstedt test a part of the routine *lumbar puncture procedure. It is used to determine whether or not the flow of cerebrospinal fluid is blocked in the spinal canal.

奎肯斯提特氏試驗 腰椎穿刺常規操作的一部分。用於測定椎管內腦脊液流動是否有阻塞。

quellung reaction a reaction in which antibodies against the bacterium *Streptococcus pneumoniae* combine with the bacterial capsule, which becomes swollen and visible to light microscopy.

莢膜腫脹反應 對具有細菌莢膜的肺炎鏈球菌產生的抗體反應。此時莢膜腫脹，在光學顯微鏡檢查時可見到。

quickening *n.* the first movement of a baby in the womb that is felt by the mother. Quickening is usually experienced after about four months of pregnancy, although it may occur up to about two months earlier. In some normal pregnancies fetal movements may never be felt.

胎動初感 母親第一次感覺到的子宮內胎兒的活動。通常約在妊娠四個月後感受到胎動初感，但也可能提早兩個月。有些正常妊娠可以從未感到胎動。

quiescent *adj.* describing a disease that is in an inactive or undetectable phase.

靜止的 形容疾病在不活動或檢查不出的時期。

quinestradol *n.* a synthetic female sex hormone (*see* oestrogen) administered by mouth to treat inflammation of the vagina, particularly after the menopause. Side-effects do not usually occur. Trade name: **Pentovis**.

雌三醇環戊醚 合成的女性激素。用於口服治療陰道炎症，尤其在絕經後。通常不發生副作用。

quinestrol *n.* a synthetic female sex hormone (*see* oestrogen) used to inhibit lactation in mothers not breast feeding. It is administered by mouth; side-effects are uncommon, though nausea and vomiting sometimes occur. Trade name: **Estrovis**.

炔雌醚 合成的女性激素。用於抑制斷奶的母親的泌乳。口服，副作用罕見，有時發生噁心與嘔吐。

quinidine *n.* a drug that slows down the activity of the heart and is administered by mouth to control abnormal and increased heart rhythm. Digestive upsets and symptoms of *cinchonism may occur as side-effects. Trade names: **Kinidin, Natisedine, Quinicardine.**

奎尼丁 減慢心臟活動的藥物。口服。用以控制心臟節律異常和增快。可能發生的副作用有消化道不適和金鷄鈉中毒的症狀。

quinine *n.* a drug formerly used to prevent and treat *malaria, now largely replaced by more effective less toxic drugs. It is administered by mouth or injection; large doses can cause severe poisoning, symptoms of which include headache, fever, vomiting, confusion and damage to the eyes and ears (*see* cinchonism).

奎寧 過去用於治療和預防瘧疾的藥物。現基本上已被毒性小且更有效的藥替代。口服或注射。大劑量可引起嚴重中毒，其症狀有頭痛、發熱、嘔吐、精神錯亂以及眼和耳的損傷。

quinism *n.* the symptoms of overdosage or too prolonged treatment with quinine. *See* cinchonism.

奎寧中毒 由於奎寧治療用藥過量或時間過長引起的症狀。

quinsy *n.* a pus-filled swelling in the soft palate around the tonsil: a complication of *tonsillitis. The patient has great difficulty in swallowing and surgical incision of the abscess may be necessary to release the collection of pus. Medical name: **peritonsillar abscess.**

扁桃體周膿腫 扁桃體炎的併發症，在扁桃體周圍軟腭內的化膿性腫脹。病人吞嚥十分困難，爲了排膿可能需要手術切開膿腫。

quotidian fever *see* malaria.

每日熱

R

R

rabbit fever *see* tularaemia.

兔熱病

rabies (hydrophobia) *n.* an acute virus disease of the central nervous system that affects all warm-blooded animals and is usually transmitted to man by a bite from an infected dog. Symptoms appear after an incubation period ranging from 10 days to over a year and include malaise, fever, difficulty in breathing, salivation, periods of intense excitement, and painful muscle spasms of the throat induced by swal-

狂犬病（恐水病） 一種中樞神經系統的急性病毒性疾病，所有溫血動物都能受累。通常是通過感染的狗咬後傳染給人。在潛伏期（10天至1年以上）後出現症狀：有全身不適、發熱、呼吸困難、流涎，有一段時間高度興奮，以及因吞嚥引起咽部痛性肌肉痙攣。疾病後

lowing. In the later stages of the disease the mere sight of water induces convulsions and paralysis; death occurs within 4–5 days.
Daily injections of rabies vaccine, together with an injection of rabies antiserum, may prevent the disease from developing in a person bitten by an infected animal. —**rabid** *adj.*

期，一旦看見水就會引起驚厥和痲痹，4～5天內死亡。每日注射狂犬病疫苗，同時注射狂犬病抗血清可以防止被感染的動物咬傷者發病。

racemose *adj.* resembling a bunch of grapes. The term is applied particularly to a compound gland the secretory part of which consists of a number of small sacs.

葡萄狀的 似一串葡萄。此詞特別用於形容其分泌部分有許多小囊腔組成的複腺。

rachi- (rachio-) *prefix denoting* the spine.

〔前綴〕 **脊柱**

rachianaesthesia *n.* *spinal anaesthesia.

脊髓麻醉

rachiotomy *n. see* laminectomy.

脊柱切開術

rachis *n. see* backbone.

脊柱

rachischisis *n. see* spina bifida.

脊柱裂

rachitic *adj.* afflicted with rickets.

佝僂病的 患有佝僂病的

rad *n.* a former unit of absorbed dose of ionizing radiation. It has been replaced by the *gray.

拉德 以往應用的離子放射吸收劑量單位，現以戈〔瑞〕代替。

radial *adj.* relating to or associated with the radius (a bone in the forearm).

橈骨的 指與橈骨（前臂的一根骨）有關的。

radial artery a branch of the brachial artery, beginning at the elbow and passing superficially down the forearm to the styloid process of the radius at the wrist. It then winds around the wrist and enters the palm of the hand, sending out branches to the fingers.

橈動脉 肱動脉的分支。起始於肘部，通過前臂的表面往下達腕部橈骨的莖突，繞過腕部並伸入手掌，分出分支到手指。

radial nerve an important mixed sensory and motor nerve of the arm, forming the largest branch of the *brachial plexus. It extends downwards behind the humerus, supplying muscles of the upper arm, to the elbow, which it supplies with branches, and then runs parallel with the radius. It supplies sensory branches to the base of the

橈神經 臂部重要的感覺和運動混合性神經。爲臂叢的粗大分支，在肱骨後方下行，支配上臂肌肉，向肘部發出分支，過肘部後與橈骨平行走行，並以感覺分支分布於拇指根部和手背側的一小部分。

thumb and a small area of the back of the hand.

radial reflex flexion of the forearm (and sometimes also of the fingers) that occurs when the lower end of the radius is tapped. It is due to contraction of the brachioradialis muscle, which is stimulated by tapping its point of insertion in the radius.

橈反射 敲打橈骨下端時引起的前臂屈曲（有時手指亦屈曲）。這是由於敲打肱橈肌在橈骨的附着點，使肱橈肌興奮而引起收縮所致。

radiation *n.* energy in the form of waves or particles, especially *electromagnetic radiation*, which includes (in order of increasing wavelength), *gamma rays, *X-rays, *ultraviolet rays, visible light, and infrared rays (radiant heat), and the particles.

輻射 以波或粒子形式發出的能量。尤指電磁輻射，它包括（按波長遞增的順序）γ 射線、X 射線、紫外線、可見光、紅外線（輻射熱）以及粒子等。

radiation sickness any acute illness caused by exposure to rays emitted by radioactive substances, e.g. X-rays or gamma rays. Very high doses cause death within hours from destructive lesions of the central nervous system. Lower doses, which may still prove fatal, cause immediate symptoms of nausea, vomiting, and diarrhoea followed after a week or more by bleeding and other symptoms of damage to the bone marrow, loss of hair, and bloody diarrhoea.

放射性疾病 由於放射性物質的射線（如 α 射線或 γ 射線）照射引起的急性病。極大劑量時可由於中樞神經系統毀壞性病變，在幾小時內引起死亡。小劑量也可以致死，可立即引起噁心、嘔吐和腹瀉，然後在一周後出現血和骨髓受損的其他症狀，以及毛髮脫落和便血。

radical treatment vigorous treatment that aims at the complete cure of a disease rather than the mere relief of symptoms. *Compare* conservative treatment.

根治療法 能幫助疾病完全痊癒的強有力的治療，而不只是緩解症狀。

radicle *n.* (in anatomy) **1.** a small *root. **2.** the initial fibre of a nerve or the origin of a vein. —**radicular** *adj.*

根 （解剖學）①細小的根。 ②神經起始部的纖維或靜脉的起端。

radiculitis *n.* inflammation of the root of a nerve. *See* polyradiculitis.

脊神經根炎 神經根發炎。

radio- *prefix denoting* **1.** radiation. **2.** radioactive substances.

〔前綴〕①**輻射** ②**放射性物質**

radioactivity *n.* disintegration of the nuclei of certain elements, with the emission of energy in the form of alpha, beta, or gamma rays. As particles are

放射性 某些元素的核蛻變時放射的呈 α 、β 或 γ 射線的能量。元素在發射出粒子時就衰變爲另一種

emitted the elements 'decay' into other elements. Naturally radioactive elements include radium and uranium. There are many artificially produced isotopes, including iodine-131 and cobalt-60, which are used in radiotherapy. *See* radioisotope. —**radioactive** *adj.*

元素。天然的放射性元素有鐳和鈾。現在有許多人工生產的同位素，如^{131}碘和^{60}鈷，可被應用於放射治療。

radioautography *n. see* autoradiography.

自體放射照像術

radiodermatitis *n.* inflammation of the skin after its exposure to ionizing radiation. This may occur after a short dose of heavy radiation (radiotherapy or atomic explosions) or to prolonged exposure to small doses, as may happen accidentally to X-ray workers. The skin becomes dry, hairless, and atrophied, losing its colouring. Infection is common.

放射性皮炎 放射性離子照射後的皮膚炎症，可以發生於短時間重照射後（放射治療或原子爆炸），或長時間的小劑量照射後，例如，偶可發生於X線工作者。皮膚變乾燥，無毛和萎縮、脫色，常發生感染。

radiograph *n.* an image produced on a film by X-rays: an X-ray picture. *See* radiography.

放射照片 由X線在膠片上構成的影像：X線像片。

radiographer *n.* a person trained in the technique of taking X-ray pictures of parts of the body. *See* radiography.

放射照像技術員 經過訓練的拍照人體各部X線像片的技術人員。

radiography *n.* the technique of examining the body by directing *X-rays through it to produce images (*radiographs*) on photographic plates or fluorescent screens. Radiography is used in the diagnosis of such disorders as broken bones, gastric ulcers, and stones in the gall bladder or kidney, when inspection from outside the body is insufficient for diagnosis. It is also widely used in dentistry for detecting dental caries, periodontal disease, periapical disease, the presence and position of unerupted teeth, and disease of the jaws.

放射照像術 用X線透射人體，在照像底板或熒光屏上形成影像的檢查技術。放射照像術用於當體外的檢查不足以作出診斷時，例如用於診斷骨折、胃潰瘍、膽囊結石或腎結石等疾病時，也廣泛用於口腔科檢查齲齒、牙周病、根尖周圍病變、有無未長出的牙齒和其位置以及頜骨病變。

radioimmunoassay *n.* the technique of using radioactive *tracers to determine the levels of particular antibodies in the blood. For example, radioactive iodine may be used to 'label' the hormone insulin. In some diabetic pa-

放射免疫測定法 應用放射性示踪劑測定血中特殊抗體的技術。例如，放射性碘可以用來"標記"胰島素。有些糖尿病患者胰島素可產生與它結合的抗

tients insulin provokes the formation of anti-insulin antibodies, which combine with the insulin. After the injection of the tracer insulin, samples of the patient's blood are analysed by *electrophoresis or *chromatography, and the antibody components of the blood are tested for the presence of radioactivity.

胰島素抗體，注射胰島素示踪劑後，用電泳法或色譜法來分析患者血標本，由於有放射性存在，就可測定血中抗體成分。

radioisotope *n.* an *isotope of an element that emits alpha, beta, or gamma radiation during its decay into another element. Artificial radioisotopes, produced by bombarding elements with beams of neutrons, are widely used in medicine as *tracers and as sources of radiation for the different techniques of *radiotherapy.

放射性同位素 一種元素的同位素。在其衰變爲另一種元素時可放射出α、β或γ射線。人工的放射性同位素是以中子流轟擊元素而產生的，在醫學上廣泛用作爲"示踪劑"和不同放射治療技術的放射源。

radiologist *n.* a doctor specialized in the interpretation of X-ray photographs for the diagnosis of disorders.

放射學家 專門從事分析X線片來診斷病變的醫師。

radiology *n.* the branch of medicine concerned with the use of radiation, including X-rays, and radioactive substances in the diagnosis and treatment of disease. *See also* radiotherapy. *Compare* radiography.

放射學 有關用X線和放射性物質診斷和治療疾病的醫學分科。

radionecrosis *n.* necrosis (death) of tissue, most commonly bone, whose ability to heal has been markedly reduced by radiotherapy for a tumour. It is easily induced by injury or surgery (such as tooth extraction) after irradiation.

放射性壞死 由於放射治療腫瘤引起的組織壞死，最常見於骨。治癒的可能性很小。容易於放射後由損傷或手術（如拔牙）引起。

radio-opaque *adj.* having the property of absorbing, and therefore being opaque to, X-rays. Radio-opaque materials, many of them containing iodine, are used as *contrast media in radiography (*see* diodone, iopanoic acid). Barium salts are also radio-opaque and used in barium 'meals' and enemas for the investigation of the digestive tract by X-rays.

不透X線的 具有吸收X線的特性所以X線不能透過的。許多含有碘的不透X線的物質作爲對比劑用於放射照像術。鋇鹽也是不透X線的，可在X線檢查消化道時用作鋇餐或鋇灌腸。

radio pill a capsule containing a miniature radio transmitter that can be swallowed by a patient. During its

放射性丸· 能被病人吞嚥的含有小型放射性傳遞器的膠囊。當通過消化道時

passage through the digestive tract it transmits information about internal conditions (acidity, etc.) that can be monitored by means of a radio receiver near the patient.

能傳遞關於內在情況（酸度等等）的信息，可被在病人身邊的放射性接受器所監測。

radioscopy *n.* examination of an X-ray image on a fluorescent screen (*see* fluoroscope).

X線透視檢查 在熒光屏前的X線影像檢查。

radiosensitive *adj.* describing certain forms of cancer cell that are particularly susceptible to radiation and are likely to be dealt with successfully by radiotherapy.

放射敏感的 描述某型癌細胞對放射線具有特殊敏感性和用放射療法時易治療成功的。

radiosensitizer *n.* a substance that increases the sensitivity of cells to radiation. The presence of oxygen and other compounds with a high affinity for electrons will increase radiosensitivity.

放射致敏物 使細胞對放射線敏感性增加的物質。對電子有高親和力的氧和其它化合物可增加放射敏感性。

radiotherapy *n.* the treatment of disease with penetrating radiation, such as X-rays, beta rays, or gamma rays, which may be produced by machines or given off by radioactive isotopes. Beams of radiation may be directed at a diseased part from a distance (*see* telecurietherapy), or radioactive material, in the form of needles, wires, or pellets, may be implanted in the body. Many forms of cancer are destroyed by radiation, the chief problem being the risk of damage to normal tissues.

放射治療 用機器或放射性同位素放出穿透性射線（X射線、β射線或γ射線）治療疾病。放射線束可經一段距離直接達病變部位，或者把放射性物質以針、導絲或小球形式埋植在體內。放射線可破壞多種癌瘤，主要的問題是有損害正常組織的危險性。

radium *n.* a radioactive metallic element that emits alpha and gamma rays during its decay into other elements. The gamma radiation is employed in *radiotherapy for the treatment of cancer. Because *radon, a radioactive gas, is released from radium, the metal must be enclosed in gas-tight containers during use. Radium is stored in lead-lined containers, which give protection from the radiation. Symbol: Ra. *See also* thorium-X.

鐳 爲一種放射金屬元素，在其衰變爲其它元素時放射α和γ射線。γ射線用在治療癌的放射療法中。由於鐳可釋放放射性氣體氡，故在應用期間必須包裝於密封氣體的容器內。鐳貯存於襯有鉛的容器內以防止放射線外射。符號：Ra。

radius *n.* the outer and shorter bone of the forearm (*compare* ulna). It partially

橈骨 爲前臂外側的短骨，它一部分圍繞尺骨，

revolves about the ulna, permitting *pronation and *supination of the hand. The head of the radius articulates with the *humerus. The lower end articulates both with the scaphoid and lunate bones of the *carpus (wrist) and with the ulna (via the *ulnar notch* on the side of the bone). —**radial** *adj.*

可以使手旋前和旋後。橈骨頭與肱骨相關節，下端與腕部舟狀骨和月狀骨相關節，並與尺骨相關節。

radix *n. see* root.

根

radon *n.* a radioactive gaseous element that is produced during the decay of *radium. Sealed in small capsules called *radon seeds*, it is used in *radiotherapy for the treatment of cancer. It emits alpha and gamma radiation. Symbol: Rn.

氡　鐳衰變過程中產生的放射性氣體元素。封存於小膠囊中叫"氡顆粒"，用於癌症的放射治療，它放射 α 與 γ 射線。

rale *n. see* crepitation.

囉音

Ramsay Hunt syndrome a form of *herpes zoster affecting the facial nerve, associated with facial paralysis and loss of taste. It also produces pain in the ear and other parts supplied by the nerve.

帶狀疱疹膝狀神經節綜合徵　一種侵犯面神經的帶狀疱疹，伴有面神經麻痹和味覺喪失。並可引起耳痛或由該神經支配的其他部位疼痛。

Ramstedt's operation *see* pyloromyotomy.

臘姆斯提特氏手術　先天幽門狹窄環狀肌切斷術。

ramus *n.* (*pl.* **rami**) **1.** a branch, especially of a nerve fibre or blood vessel. **2.** a thin process projecting from a bone, e.g. the rami of the *mandible.

①**分支**　指神經纖維或血管的分支。　②**支**　指從骨上突出的細小突起，例如下頜支。

randomized controlled trial *see* intervention study.

隨機性對照試驗

random sample a subgroup of a large population (the so-called *universe*) selected by a random process ensuring that each member of the universe has an equal chance of being included in the sample. It is sometimes *stratified* so that separate samples are drawn from each of several layers of the universe, usually on the basis of age, sex, and *social class.

隨機樣本　用隨機方法選擇的大組樣本（所謂總體）的一個分組，以確保總體的每個成員有同等的機會被選入樣本。有時採用分層抽樣。通常是根據年齡、性別和社會等級將單個樣本從總體的分層中抽出。

ranula *n.* a cyst found under the tongue, formed when the duct leading from a salivary or mucous gland is obstructed and distended.

舌下囊腫　唾液腺或黏液腺的導管阻塞和擴張形成的舌下囊腫。

raphe *n.* a line, ridge, seam, or crease in a tissue or organ, especially the line marking the junction of two embryologically distinct parts that have fused to form a single structure in the adult. For example, the *raphe of the tongue* is the furrow that passes down the centre of the dorsal surface of the tongue.

縫 組織或器官上的線、嵴、縫或皺褶，是指兩個在胚胎學上不同部分聯接的標誌線，而它在成人已融合成單一的結構。例如：舌縫是指通過舌背側正中的溝。

rarefaction *n.* thinning of bony tissue sufficient to cause decreased density of bone to X-rays, as in osteoarthritis.

疏鬆 骨組織變稀疏以致在X線上骨的密度減低，如在骨關節炎時。

rash *n.* a temporary eruption on the skin, usually typified by reddening – either discrete red spots or generalized reddening – and itching. A rash may be a local skin reaction or the outward sign of a disorder affecting the body. Rashes commonly occur with infectious diseases, such as chickenpox and measles.

皮疹 皮膚暫時性發疹，通常的特徵是發紅，可爲散在的紅斑點，也可爲全身性發紅和刺癢。皮疹可是局部皮膚的反應，或是體內病變的外表徵象。皮疹常發生於傳染病，如水痘和麻疹。

raspatory *n.* a filelike surgical instrument used for scraping the surface of bone (see illustration).

骨鋰 鋰刀樣的外科器械，用於刮鋰骨頭的表面（見圖）

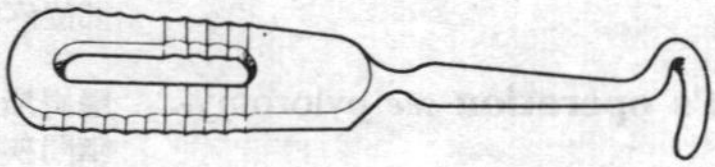

A rib raspatory
肋骨骨鋰

rat-bite fever (sodokosis) a disease, contracted from the bite of a rat, due to infection by either the bacterium *Spirillum minus*, which causes ulceration of the skin and recurrent fever, or by the fungus *Streptobacillus moniliformis*, which causes inflammation of the skin, muscular pains, and vomiting. Both infections respond well to penicillin.

鼠咬熱 由鼠咬引起的疾病。因鼠咬熱螺旋體菌感染所致，可引起皮膚潰瘍、反覆發熱。或是因念珠狀鏈球菌的眞菌所致，可引起皮膚炎症、肌肉疼痛和嘔吐。青霉素治療對兩種感染均有效。

rationalization *n.* (in psychiatry) the explanation of events or behaviour in terms that avoid giving the true reasons. For example, a patient may explain not going to a party in terms of being too tired whereas he did not go because he was afraid of meeting new people.

文飾 （精神病學）解釋某事情或行爲時避開講眞實原因的表現。例如：一病人解釋他不去參加晚會是由於他太疲乏，其實他不去的原因是怕遇見生人。

rauwolfia *n.* the dried root of the shrub *Rauwolfia serpentina*, which contains several alkaloids, including *reserpine. Rauwolfia and its alkaloids lower blood pressure and depress activity of the central nervous system. They were formerly used as tranquillizers in the treatment of mental illness but have been replaced by more effective and reliable drugs. Rauwolfia is still sometimes used to lower blood pressure.

蘿芙木 印度蘿芙木的乾根。含有數種生物鹼，如利血平。蘿芙木與其生物鹼可降血壓和抑制中樞神經系統活動。以往曾作爲安定藥物治療精神病，現已由更有效和可靠的藥物替代。但它仍被應用於降血壓。

Raynaud's disease a condition of unknown cause in which the arteries of the fingers are unduly reactive and enter spasm (*angiospasm* or *vasospasm*) when the hands are cold. This produces attacks of pallor, numbness, and discomfort in the fingers. A similar condition (*Raynaud's phenomenon*) may result from atherosclerosis, collagen diseases, ingestion of ergot derivatives, or the frequent use of vibrating tools. Gangrene or ulceration of the finger tips may result from lack of blood to the affected part. Warm gloves and antispasmodic drugs (such as phenoxybenzamine) may relieve the condition. In unresponsive cases *sympathectomy is of value.

雷諾氏病 一種原因不明的疾病，當手遇冷時，手指動脉過度反應和發生痙攣（血管痙攣），可引起手指陣發性蒼白、麻木和不適。動脉粥樣硬化、膠原病、攝入麥角衍生物，以及經常使用振動的工具也可引起類似病狀（雷諾氏現象）。因指尖缺血可引起壞疽或潰瘍。溫暖的手套和抗痙攣藥（如酚苄明）可緩解此症狀。對無效病例作交感神經切除術是有價值的。

reaction formation (in psychoanalysis) a *defence mechanism by which unacceptable unconscious ideas are replaced by the opposite conscious attitude. For instance, a man might make an ostentatious show of affection to a person for whom he has an unconscious hatred.

反應形成 （精神分析）一種防御機制，即潛意識的不能接受的想法被相反的有意識的態度所替代，例如：一個人對他在潛意識中憎恨的人可能做出誇大的愛慕表示。

reactive *adj.* describing mental illnesses that are precipitated by events in the psychological environment. For example, *reactive depression* is distinguished in this way from *endogenous depression.

反應性的 形容心理環境中的重大事件所促發的神經病。"反應性抑鬱症"就是在這方面與內原性抑鬱症有區別。

reagin *n.* a type of *antibody, formed against an allergen, that has special affinity for cell membranes and remains fixed in various tissues. Subse-

反應素 抗某種變應原的一種抗體，對細胞膜有特殊親和力，固定地留存在不同組織中。當以後再與

quent contact with the allergen causes damage to the tissue when the antigen-antibody reaction occurs. The damaged cells, particularly *mast cells, release histamine and serotonin, which are responsible for the local inflammation of an allergy or the very severe effects of anaphylactic shock (*see* anaphylaxis). Reagins belong to the IgE class of *immunoglobulins.

變應原接觸時，就發生抗原抗體反應引起組織損傷。損傷的細胞——特別是肥大細胞，釋放組織胺和5-羥色胺，引起局部的變態反應性炎症或過敏性休克等非常嚴重後果。反應素是屬於 Ig E 類的免疫球蛋白。

reamer *n.* an instrument used in *endodontics to prepare the walls of a root canal.

擴孔鑽 牙髓病時用來製備牙根管壁的工具。

receptaculum *n.* the dilated portion of a tubular anatomical part. The *receptaculum* (or *cisterna*) *chyli* is the dilated end of the *thoracic duct, into which lymph vessels from the lower limbs and intestines drain.

接受池 解剖學上管狀結構的擴張部分。乳糜池是指胸導管的擴張的終末端，下肢與腸道的淋巴管滙入其中。

receptor *n.* a cell or group of cells specialized to detect changes in the environment and trigger impulses in the sensory nervous system. All sensory nerve endings act as receptors, whether they simply detect touch, as in the skin, or chemical substances, as in the nose and tongue, or sound or light, as in the ear and eye. *See* exteroceptor, interoceptor, mechanoreceptor, proprioceptor.

感受器 能發覺環境中的改變和觸發感覺神經系統衝動的一個或一羣特異的細胞。所有感覺神經末稍都起類似感受器的作用，例如，在皮膚它們能感到觸覺，鼻與舌能感到化學物質，而耳和眼能感到聲音和光線。

recess *n.* (in anatomy) a hollow chamber or a depression in an organ or other part.

隱窩 （解剖學）器官或某部的凹窩或腔洞。

recessive *adj.* describing a gene (or its corresponding characteristic) whose effect is shown in the individual only when its *allele is the same. *Compare* dominant. —**recessive** *n.*

隱性的 形容一種基因（或它的相應特徵），這種基因的作用只有在等位基因相同的情況下才會在個體身上顯示出來。

recipient *n.* a person who receives something from a *donor, such as a blood transfusion or a kidney transplant.

受者 從供者接受某種物質者，例如輸血或腎臟移植。

record linkage the means by which information about health events from several different sources (e.g. hospital

聯鎖記錄 一種記錄方法，能將某人健康情況的幾個不同來源的信息（例

attendance, vaccination, and consultation with general practitioners) are all related to a specific individual in a common file or more usually a computerized record. This contrasts with data in which events only are recorded (*see* Hospital In-Patient Enquiry) and two separate individuals treated for the same disease cannot be distinguished from one individual treated on two separate occasions.

如：醫院的治療護理，預防注射情況，全科醫生的診治）歸併於一個共同的檔案內，或通常把記錄輸入計算機內。這與僅記錄事件的資料不同，在那種資料中不能將兩個人爲同一疾病接受治療的記錄與一個人分别兩次接受治療的記錄加以區别。

recrudescence *n.* a fresh outbreak of a disorder in a patient after a period during which its signs and symptoms had died down and recovery seemed to be taking place.

復發　病人在症狀體徵消失和似乎已康復後，經過一段時期，疾病又重新發作。

recruitment *n.* **1.** (in physiology) the phenomenon whereby an increase in the strength of a stimulus or repetition of the stimulus will stimulate increasing numbers of nerve cells to respond. **2.** the *loudness recruitment test*: a test of hearing used to distinguish deafness due to disease of the *cochlea (in the inner ear) from other causes of deafness. In cochlear deafness, while quiet sounds are heard with difficulty in the deaf ear compared with the normal one, louder sounds are heard equally well in both ears.

①**募集現象**（生理學）是指刺激强度的增加或重復刺激使更多的神經細胞受刺激而發生反應。②**復聽**　指高聲復聽試驗。一種常用於區别因耳蝸（內耳）病變引起的耳聾和其他原因的耳聾的聽力試驗。在耳蝸性耳聾時，聾側耳朵聽較輕的聲音比正常耳朵困難，較響的聲音兩耳聽得同樣清楚。

rect- (recto-) *prefix denoting* the rectum. Examples: *rectouterine* (relating to the rectum and womb); *rectovesical* (relating to the rectum and bladder).

〔前綴〕　**直腸**　例如：直腸子宮的，直腸膀胱的。

rectocele *n. see* proctocele.

直腸突出

rectosigmoid *n.* the region of the large intestine around the junction of the sigmoid colon and the rectum.

直腸乙狀結腸　在直腸與乙狀結腸連結附近的大腸部分。

rectum *n.* the terminal part of the large *intestine, about 12 cm long, which runs from the sigmoid colon to the anal canal. Faeces are stored in the rectum before defecation. —**rectal** *adj.*

直腸　大腸的終末部分，約12cm長。它始於乙狀結腸，下達肛門。在排便前糞便存於直腸。

rectus *n.* any of several straight muscles. The *rectus muscles of the orbit*

直肌　有以下幾種：眼眶的直肌是幾條眼外肌。腹

are some of the extrinsic *eye muscles. *Rectus abdominis* is a long flat muscle that extends bilaterally along the entire length of the front of the abdomen. The rectus muscles acting together serve to bend the trunk forwards; acting separately they bend the body sideways. The *rectus femoris* forms part of the *quadriceps.

直肌是沿整個腹前部兩側延伸的長而扁平的肌肉。兩條直肌共同起作用時可使軀體向前彎，一條直肌起作用時可使身體向側彎。股直肌是四頭肌的一部分。

recurrent *adj.* (in anatomy) describing a structure, such as a nerve or blood vessel, that turns back on its course, forming a loop.

回返的　（解剖學）形容一種結構如神經或血管在走行過程中折返回來形成的襻。

red blood cell *see* erythrocyte.

紅細胞

redia *n.* (*pl.* rediae) the third-stage larva of a parasitic *fluke. Rediae develop within the body of a freshwater snail and undergo a process of asexual reproduction, giving rise to many fourth-stage larvae called *cercariae. *See also* miracidium, sporocyst.

雷蚴　吸蟲類寄生蟲的第三期幼蟲。雷蚴在淡水的小螺體內發育，並進行無性生殖，產生許多第四期幼蟲，稱爲尾蚴。

reduction *n.* (in surgery) the restoration of a displaced part of the body to its normal position by manipulation or operation. The fragments of a broken bone are reduced before a splint is applied; a dislocated joint is reduced to its normal seating; or a hernia is reduced when the displaced organ or tissue is returned to its usual anatomical site.

復位術　（外科）通過手術操作將身體的錯位部分回復到正常位置。治療骨折時在用夾板前先行斷骨復位；疝氣被復位時，錯位的器官和組織就被回復至其平常的解剖位置。

reduction division the first division of *meiosis, in which the chromosome number is halved. The term is sometimes used as a synonym for the whole of meiosis.

減數分裂　性細胞成熟分裂的第一次分裂，此時染色體數減半。此術語有時用作整個成熟分裂的同義語。

reduplication *n.* doubling of the heart sounds, which may be heard in healthly individuals and shows variation with respiration due to the slightly asynchronous closure of the heart valves.

重疊音　可於健康人聽到的雙重心音，隨呼吸而變化，是由於心臟瓣膜的關閉輕度不同步所致。

reduviid *n.* any one of a group of winged insects (Reduviidae) whose mouthparts – adapted for piercing and sucking – take the form of a long

獵蝽　一組有翅的昆蟲（獵蝽科）。它的口部呈長喙狀，適於刺穿和吮吸，當不用時就卷藏在頭

proboscis that is tucked beneath the head when not in use. Some South American genera, notably *Panstrongylus*, *Rhodnius*, and *Triatoma* – the kissing bugs, are nocturnal bloodsucking insects that transmit the parasite causing *Chagas' disease in man.

的下部。有些南美種類，如錐蝽屬、紅獵蝽屬和獵蝽屬，是天然的吸血昆蟲，並將寄生蟲傳播給人引起恰加斯氏病（南美洲錐蟲病）。

Reduvius *n.* a genus of predatory bloodsucking reduviid bugs. *R. personatus*, widely distributed in Europe, normally preys upon insects but occasionally attacks man. Its bite causes various allergic symptoms, including rash (*see also* urticaria), nausea, and palpitations.

獵蝽屬 一屬食蟲的吸血昆蟲。廣泛分佈於歐洲的假裝獵蝽，通常捕食昆蟲類，但有時也侵襲人類。被咬後可引起各種過敏症狀，如皮疹、噁心或心悸。

referred pain (synalgia) pain felt in a part of the body other than where it might be expected. An abscess beneath the diaphragm, for example, may cause a referred pain in the shoulder area, while heart disorders may cause pain in the left arm and fingers. The confusion arises because sensory nerves from different parts of the body share common pathways when they reach the spinal cord.

牽涉性痛（連帶痛） 不是在病變的身體部位發生的疼痛感覺。例如：膈下膿腫可引起肩部牽涉性疼痛，心臟病可引起左臂和手指疼痛，引起這種感覺上錯亂的原因是由於身體不同部位的感覺神經經過共同的通路到達脊髓。

reflex *n.* an automatic or involuntary activity brought about by relatively simple nervous circuits, without consciousness being necessarily involved. Thus a painful stimulus such as a pinprick will bring about the reflex of withdrawing the finger before the brain has had time to send a message to the muscles involved. *See* conditioned reflex, patellar reflex, plantar reflex.

反射 由比較簡單的神經回路引起而不需意識參與的一種不隨意的自主性活動。例如針刺這樣的疼痛刺激，在大腦輸送信息到有關的肌肉之前就引起手指回縮反射。

reflex arc the nervous circuit involved in a *reflex, being at its simplest a sensory nerve with a receptor, linked at a synapse in the brain or spinal cord with a motor nerve, which supplies a muscle or gland (see illustration). In a simple reflex (such as the *patellar reflex) only two neurones may be involved, but in other reflexes there may be several *interneurones in the arc.

反射弧 參與一個反射的神經回路，其最簡單的是，一個連接感受器的感覺神經，與支配肌肉或腺體的運動神經在大腦或脊髓內形成突觸連接（見圖）。在一個簡單反射中（例如膝反射）可能有兩個神經元參加，但另一些反射的反射弧中可有幾個中間神經元。

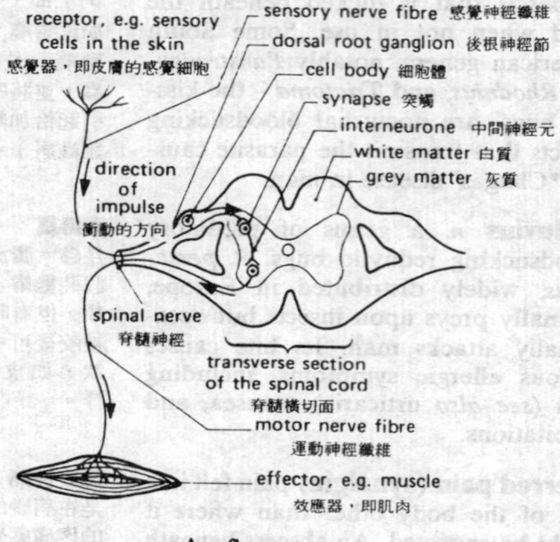

A reflex arc
反射弧

reflux *n.* a backflow of liquid, against its normal direction of movement. *See also* (reflux) oesophagitis, vesicoureteric reflux.

反流 液體的逆流，與其正常運動方向相反。

refraction *n.* **1.** the change in direction of light rays when they pass obliquely from one transparent medium to another, of a different density. Refraction occurs as light enters the eye, when it passes from air to the media of the eye, i.e. cornea, aqueous humour, lens, and vitreous humour, to come to a focus on the retina. Errors of refraction, in which light rays do not come to a focus on the retina due to defects in the refracting media or shape of the eyeball, include astigmatism and long- and short-sightedness. **2.** determination of the power of refraction of the eye. This gives the degree to which the eye differs from normal, which determines whether or not the patient needs glasses and, if so, how strong they should be.

①**折射** 當光線通過一個透明介質斜向射入另一個不同密度的介質時發生的光線方向改變。光線進入眼睛時發生折射，當它通過眼睛的介質，即角膜、眼房水、晶狀體和玻璃體，到達視網膜時，形成一個聚光點。屈光不正時，由於折射介質或眼球外形有缺損，光線不能在視網膜上形成聚光點，如散光、遠視和近視。 ②**驗光**眼睛折射力的測定。可以得知眼睛和正常相差的程度，並可測定患者是否需配眼鏡，以及眼鏡的度數。

refractometer *n. see* optometer.

屈光計

refractory *adj.* unresponsive: applied to a condition that fails to respond satisfactorily to a given treatment.

難治的 治療無效的，指治療未獲得滿意療效的狀況。

refractory period (in neurology) the time of recovery needed for a nerve cell that has just transmitted a nerve impulse or for a muscle fibre that has just contracted. During the refractory period a normal stimulus will not bring about excitation of the cell, which is undergoing *repolarization.

不應期 （神經病學）神經細胞剛傳遞神經衝動或肌肉纖維剛收縮後需要的復原時間。在不應期內，正常的刺激將不會引起正處於復極狀態的細胞興奮。

refrigeration *n.* lowering the temperature of a part of the body to reduce the metabolic activity of its tissues or to provide a local anaesthetic effect.

降溫 爲減少組織的代謝活動或產生局部麻醉作用而降低身體某部分的溫度。

regimen *n.* (in therapeutics) a prescribed systematic form of treatment, such as a diet, course of drugs, or special exercises, for curing disease or improving health.

治療（療養）方案 （治療學）爲治療疾病或改善健康而規定的系統治療方式，如膳食、藥物療程或特殊的鍛煉。

Regional Health Authority *see* National Health Service.

地區保健局

regional ileitis *see* Crohn's disease.

局限性回腸炎

Regional Manpower Committee *see* manpower committee.

地區人力委員會

Regional Medical Committee *see* medical committee.

地區醫學委員會

Regional Medical Officer *see* community physician.

地區主管醫師

registrar *n.* (in a hospital) an experienced physician or surgeon responsible for the care of a number of patients with the assistance of junior doctors, whom he instructs. A registrar may work with one or more senior surgeons, physicians, or *consultants.

副主任醫師 （醫院內）有經驗的內科醫師或外科醫師，他指導低年醫師作爲其助手，負責治療一定數量的病人。一個副主任醫師可與一個或更多的高年外科醫師、內科醫師或經治醫師共同工作。

regression *n.* **1.** (in psychiatry) reversion to a more immature level of functioning. The term may be applied to the state of a patient in hospital who becomes incontinent and demanding. It may also be applied to a single psychological function; for example, psychoanalysts speak of the *libido regressing to an early stage of development. **2.** the stage of a disease during which the

①**退化** （精神病學）倒退至較不成熟的功能水平。此術語可用於住院病人處於失控和要求過分的狀態，也可應用於單一的心理學功能方面，例如，精神分析學家所提到的性慾退化至早期發育的階段。 ②**消退** 疾病症狀與體徵消失，病人處於恢復時期。

signs and symptoms disappear and the patient recovers.

regurgitation *n.* **1.** the bringing up of undigested material from the stomach to the mouth (*see* vomiting). **2.** the flowing back of a liquid in a direction opposite to the normal one, as when blood surges back through a defective valve in the heart after the heart has contracted.

①**反胃** 不消化的食物從胃吐至口腔。 ②**回流** 液體向與正常相反的方向回流。如心臟收縮後，血液通過缺損的瓣膜向回流。

rehabilitation **1.** (in *physical medicine) the treatment of an ill, injured, or disabled patient by massage, electrotherapy, and graduated exercises to restore normal health and functions or to prevent the disability from getting worse. **2.** any means for restoring the independence of a patient after diseases or injury, including employment retraining.

康復 ①（理療學）用按摩、電療和逐漸鍛煉的方法治療疾病、外傷或殘疾人，使恢復正常的健康和功能，或預防因病情惡化而造成殘廢。 ②使病人於病後或外傷後恢復獨立生活的各種方法，包括就業的再訓練。

reimplant (replant) *vb.* to reinsert a tooth into its socket after its accidental or deliberate removal.

再植術 在意外掉牙或有意拔牙後將牙齒再植入牙槽內。

reinforcement *n.* (in psychology) the strengthening of a conditioned reflex (*see* conditioning). In classical conditioning this takes place when a conditioned stimulus is presented simultaneously with – or just before – the unconditioned stimulus. In operant conditioning it takes place when a pleasurable event (or *reinforcer*), such as a reward, follows immediately after some behaviour. The *reinforcement schedule* governs how often and when such behaviour is rewarded. Different schedules produce different effects on behaviour.

强化 （心理學）指條件反射的强化。在經典的條件反射中，當條件刺激與非條件刺激同時出現，或稍早一些出現時，就可發生强化。在操作式條件反射時，强化作用發生在緊跟某行動之後立即給以愉快的事物（或强化劑）時，例如給與獎賞。强化的方案規定對這些行為的獎賞次數和時間。不同的方案對行為產生不同的效應。

Reissner's membrane the membrane that separates the scala vestibuli and the scala media of the *cochlea of the ear.

前庭膜 將耳蝸前庭階和中階分隔的膜。

Reiter's syndrome a disease of men involving diarrhoea, inflammation of the urethra (*see* urethritis) and conjunctiva (*see* conjunctivitis), and arthritis.

萊特爾氏綜合徵 有腹瀉、尿道炎、結膜炎和關節炎的一種疾病。皮膚上可發生角化區。症狀和淋

Horny areas may develop on the skin. The symptoms resemble those of *gonorrhoea. No causative agent has been positively identified, although a virus may be implicated.

病相似。病因未能確定，但可能與病毒有關。

relapse *n.* a return of disease symptoms after recovery had apparently been achieved or the worsening of an apparently recovering patient's condition during the course of an illness.

復發 指疾病明顯痊癒後，症狀又重新發生，或者在疾病過程中病人情况明顯恢復時又惡化。

relapsing fever an infectious disease caused by bacteria of the genus *Borrelia*, which is transmitted by ticks or lice and results in recurrent fever. The first episode of fever occurs about a week after infection: it is accompanied by severe headache and aching muscles and joints and lasts 2–8 days. Subsequent attacks are milder and occur at intervals of 3–10 days; untreated, the attacks may continue for up to 12 weeks. Treatment with antibiotics, such as tetracycline or chloramphenicol, is effective.

回歸熱 包柔氏螺旋體屬細菌引起的傳染病，由壁蝨或蝨子傳播，並引起反復的發熱。第一次發熱大約發生於感染後一週，伴有頭痛、肌肉痛和關節痛，並持續2～8天。隨後的發作稍輕，間隔3～10天。若不治療，疾病可持續12週。用抗生素治療有效，如四環素或氯黴素。

relative analgesia a sedation technique, used particularly in dentistry, in which a mixture of *nitrous oxide and oxygen is given. The patient remains conscious throughout; the technique is used to supplement local anaesthesia in nervous patients.

相對止痛法 一種鎮靜方法，特别應用於牙科，即給與氧化亞氮和氧混合劑，病人始終保持意識清醒。此方法用於神經質病人，作爲局部麻醉的輔助手段。

relaxant *n.* an agent that reduces tension and strain, particularly in muscles (*see* muscle relaxant).

鬆弛劑 主要減輕肌肉緊張和勞損的一種藥物。

relaxation *n.* (in physiology) the diminution of tension in a muscle, which occurs when it ceases to contract: the state of a resting muscle.

鬆弛 （生理學）肌肉緊張的減輕，發生於肌肉收縮停止時：肌肉休息狀態。

relaxation therapy treatment by teaching a patient to decrease his anxiety by reducing the tone in his muscles. This can be used by itself to help people cope with stressful situations or as a part of *desensitization to specific fears.

鬆弛療法 教病人通過減低肌肉緊張度來減輕病人的憂慮。人們可以用此方法幫助自己對付緊張狀况，或者減少對特殊事物懼怕的敏感性。

relaxin *n.* a hormone, secreted by the placenta in the terminal stages of pregnancy, that causes the neck (cervix) of the womb to dilate and prepares the womb for the action of *oxytocin during labour.

弛緩素 妊娠末期胎盤所分泌的一種激素，它可使子宮頸擴張，並使子宮對分娩時催產素的作用有所準備。

reline *n.* the procedure by which the fitting surface of a denture is rebased to make it fit a jaw that has undergone resorption since the denture was originally made. The procedure is often necessary for dentures that were fitted immediately after extraction of the teeth.

托牙墊底術 一種牙科技術，將假牙的吻合面重新墊底，以便與原先假牙配成後又發生骨質吸收的頜骨相符合。對拔牙後立即安裝的假牙常需要這種技術。

rem *n.* roentgen equivalent man: a former unit dose of ionizing radiation equal to the dose that gives the same biological effect as that due to one roentgen of X-rays. The rem has been replaced by the *sievert.

雷姆 人體倫琴當量，是過去用的電離輻射單位，相等於一個倫琴X線所產生的同樣生物效應的劑量。雷姆現已被希〔沃特〕(SV)所代替。

REM rapid eye movement: describing a stage of *sleep during which the muscles of the eyeballs are in constant motion behind the eyelids. People woken up during this stage of sleep generally report that they were dreaming at the time.

眼球快速運動 描述睡眠的一個時相，此時眼球在眼瞼後不斷地運動。從該睡眠時相醒來的人往往訴說他們此時正在做夢。

remedial profession any profession (including occupational therapy, physiotherapy and speech therapy) in which the therapists use their skills to assist those with *handicap to achieve living and working standards as near normal as possible.

治療性職業 （包括職業性治療、理療和語言治療）治療學家用他們的技術去幫助殘疾人獲得盡可能近似正常的生活和工作水平。

remission *n.* a lessening in the severity of symptoms or their temporary disappearance during the course of an illness.

緩解 疾病過程中的症狀減輕或暫時消失。

remittent fever *see* fever.

弛張熱

Remploy *n.* (in Britain) a nationally financed system of sheltered employment for those with severe *handicap in specially designed workshops managed and financed by the Department of Employment. Limited numbers of able-bodied craftsmen are included on the

殘疾人就業保障 （在英國）由國家撥款保護嚴重殘疾人就業的制度。他們在專門設計的工場中就業，這種工場由就業部門管理和提供資金。為了幫助管理、監督和開展一些

payroll to assist with administration and supervision and also to carry out tasks that would be potentially dangerous for those with handicap. Goods produced (especially furniture and luggage) are sold on the open market.

對殘疾人可能有危險的工作，在就業人員中還包括有少數體格健全的手藝人。生產的產品（主要是家俱和皮箱）在公開市場上出售。

renal *adj.* relating to or affecting the kidneys.

腎的 與腎臟相關或影響腎臟的。

renal artery either of two large arteries arising from the abdominal aorta and supplying the kidneys. Each renal artery divides into an anterior and a posterior branch before entering the kidney.

腎動脉 來源於腹主動脉的供應腎臟的兩根大動脉，每一側腎動脉在入腎前分爲前支與後支。

renal cell carcinoma *see* hypernephroma.

腎細胞癌

renal tubule (uriniferous tubule) the fine tubular part of a *nephron, through which water and certain dissolved substances are reabsorbed back into the blood.

腎小管 腎單位的細管狀部分，水分與一些溶解的物質通過時被吸收入血液。

reni- (reno-) *prefix denoting* the kidney.

〔前綴〕 **腎〔臟〕**

renin *n.* a substance released into the blood by the kidney in response to stress. It reacts with a substrate from the liver to produce *angiotensin, which causes constriction of blood vessels and thus an increase in blood pressure. Excessive production of renin results in the syndrome of renal *hypertension.

腎素 腎臟對應激狀態起反應而釋放至血液的物質。它與肝臟產生的一種酶底物起反應而生成血管緊張素，後者引起血管收縮而增高血壓。腎素形成過多就會引起腎性高血壓綜合徵。

rennin *n.* an enzyme produced in the stomach that coagulates milk. It is secreted by the gastric glands in an inactive form, *prorennin*, which is activated by hydrochloric acid. Rennin converts caseinogen (milk protein) into insoluble casein in the presence of calcium ions. This ensures that the milk remains in the stomach, exposed to protein-digesting enzymes, for as long as possible. Rennin is present in the largest amounts in the stomachs of young mammals.

凝乳酶 一種在胃內產生的凝固牛乳的酶。胃腺分泌的是無活性的前凝乳酶，後者被鹽酸激活，在鈣離子參與下可使酪蛋白原（牛乳蛋白）轉換成不溶解的酪蛋白。這可保證牛乳在胃內停留，使其受蛋白消化酶作用的時間盡可能長些。在年輕的哺乳動物的胃內有大量的凝乳酶。

renography *n.* the radiological study of the kidneys by a *gamma camera

腎造影術 將某種在腎臟濃集和由腎排泄的放射性

following the intravenous injection of a radioactive substance, which is concentrated and excreted by the kidneys. The radioactive isotope (usually *technetium-131) emits gamma rays, which are recorded by the camera positioned over the kidneys. The resultant graph of each kidney gives information regarding function and rate of drainage.

物質由靜脉注射後，用γ照相機對腎臟進行放射學研究。放射性同位素（通常是[131]鍀）放射出γ射線，由位於腎臟上面的照像機記錄下來。對每個腎臟描繪的結果提供關於腎臟功能和排泄率的資料。

reovirus *n.* one of a group of small RNA-containing viruses that infect both respiratory and intestinal tracts without producing specific or serious diseases (and were therefore termed *r*espiratory *e*nteric *o*rphan viruses). *Compare* echovirus.

呼吸道腸道病毒 一組感染呼吸道和腸道含核糖核酸的小病毒。不引起特異性或嚴重的疾病（所以名爲呼吸道和腸道孤兒病毒）。

replacement bone a bone that is formed by replacing cartilage with bony material.

軟骨成骨 由軟骨被骨質取代而形成的骨。

replant *vb. see* reimplant.

再植入

replication *n.* the process by which *DNA makes copies of itself when the cell divides. The two strands of the DNA molecule unwind and each strand directs the synthesis of a new strand complementary to itself (see illustration).

複製 細胞分裂時脫氧核糖核酸自己複製的過程。脫氧核糖核酸分子的兩個鏈分開，每個鏈合成一個與自己互補的新鏈（見圖）。

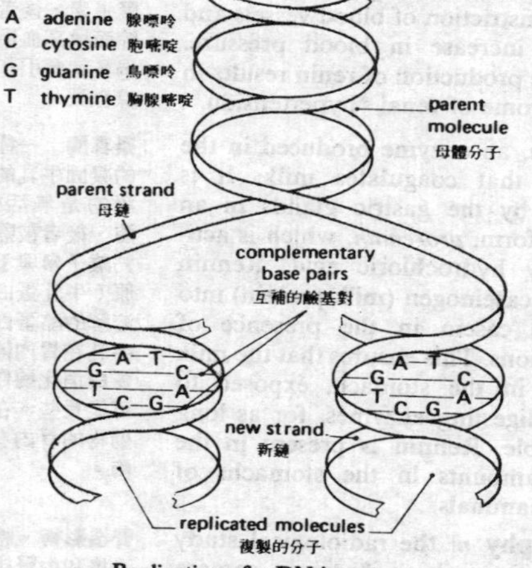

Replication of a DNA molecule
脫氧核糖核酸分子的複製

repolarization *n.* the process in which the membrane of a nerve cell returns to its normal electrically charged state after a nerve impulse has passed. During the passage of a nerve impulse a temporary change in the molecular structure of the membrane allows a surge of ions across the membrane (*see* action potential). During repolarization ions diffuse back to restore the charge and the nerve becomes ready to transmit further impulses. *See* refractory period.

復極化 神經衝動過後，神經細胞膜恢復正常帶電狀態的過程。在神經衝動通過期間，細胞膜分子結構有短暫的改變，可使大量離子通過細胞膜。在復極化時，離子向回擴散以恢復帶電，於是神經又為傳遞下一個衝動作好準備。

repositor *n.* an instrument used to return a displaced part of the body – for instance, a prolapsed womb – to its normal position.

復位器 用來恢復身體錯位部分的器械。例如將脫垂的子宮回復到正常位置。

repression *n.* (in *psychoanalysis) the process of excluding an unacceptable wish or an idea from conscious mental life. The repressed material continues to control behaviour and may give rise to symptoms. One goal of psychoanalysis is to return repressed material to conscious awareness so that it may be dealt with rationally.

壓抑 （精神分析）從有意識的精神生活中排除某種不能接受的願望和思想的過程。這種被壓抑的意識內容繼續控制行為，並可能引起症狀。精神分析的一個目的是將被壓抑的內容從潛意識回復到意識中，以便能合理地對待它。

reproduction rate *see* fertility rate.

生育率

reproductive system the combination of organs and tissues associated with

生殖系統 與生殖過程有關的器官和組織。男性有

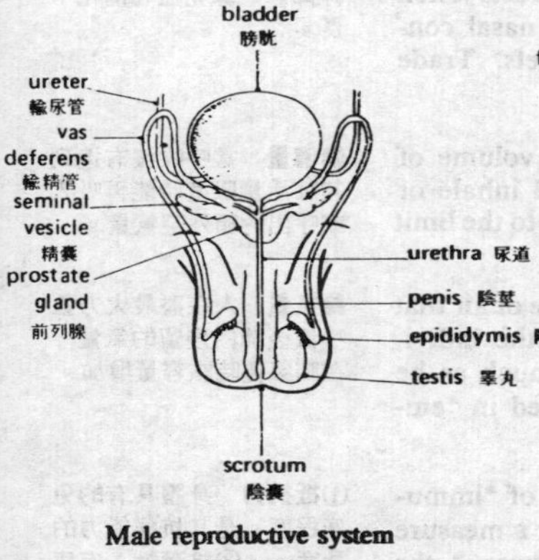

Male reproductive system
男性生殖系統

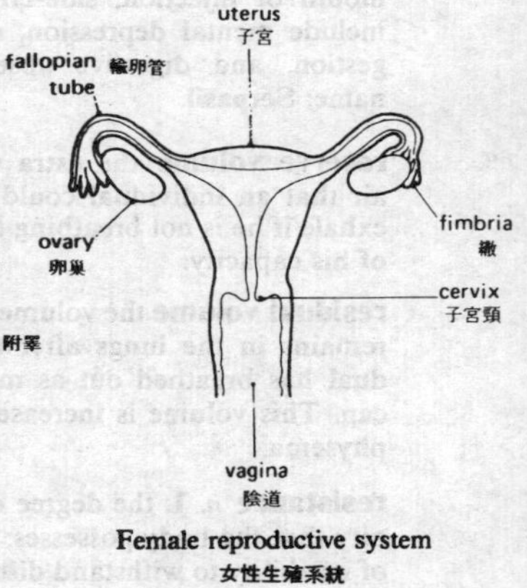

Female reproductive system
女性生殖系統

the process of reproduction. In males it includes the testes, vasa deferentia, prostate gland, seminal vesicles, urethra, and penis; in females it includes the ovaries, Fallopian tubes, womb (uterus), vagina, and vulva. (See illustration.)

睪丸、輸精管、前列腺、精囊、尿道和陰莖。女性包括有卵巢、輸卵管、子宮、陰道和外陰。（見圖）

resection *n.* surgical removal of a portion of any part of the body. For example, a section of diseased intestine may be removed and the healthy ends sewn together. A *submucous resection* is removal of part of the cartilage septum (central division) of the nose that has become deviated, usually by injury. *Transurethral resection* (*TUR*, *resection of the prostate*) – an operation performed when the prostate gland becomes enlarged – involves removal of the gland through the urethra using an instrument called a *resectoscope*.

切除術 將身體的任何一部分切除的手術。例如，可以將一段病變的腸管切除，將健康的末端互相縫合。黏膜下切除術，是將鼻中隔軟骨彎曲（通常由於損傷引起）部分切除的手術。經尿道切除術（前列腺切除術），是前列腺肥大時進行的一種手術，用一種叫作前列腺切除器的器械經尿道切除腺體。

resectoscope *n.* a type of surgical instrument (an *endoscope) used in resection of the prostate or in the removal of bladder tumours.

前列腺切除器 一種外科器械（一種內窺鏡），用於切除前列腺或切除膀胱腫瘤。

reserpine *n.* a drug extracted from *rauwolfia and used to lower high blood pressure and, occasionally, to relieve anxiety. It is administered by mouth or injection; side-effects often include mental depression, nasal congestion, and digestive upsets. Trade name: **Serpasil**.

利血平 從蘿芙木中提取的藥物，通常用於降血壓，有時用於減輕焦慮。口服或注射，副作用有精神抑鬱、鼻充血和消化不良。

reserve volume the extra volume of air that an individual could inhale or exhale if he is not breathing to the limit of his capacity.

儲備量 當呼吸沒有達到其肺活量限度時能再吸入或呼出的額外空氣量。

residual volume the volume of air that remains in the lungs after the individual has breathed out as much as he can. This volume is increased in *emphysema.

餘氣量 人在盡最大力量呼氣後肺內殘留的氣量，在肺氣腫時該容量增加。

resistance *n.* **1.** the degree of *immunity that the body possesses: a measure of its ability to withstand disease. **2.** the

①**抵抗力** 身體具有的免疫程度。是其抗病能力的量度。 ②**抗藥性** 疾病

degree to which a disease or disease-causing organism remains unaffected by antibiotics or other drugs.

或致病細菌不受抗生素或其它藥物影響的程度。

resolution *n.* **1.** the stage during which inflammation gradually disappears. **2.** the degree to which individual details can be distinguished by the eye, as through a *microscope.

①**消散** 炎症逐漸消失的階段。 ②**清晰度** 用肉眼和通過顯微鏡可辨別細微結構的程度。

resorcinol *n.* a drug that causes the skin to peel. It is applied to the skin in ointments to treat such conditions as acne, and used in hair lotions for dandruff. If the drug is absorbed into the body, it causes underactivity of the thyroid gland (myxoedema) and convulsions.

雷鎖辛 使皮膚脫皮的藥物，以軟膏用於皮膚治療（例如痤瘡），和用於治頭皮屑的頭髮洗劑。此藥若吸入人體內會引起甲狀腺功能低下（黏液水腫）和驚厥。

resorption *n.* loss of substance through physiological or pathological means.

吸收 物質通過生理或病理機制而消失。

respiration *n.* the process of gaseous exchange between an organism and its environment. This includes both *external respiration*, which involves *breathing, in which oxygen is taken up by the capillaries of the lung *alveoli and carbon dioxide is released from the blood, and *internal respiration*, during which oxygen is released to the tissues and carbon dioxide absorbed by the blood. Blood provides the transport medium for the gases between the lungs and tissue cells. In addition, it contains a pigment, *haemoglobin, with special affinity for oxygen. Once inside the cell oxygen is utilized in metabolic processes resulting in the production of energy (*see* ATP), water, and waste materials (including carbon dioxide). *See also* lung. —**respiratory** *adj.*

呼吸 機體與環境之間氣體交換的過程。有外呼吸和內呼吸。外呼吸時肺泡毛細管攝取氧，並將二氧化碳從血液中釋放出來。內呼吸時氧被釋放至組織，而二氧化碳被血液吸收。血液成爲了肺與組織細胞的氣體運輸介質。此外，它含有的色素（血紅蛋白）與氧有特殊的親和力。在產生能量、水和廢物（包括二氧化碳）的代謝過程中細胞內的氧就被利用。

respirator *n.* **1.** a device used to maintain the breathing movements of paralysed patients. In the *positive-pressure respirator* air is blown into the patient's lungs via a tube passed either through the mouth into the trachea or through a *tracheostomy. Air is released from the lungs when the pressure from the respirator is relaxed

①**呼吸器** 用於維持麻痹病人呼吸運動的裝置。用正壓呼吸器時，空氣吸入肺內是通過口腔或氣管切開經管子進入氣管。當呼吸器的壓力降低時，空氣就從肺排出。鐵肺是呼吸機的一種類型，病人除頭部外是關閉在一個不漏氣

The *iron lung* is a type of respirator in which the patient is enclosed, except for the head, in an airtight container in which the air pressure is decreased and increased mechanically. This draws air into and out of the lungs, through the normal air passages. The *cuirass respirator* works on a similar principle, but leaves the limbs free. 2. a face mask for administering oxygen or other gas or for filtering harmful fumes, dust, etc. *See also* artificial respiration.

的容器中，容器中空氣壓力機械地減壓和增壓，通過正常的氣道將空氣吸入肺內或從肺排出。胸甲式呼吸器的功能原則相似，只是肢體可以活動。 ② **呼吸罩** 用於吸氧或其他氣體的面罩，或用於過濾有害煙氣和灰塵。

respiratory distress syndrome (hyaline membrane disease) the condition of a newborn infant in which the lungs are imperfectly expanded. Initial inflation and normal expansion of the lungs requires the presence of a substance (*surfactant) that reduces the surface tension of the air sacs (alveoli). The condition is most common and serious among premature infants (especially between the 32nd and 37th weeks of gestation), in whom *surfactant is liable to be deficient. Breathing is rapid, laboured, and shallow, and microscopic examinations of lung tissue in fatal cases has revealed the presence of *hyaline material in the collapsed air sacs. The condition is treated by careful nursing, intravenous fluids, and oxygen, with or without positive pressure by a *respirator.

呼吸窘迫綜合徵（透明膜病變） 新生嬰兒肺未完全擴張的疾病。肺部最初的充氣和正常擴張需有表面活性物質存在，它能減低肺泡的表面張力。此綜合徵最常發生在早產嬰兒（尤其是在妊娠期第32週至37週之間），其病情也最嚴重，因爲在此時期容易缺乏表面活性物質。呼吸淺速而費力。顯微鏡檢查死亡病例的肺組織時，發現萎陷的肺泡中有透明物質。此症的治療是精心護理，靜脉輸液和給氧，可用正壓呼吸機。

respiratory quotient (RQ) the ratio of the volume of carbon dioxide transferred from the blood into the alveoli to the volume of oxygen absorbed into the alveoli. The RQ is usually about 0.8 because more oxygen is taken up than carbon dioxide excreted.

呼吸商 由血液向肺泡內運送的二氧化碳容積與吸收到肺泡內的氧氣容積之比。呼吸商（RQ）通常約爲0.8，因爲氧的攝取比二氧化碳排泄的多些。

respiratory syncytial virus (RSV) a paramyxovirus (*see* myxovirus) that causes infections of the nose and throat. It is a major cause of bronchiolitis and pneumonia in young children. In tissue

呼吸合胞體病毒 一種副黏病毒，可引起鼻與喉的感染。是少年兒童肺炎與細支氣管炎的主要病因。在病毒感染的組織培養

cultures infected with the virus, cells merge together to form a conglomerate (*syncytium*).

中，細胞融合在一起形成一團塊狀。

respiratory system the combination of organs and tissues associated with *breathing. It includes the nasal cavity, pharynx, larynx, trachea, bronchi, bronchioles, and lungs and also the diaphragm and other muscles associated with breathing movements.

呼吸系統 與呼吸有關的器官和組織的總稱，包括鼻腔、咽、喉、氣管、支氣管、細支氣管和肺，還有膈肌以及其他與呼吸運動有關的肌肉。

response *n.* the way in which the body or part of the body reacts to a *stimulus. For example, a nerve impulse may produce the response of a contraction in a muscle that the nerve supplies.

應答（反應） 身體或其一部分對刺激發生反應的方式。例如，某一神經衝動可以引起其所支配的肌肉收縮反應。

restiform body a thick bundle of nerve fibres that conveys impulses from tracts in the spinal cord to the cortex of the anterior and posterior lobes of the cerebellum.

繩狀體 一個粗的神經纖維束，可將衝動自脊髓束傳送至小腦前葉和後葉的皮層。

resting cell a cell that is not undergoing division. *See* interphase.

休止細胞 不進行分裂的細胞。

restoration *n.* (in dentistry) any type of dental *filling or *crown, which is aimed at restoring a tooth to its normal form, function, and appearance.

修復 （牙科學）各種類型的牙齒充填或裝冠，使牙齒恢復正常形狀、功能和外觀。

retainer *n.* (in dentistry) **1.** a component of a partial *denture that keeps it in place. **2.** an *orthodontic appliance that holds the teeth in position. **3.** a component of a *bridge that is fixed to a natural tooth.

①**固位體** （牙科學）局部托牙的一個組成部分，可使假牙保持適當位置。②**矯正器** 正畸的器械，使牙齒保持在適當位置。③固定在一個天然牙齒上的橋基的組成部分。

retardation *n.* the slowing up of a process. The term *mental retardation* is used as a synonym for mental *subnormality; it implies that the subnormality is regarded as a delay in development rather than a qualitative defect. *Psychomotor retardation* is a marked slowing down of activity and speech, which can reach a degree where a patient can no longer care for himself. It is a symptom of severe *depression.

遲緩 某一過程的減慢。術語“精神發育遲緩”是用作爲“精神低常”狀態的同義詞，它的含義是認爲低常狀態是由於發育上的延遲，而不是本質上的缺陷。“精神運動遲緩”是指活動和語言明顯的緩慢，可達到病人不再關心自己的程度。這是嚴重抑鬱症的一個症狀。

retching *n.* repeated unavailing attempts to vomit.

乾嘔 反復的無效的嘔吐企圖。

rete *n.* a network of blood vessels, nerve fibres, or other strands of interlacing tissue in the structure of an organ. The *rete testis* is a network of tubules conducting sperm from the seminiferous tubules of the *testis to the vasa efferentia.

網 一個器官結構中的血管、神經纖維的網絡，或者交織的索條，“睪丸網”是將精液從睪丸的細精管傳送至輸出小管的小管網絡。

retention *n.* inability to pass urine, which is retained in the bladder. The condition may be acute and painful or chronic and painless. The commonest cause is enlargement of the prostate gland in men, although many other conditions may result in obstruction of bladder outflow. Retention is relieved by catheter drainage of the bladder before dealing with the underlying problem.

瀦留 尿存留在膀胱而不能排出。這種狀況可以是急性的疼痛的，也可是慢性的無痛性的。最常見的原因是男子的前列腺肥大，也有許多其它情況可以引起膀胱排尿的阻塞。在處理其原發疾病之前，先作膀胱導尿以解除瀦留。

retention appliance *see* dental appliance.

固位矯正器械

retention defect (in psychology) a memory defect in which items that have been registered in the memory are lost from storage. It is a feature of *dementia.

記憶缺損 （精神病學）一種記憶力的缺失。在記憶中儲存的項目被遺忘，這是痴呆的特徵。

reticular activating system the system of nerve pathways in the brain concerned with the level of consciousness – from the states of sleep, drowsiness, and relaxation to full alertness and attention. The system integrates information from all of the senses and from the cerebrum and cerebellum and determines the overall activity of the brain and the autonomic nervous system and patterns of behaviour during waking and sleeping.

網狀激活系統 大腦內神經通道的系統，與意識水平有關：從睡眠、瞌睡和鬆弛狀態至完全警覺和注意狀態。這個系統把來自所有感覺和來自大腦與小腦的信息整合起來，並決定腦和自主神經系統總體的活動以及在清醒和睡眠期間的行爲方式。

reticular fibres microscopic, almost nonelastic, branching fibres of *connective tissue that join together to form a delicate supportive meshwork around blood vessels, muscle fibres, glands, nerves, etc. They are composed of a collagen-like protein (*reticulin*) and are

網狀纖維 顯微鏡下呈分支狀、幾乎沒有彈性的結締組織纖維。相互交聯，環繞於血管、肌肉纖維、腺體、神經等周圍，形成一個纖細的支持性網絡。它們是由類似膠原的蛋白

particularly common in lymph nodes, the spleen, liver, kidneys, and muscles.

（網硬蛋白）組成，特別多存在於淋巴結、脾臟、胃臟與肌肉。

reticular formation a network of nerve pathways and nuclei throughout the *brainstem, connecting motor and sensory nerves to and from the spinal cord, the cerebellum and the cerebrum, and the cranial nerves. It is estimated that a single neurone in this network may have synapses with as many as 25,000 other neurones.

網狀結構 神經通路和神經核所構成的網。它遍佈於腦中，連接通向和來自脊髓、小腦與大腦的運動和感覺神經以及顱神經，估計在這個網狀結構中，一個神經元可與25000個其它神經元形成突觸。

reticulin *n.* a protein that is the major constituent of *reticular fibres.

網硬蛋白 構成網狀纖維主要成分的一種蛋白。

reticulocyte *n.* an immature red blood cell (erythrocyte). Reticulocytes may be detected and counted by staining living red cells with certain basic dyes that result in the formation of a blue precipitate (*reticulum*) within the reticulocytes. They normally comprise about 1% of the total red cells and are increased (*reticulocytosis*) whenever the rate of red cell production increases.

網狀細胞 一種未成熟的紅細胞，可用某種鹼性染色劑使活的紅細胞染色的方法來測定和計數網狀細胞。此種染色可在網狀細胞內形成藍色沉淀（網狀組織）。約爲正常紅細胞總數的1%，每當紅細胞生成加速時，它就增加（網狀細胞增多）。

reticulocytosis *n.* an increase in the proportion of immature red blood cells (reticulocytes) in the bloodstream. It is a sign of increased output of new red cells from the bone marrow.

網狀細胞增多 血液中未成熟的紅細胞（網狀細胞）比例增多。這是骨髓新紅細胞生成增多的徵象。

reticuloendothelial system (RES) a community of cells – *phagocytes – spread throughout the body. It includes *macrophages and *monocytes. The RES is concerned with defence against microbial infection and with the removal of worn-out blood cells from the bloodstream. *See also* spleen.

網狀內皮系統 由吞噬細胞組成的體系，分佈於全身，包括巨噬細胞和單核細胞。網狀內皮系統與對細菌感染的抵抗力和清除血液中的衰老血細胞有關。

reticuloendotheliosis (histiocytosis X) *n.* overgrowth of cells of the *reticuloendothelial system, causing either isolated swelling of the bone marrow (*eosinophilic granuloma*) or destruction of the bones of the skull (*Hand-Schüller-Christian disease*). The most acute form, starting in infancy and usually rapidly fatal, is associated with tumours

網狀內皮組織增生（組織細胞增多症） 網狀內皮系統細胞的過度增生，既可引起骨髓弧立的腫脹（嗜酸性肉芽腫），也可導至顱骨的破壞（漢-許-克三氏病）。最多見的急性型（累-賽二氏病）發生於嬰兒，並往往迅速導

containing histiocytes in the internal organs (*Letterer-Siwe disease*).

至死亡，該病與內臟組織細胞腫瘤有關。

reticulosis *n.* abnormal overgrowth, usually malignant, of any of the cells of the lymphatic glands or the immune system. *See* lymphoma, Hodgkin's disease, Burkitt's tumour.

網狀細胞增多症　淋巴腺或免疫系統任何細胞的異常過度增多，往往是惡性的。

reticulum *n.* a network of tubules or blood vessels. *See* endoplasmic reticulum, sarcoplasmic reticulum.

網　小管或血管的網絡。

retin- (retino-) *prefix denoting* the retina. Example: *retinopexy* (fixation of a detached retina).

〔前綴〕 **視網膜**　例如視網膜固定術（使剝離的視網膜固定）。

retina *n.* the light-sensitive layer that lines the interior of the eye. The outer

視網膜　覆蓋於眼睛內部的感光層。視網膜的外側

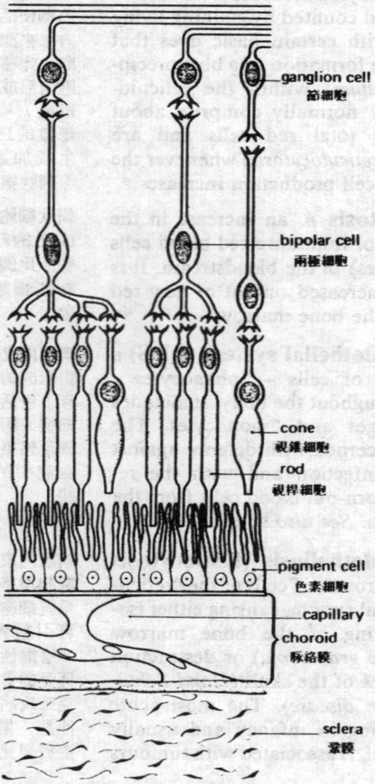

The structure of the retina

視網膜結構

part of the retina, next to the *choroid, is pigmented to prevent the passage of light. The inner part, next to the cavity of the eyeball, contains *rods and *cones (light-sensitive cells) and their associated nerve fibres (see illustration). A large number of cones is concentrated in a depression in the retina at the back of the eyeball called the *fovea. —**retinal** *adj.*

部分鄰接脉絡膜，有色素沉着可防止光線通過，靠眼球腔的內側部分含有視桿細胞和視錐細胞（感光細胞），它們與神經纖維相連（見圖），大量視錐細胞集中於眼球後部的視網膜凹陷處（稱之爲“凹”）。

retinaculum *n.* (*pl.* **retinacula**) a thickened band of tissue that serves to hold various tissues in place. For example, *flexor retinacula* are found over the flexor tendons in the wrist and ankle.

支持帶 使各種組織保持適當位置的一條粗帶。例如：位於腕和踝的屈肌腱的屈肌支持帶。

retinal (retinene) *n.* the aldehyde of retinol (*vitamin A). *See also* rhodopsin.

視黃醛（維生素A醛） 維生素A（視黃醇）的醛。

retinene *n. see* retinal.

維生素A醛

retinitis *n.* inflammation of the retina. In practice, the term is often used for conditions not strictly inflammatory; for example *retinitis pigmentosa*, a noninflammatory hereditary condition involving progressive degeneration of the retina. For such conditions the term *retinopathy is becoming more widely used.

視網膜炎 視網膜的炎症。實際上此術語並非常用於眞正的炎症。例如色素性視網膜炎，是進行性視網膜退變的非炎症遺傳性疾病。現在對這類情況更廣泛應用視網膜病這名詞。

retinoblastoma *n.* a rare malignant tumour of the retina, occurring in infants.

成視網膜細胞瘤 一種少見的發生於嬰兒的視網膜惡性腫瘤。

retinol *n. see* vitamin A.

視黃醇

retinopathy *n.* any disorder of the retina resulting in impairment or loss of vision. It is usually due to damage to the blood vessels of the retina, occurring (for example) as a complication of diabetes (*diabetic retinopathy*) or high blood pressure.

視網膜病 引起視力減弱或喪失的任何一種視網膜病變。常由於視網膜血管病變引起，如高血壓或糖尿病的併發症（糖尿病性視網膜病）。

retinoscope *n.* an instrument used to determine the power of *refraction of the eye. It is held in the hand and casts a beam of light into the subject's eye. The examiner looks along the beam and sees the shadows it produces in the

視網膜鏡 一種用於測定眼睛折光力的器械。用手持鏡，並投射一束光線到被檢者眼睛裏。檢查者沿着光束查看，可看到被檢者瞳孔內產生的光影，當

subject's pupil. By interpreting the way the shadows move when he moves the instrument, and by altering them by lenses held in his other hand near the subject's eye, he is able to detect long- or short-sightedness or astigmatism and to determine its degree. —**retinoscopy** *n.*

移動器械時光影也移動。觀察光影移動情況作出解釋，同時以另一手持鏡片改變光影，可以測出遠視、近視或散光，並能測出度數。

retraction *n.* **1.** (in obstetrics) the permanent shortening of the muscle fibres of the womb wall that occurs each time they contract during labour. **2.** (in dentistry) the drawing back of one or more teeth into a better position by an *orthodontic appliance.

縮回 ①（婦科）分娩期子宮每次收縮時，發生子宮壁肌纖維持久性的縮短。②（牙科）用正畸矯正器將一個或幾個牙齒縮回到較好的位置。

retraction ring 1. a depression on the surface of the womb that may be detected during labour by applying the hand to the lower part of the abdomen. It occurs in the region of the neck (cervix) of the womb when the circular muscle fibres fail to relax and it indicates the presence of a constriction around the womb, which tends to prevent the infant from emerging into the cervical canal. Also called: **Bandl's ring**. **2.** the dividing line between the upper contracting part of the womb in labour and the lower dilating part.

子宮收縮環 ①分娩期間用手放在下腹部可以觸知的子宮表面的凹陷。發生於子宮頸區環狀肌纖維不能鬆弛時，這提示子宮有一個縮窄圈，它往往阻止胎兒下降至子宮頸管，也稱"班都氏環" ②在分娩期間子宮上方收縮部分與下方擴張部分之間的界線。

retractor *n.* a surgical instrument used to expose the operation site by drawing aside the cut edges of skin, muscle, or other tissues. There are several types of retractors for different operations (see illustration).

牽開器 將切開的皮膚、肌肉或其他組織拉向旁邊，使手術部位暴露的外科器械。不同手術有幾種不同類型的牽開器（見圖）。

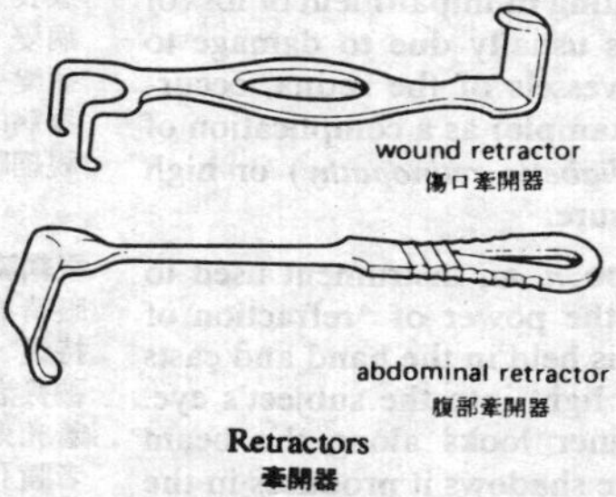

Retractors
牽開器

retro- *prefix denoting* at the back or behind. Examples: *retrobulbar* (at the back of the eyeball); *retroperitoneal* (behind the peritoneum).

〔前綴〕 **後** 例如球後（眼球的背後）、腹膜後（腹膜的後方）。

retrobulbar neuritis (optic neuritis) inflammation of the optic nerve behind the eye, causing increasingly blurred vision. When the inflammation involves the first part of the nerve and can be seen at the optic disc, it is called *optic papillitis*. Retrobulbar neuritis is one of the symptoms of multiple sclerosis but it can also occur as an isolated lesion, in the absence of any other involvement of the nervous system, with the patient recovering vision completely.

球後視神經炎（視神經炎） 眼睛後部視神經的炎症，引起進行性的視力模糊。當炎症侵犯神經的第一部分，並能在視乳頭看到時，稱爲視神經乳頭炎。球後視神經炎是多發性硬化症的症狀之一，但也可作爲單獨的病變發生，而無任何其它的神經系統病變，這種病人的視力可完全恢復。

retroflexion *n.* the bending backward of an organ or part of an organ, especially of the upper part of the womb (*uterine retroflexion*) in relation to the lower part (cervix).

後屈 指一個器官或器官的一部分向後彎曲，特別指子宮上部相對於子宮下部（子宮頸）的向後彎曲（子宮後屈）。

retrograde *adj.* going backwards, or moving in the opposite direction to the normal. (*See* (retrograde) pyelography.) *Retrograde amnesia* is a failure to remember events immediately preceding an illness or injury.

逆行的 向後或與正常相反的方向移動（見逆行腎盂造影）。逆行性遺忘是對患病或受傷前剛發生的事件失去記憶。

retropulsion *n.* a compulsive tendency to walk backwards. It is a symptom of *parkinsonism.

後退步態 一種强迫性向後走的傾向。是帕金森氏症的一種症狀。

retrospective study a backward-looking review of the characteristics of a group of individuals in relation to morbidity, embracing some aspects of *cross-sectional and/or *case control studies. The term is sometimes loosely used as a synonym for such studies.

回顧性研究 對一組人羣有關發病率特點的回顧性總結，包括一些正交設計的或病例對照方面的研究。此名詞有時廣義地作爲上述研究的同義詞。

retroversion *n.* the backward inclination of an organ, especially of the womb (*uterine retroversion*), when it is tipped back so that the neck (cervix) points towards the pubic symphysis (the bone under the pubic hair).

後傾 一個器官的向後傾斜。特指子宮（子宮後傾）向後傾斜，子宮頸朝向耻骨聯合（在陰毛下面的骨塊）。

retrovirus *n.* an RNA-containing virus that can transfer its genetic material

反轉病毒 一種含核糖核酸的病毒，能將遺傳物質

into the DNA of its host's cells. Retroviruses have been implicated in the development of some cancers.

轉移到其宿主細胞的脫氧核糖核酸中去。在有些癌病發生中有反轉病毒。

retrusion *n.* (in dentistry) **1.** backward movement of the lower jaw. **2.** a malocclusion in which some of the teeth are further back than usual. *Compare* protrusion.

後移 （牙科學）①下頜向後移。②錯位咬合，即有些牙齒比通常更向後。

rhabdomyoma *n.* a rare benign tumour of skeletal muscle or heart muscle.

橫紋肌瘤 骨骼肌或心肌的一種罕見的良性腫瘤。

rhabdomyosarcoma *n.* a malignant tumour originating in, or showing the characteristics of, striated muscle. *Pleomorphic rhabdomyosarcoma* occurs in late middle age, in the muscles of the limbs. *Embryonal rhabdomyosarcomas*, affecting infants, children, and young adults, are classified as *botryoid* (in the vagina, bladder, ear, etc.), *embryonal* (most common in the head and neck, particularly the orbit); and *alveolar* (at the base of the thumb). The pleomorphic and alveolar types respond poorly to treatment; botryoid tumours are treated with a combination of radiotherapy, surgery, and drugs. The embryonal type, if treated at an early stage, can often be cured with a combination of radiotherapy and drugs (including vincristine, actinomycin-D, and cyclophosphamide).

橫紋肌肉瘤 一種起源於橫紋肌或具有橫紋肌特徵的惡性腫瘤。多形性橫紋肌肉瘤發生於中晚年齡，在四肢肌肉。胚胎型橫紋肌肉瘤侵犯嬰兒，兒童及青年，可分爲葡萄簇狀的（在陰道、膀胱、耳等處），胚胎型的（最常見於頭、頸部，尤其是眼眶部），以及小泡狀的（在拇指的根部）。多形性的與小泡狀這兩型的治療效果差。葡萄簇狀的腫瘤可用放射治療、外科手術和藥物的聯合治療。若能在早期採取放射治療和藥物（如長春新鹼、放線菌素D和環磷醯胺）的聯合療法，則胚胎型的經常能治癒。

rhagades *pl. n.* cracks or long thin scars in the skin, particularly around the mouth or other areas of the body subjected to constant movement. The fissures around the mouth and nose of babies with congenital syphilis eventually heal to form rhagades.

皸裂 皮膚的裂口或細長的瘢痕，尤其發生在經常活動的口周和身體其他部位，先天性梅毒的嬰兒口鼻周圍的裂隙最後癒合而形成皸裂。

rheo- *prefix denoting* **1.** a flow of liquid. **2.** an electric current.

〔前綴〕 **①流動的液體 ②電流**

rhesus factor (Rh factor) a group of *antigens that may or may not be present on the surface of the red blood cells; it forms the basis of the rhesus blood group system. Most people have

Rh因子 可存在或不存在於紅細胞表面的一組抗原，它形成Rh血型系統的基礎，大多數人有Rh因子，即他們是Rh陽性

the rhesus factor, i.e. they are *Rh-positive*. People who lack the factor are termed *Rh-negative*. Incompatibility between Rh-positive and Rh-negative blood is an important cause of blood transfusion reactions and *haemolytic disease of the newborn. *See also* blood group.

者。無Rh因子者稱爲Rh陰性者。Rh陽性與Rh陰性血液的不相容性是輸血反應和新生兒溶血性疾病的一個重要原因。

rheumatic fever (acute rheumatism) a disease affecting mainly children and young adults that arises as a delayed complication of infection of the upper respiratory tract with haemolytic streptococci (*see* Streptococcus). The main features are fever, arthritis progressing from joint to joint, reddish circular patches on the skin, small painless nodules formed on bony prominences such as the elbow, abnormal involuntary movements of the limbs and head (*chorea), and inflammation of the membrane surrounding the heart. The condition may progress to *chronic rheumatic heart disease*, with scarring and chronic inflammation of the heart and its valves leading to heart failure, murmurs, and damage to the valves. The initial infection is treated with antibiotics (e.g. penicillin) and bed rest, with aspirin for the joint pain.

風濕熱(急性風濕病) 主要侵犯兒童與年輕人的疾病，起因是上呼吸道溶血性鏈球菌感染的遲發併發症。主要特徵是發熱、進行性游走性關節炎、皮膚環形紅斑，在骨的突出部位如肘部形成小的無痛性結節，肢體和頭部有異常的不自主活動(舞蹈病)，以及心包膜炎症。這種病變可以進展爲慢性風濕性心臟病，伴有心臟和其瓣膜的瘢痕形成和慢性炎症，導致心臟衰竭、雜音和瓣膜損害。最初感染時用抗生素(青黴素)治療，臥床休息和用阿司匹林治療關節疼痛。

rheumatism *n.* any disorder in which aches and pains affect the muscles and joints. *See* rheumatoid arthritis, rheumatic fever, osteoarthritis, gout.

風濕病 肌肉和關節受累而疼痛的病變。如類風濕性關節炎、骨關節炎、痛風。

rheumatoid arthritis a form of *arthritis that is the second most common rheumatic disease (after *osteoarthritis). It typically involves the joints of the fingers, wrists, feet, and ankles and often the hips and shoulders: the joints are affected symmetrically and there is a considerable range of severity. The condition is diagnosed by a blood test, which shows the presence of the *rheumatoid factor*, and by X-rays revealing typical changes (*rheumatoid erosions*) around the affected joints.

類風濕性關節炎 關節炎的一種類型，這是第二位常見的風濕性疾病(在骨關節炎之後)，典型的是侵犯指、腕、足、踝等關節，並常有髖和肩關節。關節的侵犯是對稱性的，並且其嚴重度很不相同。可通過查血診斷此病，血中有類風濕因子。X線可顯示受侵犯關節周圍有典型的改變(類風濕性侵蝕)。

A wide variety of treatments, usually based on anti-inflammatory analgesics, provide relief of symptoms. The condition may resolve spontaneously and often undergoes periods of remission of symptoms.

有廣泛多樣的治療方法，通常用消炎止痛藥，能使症狀減輕。此病可自發緩解，並常常有症狀緩解期。

rheumatology *n.* the medical specialty concerned with the diagnosis and management of disease involving joints, tendons, muscles, ligaments, and associated structures. *See also* physical medicine. —**rheumatologist** *n.*

風濕病學 關於診斷和治療關節、肌腱、肌肉、韌帶和有關結構疾病的醫學專業。

rhexis *n.* the breaking apart of a blood vessel, organ, or tissue.

破裂 血管、器官或組織的破碎分離。

Rh factor *see* rhesus factor.

Rh 因子

rhin- (rhino-) *prefix denoting* the nose.

〔前綴〕 **鼻**

rhinencephalon *n.* the parts of the brain, collectively, that in early stages of evolution were concerned mainly with the sense of smell. The rhinencephalon includes the olfactory nerve, olfactory tract, and the regions now usually classified as belonging to the *limbic system.

嗅腦 大腦的一部分，在發育早期主要與嗅覺有關。嗅腦包括嗅神經、嗅束和嗅區，後者現在分類歸於邊緣系統。

rhinitis *n.* inflammation of the mucous membrane of the nose. It may be caused by virus infection (*acute rhinitis*; *see* (common) cold) or an allergic reaction (*allergic rhinitis*; *see* hay fever). In *atrophic rhinitis* the mucous membrane becomes thinned and fragile; in *chronic catarrhal rhinitis* there is overgrowth of, and increased secretion by, the membrane.

鼻炎 鼻黏膜的炎症，可由病毒感染引起（急性鼻炎）或因變態反應所致（過敏性鼻炎），萎縮性鼻炎時鼻黏膜變薄和脆。慢性卡他性鼻炎時，鼻黏膜肥大並且分泌增加。

rhinolith *n.* a stone (calculus) in the nose.

鼻石 鼻內的結石。

rhinology *n.* the branch of medicine concerned with disorders of the nose and nasal passages.

鼻科學 關於鼻和鼻通道病變的醫學分支。

rhinomycosis *n.* fungal infection of the lining of the nose.

鼻眞菌病 鼻腔內的眞菌感染。

rhinophyma *n.* permanent redness and swelling of the nose. It commonly

肥大性酒皶鼻 鼻子持久性發紅和腫脹，常常與紅

occurs with *rosacea, in which the characteristic nodular swelling may produce grotesque deformity. Surgery may be necessary for cosmetic purposes.

斑痤瘡一起發生，有特徵性的小結節狀腫脹，可引起奇形怪狀的變形，為整容目的可能需要做手術。

rhinoplasty *n.* reparative or cosmetic surgery of the nose, sometimes by the repair of a defect with tissue (skin or bone) taken from elsewhere in the body.

鼻成形術 鼻部的修補或整容手術，有時從自體其他部位取組織（皮膚或骨）來修補缺損。

rhinorrhoea *n.* a persistent watery mucous discharge from the nose, as in the common cold.

鼻溢 鼻腔持續地流出稀薄的黏液，如發生在感冒時。

rhinoscleroma *n.* the formation of nodules in the interior of the nose and *nasopharynx, which become thickened. It is caused by bacterial infection (with *Klebsiella rhinoscleroma*).

鼻硬結 鼻與鼻部內側形成結節並增厚，此乃由細菌感染引起（克雷白氏桿菌性鼻硬結）。

rhinoscopy *n.* examination of the interior of the nose.

鼻鏡檢查 鼻內部的檢查。

rhinosporidiosis *n.* an infection of the mucous membranes of the nose, larynx, eyes, and genitals that is caused by the fungus *Rhinosporidium seeberi* and is characterized by the formation of tiny growths called *polyps. It occurs most commonly in Asia.

鼻孢子蟲病 由鼻孢子蟲屬菌引起的鼻黏膜、喉、眼睛和生殖器的感染，其特徵是形成息肉（很小的增生物）。這種病在亞洲最常見。

rhinovirus *n.* any one of a group of RNA-containing viruses that cause respiratory infections in man resembling the common cold. They are included in the *picornavirus group.

鼻病毒 一種含核糖核酸病毒，引起類似感冒的呼吸道感染，屬細小核糖核酸病毒組。

Rhipicephalus *n.* a genus of hard *ticks widely distributed in the tropics. The dog tick (*R. sanguineus*) can suck the blood of man and is commonly involved in the transmission of diseases caused by rickettsiae (*see* typhus).

扇頭蜱屬 廣泛分佈於熱帶的硬蜱屬，犬蜱（血紅扇頭蜱）可吸吮人的血液，並傳播立克次氏體引起的疾病。

rhiz- (rhizo-) *prefix denoting* a root. Example: *rhizonychia* (the root of a nail).

〔前綴〕 **根** 例如甲根。

rhizotomy *n.* a surgical procedure in which selected nerve roots are cut at the point where they emerge from the

脊神經根切斷術 選擇性地切斷從脊髓出來的神經根的外科手術。脊神經後

spinal cord. In *posterior rhizotomy* the posterior (sensory) nerve roots are cut for the relief of intractable pain in the organs served by these nerves. An *anterior rhizotomy* – the cutting of the anterior (motor) nerve roots – is sometimes done for the relief of severe muscle spasm.

根切斷術是切斷感覺神經根，以減輕它所支配的臟器的頑固性疼痛。脊神經前根切斷術是切斷運動神經根，有時是爲減輕嚴重的肌肉痙攣。

Rhodnius *n.* a genus of large blood-sucking bugs (*see* reduviid). *R. prolixus* is important in the transmission of *Chagas' disease in Central America and the northern part of South America.

紅獵蝽屬　一種大型的吸血昆蟲屬，在中美洲和南美洲中部，長紅獵蝽對恰加斯氏病（錐蟲病）的傳播起重要作用。

rhodopsin (visual purple) *n.* a pigment in the retina of the eye, within the *rods, consisting of *retinal* – an aldehyde of retinol (*vitamin A) – and a protein. The presence of rhodopsin is essential for vision in dim light. It is bleached in the presence of light and this stimulates nervous activity in the rods.

視紫質　眼睛視網膜的一種色素，在視網膜視桿細胞內，由視黃醛（維生素A醛）和一種蛋白質組成。視紫質的存在對在光線暗淡時的視覺是所必需的，當有亮光時它就脫色，此時就刺激了視桿細胞中的神經活性。

rhombencephalon *n. see* hindbrain.

菱腦

rhomboid *n.* either of two muscles (*rhomboid major* and *rhomboid minor*) situated in the upper part of the back, between the backbone and shoulder blade. They help to move the shoulder blade backwards and upwards.

菱形肌　位於背部上方在脊柱與肩胛骨之間的兩塊肌肉（大菱形肌和小菱形肌）。它們幫助肩胛骨向後和向上活動。

rhonchus *n.* (*pl.* **rhonchi**) an abnormal musical noise produced by air passing through narrowed bronchi. It is heard through a stethoscope, usually when the patient breathes out.

乾囉音　空氣通過狹窄的支氣管產生的一種異常的音樂性噪音，通常當病人呼氣時通過聽診器可聽到。

rhythm method a contraceptive method in which sexual intercourse is restricted to the *safe period* at the beginning and end of the *menstrual cycle. The safe period is calculated either on the basis of the length of the menstrual cycle or by reliance on the change of body temperature that occurs at ovulation. A third possible indicator is the change that occurs with ovulation in the stickiness of the mucus at the

安全期避孕法　一種將性交限制在月經周期前和末的"安全期"避孕方法。安全期的計算可據月經周期的時間，或依據排卵時體溫的變化。第三種可能的提示是排卵同時子宮頸黏液黏性的改變。此方法的可靠性是依賴於婦女有規律的月經周期，但其失敗率高於用工具的避孕

neck (cervix) of the womb. The method depends for its reliability on the woman having uniform regular periods and its failure rate is higher than with mechanical methods, approaching 25 pregnancies per 100 woman-years.

法。每100個婦女-年有25個妊娠。

rib *n.* a curved, slightly twisted, strip of bone forming part of the skeleton of the thorax, which protects the heart and lungs. There are 12 pairs of ribs. The head of each rib articulates with one of the 12 thoracic vertebrae of the backbone; the other end is attached to a section of cartilage (*see* costal cartilage). The first seven pairs – the *true ribs* – are connected directly to the sternum by their costal cartilages. The next three pairs – the *false ribs* – are attached indirectly: each is connected by its cartilage to the rib above it. The last two pairs of ribs – the *floating ribs* – end freely in the muscles of the body wall. Anatomical name: **costa.**

肋骨 彎曲呈輕度弓形的細長骨，形成胸廓骨骼的一部分，保護心臟和兩肺。肋骨有12對，每根肋骨頭與脊柱的12個胸椎之一相連接。另一端連接一段軟骨。第1～7對肋骨謂眞肋，直接以其肋軟骨和胸骨相連接，以後3對假肋不與胸骨連接，而借助軟骨與其上面的肋骨相連接。最後兩對肋骨稱浮肋，前端游離於胸壁的肌肉中。

riboflavin *n. see* vitamin B_2.

核黃素 維生素B_2。

ribonuclease *n.* an enzyme, located in the *lysosomes of cells, that splits RNA at specific places in the molecule.

核糖核酸酶 含於細胞溶酶體中的酶，它使核糖核酸在分子的特殊位置上分裂。

ribonucleic acid *see* RNA.

核糖核酸

ribose *n.* a pentose sugar (i.e. one with free carbon atoms) that is a component of *RNA and several coenzymes. Ribose is also involved in intracellular metabolism.

核糖 一種戊糖（即有自由碳原子的糖），是核糖核酸和幾種輔酶的成分。核糖也參與細胞內的代謝。

ribosome *n.* a particle, consisting of RNA and protein, that occurs in cells and is the site of protein synthesis in the cell (*see* translation). Ribosomes are either attached to the *endoplasmic reticulum or free in the cytoplasm as *polysomes. —**ribosomal** *adj.*

核糖體，核糖核蛋白體 細胞內由核糖核酸和蛋白質組成的一種顆粒，並是細胞內蛋白質合成的場所。核糖體可附着在內質網上，或以多核糖體的形式游離在細胞漿內。

ricin *n.* a highly toxic albumin obtained from castor-oil seeds (*Ricinus communis*) that inhibits protein synthesis and becomes attached to the surface of cells, resulting in gastroenteritis,

蓖麻毒蛋白 從蓖麻籽中提取的高毒性白蛋白，它抑制蛋白合成，並結合於細胞表面引起胃腸炎、肝淤血和黃疸，以及心血管

hepatic congestion and jaundice, and cardiovascular collapse. It is lethal to most species, even in minute amounts (1 μg/kg body weight); it is most toxic if injected intravenously or inhaled as fine particles.

性虛脫。多數品種，即使是極小劑量（1 μ g/kg 體量）亦可致死亡。靜脈注射或以細小顆粒吸入時毒性最大。

rickets *n.* a disease of children in which the bones do not harden and are malformed due to a deficiency of *vitamin D. Without vitamin D not enough calcium salts are deposited in the bones to make them rigid. They are therefore softer than normal and bend out of shape. *See also* osteomalacia. *Renal rickets* is due to impaired kidney function: the bones are malformed as bone-forming minerals are excreted in the urine.

佝僂病 由於缺乏維生素D使骨變軟和變形的兒童疾病。因缺乏維生素D，無足夠使骨變硬的鈣鹽沉積在骨內，因此骨骼比正常的軟，並形狀彎曲。腎性佝僂病是由於腎功能受損害，骨骼變形是由於形成骨的礦物質由尿排出所致。

rickettsiae *pl. n.* (*sing.* **rickettsia**) a group of very small nonmotile spherical or rodlike parasitic organisms. They resemble bacteria in their cellular structure and method of asexual reproduction, but – like viruses – they cannot reproduce outside the bodies of their hosts. Rickettsiae infect arthropods (ticks, mites, etc.), through whom they can be transmitted to mammals (including man), in which they can cause severe illness. The species *Rickettsia akari* causes *rickettsial pox; *R. conori*, *R. mooseri*, *R. prowazeki*, *R. quintana*, and *R. tsutsugamushi* cause different forms of *typhus, and *R. rickettsii* causes *Rocky Mountain spotted fever. *See also* Coxiella. —**rickettsial** *adj.*

立克次氏體 一組很小的不運動的球形的或棒狀的寄生性微生物。在細胞結構和無性生殖方面與細菌相似，但它們不能在宿主的體外繁殖，這點又與病毒相似。立克次氏體感染節肢動物（蟎、蜱等），通過它們傳播到哺乳動物（包括人在內），並可引起人的嚴重疾病。小蛛立克次氏體可引起立克次氏體痘，康諾爾氏立克次氏體、莫塞爾氏立克次氏體、普氏立克次氏體，五日熱立克次氏體以及恙蟲熱立克次氏體引起不同類型的斑疹傷寒，立氏立克次氏體引起落基山斑疹熱。

rickettsial pox a disease of mice caused by the microorganism *Rickettsia akari* and transmitted to man by mites: it produces chills, fever, muscular pain, and a rash similar to that of *chickenpox. The disease is mild and runs its course in 2–3 weeks. *See also* typhus.

立克次氏體痘 由微生物小蛛立克次氏體引起的鼠病，由蟎傳播給人，引起寒戰、發熱、肌痛以及與水痘相似的皮疹。此病經過輕，病程爲2～3週。

ridge *n.* **1.** (in anatomy) a crest or a long narrow protuberance, e.g. on a bone. **2.** (in dental anatomy) *see* alveolus.

嵴 ①（解剖學）骨頭上一條長而窄的隆起。②（牙科解剖）指齒槽嵴。

rifampicin *n.* an *antibiotic used to treat various infections, particularly tuberculosis. It is administered by mouth; digestive upsets and sensitivity reactions sometimes occur. Trade names: **Rifadin, Rimactane**.

利福平 用於治療各種感染，特別是結核病的抗生素，爲口服藥，有時可發生消化道不適和過敏反應。

rifamycin *n.* an *antibiotic used to treat certain infections, particularly tuberculosis. It is administered by injection, inhalation, or in a solution applied to the infected area. Side-effects are uncommon.

利福黴素 治療某種感染，尤其是結核病的抗生素。用於注射、吸入或製成溶液用於感染部位。副作用少見。

Rift Valley fever a virus disease of East Africa transmitted from animals to man by mosquitoes and causing symptoms resembling those of *influenza.

裂穀熱 非洲的一種病毒性疾病，通過蚊子從動物傳播給人，其症狀酷似流感。

rigidity *n.* (in neurology) resistance to the passive movement of a limb that persists throughout its range. It is a symptom of *parkinsonism. A smooth resistance is called *plastic* or *lead-pipe rigidity* while intermittent resistance is called *cogwheel rigidity*. *Compare* spasticity.

强直 （神經病學）整個肢體對被動運動的持續性抵抗。這是帕金森氏徵的一種症狀。呈均勻抵抗的强直稱爲可塑性的或鉛管樣强直，而呈間斷性抵抗的强直稱爲齒輪狀强直。

rigor *n.* **1.** an abrupt attack of shivering and a sensation of coldness, accompanied by a rapid rise in body temperature. This often marks the onset of a fever and may be followed by a feeling of heat, with copious sweating. **2.** *see* rigor mortis.

①**寒戰** 突然的戰慄發作和寒冷感，伴有體溫急劇升高。常爲發熱開始的徵兆，隨後可能有熱的感覺，並大量出汗。②**屍僵**

rigor mortis the stiffening of a body that occurs within some eight hours of death, due to chemical changes in muscle tissue. It starts to disappear after about 24 hours.

屍僵 死亡約8小時內出現的屍體僵硬。由於肌肉組織內的化學變化所致。在約24小時後開始消失。

rima *n.* (in anatomy) a cleft. The *rima glottidis* (or glottis) is the space between the vocal cords.

裂 （解剖學）一種裂隙，聲門裂（或聲門）是聲帶之間的空隙。

rimiterol *n.* a drug, similar to *isoprenaline, used as a *bronchodilator to relieve asthma and chronic bronchitis. It is administered by inhalation; side-effects, following large doses, may in-

哌喘定 與異丙腎上腺素相似的藥物，作爲支氣管擴張劑用於減輕哮喘和慢性支氣管炎。用於吸入，大劑量的副作用可有頭

clude dizziness, fainting, tremor, anxiety, and fast heart rate. Trade name: **Pulmadil**.

暈、暈厥、震顫、焦慮和心率快。

ring *n.* (in anatomy) *see* annulus.

環

Ringer's solution (Ringer's mixture) a clear colourless *physiological solution of sodium chloride (common salt), potassium chloride, and calcium chloride prepared with recently boiled pure water. The osmotic pressure of the solution is the same as that of blood serum. Ringer's solution is used for maintaining organs or tissues alive outside the animal or human body for limited periods. Sterile Ringer's solution is injected intravenously to treat dehydration.

林格氏溶液 透明無色的生理性溶液，爲氯化鈉、氯化鉀和氯化鈣溶於新鮮煮沸的純淨水製成。其滲透壓與血漿相同，可用於維持器官或組織在動物或人體外存活一定時間。靜脉注射無菌的林格氏液可治療脫水。

ringworm (tinea) *n.* a fungus infection of the surface of the skin, particularly the scalp and feet, and occasionally of the nails. Ringworm is caused by various species of the fungi *Microsporum*, *Trichophyton*, and *Epidermophyton* and it also affects animals: a source of infection for man. Ringworm is highly contagious and can be spread by direct contact or via infected materials. As its name suggests, the infection is ringlike and it causes intense itching. The commonest form of ringworm is *athlete's foot* (*tinea pedis*), which affects the skin between the toes. Another common type is ringworm of the scalp (*tinea capitis*), of which there is a severe form – *favus. Ringworm also affects the skin under a beard (*tinea barbae*). The disease is treated with antifungal agents taken by mouth (such as griseofulvin) or applied locally.

癬 皮膚表面的眞菌感染，易發於頭皮和足部，有時在指甲。由各種不同眞菌引起，有小孢子菌屬、髮癬菌和表皮癬菌屬。它也可侵犯動物，成爲人類感染的一個來源。癬有高度接觸傳染性，可由接觸傳染或通過被污染物而傳播。感染後引起奇癢。最常見的癬病類型是脚癬，侵犯脚趾間的皮膚。另一種常見類型是頭皮癬（頭癬），嚴重型是黃癬。癬病也可發生於鬍鬚下的皮膚（鬚癬）。此病治療是口服或局部應用抗眞菌劑（例如灰黃黴素）。

Rinne's test a test to determine whether *deafness is conductive or perceptive. A vibrating tuning fork is held first in the air, close to the ear, and then with its base placed on the bone (mastoid process) behind the ear. If the sound conducted by air is heard for a longer time than the sound conducted

林尼氏試驗 測定耳聾是傳導性或感音性的一種試驗。先將一振動的音叉持近耳邊，然後將音叉底部放在耳後的骨上（乳突），若由空氣傳導的聲音聽到時間長於骨傳導的聲音，則試驗爲陽性，爲

by bone the test is positive and the deafness perceptive; a negative result, when the sound conducted by the bone lasts longer, indicates conductive deafness.

感音性耳聾。若骨傳導的聲音持續時間長，則結果爲陰性，提示爲傳導性耳聾。

risk factor an attribute (such as a habit (e.g. cigarette smoking) or exposure to some environmental hazard) that leads the individual concerned to have a greater likelihood of developing an illness. The relationship is one of probability and as such can be distinguished from a *causal agent.

危險因素 導至某些人很可能患病的一種因素（例如一種習慣——吸烟，或接觸某些環境的公害）。這種因素是指一種可能性，與致病因素有所區別。

risk register a list of infants who have experienced some event in their obstetric and/or perinatal history known to be correlated with a higher than average likelihood of serious abnormality. Such children are subjected to extra surveillance. Problems associated with risk registers include limiting the designation of predisposing conditions so as to contain the number on the register within reasonable proportions and ensuring that children not on the register receive adequate surveillance.

危險登記 爲一種嬰兒登記表，登記嬰兒在產科和/或圍產期病史中發生的某些重要情況，這些情況發生嚴重畸形的可能性比正常高。這類兒童受到特別監察。危險登記所帶來的問題，一是爲使登記表上的數字控制在合理比例內，對潛在危險情況不能充分顯示；二是不能保證沒有登記的兒童接受適當的監察。

risus sardonicus an abnormal grinning expression resulting from involuntary prolonged contraction of facial muscles, as seen in *tetanus.

痙笑 不正常的咧嘴而笑的表情，由於面肌持續的不隨意收縮引起，如見於破傷風。

river blindness *see* onchocerciasis.

河盲病

RNA (ribonucleic acid) a *nucleic acid, occurring in the nucleus and cytoplasm of cells, that is concerned with synthesis of proteins (*see* messenger RNA, ribosome, transfer RNA, translation). In some viruses RNA is the genetic material. The RNA molecule is a single strand made up of units called *nucleotides.

核糖核酸 存在於細胞核與胞漿內的一種核酸，與蛋白質合成有關。有些病毒的核糖核酸是遺傳性物質。核糖核酸分子是由許多核苷酸單位組成的單鏈。

Rocky Mountain spotted fever (spotted fever, tick fever) a disease of rodents and other small mammals in the USA caused by the microorganism *Rickettsia rickettsii* and transmitted to man by ticks. Symptoms include fever,

落基山斑疹熱（斑疹熱、蜱熱） 美國嚙齒動物和一些小哺乳動物的疾病，由立氏立克次氏體引起，並通過蜱傳播給人。症狀有發熱、肌痛，並有類似麻疹

muscle pains, and a profuse reddish rash like that of measles. If untreated the disease may be fatal, but treatment with tetracycline or chloramphenicol is effective. *See also* typhus.

的彌散性紅色皮疹，此病若不治療可以致死。四環素或氯黴素治療有效。

rod *n.* one of the two types of light-sensitive cells in the *retina of the eye (*compare* cone). The human eye contains about 125 million rods, which are necessary for seeing in dim light. They contain a pigment, *visual purple* (*rhodopsin*), which is broken down (bleached) in the light and regenerated in the dark. Breakdown of visual purple gives rise to nerve impulses; when all the pigment is bleached (i.e. in bright light) the rods no longer function. *See also* dark adaptation, light adaptation.

視桿細胞 視網膜內兩種感光細胞之一，人的眼睛有125,000,000個在光線暗淡時看東西所需的視桿細胞。其中有一種色素稱為視紫質，它在亮光中破壞（脫色）而在黑暗中再生。視紫質破壞時引起神經衝動，當所有色素都脫色時（即在明亮光線中）則視桿細胞不再起作用。

rodent ulcer a slow-growing malignant tumour of the face, usually at the edge of the eyelids, lips, or nostrils. Rodent ulcers occur in middle age or later; if untreated, they destroy skin muscle and bone but they do not spread to other parts of the body. Europeans persistently exposed to hot sun may develop the disease and it is a complication of chronic *radiodermatitis. It can be treated by surgery or radiotherapy. Medical name: **basal cell carcinoma**.

侵蝕性潰瘍 面部生長緩慢的惡性腫瘤，常在眼瞼緣、口唇或鼻孔出現。侵蝕性潰瘍發生於中年或中年以後。若未經治療，則可破壞皮膚、肌肉和骨，但不向身體其它部分播散。歐洲人持久地曝曬於熾熱陽光後可以發生此病。此病也是慢性放射性皮炎的併發症。可用手術和放射治療，醫學名詞：基底細胞癌。

roentgen *n.* a unit of exposure dose of X- or gamma-radiation equal to the dose that will produce 2.58×10^{-4} coulomb on all the ions of one sign, when all the electrons released in a volume of air of mass 1 kilogram are completely stopped.

倫琴 X或γ輻射劑量的單位：在質量為1000克的空氣中，當所有的電子停止釋放時輻射所產生的同符號離子的全部電荷量為2.58×10^{-4}庫倫。

roentgenology *n.* the study of the applications of X-rays (roentgen rays) in medicine.

X線學 醫學上對X線應用的研究。

role playing acting out another person's expected behaviour, usually in a contrived situation, in order to understand them better. It is used in family psychotherapy, in teaching social skills

扮演角色 通常在預先計劃好的情況下，做出別人所預期的行為，以便使人更好地了解他們。此法用於家庭精神療法，教給病

to patients, and also in the training of psychiatric (and other) staff.

人社交技能，也可用於訓練精神病學（或其他的）工作人員。

Romaña's sign an early clinical sign of *Chagas' disease, appearing some three weeks after infection. There is considerable swelling of the eyelids of one or both eyes. This may be due to the presence of the parasites causing the disease but it may also be an allergic reaction to the repeated bites of their insect carriers.

羅曼尼亞氏徵（偏側性瞼結膜炎） 恰加斯氏病（南美洲錐蟲病）的早期臨床體徵，在感染後三週出現。一側或雙側眼瞼有明顯腫脹。可能是由於致病寄生蟲引起，但也可能是病媒昆蟲反復叮咬後的過敏反應。

Romanowsky stains a group of stains used for microscopical examination of blood cells, consisting of variable mixtures of thiazine dyes, such as azure B, with eosin. Romanowsky stains give characteristic staining patterns, on the basis of which blood cells are classified. The group includes the stains of Leishmann, Wright, May-Grunwald, Giemsa, etc.

羅曼諾夫斯基染劑 用於顯微鏡檢查血細胞的一組染劑。由噻嗪類染劑（如天藍B)與曙紅組成的各種不同的混合劑。羅曼諾夫斯基染劑可以染出特徵性的染片，在這種染片上可做血細胞分類。這類染劑包括有利什曼氏、瑞氏、梅-格二氏、吉姆薩氏染劑。

Romberg's sign evidence of a sensory disorder affecting those nerves that transmit information to the brain about the position of the limbs and joints and the tension in the muscles. The patient is asked to stand upright. Romberg's sign is positive if he maintains his posture when his eyes are open but sways and falls when his eyes are closed.

羅姆伯格氏徵 向大腦傳遞有關肢體和關節位置及肌肉張力信息的一些神經發生感覺障礙的徵象。要求病人站直，若睜眼時能維持他的姿勢，而閉眼時就搖晃和摔倒，則爲羅姆伯格氏徵陽性。

rongeur *n.* powerful biting forceps for cutting tissue, particularly bone.

咬骨鉗 能切斷組織和骨頭的有力的咬鉗。

root *n.* **1.** (in neurology) a bundle of nerve fibres at its emergence from the spinal cord. The 31 pairs of *spinal nerves have two roots on each side, an anterior root containing motor nerve fibres and a posterior root containing sensory fibres. The roots merge outside the cord to form mixed nerves. **2.** (in dentistry) the part of a *tooth that is not covered by enamel and is normally

根 ①（神經病學）從脊髓發出處的一束神經纖維。31對脊神經每一對有左右兩個根。前根有運動神經纖維，後根有感覺纖維。兩神經根在脊髓外合併形成混合神經。 ②（牙科學）牙齒無釉質遮蓋的部分，正常時借助牙周纖維與牙槽骨連接。

attached to the alveolar bone by periodontal fibres. **3.** the origin of any structure, i.e. the point at which it diverges from another structure. Anatomical name: **radix**.

③某種結構的起始部，即從其它結構分出之點。

root filling 1. the final stage of *root treatment, in which the prepared canal inside a tooth root is filled with a suitable material. **2.** the material used to fill the canal in the root, usually a core of *gutta-percha with a thin coating of sealing cement.

①**牙根充填**　根管治療的最後階段，用適當的物質充填在準備好的牙根根管內。　②**填料**　用於充填牙根的物質，通常其中心是馬來乳膠，外面包有一層薄的水門汀封閉劑。

root induction (in *endodontics) a procedure to allow continued root formation in an immature tooth with a damaged pulp.

根誘導　（牙髓病學）使牙髓損壞的未成熟牙能繼續形成牙根的方法。

root treatment (in *endodontics) the procedure of removing the remnants of the pulp of a tooth, cleaning and shaping the canal inside the tooth, and filling the root canal (*see* root filling). The entire treatment usually extends over several visits. It is used to treat toothache and apical abscesses.

根管治療　（牙髓病學）去除殘留的牙髓，使牙內根管清潔和成形，並作根管充填。全部的治療通常需要幾次，此法用於治療牙痛和根尖膿腫。

Rorschach test a test to measure aspects of personality, consisting of ten inkblots, half of which are in various colours and the other half in black and white. The responses to the different inkblots are used to derive hypotheses about the subject. The use of the test for the diagnosis of brain damage is no longer generally supported. *See also* projective test.

羅夏氏試驗　測定個性的一種試驗，由10種墨蹟組成，其中半數是不同顏色的，另一半是黑白的。用對不同墨蹟的反應來得知關於病人的思想。用這種試驗診斷大腦損害已經不再得到廣泛支持。

rosacea *n.* a skin disease of the face in which the blood vessels enlarge, giving the cheeks and nose a flushed appearance. The cause is uncertain but irritant foods or drinks or too much alcohol may play a part, and extremes of climate may aggravate the condition. The nose may enlarge (*see* rhinophyma). Rosacea usually occurs after the age of 30 and affects women more often than men, with the menopause sometimes acting as a trigger.

酒皶鼻　由於血管擴張引起面頰和鼻部發紅的面部皮膚病。病因不明，但刺激性食物和飲料或過度飲酒可能起一定作用。極壞的氣候也可加重病情，鼻可肥大。酒皶鼻通常發生在30歲以後，女性多於男性，有時絕經可激發。

roseola *n.* any rose-coloured rash, such as occurs in measles, the secondary stage of syphilis, or typhoid fever.

玫瑰疹 玫瑰色的皮疹，例如見於麻疹、梅毒的第二期或腸傷寒時。

rostellum *n.* (*pl.* **rostella**) a mobile and retractable knob bearing hooks, present on the head (scolex) of certain *tapeworms, e.g. *Taenia* and *Echinococcus*.

頂突 某些縧蟲頭節上可動的和能回縮的帶鈎的凸起，如縧蟲和棘球屬。

rostrum *n.* (*pl.* **rostra**) (in anatomy) a beaklike projection, such as that on the sphenoid bone. —**rostral** *adj.*

喙 （解剖學）一個鳥嘴狀的突起物，例如蝶骨上的喙。

rotator *n.* a muscle that brings about rotation of a part. The *rotatores* are small muscles situated deep in the back between adjacent vertebrae. They help to extend and rotate the vertebrae.

回旋肌 使某部位旋轉的肌肉。回旋肌是位於背深部兩個鄰近脊椎之間的小肌肉，可幫助脊柱伸直和旋轉。

Rothera's test a method of testing urine for the presence of acetone or acetoacetic acid: a sign of *diabetes mellitus. Strong ammonia is added to a sample of urine saturated with ammonium sulphate crystals and containing a small quantity of sodium nitroprusside. A purple colour confirms the presence of acetone or acetoacetic acid.

羅瑟雷氏試驗 測定尿內存在丙酮或乙醯乙酸的方法。尿內有丙酮或乙醯乙酸是糖尿病的一種徵象。將濃氨水加入飽含硫酸銨結晶和含有小量硝普鈉的尿標本中，出現紫色就可肯定有丙酮或乙醯乙酸。

Roth spot a pale area surrounded by haemorrhage sometimes seen in the retina, with the aid of an *ophthalmoscope, in those who have bacterial endocarditis, septicaemia, or leukaemia.

羅特氏斑 有時借檢眼鏡能在視網膜上見到的周圍出血的蒼白區。發生於細菌性心內膜炎、敗血症或白血病。

roughage *n. see* dietary fibre.

粗糙食物

rouleau *n.* (*pl.* **rouleaux**) a cylindrical structure in the blood formed from several red blood cells piled one upon the other and adhering by their rims.

紅細胞錢串 血液內由若干紅細胞互相重疊，其邊緣黏連而形成的圓柱樣結構。

round window *see* fenestra (rotunda).

圓窗

roundworm *n. see* nematode.

蛔蟲

-rrhagia (-rrhage) *suffix denoting* excessive or abnormal flow or discharge from an organ or part. Examples: *haemorrhage* (excessive bleeding); *menorrhagia* (excessive menstrual flow).

〔後綴〕**流出** 意指有某種液體從某器官或身體某部過多的或異常的流出或排出。例如：出血（過多的流出血液），月經過多（過多的流出經血）

-rrhaphy *suffix denoting* surgical sewing; suturing. Example: *herniorrhaphy* (of a hernia).

〔後綴〕**縫合術**　指外科的縫合、縫術，例如疝修補術。

-rrhexis *suffix denoting* splitting or rupture of a part.

〔後綴〕**裂**　指某部位的裂或破裂。

-rrhoea *suffix denoting* a flow or discharge from an organ or part. Example: *rhinorrhoea* (from the nose).

〔後綴〕**溢**　指從某器官或部位流出或排出液體，例如鼻溢（從鼻流出）。

RSV *see* respiratory syncytial virus.

魯斯氏肉瘤病毒

rubber dam (in dentistry) a sheet of rubber used to isolate one or more teeth during treatment.

橡皮障　（牙科學）用於在治療時隔開一個或更多牙齒的一片橡皮。

rubefacient *n.* an agent that causes reddening and warming of the skin. Rubefacients are often used as *counterirritants for the relief of muscular pain.

發紅藥　一種使皮膚發紅和發熱的藥物，發紅藥常被用做為抗刺激劑，以減輕肌肉疼痛。

rubella *n. see* German measles.

風疹

rubeola *n. see* measles.

麻疹

rubidium-81 *n.* an artificial radiactive isotope that has a half-life of about four hours and decays into the radioactive gas *krypton-81m, emitting radiations as it does so.

^{81}銣　一種人工放射性同位素，其半衰期約4小時，衰變爲放射性氣體^{81m}氪，同時放出射線。

rubor *n.* redness: one of the classical signs of inflammation in a tissue, the other three being *calor (heat), *dolor (pain) and *tumor (swelling). The redness of inflamed tissue is due to the increase in size of the small blood vessels in the area, which therefore contain more blood.

發紅　組織炎症的典型症狀之一，其它三個症狀是灼熱、疼痛和腫脹。炎症組織發紅的原因是局部小血管擴張，所以含血增多。

rubrospinal tract a tract of *motor neurones that extends from the mid-

紅核脊髓束　運動神經元的傳導束，從中腦到達脊

brain down to different levels in the spinal cord, carrying impulses that have travelled from the cerebral and cerebellar cortex via the nucleus ruber (red nucleus). The tract plays an important part in the control of skilled and dextrous movements.

髓的不同水平，傳遞來自大腦、小腦皮層並通過紅核的衝動。該束的重要作用是管理熟練和靈巧的運動。

ruga *n.* (*pl.* **rugae**) a fold or crease, especially one of the folds of mucous membrane that line the stomach.

皺褶（襞） 特別指胃內黏膜皺襞。

rumination *n.* (in psychiatry) an obsessional type of thinking in which the same thoughts or themes are experienced repetitively, to the exclusion of other forms of mental activity. The patient commonly feels depressed and guilty after rumination. Rumination may be distinguished from morbid preoccupation in that the thoughts are irrational and resisted by the patient; they often involve abhorrent or aggressive feelings about events in the remote past and are accompanied by a lack of confidence in memory.

反復思考（沉思） 精神病學）指一種不能擺脫的思想，即總是在重複體驗同樣的思想或問題而排斥了其它類型的精神活動。病人在沉思後往往覺得憂鬱和自疚。沉思與病態偏見、成見、出神的區別，在於其思想是不合理的，並爲病人所反抗，他們常常對很久以前發生的事件有厭惡憤怒和仇恨的感情，並對記憶缺乏信任。

rupture 1. *n. see* hernia. **2.** *n.* the bursting apart or open of an organ or tissue; for example, the splitting of the membranes enclosing an infant during childbirth. **3.** *vb.* (of tissues, etc.) to burst apart or open.

破裂 ①見"疝氣"。②器官或組織的破裂或裂開，例如，分娩時包住嬰兒的羊膜破裂。 ③（組織的）破裂或裂開。

Russian spring-summer encephalitis an influenza-like viral disease that affects the brain and nervous system and occurs in Russia and central Europe. It is transmitted to man either through the bite of forest-dwelling ticks of the species *Ixodes persulcatus* or by drinking the milk of infected goats. Infection of the meninges results in paralysis of the limbs and of the muscles of the neck and back. The disease, which is often fatal, can be prevented by vaccination.

蘇聯春夏型腦炎 侵犯大腦和神經系統的一種流感樣的病毒性疾病。發生在蘇聯和中歐。通過棲息於森林中的全溝硬蜱叮咬或飲用感染的山羊奶而傳播於人。腦膜感染可引起肢體癱瘓，以及頸部和背部肌肉麻痹。該病常爲致死性，但可通過接種進行預防。

Ryle's tube a thin flexible tube of rubber or plastic, inserted through the mouth or nose of a patient and used for

賴爾氏管 一種橡膠或塑料的可曲性細管，通過病人的口腔或鼻腔插入胃

withdrawing fluid from the stomach or giving a test meal.

內，用於抽吸胃內液體或注入試餐。

S

S

Sabin vaccine an oral vaccine against poliomyelitis, prepared by culture of the virus under special conditions so that it loses its virulence (i.e. it becomes attenuated) but retains its ability to stimulate antibody production.

薩賓氏疫苗 一種脊髓灰質炎口服疫苗。係在特殊條件下培養病毒製成的。使病毒失去致病力（減毒），而仍保留其刺激產生抗體的能力。

sac *n.* a pouch or baglike structure. Sacs can enclose natural cavities in the body, e.g. in the lungs (*see* alveolus) or in the *lacrimal apparatus of the eye, or they can be pathological, as in a hernia.

囊 小袋或口袋樣結構。在體內圍成自然的洞腔。如肺泡或眼的淚器，或是病理性的，如疝。

sacchar- (saccharo-) *prefix denoting* sugar.

〔前綴〕 **糖**

saccharide *n.* a carbohydrate. *See also* disaccharide, monosaccharide, polysaccharide.

糖 一種碳水化合物。

saccharine *n.* a sweetening agent. Saccharine is 400 times as sweet as sugar and has no energy content. It is very useful as a sweetener in diabetic and low-calorie foods. Saccharine is destroyed by heat and is not therefore used in cooking.

糖精 一種甜味劑。比糖甜400倍，但不產生能量。常用作糖尿病或低卡食物的甜味劑。糖精受熱破壞，故不用於烹調。

Saccharomyces *n. see* yeast.

酵母屬

saccule (sacculus) *n.* the smaller of the two membranous sacs within the vestibule of the ear: it forms part of the membranous *labyrinth. It is filled with fluid (endolymph) and contains a *macula. This responds to gravity and relays information to the brain about the position of the head.

球囊 耳的前庭內兩個膜囊中的較小者。形成部分膜迷路。球囊內充滿液體（內淋巴），並含有平衡斑，可對重力作出反應，將頭部位置改變的信息轉遞給腦。

saccus *n.* a sac or pouch. The *saccus endolymphaticus* is the small sac connected to the saccule and utricle of the inner ear by the *endolymphatic duct.

囊 小袋。內淋巴囊是由內淋巴管連接內耳的球囊和橢圓囊的一個小囊。

sacralization *n.* abnormal fusion of the fifth lumbar vertebra with the sacrum.

骶骨融合 第五腰椎與骶骨的異常融合。

sacral nerves the five pairs of *spinal nerves that emerge from the spinal column in the sacrum. The nerves carry sensory and motor fibres from the upper and lower leg and from the anal and genital regions.

骶神經 從骶骨脊柱穿出的五對脊神經。含有支配大、小腿以及肛門和生殖器部位的感覺和運動纖維。

sacral vertebrae the five vertebrae that are fused together to form the *sacrum.

骶椎 融合在一起組成骶骨的五塊椎骨。

sacro- *prefix denoting* the sacrum. Examples: *sacrococcygeal* (relating to the sacrum and coccyx); *sacrodynia* (pain in); *sacroiliac* (relating to the sacrum and ilium).

〔前綴〕 **骶，骶骨** 如骶尾骨的，骶骨痛，骶髂骨的。

sacroiliitis *n.* inflammation of the sacroiliac joint. Involvement of both joints is a common feature of ankylosing *spondylitis and associated rheumatic diseases, including *Reiter's syndrome and *psoriatic arthritis. The resultant low back pain and stiffness may be alleviated by rest and analgesics.

骶髂關節炎 骶髂關節發炎。累及兩側骶髂關節是强直性脊椎炎和兼有風濕性疾病的關節炎，包括萊特爾氏綜合徵和銀屑病患者的關節炎常見的特徵。本病引起的腰骶部疼痛和强直可通過休息與服止痛藥獲得緩解。

sacrum *n.* (*pl.* **sacra**) a curved triangular element of the *backbone consisting of five fused vertebrae (*sacral vertebrae*). It articulates with the last lumbar vertebra above, the coccyx below, and the hip bones laterally. *See also* vertebra. —**sacral** *adj.*

骶骨 由五塊融合的椎骨（骶椎）組成的一個彎曲的三角形的脊柱部分。上部與最下一塊腰椎，下部與尾骨，側部與髖骨形成關節。

saddle joint a form of *diarthrosis (freely movable joint) in which the articulating surfaces of the bones are reciprocally saddle-shaped. It occurs at the carpometacarpal joint of the thumb.

鞍狀關節 一種可動關節（可自由活動的關節）。兩骨的關節面呈鞍狀連接。見於拇指的腕掌關節。

sadism *n.* sexual excitement in response to inflicting or thinking about inflicting pain upon other people. *See also* masochism, perversion. —**sadist** *n.* —**sadistic** *adj.*

施虐狂 使他人痛苦，或想到使人痛苦就能獲得的性興奮。

safe period the days in each *menstrual cycle when conception is least likely. Ovulation generally occurs at the midpoint of each cycle, and in women with regular periods it is possible to calculate the days at the beginning and end of the cycle when coitus is unlikely to result in pregnancy. *See* rhythm method.

安全期 在每次月經周期內受孕可能最小的日期。排卵通常發生於每個周期的中期。對於經期有規律的婦女，可算出周期開始時和終止時性交不會導至懷孕的日期。

safranin (safranine) *n.* a group of water- and alcohol-soluble basic dyes used to stain cell nuclei and as counterstains for Gram-negative bacteria.

藏紅 一組鹼性染劑。溶於水和酒精。用於染細胞核，並用作革蘭氏陰性細菌的複染劑。

sagittal *adj.* describing the dorsoventral plane that extends down the long axis of the body, dividing it into right and left halves (see illustration).

矢狀的 用以描述背腹側平面的。此平面沿身體的長軸將身體分成左右兩半（見圖）。

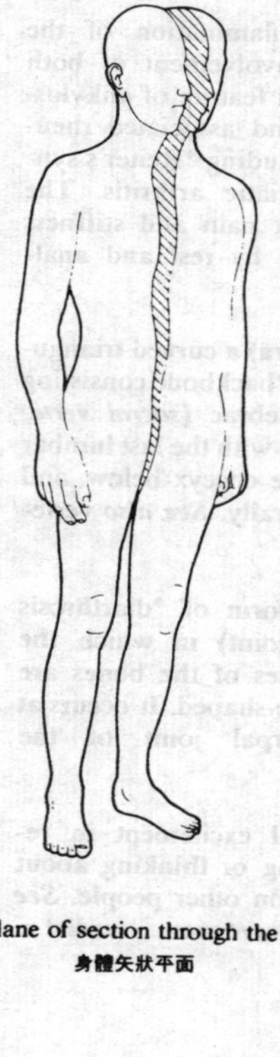

Sagittal plane of section through the body

身體矢狀平面

sagittal suture *see* suture (def. 1).

矢狀縫

salbutamol *n.* a drug, similar to *isoprenaline, used as a *bronchodilator to relieve asthma, chronic bronchitis, and emphysema. It is administered by mouth, injection, or inhalation; side-effects may include dizziness, tremor, and fast heart rate, particularly after large doses. Trade name: **Ventolin**.

沙丁胺醇 一種與異丙腎上腺素近似的藥物。用作支氣管擴張劑，治療哮喘、慢性支氣管炎和肺氣腫。口服、注射或噴霧吸入。副作用可有眩暈、肌肉震顫、心率加快，大劑量使用時尤爲多見。商品名：舒喘靈。

salicylamide *n.* an analgesic drug with effects and uses similar to those of *aspirin. It is administered by mouth and may cause dizziness, sweating, and digestive upsets at high doses. Trade name: **Salimed**.

水楊酸胺 一種鎮痛劑。其作用和用途與阿司匹林近似。口服。大劑量時可有眩暈、出汗和胃腸道不適。

salicylic acid a drug that causes the skin to peel and destroys bacteria and fungi. It is applied to the skin to treat ulcers, dandruff, eczema, psoriasis, warts, and corns. Skin sensitivity reactions may occur after continued use.

水楊酸 一種可使表皮脫落、殺滅細菌和黴菌的藥物。塗搽於皮膚治療潰瘍、頭垢、濕疹、銀屑病、疣和雞眼。連續使用可有皮膚過敏反應。

salicylism *n.* poisoning due to an overdose of aspirin or other salicylate-containing compounds. The main symptoms are headache, dizziness, ringing in the ears (tinnitus), disturbances of vision, vomiting, and – in severe cases – delirium and collapse. There is often severe *acidosis.

水楊酸中毒 過量阿司匹林或其他含有水楊酸鹽的藥物引起的中毒。主要症狀有頭痛、眩暈、耳鳴、視力減退、嘔吐，嚴重者可有譫妄和虛脫，並常有嚴重酸中毒。

saline (normal saline) *n.* a solution containing 0.9% sodium chloride. Saline may be used clinically as a diluent for drugs administered by injection and as a plasma substitute.

鹽水（生理鹽水） 含0.9%氯化鈉的水溶液。臨床上用作注射劑的稀釋液和血漿代用品。

saliva *n.* the alkaline liquid secreted by the *salivary glands and the mucous membrane of the mouth. Its principal constituents are water, mucus, buffers, and enzymes (e.g. amylase). The functions of saliva are to keep the mouth moist, to aid swallowing of food, to minimize changes of acidity in the mouth, and to digest starch. —**salivary** *adj.*

唾液 由唾液腺和口腔黏膜分泌的鹼性液體。主要成分有水、黏液、緩衝物質和酶（如澱粉酶）。其作用是使口腔保持潮濕，帮助吞嚥食物，使口腔酸度變化減到最低限度，以及消化澱粉。

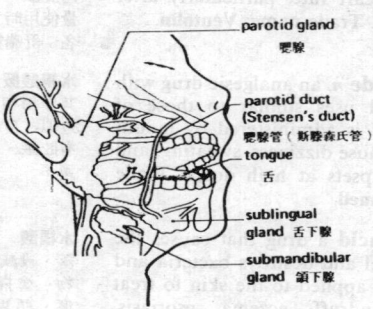

salivary gland a gland that produces *saliva. There are three pairs of salivary glands: the *parotid glands, *sublingual glands, and *submandibular glands (see illustration). They are stimulated by reflex action, which can be initiated by the taste, smell, sight, or thought of food.

唾液腺 產生唾液的腺體。有三對唾液腺：腮腺、舌下腺和頷下腺（見圖）。其分泌由味覺、嗅覺、視覺或想到食物的反射作用所引起。

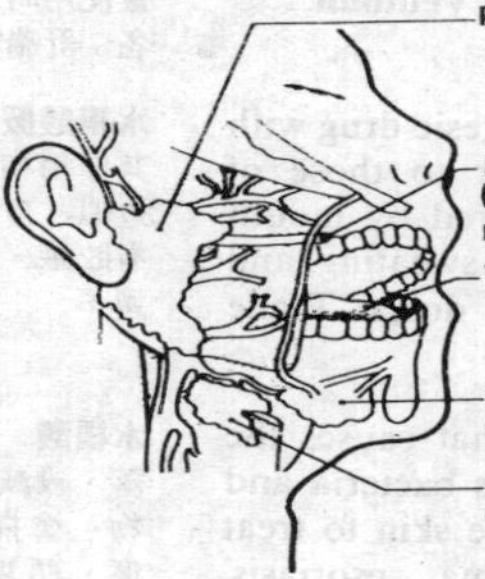

Salivary glands
唾液腺

salivation *n.* the secretion of saliva by the salivary glands of the mouth, increased in response to the chewing action of the jaws or to the thought, taste, smell, or sight of food. A small but regular flow of saliva is maintained to promote cleanliness in the mouth even when food is not being eaten. *See also* ptyalism.

流涎 由口腔唾液腺產生的唾液分泌現象。當咀嚼或者想到、嚐到、聞到或見到食物時，分泌即增加。即使沒有進食，仍有小量唾液有規律地分泌，以保持口內清潔。

Salk vaccine a vaccine against poliomyelitis, formed by treating the virus with formalin, which prevents it from causing disease but does not impair its ability to stimulate antibody production. It is administered by injection.

索爾克氏疫苗 一種抗脊髓灰質炎疫苗。用福爾馬林處理病毒製成。疫苗病毒不會致病，但不影響其刺激抗體產生的能力。注射用。

Salmonella *n.* a genus of Gram-negative motile rodlike bacteria that inhabit the intestines of animals and man and cause disease. They ferment glucose, usually with the formation of gas. The species *S. paratyphi* causes *paratyphoid fever, and *S. typhi* causes

沙門氏菌屬 一種革蘭氏陰性菌屬。桿狀，能運動。侵犯動物和人的腸道而致病。能發酵葡萄糖產生氣體。副傷寒沙門氏菌引起副傷寒，傷寒沙門氏菌引起腸傷寒。其他沙門

*typhoid fever. Other species of *Salmonella* cause *food poisoning, gastroenteritis, and septicaemia.

氏菌引起食物中毒、胃腸炎和敗血症。

salmonellosis *n.* an infestation of the digestive system by bacteria of the genus *Salmonella. See also* food poisoning.

沙門氏菌病 由沙門氏菌屬細菌引起的胃腸道感染。

salping- (salpingo-) *prefix denoting* **1.** the Fallopian tube. **2.** the auditory tube (meatus).

〔前綴〕 ①**輸卵管** ②**咽鼓管**

salpingectomy *n.* the surgical removal or cutting of a Fallopian tube. The operation involving both tubes is a permanent and completely effective method of contraception (*see* sterilization) since it prevents the egg cells passing from the ovaries to the womb.

輸卵管切除術 外科切除輸卵管。手術切除兩側輸卵管是永久性的和完全有效的避孕方法。使卵子不能從卵巢進入子宮。

salpingitis *n.* inflammation of a tube, most commonly applied to inflammation of one or both of the Fallopian tubes caused by bacterial infection spreading from the vagina or womb or carried in the blood. In *acute salpingitis* there is a sharp pain in the lower abdomen, which may be mistaken for that of appendicitis, and the infection may spread to the membrane lining the abdominal cavity (*see* peritonitis). In severe cases the tubes may become blocked with scar tissue and the patient will be unable to conceive. The condition is treated with antibiotics or by surgical removal of the diseased tube(s).

輸卵管炎 輸卵管炎症。見於一側或兩側。係由經陰道或子宮或血液傳播的細菌感染引起。急性輸卵管炎時下腹部有劇烈疼痛，常誤診爲闌尾炎。感染可傳播至腹膜。在嚴重病例，輸卵管可被瘢痕組織阻塞，患者不能再受孕。治療：用抗生素或切除病側輸卵管。

salpingography *n.* *radiography of one or both Fallopian tubes after a *radio-opaque substance has been introduced into them via an injection into the womb.

輸卵管造影術 對一側或兩側輸卵管進行X線造影的技術。經由子宮注射造影劑。

salpingo-oophoritis (salpingo-oothecitis) *n.* inflammation of a Fallopian tube and an ovary.

輸卵管卵巢炎 輸卵管和卵巢的炎症。

salpingo-oophorocele (salpingo-oothecocele) *n.* hernia involving a Fallopian tube and an ovary.

輸卵管卵巢疝 累及輸卵管和卵巢的疝。

salt depletion excessive loss of sodium chloride (common salt) from the body. This may result from sweating, persistent vomiting or diarrhoea, or loss of fluid in wounds. The main symptoms are muscular weakness and cramps. Miners and workers in hot climates are particularly at risk, and salt tablets are often taken as a preventive measure.

缺鹽 身體過度喪失氯化物（食鹽）。可由出汗、頑固性嘔吐或腹瀉，或創傷丟失液體所致。主要症狀爲肌肉無力或痙攣。礦工和勞工們在炎熱氣候下尤爲危險。常以服用鹽片作爲預防措施。

Samaritans *n.* a British voluntary organization providing a telephone service for the suicidal and despairing. Started in 1953 by the Rev. Chad Varah in the cellars of a London church (St. Stephens, Walbrook) with one telephone, it now has over 170 branches throughout the country manned by some 20,000 volunteers. It offers a nonprofessional, confidential, and (if required) anonymous service at all hours. Samaritans will listen for as long as they are needed and the service is free. They offer little advice, believing that their clients will be helped to make their own decisions by talking to someone who cares. They also offer a befriending service to support exceptionally distressed clients through a serious crisis.

撒瑪利亞社 英國的一個爲自殺者和絕望者提供電話服務的志願組織。始於1953年，由查德·瓦拉大法師在倫敦教堂的地下室設立一個電話。至今全國已有170個以上分支，約20000名志願者。該組織不分晝夜提供非職業性的、保密的和（如需要的話）匿名的服務。當有人求助於他們時，他們會耐心傾聽，而其服務是不收費的。他們很少給求助者出主意，相信求助者同關懷他的人交談後會得到幫助，作出自己的決定。他們也給遭遇嚴重危機而格外痛苦的求助人提供友好的援助服務。

sanatorium *n.* **1.** a hospital or institution for the rehabilitation and convalescence of patients of any kind. **2.** an institution for patients who have suffered from pulmonary tuberculosis.

療養院 ①使各類病人康復的醫院或機構。②爲肺結核病人設置的機構。

sandfly *n.* a small hairy fly of the widely distributed genus *Phlebotomus*. Adult sandflies rarely exceed 3 mm in length and have long slender legs. The blood-sucking females of certain species transmit various diseases, including *leishmaniasis, *sandfly fever, and *bartonellosis.

白蛉 一種多毛的白蛉屬微小昆蟲。分布很廣。成蟲的長度很少超過3mm，腿細長。有某幾種吸血的雌白蛉傳播多種疾病，包括利什曼病、白蛉熱和巴爾通氏體病。

sandfly fever (Pappataci fever) a viral disease transmitted to man by the bite of the sandfly *Phlebotomus papatasii*. Sandfly fever occurs principally in countries surrounding the Persian Gulf

白蛉熱 一種病毒病。由巴氏白蛉叮咬人而傳播。主要發生於波斯灣和熱帶地中海周圍的國家。在較暖的月份內出現，爲時不

and the tropical Mediterranean; it occurs during the warmer months, does not last long, and is never fatal. Symptoms resembie those of influenza. There is no specific treatment apart from aspirin and codeine to relieve the symptoms.
長，不致命。症狀同流感。除用阿司匹林和可待因減輕症狀外，無特殊治療。

sangui- (sanguino-) *prefix denoting* blood.
〔前綴〕 **血**

sanguineous *adj.* **1.** containing, stained, or covered with blood. **2.** (of tissues) containing more than the normal quantity of blood.
①**血性** 含血的，染血的，或被血覆蓋的。 ②**多血的** 含有超過正常量血液的（組織）。

sanies *n.* a foul-smelling watery discharge from a wound or ulcer, containing serum, blood, and pus.
腐膿液 有惡臭味的水樣排出物。由傷口或潰瘍流出，含有血清、血和膿。

saphena *n. see* saphenous vein.
隱靜脉

saphenous nerve a large branch of the *femoral nerve that arises in the upper thigh, travels down on the inside of the leg, and supplies the skin from the knee to below the ankle with sensory nerves.
隱神經 股神經的一個大分支。起於大腿上部，沿小腿內側下行。其感覺纖維分佈於膝至踝以下的皮膚。

saphenous vein (saphena) either of two superficial veins of the leg, draining blood from the foot. The *long saphenous vein* – the longest vein in the body – runs from the foot, up the medial side of the leg, to the groin, where it joins the femoral vein. The *short saphenous vein* runs up the back of the calf to join the popliteal vein at the back of the knee.
隱靜脉 小腿的兩條淺靜脉。均收集足背淺靜脉的血液。大隱靜脉——體內最長的靜脉——從足背沿小腿內側上行至腹股溝，注入股靜脉。小隱靜脉沿腓腸肌背面上行，在膕窩處注入膕靜脉。

sapr- (sapro-) *prefix denoting* **1.** putrefaction. **2.** decaying matter.
〔前綴〕 **腐** ①腐爛。②腐朽物質。

sapraemia *n.* blood poisoning by toxins of saprophytic bacteria (bacteria living on dead or decaying matter). *Compare* pyaemia, septicaemia, toxaemia.
腐血症 血中毒。由腐物寄生菌（靠屍體或腐爛物質生活的細菌）的毒素引起。

saprophyte *n.* any free-living organism that lives and feeds on the dead and putrefying tissues of animals or plants. *Compare* parasite. —**saprophytic** *adj.*
腐生物 任何靠動物和人的屍體和腐爛組織營養而生活的微生物。

sarc- (sarco-) *prefix denoting* **1.** flesh or fleshy tissue. **2.** muscle.

〔前綴〕 ①**肉** 肉樣組織。 ②**肌**

sarcocele *n.* an obsolete term for a fleshy tumour (sarcoma) of the testis.

睪丸肉樣腫 睪丸肉瘤的舊稱。

Sarcocystis *n.* a genus of parasitic protozoans (*see* Sporozoa) that infect birds, reptiles, and herbivorous mammals. *S. lindemanni*, which occasionally infects man, forms cylindrical cysts (*sarcocysts*) in the muscle fibres. In heavy infections these cysts can cause tissue degeneration and so provoke muscular pain and weakness. Sarcocysts have, in the few positively diagnosed cases, been located in the heart muscles, arm muscles, and larynx.

肉孢子蟲屬 寄生原蟲的一屬。感染鳥類、爬蟲類和食草的哺乳動物。林德曼氏肉孢子蟲偶可感染人，在肌組織內形成圓筒狀包囊（肉孢子蟲囊）。嚴重感染時包囊可導至組織變性，引起肌肉疼痛無力。少數確診病例見有肉孢子蟲囊位於心肌、臂肌和喉內。

sarcoid 1. *adj.* fleshy. **2.** *n.* a fleshy tumour.

①**肉樣的** ②**肉樣瘤，類肉瘤**

sarcoidosis *n.* a chronic disorder of unknown cause in which the lymph nodes in many parts of the body are enlarged and small fleshy nodules (*see* granuloma) develop in the lungs, liver, and spleen. The skin, nervous system, and the eyes and salivary glands are also commonly affected (*see* uveoparotitis), and the condition has features similar to *tuberculosis. Recovery is complete with minimal after-effects in two-thirds of all cases.

肉樣瘤病，類肉瘤病 一種病因未明的慢性疾患。體內許多部位的淋巴結都腫大，並在肺、肝和脾內生長小的肉樣結節。皮膚、神經系統、眼和唾液腺亦常受累。其症狀與結核有相似的特徵。可完全痊癒，僅三分之二的病例有極輕微的後遺症。

sarcolemma *n.* the cell membrane that encloses a muscle cell (muscle fibre).

肌膜 包被肌細胞（肌纖維）的細胞膜。

sarcoma *n.* any *cancer of connective tissue. These tumours may occur in any part of the body, as they arise in the tissues that make up an organ rather than being restricted to a particular organ. They can arise in fibrous tissue, muscle, fat, bone, cartilage, synovium, blood and lymphatic vessels, and various other tissues. *See also* chondrosarcoma, fibrosarcoma, leiomyosarcoma, liposarcoma, lymphangiosarcoma, osteosarcoma, rhabdomyosarcoma. —**sarcomatous** *adj.*

肉瘤 任何結締組織的惡性腫瘤。肉瘤發生於構成器官的組織中，並非局限於某一種器官，因此可發生於體內任何部位。肉瘤可發生於纖維組織、肌肉、脂肪、骨、軟骨、滑膜、血管、淋巴管及其他各種組織。

sarcoma botryoides *see* carcinosarcoma.

葡萄樣肉瘤

sarcomatosis *n.* *sarcoma that has spread widely throughout the body, most commonly through the bloodstream. It is treated with drugs, typically one or a combination of the following: cyclophosphamide, vincristine, actinomycin-D, methotrexate, or doxorubicin.

肉瘤病 肉瘤已遍及全身的疾患。以通過血流傳播最爲常見。治療：通過單獨或聯合使用下列藥物：環磷醯胺、長春新鹼、放射菌素D、甲氨蝶呤或阿黴素。

sarcomere *n.* one of the basic contractile units of which *striated muscle fibres are composed.

肌原纖維節 組成橫紋肌纖維的一個基本收縮單位。

Sarcophaga *n.* a genus of widely distributed non-bloodsucking flies, the flesh flies. Maggots are normally found in carrion or excrement but occasionally females will deposit their eggs in wounds or ulcers giving off a foul-smelling discharge; the presence of the maggots causes a serious *myiasis. Rarely, maggots may be ingested with food and give rise to an intestinal myiasis.

麻蠅屬 一種不吸血的蠅屬。或稱肉蠅。分佈甚廣。通常在腐肉或糞便中找到蛆。偶見雌蠅排卵於傷口或潰瘍內，產生惡臭的排出物。蛆的存在可致嚴重的蠅蛆病。罕見蛆被攝食而引起腸道蛆病。

sarcoplasm (myoplasm) *n.* the cytoplasm of muscle cells.

肌質（肌漿） 肌細胞的胞漿。

sarcoplasmic reticulum an arrangement of membranous vesicles and tubules found in the cytoplasm of striated muscle fibres. The sarcoplasmic reticulum plays an important role in the transmission of nervous excitation to the contractile parts of the fibres.

肌質網 由膜小泡和膜小管排列組成。見於橫紋肌纖維的胞漿內。對傳遞神經興奮信息至肌的收縮纖維起重要作用。

Sarcoptes *n.* a genus of small oval mites. The female of *S. scabiei*, the human itch mite, tunnels into the skin, where it lays its eggs. The presence of the mites causes severe irritation, which eventually leads to *scabies.

疥蟎屬 一種小的橢圓形蟎屬。雌性疥蟎，即人疥蟎，穿入皮膚挖成隧道，在該處產卵。疥蟎引起嚴重的皮膚刺激，最終導至疥瘡。

sarcostyle *n.* a bundle of muscle fibrils.

肌柱 一束肌纖維。

sartorius *n.* a narrow ribbon-like muscle at the front of the thigh, arising from the anterior superior spine of the ilium and extending to the tibia, just below

縫匠肌 一塊窄的帶狀肌肉。位於大腿前面，起自髂前上棘，延伸至脛骨，緊靠膝下方。是體內最長

the knee. The longest muscle in the body, the sartorius flexes the leg on the thigh and the thigh on the abdomen.

的肌肉，使小腿彎向大腿，大腿彎向腹部。

satyriasis *n.* an extreme degree of promiscuous heterosexual activity in men. *Compare* nymphomania.

求雌狂 男人的一種極度亂交異性的活動。

saucerization *n.* **1.** an operation in which tissue is cut away from a wound to form a saucer-like depression. It is carried out to facilitate healing and is commonly used to treat injuries or disorders in which bone is infected. **2.** the concave appearance of the upper surface of a vertebra that has been fractured by compression.

①**碟形手術** 一種從傷口切除組織形成碟狀凹陷的手術。這種手術有利於傷口癒合，通常用以治療損傷或骨受感染的疾患。②**碟形凹陷** 椎骨受壓骨折，上方椎面呈凹形。

Sayre's jacket a plaster of Paris cast shaped to fit around and support the backbone. It is used in cases where the vertebrae have been severely damaged by disease, such as tuberculosis.

塞爾氏背心 一種圓柱形石膏夾。用以支持脊柱。當椎骨由於疾病，如結核，而嚴重損壞時使用之。

scab *n.* a hard crust of dried blood, serum, or pus that develops during the body's wound-healing process over a sore, cut, or scratch.

痂 由乾涸的血、血清或膿結成的硬殼。係潰瘍、切割傷或抓傷在傷口癒合過程中產生的。

scabicide *n.* a drug that kills the mites causing *scabies.

殺疥蟎藥 一種殺滅引起疥瘡的蟎的藥物。

scabies *n.* a skin infection caused by the itch mite, **Sarcoptes scabiei*. Scabies is typified by severe itching (particularly at night), red papules, and often secondary infection. The female mite tunnels in the skin to lay her eggs and the newly hatched mites pass easily from person to person by contact. The intense itching is caused by the mite's secretion. Commonly infected areas are the groin, penis, nipples, and the skin between the fingers. Local treatment is with hexachlorophane or benzyl benzoate creams, which kill the mites. All members of a family may need treatment, and clothing and bedding should be disinfested.

疥瘡 一種由疥蟎引起的皮膚感染。其徵象爲奇癢（尤在夜間），有紅色丘疹，常繼發感染。雌蟎穿入皮膚挖成隧道，在該處產卵。新孵化的蟎極易經人與人的接觸而傳播。強烈的瘙癢由蟎的分泌物引起。通常感染的部位有腹股溝、陰莖、乳頭和手指間的皮膚。患部用六氯酚或苯甲酸苄脂乳劑殺滅疥蟎。家庭中所有成員都需治療，衣服和被褥要消毒。

scala *n.* one of the spiral canals of the *cochlea. The *scala media* (*cochlear duct*) is the central membranous canal,

階 爲耳蝸螺旋管的一種。中階（蝸管）是中央的膜管，含有耳蝸的感覺

containing the sensory apparatus of the cochlea; the *scala vestibuli* and *scala tympani* are the two bony canals of the cochlea.

器；前庭階和鼓階是耳蝸的兩個骨蝸管。

scald *n.* a *burn produced by a hot liquid or vapour, such as boiling water or steam.

燙傷 由熱的液體或蒸汽所致的燒傷。如沸水或水蒸氣。

scale 1. *n.* any of the flakes of dead epidermal cells shed from the skin. **2.** *vb.* to scrape deposits of calculus (tartar) from the teeth (*see* scaler).

①**鱗屑** 皮膚脫落的絮片或死亡的表皮細胞。 ②**刮治** 從牙齒刮除牙石的手術。

scalenus *n.* one of four paired muscles of the neck (*scalenus anterior*, *medius*, *minimus*, and *posterior*), extending from the cervical (neck) vertebrae to the first and second ribs. They are responsible for raising the first and second ribs in inspiration and for bending the neck forward and to either side.

斜角肌 頸部的四對肌肉（前斜角肌、中斜角肌、小斜角肌和後斜角肌）。起自頸椎，止於第1和第2肋。可上提第1、2肋，以助吸氣。可使頸前屈或向兩邊側屈。

scalenus syndrome (thoracic outlet syndrome) the group of symptoms caused by the scalenus anterior muscle compressing the subclavian artery and the lower roots of the brachial plexus against the fibrous and bony structures of the outlet of the upper thoracic vertebrae. Loss of sensation, wasting, and vascular symptoms may be found in the affected arm.

前斜角肌綜合徵（頸胸出口區綜合徵） 鎖骨下動脉以及臂叢下幹在前斜角肌與頸胸出口區的骨組織、纖維組織之間受到壓迫所引起的一組症狀。患側臂可有感覺喪失、消瘦和血管的症狀。

scaler *n.* an instrument for removing calculus from the teeth. It may be a hand instrument or one energized by rapid ultrasonic vibrations.

刮器 一種用以刮除齒上牙石的器械。這種刮器可以是用手操作的，或是以快速超聲振動爲能量的。的。

scalpel *n.* a small pointed surgical knife used by surgeons for cutting tissues. It has a straight handle with detachable disposable blades of different shapes.

解剖刀 一種小的帶尖頭的外科刀。外科醫生用以切割組織。這種刀有一個直的刀柄，並裝有可拆卸的、用後即可丟棄的各式刀片。

scanning speech a disorder of articulation in which the syllables are inappropriately separated and equally stressed. It is caused by disease of the cerebellum or its connecting fibres in the brainstem.

斷續言語 一種言語障礙。音節被不適當地隔開，並同等地重讀。係由於小腦疾病或小腦與腦幹的連接纖維發生障礙所致。

scaphocephaly *n.* an abnormally long and narrow skull due to premature closure of the suture between the two parietal bones, along the top of the skull. It is usually associated with mental retardation. —**scaphocephalic** *adj.*

舟狀頭 一種異常長而狹的頭顱。由於顱頂兩塊頂骨間的骨縫過早閉合所致。通常伴有精神發育遲緩。

scaphoid bone a boat-shaped bone of the wrist (*see* carpus). It articulates with the trapezium and trapezoid bones in front and with the radius behind.

舟狀骨 腕部的一塊船形小骨。前面與大多角骨和小多角骨，後面與橈骨形成關節。

scapul- (scapulo-) *prefix denoting* the scapula.

〔前綴〕 **肩胛**

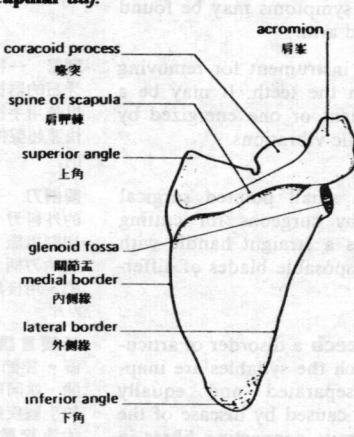

scapula *n.* (*pl.* **scapulas** *or* **scapulae**) the shoulder blade: a triangular bone, a pair of which form the back part of the shoulder girdle (see illustration). The *spine* on its dorsal (back) surface ends at the *acromion process* at the top of the shoulder. This process turns forward and articulates with the collar bone (*clavicle) at the *acromioclavicular joint*; it overhangs the *glenoid fossa*, into which the humerus fits to form the socket of the shoulder joint. The *coracoid process* curves upwards and forwards from the neck of the scapula and provides attachment for ligaments and muscles. —**scapular** *adj.*

肩胛骨 肩部的一塊三角形扁骨。一對肩胛骨形成肩胛帶的背側部分（見圖）。背側面的骨嵴末端止於肩最高點的肩峯。肩峯轉向前面與鎖骨形成肩鎖關節。肩鎖關節位於肩關節盂的上方。肱骨頭插入盂內形成肩關節的球窩。喙突從肩胛頸的上前方彎曲突出，其上有肌肉和韌帶附着。

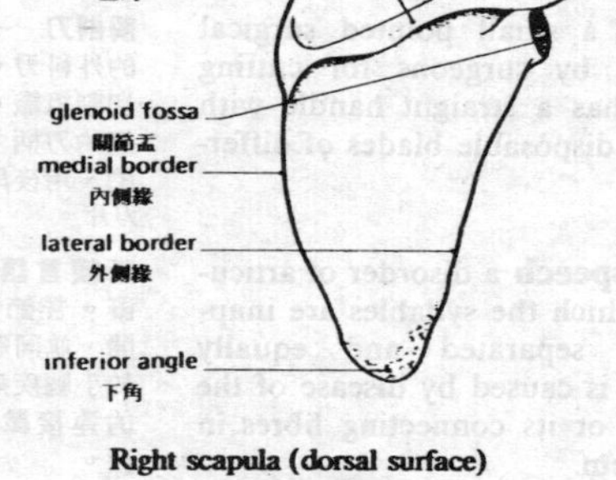

Right scapula (dorsal surface)
右肩胛骨（背面）

scar *n. see* cicatrix.
瘢痕

scarification *n.* the process of making a series of shallow cuts or scratches in the skin to allow a substance to penetrate the body. This is commonly performed during vaccination against smallpox; the vaccine is administered as a droplet left in contact with the scarified area.
劃痕 通過在皮膚上劃幾條淺的切口或痕道使某一物質得以透入體內的方法。常用於接種牛痘以預防天花，痘苗滴於劃痕部位。

scarlatina *n. see* scarlet fever.
猩紅熱

scarlet fever a highly contagious disease, mainly of childhood, caused by bacteria of the genus **Streptococcus*. It is transmitted either from a patient or carrier (by coughing) or through contaminated milk. Symptoms commence 2–4 days after exposure and include fever, sickness, sore throat, and a widespread scarlet rash that spreads from the armpits and groin to the neck, chest, back, and limbs and also affects the tongue. Treatment with antibiotics shortens the disease and prevents such complications as ear and kidney infections and swollen neck glands. An infection usually confers life-long immunity. Medical name: **scarlatina**. *Compare* German measles.
猩紅熱 一種具有高度傳染性的疾病。主要感染兒童，係鏈球菌屬的細菌所致。此病由病人或帶菌者（經咳嗽），或由污染的牛奶傳播。感染後2～4日出現症狀。有發燒、噁心、咽喉炎，以及從腋部和腹股溝遍及頸、胸、背和四肢的猩紅色皮疹，舌面上也可出現。用抗生素治療可縮短病程，並預防合併症的發生，如耳和腎的感染及頸淋巴腺腫大。一次感染通常獲得終身免疫。

Scarpa's triangle *see* femoral triangle.
斯卡帕氏三角

scat- (scato-) *prefix denoting* faeces.
〔前綴〕 糞

scatter diagram (in statistics) *see* correlation.
點圖 （用於統計學）

Schick test a test to determine whether a person is susceptible to diphtheria. A small quantity of diphtheria toxin is injected under the skin; a patch of reddening and swelling shows that the person has no immunity and – if at particular risk – should be immunized.
錫克氏試驗 檢查對白喉是否易感的試驗。用小量白喉毒素注於皮下，出現紅腫斑表示無免疫力，對處於有感染危險的人必須進行免疫接種。

Schiff's reagent aqueous *fuchsin solution decolourized with sulphur dioxide. A blue coloration develops in the presence of aldehydes.
希夫氏試劑 品紅水溶液，用二氧化硫作脫色劑。有醛類存在時即出現藍色。

Schilling test a test used to assess a patient's capacity to absorb vitamin B_{12} from the bowel. Radioactive vitamin B_{12} is given by mouth and urine collected for 24 hours. A normal individual will excrete at least 10% of the original dose over this period; a patient with *pernicious anaemia will excrete less than 5%.

希林氏試驗 檢查腸道對維生素 B_{12}的吸收能力的試驗。口服放射性維生素 B_{12}，並收集24小時尿。正常人在這期間至少排出原劑量的10%，患惡性貧血的病人僅排出不足5%。

schindylesis *n.* a form of *synarthrosis (immovable joint) in which a crest of one bone fits into a groove of another.

嵌合連接 不動關節的一種連接形式。在這種關節內，一骨之鋭緣插入另一骨之深溝中。

-schisis *suffix denoting* a cleft or split.

〔後綴〕 **裂口，裂縫**

schism *n.* a disorder of relationships within a family, in which parents quarrel and children are made to take sides. It was proposed as a cause of later schizophrenia in the children, but is more likely to be a nonspecific cause of psychological vulnerability.

分裂 家庭內的一種混亂關係。父母爭吵，子女被迫參與袒護一方。人們曾認爲這是兒童日後患精神分裂症的一個病因，但這更可能是精神創傷的一個非特異性病因。

schisto- *prefix denoting* a fissure; split.

〔前綴〕 **分裂，裂縫**

schistoglossia *n.* fissuring of the tongue. Congenital fissures are transverse, whereas those due to disease (such as syphilis) are usually longitudinal.

舌裂 舌的裂隙。先天性舌裂是横向的，而因病（如梅毒）所致的舌裂常是縱向的。

Schistosoma (Bilharzia) *n.* a genus of blood *flukes, three species of which are important parasites of man causing one of the most serious of tropical diseases (*see* schistosomiasis). *S. japonicum* is common in the Far East; *S. mansoni* is widespread in Africa, the West Indies, and South and Central America; and *S. haematobium* occurs in Africa and the Middle East.

血吸蟲屬（裂體吸蟲屬） 一種血內吸蟲屬。此屬中有三種是人的重要寄生蟲，可引起一種極爲嚴重的熱帶病。日本血吸蟲常見於遠東，曼森氏血吸蟲廣泛傳播於非洲、西印度羣島及中美與南美，埃及血吸蟲見於非洲和中東。

schistosomiasis (bilharziasis) *n.* a tropical disease caused by blood flukes of the genus *Schistosoma*. Eggs present in the stools or urine of infected people undergo part of their larval development within freshwater snails living in water contaminated with human sewage. The disease is contracted when *cercaria larvae, released from the

血吸蟲病（裂體吸蟲病） 一種熱帶病。由血吸蟲屬的住血吸蟲引起。蟲卵存在於受感染者的糞和尿內，隨人的排泄物流入水中。幼蟲的發育有一部分在淡水釘螺中進行。尾蚴離開釘螺，穿入在污染水沐浴的人的皮膚內，使感

snails, penetrate the skin of anyone bathing in infected water. Adult flukes eventually settle in the blood vessels of the intestine (*S. mansoni* and *S. japonicum*) or bladder (*S. haematobium*); the release of their spiked eggs causes anaemia, inflammation, and the formation of scar tissue. Additional intestinal symptoms are diarrhoea, dysentery, enlargement of the spleen and liver, and cirrhosis of the liver. If the bladder is affected, blood is passed in the urine and cystitis and cancer of the bladder may develop. The disease is treated with various drugs, including *stibophen and other antimony-containing preparations and *niridazole.

染致病。成蟲最終棲居於腸內血管中（曼森氏血吸蟲和日本血吸蟲）或膀胱中(埃及血吸蟲)。成蟲下卵呈窩狀堆積在一起，可導至貧血、炎症，以及形成瘢痕組織。此外腸道症狀有腹瀉、痢疾、脾和肝腫大，以及肝硬變。如膀胱受累，可見血尿，並可能發生膀胱炎和膀胱惡性腫瘤。此病可用多種藥物治療，包括銻波芬和其他含銻的製劑，以及硝噻唑唑。

schiz- (schizo-) *prefix denoting* a split or division.

〔前綴〕 **裂，分裂**

schizogony *n.* a phase of asexual reproduction in the life cycle of a sporozoan (protozoan parasite) that occurs in the liver or red blood cells. The parasite grows and divides many times to form a *schizont*, which contains many *merozoites. The eventual release of merozoites of **Plasmodium*, the malaria parasite, from the blood cells produces fever in the patient.

裂殖生殖 孢子蟲（寄生原蟲）生活史中的無性生殖期。發生於肝或紅細胞內。原蟲生長並多次分裂，形成裂殖體，含有許多裂殖子。瘧原蟲裂殖子從紅細胞內釋放出來，導至病人發燒。

schizoid personality a personality characterized by solitariness, emotional coldness to others, excessive introspection, and eccentricity of behaviour. Some schizophrenics have this personality before their illness, but most schizoid personalities do not become schizophrenic. *See* personality disorder.

精神分裂樣人格 一種以孤獨、對他人冷漠、極度內省傾向、行爲乖僻爲特徵的人格。有些精神分裂症患者在其得病前即有這樣的人格，但大多有精神分裂樣人格者並沒有成爲精神分裂症患者。

schizont *n.* one of the stages that occurs during the asexual phase of the life cycle of a sporozoan. *See* schizogony.

裂殖體 孢子蟲生活史中無性生殖階段的一期。

schizonticide *n.* any agent used for killing *schizonts.

殺裂殖體劑 殺滅裂殖體的藥物。

schizophrenia *n.* a severe mental disorder (or group of disorders) character-

精神分裂症 一種嚴重的精神疾病（或一組精神障

ized by a disintegration of the process of thinking, of contact with reality, and of emotional responsiveness. *Delusions and *hallucinations (especially of voices) are usual features, and the patient usually feels that his thoughts, sensations, and actions are controlled by, or shared with, others. He becomes socially withdrawn and loses energy and initiative. The main types of schizophrenia are *simple*, in which increasing social withdrawal and personal ineffectiveness are the major changes; *hebephrenic*, which starts in adolescence or young adulthood (*see* hebephrenia); *paranoid*, characterized by prominent delusions; and *catatonic*, with marked motor disturbances (*see* catatonia). Schizophrenia commonly – but not inevitably – runs a progressive course. The prognosis has been improved in recent years with drugs such as *phenothiazines and vigorous psychological and social management and rehabilitation. There are strong genetic factors in the causation, and environmental stress can precipitate illness. —**schizophrenic** *adj.*

礙）。其特徵爲：在思維過程、接觸現實和情感反應上有分裂現象。妄想和幻覺（尤其聽幻覺）也是常見的徵象。患者經常感到其思想、感覺和行動是受他人控制或與他人分擔的。患者迴避與外界交往、喪失活力和進取精神。精神分裂症的主要類型有：單純型，主要症狀爲與外界交往漸漸減少，活動能力日益減低；青春期痴呆型，始發於青春期或青年時期；妄想狂型，有突出的妄想特徵；緊張型，有明顯的運動障礙。精神分裂症通常——但並非必定——表現爲進行性病程。近年來用吩噻嗪類藥物治療，用强有力的心理和環境治療，以及用康復治療，使預後已有改進。精神分裂症的病因有明顯的遺傳因素，而環境壓力能助長其發病。

Schlemm's canal a channel in the eye, at the junction of the cornea and the sclera, through which the aqueous humour drains.

施累姆氏管 眼內的一個管道。位於角膜和鞏膜接合處。房水經此管向靜脉回流。

Schönlein-Henoch purpura a blood disease that affects young children; its cause is not known. It is characterized by a purple skin rash due to bleeding into the skin from defective capillaries; abdominal pain; and kidney disturbance. Spontaneous recovery is the usual outcome. *See also* purpura.

舍-亨二氏紫癜 一種侵犯幼兒的血液病。病因未明。其特徵爲皮膚出現紫色皮疹，係因病損的毛細血管出血滲入皮膚所致，腹痛，以及腎功能紊亂。通常自行恢復。

school health service (in Britain) a service concerned with the early detection of physical, mental, and emotional abnormalities in schoolchildren and their subsequent treatment and surveillance. The service was formerly based on an ideal of three examinations at 5,

學校衛生服務 （在英國）對學齡兒童的一種服務項目。目的是早日查出學童身體的、智力的和感情的異常，繼而給以治療和監視。這種服務早先的設想是由地方教育當局專

11, and 15 years by doctors and nurses specially employed by the Local Education Authority (LEA). It has now been changed to a system of selective examinations based on recommendations by teachers, *school nurses, or parental requests. The service is now the responsibility of the District Health Authority, but ascertainment and responsibility for allocation to *special schools remain the responsibility of the LEA.

門僱用醫師和護士對5、11、15歲的學童做三次檢查。現已改為根據教師和學校護士的建議以及家長的請求對學童進行選擇性檢查的制度。這種服務工作現由地段保健局負責，但對專門學校的確定和撥款，仍由地方教育當局負責。

school nurse a member of the *school health service who conducts routine examinations and/or treats minor ailments. *Health visitors may sometimes work in this capacity but State Registered and State Enrolled Nurses may also perform these tasks.

學校護士 學校保健服務系統的一個成員。擔任常規檢查及/或治療小傷小病的工作。保健員有時也擔任此項工作，而在政府注册或擔任公職的護士也可執行這些任務。

Schwann cells the cells that lay down the *myelin sheath around the axon of a medullated nerve fibre. Each cell is responsible for one length of axon, around which it twists as it grows, so that concentric layers of membrane envelop the axon. The gap between adjacent Schwann cells forms a *node of Ranvier.

許旺氏細胞 有髓神經纖維內的一種帶髓鞘細胞。其髓鞘鋪於神經纖維的軸突周圍。每一細胞包繞一段軸突，並沿軸突周圍纏繞生長，使鞘膜的同心層得以包裹軸突。鄰近的兩個許旺氏細胞間的裂縫形成一個郎飛氏結。

Schwannoma *n. see* neurofibroma.

神經鞘瘤

sciatica *n.* pain felt down the back and outer side of the thigh, leg, and foot. It is usually caused by degeneration of an intervertebral disc, which protrudes laterally to compress a lower lumbar or an upper sacral spinal nerve root. The onset may be sudden, brought on by an awkward lifting or twisting movement. The back is stiff and painful. There may be numbness and weakness in the leg. Bed rest will often relieve the pain but any persistence of numbness or weakness is an indication for surgical treatment.

坐骨神經痛 沿後腰、大腿外側、小腿直至足部的一種疼痛。常因某一椎間盤的退行性病變所致。椎間盤向側面突出，壓迫下部腰椎或上部骶椎的一條脊神經根。坐骨神經痛的發作可以是突然的，由一次不靈便的抬腿或扭轉活動引起。後腰部僵直且疼痛，腿部麻木無力。臥床休息常可減輕疼痛。如麻木無力持久不癒，則是外科治療的一個徵兆。

sciatic nerve the major nerve of the leg and the nerve with the largest diameter. It runs down behind the thigh from the lower end of the spine; above

坐骨神經 腿部的主要神經，也是體內直徑最大的神經。起自脊柱下部末端，沿大腿後面下行至膝

the knee joint it divides into two main branches, the *tibial* and *common peroneal nerves*, which are distributed to the muscles and skin of the lower leg.

關節上方，分成兩個主支，即脛神經和腓總神經，支配小腿的肌肉和皮膚。

scintigram *n.* a diagram showing the distribution of radioactive *tracer in a part of the body, produced by recording the flashes of light given off by a *scintillator as it is struck by radiation of different intensities. By scanning the body, section by section, a 'map' of the radioactivity in various regions is built up, aiding the diagnosis of cancer or other disorders. Such a record is known as a *scintiscan*.

閃爍圖 一種顯示身體某一部位放射性示踪物分佈情況的圖形。閃爍體受不同强度的放射線碰撞，可產生各種熒光，錄製下來即成閃爍圖。對身體分段掃描，製成各部位的放射性"地圖"，有助於診斷惡性腫瘤或其他疾患。這樣一種檢查稱爲閃爍掃描。

scintillascope *n.* the instrument used to produce a *scintigram. It incorporates a *scintillator, a device to magnify the fluorescence produced in it by radiations, and a means of recording the results, often aided by a computer. *See also* gamma camera.

閃爍鏡 用以產生閃爍圖的儀器。它由下列部件合併組成：一個閃爍器，一個把由射線產生的熒光放大的裝置，一個記錄器，常附有電子計算機。

scintillation counter (scintimeter) a device to measure and record the fluorescent flashes in a *scintillator exposed to high-energy radiation, as in a *scintillascope.

閃爍計數器 一個測量和記錄熒光的裝置。此裝置安裝在暴露於高能量射線的閃爍器內，同樣可安裝在閃爍鏡內。

scintillator *n.* a substance that produces a fluorescent flash when struck by high-energy radiation, such as beta or gamma rays. In medicine the most commonly used scintillator is a crystal of thallium-activated sodium iodide. The fluorescence, magnified by a phototube multiplier, may be recorded photographically or electronically during the production of a *scintigram or scintiscan.

閃爍體 一種接受高能量射線，如β或γ射線碰撞後可發生熒光的物質。在醫學上最常用的閃爍體是鉈激活的碘化鈉的結晶體。熒光被光電管倍增器放大，採用照像或電子技術製成閃爍圖或進行閃爍掃描。

scintiscan *n. see* scintigram.

閃爍掃描

scirrhous *adj.* describing carcinomas that are stony hard to the touch. Such a carcinoma (for example of the breast) is known as a *scirrhus*.

硬癌的 描述摸着如同石頭一樣堅硬的癌。這樣的癌（如乳癌）被稱爲硬癌。

scissor leg a disability in which one leg becomes permanently crossed over

剪形腿 一種殘疾。由於腿部內收肌處於强直狀

the other as a result of spasticity of its *adductor muscles. The condition occurs in children with brain damage and in adults after strokes. A *tenotomy sometimes reduces the degree of disability.

態，致使這條腿永遠交叉於另一腿的上方。這種情況發生於腦損傷的兒童和中風後的成人。施行腱切斷術有時可使殘疾不同程度地復原。

scissura (scissure) *n.* a cleft or splitting, such as the splitting of the tip of a hair or the splitting open of tissues when a hernia forms.

分裂　裂開或裂口。如毛髮的尖端裂開，或疝形成時的組織裂口。

scler- (sclero-) *prefix denoting* **1.** hardening or thickening. **2.** the sclera. **3.** sclerosis.

〔前綴〕 ①**變硬，變厚** ②**鞏膜** ③**硬化**

sclera (sclerotic coat) *n.* the white fibrous outer layer of the eyeball. At the front of the eye it becomes the cornea. *See* eye. —**scleral** *adj.*

鞏膜　眼球的白色纖維外層。在眼的前部成爲角膜。

sclerectomy *n.* an operation in which a portion of the sclera (the outer white layer of the eyeball) is removed.

鞏膜切除術　一種部分切除鞏膜（眼球的白色外層）的手術。

scleritis *n.* inflammation of the sclera (the white of the eye).

鞏膜炎　鞏膜（眼的白色部分）的炎症。

scleroderma *n.* persistent hardening and contraction of the body's connective tissue. It can affect any part, including the skin, heart, kidney, lung, or oesophagus (gullet). Scleroderma may be localized (*see* morphoea) or it can spread slowly throughout the body, eventually causing death (there is no effective treatment). The skin is thickened and tough, often with pigmented patches.

硬皮病　身體結締組織持久地硬化和收縮。可侵犯身體的任何部分，包括皮膚、心、腎、肺或食道（咽喉）。硬皮病可以是局限性的，或可緩慢地遍及全身，最終導至死亡（尚無有效的治療）。皮膚變厚變粗，常有色素沉着斑。

scleroma *n.* a hardened patch of skin or mucous membrane, consisting of *granulation tissue.

硬結　皮膚或黏膜的一塊變硬的斑。由肉芽組織組成。

scleromalacia *n.* thinning of the sclera (white of the eye) as a result of inflammation. The involved area becomes bluish in colour. Sometimes the sclera fades away completely in an area, and the underlying tissue (usually the cili-

鞏膜軟化　鞏膜（眼的白色部分）變薄。係炎症的結果。受累處顏色變藍。有時鞏膜有一部分完全消失，其下層的組織（通常是睫狀體）膨出於結膜

ary body) bulges beneath the conjunctiva. This state is known as *scleromalacia perforans*.

下。這種狀况稱爲穿通性鞏膜軟化。

scleronychia *n.* hardening and thickening of the nails.

指(趾)甲硬化 指(趾)甲變硬變厚。

sclerosis *n.* hardening of tissue, usually due to scarring (fibrosis) after inflammation. It can affect the lateral columns of the spinal cord and the medulla of the brain (*amyotrophic lateral sclerosis*), causing progressive muscular paralysis (*see* motor neurone disease). It can also occur in scattered patches throughout the brain and spinal cord (*see* multiple sclerosis) or in the walls of the arteries (*see* arteriosclerosis, atherosclerosis). *See also* tuberous sclerosis.

硬化 組織變硬。通常由於炎症後瘢痕形成(纖維化)所致。硬化可累及脊髓側索和延髓(肌萎縮性脊髓側索硬化),引起進行性肌麻痹。硬化也可在腦和脊髓中到處發生,有散發性斑塊形成,或可發生於動脉壁。

sclerotherapy *n.* treatment of varicose veins by the injection of an irritant solution. This causes thrombophlebitis, which encourages obliteration of the varicose vein by thrombosis and subsequent scarring.

硬化療法 用注射一種刺激性溶液治療靜脉曲張的方法。此療法能引起血栓性靜脉炎,導至血栓形成,繼而結成瘢痕,而使曲張的靜脉得以閉塞。

sclerotic 1. (*or* **sclerotic coat**) *n. see* sclera. **2.** *adj.* affected with *sclerosis.

①鞏膜的(或鞏膜) ②硬化的

sclerotome *n.* **1.** a surgical knife used in the operation of *sclerotomy. **2.** (in embryology) the part of the segmented mesoderm (*see* somite) in the early embryo that gives rise to all the skeletal tissue of the body. The vertebrae and ribs retain the segmented structure, which is lost in the skull and limbs.

①鞏膜刀 一種外科刀。用於鞏膜切開手術。 **②生骨節** (胚胎學)胚胎早期中胚層的體節部分。身體所有的骨骼組織來源於此體節。脊椎和肋仍保留分節的結構,而在頭顱和四肢已消失。

sclerotomy *n.* an operation in which an incision is made in the sclera (white of the eye).

鞏膜切開術 在鞏膜(眼的白色部分)上作一切口的一種手術。

scolex *n.* (*pl.* **scolices**) the head of a *tapeworm. The presence of suckers and/or hooks on the scolex enables the worm to attach itself to the wall of its host's gut.

頭節 絛蟲的頭。頭節上有吸盤和/或鈎,使絛蟲得以附着在宿主的腸壁上。

scoliosis *n.* lateral (sideways) deviation of the backbone, caused by con-

脊柱側凸 脊柱向側面偏斜。由先天的或後天的脊

genital or acquired abnormalities of the vertebrae, muscles, and nerves. Treatment is with spinal braces and, in cases of severe deformity, surgical correction by fusion or *osteotomy. *See also* kyphosis, kyphoscoliosis.

柱、肌肉、神經異常所致。用穿戴背甲治療。如畸形嚴重，可作骨融合或骨切開的手術矯正。

-scope *suffix denoting* an instrument for observing or examining. Example: *gastroscope* (instrument for examining the stomach).

〔後綴〕 **鏡** 一種用以觀察或檢查的儀器。如胃鏡（檢查胃的儀器）。

scopolamine *n. see* hyoscine.

東莨菪鹼

scorbutic *adj.* affected with scurvy.

壞血病的

scoto- *prefix denoting* darkness.

〔前綴〕 **盲，暗**

scotoma *n.* (*pl.* **scotomata**) a small area of abnormally decreased or absent vision in the visual field, surrounded by normal sight. All people have a *blind spot in the visual field of each eye due to the small area of retina occupied by the optic disc, which is not sensitive to light. Similar islands of total visual loss in other parts of the field are referred to as *absolute scotomata*. A *relative scotoma* is a spot where the vision is decreased but still present.

盲點 視野內光感異常減弱或完全缺損的一個小點。其周圍區域的光感正常。任何人每隻眼的視野內都有一個盲點。這是由於視網膜上這個小點被無感光作用的視乳頭盤佔有而形成的。在視網膜其他部分出現的光感完全缺損的相似小島，稱爲絕對盲點；而光感只是減弱但仍然存在的，則稱爲相對盲點。

scotometer *n.* an instrument used for mapping defects in the visual field. *See also* campimetry, perimeter.

暗點計 一種用於繪出視野光感缺損的部位與大小的儀器。

scotopic *adj.* relating to or describing conditions of poor illumination. For example, *scotopic vision* is vision in dim light in which the *rods of the retina are involved (*see* dark adaptation).

暗視的 描述微弱照明條件下視力的。例如：暗視力是弱光線下的視力，視網膜的視桿細胞在弱光線下起作用。

screening test a simple test carried out on a large number of apparently healthy people to separate those who probably have a specified disease from those who do not. Examples are mass X-rays and cervical smears. Limitations depend on the severity and *frequency distribution of the disease and the efficiency and availability of treatment.

過篩檢查 在大數量外表健康的人羣中對某種疾病進行普查的一種簡易的方法。如X線胸片和子宮頸塗片普查。本法的適用範圍取決於該病的嚴重程度，發病率的分佈情況以及治療的效果和可靠程度。還要考慮的其他因素

Other factors to be taken into account are the safety, convenience, cost, and *sensitivity of the test.

有安全、方便、價廉和檢查方法的敏感程度。

scrofula *n.* *tuberculosis of lymph nodes, usually those in the neck, causing the formation of abscesses. Untreated, these burst through the skin and form running sores, which leave scars when they heal. Treatment with antituberculous drugs is effective. The disease, which is now rare, most commonly affects young children. —**scrofulous** *adj.*

瘰癧 淋巴結結核。通常見於頸部淋巴結。引起膿腫形成。如不治療，膿腫穿過皮膚破裂，形成一匍行性潰瘍，癒合後留下瘢痕。用抗結核藥治療有效。此病最常感染兒童，現已少見。

scrofuloderma *n.* tuberculosis of the skin in which the skin breaks down over suppurating tuberculous glands, with the formation of irregular-shaped ulcers with blue-tinged edges. Treatment is with antituberculous drugs, to which scrofuloderma responds better than *lupus vulgaris, another type of skin tuberculosis.

皮膚瘰癧 皮膚結核。患處皮膚潰爛、覆有化膿的結核性腺體，形成帶有藍色邊緣、形狀不規則的潰瘍。用抗結核藥治療，其對皮膚瘰癧的療效高於對尋常狼瘡（另一類型的皮膚結核）的療效。

scrotum *n.* the paired sac that holds the testes and epididymides outside the abdominal cavity. Its function is to allow the production and storage of spermatozoa to occur at a lower temperature than that of the abdomen. Further temperature control is achieved by contraction or relaxation of muscles in the scrotum. —**scrotal** *adj.*

陰囊 一對在腹腔外容納睾丸和附睾的囊。其作用是使得精子在溫度較腹腔內為低的條件下生產和貯存。更進一步的溫度控制由陰囊肌肉的收縮和鬆弛來完成。

scrub typhus (tsutsugamushi disease) a disease, widely distributed in SE Asia, caused by the parasitic microorganism *Rickettsia tsutsugamushi* and transmitted to man through the bite of mites. Only larval mites of the genus **Trombicula* are involved as vectors. Symptoms include headache, chills, high temperature (104°F), a red rash over most of the body, a cough, and delirium. A small ulcer forms at the site of the bite. Scrub typhus is treated with tetracycline antibiotics. *See also* rickettsiae, typhus.

恙蟲病 一種廣泛分佈於東南亞的疾病。由寄生微生物恙蟲熱立克次氏體引起。通過螨的叮咬傳播給人。只有恙螨屬的蚴螨起到媒介作用。症狀包括頭痛、寒顫、高燒(104°F)、身體的大部分起紅疹、咳嗽以及譫妄。在螨叮咬處有小的潰瘍形成。本病用四環素類抗生素治療。

scruple *n.* a unit of weight used in pharmacy. 1 scruple = 1.295 g (20 grains). 3 scruples = 1 drachm.

英分，吩 藥衡單位。1英分＝1.295克（20英喱）。3英分＝1英錢（打蘭）。

sculpting *n.* a technique of family psychotherapy, in which all the family members are seen together and one member is asked to arrange the others' physical positions to express their relationships and feelings. *See also* group therapy.

塑雕療法 一種家庭心理治療技術。全部家庭成員聚集在一起，要求其中一個成員來擺佈其他成員的姿態，以表達他們的相互關係和感情。

scurf *n. see* dandruff.

頭皮屑，皮屑

scurvy *n.* a disease that is caused by a deficiency of *vitamin C (ascorbic acid). It results from the consumption of a diet devoid of fresh fruit and vegetables. The first sign of scurvy is swollen bleeding gums. This may be followed by subcutaneous bleeding and the opening of previously healed wounds; prolonged deficiency of the vitamin may eventually lead to death. Treatment with vitamin C soon reverses the effects.

壞血病 維生素C（抗壞血酸）缺乏引起的一種疾病。由於飲食內缺乏新鮮水菓和蔬菜所引起。壞血病的第一個體徵是牙齦腫脹、出血。繼而出現皮下出血或先前已癒合的傷口重新裂開。長期維生素缺乏可以最後導至死亡。如用維生素C治療則可迅速逆轉其病理過程。

scybalum *n.* a lump or mass of hard faeces.

硬糞塊 成團或成塊的硬糞。

seasickness *n. see* travel sickness.

暈船

sebaceous cyst (steatoma, wen) a cyst arising in an oil-secreting (sebaceous) gland of the skin. It may grow to a considerable size and be filled with yellowish cheesy sebum, which sometimes becomes infected. Sebaceous cysts are found most commonly on the scalp, scrotum, and vulva and rarely occur before puberty. Treatment is by surgical excision.

皮脂囊腫，粉瘤，脂瘤 一種在皮脂腺中產生的囊腫。它可以長成相當巨形的腫物，內部充滿淡黃色乾酪樣皮脂。有時可繼發感染。最常見於頭皮、陰囊、女性外陰部。青春期前很少發生。治療：手術切除。

sebaceous gland any of the simple or branched glands in the *skin that secrete an oily substance, *sebum. They open into hair follicles and their secretion is produced by the disintegration of their cells. Some parts of the skin have many sebaceous glands, others

皮脂腺 皮膚中分泌油性物質（皮脂）的、分支或不分支的腺體。皮脂腺開口於毛囊中，其細胞分解後即成爲其分泌物。某些部位的皮膚具有許多皮脂腺，另些部位則幾乎沒

few. Activity varies with age: the glands are most active at puberty.

有。皮脂腺的活動隨年齡而異，在青春期其活動最旺盛。

seborrhoea *n.* excessive secretion of sebum by the *sebaceous glands. The glands are enlarged, especially beside the nose and other parts of the face. The condition predisposes to acne and is common at puberty, usually lasting for a few years. Seborrhoea is sometimes associated by a kind of *eczema (seborrhoeic dermatitis). —**seborrhoeic** *adj.*

〔皮〕脂溢　皮脂腺分泌過多的皮脂。腺體常腫大，鼻子附近和面部其它部位的腺體腫大尤爲明顯。常發生於青春期。易引起痤瘡。可持續幾年。皮脂溢有時和一種濕疹同時存在（脂溢性皮炎）。

sebum *n.* the oily substance secreted by the *sebaceous glands and reaching the skin surface through small ducts that lead into the hair follicles. Sebum provides a thin film of fat over the skin, which slows the evaporation of water; it also has an antibacterial effect.

皮脂　皮脂腺所分泌的油性物質。它可通過引向毛囊的小導管抵達皮膚表面。皮脂在皮膚表面形成一層薄膜，使水分蒸發減慢。它尙具有一種抗菌作用。

second *n.* the *SI unit of time, equal to the duration of 9,192,631,770 periods of the radiation corresponding to the transition between two hyperfine levels of the ground state of the caesium-133 atom. This unit is now the basis of all time measurements. Symbol: s.

秒　時間的國際單位。等於基態下^{133}原子銫兩個精度之間放射周期的9,192,631,700倍。本制是現代計時的基礎。符號：s。

secondary medical care *see* general practitioner.

二級醫療保健

secondary prevention the avoidance or alleviation of the serious consequences of disease by early detection. Best known methods include routine examinations, as in *child health clinics and the *school health service, or *screening tests applied to populations regarded as having a high risk of contracting specific diseases.

二級預防　避免或減輕早期發現的疾病的嚴重後果。公認的最佳方法包括諸如在兒童保健所和學校衞生室內進行的常規檢查，或對被認爲可能罹患某些特殊疾病的高危人羣進行篩選性檢查。

secondary sexual characteristics the physical characteristics that develop after puberty as a result of sexual maturation. In boys they include the growth of facial and pubic hair and the breaking of the voice. In girls they include the growth of pubic hair and the development of the breasts.

第二性徵　青春期後身體發育的性別特徵。它是性成熟的結果。男孩的第二性徵包括有鬍鬚和陰毛的生長，發聲的變調。女孩的第二性徵包括有陰毛生長和乳房發育。

secretagogue *n.* a substance that stimulates secretion. An example is *pentagastrin, which stimulates the secretion of gastric juice.

促分泌的，促分泌劑 一種刺激乳腺分泌的物質。如五肽胃泌素，它刺激胃液分泌。

secretin *n.* a hormone secreted from the small intestine (duodenum) when acidified food leaves the stomach. It stimulates the secretion of relatively enzyme-free alkaline juice by the pancreas (*see* pancreatic juice) and of bile by the liver.

分泌素，腸促胰液素 酸化食物離開胃時，小腸（十二指腸）分泌的一種激素。分泌素刺激胰腺，分泌含酶較少的鹼性液體，並刺激肝臟分泌膽汁。

secretion *n.* **1.** the process by which a gland isolates constituents of the blood or tissue fluid and chemically alters them to produce a substance that it discharges for use by the body or excretes. The principal methods of secretion – *apocrine, *holocrine, and *merocrine – are illustrated in the diagram. **2.** the substance that is produced by a gland.

①**分泌** 某一腺體將血液或組織液中某些成分離析出來的過程。同時使這些成分發生化學變化，使之產生一種物質爲機體所利用或排出體外。分泌的主要方式有：頂泌、全泌和局泌三種（見圖）。②**分泌物** 腺體所分泌的物質。

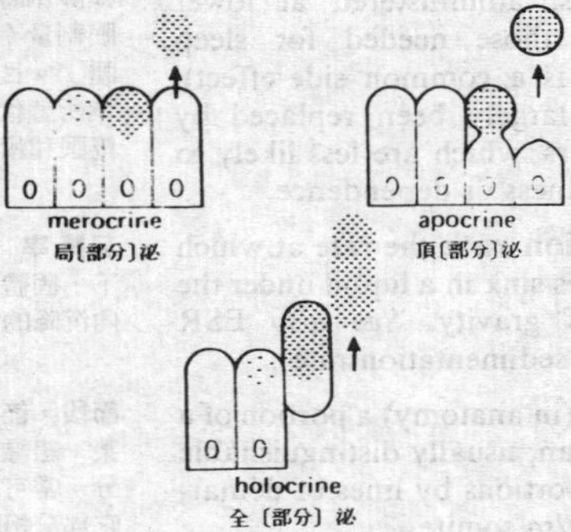

Methods of secretion
分泌方式

secretor *n.* a person in whose saliva and other body fluids are found traces of the water-soluble A, B, or O agglutinogens that determine *blood group.

血型物質分泌者 在唾液和其它體液中有決定A、B、O血型微量水溶性凝集原的人。

section 1. *n.* (in surgery) the act of cutting (the cut or division made is also called a section). For example, an *abdominal section* is performed for surgical exploration of the abdomen (*see* laparotomy). A *transverse section* is a

①**切開〔術〕，切〔斷〕面** （外科）切割動作（切口也用此詞）。如外科剖腹探查就是一種腹部切開術。對一個組織結構的長軸作一垂直切口叫做橫

cut made at right angles to a structure's long axis. *See also* Caesarean section. **2.** *n.* (in microscopy) a thin slice of the specimen to be examined under a microscope. **3.** *vb.* to issue an order for *compulsory admission to a psychiatric hospital under the appropriate section of the *Mental Health Act.

切。 **②切片** （顯微鏡檢查）顯微鏡下檢查的一種薄標本切片。 ③（動詞）根據精神保健法令相應條文發佈强制性住入精神病醫院的指令。

secundigravida *n.* a woman who has been pregnant twice.

孕$_2$ 曾妊娠兩次的婦女。

secundipara *n.* a woman who has been pregnant at least twice and who has given birth to an infant capable of survival after each of two pregnancies.

產$_2$ 至少妊娠過兩次的婦女，兩次妊娠生下的嬰兒均存活。

sedation *n.* the production of a restful state of mind, particularly by the use of drugs (*see* sedative).

鎮靜〔作用〕 產生心情平靜狀態的作用。特別於服用某些藥物以後。

sedative *n.* a drug that has a calming effect, relieving anxiety and tension. Sedatives are *hypnotic drugs, such as *barbiturates, administered at lower doses than those needed for sleep (drowsiness is a common side-effect). They have largely been replaced by *tranquillizers, which are less likely to cause drowsiness or dependence.

鎮靜劑 一種具有鎮定並緩減焦慮和緊張作用的藥物。巴比妥類安眠藥用作鎮靜劑時，用量應小於催眠劑量（常見副作用爲倦睡）。目前它們已被安定劑所替代。後者較少引起倦眠和賴藥性。

sedimentation rate the rate at which solid particles sink in a liquid under the influence of gravity. *See also* ESR (erythrocyte sedimentation rate).

沉降率 在重力的影響下，固體微粒在一種液體內沉降的速率。

segment *n.* (in anatomy) a portion of a tissue or organ, usually distinguishable from other portions by lines of demarcation. *See also* somite.

節段，節片 （解剖學）某一組織或器官的一個部分。常可根據分界線和其它部分相區別。

sella turcica a depression in the body of the sphenoid bone that encloses the pituitary gland.

蝶鞍 包藏垂體腺的蝶骨體的凹陷部分。

semeiology *n. see* symptomatology.

症狀學

semen (seminal fluid) *n.* the fluid ejaculated from the penis at sexual climax. Each ejaculate may contain 300–500 million sperms suspended in a fluid secreted by the *prostate gland and *seminal vesicles with a small contribution from *Cowper's glands. It

精液 性慾高潮時陰莖內射出的液體。一次射精可含有3～5億個精子，混懸在前列腺液、精囊液和一小部分庫珀氏腺分泌液內。精液內含有的果糖可向精子提供能量；含有的

contains fructose, which provides the sperms with energy, and *prostaglandins, which affect the muscles of the womb and may therefore assist transport of the sperms. —**seminal** *adj.*

前列腺素能影響子宮肌肉從而協助精子的移動。

semi- *prefix denoting* half.

〔前綴〕 半

semicircular canals three tubes that form part of the membranous *labyrinth of the ear. They are concerned with balance and each canal registers movement in a different plane. At the base of each canal is a small swelling (an *ampulla*), which contains a *crista. When the head moves the fluid (endolymph) in the canals presses on the cristae, which register the movement and send nerve impulses to the brain.

半規管 形成內耳的膜迷路部分的三個小管。它們涉及身體平衡，每個半規管感受不同平面的運動。每個半規管的基部有一個小的隆起（壺腹），內含有一個嵴。當頭部動作移動半規管內液體（內淋巴）壓迫這些嵴時，嵴感知這一運動，並把神經衝動傳入大腦。

semilunar cartilage one of a pair of crescent-shaped cartilages in the knee joint situated between the femur and tibia.

關節半月板 位於股骨和脛骨之間膝關節內的一對月牙形軟骨中的一個。

semilunar valve either of the two valves in the heart situated at the origin of the aorta (*aortic valve*) and the pulmonary artery (*pulmonary valve*). Each consists of three flaps (cusps), which maintain the flow of blood in one direction.

半月瓣 位於心臟主動脈根部（主動脈瓣）和肺動脈根部（肺動脈瓣）的瓣膜。每個瓣膜由三片（瓣尖）組成。使血流保持向一個方向流動。

seminal vesicle either of a pair of male accessory sex glands that open into the vas deferens before it joins the urethra. The seminal vesicles secrete most of the liquid component of *semen.

精囊 男性性腺附屬器。它開口於連接尿道之前的輸精管。大部精液成分由精囊分泌。

seminiferous tubule any of the long convoluted tubules that make up the bulk of the *testis.

輸精小管，細精管 組成睾丸大部分的卷曲細長小管。

seminoma *n.* a malignant tumour of the testis, appearing as a swelling, often painless, in the scrotum. It tends to occur in an older age group than the *teratomas. The best treatment for localized disease is surgery involving removal of the testis (*see* orchidectomy). Secondary tumours in the lungs

精原細胞瘤 一種睾丸的惡性腫瘤。它表現爲陰囊腫大，無痛。它常出現於較畸胎瘤更大的年齡組。睾丸切除術是局限性病變的最佳療法。腫瘤轉移至肺時可用環磷醯胺靜注治療，隨後以小劑量肺部放

can be treated with intravenous cyclophosphamide followed by low-dose irradiation to the lungs. A similar tumour occurs in the ovary (*see* dysgerminoma).

射療法補充之。卵巢也可有類似腫瘤。

semipermeable membrane a membrane that allows the passage of some molecules but not others. *Cell membranes are semipermeable. Semipermeable membranes are used clinically in *haemodialysis for patients with kidney failure.

半透膜 允許某些分子通過而不允許其它分子通過的膜。細胞膜是半透膜。臨床利用半透膜作腎功能衰竭患者的血液透析之用。

semiprone *adj.* describing the position of a patient lying face downwards, but with one or both knees flexed to one side so that the body is not lying completely flat. *Compare* prone, supine.

半俯臥位 描述一種俯臥病人的體位。其一個或兩個膝關節向一邊屈曲。因此其軀體並非完全平臥。

senescence *n.* the condition of ageing, which is often marked by a decrease in physical and mental abilities. —**senescent** *adj.*

衰老 機體的老化狀態。常以體力和精力減退爲標誌。

senile dementia loss of the intellectual faculties, beginning for the first time in old age. *See also* dementia.

老年性痴呆 老年開始出現的智力喪失。

senior house officer *see* consultant.

主治醫師

senna *n.* the dried fruits of certain shrubs of the genus *Cassia*, used as an irritant *laxative to relieve constipation and to empty the bowels before X-ray examination. It is administered by mouth; side-effects do not usually occur, but severe diarrhoea may follow large doses.

番瀉葉 某些番瀉屬灌木的乾葉。係一種刺激性輕瀉劑，用以減輕便祕或X線檢查前排空大腸。口服。一般無副作用。但大劑量可引起嚴重腹瀉。

sensation *n.* a feeling: the result of messages from the body's sensory receptors registering in the brain as information about the environment. Messages from *exteroceptors are interpreted as specific sensations – smell, taste, temperature, pain, etc. – in the conscious mind. Messages from *interoceptors, however, rarely reach the consciousness to produce sensation.

感覺 來自感覺器的信號作爲環境的信息被大腦感知的結果。來自外感受器的信號在人的意識中產生特異性感覺——嗅覺、味覺、溫覺、痛覺等。來自內感受器的信號，罕有到達意識產生感覺的。

sense *n.* one of the faculties by which the qualities of the external environment are appreciated – sight, hearing, smell, taste, or touch.

〔感〕覺　一種鑑別外界環境的質的能力——視覺、聽覺、嗅覺或觸覺。

sense organ a collection of specialized cells (*receptors), connected to the nervous system, that is capable of responding to a particular stimulus from either outside or inside the body. Sense organs can detect light (the eyes), heat, pain, and touch (the skin), smell (the nose), and taste (the taste buds).

感覺器官　一些特異性細胞的集合體（感受器）。它與神經系統相連接，回答來自體內外某一特定的刺激。感覺器官可察覺光綫（眼）、熱、痛和觸（皮膚），氣味（鼻）和味道（味蕾）。

sensibility *n.* the ability to be affected by, and respond to, changes in the surroundings (*see* stimulus). Sensibility is a characteristic of cells of the nervous system.

感受性　感受並回答周圍環境變化的能力。感受性是神經系統細胞的一個特徵。

sensitive *adj.* possessing the ability to respond to a *stimulus. The cells of the retina, for example, are sensitive to the stimulus of light and respond by sending nerve impulses to the brain. Other *receptors are sensitive to different specific stimuli, such as pressure or the presence of chemical substances.

能感受的，敏感的　具有對一個刺激發生反應的能力。如視網膜細胞對光刺激是能感受的，且能發生反應——將神經衝動傳到大腦。其它不同的感受器感受各種不同的特異性刺激，諸如壓力或各種化學性刺激。

sensitivity *n.* (in preventive medicine) a measure of the reliability of a *screening test based on the proportion of people with a specific disease who react positively to the test (the higher the sensitivity the fewer false negatives). This contrasts with *specificity*, which is the proportion of people free from disease who react negatively to the test (i.e. the higher the specificity the fewer the false positives). Though these are theoretically independent variables, most screening tests are so designed that if the sensitivity is increased the specificity is reduced and the number of false positives may rise to wasteful proportions.

敏感性　（預防醫學）篩選試驗可靠性的一種量度。根據某一特異疾病患者中該試驗呈陽性反應的百分數而定（敏感性越高，假陰性越少）。相反，特異性則指在無病的人羣中該試驗呈陰性的百分數（即特異性越高，假陽性越少）。雖然，在理論上，這些都是獨立的度量，但實際上大多數篩選試驗的設計均相同，如果敏感性增加，特異性即降低，因而假陽性率增加，造成浪費。

sensitization *n.* **1.** alteration of the responsiveness of the body to the presence of foreign substances. In the devel-

①**致敏〔感作用〕**　機體對異物反應的改變。在形成過敏過程中，機體被某一

opment of an *allergy, an individual becomes sensitized to a particular allergen and reaches a state of *hypersensitivity. The phenomena of sensitization are due to the production of antibodies. **2.** (in behaviour therapy) a form of *aversion therapy in which anxiety-producing stimuli are associated with the unwanted behaviour. In *covert sensitization* the behaviour and an unpleasant feeling (such as disgust) are evoked simultaneously by verbal cues.

特殊過敏原致敏，而進入過敏狀態。抗體形成是致敏現象的原因。②**致過敏，敏感化**（行爲療法）厭惡療法的一種形式，是把產生焦慮的刺激與不良的行爲聯繫起來。隱性致過敏是通過語言暗示，在一種不良行爲的同時喚起一種不愉快感覺（如厭惡）。

sensory *adj.* relating to the input division of the nervous system, which carries information from *receptors throughout the body towards the brain and spinal cord.

感覺的 和神經系統傳入部分有關的。它把遍及全身感受器得到的信息帶給大腦和脊髓。

sensory cortex the region of the *cerebral cortex responsible for receiving incoming information relayed by sensory nerve pathways from all parts of the body. Different areas of cortex correspond to different parts of the body and to the various senses. *Compare* motor cortex.

感覺皮層 大腦皮層中，負責接受感覺神經通路從全身各部分輾轉傳入的信息的區域。不同的大腦皮層區和機體不同部位、各種不同感覺相對應。

sensory nerve a nerve that carries information inwards, from an outlying part of the body towards the central nervous system. Different sensory nerves convey information about temperature, pain, touch, taste, etc., to the brain. *Compare* motor nerve.

感覺神經 把信息從機體外圍部位傳向中樞神經系統的神經。不同的感覺神經分別向大腦轉運溫、痛、觸、味等感覺。

separation anxiety a state of distress and fear at the prospect of leaving secure surroundings, such as is experienced by some children when they must leave parents to go to school. It is often caused by insecure *attachment.

分離焦慮 對於將要離開安全可靠的環境感到苦悶和恐懼的狀態。如某些兒童必須離開家長去上學的感受。它常由於不可靠的依附所引起。

sepsis *n.* the putrefactive destruction of tissues by disease-causing bacteria or their toxins.

膿毒病，膿毒症 致病菌或其毒素引起的組織腐敗性破壞。

sept- (septi-) *prefix denoting* **1.** seven. **2.** (*or* **septo-**) a septum, especially the nasal septum. **3.** sepsis.

〔前綴〕 ①**七** ②**中隔** 尤指鼻中隔。 ③**膿毒症**

septal defect a hole in the partition (septum) between the left and right halves of the heart. This abnormal communication is congenital due to an abnormality of heart development in the fetus. It may be found between the two atria (*atrial septal defect*) or between the ventricles (*ventricular septal defect*). A septal defect permits abnormal circulation of blood from the left side of the heart, where pressures are higher, to the right. This abnormal circulation is called a *shunt* and results in excessive blood flow through the lungs. *Pulmonary hypertension develops and *heart failure may occur with large shunts. A heart *murmur is normally present. Large defects are closed surgically but small defects do not require treatment.

間隔缺損 心臟左右半側之間的間隔上的一個洞口。這一異常交通口來源于胎兒期心臟的先天性發育畸形。洞口可位於兩個心房間（房間隔缺損）或位於兩個心室間（室間隔缺損）。間隔缺損的存在引起血液從壓力較高的左側流向右側，產生異常血循。此種異常血循叫做分流。它導至大量血流通過肺臟。大量分流情況下可發生肺動脉高壓和心力衰竭。通常有心臟雜音存在。大的缺損應外科修補，但小缺損不需治療。

septic *adj.* relating to or affected with *sepsis.

膿毒性的 與膿毒症有關的，或罹患膿毒症的。

septicaemia *n.* widespread destruction of tissues due to absorption of disease-causing bacteria or their toxins from the bloodstream. The term is also used loosely for any form of *blood poisoning. *Compare* pyaemia, sapraemia, toxaemia.

敗血病，敗血症 血流內致病菌或致病毒素的吸收引起組織的廣泛破壞。

Septrin *n. see* co-trimoxazole.

複方新諾明，塞潑亭

septum *n.* (*pl.* **septa**) a partition or dividing wall within an anatomical structure. For example, the *atrioventricular septum* divides the atria of the heart from the ventricles. —**septal** *adj.* —**septate** *adj.*

間隔 某解剖結構中的分隔部分。如心房和心室之間的房室隔。

sequela *n.* (*pl.* **sequelae**) any disorder or pathological condition that results from a preceding disease or accident.

後遺症，後發病 任何由先前的疾病或意外事故所造成的功能障礙或病理狀態。

sequestration *n.* the formation of a fragment of dead bone (*see* sequestrum) and its separation from the surrounding tissue.

死骨形成 形成死骨片並和周圍組織分離。

sequestrectomy *n.* surgical removal of a *sequestrum.

死骨切除術 切除死骨片的手術。

sequestrum *n.* (*pl.* **sequestra**) a portion of dead bone formed in an infected bone in chronic *osteomyelitis. It is surrounded by an envelope (*involucrum*) of sclerotic bone and fibrous tissue and can be seen as a dense area within the bone on X-ray. It can cause irritation and the formation of pus, which may discharge through a *sinus, and is usually surgically removed (*sequestrectomy*).

死骨〔片〕 慢性骨髓炎患者骨感染時形成的死骨的一部分。它的周圍常被硬化性骨質和纖維組織所包裹（死骨包殼），X綫照片上骨質內有緻密區。它可引起刺激性疼痛和膿液形成。膿可由竇道流出，常需手術切除（死骨切除術）。

ser- (sero-) *prefix denoting* **1.** serum. **2.** serous membrane.

〔前綴〕 ① 血清 ② 漿〔液〕膜

serine *n. see* amino acid.

絲氨酸

serofibrinous *adj.* describing an exudate of serum that contains a high proportion of the protein fibrin.

漿液纖維蛋白性的 描述含有大量纖維蛋白的漿液性滲出物。

serology *n.* the study of blood serum and its constituents, particularly their contribution to the protection of the body against disease. *See* agglutination, complement fixation, precipitin. —**serological** *adj.*

血清學 研究血清及其成分的科學。尤其研究其保護機體抵抗疾病的作用。

seropus *n.* a mixture of serum and pus, which forms, for example, in infected blisters.

漿液性膿 漿液和膿的混合物。例如於感染性水疱內形成的混合物。

serosa *n. see* serous membrane.

漿膜

serositis *n.* inflammation of a *serous membrane, such as the lining of the thoracic cavity (pleura). *See* polyserositis.

漿膜炎 漿膜的炎症。如覆蓋於胸腔內面的膜（胸膜）的炎症。

serotherapy *n.* the use of serum containing known antibodies (*see* antiserum) to treat a patient with an infection or to confer temporary passive *immunity upon a person at special risk. The use of antisera prepared in animals carries its own risks (for example, a patient may become hypersensitive to horse protein); the risk is reduced if the serum is taken from an immune human being.

血清療法 應用含有已知抗體的血清，治療某種感染患者。或給予某一高危患者的暫時性被動免疫。應用動物製備的抗血清可帶來它本身的危險性（如某些患者可對馬的血清蛋白過敏）。

serotonin (5-hydroxytryptamine) *n.* a compound widely distributed in the tissues, particularly in the blood plate-

五羥色胺 廣泛分佈於組織中的一種化合物。在血小板、小腸壁和中樞神經

lets, intestinal wall, and central nervous system. It is thought to play a role in inflammation similar to that of *histamine and it also possibly acts as a *neurotransmitter, especially concerned with the process of sleep.

系統內的含量較多。在炎症中它被認爲和組織胺起相似的作用。它也可能起神經介質的作用，尤其是參與睡眠過程的神經介質。

serotype *n.* a category into which material is placed based on its serological activity, particularly in terms of the antigens it contains or the antibodies that may be produced against it. Thus bacteria of the same species may be subdivided into serotypes that produce slightly different antigens. The serotype of an infective organism is important when treatment or prophylaxis with a vaccine is being considered.

血清型 根據血清活性，尤其根據所含抗原或抗體物質所作的血清分類。因此，同種細菌可分爲抗原稍有不同的若干種血清型。當考慮應用一種疫苗作爲治療或預防時，對感染性病原體的血清型的選擇是重要的。

serous *adj.* **1.** relating to or containing serum. **2.** resembling serum or producing a fluid resembling serum.

血清的，漿液的 ①與血清（漿液）有關的，或含有血清（漿液）的。 ②與血清（漿液）相似的，或產生類似血清（漿液）的液體的。

serous membrane (serosa) a smooth transparent membrane, consisting of *mesothelium and underlying elastic fibrous connective tissue, lining certain large cavities of the body. The *peritoneum of the abdomen, *pleura of the chest, and *pericardium of the heart are all serous membranes. Each consists of two portions: the *parietal* portion lines the walls of the cavity, and the *visceral* portion covers the organs concerned. The two are continuous, forming a closed sac with the organs essentially outside the sac. The inner surface of the sac is moistened by a thin fluid derived from blood serum, which allows frictionless movement of organs within their cavities. *Compare* mucous membrane.

漿膜 光滑而透明的膜。它由間皮及其下面的彈性結締組織組成，覆蓋於某些巨大體腔的表面。腹膜、胸膜和心包膜均係漿膜。每一漿膜由兩個部分組成：壁層組成腔的外壁，臟層覆蓋所在的臟器。壁層和臟層互相連續，構成一個密封的囊袋。其臟器位於這一囊袋之外。囊袋的內面常由來自血清的一薄層液體所濕潤，以便腔內臟器活動時不產生摩擦。

serpiginous *adj.* having an indented or wavy margin: applied to certain skin lesions.

匐行的 具有鋸齒形或波浪形邊緣的。常用以描述某些皮膚病變。

serratus *n.* any of several muscles arising from or inserted by a series of

鋸肌 起始部或附着部呈一連串鋸齒狀的肌肉。如

processes that resemble the teeth of a saw. An example is the *serratus anterior*, a muscle situated between the ribs and shoulder blade in the upper and lateral parts of the thorax. It is the chief muscle responsible for pushing and punching movements.

前鋸肌位於胸廓上部肋骨和肩胛骨之間，是司推擊動作的主要肌肉。

Sertoli cells cells found in the walls of the seminiferous tubules of the *testis. Compared with the germ cells they appear large and pale. They anchor and probably nourish the developing germ cells, especially the *spermatids, which become partly embedded within them.

塞爾托利氏細胞，足細胞 睾丸輸精小管（細精管）的壁細胞。與生殖細胞相比，形態大且蒼白。它們支持並可能營養正在發育中的生殖細胞，尤其是精細胞。部分精細胞包埋其中。

serum (blood serum) *n.* the fluid that separates from clotted blood or blood plasma that is allowed to stand. Serum is essentially similar in composition to *plasma but lacks fibrinogen and other substances that are used in the coagulation process.

血清 從凝血塊或血漿中分離出來的液體。血清和血漿的成分基本相似，只是血清內缺乏纖維蛋白原和其它凝血過程中被消耗的物質。

serum hepatitis *see* hepatitis.

血清性肝炎

serum sickness a reaction that sometimes occurs 7–12 days after injection of a quantity of foreign serum, such as horse serum used in the preparation of antitetanus injections. The usual symptoms are rashes, fever, joint pains, and enlargement of the lymph nodes. The reaction is due to the presence of antigenic material still in the circulation by the time that the body has started producing antibodies against it; it is therefore a form of delayed *hypersensitivity reaction. The condition is rarely serious.

血清病 有時在注射一定量的異體蛋白後7～12天出現的一種反應。如注射抗破傷風製劑中的馬血清時。常見症狀爲：皮疹、發熱、關節痛和周圍淋巴結腫大。反應的機理是機體開始產生抗體的時候，血循內仍有抗原性物質。因此，它是遲發性過敏反應的一種，此病嚴重者罕見。

sesamoid bone an oval nodule of bone that lies within a tendon and slides over another bony surface. The patella (kneecap) and certain bones in the hand and foot are sesamoid bones.

籽骨 位於肌腱之中，而在另一骨面滑動的卵圓形骨結節。髕骨（膝蓋骨）以及某些手足骨均係籽骨。

sessile *adj.* (of a tumour) having no stalk.

無柄的，無蒂的，固着的 無蒂的（腫瘤）。

seton *n.* an outmoded form of treatment in which a thread was passed

掛線，串線 一種過時的療法。將一根線穿過一塊

through a pinch of skin and tied in a loop. This acted as a counterirritant to pain elsewhere and produced a running sore thought to be useful for the drainage of harmful materials from the body.

皮膚，並打成結。它可起到減少別處疼痛的作用。同時產生一個膿瘡，據認爲這可以把有害物質引流出體外。

sex chromatin *chromatin found only in female cells and believed to represent a single X chromosome in a nondividing cell. It can be used to discover the sex of a baby before birth by examination of cells obtained by *amniocentesis. There are two main kinds: (1) the *Barr body*, a small object that stains with basic dyes, found on the edge of the nucleus just inside the nuclear membrane; (2) a drumstick-like appendage to the nucleus in neutrophils (a type of white blood cell).

性染色質 只存在於雌性細胞內的染色質。據信，它在一個未分裂細胞內代表單一X染色體。檢查羊膜穿刺獲得的細胞中有無性染色質，可在嬰兒出生前鑑定其性別。它有兩個主要類別：①巴爾體，呈鹹性染色的小體，緊貼於細胞核膜的內側。②中性白細胞核內的鼓槌狀附件。

sex chromosome a chromosome that is involved in the determination of the sex of the individual. Women have two *X chromosomes; men have one X chromosome and one *Y chromosome. *Compare* autosome.

性染色體 決定個體性別的染色體。女性有兩個X染色體；男性有一個X染色體和一個Y染色體。

sex hormone any steroid hormone, produced mainly by the ovaries or testes, that is responsible for controlling sexual development and reproductive function. *Oestrogens and *progesterone are the female sex hormones; *androgens are the male sex hormones.

性激素 主要由卵巢或睾丸分泌的固醇類激素。它負責性發育和生殖功能的控制。雌激素和黃體酮係雌性激素；雄激素係雄性激素。

sex-limited *adj.* describing characteristics that are expressed differently in the two sexes but are controlled by genes not on the sex chromosomes, e.g. baldness in men.

限性的 在兩性中表現出不同特徵，但只受性染色體以外的基因控制的，如男性禿頭。

sex-linked *adj.* describing genes (or the characteristics controlled by them) that are carried on the sex chromosomes, usually the *X chromosome. The genes for certain disorders, e.g. *haemophilia, are carried on the X chromosome. Since these sex-linked genes are *recessive, men are more likely to have the diseases since they have only one X chromosome; women

伴性的(性連鎖) 描述由性染色體(通常由X染色體)攜帶的某些基因(或受這些基因控制的)特徵。某些疾病，如血友病，其基因由X染色體攜帶。由於這些連鎖的基因是隱性的，而男性只有一個X染色體，所以罹患這些疾病的機會較多。女性

can carry the genes but their harmful effects are usually masked by the dominant (normal) alleles on their second X chromosome.

雖也能攜帶這些基因，但其有害作用常被其第二個X染色體上的顯性（正常）等位基因掩蔽。

sexology *n.* the study of sexual matters, including anatomy, physiology, behaviour, and techniques.

性學 研究性的科學。包括研究解剖學、生理學、行爲學和性技術。

sex ratio the proportion of males to females in a population, usually expressed as the number of males per 100 females. The *primary sex ratio*, at the time of fertilization, is in theory 50% male. The *secondary sex ratio*, found at birth, usually indicates slightly fewer girls than boys.

兩性比率，性〔別〕比率 人羣中的男女比例。通常用每100個女性有多少男性來表示。在理論上，受精期的最初性比率是50%爲男性。出生時的實際比率常表明女嬰稍少於男嬰。

sextigravida *n.* a woman who has been pregnant six times.

孕$_6$ 曾妊娠六次的婦女。

sextipara *n.* a woman who has been pregnant at least six times and who has given birth to an infant capable of survival after each of six pregnancies.

產$_6$ 至少妊娠六次的婦女，而且六次妊娠均產下存活的嬰兒。

sexual abuse sexual activity by an adult involving a child. *See also* paedophilia.

性濫用 成人對兒童的性行爲。

SGOT serum glutamic oxaloacetic transaminase. *See* glutamic oxaloacetic transaminase.

血清穀草轉氨酶 血清穀〔氨酸〕草〔醯乙酸〕轉氨酶。

SGPT *n.* serum glutamic pyruvic transaminase. *See* glutamic pyruvic transaminase.

血清穀丙轉氨酶 血清穀〔氨酸〕丙〔酮酸〕轉氨酶。

shaking palsy an archaic name for *parkinsonism.

震顫麻痹 帕金森氏病的原始名稱。

shaping *n.* a technique of *behaviour modification used in the teaching of complex skills or in encouraging rare forms of behaviour. At first the therapist rewards actions that are similar to the desired behaviour; thereafter the therapist rewards successively closer approximations, until eventually only the desired behaviour is rewarded and thereby learned.

塑造療法 一種改變行爲的技術，用以教授某些複雜技能或鼓勵某些罕見的行爲方式。首先，治療師對於患者所做的與預期行爲相似的動作給予獎勵；而後對一次比一次更加近似的動作給予報償，直到最後做出完全與預期符合的行爲，終於學會它。

sheath *n.* (in anatomy) the layer of connective tissue that envelops structures such as nerves, arteries, tendons, and muscles.

鞘 （解剖學）包被神經、動脉、腱和肌肉的結締組織層。

sheltered housing specially converted (or adapted) accommodation, often in the form of a flatlet, designed to meet the special needs of the elderly who are capable of self-care. A warden is generally in attendance. The extent to which meals and other services are provided on a continuous basis varies; so too in Britain does the *per capita* payment from the appropriate social service department.

老人公寓 一種經過改建（或適應某種目的）的特殊住所。通常爲生活能自理的老人們的特殊需要設計成小套間的形式。一般配備有一名管理員。連續不斷供應膳食和其它服務項目因地而異。在英國，爲每一位來此居住的老人從相應社會服務部門支出的經費亦因人而異。

Shigella *n.* a genus of nonmotile rodlike Gram-negative bacteria normally present in the intestinal tract of warm-blooded animals and man. They ferment carbohydrates without the formation of gas. Some species are pathogenic. *S. dysenteriae* is associated with bacillary *dysentery.

志賀氏〔桿〕菌屬 熱血動物和人類腸道內正常存在的、無運動的、革蘭氏陰性桿狀菌。它們使碳水化合物發酵，不產氣。若干種有致病性。痢疾志賀氏菌能引起細菌性痢疾。

shigellosis *n.* an infestation of the digestive system by bacteria of the genus *Shigella*, causing bacillary *dysentery.

志賀氏菌病，志賀氏菌痢疾 志賀氏菌屬細菌所引起的消化道感染，即細菌性痢疾。

shingles *n.* herpes zoster (*see* herpes).

帶狀疱疹

shock *n.* the condition associated with circulatory collapse, when the arterial blood pressure is too low to maintain an adequate supply of blood to the tissues. The patient has a cold sweaty pallid skin, a weak rapid pulse, irregular breathing, dry mouth, dilated pupils, and a reduced flow of urine.
Shock may be due to a decrease in the volume of blood, as occurs after internal or external *haemorrhage, dehydration, burns, or severe vomiting or diarrhoea. It may be caused by reduced activity of the heart, as in coronary thrombosis, myocardial infarction, or pulmonary embolism. It may also be due to widespread dilation of the veins so that there is insufficient blood to fill them. This may be caused by the

休克 動脉壓太低，難於維持足夠血液供應機體組織時所出現的循環衰竭狀態。患者皮膚蒼白、出冷汗、脉搏快而弱、呼吸不規則、口乾、瞳孔擴大以及尿量減少。
休克可由血容量減少引起。如內出血、外出血、脫水、燒傷、嚴重嘔吐或腹瀉。它也可由心臟活動力減低引起。如冠狀動脉血栓形成、心肌梗塞或肺栓塞。它也可由靜脉普遍擴張，靜脉內血液充盈不足引起。其原因有：血流內有細菌存在（菌血症性休克）；嚴重過敏反應（過敏性休克）；藥物過

presence of bacteria in the bloodstream (*bacteraemic shock*), a severe allergic reaction (*anaphylactic shock*: *see* anaphylaxis), overdosage with such drugs as narcotics or barbiturates, or the emotional shock due to a personal tragedy or disaster (*neurogenic shock*). Sometimes shock may result from a combination of any of these causes, as in *peritonitis. The treatment of shock is determined by the cause.

量，如痳醉藥或巴比妥類；或因某一悲劇事件或災難所引起情緒性休克（神經性休克）。有時，休克可由上述幾種不同原因的組合所引起，如腹膜炎。休克的治療取決於其病因。

short-sightedness *n. see* myopia.

近視

shoulder girdle (pectoral girdle) the bony structure to which the bones of the upper limbs are attached. It consists of the right and left *scapulas (*shoulder blades*) and clavicles (collar bones).

上肢帶（胸帶） 上肢骨附着的骨骼結構。它由左右肩胛骨和鎖骨組成。

shunt *n.* (in medicine) a passage connecting two anatomical channels and diverting blood from one to the other. It may occur as a congenital abnormality or be surgically created. *See also* anastomosis.

分流 （醫學）連接兩個解剖管腔的通道，使血液改道從一個腔流向另一個腔。它可以是先天性畸形或由分流手術形成。

sial- (sialo-) *prefix denoting* **1.** saliva. **2.** a salivary gland.

〔前綴〕 **①涎，唾液** **②涎腺，唾液腺**

sialadenitis *n.* inflammation of a salivary gland.

涎腺炎 涎（唾液）腺的炎症。

sialic acid an amino sugar. Sialic acid is a component of some *glycoproteins, *gangliosides, and bacterial cell walls.

涎（唾液）酸 一種氨基酸。涎酸是某些糖蛋白、神經節苷脂和菌細胞壁的成分。

sialogogue *n.* a drug that promotes the secretion of saliva. *Parasympathomimetic drugs have this action.

催涎劑 促進唾液腺分泌的藥物。擬副交感神經藥有此作用。

sialography (ptyalography) *n.* X-ray examination of the salivary glands, after introducing a quantity of radio-opaque material into the ducts of the salivary glands in the mouth. It enables the presence of any obstruction to be detected.

涎管〔X線〕造影術 把不透射線的物質注入口內涎（唾液）腺導管內所作的涎腺X線檢查。它能檢出涎管內存在的阻塞。

sialolith *n.* a stone (calculus) in a salivary gland or duct, most often the duct of the submaxillary gland. The flow of saliva is obstructed, causing swelling and intense pain.

涎石 存在於唾液腺或其導管內，尤其常見於頷下腺導管內的石頭（結石）。唾液腺的分泌液受阻塞，引起腺體腫脹和劇痛。

sialorrhoea *n. see* ptyalism.

流涎，多涎

Siamese twins identical twins that are physically joined together at birth. The condition ranges from twins joined only by the umbilical blood vessels (i.e. *allantoido-angiopagous twins*) to those in whom conjoined heads or trunk are inseparable.

塞米斯氏雙胎 生下時呈連體的單卵雙胎。包括臍血管相連（即尿囊血管雙胎）、頭部或驅幹相連等各種情況。

sib *n. see* sibling.

血親，同胞

sibilant *adj.* whistling or hissing. The term is applied to certain abnormal sounds heard through a stethoscope.

咝音的 笛音或嘶嘶聲。聽診器聽到的某些異常音所用的術語。

sibling (sib) *n.* one of a number of children of the same parents, i.e. a brother or sister.

同胞 同一父母的子女中的一個，即兄弟或姊妹。

sickle-cell disease (drepanocytosis) *n.* a hereditary blood disease that affects negroes. It is characterized by the production of an abnormal type of *haemoglobin – *sickle-cell haemoglobin* (*Hbs*) – in the red blood cells. Hbs becomes insoluble when the blood is deprived of oxygen and precipitates, forming elongated crystals that distort the blood cell into the characteristic sickle shape: this process is known as *sickling*. Sickle cells are rapidly removed from the circulation, leading to anaemia. There is no satisfactory treatment, but patients with this disease are resistant to infection with *Plasmodium falciparum*, which causes a serious form of malaria.

鐮狀細胞病（貧血） 黑人罹患的一種遺傳性血液病。其特徵爲紅血球內產生的一種異常血紅蛋白，即鐮狀細胞血紅蛋白。當血液失氧以後此種血紅蛋白變爲不溶性而沉澱，形成細長狀結晶，使紅細胞變成特殊的鐮刀形。這一過程被稱之爲鐮狀形成。鐮狀細胞很快從血循環中被除去，導至貧血。尙無滿意的療法。但此種患者能耐受惡性瘧原蟲感染。後者是瘧疾的一種嚴重型。

sickling *n. see* sickle-cell disease.

鐮狀化，鐮狀形成

sickness benefit (in Britain) weekly payments made to those who are unable to work through illness, provided they have made the necessary number of consecutive contributions under the

疾病津貼 （英國）按照國家保險條例規定，每週向因病不能工作的人支付津貼，條件是這些人已經作出過一定數量的連續性

terms of the National Insurance Act. The rate is higher for married men and there is also increased payment for each dependent child. Those who claim may do so initially on the basis of a personal affidavit. However, in the long term they are required to provide supporting evidence of incapacity, normally a *medical certificate provided by their general practitioner. Those who do not qualify may be eligible for similar payments as supplementary benefits under the terms of the *National Assistance Act. When incapacity arises from an injury at work or through contact with toxic substances (e.g. lead) at work, payment is made at a higher rate and there is also no qualifying period (*injury benefit*). The same conditions apply to those incapacitated by certain industrial diseases where the nature of the work is a recognized hazard (e.g. tuberculosis in mortuary attendants).

貢獻。已婚者的津貼較高。對不能獨立生活的兒童的支付額也較高。對那些要求津貼的且已很早塡寫個人申請書的人，他們應提供在長時間內不能工作的有力證據。正常情況下，需要一個由他們的全科醫師開具的疾病證明。對那些不具備條件申請津貼的人，則可根據國家救濟條例的條款得到類似的補助性津貼。凡由於工作中受傷或接觸有毒物質（如鉛）而喪失工作能力，津貼應有所增加，且無須通過資格審定期（工傷津貼）。上述情況同樣適用於工作性質公認有危險的某些職業病（如停屍間工作人員的結核病）。

side-effect *n.* an unwanted effect produced by a drug in addition to its desired therapeutic effects. Side-effects are often undesirable and may be harmful.

副作用　某一藥物除了預料到的治療作用以外，尙產生一些無用的作用。副作用常是令人討厭的，且可能是有害的。

sidero- *prefix denoting* iron.

〔前綴〕 **鐵**

sideroblast *n.* a red blood cell precursor (*erythroblast) in which iron-containing granules can be demonstrated by suitable staining techniques. Sideroblasts may be seen in normal individuals and are absent in iron deficiency. A certain type of anaemia (*sideroblastic anaemia*) is characterized by the presence of abnormal *ringed sideroblasts*. —**sideroblastic** *adj.*

鐵粒幼紅細胞　紅細胞的前體（成紅細胞）。適當的染色技術可顯示該細胞內有含鐵顆粒。鐵粒幼紅細胞存在於正常人。不存在於鐵缺乏患者。出現異形環圈狀鐵粒幼紅細胞是某些貧血型的特徵。

siderocyte *n.* a red blood cell in which granules of iron-containing protein (*Pappenheimer bodies*) can be demonstrated by suitable staining techniques. These granules are normally removed by the spleen and siderocytes are characteristically seen when the spleen is absent.

高鐵紅細胞　用適當染色技術可顯示含鐵蛋白顆粒（帕彭海默小體）的一種紅細胞。正常情況下，這些顆粒由脾清除。如脾缺失，則可看到特徵性高鐵紅細胞。

sideropenia *n.* iron deficiency. This may result from dietary inadequacy; increased requirement of iron by the body, as in pregnancy or childhood; or increased loss of iron from the body, usually due to chronic bleeding. The most important manifestation of iron deficiency is *anaemia, which is readily corrected by iron therapy.

鐵〔質〕缺乏〔症〕 可因飲食內缺少鐵元素，或因機體對鐵的需要增加所致。如姙娠或兒童期；或因機體失鐵增多，但一般多因慢性失血所致。貧血是鐵缺乏的最重要表現。此種貧血可迅速被鐵劑治療糾正。

siderosis *n.* the deposition of iron oxide dust in the lungs, occurring in silver finishers, arc welders, and haematite miners. Iron oxide itself is inert, but pulmonary *fibrosis may develop if fibrogenic dusts such as silica are also inhaled.

肺鐵末沉着病，鐵塵肺 氧化鐵塵末在肺內沉着。見於銀器精製工、電弧焊工和赤鐵礦工。氧化鐵本身無致病性，但是，如果與致纖維化粉塵（如與硅塵）同時吸入，則可發展爲肺纖維化。

siemens *n.* the *SI unit of electrical conductance, equal to the conductance between two points on a conductor when a potential difference of 1 volt between these points causes a current of 1 ampere to flow between them. Symbol: S.

西〔門子〕 電導的國際單位。當一導體的兩點之間1伏電位差引起1安培的電流時即等於1西〔門子〕單位。符號：S。

sievert *n.* the *SI unit of dose equivalent, being the dose equivalent when the absorbed dose of ionizing radiation multiplied by the stipulated dimensionless factors is $1\ J\ kg^{-1}$. As different types of radiation cause different effects in biological tissue a weighted absorbed dose, called the dose equivalent, is used in which the absorbed dose is modified by multiplying it by dimensionless factors stipulated by the International Commission on Radiological Protection. The sievert has replaced the *rem. Symbol: Sv.

希〔沃特〕 劑量當量的國際單位。當電離輻射的吸收劑量乘以規定的無量綱因子是1焦耳千克$^{-1}$時，即爲1希〔沃特〕。因爲不同類型的輻射在生物體組織中引起不同的效應，故使用加權的吸收劑量，即所謂劑量當量。劑量當量是吸收劑量乘以國際放射防護委員會規定的無量綱因子的乘積。舊名稱雷姆已爲希〔沃特〕所代替。符號：Sv。

sigmoid- *prefix denoting* the sigmoid colon. Example: *sigmoidotomy* (incision into).

〔前綴〕 **乙狀結腸** 例如乙狀結腸切開。

sigmoid colon (sigmoid flexure) the S-shaped terminal part of the descending *colon, which leads to the rectum.

乙狀結腸（乙狀腸曲） 降結腸的S形終末部分，和直腸相接。

sigmoidectomy *n.* removal of the sigmoid colon by surgery. It is performed

乙狀結腸切除術 手術切除乙狀結腸。切除的原因

for tumours, severe *diverticular disease, or for an abnormally long sigmoid colon that has become twisted (*see* volvulus).

有腫瘤，嚴重憩室性疾病，或因乙狀結腸異常冗長所引起的腸扭轉。

sigmoidoscope *n.* an instrument inserted through the anus in order to inspect the interior of the rectum and sigmoid colon. In its commonest form it consists of a steel or chrome tube, 25 cm long and 3 cm in diameter, with some form of illumination and a bellows to inflate the bowel.

乙狀結腸鏡 一種通過肛門插入直腸和乙狀結腸內的器械。最常用的由鋼管或電鍍金屬管組成。長25cm，內徑3cm，附有照明裝置和一個手用吹氣器，給結腸充氣。

sigmoidoscopy *n.* examination of the rectum and sigmoid colon with a *sigmoidoscope. It is used in the investigation of diarrhoea or rectal bleeding, particularly to detect colitis or cancer of the rectum. A general anaesthetic is sometimes given, especially if the procedure is expected to be painful or uncomfortable.

乙狀結腸鏡檢查 使用乙狀結腸鏡作直腸和乙狀結腸檢查。用以檢查腹瀉或直腸出血。特別是用以檢出結腸炎或直腸癌。有時應予全身麻醉，尤其如果事先預料到這一檢查給患者帶來痛苦或不適時。

sign *n.* an indication of a particular disorder that is observed by a physician but is not apparent to the patient. *Compare* symptom.

體徵 由醫師觀察到的一種特殊病徵，但患者自己並不覺察。

significance *n.* (in statistics) a relationship between two groups of observations indicating that the difference between them (e.g. between the percentages of smokers and nonsmokers respectively who die from lung cancer) is unlikely to have occurred by chance alone. An assumption is made that there is no difference between the two populations from which the two groups come (*null hypothesis*). This is tested, and a calculation indicating that there is a *probability* of less than 5% ($P<0.05$) that the observed difference or a larger one could have arisen by chance is regarded as being *statistically significant* and the null hypothesis is rejected. Some tests are *parametric*, based on the assumption that the range of observations are distributed by chance in a *normal* or *Gaussian distribution*, with 95% within two *standard

顯著性 （統計學）兩組觀察值之間的相互關係，表明其差別不會是偶然發生的（如死於肺癌的患者中，吸煙者和非吸煙者的兩個組百分數之間的關係）。假設這兩組觀察值所屬的兩個羣體之間沒有差別（零假設或無效假設）。經過檢驗、計算表明，這一被觀察到的差別（或更大些的差別）是偶然發生的這種可能性小於5%（$P<0.05$），被認爲有統計學顯著性，於是零假設就被否定。有些檢驗是參數性的，基於如下假定：觀察值的頻數范圍呈隨機的正態分佈（或高斯分佈），分佈於平均值的兩個標準差之間的佔95%（“t”檢驗，常用於兩均

deviations of the *mean (*Student's t test* to compare means). Nonparametric tests (*Mann-Whitney U tests*) make no assumptions about distribution patterns. *See also* frequency distribution, standard error.

數的比較）。非參數性檢驗則對於分佈態不作假設。

silicosis *n.* a lung disease – a form of *pneumoconiosis – produced by inhaling silica dust particles. It affects workers in mineral mining, quarrying, stone dressing, sand blasting, and boiler scaling. Silica stimulates *fibrosis of lung tissue, which produces progressive breathlessness and considerably increased susceptibility to tuberculosis (but not to lung cancer).

矽肺，硅肺，石末沉着病 肺塵埃沉着病（塵肺）的一種類型。由吸入二氧化硅粒引起。採礦工人、採石工人、石器修琢工易罹患此病。二氧化硅刺激肺組織形成纖維化，產生進行性呼吸困難，顯著增加對肺結核的易感性（但不增加對肺癌的易感性）。

silver nitrate a salt of silver with *caustic, *astringent, and *disinfectant properties. It is applied in solutions or creams to destroy warts and to treat skin injuries, including burns. Continued application discolours the skin black, and ingestion of silver nitrate may cause severe poisoning.

硝酸銀 銀的一種鹽類。具有腐蝕、收斂、消毒等性能。其溶液或乳霜可用以消除疣，治療包括燒傷在內的皮膚創傷。連續使用可使黑色皮膚脫色。吞服硝酸銀可引起嚴重中毒。

Simmond's disease loss of sexual function, loss of weight, and other features of failure of the pituitary gland (*hypopituitarism) occurring in women after childbirth complicated by bleeding (postpartum haemorrhage).

西蒙氏病 性機能喪失、體重減輕和有其它垂體腺機能衰竭徵象（垂體機能減退症）的疾病。見於產時或產後出血的婦女。

Simulium *n. see* black fly.

蚋屬

sinew *n.* a tendon.

腱

singultus *n. see* hiccup.

呃逆的

sinistr- (sinistro-) *prefix denoting* left or the left side.

〔前綴〕 **左，左側的**

sino- (sinu-) *prefix denoting* **1.** a sinus. **2.** the sinus venosus.

〔前綴〕 ① **竇** ② **靜脈竇。**

sinoatrial node (SA node) the pacemaker of the heart: a microscopic area of specialized cardiac muscle located in the upper wall of the right atrium near the entry of the vena cava. Fibres of the SA node are self-excitatory, contracting rhythmically at around 70 times per minute. Following each contraction,

竇房結（SA結） 心臟起搏點：位於上腔靜脈入口附近右房壁上部的特殊心肌的顯微鏡下結構。竇房結纖維具有自主應激性。每分鐘呈70次左右規律性收縮。隨着每次收縮，衝動經心房肌向竇房

the impulse spreads throughout the atrial muscle and into fibres connecting the SA node with the *atrioventricular node. The SA node is supplied by fibres of the autonomic nervous system; impulses arriving at the node accelerate or decrease the heart rate.

結和房室結之間的纖維傳遞。竇房結的神經分佈來自植物神經系統。衝動抵達竇房結，使心率加速或減慢。

sinus *n.* **1.** an air cavity within a bone, especially any of the cavities within the bones of the face or skull (*see* paranasal sinus). **2.** any wide channel containing blood, usually venous blood. *Venous sinuses* occur, for example, in the dura mater and drain blood from the brain. **3.** a pocket or bulge in a tubular organ, especially a blood vessel; for example, the *carotid sinus. **4.** an infected tract leading from a focus of infection to the surface of the skin or a hollow organ. *See* pilonidal sinus.

竇，竇道 ①骨內含氣腔，尤指面頰骨或頭顱骨內的含氣腔。 ②含有血液（通常是靜脈血）的寬大管腔。如硬腦膜內的靜脈竇可從大腦引流血液。③在一個管狀器官，尤其是在血管內出現的一個小袋膨出，如頸動脈竇。④感染性病竈通向體表或一個中空臟器的感染性通道。

sinus arrhythmia a normal variation in the heart rate, which accelerates slightly on inspiration and slows on expiration. It is common in healthy individuals.

竇性心律不齊 心率的正常變異。吸氣時輕度增快，呼氣時變慢。一般見於健康者。

sinusitis *n.* inflammation of one or more of the mucous-lined air spaces in the facial bones that communicate with the nose (the paranasal sinuses). It is often caused by infection spreading from the nose. Symptoms include headache and tenderness over the affected sinus, which may become filled with a purulent material that is discharged through the nose. In persistent cases treatment may require the affected sinus to be washed out or drained by a surgical operation.

竇炎 與鼻腔相通的面頰骨內的一個或一個以上的含氣黏膜腔（副鼻竇）的炎症。通常由鼻腔的感染蔓延引起。症狀有頭痛、鼻竇部壓痛；可被膿性物質充塡，膿性物質可從鼻腔流出。頑固病例需作病竇冲洗治療或手術引流治療。

sinusoid *n.* a small blood vessel found in certain organs, such as the adrenal gland and liver. Large numbers of sinusoids occur in the liver. They receive oxygen-rich blood from the hepatic artery and nutrients from the intestines via the portal vein. Oxygen and nutrients diffuse through the capillary walls into the liver cells. The sinusoids

竇狀隙 腎上腺和肝臟等若干臟器內的小血管。肝臟內可有大量竇狀隙。它們從肝動脈內接受含氧血液，通過門脉從腸內接受營養。氧和營養素經毛細血管管壁瀰散滲入肝細胞。竇狀隙內的血液由肝靜脈引流。

are drained by the hepatic veins. *See also* portal system.

靜脈竇 胚胎期心臟的一個腔室，它同時接受幾條靜脈的血液。在成年期的心臟中它成爲右房的一部。

sinus venosus a chamber of the embryonic heart that receives blood from several veins. In the adult heart it becomes part of the right atrium.

siphonage *n.* the transfer of liquid from one container to another by means of a bent tube. The procedure is used in gastric *lavage, when the stomach is filled with water through a funnel and rubber tube, and the tube is then bent downwards to act as a siphon and empty the stomach of its contents.

虹吸法 用一根曲管把液體從一容器轉移到另一容器。本法可用以作洗胃術。通過一個漏斗和橡皮管把水灌入胃內，而後把橡皮管向下彎垂，起到一種虹吸作用，把胃內容物排空。

Siphunculina *n.* a genus of flies. *S. funicola*, the eye fly of India, feeds on the secretions of the tear glands and in landing on or near the eyes contributes to the spread of *conjunctivitis.

眼蠅 蠅的一個屬。印度眼蠅以淚腺的分泌物爲食物，寄生於眼內或眼附近，傳播結膜炎。

sirenomelia *n. see* sympodia.

〔無足〕並腿畸形

sito- *prefix denoting* food.

〔前綴〕 **食物**

sitz bath a fairly shallow hip bath in which the person is seated. Sitz baths of cold and hot water, rapidly alternated, were formerly used for the treatment of a variety of sexual disorders.

坐浴 一種淺水臀部坐浴。從前曾用冷水和熱水快速交替以治療各種性慾障礙。

SI units (Système International d'Unités) the internationally agreed system of units now in use for all scientific purposes. Based on the metre-kilogram-second system, SI units have seven base units and two supplementary units. Measurements of all other physical quantities are expressed in derived units, consisting of two or more base units. Tables 1 and 2 (Appendix) list the base units and the derived units having special names; all these units are defined in the dictionary.
Decimal multiples of SI units are expressed using specified prefixes; where possible a prefix representing 10 raised to a power that is a multiple of three

國際單位 （單位的國際制）目前在科學上所使用的都是國際單位制。根據米-公斤-秒制，國際單位共有7個基本單位和兩個增補單位。所有其它的物量的測定都是上述的導出單位。它由二個或二個以上基本單位組成。各種基本單位和具有專門名稱的導出單位均列於表1和表2（見附錄）中。所有這些單位的含義均可在本字典中查到。
以10進制爲基礎的各種倍數的國際單位均用不同的專門前綴來表示，如果表

should be used. Prefixes are listed in Table 3 (Appendix).

達一個10^3的數字，就應該用一個特殊的前綴。各種前綴列於表3（見附錄）。

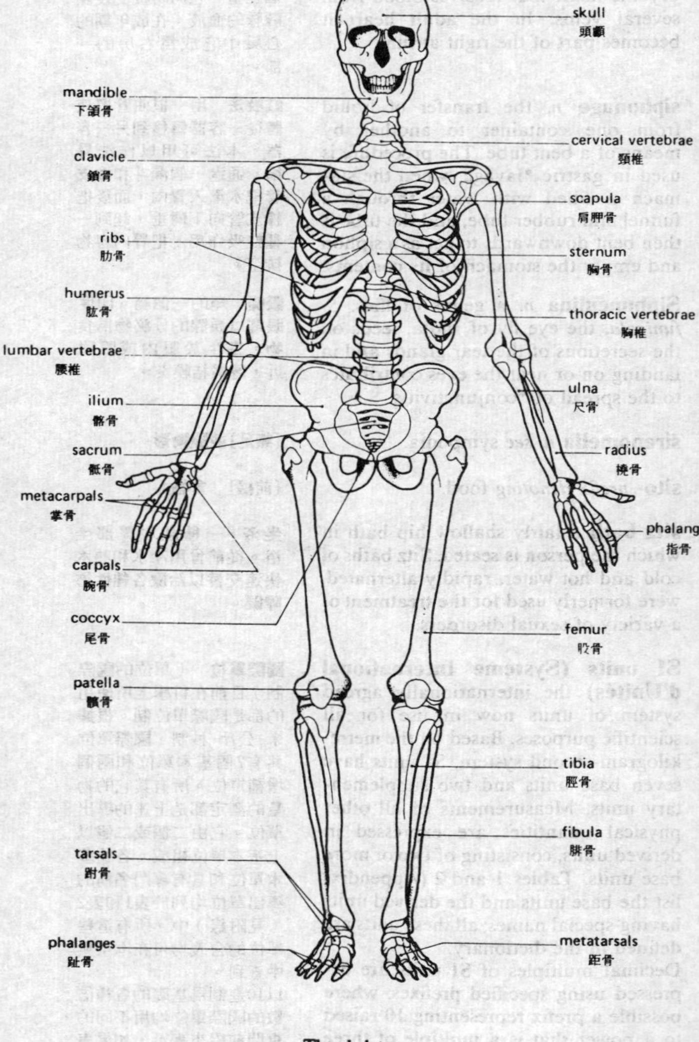

The skeleton
骨骼

Sjögren's syndrome a condition in which the patient complains of a dry mouth, caused by wasting of the salivary glands. It is associated with rheumatoid arthritis and dryness of the eyes.

斯耶格倫氏綜合徵，乾燥綜合徵 患者主訴因唾液腺耗竭而口乾，並伴類風濕性關節炎和兩眼乾燥的一種疾病。

skatole (methyl indole) *n.* a derivative of the amino acid tryptophan, excreted in the urine and faeces.

糞臭素（甲基吲哚） 在尿和糞內排泄的一種氨基酸色氨酸的衍化物。

skeletal muscle *see* striated muscle.

骨骼肌

skeleton *n.* the rigid framework of connected *bones that gives form to the body, protects and supports its soft organs and tissues, and provides attachments for muscles and a system of levers essential for locomotion. The 206 named bones of the body are organized into the *axial skeleton* (of the head and trunk) and the *appendicular skeleton* (of the limbs). (See illustration.) —**skeletal** *adj.*

骨骼 許多骨連接在一起的堅硬框架。它構成身體的外形，保護並支撑着體內柔軟的臟器和組織，它提供肌肉的附着點和一個爲運動所必要的杠桿系統。機體共有206塊有名稱的骨組成中軸骨骼（頭顱和軀幹）以及附屬骨骼（四肢）（見圖）。

skew *n.* a disorder of relationships within a family, in which one parent is overpowering and the other is submissive and there is a general avoidance of anxiety-provoking situations. It was proposed as a specific cause of schizophrenia in the children, but this has not been confirmed.

反常家庭 家庭內部關係的反常。父母的一方專制，另一方順從。兒童經常需要迴避這種引起焦慮的處境。曾認爲這是兒童精神分裂症的一種特異性病因，但尚未確定。

skew deviation a rare condition of the eyes in which one eye turns down and inwards while the other turns up and outwards. It is sometimes seen in disorders of the *cerebellum.

偏斜視 罕見的一種眼病：一眼球向下向內側轉動時，另一眼球却向上或向外側轉動。本病有時可見於小腦疾患。

skia- *prefix denoting* shadow.

〔前綴〕**影**（尤指X線的）

skiagram *n.* a 'shadow-photograph', such as an X-ray photograph produced in radiography. —**skiagraphy** *n.*

影像〔照〕片 一張影像照片。如X線拍攝的X線照片。

skin *n.* the outer covering of the body, consisting of an outer layer, the *epidermis, and an inner layer, the *dermis (see illustration). Beneath the dermis is a layer of fatty tissue. The skin has several functions. The epidermis protects the body from injury and from invasion by parasites. It also helps to prevent the body from becoming dehy-

皮膚 身體外面的覆蓋物。它由外層的表皮和內層的眞皮組成（見圖）。眞皮下有一層脂肪組織。皮膚有多種功能。表皮保護機體免受創傷和寄生虫的侵襲。同時也協助機體預防脫水。皮膚內能豎立的汗毛、汗腺和毛細血管

drated. The combination of erectile hairs, *sweat glands, and blood capillaries in the skin form part of the temperature-regulating mechanism of the body. When the body is too hot, loss of heat is increased by sweating and by the dilation of the capillaries. When the body is too cold the sweat glands are inactive, the capillaries contract, and a layer of air is trapped over the epidermis by the erected hairs. The skin also acts as an organ of excretion (by the secretion of *sweat) and as a sense organ (it contains receptors that are sensitive to heat, cold, touch, and pain). The layer of fat underneath the dermis can act as a reservoir of food and water. Anatomical name: **cutis**.

構成體溫調節機制的一個部分。當機體太熱時，加強出汗，擴張毛細血管以增加散熱。當機體太冷時，汗腺停止工作，毛細血管收縮，汗毛豎起，把一層空氣吸附在表皮上。皮膚也是一個分泌器官（分泌汗腺）和感覺器官（它含有對冷熱和觸痛覺的感受器）。眞皮底下的脂肪層具有營養物和水分貯藏庫的功能。

skin graft a portion of healthy skin cut from one area of the body and used to cover a part that has lost its skin, usually as a result of injury, burns, or operation. A skin graft is normally taken from another part of the body of the same patient (an *autograft), but occasionally skin may be grafted from one person to another as a temporary healing measure (a *homograft). The full thickness of skin may be taken for a graft (*see* flap) or the surgeon may use three-quarters thickness, thin sheets of skin (*see* Thiersch's graft), or a pinch skin graft. The type used depends on the condition and size of the damaged area to be treated.

移植皮片 從身體某部分切下一塊健康皮膚用以覆蓋缺損皮膚部分。此種缺損通常由皮膚創傷、灼傷或手術造成。正常情況下，移植皮片取自自身的另一部位皮膚（自體移植）。偶爾，作爲暫時性治療措施，移植皮片取自另一人的皮膚（同種移植）。移植皮片應取足夠厚度。外科醫師也可用¾厚度的皮膚、或紙片樣薄皮片或點狀植皮片。植皮類型取決於損傷皮膚的狀況和面積。

skull *n.* the skeleton of the head and face, which is made up of 22 bones. It can be divided into the cranium, which encloses the brain, and the face (including the lower jaw (mandible)). (See illustration.) The *cranium* consists of eight bones. The frontal, parietals (two), occipital, and temporals (two) form the vault of the skull (*calvaria*) and are made up of two thin layers of compact bone separated by a layer of spongy bone (*diploë*). The remaining bones of the cranium – the sphenoid and ethmoid – form part of its base.

頭顱 頭和面的骨骼，由22塊骨組成。它可分爲頭顱骨（包住大腦）和面骨（包括下頜骨）（見圖）。顱骨由8塊骨組成。額骨、頂骨（兩塊）、枕骨和顳骨（兩塊）共同形成頭顱的穹窿（顱蓋）。所有顱骨均由兩層緻密骨質組成，兩層之間被一層海綿狀骨質所分開（板障）。其餘的蝶骨和篩骨組成顱骨的基底部。其它組成面部的14塊

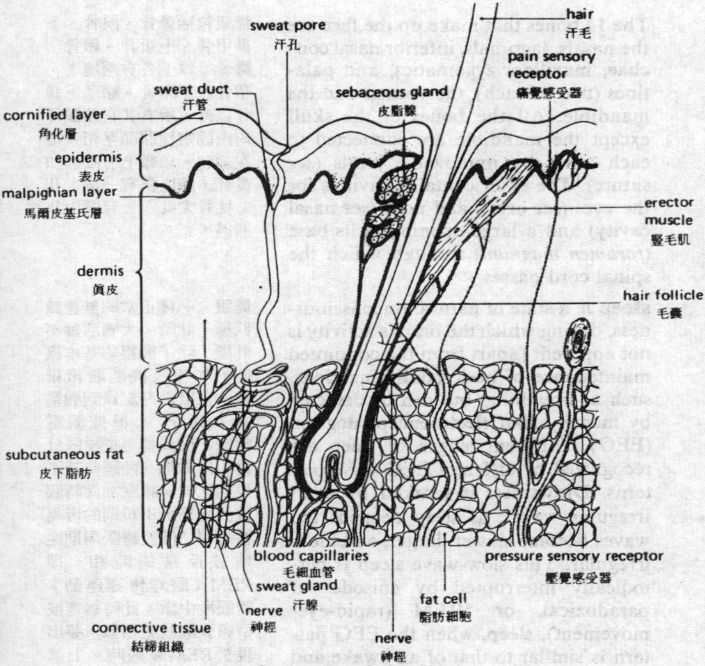

Section through the skin
皮膚切面示意圖

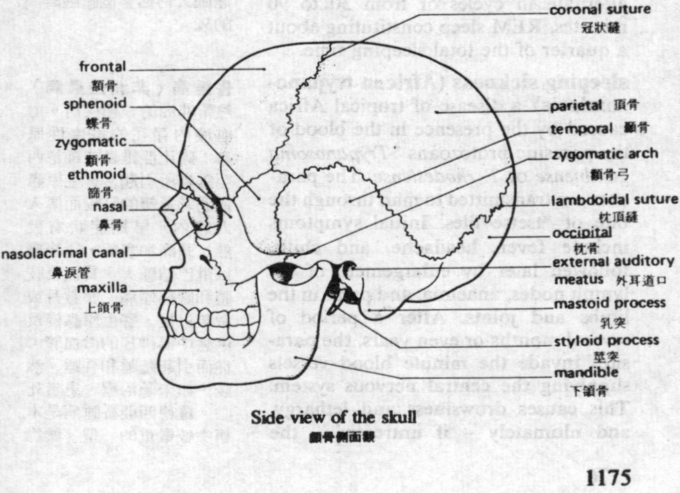

Side view of the skull
顱骨側面觀

The 14 bones that make up the face are the nasals, lacrimals, inferior nasal conchae, maxillae, zygomatics, and palatines (two of each), the vomer, and the mandible. All the bones of the skull except the mandible are connected to each other by immovable joints (*see* suture). The skull contains cavities for the eyes (*see* orbit) and nose (*see* nasal cavity) and a large opening at its base (*foramen magnum*) through which the spinal cord passes.

骨頭包括鼻骨、淚骨、下鼻甲骨、上頜骨、顴骨、腭骨（以上各有兩塊）、犁骨和下頜骨。除了下頜骨以外，所有其它頭顱骨均由固定性關節互相連接在一起。頭顱上有眼眶和鼻孔，顱底部有一個大孔（枕骨大孔），脊髓由此通過。

sleep *n.* a state of natural unconsciousness, during which the brain's activity is not apparent (apart from the continued maintenance of basic bodily functions, such as breathing) but can be detected by means of an electroencephalogram (EEG). Different stages of sleep are recognized by different EEG wave patterns. Drowsiness is marked by short irregular waves; as sleep deepens the waves become slower, larger, and more irregular. This slow-wave sleep is periodically interrupted by episodes of paradoxical, or *REM (rapid-eye-movement), sleep, when the EEG pattern is similar to that of an awake and alert person. Dreaming occurs during REM sleep. The two states of sleep alternate in cycles of from 30 to 90 minutes, REM sleep constituting about a quarter of the total sleeping time.

睡眠 一種正常的無意識狀態。此時，大腦活動不外顯（除了機體的基本機能，如呼吸機能繼續維持），但仍可記錄到腦電圖（EEG）。根據腦電圖的不同波型可把睡眠分爲不同的期。瞌睡時是不規則低波。睡眠加深時腦電波變爲更不規則的慢高波。這一慢波睡眠周期性地被反常的時相，即REM（眼球快速運動）睡眠所中斷。此時腦電波型與覺醒狀態相似。夢出現於REM睡眠時。上述兩種睡眠狀態每隔30～90分呈周期性交替。REM睡眠大約佔整個睡眠時間的¼。

sleeping sickness (African trypanosomiasis) a disease of tropical Africa caused by the presence in the blood of the parasitic protozoans **Trypanosoma gambiense* or *T. rhodesiense*. The parasites are transmitted to man through the bite of *tsetse flies. Initial symptoms include fever, headache, and chills, followed later by enlargement of the lymph nodes, anaemia, and pains in the limbs and joints. After a period of several months or even years, the parasites invade the minute blood vessels supplying the central nervous system. This causes drowsiness and lethargy, and ultimately – if untreated – the

昏睡病（非洲錐蟲病） 熱帶非洲的一種疾病。由血液內存在的寄生性原蟲：岡比亞錐蟲或羅德西亞錐蟲所引起。寄生原蟲通過彩彩蠅的叮咬而傳入人體內。早期症狀有發熱、頭痛和寒顫，隨後繼以淋巴結腫大、貧血及肢體和關節疼痛。歷數月或數年以後，寄生原蟲侵及供應中樞神經的微血管，從而引起瞌睡和昏睡。然後，如未予治療，患者死亡。羅德西亞昏睡病是本病中較嚴重的一型。藥物

patient dies. Rhodesian sleeping sickness is the more virulent form of the disease. The drugs *suramin and pentamidine are used to treat the early curable stages of sleeping sickness; drugs containing arsenic (*see* tryparsamide) are administered after the brain is affected. Eradication of tsetse flies helps prevent spread of the infection.

蘇拉明、戊氧苯脒可用以治療早期可治型昏睡病。如大腦被侵及以後，則使用含砷製劑。彩彩蠅的徹底撲滅有助於預防這一感染性疾病的傳播。

sleep-walking *n. see* somnambulism.

夢行

sling *n.* a bandage arranged to support and rest an injured limb so that healing is not hindered by activity. The most common sling is a *triangular bandage tied behind the neck to support the weight of a broken arm. The arm is bent at the elbow and held across the body.

懸帶　懸吊的繃帶。用以支撐和固定一個受傷的肢體，以免動作妨礙痊癒。三角繃帶最爲常用。它懸吊在頸後，以支撐傷臂的重量。上肢的肘部屈曲，手托在身體的一邊。

slipped disc a colloquial term for a *prolapsed intervertebral disc.

滑出盤　椎間盤脫出的俗稱。

slit lamp a device for providing a narrow beam of light, used in conjunction with a special microscope. It can be used to examine minutely the structures within the eye, one layer at a time.

裂隙燈　一種產生一個窄光束並和一架專門顯微鏡相連接的裝置。用以檢查眼內細微結構，每次檢查一個層次。

slough *n.* dead tissue, such as skin, that separates from healthy tissue after inflammation or infection.

腐肉　壞死的組織。如一塊皮膚在一次炎症或感染以後，和正常組織呈分離狀態。

smallpox *n.* an acute infectious virus disease causing high fever and a rash that scars the skin. It is transmitted chiefly by direct contact with a patient. Symptoms commence 8–18 days after exposure and include headache, backache, high fever, and vomiting. On the third day, as the fever subsides, red spots appear on the face and spread to the trunk and extremities. Over the next 8–9 days all the spots (macules) change to pimples (papules), then to pea-sized blisters that are at first watery (vesicles) but soon become pus-filled (pustules). The fever returns, often causing delirium. On the eleventh or twelfth day the rash and fever abate. Scabs formed by

天花　一種急性病毒性感染。可引起高熱和使皮膚形成疤痕的皮疹。主要由於和患者直接接觸而被傳染。接觸後第8～18天開始出現症狀。包括頭痛、背痛、高熱和嘔吐。發病第三天在高熱減退時，臉部開始出現紅斑，且向軀幹和四肢蔓延。再經過8～9天，全部斑點變成爲膿疱丘疹，而後變爲豆大的疱疹，起初爲水疱，不久即變爲膿疱。體溫重新上升，常伴譫妄。第11～12天，皮疹和體溫消退。膿疱乾燥結痂，7～20天以後

drying out of pustules fall off 7–20 days later, leaving permanent scars. The patient remains infectious until all scabs have been shed. Most patients recover but serious complications such as nephritis or pneumonia may develop. Treatment with *thiosemicarbazone is effective. An attack usually confers immunity; immunization against smallpox has now totally eradicated the disease. Medical name: **variola**. *See also* alastrim, cowpox.

脫落，造成永久性疤痕。患者的感染狀態持續至全部痂脫落爲止。大部患者可恢復健康。唯可發生某些嚴重併發症，諸如腎炎或肺炎。氨硫脲治療有效。一次感染常可終身免疫。目前，抗天花免疫接種（種痘）已徹底消滅了此病。

smear *n.* a specimen of tissue or other material taken from part of the body and smeared on a microscope slide for examination. *See* cervical smear.

塗片 從身體某一部分取下的組織或其他材料的標本，塗成顯微鏡薄片，以供檢查。

smegma *n.* the secretion of the glands of the foreskin (*prepuce), which accumulates under the foreskin and has a white cheesy appearance. It becomes readily infested by a harmless bacterium that resembles the tubercle bacillus.

陰垢 包皮腺的分泌物。在包皮內積累，呈白色奶酪樣外觀。它很易沾染一種類似於結核桿菌的無害細菌。

smooth muscle (involuntary muscle) muscle that produces slow long-term contractions of which the individual is unaware. Smooth muscle occurs in hollow organs, such as the stomach, intestine, blood vessels, and bladder. It consists of spindle-shaped cells within a

平滑肌（非隨意肌） 一種肌肉，能產生緩慢的長時間的收縮，本人却不覺察。平滑肌存在於各種中空臟器，如胃、腸、血管和膀胱。它由結締組織網內的許多梭狀細胞（見

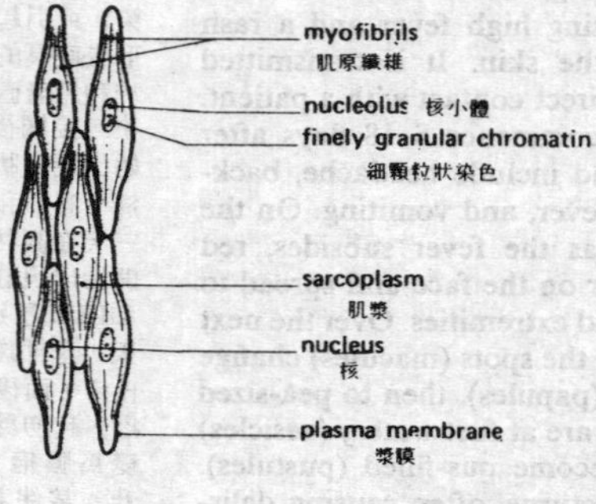

Arrangement of smooth muscle cells
平滑肌細胞排列

network of connective tissue (see illustration) and is under the control of the autonomic nervous system. *Compare* striated muscle.

圖）組成，由植物神經系統控制。

snare *n.* an instrument consisting of a wire loop designed to remove polyps, tumours, and other projections of tissue, particularly those occurring in body cavities (see illustration). The loop is used to encircle the base of the tumour and is then pulled tight. *See also* diathermy.

勒除器 由鋼絲套圈組成的器械。用以除去存在於體腔的息肉、腫瘤和其它隆突組織（見圖）。用套圈套住腫瘤的基部，而後把圈套收緊。

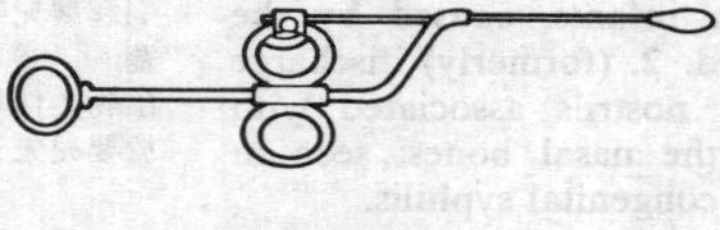

A nasal snare
鼻勒除器

sneeze 1. *n.* an involuntary violent reflex expulsion of air through the nose and mouth provoked by irritation of the mucous membrane lining the nasal cavity. **2.** *vb.* to produce a sneeze.

噴嚏 ①鼻腔內的黏膜受刺激而引起一種非隨意性强烈反射，將空氣從鼻腔和口腔噴出。 ②使產生噴嚏動作。

Snellen chart the commonest chart used for testing sharpness of distant vision (*see* visual acuity). It consists of rows of capital letters, called *test types*, the letters of each row becoming smaller down the chart. The large letter at the top is of such a size that it can be read by a person with normal sight from a distance of 60 metres. A normally sighted person can read successive lines of letters from 36, 24, 18, 12, 9, 6, and 5 metres respectively, There is sometimes a line for 4 metres. The subject sits 6 metres from the chart and one eye is tested at a time. If he can only read down as far as the 12-metre line the visual acuity is expressed as 6/12. Normally sighted people can read the 6-metre line, i.e. normal acuity is 6/6, and many people read the 5-metre line with ease. A smaller chart on the same principle is available for testing near vision.

斯力倫氏視力表 用以測量遠〔距〕視力敏鋭度的最常用表。它由數排大寫字母組成。表的下方每一排字母小於上排的字母。最上方的大字母可由一個正常視力的人從60米以外讀認。一個正常視力的人可以分別從36、24、18、12、9、6和5米外讀出第一排以下相應各排的字母。有時每排也可相差4米。被檢者也可以在離表6米處每次用一隻眼睛測試。如果只能讀出12米這一排字母，那末其視敏度可用$\frac{6}{12}$表示。正常人被檢時應能讀出6米這一排字母，即正常視敏度應爲$\frac{6}{6}$。很多人可以容易地讀出這一排字母。一種與以上原理相同的類似小表可供近距視力測試。

snore 1. *vb.* to breathe in such a way as to cause vibration of the soft palate of the roof of the mouth, resulting in a hoarse noise. Snoring usually occurs during sleep. **2.** *n.* the sound made by breathing in this way.

①**打鼾** 引起口腔頂部軟腭振動的一種呼吸方式。它產生一種噪音。打鼾通常發生於睡眠時。 ②**鼾聲** 以這種方式呼吸所發出的聲音。

snow blindness a painful disorder of the cornea of the eye due to excessive exposure to ultraviolet light reflected from the snow. Recovery usually follows within 24 hours of covering the eyes.

雪盲 過度暴露於雪反射的紫外線而致眼角膜產生的疼痛性疾患。眼睛覆蓋後，通常於24小時內恢復。

snuffles *n.* **1.** partial obstruction of breathing in infants, caused by the common cold. **2.** (formerly) discharge through the nostrils associated with necrosis of the nasal bones: seen in infants with congenital syphilis.

嬰兒鼻塞 ①由普通感冒引起嬰兒呼吸道的部分阻塞。 ②（舊稱）鼻孔流出物內伴壞死性鼻骨：見於嬰兒先天性梅毒。

social class any one of the subdivisions of the population made by the Office of Population Censuses and Surveys based on occupation, as indicated in the ten-yearly census. Such groupings are intended to stratify the population according to standard of living and income (married women and children up to school-leaving age are classified in accordance with the occupation of husband/father). Five classes are recognized: I professional/self employed; II administrative; III (non-manual) clerical and (manual) skilled manual workers; IV semi-skilled; V unskilled. An alternative subdivision into *socio-economic groups* is believed by many sociologists to reflect employment grades more accurately, but it is more complicated and tends to be less generally applied.

社會階層 在人口調查局每10年進行的一次調查中根據職業劃分的人口詳細分類之一。按照生活水平和收入（已婚婦女或在學兒童的分類，依據其丈夫或父親）把人口分成5個階層：Ⅰ專業人員或自由職業者；Ⅱ行政管理人員；Ⅲ（非體力）職員及熟練體力工人；Ⅳ半熟練工人；Ⅴ非熟練工人。另一種分類是把人羣分成若干社會經濟羣。許多社會學家認為此種分類法能更正確地反映職業等級。但此法較複雜，一般不被採納。

social medicine *see* community medicine.

社會醫學

social services advice and practical help with problems due to social circumstances. Every local authority is responsible for establishing and starting a social service department, though block exchequer grants meet some of

社會服務 對具有由社會環境引起問題的人提供建議或實際幫助。每一地方政府儘管經費有困難，應有責任建立一個社會服務部。在這些部門接受過專

the costs. An increasing proportion of the *social workers* in these departments are professionally trained. The present policy is to train generic social workers, but there are special social workers with medical and psychiatric training who are seconded for work in hospitals (*see* medical social worker). Social workers assess eligibility of clients for such social services as home helps and meals on wheels or refer them to the appropriate statutory or voluntary services. *Case work* involves identifying the cause of the client's problem and, where appropriate, advising how best to correct it and/or adapt to the circumstances.

業訓練的社工人員的比例要提高。目前的方針是培訓一般社工人員。但還有一些接受過醫學和心理學訓練的專門社工人員。他們充當醫院工作的副手。社工人員審定申請者（當事人）的合格條件，並向他們提供家務幫助、運送上門膳食，或指點他們到適當的法定機構或民辦機構去申請。對申請者情況的個案調查工作涉及核實申請的理由，並適當地給予如何解決這些問題及/或適應環境的建議。

social worker *see* social services.

社工人員

socio-economic group *see* social class.

社會經濟羣

socket *n.* (in anatomy) a hollow or depression into which another part fits, such as the cavity in the alveolar bone of the jaws into which the root of a tooth fits. *See also* dry socket.

槽，臼，窩 （解剖學）一個中空或凹陷結構，其中有其它組織充塡。例如上下頜骨的牙槽骨的孔穴由牙根充塡。

sodium *n.* a mineral element and an important constituent of the human body (average sodium content of the adult body is 4000 mmol). Sodium controls the volume of extracellular fluid in the body and maintains the acid-base balance. It also helps maintain electrical potentials in the nervous system and is thus necessary for the functioning of nerves and muscles. Sodium is contained in most foods and is well absorbed, the average daily intake in the UK being 200 mmol. The amount of sodium in the body is controlled by the kidneys. An excess of sodium leads to the condition of *hypernatraemia*, which often results in *oedema. This may develop in infants fed on bottled milk, which has a much higher sodium content than human milk. Since babies are less able to

鈉 一種無機元素。也是人體的一個重要成分（成人體內平均含鈉4000毫克分子）。鈉控制機體細胞外液容量，維持酸鹼平衡。它亦參與神經系統電位差的維持，因而它爲神經、肌肉功能所必需。大部分食物內均含有鈉，且吸收良好。英國人每日鈉攝取量爲200毫克分子。體內總鈉量由腎臟控制。鈉過多可導至高鈉血症，常能引起水腫。由於牛奶含鈉量遠高於人奶，因此，高鈉血症可發生於牛奶餵養的嬰幼兒。嬰兒從體內排鈉能力遜於成人，因此嬰兒的高鈉飲食餵養可以引起脫水。鈉也參與高血壓的發病。高鈉飲食

remove sodium from the body than adults the feeding of a high-sodium diet to babies is dangerous and may lead to dehydration. Sodium is also implicated in hypertension: a high-sodium diet is thought to increase the risk of hypertension in later life.

被認爲能增加後半生的高血壓危險。

sodium aminosalicylate a drug with effects and uses similar to those of *para-aminosalicylic acid. Trade name: **Paramisan**.

氨基水楊酸鈉 一種與對氨水楊酸作用和用途相似的藥物。

sodium bicarbonate a salt of sodium that neutralizes acid and is used to treat stomach and digestive disorders, *acidosis, and sodium deficiency. It is administered by mouth or injection; high doses may cause digestive upsets. *See also* antacid.

碳酸氫鈉 一種能中和酸的鈉鹽。用以治療胃腸道疾病、酸中毒和鈉缺乏症。可供口服或注射。大劑量可引起消化道不適感。

sodium fluoride a salt of sodium used to prevent tooth decay. It is administered by mouth or applied to the teeth as paste or solution. Taken by mouth, it may cause digestive upsets and large doses may cause fluorine poisoning. *See also* fluoridation.

氟化鈉 一種用以預防齲齒的鈉鹽。口服或以其膏劑或溶液直接塗敷牙齒。口服時可以引起消化道不適感。大劑量口服則可引起氟中毒。

sodium fusidate an *antibiotic used mainly to treat infections caused by **Staphylococcus*. It is administered by mouth or injection or applied in an ointment for skin infections; common side-effects are mild digestive upsets. Trade name: **Fucidin**.

梭鏈孢酸鈉，褐霉酸鈉 一種主要用以治療葡萄球菌引起的感染的抗生素。可供口服或注射。皮膚感染時則用油膏制劑。常見副作用爲消化道不適感。

sodium hydroxide (caustic soda) a powerful alkali in widespread use as a cleaning agent. It attacks the skin, causing severe chemical burns that are best treated by washing the area with large quantities of water. When swallowed it causes burning of the mouth and throat, which should be treated by giving water, milk, or other fluid to dilute the stomach contents and by gastric lavage.

氫氧化鈉（苛性鈉） 一種廣泛用作清潔劑的强鹼。它强烈刺激皮膚，可引起皮膚化學性灼傷。此時最好用大量的水清洗創面。如果係吞下後引起的口腔和喉部灼傷，此時的治療應包括飲水和牛奶或其它飲料，旨在使胃內容物稀釋，並進行洗胃治療。

sodium nitrite a sodium salt used, with sodium thiosulphate, to treat cyan-

亞硝酸鈉 一種鈉鹽。和硫代硫酸鈉合用治療氰化

ide poisoning. It is administered by injection and may cause digestive upsets, dizziness, headache, fainting, and cyanosis. It also has effects similar to *glyceryl trinitrate and has been used to treat angina.

物中毒。供注射用。可引起消化道不適感、頭暈、頭痛、暈厥和紫紺。它尚具有和硝酸甘油相似的作用，因而它可用於治療心絞痛。

sodium salicylate a drug with actions and side-effects similar to those of *aspirin. It is used mainly to treat rheumatic fever. Trade name: **Entrosalyl**.

水楊酸鈉 一種和阿司匹林作用和副作用相似的藥物。它主要用以治療風濕熱。

sodium thiosulphate a salt of sodium used, with *sodium nitrite, to treat cyanide poisoning. It is administered by intravenous injection.

硫代硫酸鈉 一種鈉鹽。與亞硝酸鈉合用治療氰化物中毒。供靜脈注射。

sodium valproate an *anticonvulsant drug used to treat all types of epilepsy. It is administered by mouth; side-effects may include digestive upsets, drowsiness, and muscle incoordination. Trade name: **Epilim**.

丙戊酸鈉 用以治療各類癲癇的抗痙藥。供口服。副作用包括消化道不適感，倦眠和肌肉共濟失調。

sodokosis *n. see* rat-bite fever.

鼠咬熱

sodomy *n.* sexual intercourse using the anus. This may be homosexual, heterosexual, or between man and beast. *See also* perversion.

雞奸，獸奸 通過肛門性交。可在同性、異性或人獸間進行。

soft sore (chancroid) a venereal disease caused by the bacterium *Haemophilus ducreyi*, resulting in enlargement and ulceration of lymph nodes in the groin. Treatment with sulphonamides is effective.

軟下疳 一種杜克雷氏嗜血桿菌引起的性病。它導至腹股溝淋巴結腫大和潰瘍。磺胺類藥物治療有效。

solarium *n.* a room in which patients are exposed to either sunlight or artificial sunlight (a blend of visible light and infrared and ultraviolet radiation directed from special lamps).

日光浴室 患者接受太陽光或人工太陽光照射的房間（人工太陽光由專門的燈發出的可視光、紅外線和紫外線輻射的混合光組成）。

solar plexus (coeliac plexus) a network of sympathetic nerves and ganglia high in the back of the abdomen.

腹腔〔神經〕叢 一種交感神經和神經節的網狀結構。位於腹腔的後上部。

soleus *n.* a broad flat muscle in the calf of the leg, beneath the *gastrocnemius

比目魚肌 小腿後部的一個寬而扁平的肌肉。位於

muscle. The soleus flexes the foot, so that the toes point downwards.

腓腸肌的下層。比目魚肌可使足向後屈，趾尖朝下。

soma *n.* **1.** the entire body excluding the germ cells. **2.** the body as distinct from the mind.

體，軀體 ①指生殖細胞以外的整個身體。 ②指和精神有區別的軀體。

somat- *prefix denoting* **1.** the body. **2.** somatic.

〔前綴〕 ①**身體** ②**軀體的**

somatic *adj.* **1.** relating to the nonreproductive parts of the body. A somatic mutation cannot be inherited. **2.** relating to the body wall (i.e. excluding the viscera), e.g. somatic *mesoderm. *Compare* splanchnic. **3.** relating to the body rather than the mind.

身體的，軀體的，體壁的 ①與身體非生殖部分有關的。軀體的突變不能被遣傳。 ②與體壁有關的（即內臟除外）。如體壁中胚層。 ③與軀體有關而與精神無關的。

somatopleure *n.* the body wall of the early embryo, which consists of a simple layer of ectoderm lined with mesoderm. The amnion is a continuation of this structure outside the embryo. *Compare* splanchnopleure.

胚體壁（外胚層和體壁中胚層） 早期胚胎的體壁。它是由外胚層和中胚層組成的一個單一層。羊膜是這一結構在胚胎外的繼續。

somatotrophin *n. see* growth hormone.

促生長素

somatotype *n. see* body type.

體型，體式

somite *n.* any of the paired segmented divisions of *mesoderm that develop along the length of the early embryo. The somites differentiate into voluntary muscle, bones, connective tissue, and the deeper layers of the skin (*see* dermatome, myotome, sclerotome).

體節 沿着早期胚胎的長度發育的中胚層的任一成對的節段。體節可區分爲隨意肌、骨、結締組織和皮膚較深層組織。

somnambulism (noctambulation) *n.* sleep-walking: walking about and performing other actions in a semiautomatic way during sleep without later memory of doing so. It is common during childhood and may persist into adult life. It can also arise spontaneously, as the result of stress or hypnosis. —**somnambulistic** *adj.*

夢行〔症〕 睡眠中起來行走或做出其它一些半自主的動作，而事後不能記起做過的事情。一般常見於兒童期，並可持續到成年期。亦可在應激或催眠狀態中自發產生。

somniloquence *n.* talking in one's sleep. *See also* somnambulism.

夢囈，夢語 夢中講話。

somnolism *n.* a hypnotic trance. *See* hypnosis.

催眠狀態 一種催眠性迷睡狀態。

sonoplacentography *n.* the technique of using *ultrasound waves to determine the position of the placenta during pregnancy. This has the advantage over using X-rays that the fetus is not subjected to possibly harmful radiation.

超聲胎盤造影術 妊娠期間，應用超聲波確定胎盤位置的一種技術。因爲胎兒不能耐受可能有害的放射，所以此技術比X線造影術優越。

sonotopography *n.* the use of *ultrasound waves to determine the position of structures within the body, such as the position of a fetus within the womb or the midline of the brain within the skull.

超聲斷層檢查術 應用超聲波檢查體內各種結構的位置，如胎兒在子宮內的位置或顱內大腦中線的位置。

soporific *n. see* hypnotic.

催眠的，催眠藥

sorbitol *n.* a carbohydrate with a sweet taste, used by diabetics as a substitute for cane sugar. It is also used in disorders of carbohydrate metabolism and in drip feeding. It is administered by mouth or injection; large doses taken by mouth may cause digestive upsets.

山梨〔糖〕醇 一種帶有甜味的碳水化合物。糖尿病患者用作蔗糖的代替物。它亦用於碳水化物代謝障礙和滴注餵養患者。供口服或注射。大劑量口服可以引起消化道不適感。

sordes *pl. n.* the brownish encrustations that form around the mouth and teeth of patients suffering from fevers.

口垢 發熱患者口腔和牙齒附近形成的帶褐色痂皮。

sore *n.* a lay term for any ulcer or other open wound of the skin or mucous membranes, which may be caused by injury or infection. *See also* bedsore, soft sore.

瘡，潰瘍 皮膚或黏膜的各種潰瘍或開放性傷口的一個俗稱。它們可由外傷或感染引起。

sore throat pain at the back of the mouth, commonly due to bacterial or viral infection of the tonsils (*tonsillitis) or the pharynx (*pharyngitis). If infection persists the lymph nodes in the neck may become tender and enlarged (cervical adenitis).

咽喉痛 口腔後壁痛，一般常由扁桃體（扁桃體炎）或咽（咽炎）的細菌性或病毒性感染引起。如感染持續存在，則頸部淋巴結可腫大和觸痛（頸淋巴腺炎）。

sotalol *n.* a drug (*see* beta blocker) used to treat abnormal heart rhythm, angina, and high blood pressure and to relieve symptoms in *thyrotoxicosis. It is administered by mouth or injection; side-effects may include digestive upsets, tiredness, and dizziness. Trade names: **Beta-Cardone, Sotacor.**

甲磺胺心定 一種用以治療心律失常、心絞痛和高血壓的藥物。並可緩解甲狀腺毒症。供口服或注射。副作用有消化道不適感、乏力和頭暈。商品名：心得怡。

souffle *n.* a soft blowing sound heard through the stethoscope, usually produced by blood flowing in vessels.

雜音，吹氣音 用聽診器聽到的一種柔和吹風樣音。通常由於血管內血液流動所產生。

sound (in surgery) **1.** *n.* a long rodlike instrument, often with a curved end, used to explore body cavities (such as the bladder) or to dilate *strictures in the urethra or other canals. **2.** *vb.* to explore a cavity using a sound.

探子（外科） ①一種長杜樣器械，末端常有一個彎曲。常用以探查體腔（如膽囊與膀胱）或用以擴張狹窄的尿道或其它管腔。②用探子探查某一個腔孔。

Southey's tubes fine-calibre tubes for insertion into subcutaneous tissue to drain excess fluid. They are rarely used in practice today.

騷錫氏管 用以插入皮下組織引流多餘體液的細口徑管。實際上目前已很少使用。

space maintainer an orthodontic appliance that maintains an existing space in the dentition.

牙間隙保持器 牙正畸器械，它保持牙列間隙的存在。

Spanish fly the blister beetle, *Lytta vesicatoria*: source of the irritant and toxic chemical compound *cantharidin.

西班牙蠅，斑蝥，歐芫菁 起疱甲蟲。具有刺激性和毒性，是複方斑蝥素製劑的來源。

sparganosis *n.* a disease caused by the migration of certain tapeworm larvae (*see* Sparganum) in the tissues beneath the skin, between the muscles, and occasionally in the viscera and brain. The larvae, which normally develop in frogs and reptiles, are accidentally transferred to man by eating the uncooked flesh of these animals or by drinking water contaminated with minute crustaceans infected with the tapeworm larvae. The larvae cause inflammation, swelling, and fibrosis of the tissues. Treatment of the condition, common in the Far East, involves intravenous injections of neosalvarsan and surgical removal of the larvae.

裂頭蚴病 某種絛蟲的幼蟲移行所引起的疾病。幼蟲存在於皮下組織、肌肉間，偶見於內臟和大腦內。正常情況下，這些幼蟲在蛙和爬行動物體內發育。偶然傳播給人的途徑是吃了這些未煮熟的宿主動物的肉，或飲用了含有被絛蟲幼蟲污染的甲殼綱動物的飲料。幼蟲可引起機體組織的炎症、腫脹和纖維化。遠東地區常用的治療是靜注新灑爾佛散（九一四）以及手術取出幼蟲。

Sparganum *n.* the larvae of certain tapeworms, including species of **Diphyllobothrium* and *Spirometra*, which may accidentally infect man (*see* sparganosis). They are actually *plerocercoids, but the generic name *Sparganum*

裂頭蚴屬 某些絛蟲幼蟲，包括裂頭絛蟲和疊宮絛蟲。實際上，它們是全尾裂頭蚴，但通俗地稱它們爲裂頭蚴屬，因它們不能發育爲成蟲，而又無法

is given to them since they fail to develop into adults and definite classification of the species is not possible from the larvae alone.

單獨根據幼蟲作出蟲種的明確分類。

spasm *n.* a sustained involuntary muscular contraction, which may occur either as part of a generalized disorder, such as a *spastic paralysis, or as a local response to an otherwise unconnected painful condition. *Carpopedal spasm* affects the muscles of the hands and feet and is caused by a deficiency of available calcium in the body.

痙攣 肌肉呈持久不隨意收縮。可爲全身性疾病的一個部分，如痙攣性麻痹；也可爲對另一不相關疼痛狀態產生的局部反應。手足痙攣可侵及手足肌肉，它由體內鈣缺乏引起。

spasmo- *prefix denoting* spasm.

〔前綴〕 **痙攣**

spasmodic *adj.* occurring in spasms or resembling a spasm.

痙攣的 痙攣引起的，或與痙攣類似的。

spasmolytic *n.* a drug that relieves spasm of smooth muscle, e.g. *aminophylline, *papaverine, or *piperidolate. Spasmolytics may be used as *bronchodilators to relieve spasm in bronchial muscle, to stimulate the heart in the treatment of angina, or to relieve colic due to spasm of the digestive system.

解痙劑，鎮痙劑 一種緩解平滑肌痙攣的藥物。如氨茶鹼、罌粟鹼或二苯哌酯。解痙劑可用作支氣管擴張劑，緩解支氣管肌的痙攣，在心絞痛治療中它興奮心臟，或用於緩解消化系痙攣引起的腸絞痛。

spasmus nutans a combination of symptoms including a slow nodding movement of the head, *nystagmus (involuntary movements of the eyes), and spasm of the neck muscles. It affects infants and it normally disappears within a year or two.

點頭狀痙攣 一組混合症狀，包括緩慢點頭動作、眼球震顫（眼球的非隨意運動）和頸部肌肉痙攣。它侵及嬰幼兒。正常情況下1至2年內症狀消失。

spastic colon *see* irritable bowel syndrome.

痙攣性結腸

spasticity *n.* resistance to the passive movement of a limb that is maximal at the beginning of the movement and gives way as more pressure is applied. It is a symptom of damage to the corticospinal tracts in the brain or spinal cord. It is usually accompanied by weakness in the affected limb (*see* spastic paralysis). *Compare* rigidity.

痙攣狀態，强直〔狀態〕 對肢體被動性動作的抵抗。動作開始時抵抗最强，需要較强的力量才能使之動作。它是大腦或脊髓內皮層脊髓束受損的一個症狀。常伴有病側肢體無力。

spastic paralysis weakness of a limb or limbs associated with increased

痙攣性麻痹 一個或兩個肢體無力伴反射增强。病

reflex activity. This results in resistance to passive movement of the limb (*see* spasticity). It is caused by disease affecting the nerve fibres of the corticospinal tract, which in health not only initiate movement but also inhibit the stretch reflexes to allow the movements to take place. *See* cerebral palsy.

肢對運動有抵抗。它由皮層脊髓束神經纖維的疾病所引起。正常人的皮層脊髓束不僅可使肢體運動，而且可抑制牽張反射，從而保證動作的完成。

spatula *n.* an instrument with a blunt blade used to spread ointments or plasters and, particularly in dentistry, to mix materials.

藥刀，藥鏟 一種醫療器械。有一個鈍的刀刃，用以使油膏或硬膏舖開。尤多在牙科用以調合材料。

special hospitals hospitals for the care of mentally ill patients who are also dangerous and must therefore by kept securely. There are four in the UK: Broadmoor, Rampton, Moss Side, and Carstairs. Most (but not all) patients are there compulsorily under a hospital order made by a court according to the *Mental Health Act.

專門醫院 治療精神病患者的醫院。這些患者有危險性，因此必需保持安全。在英國有4所此類醫院：布羅德穆、蘭普頓、莫斯賽德和卡斯泰爾斯。根據國家精神保健法令，大部分（但不是全部）患者應接受醫院强制管理。

Specialist in Community Medicine (SCM) *see* community physician.

公共醫學專家

special school (in Britain) an education establishment for handicapped children. The discovery and assessment (*ascertainment*) of those needing to attend a special school may occur long before school age (2 years or younger); the responsibility for deciding who attends a special school lies with the local education authority. Special schools exist for each of the following 11 groups of handicapped children: the blind, the partially sighted, the deaf, those with partial hearing, the delicate (those with such medical handicaps as congenital heart disease or cystic fibrosis), the educationally subnormal, the mentally handicapped (in which learning potential is limited and independent living may prove impossible), the maladjusted (those with behavioral difficulties), the physically handicapped (by such conditions as poliomyelitis, muscular dystrophy, or limb absence from thalidomide), the epileptic, and those with speech defects. Some special

專門學校 （英國）爲殘疾兒童辦的教育機構。應發現並確定（查明）需要在學齡前（2歲或2歲以前）進入專門學校的殘疾兒童。決定誰進入此專門學校是地方教育當局的責任。以下11個組的殘疾兒童可進此專門學校：全盲、全聾、半聾、病殘者（如先天性心臟病、囊性纖維性變）、智力遜常、精神殘疾（學習困難、不能獨立生活）、適應不良（行動困難）、軀體殘疾（如脊髓灰白質炎、肌營養不良、或因母親妊期內服用酞胺哌啶酮而致缺肢畸形）、癲癇以及語言缺陷者。若干專門學校接受以上兩種或兩種以上複雜殘疾兒童。盲童及其他嚴重殘疾兒童的教育開始於2歲，聾兒則一經發現應即開始專門教育。

schools cater for combinations of two or more of these handicaps. Special education for the blind and for those with other severe handicaps may start as early as 2 years, deaf children requiring special education from the date of discovery.

species *n.* the smallest unit used in the classification of living organisms. Members of the same species are able to interbreed and produce fertile offspring. Similar species are grouped together within one *genus.

〔物〕種　生物分類中的最小單位。某些種生物能雜交繁殖，產生能生育的後代。通常把相近種的生物歸入同一屬。

specific 1. *n.* a medicine that has properties especially useful for the treatment of a particular disease. **2.** *adj.* (of a disease) caused by a particular microorganism that causes no other disease. **3.** *adj.* of or relating to a species.

①**特效藥**　對某一特定疾病有特殊療效的藥物。②**特異性（疾病）**　某種微生物專門引起某病，而不引起其它病。③**物種的**　屬於某一物種的或與某物種有關的。

specificity *n.* (in screening tests) *see* sensitivity.

特異性，特殊性　（篩選試驗）

spectinomycin *n.* an *antibiotic used to treat various infections, particularly gonorrhoea. It is administered by injection; side-effects may include nausea, dizziness, fever, and rash. Trade name: **Trobicin**.

壯觀黴素　用以治療各種感染，尤其用以治療淋病的一種抗生素。

spectrograph *n.* an instrument (a *spectrometer or *spectroscope) that produces a photographic record (*spectrogram*) of the intensity and wavelength of electromagnetic radiations.

攝影儀　一種以攝影方法記錄電磁射綫强度和波長（光譜圖）的儀器。

spectrometer *n.* any instrument for measuring the intensity and wavelengths of visible or invisible electromagnetic radiations. *See also* spectroscope.

分光計，光譜計　測定可視和非可視性電磁射綫波長和强度的儀器。

spectrophotometer *n.* an instrument (a spectrometer) for measuring the intensity of the wavelengths of the components of light (visible or ultraviolet).

分光光度計　測定光的成分（可視光或紫外綫）的波長和强度的儀器（分光計）。

spectroscope *n.* an instrument used to split up light or other radiation into

分光鏡　用以分解光或其它射綫成爲不同波長成分

components of different wavelengths. The simplest spectroscope uses a prism, which splits white light into the rainbow colours of the visible spectrum.

的儀器。最簡單的分光鏡是用一個稜鏡把白光分解成彩虹七色的可視光譜。

specular reflection (in *ultrasonics) the reflection of sound waves from the surface of an internal structure, which can be used to produce a picture of the surface as an echogram (*see* echography). A specular reflection contrasts with vaguer diffuse echoes produced by minor differences in tissue density.

鏡面反射 （超聲〔波〕學）從體內一個結構表面反射超聲波。該表面的圖像，叫做回聲圖。它與密度差別很小的組織所產生的模糊而彌散的回聲圖形成鮮明對照。

speculum *n.* (*pl.* **specula**) a metal instrument for inserting into and holding open a cavity of the body, such as the vagina, rectum, or nasal orifice, in order that the interior may be examined (see illustration).

窺器 用以插入機體某個孔腔並保持其張開狀態的金屬器械。它可插入陰道、直腸或鼻腔，以檢查其內部情況。（見圖）。

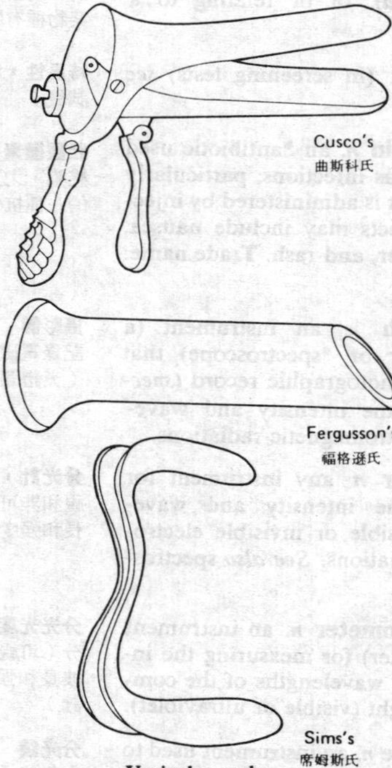

Vaginal specula
陰道窺鏡示意圖

speech therapy the rehabilitation of patients who are unable to speak coherently because of congenital causes, accidents, or illness (e.g. stroke). Speech therapists have special training in this field but are not medically registered.

語言療法 對於因先天性疾病，意外事故或病殘（如中風）而不能有條理地講話的患者的康復治療。語言治療師在此領域內曾受專門訓練，但無行醫註册執照。

sperm *n. see* spermatozoon.

精子，精液

sperm- (spermi(o)- spermo-) *prefix denoting* sperm or semen.

〔前綴〕 **精子，精液**

spermat- (spermato-) *prefix denoting* **1.** sperm. **2.** organs or ducts associated with sperm.

〔前綴〕 ①**精子，精液** ②與精子或精液有關的器官或導管

spermatic artery either of two arteries that originate from the abdominal aorta and travel downwards to supply the testes.

精索動脉 兩根精索動脉之一。它源自腹主動脉，向下走行，向睪丸供血。

spermatic cord the cord, consisting of the *vas deferens, nerves, and blood vessels, that runs from the abdominal cavity to the testicle in the scrotum. The *inguinal canal, through which the spermatic cord passes, becomes closed after the testes have descended.

精索 由輸精管、神經和血管組成。自腹腔走向陰囊內的睪丸。輸精管所經過的腹股溝管，一俟睪丸降至陰囊後即變爲閉鎖狀態。

spermatid *n.* a small cell produced as an intermediate stage in the formation of spermatozoa. Spermatids become embedded in *Sertoli cells in the testis. They are transformed into spermatozoa by the process of spermiogenesis (*see* spermatogenesis).

精細胞，精子細胞 精子形成的中間期小細胞。精〔子〕細胞在睪丸內鑲嵌於塞爾托利氏細胞之間。通過精子發生過程，精細胞轉變爲精子。

spermatocele *n.* a cystic swelling in the scrotum containing sperm. The cyst arises from the epididymis (the duct conveying sperm from the testis) and can be felt as a lump above the testis. Needle *aspiration of the cyst reveals a milky opalescent fluid containing sperm. Treatment is by surgical removal.

精子囊腫 陰囊的囊性腫脹，內含精子。囊腫來自附睪（從睪丸轉運精子的導管），附睪猶如睪丸上的一個腫塊。從囊腫中可用針吸出牛奶樣不透明液體，內含精子。手術切除治療。

spermatocyte *n.* a cell produced as an intermediate stage in the formation of spermatozoa (*see* spermatogenesis). Spermatocytes develop from spermato-

精母細胞 精子形成的中間期細胞。精母細胞發育自睪丸細精管壁上的精原細胞。根據它們發生第一

gonia in the walls of the seminiferous tubules of the testis; they are known as either *primary* or *secondary spermatocytes* according to whether they are undergoing the first or second division of meiosis.

次抑或第二次減數分裂，分別稱爲初級或次級精母細胞。

spermatogenesis *n.* the process by which mature spermatozoa are produced in the testis (see illustration). *Spermatogonia, in the outermost layer of the seminiferous tubules, multiply throughout reproductive life. Some of them divide by meiosis into *spermatocytes, which produce haploid *spermatids. These are transformed into mature spermatozoa by the process of *spermiogenesis*. The whole process takes 70–80 days.

精子發生　睪丸內成熟精子的形成過程（見圖）。

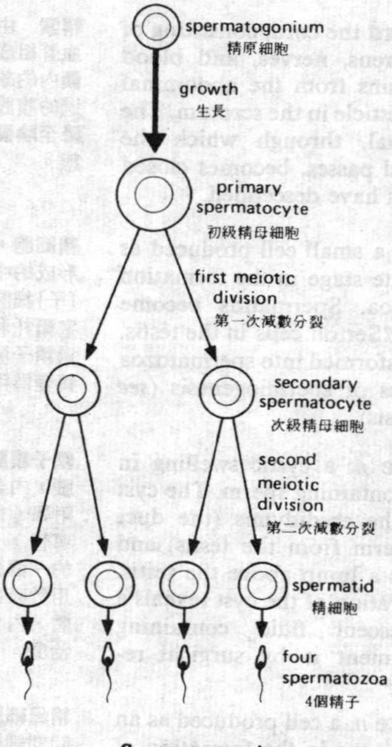

Spermatogenesis
精子發生示意圖

spermatogonium *n.* (*pl.* **spermatogonia**) a cell produced at an early stage in the formation of spermatozoa (*see* spermatogenesis). Spermatogonia first appear in the testis of the fetus but do not multiply significantly until after puberty. They act as stem cells in the walls of the seminiferous tubules, dividing continuously by mitosis and giving rise to *spermatocytes.

精原細胞 精子形成早期階段的細胞。精原細胞最早出現於胎兒睪丸內，但直到青春期才大量增殖。它位於細精管壁，起幹細胞作用。以減數分裂方式繼續分裂，產生精母細胞。

spermatorrhoea *n.* the involuntary discharge of semen without orgasm. Semen is usually produced by ejaculation at orgasm and does not normally discharge at other times. If, however, the mechanism of ejaculation is lost, spermatorrhoea may occur.

遺精，精溢 無性慾高潮下的非隨意排精。正常時在性慾高潮時射出精液，其他時間不排精。不過，如喪失射精能力，則可遺精。

spermatozoon (sperm) *n.* (*pl.* **spermatozoa**) a mature male sex cell (*see* gamete). The tail of a sperm enables it to swim, which is important as a means for reaching and fertilizing the ovum (although muscular movements of the womb may assist its journey from the vagina). *See also* acrosome, fertilization.

精子 成熟男性的性細胞。精子有尾，可以游動，這是精子接近卵子、並使卵受精的一個重要手段（子宮肌運動亦可協助它自陰道游入）。

spermaturia *n.* the presence of spermatozoa in the urine. Spermatozoa are occasionally seen on microscopic examination of the urine and their presence is not abnormal. If present in large numbers, the urine becomes cloudy, usually towards the end of micturition. Abnormal ejaculation into the bladder on orgasm (retrograde ejaculation) may occur after *prostatectomy or other surgical procedures or in neurological conditions that destroy the ability of the bladder neck to close on ejaculation.

精液尿 尿內存在精子。尿顯微鏡檢查偶可見到精子，它們的存在並非異常。如有大量精子，尿即變爲混濁，通常在尿的終末段尤爲明顯。性高潮時向膀胱內射精（逆向射精）可出現於前列腺切除術或其它術後，或某些神經系疾病以及膀胱頸部與射精有密切關係的括約肌功能損壞。

sperm count an estimate of the concentration of spermatozoa in ejaculated semen, which is used as a measure of male fertility. Between 300 million and 500 million spermatozoa in the total ejaculate is normal; less than 60 million is usually accompanied by *sterility.

精子計數 射出的精液內的精子含量測定。它作爲男性生殖能力的一種檢查。射出精液總量含精子3億至5億間爲正常，少於6千萬時通常合併不育。

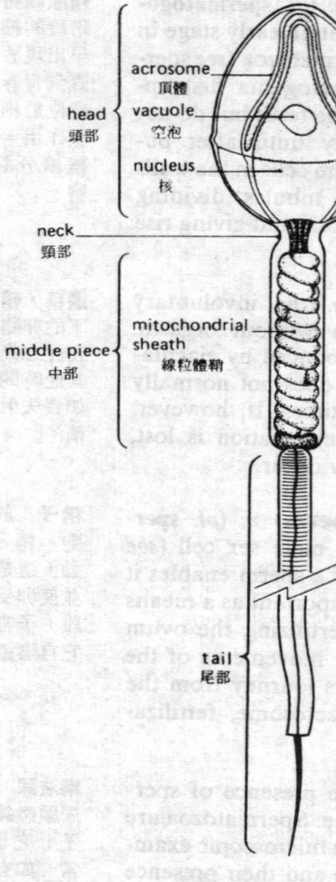

A spermatozoon
精子

spermicide *n.* an agent that kills spermatozoa. Creams and jellies containing chemical spermicides are used – in conjunction with a *diaphragm – as contraceptives. —**spermicidal** *adj.*

殺精子劑　一種殺死精子的藥物。含有化學性殺精子藥常爲霜劑或膠凍劑，與陰道隔膜共用，作爲避孕藥。

spermiogenesis *n.* the process by which spermatids become mature spermatozoa within the seminiferous tubules of the testis. *See* spermatogenesis.

精子發生　睪丸輸精管內精細胞變爲成熟精子的過程。

spheno- *prefix denoting* the sphenoid bone. Examples: *sphenomaxillary* (relating to the sphenoid and maxillary bones); *sphenopalatine* (relating to the sphenoid bone and palate).

〔前綴〕 **蝶骨**　如蝶頜的（與蝶骨和上頜骨有關的），蝶腭的（與蝶骨和腭骨有關的）。

sphenoid bone a bone forming the base of the cranium behind the eyes. It consists of a *body*, containing air spaces continuous with the nasal cavity (*see* paranasal sinus); two *wings* that form part of the orbits; and two *pterygoid processes* projecting down from the point where the two wings join the body. *See* skull.

蝶骨 位於兩眼後方，形成顱底的一塊骨頭。它由一個體和兩個翼組成。體部含氣腔，與鼻腔相通。翼組成兩個眼眶。兩個翼突自翼和體的結合點出發，向下突出。

spherocyte *n.* an abnormal form of red blood cell (*erythrocyte) that is spherical rather than disc-shaped. In blood films spherocytes appear smaller and stain more densely than normal red cells. Spherocytes tend to be removed from the blood as they pass through the spleen, resulting in anaemia. *See also* spherocytosis.

球形紅細胞 一種異形紅細胞。它呈球形，而不呈盤形。在血膜上，球形紅細胞比正常紅細胞小，且染色較濃。經過脾臟時，球形紅細胞被清除，從而導至貧血。

spherocytosis *n.* the presence in the blood of abnormally shaped red cells (*spherocytes). Spherocytosis may occur as a hereditary disorder (*hereditary spherocytosis*) or in certain haemolytic *anaemias.

球形紅細胞症 血液內存在異形紅細胞（球形紅細胞）。它可出現於某一遺傳性疾病（遺傳性球形紅細胞症）或某些溶血性貧血。

sphincter *n.* a specialized ring of muscle that surrounds an orifice. Contractions of the sphincter partly or completely close the orifice. Sphincters are found, for example, around the anus (*anal sphincter*) and at the opening between the stomach and duodenum (*pyloric sphincter*).

括約肌 體腔孔口周圍的特殊肌環。括約肌收縮可使該孔口部分地或完全閉合。如肛門周圍有括約肌（肌門括約肌）以及胃、十二指腸間開口處有括約肌（幽門括約肌）。

sphincter- *prefix denoting* a sphincter.

〔前綴〕 **括約肌**

sphincterectomy *n.* **1.** the surgical removal of any sphincter muscle. **2.** surgical removal of part of the iris in the eye at the border of the pupil.

括約肌切除術 ①手術切除括約肌。 ②手術切除瞳孔邊緣的部分虹膜。

sphincterotomy *n.* surgical division of any sphincter muscle.

括約肌切開術 手術切開某一括約肌。

sphingomyelin *n.* a *phospholipid that contains sphingosine, a fatty acid, phosphoric acid, and choline. Sphingomyelins are found in large amounts in brain and nerve tissue.

〔神經〕鞘髓磷脂 一種磷脂。它含有〔神經〕鞘氨醇、脂肪酸、磷酸和膽鹼。大腦和神經組織含有大量〔神經〕鞘髓磷脂。

sphingosine *n.* a lipid alcohol that is a constituent of sphingomyelin and cerebrosides.

〔神經〕鞘氨醇 一種脂醇，它是鞘髓磷脂和腦苷的成分。

sphygmo- *prefix denoting* the pulse.

〔前綴〕 脉，脉搏

sphygmocardiograph *n.* an apparatus for producing a continuous record of both the heart beat and the subsequent pulse in one of the blood vessels. The recording can be shown on a moving tape or on an electronic screen.

心動脉搏描記儀 一種連續記錄心搏和某一血管脉搏的儀器。記錄可由連續記錄帶或電子示波器顯示。

sphygmograph *n.* an apparatus for producing a continuous record of the pulse in one of the blood vessels, showing the strength and rate of the beats.

脉搏描記儀，脉搏計 一種連續記錄某一血管搏動的儀器。它可顯示搏動的強度和速率。

sphygmomanometer *n.* an instrument for measuring *blood pressure in the arteries. It consists of an inflatable cuff connected via a rubber tube to a column of mercury with a graduated scale. The cuff is applied to a limb (usually the arm) and inflated to exert pressure on a large artery until the blood flow stops. The pressure is then slowly released and, with the aid of a stethoscope to listen to the pulse, it is possible to determine both the systolic and diastolic pressures (which can be read on the scale).

血壓計 一種測定動脉血壓的儀器。它由一個可打氣的袖套和通過皮管連接有刻度的汞柱所組成。把袖套纏在一個肢體上（通常是上臂），打氣時對一根大動脉施加壓力，直至阻斷血流，而後，緩緩地減壓，與此同時，借助於聽診器聽取收縮壓和舒張壓（在有刻度的汞柱上讀取數字）。

sphygmophone *n.* a device to record the heart beat or pulse in the form of amplified sound waves played through a loudspeaker or earphones.

脉音聽診器 一種記錄心搏或脉搏的裝置，聲波放大後，通過喇叭或耳機播出。

sphygmoscope *n.* a device for showing the heart beat or pulse as a visible signal, especially a continuous wave signal on a cathode-ray tube.

脉波檢視器 一種以可視信號方式顯示心搏或脉搏的裝置。主要借助於一陰極射線管顯示其連續波信號。

spica *n.* a bandage wound spirally around an injured limb. At each turn it is given a twist so that the slack material is taken up at the overlap.

人字形繃帶 用繃帶呈螺旋狀綁扎一受傷肢體的傷口。每繞一圈，繃帶反折一次，使繃帶的鬆弛部分收緊，呈人字形疊蓋。

spicule *n.* a small splinter of bone.

骨針 骨的碎片。

spina bifida (rachischisis) a developmental defect in which the newborn baby has part of the spinal cord and its coverings exposed through a gap in the backbone. The symptoms may include paralysis of the legs, incontinence, and mental retardation from the commonly associated brain defect, *hydrocephalus. Spina bifida is associated with abnormally high levels of *alpha-fetoprotein in the amniotic fluid surrounding the embryo. The condition can be diagnosed at about the 16th week of pregnancy by a test on the amniotic fluid (*see* amniocentesis), so making termination of the pregnancy possible. *See also* neural tube defects.

脊柱裂 新生兒部分脊髓膜由一個裂口暴露在外的一種先天性發育缺陷。症狀有下肢麻痺、大小便失禁以及由於一般均合併大腦發育不全和腦積水而有精神發育遲緩。脊柱裂常合併胎周羊水甲胎蛋白的異常增多。大約於妊期第16週作羊水檢查可以確診。此時中止妊娠是可能的。

spinal accessory nerve *see* accessory nerve.

脊髓副神經

spinal anaesthesia 1. suppression of sensation in part of the body by the injection of a local anaesthetic into the space surrounding the spinal cord. There are two types used for surgery: *subarachnoid* and *epidural.* In the latter the anaesthetic is injected into the outer lining of the cord. The injection site for subarachnoid spinal anaesthetics is in the lumbar region of the vertebral column, the needle being inserted between the vertebrae (anywhere between the second and fifth). For epidural anaesthetics, the sacral region may also be used. The extent of the area anaesthetised depends upon the amount and strength of local anaesthetic injected. Spinal anaesthesia is useful in patients whose condition makes them unsuitable for a general anaesthetic, perhaps because of chest infection; for certain obstetric procedures; or in circumstances where a skilled anaesthetist is not readily available to administer a general anaesthetic. The technique is more commonly used in Scandinavia and the USA than in Britain. **2.** loss of sensation in part of the body as a result of injury or disease to the spinal cord. The area of the body affected depends

脊髓麻醉 ①在脊髓周圍腔隙內注射局部麻醉劑，使身體部分的感覺阻抑。外科應用的脊髓麻醉有兩類：蛛網膜下麻醉和硬膜外麻醉。後者把麻醉劑注入脊髓的外膜。蛛網膜下脊髓麻醉的注射是在脊柱的腰椎區，把針刺入椎體之間（腰Ⅱ和腰Ⅴ之間的任一椎間）。骶部也可作硬膜外麻醉。麻醉區域的範圍取決於所注射的麻醉藥劑量和强度。脊髓麻醉適用於不宜作全身麻醉者，如胸腔感染；某些產科手術；或在熟練麻醉師本人不樂於作全身麻醉的情況下。脊髓麻醉技術較普遍應用於斯堪的納維亞和美國。較少應用於英國。②由於外傷或脊髓疾患導至身體某部分的感覺缺失。感覺缺失的面積取決於病變的位置。病變的位置越是靠下方，感覺障礙越輕。

upon the site of the lesion: the lower it is in the cord the less the sensory disability.

spinal column *see* backbone.

脊柱

spinal cord the portion of the central nervous system enclosed in the vertebral column, consisting of nerve cells and bundles of nerves connecting all parts of the body with the brain. It contains a core of grey matter surrounded by white matter (see illustration). It is enveloped in three layers of membrane, the *meninges, and extends from the medulla oblongata in the skull to the level of the second lumbar vertebra. From it arise 31 pairs of *spinal nerves.

脊髓 包在脊柱內的中樞神經部分。它由神經細胞和神經束組成。它們把身體各部分與大腦相連接。其中心部分是灰質，灰質周圍係白質（見圖）。被三層脊膜包被。脊髓起至顱內的延髓，並延伸至第二腰椎水平。在走行過程中，它發出31對脊髓神經。

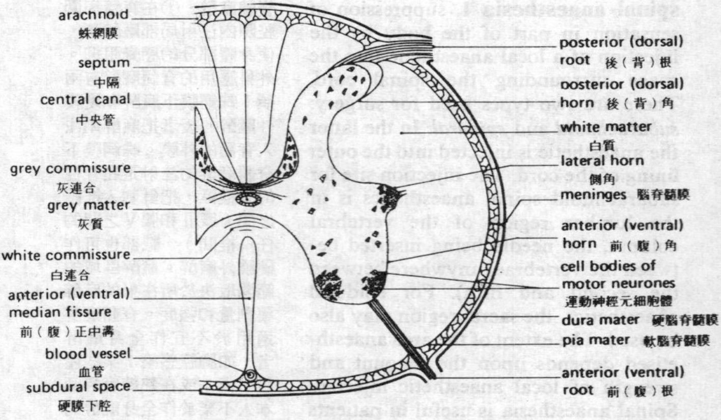

Transverse section through the spinal cord

脊髓橫斷面示意圖

spinal nerves the 31 pairs of nerves that leave the spinal cord and are distributed to the body, passing out from the vertebral canal through the spaces between the arches of the vertebrae. Each nerve has two *roots, an anterior, carrying motor nerve fibres, and a posterior, carrying sensory fibres. Immediately after the roots leave the

脊髓神經 從脊髓發出，經椎弓隙，通過椎管，分佈至全身的31對神經。每對神經有兩個根，前根含運動神經纖維；後根含感覺神經。兩個根自脊髓發出後不遠即合併。兩側各自形成混合性脊髓神經。

spinal cord they merge to form a mixed spinal nerve on each side.

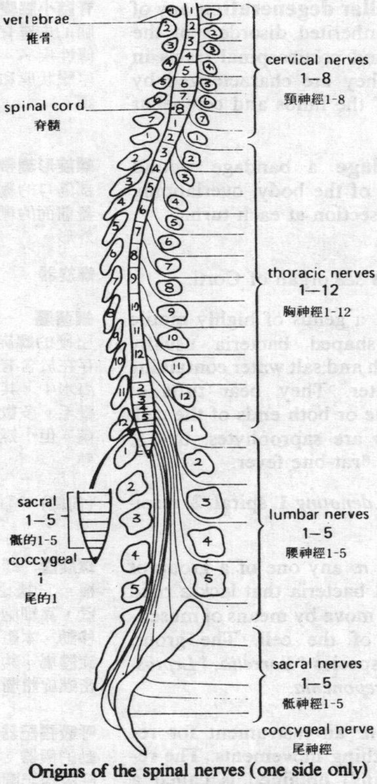

Origins of the spinal nerves (one side only)
脊髓神經起源（限於側面）

spindle *n.* a collection of fibres seen in a cell when it is dividing. The fibres radiate from the two ends (*poles*) and meet at the centre (the *equator*) giving a structure shaped like two cones placed base to base. It plays an important part in chromosome movement in *mitosis and *meiosis and is also involved in division of the cytoplasm.

梭，紡錘體　細胞分裂時細胞內細絲的集合體。從細胞兩端（極）輻射細絲，在中心集合（中緯線），形成兩個圓椎樣的結構，底對底排列。它們在有絲分裂和減數分裂的染色體運動中起重要作用，且亦涉及胞漿的分裂。

spine *n.* **1.** a sharp process of a bone. **2.** the vertebral column (*see* backbone). —**spinal** *adj.*

①**棘**　骨的尖銳突出部分。②**脊柱**

spino- *prefix denoting* **1.** the spine. **2.** the spinal cord.

〔前綴〕 ①**棘** ②**脊柱**

spinocerebellar degeneration any of a group of inherited disorders of the cerebellum and corticospinal tracts in the brain. They are characterized by *spasticity of the limbs and cerebellar *ataxia.

脊髓小腦變性 小腦和大腦的皮層脊髓束的一組遺傳性疾病。其特點爲肢體痙攣狀態和小腦性共濟失調。

spiral bandage a bandage wound round a part of the body, overlapping the previous section at each turn.

螺旋形繃帶 繞在身體某部傷口的繃帶，每圈均疊蓋前面的繃帶而呈螺旋狀外形。

spiral organ *see* organ of Corti.

螺旋器

Spirillum *n.* a genus of highly motile rigid spiral-shaped bacteria usually found in fresh and salt water containing organic matter. They bear tufts of flagella at one or both ends of the cell. Most species are saprophytes, but *S. minus* causes *rat-bite fever.

螺菌屬 一種活動力强、堅硬的螺旋形細菌。通常存在於含有有機物的新鮮海水中。其一端或兩端有鞭毛。多數係腐〔物寄〕生菌。但小螺菌能引起鼠咬熱。

spiro- *prefix denoting* **1.** spiral. **2.** respiration.

〔前綴〕 ①**螺旋** ②**呼吸**

spirochaete *n.* any one of a group of spiral-shaped bacteria that lack a rigid cell wall and move by means of muscular flexions of the cell. The group includes the species **Borrelia*, **Leptospira*, and **Treponema*.

螺旋體 螺旋形細菌的一種。它缺乏堅硬的細胞壁，靠細胞的肌性屈曲而移動。本組包括包柔氏螺旋體屬、鈎端螺旋體屬和密螺旋體屬。

spirograph *n.* an instrument for recording breathing movements. The record (a tracing) obtained is called a *spirogram*. —**spirography** *n.*

呼吸描記器 記錄呼吸運動的儀器。記錄的圖形稱呼吸描記圖。

spirometer *n.* an instrument for measuring the volume of air inhaled and exhaled. It is used in tests of *ventilation. —**spirometry** *n.*

肺量計 測量吸入和呼出空氣體積的儀器。用於肺換氣試驗。

spironolactone *n.* a synthetic *corticosteroid that inhibits the activity of the hormone *aldosterone and is used to treat heart failure, high blood pressure, and fluid retention (oedema). It is administered by mouth; side-effects may include headache, stomach upsets,

螺旋內酯 一種合成的皮質類固醇，能抑制醛固酮激素的活性，用於治療心力衰竭、高血壓和液體豬留（水腫）。口服。副作用可有頭痛、胃不適、倦眠。

and drowsiness. Trade name: **Aldactone**.

Spitz-Holter valve a one-way valve used to drain cerebrospinal fluid in order to control *hydrocephalus. The device is inserted into the ventricles of the brain and passes via a subcutaneous tunnel to drain into the right atrium.

斯皮茨-荷爾特氏瓣 一種單向開放的瓣，用於引流腦脊液以控制腦水腫。此裝置可插入腦室內，從皮下將腦脊液引流至右心房。

splanch- (splanchno-) *prefix denoting* the viscera.

〔前綴〕 **內臟**

splanchnic *adj.* relating to the viscera, e.g. splanchnic *mesoderm. *Compare* somatic (def. 2).

內臟的 與內臟有關的。例如臟壁中胚層。

splanchnic nerves the series of nerves in the sympathetic system that are distributed to the blood vessels and viscera, passing forwards and downwards from the chain of sympathetic ganglia near the spinal cord to enter the abdomen and branch profusely.

內臟神經 交感神經系統的一組神經，起始於靠近脊柱的交感神經節鏈，向前向下走行進入腹腔，發出大量分支，分佈於血管和內臟。

splanchnocranium *n.* the part of the skull that is derived from the *pharyngeal arches, i.e. the mandible (lower jaw).

臟顱 頭顱的一部分，由腮弓衍化而來，例如下頜骨。

splanchnopleure *n.* the wall of the embryonic gut, which consists of a layer of endoderm with a layer of mesoderm outside it. The yolk sac is a continuation of this structure. *Compare* somatopleure.

胚臟壁 胚腸的壁，由一層內胚層和外面的一層中胚層構成。卵黃囊即是胚臟壁的延續。

spleen *n.* a large dark-red ovoid organ situated on the left side of the body below and behind the stomach. It is enclosed within a fibrous capsule that extends into the spongy interior – the *splenic pulp* – to form a supportive framework. The pulp consists of aggregates of *lymphoid tissue (*white pulp*) within a meshwork of *reticular fibres packed with red blood cells (*red pulp*). The spleen is a major component of the *reticuloendothelial system, producing lymphocytes in the newborn and containing *phagocytes, which remove worn-out red blood cells and other

脾 大的暗紅色橢圓形器官，位於身體左側，胃的下後方。脾外包纖維囊，囊向疏鬆的內部即脾髓內延伸，形成支持網絡。脾髓由聚集成堆的淋巴樣組織（白髓）構成，淋巴組織周圍是網狀纖維網架，網眼中含有紅細胞（紅髓）。脾是網狀內皮系統的主要組成部分，在新生兒時能生成淋巴細胞，並含有吞噬細胞，後者能清除血流中的衰老紅細胞和其他異物。脾還是血液的

foreign bodies from the bloodstream. It also acts as a reservoir for blood and, in the fetus, as a source of red blood cells. Anatomical name: **lien**. —**splenic** *adj.*

貯存庫，在胚胎期是造紅細胞器官。

splen- (spleno-) *prefix denoting* the spleen. Example: *splenorenal* (relating to the spleen and kidney).

〔前綴〕 **脾** 例如脾腎的（與脾和腎有關的）。

splenectomy *n.* surgical removal of the spleen. This is sometimes necessary in the emergency treatment of bleeding from a ruptured spleen and in the treatment of some blood diseases.

脾切除術 手術切除脾。當脾破裂造成出血時，脾切除有時是必需的急救治療方法。亦用於治療某些血液病。

splenitis *n.* inflammation of the spleen. *See also* perisplenitis.

脾炎 脾的炎症。

splenium *n.* the thickest part of the *corpus callosum, rounded and protruding backwards over the thalami, the pineal body, and the midbrain.

壓部 胼胝體的最厚部，圓形，向後跨越丘腦、松果體和中腦。

splenomegaly *n.* enlargement of the spleen. It commonly occurs in *malaria, *schistosomiasis, and other disorders caused by parasites; in infections; in blood disorders, including some forms of anaemia and lack of platelets (*thrombocytopenia); in *leukaemia; and in *Hodgkin's disease. *See also* hypersplenism.

脾大 脾增大。常發生於瘧疾、血吸蟲病及其他一些寄生蟲病、傳染病、血液病（包括某些類型的貧血、血小板減少症、白血病及何傑金氏病）。

splenorenal anastomosis a method of treating *portal hypertension by joining the splenic vein to the left renal vein. *Compare* portacaval anastomosis.

脾腎靜脉吻合術 通過吻合脾靜脉和左腎靜脉治療門脉高壓症的方法。

splint *n.* a rigid support to hold broken bones in position until healing has occurred.

夾板 骨折時使用的硬性支托物，用以保持斷骨的正常位置直到痊癒。

spondyl- (spondylo-) *prefix denoting* a vertebra or the spine.

〔前綴〕 **脊椎，脊柱**

spondylitis *n.* inflammation of the synovial joints of the backbone. *Ankylosing spondylitis* is a rheumatic disease involving the backbone and sacroiliac joints (*see* sacroiliitis) and sometimes also causing arthritis in the shoulder and hip. The resultant pain and stiff-

脊椎炎 脊柱滑膜關節的炎症。强直性脊椎炎是一種風濕性疾病，侵犯脊柱、骶髂關節，有時還引起肩關節或髖關節炎症。脊柱疼痛和僵硬可用鎮痛藥和每日規律的鍛煉治

ness of the backbone are treated by analgesics and regular daily exercises. In severe cases the spine becomes completely rigid, through fusion of its joints, and *kyphosis results. *See also* ankylosis.

療。在嚴重病例脊柱可因脊柱關節融合而完全强直，結果造成脊柱後凸。

spondylolisthesis *n.* a forward shift of one vertebra upon another, due to a defect of the joints that normally bind them together. This may be congenital or develop after injury. The majority of cases in which pain is present are treated with rest and a surgical belt or corset; in a small minority, showing severe disability or pressure on nerve roots, surgical fusion may be required.

脊椎前移 脊椎逐個向前移位，係由於正常時連結脊椎的關節的缺陷所致。可爲先天性，也可發生於外傷後。大多數出現疼痛的病例可採取休息、外科束帶或背心治療。少數嚴重殘疾或神經根受壓者可能需要作關節融合手術。

spondylosis *n.* degeneration of the intervertebral discs in the cervical, thoracic, or lumbar regions of the backbone. Symptoms include pain and restriction of movement. Spondylosis produces a characteristic appearance on X-ray, including narrowing of the space occupied by the disc and the presence of *osteophytes; these features of the disease (*radiological spondylosis*) may not be accompanied by any signs and symptoms. Pain is relieved by wearing a collar (when the neck region is affected) or a surgical belt (for the lower spine), which prevents movement. Very severe cases sometimes require surgical fusion.

脊椎關節强直 脊柱頸椎、胸椎或腰椎部椎間盤變性。症狀有疼痛和運動受限。脊椎關節强直在X線檢查時呈現典型的表現：椎間盤所佔的空間變窄以及存在骨贅。這些X線所見（放射學所見的脊椎關節强直）也可不伴有任何症狀和體徵。戴領圈（頸椎受累時）或外科束帶（下位脊椎受累時）限制運動可減輕疼痛。十分嚴重的病例有時需作融合手術。

spondylosyndesis *n.* surgical fusion of the intervertebral joints of the backbone.

脊柱制動術 脊柱椎間關節的外科融合手術。

spongioblast *n.* a type of cell that forms in the early stages of development of the nervous system, giving rise to *astrocytes and *oligodendrocytes.

成膠質細胞 神經系統發育早期形成的一類細胞，以後轉化爲星形膠質細胞和少突膠質細胞。

spongioblastoma *n. see* glioblastoma.

成膠質細胞瘤

spontaneous *adj.* arising without apparent cause or outside aid. The term is applied in medicine to certain conditions, such as pathological fractures,

自發的，特發的 無明顯原因或外來因素而發生的。此詞在醫學中用於下列情況：無外傷而發生的

that arise in the absence of outside injury; also to recovery from a disease without the aid of specific treatment.

病理性骨折，疾病不經特殊治療而痊癒。

sporadic *adj.* describing a disease that occurs only occasionally or in a few isolated places. *Compare* endemic, epidemic.

散發的 指偶爾發生，或只在少數分散地區發生的疾病。

spore *n.* a small reproductive body produced by plants and microorganisms. Some kinds of spores function as dormant stages of the life cycle, enabling the organism to survive adverse conditions. Other spores are the means by which the organism can spread vegetatively. *See also* endospore.

孢子，芽胞 植物和微生物產生的一種有繁殖能力的小體。有些類型的孢子是生活週期中的休眠狀態，以使機體能在逆境中生存。另一些孢子則是機體營無性繁殖的手段。

sporicide *n.* an agent that kills spores (e.g. bacterial spores). Some disinfectants that liberate chlorine are sporicides, but most germicides are ineffective since spores are very resistant to chemical action. —**sporicidal** *adj.*

殺孢子劑 能殺死孢子（如細菌芽孢）的藥劑。某些能釋放氯的消毒劑屬於殺孢子劑，但大多數殺蟲劑不能殺死孢子，因爲孢子對化學作用有很强的抵抗力。

sporocyst *n.* the second-stage larva of a parasitic *fluke, found within the tissues of a freshwater snail. A sporocyst develops from a first stage larva (*see* miracidium) and gives rise either to the next larval stage (*see* redia) or daughter sporocysts. The latter develop directly into the final larval stage (*see* cercaria) without the intermediate redia stage.

包蚴 寄生性吸蟲的二期幼蟲，存在於淡水螺的組織內。包蚴由一期幼蟲發育而來，再發育爲雷蚴或子包蚴。子包蚴不經過中間的雷蚴期直接發育爲尾蚴。

sporogony *n.* the formation of *sporozoites during the life cycle of a sporozoan. The contents of the zygote, formed by the fusion of sex cells, divide repeatedly and eventually release a number of sporozoites. *Compare* schizogony.

孢子生殖 孢子蟲生活週期中形成子孢子的過程。由性細胞融合而成的合子反覆分裂，最後釋出許多子孢子。

sporotrichosis *n.* a chronic infection of the skin and superficial lymph nodes that is caused by the fungus *Sporotrichum schenckii* and results in the formation of abscesses and ulcers.

孢子絲菌病 一種皮膚和淺表淋巴結慢性炎症，由申克孢子絲菌引起，導至膿腫和潰瘍形成。

Sporozoa *n.* a group of parasitic Protozoa that includes **Plasmodium*, the

孢子蟲綱 一類寄生性原生動物，其中包括瘧原蟲

malaria parasite. Most sporozoans do not have cilia or flagella. Sporozoan life cycles are complex and usually involve both sexual and asexual stages. Some sporozoans are parasites of invertebrates, and the parasites are passed to new hosts by means of spores. Sporozoans that parasitize vertebrates are transmitted from host to host by invertebrates, which act as intermediate hosts. For example, the mosquito *Anopheles* is the intermediate host of *Plasmodium*.

——引起瘧疾的寄生蟲。多數孢子蟲無纖毛或鞭毛。孢子蟲的生活周期很複雜，通常既有有性繁殖期，也有無性繁殖期。有些孢子蟲寄生於無脊椎動物，以孢子形式進入新宿主。寄生於脊椎動物的孢子蟲則以無脊椎動物爲中間宿主而傳播。例如，按蚊是瘧原蟲的中間宿主。

sporozoite *n.* one of the many cells formed as a result of *sporogony during the life cyle of a sporozoan. In **Plasmodium* sporozoites are formed by repeated divisions of the contents of the *oocyst inside the body of the mosquito. The released sporozoites ultimately pass into the insect's salivary glands and await transmission to a human host at the next blood meal.

子孢子 在孢子蟲生活周期中行孢子生殖而形成的許多細胞。在蚊蟲體內，卵囊的內容物反覆分裂，形成瘧原蟲子孢子。釋出的子孢子最後進入蚊子的唾液腺，等待下一次吸血時傳入人類宿主。

spotted fever *see* cerebrospinal fever, Rocky Mountain spotted fever, typhus.

斑疹熱

sprain *n.* injury to a ligament, caused by sudden overstretching. As the ligament is not severed it gradually heals, but this may take several months. Sprains should be treated by cold compresses (ice-packs) at the time of injury, and later by restriction of activity.

扭傷 由於突然過度伸展所致的韌帶損傷。因韌帶沒有斷裂，可逐漸痊癒，但須歷時數月。治療：損傷當時用冷敷（冰袋），以後要限制活動。

Sprengel's deformity a congenital abnormality of the scapula (shoulder blade), which is small and positioned high in the shoulder. It is caused by failure of the normal development of this bone.

施普倫格氏畸形 一種先天性肩胛骨異常，表現爲肩胛骨小而高位。係肩胛骨不能正常發育所致。

sprue (psilosis) *n.* deficient absorption of food due to disease of the small intestine. *Tropical sprue* is seen in people from temperate regions who stay in tropical climates for weeks or months. It is characterized by diarrhoea (usually *steatorrhoea), inflamed tongue (glossitis), anaemia, and weight loss; the lining of the small intestine is inflamed

口炎性腹瀉 小腸疾病所致的食物吸收障礙。熱帶性口炎性腹瀉見於從溫帶地區來到熱帶數週或數月的人。其特徵爲：腹瀉（通常爲脂肪痢）、舌炎、貧血和體重下降，小腸黏膜因感染而發炎並萎縮。用抗生素和葉酸治療

and atrophied, probably because of infection. Treatment with antibiotics and *folic acid is usually effective, but the condition often improves spontaneously on return to a temperate climate. *See also* coeliac disease (nontropical sprue), malabsorption.

通常有效，病人返回溫帶後病情常自然改善。

spud *n.* a blunt needle used for removing foreign bodies embedded in the cornea of the eye.

眼科鏟 用於去除埋入眼角膜內的異物的鈍頭針。

spur *n.* a sharp projection, especially one of bone.

刺 尖鋭的突起，尤指骨上的骨刺。

sputum *n.* saliva mixed with mucus coughed up from the respiratory tract. A sputum-productive cough occurs in many conditions in which examination of the sputum for microorganisms, cells, and other substances may help diagnosis.

痰 唾液與呼吸道咳出的黏液的混合物。許多疾病時有咳嗽帶痰，此時檢查痰內微生物、細胞和其他物質有助於診斷。

squalene *n.* an unsaturated hydrocarbon (a terpene), synthesized in the body, from which *cholesterol is derived.

角鯊烯 一種體內合成的不飽和烴（萜烯），由之衍生膽固醇。

squama *n.* (*pl.* **squamae**) **1.** a thin plate of bone. **2.** a scale, such as any of the scales from the cornified layer of the *epidermis.

鱗 ①薄的骨片。 ②鱗屑，如來自表皮角質層的任何一種鱗屑。

squamo- *prefix denoting* **1.** the squamous portion of the temporal bone. **2.** squamous epithelium.

〔前綴〕 ①**顳骨鱗部** ②**鱗狀上皮**

squamous bone *see* temporal bone.

顳骨鱗部

squamous epithelium *see* epithelium.

鱗狀上皮

squint *n.* *see* strabismus.

斜視

stadium *n.* a stage in the course of a disease; for example, the *stadium invasioni* is the period between exposure to infection and the onset of symptoms.

期 疾病過程中的一個階段。例如，侵襲期指從接觸感染到症狀出現的一段時間。

stage *vb.* (in oncology) to determine the presence and site of metastases from a primary tumour in order to plan treatment. In addition to clinical examination, a variety of imaging and surgi-

分期 （腫瘤學）確定原發腫瘤是否有轉移及轉移的部位，以便制訂治療計劃。除進行臨床檢查外，還可採取各種照影和外科

cal techniques may be employed to provide a more accurate assessment.

技術以提供更爲精確的評價。

stagnant loop syndrome a condition in which a segment of the small intestine (e.g. a jejunal *diverticulum) is out of continuity with the rest of the intestine or in which progress of contents through the small intestine is delayed by an obstruction (such as a *stricture or *Crohn's disease) that allows an overgrowth of bacteria, causing *malabsorption and the passing of fatty stools (*see* steatorrhoea).

腸襻鬱滯綜合徵 一段小腸（如空腸憩室）不與小腸其餘部分通連的狀況，或者由於梗阻（如腸狹窄或克羅恩氏病）腸內容物通過小腸遲緩的狀況，其結果引起腸內細菌大量繁殖、吸收障礙和脂肪便。

stain 1. *n.* a dye used to colour tissues and other specimens for microscopical examination. In an *acid stain* the colour is carried by an acid radical and the stain is taken up by parts of the specimen having a basic (alkaline) reaction. In a *basic stain* the colour, carried by a basic radical, is attracted to parts of the specimen having an acidic reaction. *Neutral stains* have neither acidic nor basic affinities. A *contrast stain* is used to give colour to parts of a tissue not affected by a previously applied stain. A *differential stain* allows different elements in a specimen to be distinguished by staining them in different colours. **2.** *vb.* to treat a specimen for microscopical study with a stain.

①**染劑** 用於使組織和其他標本染色以進行顯微鏡檢查的染料。酸性染劑的酸基帶色，染色時標本上呈鹼性反應的部分着色。鹼性染劑的鹼基帶色，染色時標本上呈酸性反應的部分着色。中性染劑對酸性或鹼性均無親和性。此染劑用以使對先前使用的染劑不着色的部分着色。鑑別染劑可使標本的不同成分染成不同顏色以助辨認。②**染色** 用染劑處理標本以進行顯微鏡觀察。

stammering (stuttering) *n.* halting articulation with interruptions to the normal flow of speech and repetition of the initial consonants of words or syllables. It usually first appears in childhood and the symptoms are most severe when the stammerer is under any psychological stress. It is not a symptom of organic disease and it will usually respond to the re-education of speech by a trained therapist. Medical name: **dysphemia**. —**stammerer** *n.*

口吃 表現爲正常說話流暢性中斷的發音停頓，並重復開始的輔音或音節。通常始於兒童期，當口吃者處於心理緊張時表現最爲嚴重。口吃不是器質性疾病的症狀，由受過訓練的治療人員進行語言再教育，常能有所改善。

standard deviation (in statistics) a measure of the scatter of observations about their arithmetic *mean, which is calculated from the square root of the *variance* of the readings in the series.

標準差 （統計學）表示一組觀察的算術平均值的離散度的量度，由該組讀數的方差平方根求得。各觀察值與平均值的差之算

The arithmetic sum of the amounts by which each observation varies from the mean must be zero, but if these variations are squared before being summated, a positive value is obtained: the mean of this value is the variance. In practice a more reliable estimate of variance is obtained by dividing the sum of the squared deviations by one *less* than the total number of observations. *See also* significance.

術總和應爲零，但若將這些差乘平方後再相加，則得到一個正數，此數值的平均值即爲方差。事實上，求方差的較可靠的計算方法是：將離差平方之和除以觀察總數減一。

standard error (of a *mean) the extent to which the means of several different samples would vary if they were taken repeatedly from the same population. Differences between means are said to have statistical *significance when they are greater than twice the standard error of those means, since the probability of this difference or a larger one occurring by chance is less than 5%.

標準誤 從同一羣體反覆取樣時，幾個不同樣本平均值變異的範圍。當平均值之間的差別大於兩個以上標準誤時，稱爲有統計學顯著性，因爲這一差別的概率，或者說更大概率出現的機會，小於5%。

stanolone *n.* a synthetic male sex hormone with *anabolic activity, used to treat wasting diseases, such as osteoporosis and anorexia, and breast cancer. It is administered by mouth. Trade name: **Anabolex.**

雙氫睪酮 一種合成的雄性激素，有同化活性，用於治療消耗性疾病如骨質疏鬆症、厭食症和乳腺癌。口服。

St Anthony's fire a popular name for inflammation of the skin associated with ergot poisoning. *See* ergotism.

聖安東尼熱 麥角中毒時伴發的皮膚炎的俗稱。

stapedectomy *n.* surgical removal of the third ear ossicle (stapes): part of the treatment for deafness due to *otosclerosis.

鐙骨切除術 手術切除第三塊聽小骨——鐙骨，爲治療耳硬化症致聾的方法之一。

stapes *n.* a stirrup-shaped bone in the middle *ear that articulates with the incus and is attached to the membrane of the fenestra ovalis. *See* ossicle.

鐙骨 中耳內的一塊馬鐙形小骨，與砧骨相連接，貼附在前庭卵圓窗的膜上。

staphylectomy *n.* surgical removal of the uvula (the back of the soft palate).

懸壅垂切除術 手術切除懸壅垂（軟腭後部）。

Staphylococcus *n.* a genus of Gram-positive nonmotile spherical bacteria occurring in grapelike clusters. Some species are saprophytes; others parasites. Many species produce *exotoxins. The species *S. aureus* is commonly

葡萄球菌屬 一屬不具運動能力的革蘭氏陽性球形菌，以葡萄串狀出現。某些種爲腐物寄生菌，其餘爲一般寄生菌。許多種產生外毒素。金黃色葡萄球

present on skin and mucous membranes; it causes boils and internal abscesses. *S. pyogenes albus* and *S. pyogenes aureus* are associated with most suppurative infections. Other species produce toxins causing *food poisoning.

菌普遍存在於皮膚和黏膜表面，可引起癤腫和體內膿腫。白色釀膿葡萄球菌和金黃色釀膿葡萄球菌與多數化膿性感染有關。還有一些葡萄球菌產生毒素，可引起食物中毒。

staphyloma *n.* abnormal bulging of the cornea or sclera (white) of the eye. *Anterior staphyloma* is a bulging scar in the cornea to which a part of the iris is attached. It is usually the site of a healed corneal ulcer that has penetrated right through the cornea; the iris blocks the hole and prevents the further leakage of fluid from the front chamber of the eye. In *ciliary staphyloma* the sclera bulges over the ciliary body as a result of high pressure inside the eyeball. A bulging of the sclera at the back of the eye (*posterior staphyloma*) occurs in some severe cases of short-sightedness.

葡萄腫 眼角膜和鞏膜（白眼珠）的異常膨出。前葡萄腫是角膜下膨出瘢痕，其下有虹膜部分黏着。該處通常曾發生過角膜潰瘍，但已痊癒。潰瘍導至角膜穿孔，而虹膜將穿孔堵塞，防止了眼前房液繼續外溢。睫狀體葡萄腫爲鞏膜在睫狀體部位向外膨出，是眼內壓過高的結果。眼球後部鞏膜膨出（後葡萄腫）發生於某些高度近視患者。

staphylorrhaphy (palatorrhaphy, uraniscorrhaphy) *n.* surgical suture of a cleft palate.

軟腭縫合術（腭裂縫合術，腭修補術） 手術縫合腭裂。

starch *n.* the form in which *carbohydrates are stored in many plants and a major constituent of the diet. Starch consists of linked glucose units and occurs in two forms, *α-amylose* and *amylopectin*. In *α-amylose* the units are in the form of a long unbranched chain; in amylopectin they form a branched chain. The presence of starch can be detected using iodine: α-amylose gives a blue colour with iodine; amylopectin a red colour. Starch is digested by means of the enzyme *amylase. *See also* dextrin.

澱粉 碳水化合物在許多植物中的儲藏形式，也是食物的主要組成成分。澱粉由葡萄糖單位連接而成，以兩種形態存在：α-直鏈澱粉和支鏈澱粉。在α-直鏈澱粉中葡萄糖單位形成一條不分支的長鏈，在支鏈澱粉中葡萄糖形成一條分支的鏈。澱粉的存在可用碘檢測：α-直鏈澱粉遇碘呈藍色，支鏈澱粉則呈紅色。澱粉可被澱粉酶消化。

Starling's law a law stating that a muscle, including the heart muscle, responds to increased stretching at rest by an increased force of contraction when stimulated.

斯塔林定律 定律闡明：肌肉（包括心肌）靜息時被拉得越長，受刺激時的收縮力越大。

starvation *n. see* malnutrition.

飢餓

stasis *n.* stagnation or cessation of flow; for example, of blood or lymph whose flow is obstructed or of the intestinal contents when onward movement (peristalsis) is hindered.

停滯 液體流動停滯或靜止，例如血流或淋巴流被阻塞稱血液停滯或淋巴停滯；腸內容物前進運動受阻（淤滯）也稱爲停滯。

-stasis *suffix denoting* stoppage of a flow of liquid; stagnation. Example: *haemostasis* (of blood).

〔後綴〕 **停滯** 液體流動停止，例如血流停滯。

static reflex the reflex maintenance of muscular tone for posture.

靜位反射 爲保持姿勢而維持肌緊張的反射。

status asthmaticus an attack of *asthma lasting for more than 24 hours. This causes great distress and there is a risk of death from respiratory failure or exhaustion. Treatment with corticosteroid drugs may be life-saving and artificial respiration may be needed. Sedation is risky, and these cases require skilled care.

氣喘持續狀態 持續24小時以上的氣喘發作。此狀態引起巨大痛苦，並有因呼吸衰竭或耗竭導至死亡的危險。用皮質固醇類藥物治療可挽救生命，也可能需作人工呼吸。用鎭靜藥有危險性，此時須熟練的醫護。

status epilepticus the occurrence of repeated epileptic fits without any recovery of consciousness between them. Its control is a medical emergency, since prolonged status epilepticus causes a serious imbalance of the salts (electrolytes) in the body, which may lead to the patient's death. During each fit, the breathing is arrested and the body is deprived of oxygen, resulting in further damage to the brain cells.

癲癇持續狀態 反覆的癲癇發作，發作之間意識不恢復。需緊急治療予以控制，因爲癲癇持續狀態的拖延導至體內鹽類（電解質）平衡嚴重失調，從而可致病人死亡。每次發作時呼吸停止，機體得不到氧氣，進一步損傷腦細胞。

status lymphaticus enlargement of the thymus gland and other parts of the lymphatic system, formerly believed to be a predisposing cause to sudden death in infancy and childhood associated with hypersensitivity to drugs or vaccines.

淋巴體質 胸腺和其他淋巴器官增大，過去認爲是使兒童和嬰兒對藥物或疫苗敏感性過高而突然死亡的素質性原因。

steapsin *n. see* lipase.

胰脂酶

stearic acid *see* fatty acid.

脂肪酸

steat- (steato-) *prefix denoting* fat; fatty tissue.

〔前綴〕 **脂肪，脂肪組織**

steatoma *n. see* sebaceous cyst. The term is also used for any tumour of a sebaceous gland.

脂瘤 此名稱亦用於皮脂腺的各種腫瘤。

steatopygia *n.* the accumulation of large quantities of fat in the buttocks. In the Hottentots of Africa this is a normal condition, thought to be an adaptation that allows fat storage without impeding heat loss from the rest of the body.

臀脂過多 大量脂肪蓄積於臀部。此在非洲霍坦托特人爲正常現象，據認爲是一種適應性表現，脂肪蓄積於臀部可避免影響身體其他部分的散熱作用。

steatorrhoea *n.* the passage of abnormally increased amounts of fat in the faeces (more than 5 g/day) due to reduced absorption of fat by the intestine (*see* malabsorption). The faeces are pale, smell offensive, may look greasy, and are difficult to flush away.

脂肪痢 隨糞便排出的脂肪量異常增多（每日超過5克），係由於小腸吸收脂肪減少所致。大便色灰白，有臭味，外觀可以似油脂，難以沖洗乾淨。

stellate fracture a star-shaped fracture of the kneecap caused by a direct blow. The bone may be either split or severely shattered; if the fragments are displaced, the bone may need to be surgically removed (*patellectomy*).

星形骨折 直接撞擊所致的髕骨呈星形的骨折。髕骨可裂開或嚴重碎裂。如果碎骨片已移位，可能需行外科手術除去髕骨（髕骨切除術）。

stellate ganglion a star-shaped collection of sympathetic nerve cell bodies in the root of the neck, from which sympathetic nerve fibres are distributed to the face and neck and to the blood vessels and organs of the thorax.

星形神經節 頸根部交感神經細胞胞體聚集呈星形集團。從此處發出的交感神經纖維分佈於面、頸部、胸腔的血管和器官。

Stellwag's sign apparent widening of the distance between the upper and lower eyelids (the palpebral fissure) due to retraction of the upper lid and protrusion of the eyeball. It is a sign of exophthalmic *goitre.

施特爾瓦格氏徵 上瞼與下瞼間的距離（瞼裂）明顯增大，係上瞼退縮和眼球突出所致。爲突眼性甲狀腺腫的體徵。

steno- *prefix denoting* **1.** narrow. Example: *stenocephaly* (narrowness of the head). **2.** constricted.

〔前綴〕 ①**狹窄** 例如頭狹窄。 ②**收縮的**

stenopaeic *adj.* (in ophthalmology) describing an optical device consisting of an opaque disc punctured with a fine slit or hole (or holes), which is placed in front of the eye in the same position as glasses and enables sharper vision in cases of gross long- or short-sightedness or astigmatism. It reduces distortion in the image formed on the retina because it confines the light reaching the eye to

裂隙的 （眼科學）描述一種由一個其中開有一小裂縫或（一或多個）小孔的不透明圓盤構成的光學裝置。在高度遠視、近視或散光情況下，將此裝置置於眼前戴眼鏡的位置，可增加視力。它將進入眼的光線約束成爲一或幾條細束，從而使視網膜上成

one or more fine beams. The same principle is used in the pin-hole camera.

像的畸變減少。針孔攝影機亦爲同一原理。

stenosis *n.* the abnormal narrowing of a passage or opening, such as a blood vessel or heart valve. *See* aortic, mitral, pulmonary, and pyloric stenosis.

狹窄 通路或開口（如血管和心瓣膜）的異常狹窄。

stenostomia (stenostomy) *n.* the abnormal narrowing of an opening, such as the opening of the bile duct.

口狹窄 開口（如膽道口）的異常狹窄。

Stensen's duct the long secretory duct of the *parotid salivary gland.

斯坦森氏管 腮腺的長分泌導管。

stent *n.* a splint left inside the lumen of a duct at operation to aid healing of an anastomosis by draining the contents away. *J-stents* or *double J-stents* are those with a 'pig-tail' curve on one or both ends of the splint to prevent extrusion. Stents are increasingly used in the ureter to overcome obstruction by draining the renal pelvis into the bladder.

引流條 手術時置於導管腔內的條狀物，用以將內容物引流出來以促進吻合部癒合。J形或雙J形引流條爲一端或兩端呈"猪尾"樣彎曲的引流條，以防脫出。引流條常放置於輸尿管內將尿液自腎盂引流入膀胱以克服阻塞。

sterco- *prefix denoting* faeces.

〔前綴〕 **糞**

stercobilin *n.* a brownish-red pigment formed during the metabolism of the *bile pigments biliverdin and bilirubin, which are derived from haemoglobin. Stercobilin is subsequently excreted in the urine or faeces.

糞膽素 在血紅蛋白衍生的膽色素（膽綠素和膽紅素）代謝中生成的棕紅色色素。糞膽素從尿和糞中排出。

stercolith *n.* a stone formed of dried compressed faeces.

糞石 糞便乾縮形成的結石。

stercoraceous *adj.* composed of or containing faeces.

糞的 由糞組成的或含糞的。

stereognosis *n.* the ability to recognize the three-dimensional shape of an object by touch alone. This is a function of the *association areas of the parietal lobe of the brain. *See also* agnosia.

實體覺 僅靠觸覺辨認物體的三維形狀的能力。爲大腦頂葉聯絡區的一種功能。

stereoisomers *n.* compounds having the same molecular formula but different three-dimensional arrangements of their atoms. The atomic structures of stereoisomers are mirror images of each other.

立體異構體 分子式相同但原子三維結構不同的化合物。立體異構體的原子結構互呈鏡像對應。

stereoscopic vision perception of the shape, depth, and distance of an object as a result of having *binocular vision. The brain receives two distinct images from the eyes, which it interprets as a single three-dimensional image.

立體視覺 由雙眼視覺產生的對物體的形狀、厚度和距離的知覺。大腦從兩眼獲得兩個不同的映像並使之轉化爲單一的三維像。

stereotaxy *n.* a relatively recent surgical procedure in which a deep-seated area in the brain is operated upon after its position has been established very accurately by three-dimensional measurements. The operation may be performed using an electrical current or by heat, cold, or mechanical techniques. *See also* leucotomy.

立體定位法 一種較新的外科操作，係通過三維測量精確定位後施行大腦深在區域的手術。手術可用電流、高熱、冷凍或機械方法進行。

stereotypy *n.* the constant repetition of a complex action, which is carried out in the same way each time. It is seen in *catatonia and infantile *autism; sometimes it is an isolated symptom in mental *subnormality. It is more common in patients who live in institutions where they are bored and unstimulated. It can prevent a patient from carrying on normal life, and sometimes causes physical injury to the patient. Drugs, such as *phenothiazines, and behaviour therapy are sometimes used in treating the condition.

刻板症 每次都按同一方式重複完成一組動作。見於緊張症和幼兒孤獨症病人，有時爲精神低常的一個獨立症狀，更常發生於生活在單調乏味環境中的病人。刻板症可使病人不能正常生活，有時可導至身體受傷。治療用吩噻嗪之類的藥物，有時可用行爲療法。

sterile *adj.* **1.** (of a living organism) barren; unable to reproduce its kind (*see* sterility). **2.** (of inanimate objects) completely free from bacteria, fungi, viruses, or other microorganisms that could cause infection.

①（用於活的有機體）**不育的，不能繁殖的** ②（用於無生命物體）**完全無菌的**（無眞菌、病毒或其他能引起感染的微生物）

sterility *n.* inability to have children, due either to *infertility or (in someone who has been fertile) to a surgical operation (*see* sterilization). Sterility may be an incidental result of an operation done for other reasons, such as removal of the womb (*hysterectomy) for cancer.

不育 因不育症或對曾有生育力者施行外科手術所致的不能生育的狀態。不育也可能是因其他原因做手術（如因癌切除子宮）產生的後果。

sterilization *n.* **1.** a surgical operation or any other process that induces *sterility in men or women; for example, by cutting the vasa deferentia in men (*see*

①**絕育** 造成男性或女性不育的外科手術或其他方法。如切斷男性輸精管或女性輸卵管或閹割。 ②

vasectomy) and the Fallopian tubes in women (*see* salpingectomy) or by *castration. **2.** any means of rendering objects, wounds, etc., free of bacteria that would otherwise cause disease. Surgical instruments and dressings can be sterilized by being subjected to steam in an *autoclave. *Disinfectants and *antiseptics are chemicals used to destroy bacteria.

消毒　消滅物體或傷口上的致病菌的手段。外科器械和敷料可置於高壓鍋內用蒸氣消毒。殺滅細菌的化學劑包括消毒劑和滅菌劑。

stern- (sterno-) *prefix denoting* the sternum. Example: *sternocostal* (relating to the sternum and ribs).

〔前綴〕 **胸骨**　例如胸肋的（與胸骨和肋骨有關的）。

sternebra *n.* (*pl.* **sternebrae**) one of the four parts that fuse during development to form the body of the sternum.

胸骨節　共4塊，在發育過程中融合而成胸骨體。

sternocleidomastoid muscle *see* sternomastoid muscle.

胸鎖乳突肌

sternohyoid *n.* a muscle in the neck, arising from the sternum and inserted into the hyoid bone. It depresses the hyoid bone.

胸骨舌骨肌　頸部一塊起自胸骨終於舌骨的肌肉。該肌使舌骨下降。

sternomastoid muscle (sternocleidomastoid muscle) a long muscle in the neck, extending from the mastoid process to the sternum and clavicle. It serves to rotate the neck and flex the head.

胸鎖乳突肌　頸部一條長肌，起自乳突，止於胸骨和鎖骨。其功能爲轉頸和屈頭。

sternomastoid tumour a small painless nonmalignant swelling in the lower half of the *sternomastoid muscle, appearing a few days after birth. It occurs when the neck of the fetus is in an abnormal position in the womb, which interferes with the blood supply to the affected muscle, and it is most common after breech births. The tumour may cause a slight tilt of the head towards the tumour and turning of the face to the other side. This can be corrected by physiotherapy aimed at increasing all movements of the body, but without stretching the neck.

胸鎖乳突肌腫瘤　位於胸鎖乳突肌下半部的無痛性良性小腫物，在生後數日出現。由於胎頸在子宮內姿勢異常，該肌的血液供應受影響所致，在臀位分娩後最爲常見。腫瘤可使頭部向患側輕度歪斜，而面部轉向健側。可用物理療法治療，即在不牽拉頸部的情況下增強全身運動。

sternotomy *n.* surgical division of the breastbone (sternum), performed to allow access to the heart and its major vessels.

胸骨切開術 手術切開胸骨以通向心臟及其大血管。

sternum *n.* (*pl.* **sterna**) the breastbone: a flat bone, 15–20 cm long, extending from the base of the neck to just below the diaphragm and forming the front part of the skeleton of the thorax. The sternum articulates with the collar bones (*see* clavicle) and the costal cartilages of the first seven pairs of ribs. It consists of three sections: the middle and longest section – the *body* or *gladiolus* – is attached to the *manubrium at the top and the *xiphoid (or ensiform) process at the bottom. The manubrium slopes back from the body so that the junction between the two parts forms an angle (*angle of Louis* or *sternal angle*). —**sternal** *adj.*

胸骨 一塊扁骨，長15～20cm，從頸根部起直到膈下，構成胸部骨骼的前部。胸骨與鎖骨及第1～7對肋骨相關節。胸骨由三部分組成：中間部分最長，爲胸骨體，上下與胸骨柄及劍突相連。胸骨柄從胸骨體向後傾斜，在兩部的連接處形成一個角（路易斯角或胸骨角）。

sternutator *n.* an agent that produces sneezing.

催嚏劑 引起噴嚏的藥物。

steroid *n.* one of a group of compounds having a common structure based on the *steroid nucleus*, which consists of three six-membered carbon rings and one five-membered carbon ring. The naturally occurring steroids include the male and female sex hormones (*androgens and *oestrogens), the hormones of the adrenal cortex (*see* corticosteroid), *progesterone, *bile salts, and *sterols. Synthetic steroids have been produced for therapeutic purposes.

類固醇，甾類 一族有同樣的甾體（由三個六碳環和一個五碳環組成）結構的化合物。天然的類固醇包括雄性和雌性激素（雄激素和雌激素類）、腎上腺皮質激素、孕酮、膽酸鹽和固醇。現已有合成的類固醇用於治療。

sterol *n.* one of a group of *steroid alcohols. The most important sterols are *cholesterol and *ergosterol.

固醇，甾醇 類固醇中的一類。最重要的有膽固醇和麥角固醇。

stertor *n.* a snoring type of noisy breathing heard in deeply unconscious patients.

鼾息 呼吸時發出鼾聲樣的噪音，見於深度昏迷的病人。

steth- (stetho-) *prefix denoting* the chest.

〔前綴〕 **胸**

stethograph *n.* an instrument for recording chest movements during breathing. —**stethography** *n.*

胸動描記器 記錄呼吸時胸廓運動的器械。

stethometer *n.* an instrument for measuring the expansion of the chest during breathing.

胸圍計 測量呼吸時胸廓擴張程度的器械。

stethoscope *n.* an instrument used for listening to sounds within the body, such as those in the heart and lungs (*see* auscultation). A simple stethoscope usually consists of a diaphragm or an open bell-shaped structure (which is applied to the body) connected by rubber or plastic tubes to shaped earpieces for the examiner. More complicated devices may contain electronic amplification systems to aid diagnosis.

聽診器 用以聽取體內聲音（例如心音和肺呼吸音）的器械。簡單的聽診器通常由一隔膜或開口的鐘形結構（用以接觸身體），通過兩條塑料管與耳件（接觸檢查者）連接而成。複雜的聽診裝置則可含有電子放大系統以助診斷。

sthenia *n.* a state of normal or greater than normal strength. *Compare* asthenia. —**sthenic** *adj.*

强壯 體力正常或超過體力正常的狀態。

stibophen *n.* a sodium-containing salt of antimony used to treat *schistosomiasis. It is administered by injection; side-effects may include digestive upsets, slow heart rate, and anaemia.

睇波芬 一種含鈉的銻鹽，用於治療血吸蟲病。注射。副作用有消化道不適、心率減慢和貧血。

stigma *n.* (*pl.* **stigmata**) **1.** a mark that characterizes a particular disease, such as the café-au-lait spots characteristic of neurofibromatosis. **2.** any spot or lesion on the skin.

斑 ①某種疾病特有的標記，如神經纖維瘤病特有的咖啡牛乳色斑。 ②皮膚的任何斑點或病損。

stilboestrol *n.* a synthetic female sex hormone (*see* oestrogen) used to relieve menstrual disorders and symptoms of the menopause, to treat prostate and breast cancer, and to suppress lactation. It is administered by mouth or injection; side-effects are those of other synthetic oestrogens.

己烯雌酚 一種合成的女性激素，用於減輕月經紊亂和經絕期症狀，治療前列腺癌和乳腺癌，以及抑制泌乳。口服或注射。副作用與其他合成雌激素相同。

stilet (stylet, stylus) *n.* **1.** a slender probe. **2.** a wire placed in the lumen of a catheter to give it rigidity while the instrument is passed along a body canal (such as the urethra).

①**細探子** 細的探針。 ②**通管絲** 置於導管腔內的金屬絲，當導管通過身體的管道（如尿道）時使導管具有一定硬度。

stillbirth *n.* birth of a fetus that shows no evidence of life (heart beat, respira-

死產 妊娠28周後任何時刻分娩的無生命特徵（心

tion, or independent movement) at any time later than 28 weeks after conception. The number of such births expressed per 1000 births (live and still) is known as the *stillbirth rate*. Viability is deemed to start at the 28th week of pregnancy and a fetus born dead before this time is known as an *abortion or miscarriage. There is no reason why a child born alive before the 28th week should not survive if properly nurtured, though the small size will greatly increase the risk of neonatal death (*see* infant mortality rate).

跳、呼吸或自主運動）的胎兒。每1000次分娩（活產加死產）中的死產數稱爲死產率。一般認爲妊娠28周起胎兒開始有生活能力。在此以前娩出的死胎稱爲流產。雖然胎兒小會大大增加新生兒死亡的危險；但是，妊娠28周前分娩的活胎，在合理營養的條件下並非不能存活。

Still's disease chronic arthritis developing in children before the age of 16. There are several different forms of arthritis affecting children, and some authorities confine the diagnosis of Still's disease to the following: a disease of childhood marked by arthritis (often involving several joints) with a swinging fever and a transitory red rash. There is often severe illness affecting the entire body and the condition may be complicated by enlargement of the spleen and lymph nodes and inflammation of the pericardium and iris.

斯提爾氏病 16歲前兒童發生的慢性關節炎。侵襲兒童的關節炎有幾種不同的類型，有些權威學者認爲符合以下情況可診斷斯提爾氏病：兒童期得病，以關節炎（經常侵犯幾處關節）爲特徵，伴有高熱和一過性紅色皮疹。本病爲全身性疾病，病情常嚴重，並可合併脾和淋巴結腫大、心包炎以及虹膜炎。

stimulant *n.* an agent that promotes the activity of a body system or function. *Amphetamine and *caffeine are stimulants of the central nervous system.

興奮劑 刺激身體系統和功能活動的藥物。苯丙胺和咖啡因均爲中樞神經系統興奮劑。

stimulus *n.* (*pl.* **stimuli**) any agent that provokes a response, or particular form of activity, in a cell, tissue, or other structure, which is said to be *sensitive* to that stimulus.

刺激物 任何能引起對該種刺激有感受性的細胞、組織或其他結構產生反應或特定形式活動的物質。

stippling *n.* a spotted or speckled appearance, such as is seen in the retina in certain eye diseases or in abnormal red blood cells stained with basic dyes.

點彩 一種斑狀或點狀的表現，可見於某些眼病時的視網膜或用鹼性染劑染色的異常紅細胞內。

stirrup *n.* (in anatomy) *see* stapes.

鐙骨

stitch *n.* **1.** a sharp localized pain, commonly in the abdomen, associated with strenuous physical activity (such as running), especially shortly after

①**刺痛** 局部的銳痛，一般發生於腹部，與緊張的體力活動（如跑步），尤其是飯後立即活動有關。

eating. It is a form of cramp. **2.** *see* suture.
爲痛性痙攣的一種類型。②縫線

stock culture *see* culture.
存儲培養

Stokes-Adams syndrome (Adams-Stokes syndrome) attacks of temporary loss of consciousness that occur when blood flow ceases due to ventricular *fibrillation or *asystole. This syndrome may complicate *heart block. It is treated by means of a battery-operated *pacemaker.
阿-斯綜合徵 突然發生的短暫的意識喪失，係由於室性纖顫或心搏停止引起血流停滯而發生。此綜合徵可併發於心傳導阻滯。治療用電起搏器。

stoma *n.* (*pl.* **stomata**) **1.** (in anatomy) the mouth or any mouthlike part. **2.** (in surgery) the artificial opening of a tube (e.g. the colon or ileum) that has been brought to the abdominal surface (*see* colostomy, ileostomy). *Stoma therapists* are nurses specially trained in the care of these artificial openings and the appliances used with them. —**stomal** *adj.*
口 ①（解剖學）開口或任何孔樣部分。 ②（外科學）植於腹壁表面的管道（如結腸或回腸）的人工開口。造口術治療員係指經過專門訓練，能對人工造口進行護理及運用工具進行操作的護士。

stomach *n.* a distensible saclike organ that forms part of the alimentary canal between the oesophagus (gullet) and the duodenum (see illustration). It communicates with the former by means of the *cardiac orifice* and with the latter by the *pyloric sphincter*.
胃 可擴張的囊袋狀器官，是消化道中食管和十二指腸之間的部分（見圖）。胃藉賁門與食管相接，藉幽門括約肌與十二指腸相連。

The stomach lies just below the diaphragm, to the right of the spleen and partly under the liver. Its function is to continue the process of digestion that begins in the mouth. *Gastric juice, secreted by gastric glands in the mucosa, contains hydrochloric acid and the enzyme *pepsin, which contribute to chemical digestion. This – together with the churning action of the muscular layers of the stomach – reduces the food to a semiliquid partly digested mass that passes on to the duodenum.
胃位於膈下，脾的右方，部分爲肝臟所覆蓋。其功能是繼續由口腔開始的消化過程。黏膜內的胃腺分泌胃液，其中含有鹽酸和胃蛋白酶，進行化學性消化。化學性消化加上胃肌層的攪拌作用，將食物變成部分消化的半流體狀物質，然後進入十二指腸。

stomachic *n.* an agent that stimulates the secretory activity of the stomach, used as a tonic to improve the appetite.
健胃藥 刺激胃分泌活動的藥物，用作促進食慾的強壯劑。

stomat- (stomato-) *prefix denoting* the mouth.
〔前綴〕 口腔

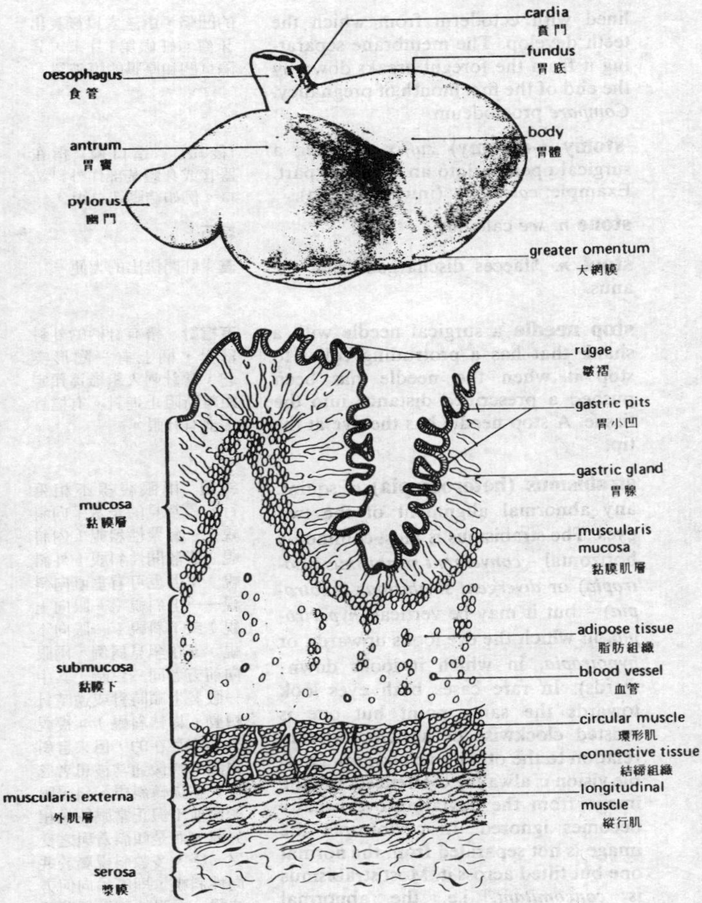

Regions of the stomach seen from the front (above); layers of the stomach wall (below)

胃的分區前面觀（上圖）；胃壁各層（下圖）

stomatitis *n.* inflammation of the mucous lining of the mouth.

口炎 口腔黏膜的炎症。

stomatology *n.* the branch of medicine concerned with diseases of the mouth.

口腔學 從事口腔疾病防治的醫學分支。

stomodeum *n.* the site of the embryonic mouth, marked by a depression

口凹 胚胎口腔所在的部位，表現爲被外胚層覆蓋

lined with ectoderm from which the teeth develop. The membrane separating it from the foregut breaks down by the end of the first month of pregnancy. *Compare* proctodeum.

的凹陷，由該處以後長出牙齒。妊娠第1月末，分隔口凹和原腸的膜破裂。

-stomy (-ostomy) *suffix denoting* a surgical opening into an organ or part. Example: *colostomy* (into the colon).

〔後綴〕 **造口術** 指在器官或身體某部作外科造口。例如結腸造口術。

stone *n. see* calculus.

結石

stool *n.* *faeces discharged from the anus.

糞 肛門排出的大便。

stop needle a surgical needle with a shank that has a protruding collar to stop it when the needle has been pushed a prescribed distance into the tissue. A stop needle has the eye at the tip.

有檔針 帶有針柄的外科縫針，柄上有一圈形突起，當針刺入組織達預定距離時阻止進針。有檔針尖部有針眼。

strabismus (heterotropia) *n.* squint: any abnormal alignment of the two eyes. The strabismus is most commonly horizontal – *convergent strabismus* (*esotropia*) or *divergent strabismus* (*exotropia*) – but it may be vertical (*hypertropia*, in which the eye looks upwards, or *hypotropia*, in which it looks downwards). In rare cases both eyes look towards the same point but one is twisted clockwise or anticlockwise in relation to the other (*cyclotropia*). Double vision is always experienced, but the image from the deviating eye usually becomes ignored. In cyclotropia the image is not separated from the normal one but tilted across it. Most strabismus is *concomitant*, i.e. the abnormal alignment of the two eyes remains fairly constant, in whatever direction the person is looking. This is usual with childhood squints. Strabismus acquired by injury or disease is usually *incomitant*, i.e. the degree of misalignment varies in different directions of gaze. *See also* cover test, heterophoria.

斜視 兩眼視線不相平行。最常見的是水平向斜視——會聚性斜視（內斜視）或散開性斜視（外斜視）；但也可有垂直向斜視——上斜視（一眼向上視）或下斜視（一眼向下視）。在罕見病例，兩眼向前方看同一點時，其中一眼發生順時針或逆時針轉動（旋轉斜視）。複視是必定存在的，但來自斜視眼的映像通常被患者忽視。在旋轉斜視，斜視眼的像並不與正常眼的像相分離，而是傾斜着與之交叉。絕大多數斜視屬於共同性斜視，即不論向何方注視，兩眼的不平行關係始終保持恒定。兒童期斜視通常是這種情況。由外傷或疾病造成的斜視則通常爲非共同性斜視，即隨着注視方向的不同，兩眼不平行的程度發生變化。

strain 1. *n.* excessive stretching or working of a muscle, resulting in pain

①**勞損** 肌肉因過度牽伸或作功而發生疼痛和腫

and swelling of the muscle. *Compare* sprain. **2.** *n.* a group of organisms, such as bacteria, obtained from a particular source or having special properties distinguishing them from other members of the same species. **3.** *vb.* to damage a muscle by overstretching.

脹。②**株** 得自一個特定來源或具有與同一種屬其他成員不同的特性的一羣有機體，如細菌株。③作動詞用時指因過度牽伸而損傷肌肉。

strangulated *adj.* describing a part of the body whose blood supply has been interrupted by compression of a blood vessel, as may occur in a loop of intestine trapped in a *hernia.

絞窄的 描述身體某部分因血管受壓致血液供應中斷的狀況，如小腸嵌入疝內可造成絞窄。

strangulation *n.* the closure of a passage, such as the main airway to the lungs (resulting in the cessation of breathing), a blood vessel, or the gastrointestinal tract.

絞窄 通路的關閉，如通向肺的主要氣道的絞窄（導至呼吸停止），血管或胃腸道的絞窄。

strangury *n.* severe pain in the urethra referred from the base of the bladder and associated with an intense desire to pass urine. It occurs when the base of the bladder is irritated by a stone or an indwelling catheter. It is also noted in patients with an invasive cancer of the base of the bladder or severe *cystitis or *prostatitis, when the strong desire to urinate is accompanied by the painful passage of a few drops of urine.

痛性尿淋瀝 從膀胱底傳向尿道的劇烈疼痛，伴有強烈尿意。發生於膀胱底受結石或留置導尿管刺激時。在膀胱底侵襲性癌、重症膀胱炎或前列腺炎病人亦可出現，表現爲强烈尿意、尿痛而僅能排出幾滴尿液。

stratum *n.* a layer of tissue or cells, such as any of the layers of the *epidermis of the skin (the *stratum corneum* is the outermost layer).

層 一層組織或細胞，如皮膚表皮各層（最外層爲角質層）。

streak *n.* (in anatomy) a line, furrow, or narrow band. *See also* primitive streak.

條，紋 （解剖學）線，溝紋，窄條。

Streptobacillus *n.* a genus of Gram-negative aerobic nonmotile rodlike bacteria that tend to form filaments. The single species, *S. moniliformis*, is a normal inhabitant of the respiratory tract of rats but causes *rat-bite fever in man.

鏈桿菌屬 一屬革蘭氏陰性、無活動能力的需氧桿狀細菌，有形成菌絲傾向。其中一株念珠狀鏈桿菌爲大鼠呼吸道正常寄生菌，但能引起人患鼠咬熱。

Streptococcus *n.* a genus of Gram-positive nonmotile spherical bacteria occurring in chains. Most species are

鏈球菌屬 一屬革蘭氏陽性、無活動能力、呈鏈狀排列的球菌。多數種爲腐

saprophytes; some are pathogenic. Many pathogenic species are *haemolytic*, i.e. they have the ability to destroy red blood cells in blood agar. This provides a useful basis for classifying the many different strains. Strains of *S. pyogenes* (the β-haemolytic streptococci) are associated with many infections, including *scarlet fever, and produce many *exotoxins. Strains of *S. viridans* (the α-haemolytic streptococci) are associated with bacterial *endocarditis. The species *S. pneumoniae* (formerly *Diplococcus pneumoniae*) – the *pneumococcus* – is associated with pneumonia. It occurs in pairs, surrounded by a capsule (*see* quellung reaction). *See also* Lancefield classification, streptokinase.

物寄生菌，有些具致病性。許多致病種爲溶血性，即具有在血瓊脂培養基中破壞紅細胞的能力。這一特性是對許多不同菌株進行分類的有用依據。一些釀膿鏈球菌株（β溶血性鏈球菌）與猩紅熱等許多傳染病有關，能產生多種外毒素。綠色鏈球菌株（β溶血性鏈球菌）則與細菌性心內膜炎有關。肺炎鏈球菌種（過去稱爲肺炎雙球菌）或肺炎球菌與肺炎有關。此菌成雙存在，外包莢膜。

streptodornase *n.* an enzyme produced by some haemolytic bacteria of the genus *Streptococcus* that is capable of liquefying pus. *See also* streptokinase.

鏈球菌脫氧核糖核酸酶 鏈球菌屬中某些溶血性鏈球菌產生的酶，能使膿液化。

streptokinase *n.* an enzyme produced by some haemolytic bacteria of the genus **Streptococcus* that is capable of liquefying blood clots. It is injected to treat blockage of blood vessels, including infarction and pulmonary embolism. It is also used in combination with streptodornase, applied topically or taken by mouth or injection, to liquefy pus and relieve inflammation. Side-effects may include digestive upsets, fever, and haemorrhage.

鏈球菌激酶 鏈球菌屬中某些溶血性鏈球菌產生的酶，能使血凝塊液化。注射可治療血管阻塞，如梗塞和肺栓塞。還可與鏈球菌脫氧核糖核酸酶聯合使用（局部外用、口服或注射）使膿液化，減輕炎症。副作用可有消化道不適、發熱和出血。

streptolysin *n.* an *exotoxin that is produced by *Streptococcus pyogenes* and destroys red blood cells.

鏈球菌溶血素 釀膿鏈球菌產生的一種外毒素，能破壞紅細胞。

Streptomyces *n.* a genus of aerobic mouldlike bacteria. Most species live in the soil, but some are parasites of animals, man, and plants; in man they cause *Madura foot. They are important medically as a source of such antibiotics as *streptomycin, *actino-

鏈黴菌屬 一屬眞菌樣需氧菌。多數種生活於土壤中，某些寄居於動物、人和植物，在人類可引起足分支菌病。此菌醫學上所以重要，乃因它們是諸如鏈黴素、放線菌素、氯黴

mycin, *chloramphenicol, and *neomycin.

素和新黴素等抗生素的來源。

streptomycin *n.* an *antibiotic, derived from the bacterium *Streptomyces griseus*, that is effective against a wide range of bacterial infections; it is administered by mouth or intramuscular injection. Streptomycin is an important drug in tuberculosis therapy but is usually given in conjunction with other drugs (e.g. *isoniazid) because bacteria soon become resistant to it. Side-effects causing ear and kidney damage may develop in some patients.

鏈黴素 由灰色鏈黴菌製取的抗生素，具有廣泛的抗細菌感染作用。口服或肌注。爲治療結核病的重要藥物，但通常與其他藥物（如異菸肼）聯合應用，因爲細菌很快對鏈黴素產生耐藥性。副作用爲某些病人可有耳和腎臟損害。

stress *n.* any factor that threatens the health of the body or has an adverse effect on its functioning, such as injury, disease, or worry. The existence of one form of stress tends to diminish resistance to other forms. Constant stress brings about changes in the balance of hormones in the body.

應激物 危及身體健康或有害於機體功能的任何因素，如外傷、疾病或憂慮。一種應激物的存在還可能導至對其他應激物的抵抗力的降低。持續的應激狀態會引起體內激素平衡失調。

stretch receptor a cell or group of cells found between muscle fibres that responds to stretching of the muscle by transmitting impulses to the central nervous system through sensory nerves. Stretch receptors are part of the *proprioceptor system necessary for the performance of coordinated muscular activity.

牽張感受器 存在於肌纖維間的一個細胞或一組細胞，能對肌肉的牽伸發生反應，將衝動通過感覺神經傳入中樞神經系統。牽張感受器是本體感受器系統的一部分，爲完成協調的肌肉活動所必需。

stretch reflex (myotatic reflex) the reflex contraction of a muscle in response to its being stretched.

牽張反射（肌伸長反射） 對肌肉牽伸而產生肌肉收縮的反射。

stria *n.* (*pl.* **striae**) (in anatomy) a streak, line, or thin band. The *striae gravidarum* are the lines that appear on the skin of the abdomen of pregnant women, due to stretching and rupture of the elastic fibres. Pinkish during pregnancy, they become white after delivery. The *stria terminalis* is a white band that separates the thalamus from the ventricular surface of the caudate nucleus in the brain.

紋 （解剖學）條紋，線，或細帶。妊娠紋是孕婦腹部皮膚上出現的條紋，係彈性纖維拉長、斷裂所致。妊娠期間的妊娠紋呈粉紅色，分娩後變爲白色。終紋是腦內將丘腦與尾狀核的腦室面隔開的白色條帶。

striated muscle a tissue comprising the bulk of the body's musculature. It is also known as *skeletal muscle*, because it is attached to the skeleton and is responsible for the movement of bones, and *voluntary muscle*, because it is under voluntary control. Striated muscle is composed of parallel bundles of multinucleate fibres (each containing many *myofibrils*), which reveal cross-banding when viewed under the microscope. This effect is due to the alternation of *actin* and *myosin* protein filaments within each myofibril (see illustration). When muscle contraction takes place, the two sets of filaments slide past each other, so reducing the length of each unit (*sarcomere*) of the myofibril. The sliding is caused by a series of cyclic reactions resulting in a change in orientation of projections on the myosin filaments; each projection is first attached to an actin filament but contracts and releases it to become reattached at a different site.

橫紋肌　構成身體肌肉系統主體的組織。因爲它附着於骨骼並負責骨的運動，又稱骨骼肌。因爲它受意志的支配，還有隨意肌之稱。橫紋肌由大量平行的多核肌纖維（每條肌纖維又含有大量肌原纖維）束組成，在顯微鏡下觀察時肌纖維呈現交錯的帶。這是由於每條肌原纖維內的肌動蛋白絲和肌凝蛋白絲交錯排列的結果。當肌肉收縮時，這兩組肌絲在相互之間滑動，使肌原纖維的每個單位（肌節）長度縮短。肌絲的滑動係由一系列週期性反應所引起，這些反應的結果是使肌凝蛋白絲上的突起發生方向的變化，每個突起先是觸及一條肌動蛋白絲，隨着收縮，脫離後者，而在另一個位置重又接觸肌動蛋白絲。

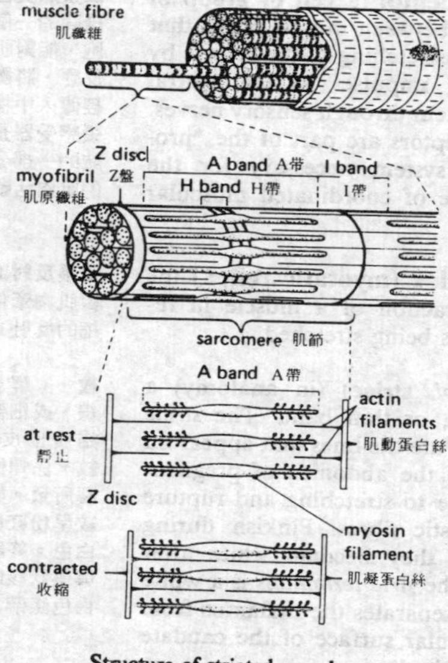

Structure of striated muscle
橫紋肌的構造

stricture *n.* a narrowing of any tubular structure in the body, such as the oesophagus (gullet), bowel, ureter, or urethra. A stricture may result from inflammation, muscular spasm, growth of a tumour within the affected part, or from pressure on it by neighbouring organs. For example, a *urethral stricture* is a fibrous narrowing of the urethra, usually resulting from injury or inflammation. The patient has increasing difficulty in passing urine and may develop *retention. The site and length of the stricture is assessed by *urethrography and urethroscopy, and treatment is by periodic dilatation of the urethra using *sounds, *urethrotomy, or *urethroplasty.

狹窄 體內任何管腔結構（如食管、腸、輸尿管或尿道）狹窄。狹窄可由受累部分的炎症、肌肉痙攣、腫瘤生長所致，也可因毗鄰器官壓迫而發生。例如，尿道狹窄是外傷或炎症所致的一種纖維性狹窄。病人排尿困難逐漸加重，可發生尿瀦留。尿道X線照影和尿道鏡檢查可確定狹窄的部位和長度。治療是每隔一定時間用探子擴張尿道，或作尿道切開術或尿道成形術。

stridor *n.* the noise heard on breathing in when the trachea or larynx is obstructed. It tends to be louder and harsher than *wheeze.

喘鳴 氣管或喉堵塞的病人呼吸時發生的響聲。其聲比喘氣響而粗糙。

strobila *n.* (*pl.* **strobilae**) the entire chain of segments that make up the body of an adult *tapeworm.

鏈體 組成絛蟲成蟲身體的整條節片鏈。

stroke (apoplexy) *n.* a sudden attack of weakness affecting one side of the body. It is the consequence of an interruption to the flow of blood to the brain. The primary disease is in the heart or blood vessels and the effect on the brain is secondary. The flow of blood may be prevented by clotting (*thrombosis*), a detached clot that lodges in an artery (*embolus*), or rupture of an artery wall (*haemorrhage*). A stroke can vary in severity from a passing weakness or tingling in a limb to a profound paralysis, coma, and death. *See also* cerebral haemorrhage.

卒中 突然發生的身體一側虛弱無力。係大腦血流障礙的結果。原發病在心臟或血管，大腦的病變是繼發的。血流受阻的原因可能是血凝塊（血栓形成）、脫落的血凝塊堵塞了動脉（栓塞）或動脉壁破裂（出血）。卒中的嚴重程度不同，輕的僅有一過性虛弱無力或肢體刺痛，重的可致深度癱瘓、昏迷以至死亡。

stroma *n.* **1.** the supportive tissue of an organ, as opposed to the functional tissue (*parenchyma*). **2.** the spongy framework of protein strands within a red blood cell in which the blood pigment haemoglobin is packed.

基質 ①器官內的支持組織。基質是與器官的功能組織（實質）相對而言的。②紅細胞內由蛋白質構成的海綿狀框架，血液色素——血紅蛋白充塡於其中。

Strongyloides *n.* a genus of small slender nematode worms that live as parasites in the small intestines of mammals. *S. stercoralis* infects the human small intestine (*see* strongyloidiasis); its larvae, which are passed out in the stools, develop quickly into infective forms.

類圓線蟲屬 一屬寄生於哺乳動物小腸內的細小線蟲。糞類圓線蟲感染人小腸，其幼蟲隨糞便排出，迅速發育爲感染型線蟲。

strongyloidiasis (strongyloidosis) *n.* an infestation of the small intestine with the parasitic nematode worm *Strongyloides stercoralis*, common in humid tropical regions. Larvae, present in soil contaminated with human faeces, penetrate the skin of a human host and may produce an itching rash. They migrate to the lungs, where they cause tissue destruction and bleeding, and then via the windpipe and gullet to the intestine. Adult worms burrow into the intestinal wall and may cause ulceration, diarrhoea, abdominal pain, nausea, anaemia, and weakness. Treatment involves use of the drugs thiabendazole and *dithiazanine.

類圓線蟲病 糞類圓線蟲寄生於小腸所致的感染，一般見於潮濕的熱帶地區。存在於人糞便污染的土壤中的幼蟲，穿透人宿主的皮膚，在皮膚上產生癢疹。幼蟲游走入肺，引起組織破壞和出血，然後經氣管和食管而進入腸內。成蟲鑽入腸壁，可引起潰瘍、腹瀉、噁心、貧血和虛弱。治療用噻苯咪唑和噻唑青胺等藥物。

strontium *n.* a yellow metallic element, absorption of which causes bone damage when its atoms displace calcium in bone. The radioactive isotope *strontium-90*, which emits beta rays, is used in radiotherapy for the *contact therapy of skin and eye tumours. Symbol: Sr.

鍶 一種黃色金屬元素，吸收後鍶原子可取代骨鈣而引起骨損害。放射性同位素^{90}鍶釋放β射線，在放射治療中用於皮膚和眼腫瘤的接觸治療。符號：Sr。

struma *n.* (*pl.* **strumae**) a swelling of the thyroid gland (*see* goitre). ***Riedel's struma*** is a rare chronic inflammation of the thyroid (*see* thyroiditis), which becomes firm and enlarged and is eventually destroyed.

甲狀腺腫 甲狀腺腫大。里德爾氏甲狀腺腫是一種少見的甲狀腺慢性炎症，其時甲狀腺變硬增大，最終破壞。

strychnine *n.* a poisonous alkaloid produced in the seeds of the East Indian tree *Strychnos nux-vomica*. In small doses it was formerly widely used in 'tonics'. Poisoning causes painful muscular spasms similar to those of tetanus; the back becomes arched (the

士的寧 東印度馬錢樹種子中產生的一種毒性生物鹼。過去在"强壯劑"中曾廣泛使用小量士的寧。中毒時引起痛性肌痙攣，類似破傷風，背部彎成弓形（此種姿勢稱爲角弓反

posture known as *opisthotonus*) and death is likely to occur from spasm in the respiratory muscles.

張），呼吸肌痙攣可能導至死亡。

Student's t test *see* significance.

T檢驗

stupe *n.* any piece of material, such as a wad of cottonwool, soaked in hot water (with or without medication) and used to apply a poultice.

熱敷布 一塊用熱水浸濕的、加或不加藥物的織物，如脫脂棉片，用於包敷泥罨劑。

stupor *n.* a condition of near unconsciousness, with apparent mental inactivity and reduced ability to respond to stimulation.

木僵 接近喪失意識的狀態，伴有明顯的精神遲鈍，對刺激反應的能力降低。

Sturge-Weber syndrome *see* angioma.

斯特季-韋勃氏綜合徵

stuttering *n. see* stammering.

口吃

St. Vitus' dance an archaic name for Sydenham's *chorea.

聖維特斯氏舞蹈 西登哈姆氏舞蹈病的舊稱。

stye *n.* acute inflammation of a gland at the base of an eyelash, caused by bacterial infection. The gland becomes hard and tender and a pus-filled cyst develops at its centre. Styes are treated by bathing in warm water or removal of the eyelash involved. Medical name: **hordeolum**.

瞼腺炎，麥粒腫 睫毛基部腺體的急性炎症，由細菌感染引起。腺體變硬有觸痛，其中心部生成一個充滿膿的囊。治療用熱敷或拔除受累睫毛。

stylet *n. see* stilet.

通管絲，細探子

stylo- *prefix denoting* the styloid process of the temporal bone. Example: *stylomastoid* (relating to the styloid and mastoid processes).

〔前綴〕 **莖突** 指顳骨的莖狀突起。例如：莖突乳突的。

styloglossus *n.* a muscle that extends from the tongue to the styloid process of the temporal bone. It serves to draw the tongue upwards and backwards.

莖突舌肌 一塊由舌走向顳骨莖突的肌肉。其功能為將舌拉向上方和後方。

stylohyoid *n.* a muscle that extends from the styloid process of the temporal bone to the hyoid bone. It serves to draw the hyoid bone backwards and upwards.

莖突舌骨肌 一塊由顳骨莖突走向舌骨的肌肉。其功能為將舌骨拉向後方和上方。

styloid process **1.** a long slender downward-pointing spine projecting from the lower surface of the *temporal

莖突 ①顳顳骨下表面上的指向下方的細長棘狀突起。為舌和舌骨的肌肉、

bone of the skull. It provides attachment for muscles and ligaments of the tongue and hyoid bone. **2.** any of various other spiny projections; occurring, for example, at the lower ends of the ulna and radius.

韌帶的附着處。 ②其他各種棘狀突起，例如見於尺骨和橈骨的下端。

stylus *n.* **1.** a pencil-shaped instrument, commonly used for applying external medication; for example, to apply silver nitrate to warts. **2.** *see* stilet.

①棒 筆形工具。一般用於外部用藥，例如用硝銀棒治療疣。 **②通管絲，細探子**

styptic *n. see* haemostatic.

止血劑

sub- *prefix denoting* **1.** below; underlying. Examples: *subcostal* (below the ribs); *sublingual* (below the tongue); *submandibular* (below the mandible). **2.** partial or slight.

〔前綴〕 ①**下** 例如肋骨下的，舌下的，下頜下的。 ②**亞** 部分的，輕度的。

subacute *adj.* describing a disease that progresses more rapidly than a *chronic condition but does not become *acute.

亞急性的 描述較慢性病進展快但尚未成爲急性的疾病。

subacute combined degeneration of the cord the neurological disorder complicating a deficiency of *vitamin B_{12} and pernicious anaemia. There is selective damage to the motor and sensory nerve fibres in the spinal cord, resulting in *spasticity of the limbs and a sensory *ataxia. It may also be accompanied by damage to the peripheral nerves and the optic nerve and by dementia. It is treated by giving vitamin B_{12} injections.

亞急性脊髓混合變性 一種合併維生素B_{12}缺乏和惡性貧血的神經系統病患。脊髓的運動和感覺神經纖維選擇地受損，引起肢體痙攣狀態和感覺性共濟失調。也可伴有周圍神經和視神經損害以及痴獃。治療爲維生素B_{12}注射。

subarachnoid haemorrhage bleeding into the subarachnoid space surrounding the brain, which causes severe headache with stiffness of the neck. The usual source of such a haemorrhage is a cerebral *aneurysm that has burst. The diagnosis is confirmed by finding blood-stained cerebrospinal fluid at *lumbar puncture. Identification of the site of the aneurysm, upon which decisions about treatment will be based, is achieved by cerebral *angiography.

蛛網膜下（腔）出血 血液流入圍繞腦的蛛網膜下腔內，引起劇烈頭痛和頸部發硬。這種出血通常源自腦動脉瘤破裂。腰椎穿刺發現血性腦脊液即可確診。作腦血管造影可確定動脉瘤的位置，據此決定如何治療。

subarachnoid space the space between the arachnoid and pia *meninges

蛛網膜下腔 腦和脊髓的蛛網膜與軟膜之間的腔

of the brain and spinal cord, containing circulating cerebrospinal fluid and large blood vessels. Several large spaces within it are known as *cisternae*.

隙，內含循環的腦脊液和大血管。蛛網膜下腔內幾個大的腔隙稱爲池。

subclavian artery either of two arteries supplying blood to the neck and arms. The right subclavian artery branches from the innominate artery; the left subclavian arises directly from the aortic arch.

鎖骨下動脉 兩條向頸和臂供血的動脉。右鎖骨下動脉爲無名動脉的分支，左鎖骨下動脉則直接由主動脉弓發出。

subclinical *adj.* describing a disease that is suspected but is not sufficiently developed to produce definite signs and symptoms in the patient.

亞臨床的 指疾病已屬可疑但尚未發展到足以產生確切症狀和體徵的狀況。

subconscious *adj.* **1.** describing mental processes of which a person is not aware. **2.** (in psychoanalysis) denoting the part of the mind that includes memories, motives, and intentions that are momentarily not present in consciousness but can more or less readily be recalled to awareness. *Compare* unconscious.

下意識的 ①指人的無意識的精神過程。 ②（精神分析）指在某瞬間處於無意識狀態但相當容易進入意識領域的思維部分，包括記憶、動機和意向。

subcutaneous *adj.* beneath the skin. A *subcutaneous injection* is given beneath the skin. *Subcutaneous tissue* is loose connective tissue, often fatty, situated under the dermis.

皮下的 皮膚下面的。皮下注射是注射到皮膚下面。皮下組織是位於眞皮下面的疏鬆結締組織，常爲脂肪組織。

subdural *adj.* below the dura mater (the outermost of the meninges); relating to the space between the dura mater and arachnoid. *See also* haematoma.

硬膜下的 硬膜（腦膜的最外層）下面的，在硬腦膜與蛛網膜之間的腔隙。

subinvolution *n.* failure of a part of the body to return to its normal size after being enlarged. In *uterine subinvolution* the womb does not revert to its normal size during the six weeks following childbirth. *Compare* hyperinvolution.

復舊不全 身體某部分增大之後不能恢復到正常大小。子宮復舊不全指分娩後6周子宮未能恢復到正常大小。

sublimation *n.* the replacement of socially undesirable means of gratifying motives or desires by means that are socially acceptable. *See also* defence mechanism, repression.

昇華 把社會所不能容忍的方式轉變爲社會可以接受的方式來使動機和慾望得到滿足。

subliminal *adj.* subconscious: beneath the threshold of conscious perception.

閾下的 下意識的，在意識知覺的閾限之下的。

sublingual gland one of a pair of *salivary glands situated in the lower part of the mouth, one on either side of the tongue. The sublingual glands are the smallest salivary glands; each gland has about 20 ducts, most of which open into the mouth directly above the gland.

舌下腺 位於口底部舌兩側的成對唾液腺。舌下腺是最小的唾液腺，每側有大約20個導管，其中多數直接在腺上方開口於口腔。

subluxation *n.* partial *dislocation of a joint, so that the bone ends are misaligned but still in contact.

不全脫位 關節部分脫位，結果骨端雖然錯位但仍保持接觸。

submandibular gland (submaxillary gland) one of a pair of *salivary glands situated below the parotid glands. Their ducts (*Wharton's ducts*) open in two papillae under the tongue, on either side of the frenulum.

下頜下腺 位於腮下方的成對唾液腺。其導管（華頓氏導管）開口於舌下舌繫帶兩側的乳頭上。

submaxillary gland *see* submandibular gland.

下頜下腺

submentovertical (SMV) *adj.* (in radiology) denoting a horizontal view of the base of the skull.

頦下水平位的 （放射學）指顱底的水平位觀察所見。

submucosa *n.* the layer of loose connective (*areolar) tissue underlying a mucous membrane; for example, in the wall of the intestine. —**submucosal** *adj.*

黏膜下層 黏膜下面的疏鬆（蜂窩狀）結締組織層，例如腸壁的黏膜下層。

subnormality *n.* a state of arrested or incomplete development of the mind. *Mental subnormality* is essentially an administrative concept, describing the state of those whose intellectual powers have failed to develop to such an extent that they are in need of care and protection. This depends in part on social circumstances, for a person who is subnormal in a demanding culture may manage well in a simpler environment. It is also known as *mental retardation*, *mental deficiency*, and *amentia*. *Intellectual subnormality* is a scientific concept, denoting the state of those whose intellectual powers fall below some point on a standardized *intelligence test. Mildly subnormal people (with an IQ of approximately 50–70) often make a good adjustment to life after special help with education. The

低常狀態 精神發育停滯或發育不全的狀態。精神低常主要是管理學概念，指那些智力發育障礙以致需要照料和保護的情況。這種情況部分與社會環境有關：一個在文化要求高的環境中的精神低常者，若在簡單的環境內可能會處理得很好。精神低常又稱精神發育遲滯、精神缺陷、智力缺陷。智力低下是一個科學概念，係指在標準智力測驗中智力低於某一水平的情況。輕度智力低下者（智商約爲50～70）經專門教育後能很好適應生活。中度或嚴重智力低下者（智商約爲20～50）常需要較多帮助，多數需長期依賴他人生活。

moderately and severely subnormal (with an IQ of approximately 20–50) usually need much more help; most are permanently dependent on other people. The profoundly subnormal (with an IQ less than about 20) usually need constant attention. There are very many causes of intellectual subnormality, including *Down's syndrome, inherited metabolic disorders, brain injury, and gross psychological deprivation; some are preventable or treatable. Good education alters the course of the handicap, but many patients need residential care in local authority homes or in hospitals.

極度低下者（智商低於20）常需要終身照料。引起智力低下狀態的原因很多，包括唐氏綜合徵、遺傳性代謝病、腦外傷、精神總體喪失等。有些是可以預防或治癒的。良好的教育可阻止這種殘疾的進程，但許多病人須在地方當局辦的療養院或醫院內住院治療。

subphrenic abscess a collection of pus in the space below the diaphragm, usually on the right side, between the liver and diaphragm. Causes include postoperative infection (particularly after the stomach or bowel have been opened) and perforation of an organ (e.g. perforated peptic ulcer). Prompt treatment by antibiotics may be effective, but more frequently the abscess requires surgical drainage.

膈下膿腫 膈肌下方積膿，通常在右側，肝與膈肌之間。病因有：術後感染（主要在切開胃腸的手術後）、器官穿孔（如消化性潰瘍穿孔）。立即給予抗生素治療可能奏效。但更多情況下膿腫須作外科引流。

substitution *n.* **1.** (in psychoanalysis) the replacement of one idea by another: a form of *defence mechanism. **2.** *symptom substitution* is the supposed process whereby removing one psychological symptom leads to another symptom appearing if the basic psychological cause has not been removed. It is controversial whether this happens.

①**替代** （精神分析）一個思想爲另一個思想所替換，是心理防禦機制的一種形式。 ②**症狀更替** 人們假設：只要基本的精神性病因存在，則一種精神症狀消除了，另一種精神症狀又會產生。是否如此，衆說紛紜。

sulphaguanidine *n. see* sulphonamide.

sulphamethizole *n. see* sulphonamide.

sulphamethoxazole *n.* a drug of the *sulphonamide group. It is taken by mouth and is effective in the treatment of infections of the respiratory tract (including bronchitis), the urinary and has become addicted by the gradual substitution of a nonaddictive drug with a similar or a sedative effect.

替代療法 用一種害處較小的藥物代替病人一直使用的另一種藥物進行治療。此法用於病人對某藥成癮或過度依賴時。通過給予作用相似或有鎮靜作用的非成癮藥物，逐漸取代病人對之成癮的藥物，從而使病人戒除“劇毒”藥物。

substrate *n.* the specific substance or substances on which a given *enzyme acts. For example, starch is the substrate for salivary amylase; RNA is the substrate for ribonuclease.

底物 酶對之起作用的一種或幾種特殊物質。例如，澱粉是唾液澱粉酶的底物；核糖核酸是核糖核酸酶的底物。

subsultus *n.* abnormal twitching or tremor of muscles, such as may occur in feverish conditions.

顫跳 肌肉的異常顫動，可發生發熱情況下。

subtertian fever a form of *malaria resulting from repeated infection by *Plasmodium falciparum* and characterized by continuous fever.

惡性瘧 由惡性瘧原蟲重複感染所致的瘧疾類型，以持續發熱爲特徵。

subthalamic nucleus a collection of grey matter, shaped like a biconvex lens, lying beneath the *thalamus and close to the *corpus striatum, to which it is connected by nerve tracts. It has connections with the cerebral cortex and several other nuclei nearby.

下丘腦核團 灰質的集團，外形如雙凸鏡，位於丘腦下方，緊靠紋狀體，並以神經束與之相連。核團與大腦皮質及附近其他一些神經核均有聯繫。

succus *n.* any juice or secretion of animal or plant origin.

汁，液 動、植物的汁液或分泌物。

succus entericus (intestinal juice) the clear alkaline fluid secreted by the glands of the small intestine. It contains mucus and digestive enzymes, including *enteropeptidase, *erepsin, *lactase, and *sucrase.

腸液 小腸腺分泌的清亮鹼性液體。內含黏液和腸肽酶、乳糖酶、蔗糖酶等消化酶。

succussion *n.* a splashing noise heard when a patient who has a large quantity of fluid in a body cavity, such as the pleural cavity, moves suddenly or is deliberately shaken.

振盪音 體腔（如胸膜腔）中有大量液體的病人突然活動或故意搖晃身體時可以聽到的一種濺水樣聲響。

sucrase *n.* an enzyme, secreted by glands in the small intestine, that catalyses the hydrolysis of sucrose into its components (glucose and fructose).

蔗糖酶 小腸腺分泌的一種酶，催化蔗糖水解爲其組成成分（葡萄糖及果糖）。

sucrose *n.* a carbohydrate consisting of glucose and fructose. Sucrose is the principal constituent of cane sugar and sugar beet; it is the sweetest of the natural dietary carbohydrates. The increasing consumption of sucrose in the last 50 years has coincided with an

蔗糖 由葡萄糖和果糖組成的碳水化合物。是甘蔗糖和甜菜糖的主要成分，天然碳水化合物性食物中最甜的一種。近50年來，隨着蔗糖消耗的增長，齲病、糖尿病、冠狀動脈性

increase in the incidence of dental caries, diabetes, coronary heart disease, and obesity.

心臟病和肥胖病等的發病率相應上升。

suction *n.* the use of reduced pressure to remove unwanted fluids or other material through a tube for disposal. Suction is often used to clear secretions from the airways of newly born infants to aid breathing. During surgery, suction tubes are used to remove blood from the area of operation.

抽吸 利用減壓原理通過導管吸出有害液體或其他物質以廢棄之。常用於清除新生嬰兒呼吸道內分泌物以助呼吸。手術中用導管抽吸手術區的血液。

sudamen *n.* (*pl.* **sudamina**) a white blister caused by sweat collecting in the sweat ducts or in the layers of the skin.

汗疹 汗液蓄積於汗腺導管或皮膚表層內所致的白色小疱。

Sudan stains a group of azo compounds used for staining fats. The group includes *Sudan I*, *Sudan II*, *Sudan III*, *Sudan IV*, and *Sudan black*.

蘇丹染液 用於脂肪染色的一組偶氮化合物，包括蘇丹Ⅰ、蘇丹Ⅱ、蘇丹Ⅲ、蘇丹Ⅳ和蘇丹黑。

Sudek's atrophy rapid development of *osteoporosis in a hand or foot, resulting from injury, infection, or malignancy.

祖德克氏萎縮 外傷、感染或惡性腫瘤所致的手或足的急性骨質疏鬆症。

sudor *n. see* sweat.

汗

sudorific *n. see* diaphoretic.

發汗劑

suffocation *n.* cessation of breathing as a result of drowning, smothering, etc., leading to unconsciousness or death (*see* asphyxia).

窒息 淹溺、煙嗆所致的呼吸停止，導至意識喪失以至死亡。

suffusion *n.* the spreading of a flush across the skin surface, caused by changes in the local blood supply.

漲紅 局部血液供應改變所致的皮膚表面泛紅現象。

sugar any *carbohydrate that dissolves in water, is usually crystalline, and has a sweet taste. Sugars are classified chemically as *monosaccharides or *disaccharides. Table sugar is virtually 100% pure *sucrose and contains no other nutrient; brown sugar is less highly refined sucrose. Sugar is used as both a sweetening and preserving agent. *See also* fructose, glucose, lactose.

糖 一切溶於水、常呈結晶態、具甜味的碳水化合物。糖在化學上分爲單糖和雙糖。方糖爲100%的純蔗糖，不含其他營養成分；紅糖爲精製度較差的蔗糖。糖用作甜味劑和保存劑。

suggestion *n.* (in psychology) the process of changing a person's beliefs, attitudes, or emotions by telling him

暗示 （心理學）使人改變其信念、態度或情緒的過程。採用的方法是告訴

that they will change. It is sometimes used as a synonym for *hypnosis. *See also* autosuggestion.

他即將發生這些變化。有時此詞用作催眠的同義詞。

suicide *n.* self-destruction as a deliberate act. Distinction is usually made between *attempted suicide*, when death is averted although the person concerned intended to kill himself (or herself), and *parasuicide, when the attempt is made for reasons other than actually killing oneself. In the UK deliberate overdosing is the commonest cause of admission to hospital medical wards and it is estimated that some 85% of attempted suicides are happy to have survived. Death by suicide in the UK declined by some 36% in the period 1963–75, contrary to the general trend in other Western countries. This fall is claimed to have resulted from the work of the *Samaritans, a voluntary suicide-prevention organization that grew into a nationwide service over this period.

自殺 蓄意進行的自我摧毁行爲。在下列兩種自殺之間須進行區別，一種是企圖自殺：當事人企圖自殺而未遂；另一種是假自殺：自殺的企圖是爲了達到某種目的而不是眞的要殺死自己。在英國，有意攝入過量藥物是收住醫院的最常見原因，幸而約85%的企圖自殺獲得生存。1963～1975年期間，英國的自殺死亡率下降了約36%，而在其他西方國家則總的趨勢相反。這種下降被認爲是“撒瑪利亞人協會”努力的成果，這是一個志願的防止自殺組織，在上述時期發展壯大，遍佈全國。

sulcus *n.* (*pl.* **sulci**) **1.** one of the many clefts or infoldings of the surface of the brain. The raised outfolding on each side of a sulcus is termed a *gyrus*. **2.** any of the infoldings of soft tissue in the mouth, for example between the cheek and the alveolus.

溝 ①大腦表面的許多裂隙和皺褶。溝兩旁凸起的褶稱回。 ②口內軟組織的皺褶，例如頰與牙槽之間的溝。

sulphacetamide *n.* a drug of the *sulphonamide group that is used in eye drops to treat such infections as conjunctivitis. Transient irritation may occur with higher doses. Trade names: **Albucid, Ocusol.**

乙醯磺胺 磺胺類藥物的一種，製成滴眼劑治療結膜炎等感染。大劑量可引起短暫的刺激症狀。

sulphadimidine *n. see* sulphonamide.

磺胺二甲嘧啶

sulphadoxine *n. see* sulphonamide.

磺胺鄰二甲氧嘧啶

sulpha drug *see* sulphonamide.

磺胺藥

sulphafurazole *n. see* sulphonamide.

磺胺異噁唑

sulphaguanidine *n. see* sulphonamide.

磺胺胍

sulphamethizole *n. see* sulphonamide.

磺胺甲噻二唑

sulphamethoxazole *n.* a drug of the *sulphonamide group. It is taken by mouth and is effective in the treatment

磺胺甲基異噁唑，新諾明 磺胺類藥物的一種。口服。治療呼吸道（如支氣

of infections of the respiratory tract (including bronchitis), the urinary and gastrointestinal tracts, and the skin. The drug is frequently administered in a combined preparation with trimethoprim (*see* co-trimoxazole (Bactrim, Septrin)). Trade name: **Gantanol**.

管炎）、泌尿道、胃腸道和皮膚感染有效。常與磺胺甲氧苄胺嘧啶製成合劑片服用。

sulphaphenazole *n. see* sulphonamide.

磺胺苯吡唑

sulphasalazine *n.* a drug of the *sulphonamide group, used in the treatment of ulcerative colitis. It is given by mouth or in the form of suppositories. The most common side-effects are nausea, loss of appetite, and raised temperature. Trade name: **Salazopyrin**.

水楊酸偶氮磺胺吡啶 磺胺類藥物的一種，用於治療潰瘍性結腸炎。口服或製成栓劑。最常見的副作用爲噁心、食慾喪失和發熱。

sulphinpyrazone *n.* a *uricosuric drug given by mouth for the treatment of chronic gout. The main side-effects are nausea and abdominal pain; the drug may also activate a latent duodenal ulcer and it should not be taken by patients with impaired kidney function. Trade name: **Anturan**.

苯磺唑酮 一種促尿酸排泄藥，口服治療慢性痛風。主要副作用爲噁心和腹痛，還可使潛在的十二指腸潰瘍發作。腎臟機能不好的病人禁用。

sulphomyxin *n.* an antibiotic, similar to *polymyxin B, given by local application or intramuscular injection to treat infections of the skin, mucous membranes, eyes, and ears caused by *Pseudomonas*. Common side-effects include flushing, dizziness, blurred vision, and weakness.

硫黏菌素 一種類似多黏菌素B的抗生素。局部應用或肌內注射，治療假單胞菌屬所致的皮膚、黏膜、眼、耳感染。常見副作用有潮紅、頭暈、視力模糊和無力。

sulphonamide (sulpha drug) *n.* one of a group of drugs, derived from sulphanilamide (a red dye), that prevent the growth of bacteria (i.e. they are bacteriostatic). Sulphonamides are usually given by mouth and are effective against a variety of infections. Most of them, including *sulphamethoxazole and *sulphaphenazole*, are rapidly absorbed from the stomach and small intestine and should be taken at frequent intervals. Some, such as *sulphadoxine* (used for leprosy and malaria) and *sulphametopyrazine* are long-acting and need be taken only once a day.

磺胺（磺胺藥） 由紅色顏料氨苯磺胺衍生的一組藥物，具有防止細菌生長（制菌）的作用。磺胺通常口服，對多種感染有效。多種磺胺，包括磺胺甲基異噁唑和磺胺苯吡唑，在口和小腸內迅速吸收，須多次間隔服用。而磺胺鄰二甲氨嘧啶（用於麻瘋和瘧疾）和磺胺甲氧吡嗪等則具長效，每天只須服用一次。另一些如磺胺脒，難以吸收，故用於治療細菌性痢疾和胃腸炎

Others, including *sulphaguanidine*, are poorly absorbed and are therefore used to treat infections of the gastrointestinal tract, such as bacillary dysentery and gastroenteritis. Prolonged use of these sulphonamides may lead to the development of resistant stains of microorganisms in the gut. Many sulphonamides are rapidly excreted and very soluble in the urine and are used to treat infections of the urinary tract; examples are *sulphadimidine*, *sulphafurazole*, and *sulphamethizole*.

等胃腸道感染。長期使用這些磺胺藥可引起腸內耐藥菌株的發展。許多磺胺迅速排泄並且易溶於尿內，故用於治療泌尿道感染，這類藥有磺胺二甲嘧啶、磺胺異噁唑和磺胺甲噻二唑等。

A variety of side-effects may occur with sulphonamide treatment, including nausea, vomiting, headache, and loss of appetite. In acute infections these are unimportant compared with the benefit produced by the drugs. More severe effects include *cyanosis, blood disorders, skin rashes, and fever. Sulphonamides should be avoided in jaundice and kidney disease and in patients allergic to these drugs. In general, patients treated with sulphonamides should avoid exposure to direct sunlight.

磺胺藥治療可產生多種副作用，如噁心、嘔吐、頭痛、食慾喪失。在急性感染時，這些作用與藥物帶來的好處相比是不足道的。遠爲嚴重的副作用有發紺、血液疾病、皮疹和發熱。磺胺在有黃疸、腎臟疾病以及對磺胺過敏的病人應避免使用。一般來說，用磺胺治療的病人應避免日光直接曝曬。

sulphone *n.* one of a group of drugs closely related to the *sulphonamides in structure and therapeutic actions. Sulphones possess powerful activity against the bacteria that cause leprosy and tuberculosis. The best known sulphone is *dapsone.

碸 結構和治療作用均與磺胺相近的一組藥物。碸類具有强大的抗痲瘋和結核病病菌的作用。氨苯碸是最著名的碸類藥。

sulphonylurea *n.* one of a group of drugs, derived from a sulphonamide, that reduce the level of glucose in the blood. These drugs are given by mouth and are used in the treatment of diabetes mellitus. They include *chlorpropamide, *tolazamide, and *tolbutamide.

磺胺醯脲 一組由磺胺衍化而成的藥物，具有降低血中葡萄糖的作用。口服，用於治療糖尿病。這類藥包括氯磺丙脲、甲磺氮䓬脲和甲磺丁脲。

sulphur *n.* a nonmetallic element that is active against fungi and parasites. It is a constituent of ointments and other preparations used in the treatment of skin disorders and infections (such as psoriasis and dermatitis).

硫 非金屬元素，具有抗眞菌和寄生蟲的作用。將硫加入軟膏和其他製劑可用於治療皮膚病和感染，如銀屑病和皮炎。

sulphuric acid a powerful corrosive acid, H_2SO_4, widely used in industry. Swallowing the acid causes severe burning of the mouth and throat and difficulty in breathing, speaking, and swallowing. The patient should drink large quantities of milk or water or white of egg; gastric lavage should not be delayed. Skin or eye contact should be treated by flooding the area with water.

硫酸 一種强腐蝕性酸，分子式爲H_2SO_4，廣泛用於工業。吞飲硫酸引起口、咽部嚴重灼傷，病人呼吸、說話、吞嚥發生困難。搶救病人須飲入大量乳、水或蛋清，立即洗胃。皮膚或眼接觸者須用水冲洗患部。

sulthiame *n.* an *anticonvulsant drug used in the treatment of severe forms of epilepsy. The drug is given by mouth and mild side-effects may develop in some patients, including muscular incoordination, loss of appetite, and headache. Trade name: **Ospolot**.

硫噻嗪 一種用於治療重型癲癇的抗驚厥藥。口服。部分病人可有輕度副作用，如肌肉共濟失調、食慾不振、頭痛。

sunburn *n.* damage to the skin by prolonged or unaccustomed exposure to the sun's rays. Sunburn may vary from reddening of the skin to the development of large painful fluid-filled blisters, which may cause shock if they cover a large area (*see* burn). Fair-skinned people are more susceptible to sunburn than others.

曬傷 長時間日光曝曬或皮膚對曝曬不適應所致的皮膚損害。對曝曬傷的表現多種多樣，從皮膚發紅到疼痛的大型水疱，後者如範圍廣泛，可致休克。皮膚細嫩者易發生曬傷。

sunstroke *n. see* heatstroke.

日射病

super- *prefix denoting* **1.** above; overlying. **2.** extreme or excessive.

〔前綴〕 **①在上，上 ②極，超**

superciliary *adj.* of or relating to the eyebrows (supercilia).

眉的 眼眉的。

superego *n.* (in psychoanalysis) the part of the mind that functions as a moral conscience or judge. It is also responsible for the formation of ideals for the *ego. The superego is the result of the incorporation of parental injunctions into the child's mind.

超我 （精神分析）在意識中具有道德感或對是非的判斷力的那一部分。同時還是自我中理想形成的決定因素。超我是父母的訓誡與孩童時代的心理相結合的結果。

superfecundation *n.* the fertilization of two or more ova of the same age by spermatozoa from different males. *See* superfetation.

同期復孕 來自不同男性的精子使同期2個或更多的卵子同時受精的現象。

superfetation *n.* the fertilization of a second ovum some time after the start

異期復孕 在已經妊娠後一段時間發生第二個卵子

of pregnancy, resulting in two fetuses of different maturity in the same womb.

受精的現象，結果子宮內有2個不同成熟程度的胎兒。

superficial *adj.* (in anatomy) situated at or close to a surface. Superficial blood vessels are those close to the surface of the skin.

淺的 （解剖學）位於或接近表面的。淺血管係指接近皮膚的血管。

superinfection *n.* an infection arising during the course of another infection and caused by a different microorganism, which is usually resistant to the drugs used to treat the primary infection. The infective agent may be a normally harmless inhabitant of the body that becomes pathogenic when other harmless types are removed by the drugs or it may be a resistant variety of the primary infective agent.

重複感染 在一種感染的過程中又發生另一種微生物感染。這種微生物通常對原發感染的治療藥物有抗藥性。這種微生物正常時可以是身體的無害棲居者，而當其他無害細菌被藥物消滅後轉變爲致病性的，或者也可以是原發感染病菌中的耐藥菌株。

superinvolution *n. see* hyperinvolution.

子宮復舊過度

superior *adj.* (in anatomy) situated uppermost in the body in relation to another structure or surface.

上的 （解剖學）位於體內其他結構或表面上部的。

supernumerary *n.* (in dentistry) an additional tooth.

額外牙 （牙科學）附加的牙。

supination *n.* the act of turning the hand so that the palm is uppermost. *Compare* pronation.

旋後 使手掌朝上的旋轉動作。

supinator *n.* a muscle of the forearm that extends from the elbow to the shaft of the radius. It supinates the forearm and hand.

旋後肌 起自肘部止於橈骨幹的前臂肌，使前臂和手旋後。

supine *adj.* **1.** lying on the back or with the face upwards. **2.** (of the forearm) in the position in which the palm of the hand faces upwards. *Compare* prone.

①**仰臥的** 仰面躺下的。②**旋後的（前臂）** 手掌面朝上的。

supplementary benefit *see* National Assistance Act (1945).

補充救濟金

suppository *n.* a medicinal preparation in solid form suitable for insertion into the rectum or vagina. *Rectal suppositories* may contain simple lubricants (e.g. glycerin); drugs that act locally in the rectum or anus (e.g. corticosteroids, local anaesthetics); or drugs that are

栓劑 一種固體型的藥物製劑，通常適用於塞入直腸或陰道內。直腸栓劑可僅含潤滑劑（如甘油）。有的藥物作用於直腸或肛門局部（如皮質類固醇，局部麻醉藥），有的吸收後

absorbed and act at other sites (e.g. *bronchodilators). *Vaginal suppositories* are used to treat some gynaecological disorders (*see* pessary).

在其他部位發生作用（如支氣管擴張藥）。陰道栓劑用於治療某些婦科疾病。

suppression *n.* **1.** the cessation or complete inhibition of any physiological activity. **2.** treatment that removes the outward signs of an illness or prevents its progress. **3.** (in psychology) a *defence mechanism by which a person consciously and deliberately ignores an idea that is unpleasant to him.

①**抑制**　生理活動的靜息或完全停止。　②**控制**　消除疾病外部體徵或防止疾病進展的治療。　③**壓制**　（心理學）一種防禦機制，個體有意識地或蓄意地忽視使他不愉快的觀念。

suppuration *n.* the formation of pus.

化膿　膿液生成。

supra- *prefix denoting* above; over. Examples: *supraclavicular* (above the clavicle); *suprahyoid* (above the hyoid bone); *suprarenal* (above the kidney).

〔前綴〕**在上，上**　例如：鎖骨上的，舌骨上的，腎上的。

supraorbital *adj.* of or relating to the area above the eye orbit.

眶上的　指眼眶上方的區域。

supraorbital reflex the closing of the eyelids when the supraorbital nerve is struck, due to contraction of the muscle surrounding the orbit (orbicularis oculi muscle).

眶上反射　叩擊眶上神經時，由於眶周圍肌（眼輪匝肌）收縮，使眼瞼閉合。

suprarenal glands *see* adrenal glands.

腎上腺

supravital staining the application of a *stain to living tissue, particularly blood cells, removed from the body.

體外活體染色　對活組織、特別是離體血細胞進行染色。

suramin *n.* a nonmetallic drug used in the treatment of *trypanosomiasis. It is usually given by slow intravenous injection. Side-effects, which vary in intensity and frequency and are related to the nutritional state of the patient, include nausea, vomiting, shock, and loss of consciousness.

蘇拉明　一種用於治療錐蟲病的非金屬藥物。通常緩慢靜脉注射。副作用發生的頻率和程度與病人的營養狀況有關，其中包括噁心、嘔吐、休克和喪失意識。

surfactant *n.* a wetting agent: a substance, such as a detergent, that reduces surface tension. A surfactant is secreted by the cells (*pneumocytes) lining the alveoli of the lungs to prevent the alveolar walls from sticking together. In its absence, as in the immature lungs of premature babies and in some diseases,

表面活性物質　濕潤劑，降低表面張力的物質，如去垢劑。鋪襯肺泡的細胞（肺細胞）分泌一種表面活性物質，防止肺泡壁黏貼在一起。在早產兒的不成熟的肺內，以及在某些疾病時，由於缺乏這種表

the lungs tend to collapse. *See* atelectasis, respiratory distress syndrome.

面活性物質，肺會發生萎陷。

surgeon *n.* a qualified medical practitioner who specializes in surgery. *See* doctor.

外科醫師 獲得行醫資格的專長外科的醫師。

surgery *n.* the branch of medicine that treats injuries, deformities, or disease by operation or manipulation. *See also* cryosurgery, microsurgery. —**surgical** *adj.*

外科學 用手術或手法操作治療外傷，畸形和疾病的醫學分支。

surgical neck the constriction of the shaft of the *humerus, below the head. It is frequently the point at which fracture of the humerus occurs.

外科頸 肱骨頭下方的骨幹縮窄部分。爲肱骨骨折的易發部位。

surgical spirit methylated spirit, usually with small amounts of castor oil and oil of wintergreen: used to sterilize the skin before surgery, injections, etc.

外科酒精 含甲醇的酒精，通常含有少量蓖麻油和冬青油。在手術、注射前用於皮膚消毒。

surrogate *n.* (in psychology) a person or object in someone's life that functions as a substitute for another person. In the treatment of sexual problems, when the patient does not have a partner to cooperate in treatment, a surrogate provided by the therapist acts as a sexual partner who gives service to the patient up to and including intercourse. According to psychoanalysts, people and objects in dreams can be surrogates for important individuals in a person's life.

替身 （心理學）在某人的生活中起代替另一人作用的人或物。在性生活障礙的治療中，如果病人沒有一個與之在治療中合作的伴侶，醫者就要提供替身作病人的性伴侶，後者服侍病人甚至與病人性交。精神分析學家認爲，一個人在夢中可以將另一人或物當作其生活中某重要人物的替身。

susceptibility *n.* lack of resistance to disease. It is partly a reflection of general health but is also influenced by vaccination or other methods of increasing resistance to specific diseases.

易感性 對疾病缺乏抵抗力。易感性部分地反映了全身健康狀況。另外，易感性也是可以改變的，如採取接種和其他方法提高對特定疾病的抵抗力。

suspensory bandage a bandage arranged to support a hanging part of the body. Examples include a sling used to hold an injured lower jaw in position and a bandage used to support the scrotum in various conditions of the male genital organs.

懸吊帶 用以支托身體懸吊部分的綳帶。例如，用以使受傷下頜保持適合位置的吊帶，患不同男性生殖器疾病時支托陰囊的綳帶等。

suspensory ligament a ligament that serves to support or suspend an organ in position. For example, the suspensory ligament of the lens is a fibrous structure attached to the ciliary processes (*see* ciliary body) by means of which the lens of the eye is held in position.

懸韌帶 支持或懸吊器官於適當位置的韌帶。例如，晶狀體懸韌帶是附着於睫狀突的纖維性結構，它使眼晶狀體保持於適當位置。

sustentaculum *n.* any anatomical structure that supports another structure. —**sustentacular** *adj.*

支持物 支持其他結構的解剖結構。

suture 1. *n.* (in anatomy) a type of immovable joint, found particularly in the skull, characterized by a minimal amount of connective tissue between the two bones. The cranial sutures include the *coronal suture*, between the frontal and parietal bones; the *lambdoidal suture*, between the parietal and occipital bones; and the *sagittal suture*, between the two parietal bones (see illustration). **2.** *n.* (in surgery) the closure of a wound or incision with material such as silk or catgut, to facilitate the healing process. There is a wide variety of suturing techniques developed to meet the differing circumstances of injuries to and incisions in the body tissues (see illustration). **3.** *n.* the material – silk, catgut, nylon, or wire – used to sew up a wound. **4.** *vb.* to close a wound by suture.

①**縫** （解剖學）一種不能動的關節類型。主要見於顱骨，其特徵爲在兩骨之間僅有極小量結締組織。顱縫包括：冠狀縫，位於額骨與頂骨之間；人字縫，位於頂骨與枕骨之間；矢狀縫，位於兩頂骨之間（見圖）。 ②**縫合術** （外科學）用絲線或腸線等材料閉合創口或切口以促進癒合過程。針對身體組織的不同損傷和切口情況，有多種多樣的縫合技術（見圖）。 ③**縫線** 絲線、腸線、尼龍線或金屬絲等用以縫合創口的材料。 ④**縫合** 用縫線閉合創口。

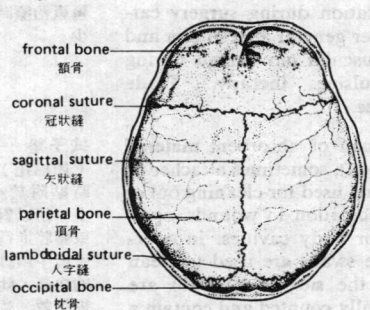

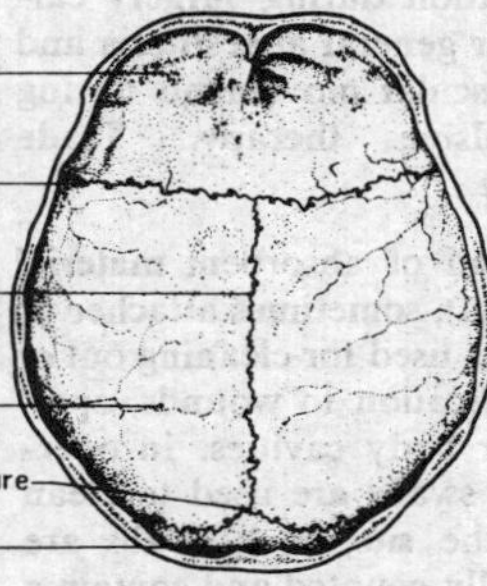

Sutures of the skull (internal surface of the vault)

顱骨諸縫（顱穹的內表面）

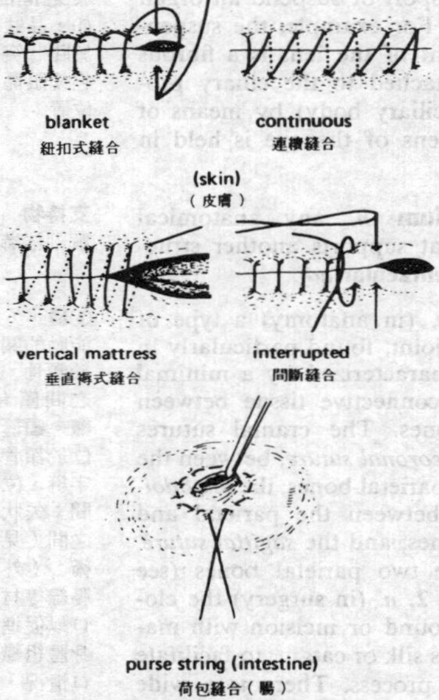

Types of surgical suture
各種外科縫合術式

suxamethonium *n.* a drug that relaxes voluntary muscle (*see* muscle relaxant). It is administered by intravenous injection and is used mainly to produce muscle relaxation during surgery carried out under general anaesthesia and to reduce muscular movements during *electroconvulsive therapy. Trade name: **Scoline**.

琥珀膽鹼 使隨意肌鬆弛的藥物。靜脈內注射。主要用途是在全身麻醉下手術時使肌肉鬆弛以及在電驚厥治療時使肌肉活動減少。

swab *n.* a pad of absorbent material (such as cotton), sometimes attached to a stick or wire, used for cleaning out or applying medication to wounds, operation sites, or body cavities. In operations, gauze swabs are used to clean blood from the site; such swabs are always carefully counted and contain a *radio-opaque 'tag' to facilitate identification should it by mischance remain in the body after operation.

拭子墊 一片吸水材料（如棉花）做的襯墊，有時貼附於小棍或金屬線上，用以對創口、手術野或體腔進行清潔或給藥。手術中用紗布墊清除局部的血液，此種紗布墊須仔細點數，並帶有不透放射線的標簽，以便萬一由於疏忽紗布墊遺留體內時於手術後利於查出。

swallowing (deglutition) *n.* the process by which food is transferred from the mouth to the oesophagus (gullet). Voluntary raising of the tongue forces food backwards towards the pharynx. This stimulates reflex actions in which the larynx is closed by the epiglottis and the nasal passages are closed by the soft palate, so that food does not enter the trachea (windpipe). Lastly, food moves down the oesophagus by *peristalsis and gravity.

吞嚥 食物從口進入食管的過程。舌的隨意升舉將食物向後推向咽部。這一刺激引起反射動作：喉被會厭遮蓋，而鼻的通道為軟腭所關閉，使食物不會進入氣管。最後，食物藉食管的蠕動和重力作用，沿食管向下移動。

sweat *n.* the watery fluid secreted by the *sweat glands. Its principal constituents in solution are sodium chloride and urea. The secretion of sweat is a means of excreting nitrogenous waste; at the same time it has a role in controlling the temperature of the body – the evaporation of sweat from the surface of the skin has a cooling effect. Therefore an increase in body temperature causes an increase in sweating. Other factors that increase the secretion of sweat include pain, nausea, nervousness, and drugs (*diaphoretics). Sweating may be reduced by colds, diarrhoea, and certain drugs. Anatomical name: **sudor**.

汗 汗腺分泌的水樣液體。其溶液中的主要成分是氯化鈉和尿素。泌汗是排出含氮廢物的一種手段，同時在體溫調節中起一定作用——汗在皮膚表面的蒸發起降溫效應。因此，體溫增高引起泌汗增加。使泌汗增多的其他因素有：疼痛、噁心、神經過敏、某些藥物（發汗藥）等。寒冷、腹瀉、某些藥物則使泌汗減少。

sweat gland a simple coiled tubular *exocrine gland that lies in the dermis of the *skin. A long duct carries its secretion (*sweat) to the surface of the skin. Sweat glands occur over most of the surface of the body; they are particularly abundant in the armpits, on the soles of the feet and palms of the hands, and on the forehead.

汗腺 皮膚眞皮內的一種卷繞狀單管外分泌腺。有一長的導管將分泌物（汗）引向皮膚表面。汗腺在體表大部分均有分佈，腋窩，脚底、手掌以及額部尤其豐富。

sycosis *n.* inflammation of the hair follicles caused by bacterial infection. It commonly affects the beard area (*sycosis barbae*) and may cause intense itching. The infection usually spreads unless treated by allowing the beard to grow and applying antibiotic ointments.

鬚瘡 細菌感染所致的毛囊炎症。一般發生於髫鬚部位，可有劇癢。除非留鬚和使用抗生素軟膏治療，感染常可擴展。

symbiosis *n.* an intimate and obligatory association between two different

共生 兩個不同種有機體（共生生物）之間親密和

species of organism (*symbionts*) in which there is mutual aid and benefit. *Compare* commensal, mutualism, parasite.

相互依存的聯合，相互之間存在着互助和互利的關係。

symblepharon *n.* a condition in which the eyelid adheres to the eyeball. It is usually the result of acid or alkali burns to the conjunctiva lining the eyelid and eyeball.

瞼球黏連 眼瞼與眼球的黏連。通常為眼瞼和眼球的結膜被酸、鹼灼傷的結果。

symbolism *n.* (in psychology) the process of representing an object or an idea by something else. Typically an abstract idea is represented by a simpler and more tangible image. Psychoanalytic theorists hold that conscious ideas frequently act as symbols for unconscious thoughts and that this is particularly evident in dreaming, in *free association, and in the formation of psychological symptoms. According to this theory, a symptom (such as difficulty in swallowing) might be a symbolic representation of an unconscious idea (such as a fantasy of oral intercourse). —**symbolic** *adj.*

象徵主義 （心理學）以某物代表某客體或觀念的過程。典型的表現是以某種較簡單和較實在的表象來代表某抽象的觀念。精神分析學說認為，意識中的觀念常常是下意識的思維的符號，這一點在夢、自由聯想和某些精神病症狀的形成中尤為明顯。根據此學說，吞嚥困難之類症狀可能是某種下意識觀念（如經口性交幻想）的象徵性的表現。

symmelia *n.* a developmental abnormality in which the legs appear to be fused.

並腿畸形 一種表現為兩腿融合的發育異常。

symmetry *n.* (in anatomy) the state of opposite parts of an organ or parts at opposite sides of the body corresponding to each other.

對稱 （解剖學）器官的相對部分或身體兩側的部分相互一致的狀況。

sympathectomy *n.* the surgical *division of sympathetic nerve fibres. It is done to minimize the effects of normal or excessive sympathetic activity. Most often it is used to improve the circulation to part of the body; less commonly to inhibit excess sweating or to relieve the *photophobia induced by an abnormally dilated pupil of the eye.

交感神經切除術 手術切斷交感神經纖維。目的是使正常或過高的交感神經活動降至最低程度。最常用於改善身體某部分的循環，其次為抑制過多的泌汗及解除眼瞳孔異常擴大所致的畏光。

sympathetic nervous system one of the two divisions of the *autonomic nervous system, having fibres that leave the central nervous system, via a chain of ganglia close to the spinal cord, in

交感神經系統 植物性神經系統兩部分之一，其纖維自中樞神經系統發出，通過近鄰脊柱的胸腰部神經節鏈繼續行進。纖維分

the thoracic and lumbar regions. Its nerves are distributed to the blood vessels, sweat glands, salivary glands, heart, lungs, intestines and other abdominal organs, and the genitals, whose functions it governs by reflex action, in balance with the *parasympathetic nervous system.

佈於血管、汗腺、唾液腺、心、肺、腸和其他腹腔器官以及生殖器，通過反射活動調節這些器官的機能，與副交感神經系統維持平衡。

sympathin *n.* the name given by early physiologists to the substances released from sympathetic nerve endings, now known to be a mixture of *adrenaline and *noradrenaline.

交感素 早期生理學家對交感神經末梢釋放的物質起的名稱，現今已知爲腎上腺素和去甲腎上腺素的混合物。

sympathoblast *n.* one of the small cells formed in the early development of nerve tissue that eventually become the neurones of the sympathetic nervous system.

成交感神經細胞 神經組織早期發育中生成的一種小細胞，最終變爲交感神經系統的神經元。

sympatholytic *n.* a drug that opposes the effects of the sympathetic nervous system. Drugs such as *guanethidine and *methyldopa block the transmission of impulses along adrenergic nerves; they are used to treat high blood pressure. Drugs such as *phentolamine, *phenoxybenzamine, and *tolazoline block alpha-adrenergic receptors, causing – in particular – dilation of peripheral blood vessels; they are used for disorders of the circulation or to lower the blood pressure. Other sympatholytic drugs are *beta blockers, which selectively block the beta-adrenergic receptors and principally affect the heart.

抗交感神經藥，交感神經阻滯藥 對抗交感神經系統效應的藥物。胍乙啶和甲基多巴等藥物具有阻斷衝動沿腎上腺素能神經傳導的作用，用於治療高血壓。酚胺唑啉、苯氧苄胺和苄唑啉等藥物阻斷 α-腎上腺素能受體，主要引起周圍血管擴張，用於治療循環障礙和降低血壓。另外一些抗交感神經藥物爲 β-阻滯劑，選擇性阻斷 β-腎上腺素能受體，主要影響心臟。

sympathomimetic *n.* a drug that has the effect of stimulating the *sympathetic nervous system. The actions of sympathomimetic drugs are *adrenergic* (resembling those of *noradrenaline). *Alpha-adrenergic* drugs, e.g. *phenylephrine, constrict blood vessels in the skin and intestine and are used in nasal decongestants; *beta-adrenergic* drugs, e.g. *salbutamol, relax bronchial smooth muscle and are used as *bronchodilators. *Ephedrine and *isopre-

擬交感神經藥 具有興奮交感神經系統效應的藥物。其作用爲腎上腺素能性，類似去甲腎上腺素。α-腎上腺素能藥物如苯腎上腺素能使皮膚和腸道血管收縮，可用於消除鼻腔充血。β-腎上腺素能藥物如舒喘靈，使支氣管平滑肌鬆弛，用作支氣管擴張藥。麻黃素和異丙腎上腺素的作用缺少選擇

naline are less selective and have both alpha- and beta-adrenergic effects; if used as bronchodilators, these drugs may have unwanted side-effects on the heart.

性，具有α和β腎上腺素能兩種效應，故當用作支氣管擴張藥時，可產生心臟方面的不良副作用。

sympathy *n.* (in physiology) a reciprocal influence exercised by different parts of the body on one another.

交感作用 （生理學）身體不同部分彼此間遭受對方的影響。

symphysiectomy *n.* removal of a part of the bone at the front of the pelvis (pubic symphysis) in order to aid childbirth.

恥骨聯合切除術 切除骨盆前部（恥骨聯合）的一部分骨以助分娩。

symphysiotomy (symphyseotomy) *n.* incision into the bone at the front of the pelvis (pubic symphysis) in order to enlarge the diameter of the birth passage and aid delivery.

恥骨聯合切開術 切開骨盆前面（恥骨聯合），擴大產道以助分娩。

symphysis *n.* **1.** a joint in which the bones are separated by fibrocartilage, which minimizes movement and makes the bony structure rigid. Examples are the *pubic symphysis* (the joint between the pubic bones of the pelvis) and the joints of the backbone, which are separated by intervertebral discs (see illustration). **2.** the line that marks the fusion of two bones that were separate at an early stage of development, such as the symphysis of the *mandible.

聯合 ①以纖維軟骨隔開兩骨而構成的關節。這種關節活動受限，骨結構變得強硬。此類關節有恥骨聯合（骨盆兩恥骨間的關節）和脊柱關節（由椎間盤隔開）（見圖）。②標誌發育早期分離的兩骨以後融合的線，如下頜聯合。

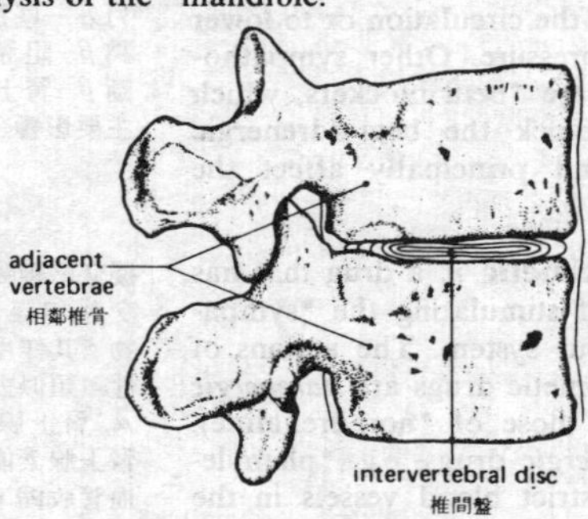

Symphysis between two vertebrae
兩椎骨間的聯合

sympodia (sirenomelia) *n.* a developmental abnormality in which there is

無足並腿畸形 兩腿融合且無足的發育異常。

fusion of the legs with absence of the feet.

symptom *n.* an indication of a disease or disorder noticed by the patient himself. A *presenting symptom* is one that leads a patient to consult a doctor. *Compare* sign.

症狀 由病人自己發現的疾病或障礙的表現。症狀是促使病人就醫的原因之一。

symptomatology (semeiology) *n.* **1.** the branch of medicine concerned with the study of symptoms of disease. **2.** the symptoms of a disease, collectively.

症狀學 ①研究疾病症狀的醫學分支。 ②某種疾病的所有症狀的總稱。

syn- (sym-) *prefix denoting* union or fusion.

〔前綴〕 **融合，聯合**

synalgia *n. see* referred pain.

連帶痛

synapse *n.* the minute gap across which *nerve impulses pass from one neurone to the next, at the end of a nerve fibre. Reaching a synapse, an impulse causes the release of a *neurotransmitter, which diffuses across the gap and triggers an electrical impulse in the next neurone. Some brain cells have more than 15,000 synapses. *See also* neuromuscular junction.

突觸 神經衝動在神經纖維末端從一神經元傳向另一神經元時所跨越的微小間隙。衝動抵達突觸時，引起神經遞質的釋放，遞質彌散越過間隙，觸發另一神經元產生電衝動。一些大腦細胞擁有15000個以上的突觸。

synarthrosis *n.* an immovable joint in which the bones are united by fibrous tissue. Examples are the cranial *sutures. *See also* gomphosis, schindylesis.

不動關節 兩骨之間以纖維組織聯合構成的無活動力的關節。例如顱骨縫。

synchilia (syncheilia) *n.* congenital fusion of the lips.

並唇畸形 先天性唇融合。

synchondrosis *n.* a slightly movable joint (*see* amphiarthrosis) in which the surfaces of the bones are separated by hyaline cartilage, as occurs between the ribs and sternum. This cartilage may become ossified in later development, as between the *epiphyses and shaft of a long bone.

軟骨結合 一種微動關節，兩骨表面以透明軟骨隔開，如肋骨與胸骨之間的關節。透明軟骨在發育晚期骨化，例如長骨骺和幹之間的軟骨。

syncope (fainting) *n.* loss of consciousness induced by a temporarily insufficient flow of blood to the brain. It commonly occurs in otherwise healthy people and may be caused by an

暈厥 由於腦部短暫血流不足所致的意識喪失。常見於健康人，可由情緒打擊、長時站立、外傷、大出血引起。發作逐漸開

emotional shock, by standing for prolonged periods, or by injury and profuse bleeding. An attack comes on gradually, with lightheadedness, sweating, and blurred vision. Recovery is normally prompt and without any persisting ill-effects.

始，伴有頭暈眼花、出汗和視力模糊。一般迅速恢復，不留任何持續的不良後果。

syncytiotrophoblast *n. see* plasmidotrophoblast.

合胞體滋養層

syncytium *n.* (*pl.* **syncytia**) a mass of *protoplasm containing several nuclei. Muscle fibres are syncytia.

合胞體 含有多個核的原漿質體。肌纖維即爲合胞體。

syndactyly *n.* congenital fusion of the fingers or toes. It varies in severity from no more than marked webbing of two or more fingers to virtually complete union of all the digits.

併指（趾）畸形 先天性指或趾的融合。其嚴重程度不等，輕者兩或多指間有不明顯的指蹼，重者所有指節完全融合。

syndesm- (syndesmo-) *prefix denoting* connective tissue, particularly ligaments.

〔前綴〕**結締組織，韌帶**

syndesmology *n.* the branch of anatomy dealing with joints and their components.

韌帶學 研究關節及其組成的解剖學分支。

syndesmophyte *n.* a vertical outgrowth of bone from a vertebra, seen in ankylosing *spondylitis, *Reiter's syndrome, and *psoriatic arthritis. Fusion of syndesmophytes across the joints between vertebrae contributes to rigidity of the spine, seen in advanced cases of these diseases.

韌帶骨贅 脊椎骨上的垂直突出物，見於强直性脊椎炎、萊特氏綜合徵和銀屑病性關節炎。椎骨間的韌帶骨贅如發生跨節融合，可致脊椎强直，見於上述疾病的嚴重病例。

syndesmosis *n.* an immovable joint in which the bones are separated by connective tissue. An example is the articulation between the bases of the tibia and fibula (see illustration).

韌帶聯合 被結締組織隔開的兩骨所形成的不動關節。例如脛骨與腓骨底之間的關節（見圖）。

syndrome *n.* a combination of signs and/or symptoms that forms a distinct clinical picture indicative of a particular disorder.

綜合徵 一些體徵和/或症狀的集合，構成代表某種特殊病患的獨特的臨床徵象。

synechia *n.* an adhesion between the iris and another part of the eye. An *anterior synechia* is between the iris and

虹膜黏連 虹膜與眼其他部分黏連。虹膜前黏連爲虹膜與角膜或鞏膜的一部

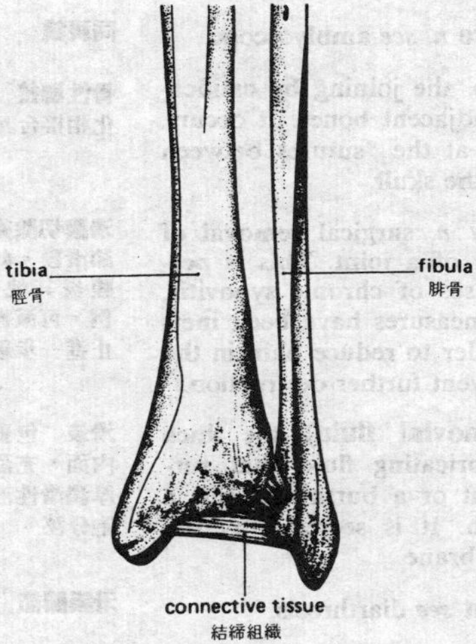

A syndesmosis
韌帶聯合

the cornea or the part of the sclera that normally hides the extreme outer edge of the iris from view. A *posterior synechia* is between the iris and the lens.

（正常時遮蔽鞏膜最外緣的部分）黏連。虹膜後黏連為虹膜與晶體黏連。

syneresis *n.* contraction of a blood clot. When first formed, a blood clot is a loose meshwork of fibres containing various blood cells. Over a period of time this contracts, producing a firm mass that seals the damaged blood vessels.

血塊凝縮　血凝塊收縮。血凝塊剛形成時為內含有各種血細胞的疏鬆網狀物，經過一段時間，血凝塊收縮，變為堅實的團塊，堵塞受損的血管。

synergist *n.* **1.** a drug that interacts with another to produce increased activity, which is greater than the sum of the effects of the two drugs given separately. For example sodium aminosalicylate and streptomycin are used together to treat tuberculosis. Some synergists may have dangerous effects, as when MAO inhibitors enhance the effects of barbiturates. **2.** a muscle that acts with an *agonist in making a particular movement. —**synergism** *n.*

①**協同劑**　與其他藥物協同作用而使活性增高的藥物，增高的程度大於兩藥物分別使用的效應的總和。例如，對氨基水楊酸鈉與鏈黴素聯合應用治療結核病。某些協同劑可有危險的效應，如單氨氧化酶抑制劑可增强巴比妥類的作用。　②**協同肌**　此肌與拮抗肌共同作用產生特定的動作。

syngraft *n. see* isograft.

同基因移植物

synoptophore *n. see* amblyoscope.

同視鏡

synostosis *n.* the joining by ossification of two adjacent bones. It occurs, for example, at the *sutures between the bones of the skull.

骨性聯接　相鄰兩骨以骨化相接合。例如顱骨縫。

synovectomy *n.* surgical removal of the synovium of a joint. This is performed in cases of chronic synovitis, when other measures have been ineffective, in order to reduce pain in the joint and prevent further destruction.

滑膜切除術　手術切除關節滑膜。此術用於慢性滑膜炎其他治療無效的病例，可減輕關節疼痛，防止進一步破壞。

synovia (synovial fluid) the thick colourless lubricating fluid that surrounds a joint or a bursa and fills a tendon sheath. It is secreted by the synovial membrane.

滑液　包裹於關節和滑囊內面，充盈腱鞘的無色稠厚潤滑性液體。由滑液細胞分泌。

synovial joint *see* diarthrosis.

滑膜關節

synovial membrane (synovium) the membrane, composed of mesothelium and connective tissue, that forms the sac enclosing a freely movable joint (*see* diarthrosis). It secretes the lubricating synovial fluid.

滑膜　由間皮和結締組織組成的膜，形成封閉的能自由活動的關節囊。滑膜分泌潤滑性的滑液。

synovioma *n.* a benign or malignant tumour of the synovial membrane. Benign synoviomas occur on tendon sheaths; malignant synoviomas (*synovial sarcomas*) may occur where synovial tissue is not normally found, e.g. in the oesophagus.

滑膜瘤　滑膜的良性或惡性腫瘤。良性者發生於腱鞘，惡性者（滑膜肉瘤）可發生於正常無滑膜組織的部位，如食管內。

synovitis *n.* inflammation of the membrane (synovium) that lines a joint capsule, resulting in pain and swelling (arthritis). It is caused by injury, infection, or rheumatic disease. Treatment depends on the underlying cause; to determine this, samples of the synovial fluid or membrane are taken for examination.

滑膜炎　覆蓋關節囊的滑膜的炎症，引起疼痛和腫脹（關節炎）。原因爲外傷、感染或風濕病。針對病因治療；爲確定病因，可取滑液或滑膜標本作檢查。

synovium *n. see* synovial membrane.

滑膜

syphilide (syphilid) *n.* the skin rash that appears in the second stage of *syphilis, usually two months to two years after primary infection. Syphi-

梅毒疹　出現於梅毒第二期（常爲原發感染後2個月至2年）的皮疹。梅毒疹成批出現，可持續數天

lides occur in crops that may last from a few days to several months. They denote a highly infectious stage of the disease.

至數月。梅毒疹標誌疾病處於高度傳染期。

syphilis *n.* a chronic venereal disease caused by the bacterium *Treponema pallidum*, resulting in the formation of lesions throughout the body. Bacteria usually enter the body during sexual intercourse, through the mucous membranes of the vagina or urethra, but they may rarely be transmitted through skin wounds or scratches. Bacteria may also pass from an infected pregnant woman across the placenta to the developing fetus, resulting in the disease being present at birth (*congenital syphilis*).
The primary symptom – a hard ulcer (*chancre) at the site of infection – forms 2–4 weeks after exposure. Neighbouring lymph nodes enlarge about two weeks later. Secondary stage symptoms appear about two months after infection and include fever, malaise, general enlargement of lymph nodes, and a faint red rash on the chest that persists for 1–2 weeks. After months or even years, the disease enters its tertiary stage with widespread formation of tumour-like masses (*gummas). Tertiary syphilis may cause serious damage to the heart and blood vessels (*cardiovascular syphilis*) or to the brain and spinal cord (*neurosyphilis*), resulting in *tabes dorsalis, blindness, and *general paralysis of the insane.
Treatment with penicillin is fully effective if administered in the early weeks of the infection. Syphilis can be diagnosed by the *Wasserman reaction. *Compare* bejel. —**syphilitic** *adj.*

梅毒 一種由蒼白密螺旋體引起的全身性慢性性病。病原體通常在性交時通過陰道或尿道黏膜侵入體內，偶爾也可通過皮膚傷口或擦傷侵入。病原體還可由妊娠婦女通過胎盤傳給發育中的胎兒，以致出生時即已患病（先天性梅毒）。
初發症狀爲一硬性潰瘍（下疳），位於感染部位，出現於與患者接觸後2～4周。約2周後，附近的淋巴結腫大。感染後約2個月出現第二期症狀，包括發熱、不適、全身淋巴結腫大，胸部出現淡紅皮疹，持續1～2周。數月或數年後，疾病進入第三期，全身廣泛出現腫瘤樣團塊（樹膠腫）。三期梅毒可嚴重損害心臟和血管（心血管梅毒）或腦和脊髓（神經梅毒），導至脊髓痨、盲瞎、全身痲痹和精神錯亂。
治療用青黴素，如在感染最初幾周使用，可獲充分療效。梅毒可用瓦色曼反應診斷。

syring- (syringo-) *prefix denoting* a tube or long cavity, especially the central canal of the spinal cord.

〔前綴〕 **管，長腔** 主要指脊髓中央管。

syringe *n.* an instrument consisting of a piston in a tight-fitting tube that is attached to a hollow needle or thin

注射器 一種器械，由針栓和一與之緊密相配的針管組成，針管上可裝一空

tube. A syringe is used to give injections, remove material from a part of the body, or to wash out a cavity, such as the outer ear.

芯針頭或細管。用於注射，從身體某部吸出物質，冲洗腔室（如冲洗外耳）。

syringobulbia *n. see* syringomyelia.

延髓空洞症

syringocystadenoma (syringoma) *n.* a multiple benign tumour of the sweat glands, which shows as small hard swellings in the skin.

汗腺腺瘤 汗腺多發性良性瘤，表現爲皮內小的硬結。

syringomyelia *n.* a disease of the spinal cord in which longitudinal cavities form within the cord in the cervical (neck) region. The centrally situated cavity (*syrinx*) is especially likely to damage the motor nerve cells and the nerve fibres that transmit the sensations of pain and temperature. Characteristically there is weakness and wasting of the muscles in the hands with a loss of awareness of pain and temperature. An extension of the cavitation into the lower brainstem is called *syringobulbia*. Cerebellar *ataxia, a partial loss of pain sensation in the face, and weakness of the tongue and palate may occur.

脊髓空洞症 一種脊髓疾病。在脊髓頸段內形成一些縱形的腔洞。位於中央的腔洞特別容易損害運動神經細胞以及傳導痛覺和溫度覺的神經纖維。典型表現爲手部肌肉無力羸瘦，疼痛和溫度感覺喪失。腔洞向上擴展到腦幹下部時稱爲延髓空洞症。可出現小腦性共濟失調，面部部分喪失痛覺，舌和腭無力。

system *n.* (in anatomy) a group of organs and tissues associated with a particular physiological function, such as the *nervous system or *respiratory system.

系統 （解剖學）聯合起來完成特定生理機能的一組器官和組織，例如神經系統、呼吸系統。

systemic *adj.* relating to or affecting the body as a whole, rather than individual parts and organs.

系統的，全身的 影響全身而非個別部分或器官的。

systemic circulation the system of blood vessels that supplies all parts of the body except the lungs. It consists of the aorta and all its branches, carrying oxygenated blood to the tissues, and all the veins draining deoxygenated blood into the vena cava. *Compare* pulmonary circulation.

體循環 供應除肺以外身體各部的血管系統。由主動脉及其所有分支（輸送氧合血到組織）以及全部靜脉（將脫氧的血液引入腔靜脉）所組成。

systole *n.* the period of the cardiac cycle during which the heart contracts. The term usually refers to *ventricular systole*, which lasts about 0.3 seconds.

收縮期 心動周期中的心收縮階段。本詞通常指心室收縮期，持續約0.3秒。心房收縮期持續約0.1秒。

Atrial systole lasts about 0.1 seconds. —**systolic** *adj.*

systolic pressure *see* blood pressure. **收縮壓**

T

T

tabes dorsalis (locomotor ataxia) a form of neurosyphilis occurring 5–20 years after the original venereal infection. The infecting organisms progressively destroy the sensory nerves. Severe stabbing pains in the legs and trunk, an unsteady gait, and loss of bladder control are common. Some patients have blurred vision caused by damage to the optic nerves. Penicillin is used to arrest the progression of this illness. *See also* syphilis, general paralysis of the insane.

脊髓痨（運動性共濟失調） 初次感染性病後經過5～20年發生的一型神經梅毒。梅毒的病原體進行性地破壞感覺神經。腿部和軀幹有嚴重的刺痛，步態不穩，並常有膀胱失控。有些病人因視神經損害引起視力模糊。可用青黴素阻止此病的發展。

tablet *n.* (in pharmacy) a small disc containing one or more drugs, made by compressing a powdered form of the drug(s). It is taken by mouth.

片劑 （藥學）以粉劑壓縮製成的含一種或多種藥的小圓片。用於口服。

tabo-paresis *n.* a late effect of syphilitic infection of the nervous system in which the patient shows features of *tabes dorsalis and *general paralysis of the insane.

脊髓痨性麻痹性痴呆 梅毒神經系統感染的遲發反應，病人有脊髓痨特徵，並有精神病性的全身癱瘓。

TAB vaccine a combined vaccine used to produce immunity against the diseases typhoid, paratyphoid A, and paratyphoid B.

傷寒副傷寒菌苗 用於產生免疫以抵抗傷寒、副傷寒A和副傷寒B的一種聯合疫苗。

tachy- *prefix denoting* fast; rapid.

〔前綴〕 **快速**

tachycardia *n.* an increase in the heart rate above normal. *Sinus tachycardia* may occur normally with exercise or excitement or it may be due to illness, such as fever. *Arrhythmias may also produce tachycardia (*ectopic tachycardia*).

心動過速 心率增加超過正常。竇性心動過速可發生於體育鍛煉或情緒激動時，或因疾病引起，例如發熱。心律失常時也可發生心動過速（異位性心動過速）。

tachyphrasia *n.* rapid and voluble speech, such as that encountered in *mania.

言語快速 快速和滔滔不絕的講話，例如發生於躁狂時。

tachyphrenia *n.* excessive rapidity of the mental processes, as in *mania.

精神活動過速 精神活動過度地快速，見於躁狂時。

tachyphylaxis *n.* a falling-off in the effects produced by a drug during continuous use or constantly repeated administration, common in drugs that act on the nervous system.

快速減敏 藥物繼續應用或經常重複應用時發生效果的減退，常見於作用於神經系統的藥物。

tachypnoea *n.* rapid breathing.

呼吸急促 快速的呼吸。

tactile *adj.* relating to or affecting the sense of touch.

觸覺的 與觸覺有關或影響觸覺的。

taenia *n.* (*pl.* **taeniae**) a flat ribbon-like anatomical structure. The *taeniae coli* are the longitudinal ribbon-like muscles of the colon.

帶 扁平的帶狀解剖結構，結腸帶是結腸的縱形帶狀肌肉。

Taenia *n.* a genus of large tapeworms, some of which are parasites of the human intestine. The 4–10 m long beef tapeworm, *T. saginata*, is the commonest tapeworm parasite of man. Its larval stage (*see* cysticercus) develops within the muscles of cattle and other ruminants, and man becomes infected on eating raw or undercooked beef. *T. soleum*, the pork tapeworm, is 2–7 m long. Its larval stage may develop not only in pigs but also in man, in whom it may cause serious disease (*see* cysticercosis). *See also* taeniasis.

絛蟲屬 一屬大型絛蟲，有些寄生於人的腸道。牛肉絛蟲是最常見的寄生於人的絛蟲。幼蟲期是在牛和其它反芻動物的肌肉中發育。而人是在食入生的或半熟的牛肉後被感染。豬肉絛蟲長 2～7 米，幼蟲期不僅可在豬並且也在人身上發育，並可引起嚴重疾病。

taeniacide (taenicide) *n.* an agent that kills tapeworms.

殺絛蟲劑 殺死絛蟲的藥物。

taeniafuge *n.* an agent, such as *dichlorophen, that eliminates tapeworms from the body of their host.

驅絛蟲劑 可以將絛蟲從宿主的體內驅除的一種藥物，例如雙氯酚。

taeniasis *n.* an infestation with tapeworms of the genus **Taenia*. Man becomes infected with the adult worms following ingestion of raw or undercooked meat containing the larval stage of the parasite. The presence of a worm in the intestine may occasionally give rise to increased appetite, hunger pains,

絛蟲病 絛蟲的感染。人在食入生的或半熟的帶有絛蟲幼蟲的肉後，成爲成蟲感染者，有時腸道內有此蟲寄生時，可使食慾增加，出現飢餓性疼痛、虛弱及體重下降。可用各種不同驅腸蟲劑以驅蟲，其

weakness, and weight loss. Worms are expelled from the intestine using various *anthelmintics, including niclosamide, dichlorophen, and quinacrine hydrochloride. *See also* cysticercosis.

中有氯硝柳胺、雙氯酚和鹽酸阿的平。

Tagamet *n. see* cimetidine.

甲氰咪胍

tal- (talo-) *prefix denoting* the ankle bone (talus).

〔前綴〕 **距骨**

talipes *n. see* club-foot.

畸形足

talus (astragalus) *n.* the ankle bone. It forms part of the *tarsus, articulating with the tibia above, with the fibula to the lateral (outer) side, and with the calcaneus below.

距骨 組成跗骨的一部分，上方與脛骨相關節，外側與腓骨相關節，下方與跟骨相關節。

tambour *n.* a recording drum consisting of an elastic membrane stretched over one end of a cylinder. It is used in various instruments for recording changes in air pressure.

氣鼓 一種鼓形記錄器。在圓筒的一端，張以彈性膜而成。用於記錄氣體壓力改變的各種儀器上。

tamoxifen *n.* a drug used in the treatment of advanced breast cancer. It combines with hormone receptors in the tumour to inhibit the effect of oestrogens. Side-effects are uncommon but include facial flushing, tumour pain, and hypercalcaemia. Trade name: **Nolvadex.**

三苯氧胺 治療進展型乳腺癌的藥物。它與腫瘤的激素感受器結合以抑制雌激素的作用。副作用不常見，但可有面紅、腫瘤疼痛和高血鈣。

tampon *n.* a pack of gauze, cotton wool, or other absorbent material used to plug a cavity or canal in order to absorb blood or secretions. A vaginal tampon is commonly used by women to absorb the menstrual flow.

塞子 填塞腔或管道以吸收血液或分泌液的一團紗布、藥棉或者其它有吸收力的材料。陰道塞子通常是被婦女用於吸收月經血液的。

tamponade *n.* **1.** the insertion of a tampon. **2.** abnormal pressure on a part of the body; for example, as caused by the presence of excessive fluid between the pericardium (sac surrounding the heart) and the heart.

填塞 ①將塞子插入。②身體某部不正常的壓迫。例如：由於心包膜（包住心臟的囊）和心臟之間液體過多所引起。

tantalum *n.* a rare heavy metal used in surgery as it is easily moulded and does not corrode. For example, tantalum sutures and plates are used for repair of defects in the bones of the skull. Symbol: Ta.

鉭 一種稀有重金屬。由於它易於鑄造和不被腐蝕而在外科應用，例如：鉭製的縫線或板用於修補顱骨缺損。

tapetum *n.* **1.** a layer of specialized reflecting cells in the *choroid behind the retina of the eye. **2.** a band of nerve fibres that form the roof and wall of the lower posterior part of the *corpus callosum.

毯 ①眼睛視網膜後脉絡膜裏一層特殊反射性細胞。②構成胼胝體下後部分的頂部和壁部的一束神經纖維。

tapeworm *n.* any of a group of flatworms that have a long thin ribbon-like body and live as parasites in the intestines of man and other vertebrates. The body of a tapeworm consists of a head (*scolex*), a short neck, and a *strobila* made up of a chain of separate segments (*proglottides*). Mature proglottides, full of eggs, are released from the free end of the worm and pass out in the host's stools. Eggs are then ingested by an intermediate host, in whose tissues the larval stages develop (*see* plerocercoid, cysticercus, hydatid). Man is the primary host for some tapeworms (*see* Taenia, Hymenolepis). However, other genera are also medically important (*see* Diphyllobothrium, Dipylidium, Echinococcus).

縧蟲 一組細長帶狀的扁形蟲類，寄生於人或其它脊椎動物的腸道。縧蟲分爲頭部、短的頸部和由許多節段（節片）構成的鏈狀體部。成熟的節片充滿蟲卵，並從成蟲的游離端釋放出來，在宿主的大便中排出。然後蟲卵被中間宿主攝入，在它的組織中發育爲幼蟲。人是有些縧蟲的終宿主（如豬肉縧蟲、牛肉縧蟲、膜殼縧蟲），但是另一些種類的縧蟲同樣也有醫學上的重要性。

tapotement *n.* a technique used in *massage in which a part of the body is struck rapidly and repeatedly with the hands. Tapotement of the chest wall in bronchitic patients often helps to loosen mucus within the air passages so that it can be coughed up.

叩撫法 一種按摩的方法，用手迅速與重復地擊打身體某部，於支氣管炎病人施行胸壁叩撫法，有助於氣道內的黏液鬆解、使之易被咳出。

tapping *n. see* paracentesis.

穿刺放液法

target cell (in haematology) an abnormal form of red blood cell (*erythrocyte) in which the cell assumes the ringed appearance of a 'target' in stained blood films. Target cells are a feature of several types of anaemia, including those due to iron deficiency and abnormalities in haemoglobin structure.

靶形細胞 （血液病學）一種不正常形狀的紅細胞，在染色的血片中這種細胞呈現爲靶環狀。靶形細胞是幾種類型貧血的特徵，例如由於缺鐵和血紅蛋白結構異常引起的貧血。

target organ the specific organ or tissue upon which a hormone, drug, or other substance acts.

靶器官 被激素、藥物或其它物質作用的特異器官和組織。

tars- (tarso-) *prefix denoting* **1.** the ankle; tarsal bones. **2.** the edge of the eyelid.

〔前綴〕 ①**跗骨** 踝下部的幾塊足骨。 ②**眼瞼緣**

tarsal 1. *adj.* relating to the bones of the ankle and foot (*tarsus). **2.** *adj.* relating to the eyelid, esp. to its supporting tissue (tarsus). **3.** *n.* any of the bones forming the tarsus.

①**跗骨的** 踝關節下部諸骨的。 ②**眼瞼的** 尤指其支持組織（瞼板的）。 ③**跗骨**

tarsalgia *n.* aching pain arising from the tarsus in the foot.

跗骨痛 跗骨發生的疼痛。

tarsal glands *see* meibomian glands.

瞼板腺

tarsectomy *n.* **1.** surgical excision of the tarsal bones of the foot. **2.** surgical removal of a section of the tarsus of the eyelid.

①**跗骨切除術** 切除跗骨的手術。 ②**瞼板切除術** 切除瞼板的手術。

tarsitis *n.* inflammation of the eyelid.

瞼板炎 眼瞼發炎。

tarsoplasty *n. see* blepharoplasty.

瞼成形術

tarsorrhaphy *n.* an operation in which the upper and lower eyelids are joined together, either completely or along part of their length. It is performed to protect the cornea or to allow a corneal injury to heal.

瞼縫合術 將上下眼瞼縫在一起的手術。或完全縫合或縫其長度的一部分。其目的是保護角膜，或使角膜的損傷癒合。

tarsus *n.* (*pl.* **tarsi**) **1.** the seven bones of the ankle and proximal part of the foot (see illustration). The tarsus articulates with the metatarsals distally and with the tibia and fibula proximally. **2.** the firm fibrous connective tissue that forms the basis of each eyelid.

①**跗骨** 位於踝關節下部和足部近端的幾塊骨（見圖）。跗骨遠端與蹠骨相聯接，近端與脛骨和腓骨相接。②**瞼板** 構成眼瞼主要成分的堅韌的纖維性結締組織。

tartar *n.* an obsolete term for *calculus, the hard deposit that forms on the teeth.

牙石 牙齒上形成的硬的沉積物。爲廢用詞。

tartar emetic *see* antimony potassium tartrate.

吐酒石 酒石酸銻鉀。

taste *n.* the sense for the appreciation of the flavour of substances in the mouth. The sense organs responsible are the *taste buds on the surface of the

味覺 辨別口腔內物質味道的感覺。這種感覺器官是舌表面的味蕾。當口腔內食物在唾液裏溶解時，

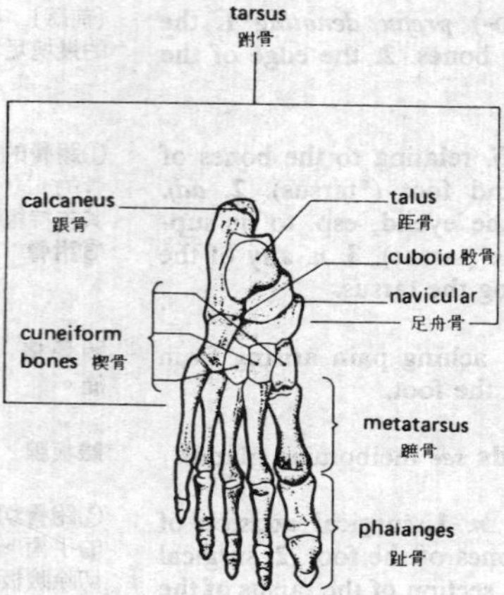

Bones of the right ankle and foot
右踝和右足骨

*tongue, which are stimulated when food dissolves in the saliva in the mouth. It is generally held that there are four basic taste sensations – sweet, bitter, sour, and salt – but two others – alkaline and metallic – are sometimes added to this list.

它就被刺激。通常認爲有四種主要味覺——甜、苦、酸和鹹，但另外二種味，即鹼味和金屬味有時也算兩種味覺。

taste buds the sensory receptors concerned with the sense of taste (see illustration). They are located in the epithelium that covers the surface of the *tongue, lying in the grooves around the papillae, particularly the circumvallate papillae. Taste buds are also present in the soft palate, the epiglottis, and parts of the pharynx. When a taste cell is stimulated by the presence of a dissolved substance impulses are sent via nerve fibres to the brain. From the anterior two-thirds of the tongue impulses pass via the facial nerve. The taste buds in the posterior third of the tongue send impulses via the glossopharyngeal nerve.

味蕾 與味覺有關的感覺感受器（見圖），它位於舌表面的上皮內，舌乳頭（尤其是輪廓乳頭）週圍的溝裏。味蕾也存在於軟腭、會厭和咽的一部分。當味覺細胞被溶解的食物刺激後，衝動就通過神經纖維傳送至大腦。舌前三分之二的衝動通過面神經，舌後三分之一的味蕾是通過舌咽神經傳送衝動的。

taurine *n.* an amino acid that is a constituent of the *bile salt tauroch-

牛磺酸 一種氨基酸，爲牛磺膽酸鹽的組成成分，

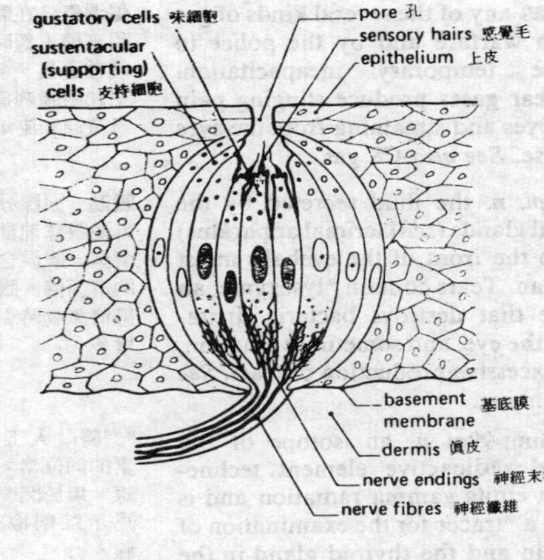

Structure of a taste bud
味蕾的結構

late and also functions as a *neurotransmitter in the central nervous system.

在中樞神經系統中也起神經遞質的作用。

taurocholic acid *see* bile acids.

牛磺膽酸

taxis *n.* (in surgery) the returning to a normal position of displaced bones, organs, or other parts by manipulation only, unaided by mechanical devices.

整復法 （外科）僅用手法而不用器械使錯位的骨、器官或其它部分回復到正常位置。

Tay-Sachs disease (amaurotic familial idiocy) an inherited disorder of lipid metabolism (*see* lipidosis) in which abnormal accumulation of lipid in the brain leads to blindness, mental retardation, and death in infancy. The gene responsible for the disorder is *recessive, and the disease can now be largely prevented by genetic counselling in communities known to be affected.

家族黑矇性白痴 遺傳性脂肪代謝障礙。脂肪在大腦異常蓄積，引起失明，精神發育遲滯，並在嬰兒期死亡。這種病變的基因是隱性遺傳的。由於在已知患病人羣中開展遺傳諮詢，目前此病基本上得到預防。

TCP *Trade name*. a solution of trichlorphenol: an effective *antiseptic for minor skin injuries and irritations. It may also be used as a gargle for colds and sore throats.

三氯苯酚 三氯苯酚溶液的商品名。是皮膚輕微損傷和刺激的有效抗菌劑，也可作爲含漱劑用於感冒和咽痛。

tear gas any of the several kinds of gas used in warfare and by the police to produce temporary incapacitation. Most tear gases produce stinging pain in the eyes and streaming from the eyes and nose. *See also* CS gas.

催淚氣 在戰爭中或警察用來使人暫時失去能力的幾種毒氣。多數催淚氣可引起眼睛刺痛，並從眼和鼻流淚和流涕。

tears *pl. n.* the fluid secreted by the lacrimal glands (*see* lacrimal apparatus) to keep the front of the eyeballs moist and clean. Tears contain *lysozyme, an enzyme that destroys bacteria. Irritation of the eye, and sometimes emotion, cause excessive production of tears. *See also* blinking.

眼淚 淚腺分泌的液體。可使眼球前部保持濕潤和清潔。眼淚含有消滅細菌的溶菌酶。眼睛受刺激和感情激動時引起眼淚分泌增多。

technetium-99m *n.* an isotope of the artificial radioactive element technetium. It emits gamma radiation and is used as a *tracer for the examination of the brain and the thyroid gland in the technique of scintigraphy.

^{99m}鍀 人工放射性鍀元素的同位素。它發射γ射線。用於閃爍照相，可作爲示踪劑檢查腦和甲狀腺。

tectospinal tract a tract that conveys nerve impulses from the midbrain, across the midline as it descends, to the spinal cord in the cervical (neck) region. It contains important *motor neurones.

頂蓋脊髓束 傳遞神經衝動的傳導束，自中腦經過中線下降達頸髓部位，它包含有重要的運動神經元。

tectum *n.* the roof of the *midbrain, behind and above the *cerebral aqueduct. From the nerve tissue protrude two pairs of rounded swellings called the *superior* and *inferior colliculi*, which contain cells concerned with reflexes involving vision and hearing, respectively.

頂蓋 中腦的頂部，在大腦導水管的後上方。從神經組織突出兩對圓形的隆起稱爲上丘和下丘，其中分別含有與視覺和聽覺反射有關的細胞。

teeth *pl. n. see* tooth.

牙

tegmen *n.* (*pl.* **tegmina**) a structure that covers an organ or part of an organ. For example the *tegmen tympani* is the bony roof of the middle ear.

蓋 遮蓋一器官或器官一部分的結構。例如鼓室蓋是中耳的頂部。

tegmentum *n.* the region of the *midbrain below and in front of the *cerebral aqueduct. It contains the nuclei of several cranial nerves, the *reticular formation, and other ascending and descending nerve pathways linking the forebrain and the spinal cord.

大腦脚蓋 大腦導水管前下方的中腦部位，其中包含有幾種顱神經核、網狀結構和聯接前腦和脊髓的其他上行的神經通路。

teichopsia *n.* shimmering coloured lights, accompanied by blank spots in the visual field (*transient scotomata*), often seen by sufferers at the beginning of an attack of migraine.

閃光暗點　感覺有色光線閃爍伴有視野空白點（短暫的暗點），常見於偏頭痛發作開始的患者。

tel- (tele-, telo-) *prefix denoting* **1.** end or ending. **2.** distance.

〔前綴〕 ①**末端**　②**距離**

tela *n.* any thin weblike tissue, particularly the *tela choroidea*, a folded double layer of *pia mater containing numerous small blood vessels that extends into several of the *ventricles of the brain.

組織　薄的蛛網狀組織，尤指脉絡組織，爲折疊雙層的含有很多小血管的軟腦膜，並延伸至大腦的一些腦室中去。

telangiectasis (*pl.* **telangiectases**) a localized collection of distended blood capillary vessels. It is recognized as a red spot, sometimes spidery in appearance, that blanches on pressure. Telangiectases may be found in the skin or the lining of the mouth, gastrointestinal, respiratory, and urinary passages. The condition in which multiple telangiectases occur is termed *telangiectasia*. It may be seen as an inherited condition associated with a bleeding tendency (*haemorrhagic telangiectasia*). Accessible bleeding telangiectases (e.g. in the nose) may be obliterated by cauterization.

毛細血管擴張　局部擴張的毛細血管的聚集。看起來像是紅的斑點，有時似蜘蛛狀，壓迫後褪色。毛細血管擴張可以發生在皮膚，或在口腔、胃腸道、呼吸道和尿路的內面。有多發性毛細血管擴張的症狀時稱之爲毛細血管擴張症。可以認爲是一種有出血傾向的遺傳性疾病。易出血的毛細血管擴張（如在鼻腔）可用燒灼法使血管閉塞。

telangiitis *n.* inflammation of the smallest blood vessels (*see* angiitis).

毛細血管炎　最小的血管發炎。

teleceptor *n.* a sensory *receptor that is capable of responding to distant stimuli. An example is the eye, which is capable of detecting changes and happenings at a great distance, unlike touch receptors, which require close contact.

距離感受器　可對距離較遠的刺激發生反應的感覺感受器。例如眼睛，它能察覺遠距離的變化和事件，這與需緊密接觸的觸覺感受器不同。

telecurietherapy *n.* a form of *radiotherapy in which penetrating radiation is directed at a patient from a distance. Originally radium was used as the radiation source; today artificial radioactive isotopes, such as cobalt-60, are used.

遠距離治療　放射治療的一種類型，即穿透性射線從一段距離外對着病人。原先曾用鐳作放射源，如今採用人工的放射性同位素，如 ^{60}鈷。

telegony *n.* the unsubstantiated theory that mating with one male has an effect on the offspring of later matings with other males.

前父遺傳 一種虛幻的假設，指與一個男子結過婚會影響與另一個男人結婚的後代。

telencephalon *n. see* cerebrum.

端腦

teleradiography *n.* a form of *radiography in which the X-ray source is situated about 2 metres from the patient, which produces X-ray pictures with less distortion.

遠距X線照像術 將X射線源置於距患者約2米遠的一種X射線照像術，所得到的X線像很少失真。

telocentric *n.* a chromosome in which the centromere is situated at either of its ends. —**telocentric** *adj.*

端着絲粒 着絲粒位於兩側末端的一種染色體。

telodendron *n.* one of the branches into which the *axon of a neurone divides at its destination. Each telodendron finishes as a terminal *bouton*, which takes part in a *synapse or a *neuromuscular junction.

終樹突 神經元的軸索在其終點分成的分支，每個終樹突的最末端似一個終鈕，它參與形成突觸或神經肌肉接頭。

telophase *n.* the final stage of *mitosis and of each of the divisions of *meiosis, in which the chromosomes at each end of the cell become long and thin and the nuclear membrane reforms around them. The cytoplasm begins to divide.

末期 有絲分裂的最後期和減數分裂的每次分裂的最末期。此時染色體在細胞兩端變得長而細，並在其周圍重新形成核膜，細胞漿開始分裂。

temple *n.* the region of the head in front of and above each ear.

顳部 頭部耳前上方的部位。

temporal *adj.* of or relating to the temple.

顳的 有關顳部的。

temporal arteritis *see* arteritis.

顳動脈炎

temporal artery a branch of the external carotid artery that supplies blood mainly to the temple and scalp.

顳動脈 頸內動脈的分支，其血液主要供應顳部和頭皮。

temporal bone either of a pair of bones of the cranium. The *squamous* portion forms part of the side of the cranium. The *petrous* part contributes to the base of the skull and contains the middle and inner ears. Below it are the *mastoid process, *styloid process, and zygomatic process (*see* zygomatic arch). *See also* skull.

顳骨 頭顱兩側的一對骨。其鱗狀部構成顱骨的側面部分，岩部構成頭顱的基底部，並包括了中耳和內耳，其下方是乳突、莖突和顴突。

temporalis *n.* a fan-shaped muscle situated at the side of the head, extend-

顳肌 位於頭部側面的扇形肌肉，起自顳窩到達下

ing from the temporal fossa to the mandible. This muscle lifts the lower jaw, thus closing the mouth.

頜骨。該肌肉能抬舉下頜使嘴關閉。

temporal lobe one of the main divisions of the *cerebral cortex in each hemisphere of the brain, lying at the side within the temple of the skull and separated from the frontal lobe by a cleft, the *lateral sulcus*. Areas of the cortex in this lobe are concerned with the appreciation of sound and spoken language.

顳葉 大腦兩半球皮層的主要部分之一，位於頭顱兩側顳部內，並由一裂將其與額葉分開。該葉的皮層區與聲音和語言的刺激有關。

temporal lobe epilepsy *see* epilepsy.

顳葉癲癇

temporo- *prefix denoting* **1.** the temple. **2.** the temporal lobe of the brain.

〔前綴〕 ①**顳部** ②**大腦顳葉**

temporomandibular joint the articulation between the *mandible and the *temporal bone: a hinge joint (*see* ginglymus).

顳下頜關節 下頜骨與顳骨之間的關節，是屈戌關節。

temporomandibular joint syndrome a condition in which the patient has painful temporomandibular joints, tenderness in the muscles that move the jaw, clicking of the joints, and limitation of jaw movement.

顳下頜關節綜合徵 病人有顳下頜關節疼痛，下頜運動的肌肉有觸痛，關節有卡噠聲以及下頜活動受限等病狀。

tenaculum *n.* **1.** a sharp wire hook with a handle. The instrument is used in surgical operations to pick up pieces of tissue or the cut end of an artery. **2.** a band of fibrous tissue that holds a part of the body in place.

①**把持鈎** 銳利的金屬絲鈎，有柄，用於外科手術要提起一塊組織時或切割一動脉終端時。 ②**支持體** 將身體組織某部維持於適當位置的纖維組織帶。

tendinitis *n.* inflammation of a tendon. It occurs most commonly after excessive overuse but is sometimes due to bacterial infection (e.g. *gonorrhoea), or a generalized rheumatic disease (e.g. *rheumatoid arthritis, ankylosing spondylitis). Treatment is by rest, achieved sometimes by splinting the adjacent joint, and corticosteroid injection into the tender area around the tendon. Tendinitis at the insertion of the supraspinatus muscle is a frequent cause of pain and restricted movement in the shoulder. *See also* tennis elbow. *Compare* tenosynovitis.

腱炎 肌腱發炎。最常發生於運動過度後，但有時可由於細菌感染（如淋病）或全身性風濕性疾病（即類風濕性關節炎，强直性脊椎炎）引起。治療：休息，有時用夾板固定鄰近關節，於肌腱周圍壓痛區注射皮質類固醇。岡上肌肌肉附着處腱炎是肩痛的常見原因，並使肩活動受限。

tendon *n.* a tough whitish cord, consisting of numerous parallel bundles of collagen fibres, that serves to attach a muscle to a bone. Tendons are inelastic but flexible; they assist in concentrating the pull of the muscle on a small area of bone. Some tendons are surrounded by *tendon sheaths* – these are tubular double-layered sacs lined with synovial membrane and containing synovial fluid. Tendon sheaths enclose the flexor tendons at the wrist and ankle, where they minimize friction and facilitate movement. *See also* aponeurosis. —**tendinous** *adj.*

肌腱 許多平行的膠原纖維束構成的堅韌白色索帶。它的作用是使肌肉連接於骨上。肌腱無彈性但可彎曲，它可協助將肌肉的牽拉力集中在骨的一小區域上，有些肌腱外包腱鞘，腱鞘是管形雙層腔，內襯滑膜，含有滑液，腱鞘包住腕和踝的屈肌肌腱，可減少摩擦和易於活動。

tendon organ (Golgi tendon organ) a sensory *receptor found within a tendon that responds to the tension or stretching of the tendon and relays impulses to the central nervous system. Like stretch receptors in muscle, tendon organs are part of the *proprioceptor system.

腱感受器（高爾基氏腱器） 存在於肌腱內的感覺感受器，接受肌腱的張力和牽張的刺激，並向中樞神經系統傳送衝動。與肌肉的牽張感受器相似，腱感受器是本體感受器系統的一部分。

tendovaginitis (tenovaginitis) *n.* inflammatory thickening of the fibrous sheath containing one or more tendons, usually caused by repeated minor injury. It usually occurs at the back of the thumb (*de Quervain's tendovaginitis*) and results in pain on wringing the wrists. Treatment is by rest, injection of cortisone into the tendon sheath, and, if these fail, surgical incision of the sheath.

腱鞘炎 一個或一個以上肌腱纖維鞘的炎症性增厚，通常是因反覆輕微損傷引起，常發生在拇指背面，在擰手腕時引起疼痛。治療：休息，腱鞘內注射皮質激素，若無效可手術切開腱鞘。

tenesmus *n.* a sensation of the desire to defecate, which is continuous or recurs frequently, without the production of significant amounts of faeces (often small amounts of mucus or blood alone are passed). This uncomfortable symptom may be due to *proctitis, prolapse of the rectum, rectal tumour, or *irritable bowel syndrome.

裏急後重 持續的或頻繁重複的便意感而無足夠量的大便（常僅排出小量黏液和血），這種不適症狀可能因直腸炎、直腸脫垂、直腸腫瘤或腸道激惹綜合徵引起。

tennis elbow a painful inflammation of the tendon at the outer border of the elbow, caused by overuse of the forearm muscles. Treatment is by rest,

撓肱骨黏液囊炎（網球肘） 肘部外緣肌腱疼痛性炎症，是由於前臂肌肉應用過度引起。治療：休

massage, and local corticosteroid injection. *See also* tendinitis.

息、按摩和局部皮質類固醇注射。

teno- *prefix denoting* a tendon.

〔前綴〕 **腱**

Tenon's capsule the fibrous tissue that lines the orbit and surrounds the eyeball.

特農氏囊（眼球囊） 覆蓋在眼眶內面包繞眼球的纖維組織。

tenoplasty *n.* surgical repair of a ruptured or severed tendon.

腱成形術 外科修復破裂的或嚴重損傷的肌腱。

tenorrhaphy *n.* the surgical operation of uniting the ends of divided tendons by suture.

腱縫合術 用縫合法將肌腱裂開端連接的外科手術。

tenosynovitis (peritendinitis) *n.* inflammation of a tendon sheath, producing pain, swelling, and an audible creaking on movement. It may result from a bacterial infection or occur as part of a rheumatic disease causing *synovitis.

腱鞘炎 腱鞘的炎症，引起疼痛、腫脹，並在活動時可聽到吱嘎聲。可因細菌感染引起，或是引起滑膜炎的風濕性疾病的一部分。

tenotomy *n.* surgical *division of a tendon. This may be necessary to correct a joint deformity caused by tendon shortening or to reduce the imbalance of forces caused by an overactive muscle in a spastic limb. *See also* scissor leg.

腱切斷術 切斷肌腱的手術。為糾正因肌腱短縮所引起的關節畸形，或使痙攣的肢體減輕肌肉力量的不平衡時，可能需做這種手術。

tenovaginitis *n. see* tendovaginitis.

腱鞘炎

tensor *n.* any muscle that causes stretching or tensing of a part of the body.

張肌 使身體某部伸長或緊張的肌肉。

tent *n.* **1.** an enclosure of material (usually transparent plastic) around a patient in bed, into which a gas or vapour can be passed as part of treatment. An *oxygen tent* is relatively inefficient as a means of administering oxygen; a face mask or intranasal oxygen are used where possible. **2.** a piece of dried vegetable material, usually a seaweed stem, shaped to fit into an orifice, such as the cervical canal. As it absorbs moisture it expands, providing a slow but forceful means of dilating the orifice.

①**帷帳** 臥床病人周圍的圍帳（通常是用透明的塑料做的）。可充入氣體或蒸氣，作為治療的一部分。氧氣帳是效率比較低的給氧方法，如有可能則用面罩或鼻管吸氧。 ②**塞條** 一片乾的植物材料，通常是海藻莖。使其形狀適合於進入管口，例如子宮頸管。由於它能吸收水分而擴張，可作為緩慢的但強有力的擴張管口的方法。

tentorium *n.* a curved infolded sheet of *dura mater that dips inwards from the

幕 硬腦膜彎曲折疊而形成的覆蓋物。它從顱骨內

skull and separates the cerebellum below from the occipital lobes of the cerebral hemispheres above.

傾斜延伸，並將下面的小腦與上面的大腦半球枕葉分隔開。

terat- (terato-) *prefix denoting* a monster or congenital abnormality.

〔前綴〕 **畸胎，先天性異常**

teratogen *n.* any substance, agent, or process that induces the formation of developmental abnormalities in a fetus. Known teratogens include such drugs as *thalidomide and alcohol; such infections as German measles and cytomegalovirus; and irradiation with X-rays and other ionizing radiation. *Compare* mutagen. —**teratogenic** *adj.*

致畸形物 導至胎兒發育畸形的物質、藥物或過程。已知的致畸形物有：藥物，如反應停和乙醇；某些感染，如風疹和巨細胞病毒；以及X線和其他電離輻射的照射等。

teratogenesis *n.* the process leading to developmental abnormalities in the fetus.

畸形形成 導至胎兒期發育異常的過程。

teratology *n.* the study of developmental abnormalities and their causes.

畸形學 對發育異常及其原因的研究。

teratoma *n.* a tumour composed of a number of tissues not usually found at that site. Teratomas most frequently occur in the testis and ovary, possibly derived from remnants of embryological cells that have the ability to differentiate into many types of tissue. *Malignant teratoma of the testis* is found in young men: it is most common in the undescended testis. Like *seminoma, it frequently occurs as a painless swelling of one testis (pain is not a good indication that the swelling is benign). Treatment is by *orchidectomy avoiding an incision into the scrotum. The tumour can spread to lymph nodes, lungs, and bone, treatment of which may involve the use of radiotherapy and drugs such as vinblastine, bleomycin, and platinum compounds. Teratomas often produce *alpha-fetoprotein, beta human chorionic gonadotrophin, or both; the presence of these substances in the blood is a useful indication of the amount of tumour and the effect of treatment.

畸胎瘤 由許多不常見於該部位的組織所構成的腫瘤。畸胎瘤最常發生在睾丸和卵巢，可能來源於殘餘的胚胎細胞，它能分化爲多種類型的組織。睾丸惡性畸胎瘤見於年輕人，最常發生於未下降的睾丸，與精原細胞瘤類似，常表現爲一側睾丸無痛性腫脹（疼痛不是惡性腫瘤的可靠指標）。治療是作避免切開陰囊的睾丸切除術。該腫瘤可播散到淋巴結、肺和骨。治療可以採用放射治療和藥物，如長春鹼、爭光黴素和鉑化合物。畸胎瘤常產生甲胎蛋白，β-人絨毛膜促性腺激素或兩者都有。這些物質在血液中存在是腫瘤大小和治療效果的有意義的指標。

terbutaline *n.* a *bronchodilator drug used in the treatment of asthma, bron-

叔丁喘寧 治療哮喘、支氣管炎和其它呼吸系病變

chitis, and other respiratory disorders. It may be given by mouth, injection, or inhalation; common side effects include nervousness and dizziness. Trade name: **Bricanyl**.

的支氣管擴張藥。可以口服、注射或吸入，常見的副作用有神經激動和頭暈。

teres *n.* either of two muscles of the shoulder, extending from the scapula to the humerus. The *teres major* draws the arm towards the body and rotates it inwards; the *teres minor* rotates the arm outwards.

圓肌 肩部的兩塊肌肉，從肩胛骨到肱骨。大圓肌使上臂內收並內旋，小圓肌使上臂外旋。

terpene *n.* any of a group of unsaturated hydrocarbons many of which are found in plant oils and resins and are responsible for the scent of these plants (e.g. mint). Larger terpenes include vitamin A, squalene, and the carotenoids.

萜 一組未飽和的碳氫化合物，多數存在於植物油和樹脂，並具有這些植物的香味（如薄荷）。較大的萜類有維生素A、鯊烯以及類胡蘿蔔素。

Terramycin *n. see* oxytetracycline.

土黴素

tertian fever *see* malaria.

間日瘧

tertigravida (trigravida) *n.* a woman who has been pregnant three times.

孕$_3$ 曾妊娠 3 次的婦女。

tertipara (tripara) *n.* a woman who has been pregnant at least three times and who has given birth to an infant capable of survival after each of three pregnancies.

產$_3$ 至少妊娠 3 次的婦女，並每次所生的嬰兒均能存活。

tesla *n.* the *SI unit of magnetic flux density, equal to a density of 1 weber per square metre. Symbol: T.

特〔斯拉〕 磁通量密度的國際單位，相當於每平方米 1 韋〔伯〕的密度。符號：T。

testicle *n.* either of the pair of male sex organs within the scrotum. It consists of the *testis and its system of ducts (the vasa efferentia and epididymis).

睾丸 陰囊內一對男性性器官。它包括有睾丸與輸精管道系統（輸精管與附睾）。

testis *n.* (*pl.* **testes**) either of the pair of male sex organs that produce spermatozoa and secrete the male sex hormone *androgen under the control of *gonadotrophins from the pituitary gland. The testes of the fetus form within the abdomen but descend into the *scrotum in order to maintain a lower temperature that favours the pro-

睾丸 一對男性性器官，能產生精子和在垂體促性腺激素控制下分泌男性激素——雄性素。胎兒時睾丸在腹腔內形成，但以後下降至陰囊以保持有利於精子產生和貯存的較低溫度，睾丸由長而紆曲的細精管構成（見圖）。精

duction and storage of spermatozoa. The bulk of the testis is made up of long convoluted *seminiferous tubules* (see illustration), in which the spermatozoa develop (*see* spermatogenesis). The tubules also contain *Sertoli cells, which may nourish developing sperm cells. Spermatozoa pass from the testis to the *epididymis to complete their development. The *interstitial* (*Leydig*) *cells*, between the tubules, are the major producers of androgen.

子在細精管發育，細精管也有滋養細胞，它能營養正在發育的精子。精子通過睾丸到達附睾，完成了它的發育過程。在細精管之間的間質細胞是分泌雄性素的主要細胞。

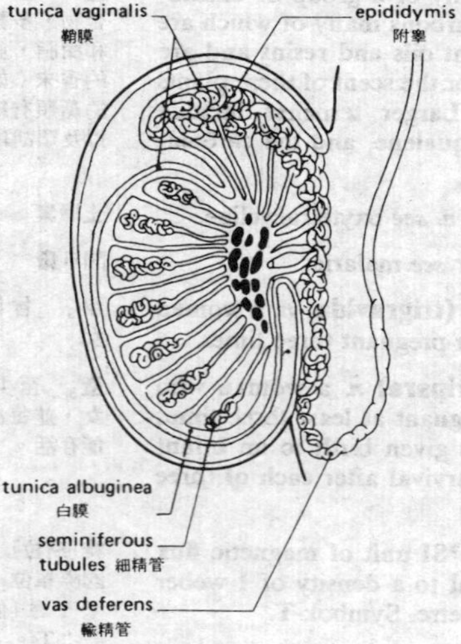

Longitudinal section through a testis
睾丸的縱切面

test meal a standard meal given to stimulate secretion of digestive juices, which can then be withdrawn by tube and measured as a test of digestive function. A *fractional test meal* was a gruel preparation to stimulate gastric secretion, whose acid content was measured. This has been replaced by tests using histamine or pentagastrin as secretory stimulants. The *Lundh test meal* is a meal of oil and protein to stimulate pancreatic secretion, which is withdrawn from the duodenum and its

試餐 刺激消化液分泌的標準膳食。進試餐後用管子抽吸消化液，並作測定，可作為消化功能的一種試驗。功能性試餐是一種糊劑，用來刺激胃分泌，並測定其酸含量。此種試餐已被分泌刺激劑組織胺或五肽胃泌素試驗所替代。朗得氏試餐是一種油和蛋白組成的膳食，用於刺激胰腺分泌，從十二指腸抽吸出胰液，並測定

trypsin content measured as a test of pancreatic function.

其胰蛋白酶含量，為檢查胰腺功能的一種試驗。

testosterone *n.* the principal male sex hormone (*see* androgen).

睾酮 主要的男性激素。

test-tube baby a baby born to a woman as a result of fertilization of one of her ova by her husband's sperm outside her body (*in vitro fertilization*). This technique, pioneered in Britain, resulted in the birth of a live baby girl in July 1978. It is useful when the woman has blocked Fallopian tubes or some similar defect in the reproductive system. The mother-to-be is given a short course of hormones, causing several ova to mature at the same time. Several ova are removed using a *laparoscope. The ova are mixed with sperm in a culture medium and incubated until the *blastocyst forms. The blastocyst is then implanted in the mother's womb and the pregnancy continues normally thereafter.

試管嬰兒 婦女的卵子和其丈夫的精子在體外受精（試管受精）結果而誕生的嬰兒。此方法始創於美國，於 1978 年 7 月分娩一活嬰。此方法用於婦女有輸卵管阻塞或生殖系統有某些類似的缺陷時。給未來的母親短療程的激素，使幾個卵同時成熟，用腹腔鏡將幾個卵取出，將卵和精子在培養基裏混合並孵化，直至胚泡形成，將胚泡植入於母體子宮內，然後妊娠就正常地繼續。

tetan- (tetano-) *prefix denoting* **1.** tetanus. **2.** tetany.

〔前綴〕 ①**破傷風** ②**手足搐搦**

tetanolysin *n.* a toxin produced by tetanus bacilli in an infected wound, causing the local destruction of tissues.

破傷風溶解毒素 破傷風桿菌在感染的傷口產生的毒素。引起組織局部破壞。

tetanospasmin *n.* a toxin produced by tetanus bacilli in an infected wound. The toxin diffuses along nerves, causing paralysis, and may reach the spinal cord and brain, when it causes violent muscular spasms and the condition of lockjaw.

破傷風痙攣毒素 破傷風桿菌在感染的傷口產生的毒素。此毒素沿神經瀰散，造成癱瘓，並可到達脊髓和大腦，引起肌肉劇烈痙攣和牙關緊閉症狀。

tetanus (lockjaw) *n.* an acute infectious disease, affecting the nervous system, caused by the bacterium *Clostridium tetani*. Infection occurs by contamination of wounds by bacterial spores. Bacteria multiply at the site of infection and produce a toxin that irritates nerves so that they cause spasmodic contraction of muscles. Symptoms appear 4–25 days after infection and consist of muscle stiffness, spasm,

破傷風 破傷風梭狀芽胞桿菌引起的侵犯神經系統的急性傳染病。由於細菌芽胞接觸傷口而引起感染。細菌在感染部位繁殖，並產生毒素刺激神經，因而引起肌肉痙攣性收縮。感染後 4～25 天出現症狀，有肌肉僵硬、痙攣，然後發生强直，先是在下頷和頸部，以後是在

and subsequent rigidity, first in the jaw and neck then in the back, chest, abdomen, and limbs; in severe cases the spasm may affect the whole body, which is arched backwards (*see* opisthotonos). High fever, convulsions, and extreme pain are common. If respiratory muscles are affected, a *tracheostomy is essential to avoid death from asphyxia. Mortality is high in untreated cases but prompt treatment with penicillin and antitoxin is effective. An attack does not confer immunity. Immunization against tetanus is effective but temporary. —**tetanic** *adj.*

背部、胸部和四肢。在嚴重病例痙攣可侵犯全身。背向後彎曲呈弓形。常有高熱、驚厥和劇烈疼痛。若呼吸肌受侵犯時，爲了避免窒息死亡很重要的是做氣管切開。不治療的病例死亡率很高，但迅速果斷地應用青黴素和抗毒素治療是有效的。一次患病後不產生免疫。抗破傷風的免疫法是有效的，但效果是暫時的。

tetany *n.* spasm and twitching of the muscles, particularly those of the face, hands, and feet. Tetany is caused by a reduction in the blood calcium level, which may be due to underactive parathyroid glands, rickets, or *alkalosis.

手足搐搦 肌肉痙攣和抽動，特別是面部、手和足的肌肉。手足搐搦是因血鈣水平減低而引起，而血鈣低可能是由於甲狀旁腺功能低下、佝僂病或鹼中毒。

tetra- *prefix denoting* four.

〔前綴〕 **四**

tetrachloroethylene *n.* an *anthelmintic drug used in the treatment of hookworm disease. It is given by mouth. Toxic side-effects are rare, but vertigo and headache frequently occur and patients with severe anaemia may collapse during treatment.

四氯乙烯 治療鈎蟲病的驅腸蟲劑，用於口服。毒性副作用少見，但常發生頭暈和頭痛，有嚴重貧血的病人治療期間可能發生虛脫。

tetracycline *n.* **1.** one of a group of *antibiotic compounds derived from cultures of *Streptomyces* bacteria. These drugs, which include *chlortetracycline, doxycycline, *oxytetracycline, and tetracycline, are effective against a wide range of bacterial infections. They are usually given by mouth to treat various conditions, including respiratory-tract infections, syphilis, and acne. Side-effects such as nausea, vomiting, and diarrhoea are fairly common. In addition, suppression of normal intestinal bacteria may make the patient susceptible to infection with tetracycline-resistant organisms. Tetracyclines

①**四環素族** 從鏈球菌屬培養液中取得的一組抗菌化合物。這類藥物包括有金黴素、强力黴素、土黴素和四環素，對廣譜細菌感染有效，通常用於口服治療各種疾病，如呼吸道感染，梅毒和痤瘡。較常發生的副作用有噁心，嘔吐與腹瀉。此外，正常腸道細菌被四環素族抑制後，病人易受抗藥性細菌感染。妊娠4個月後不應服用四環素，對於幼兒也要避免應用，以防止恒牙被染成難看的顏色。②

should not be administered after the fourth month of pregnancy and their use should be avoided in young children to prevent unsightly staining of the permanent teeth. **2.** a particular antibiotic of the tetracycline group. Trade names: **Achromycin, Steclin.**

四環素 專指四環素族中一種特殊的抗生素。

tetrad *n.* (in genetics) **1.** the four cells resulting from meiosis after the second telophase. **2.** the four chromatids of a pair of homologous chromosomes (*see* bivalent) in the first stage of meiosis.

①**四裂體** （遺傳）第二次減數分裂末期後形成的四個細胞。 ②**四分體** 在減數分裂第一期時一對同源染色體的四個染色體單體。

tetradactyly *n.* a congenital abnormality in which there are only four digits on a hand or foot.

四指（趾） 手或脚僅有四指（趾）的先天性異常。

tetrahydrocannabinol *n.* a derivative of marijuana that has antiemetic activity and also produces euphoria. These two properties are utilized in the prevention of chemotherapy-induced sickness.

四氫大麻酚 大麻的衍生物，有止嘔作用，並能產生欣快感，可以這兩種特性防治化療引起的嘔吐。

tetrahydrozoline *n.* a drug that constricts blood vessels and is used as a nasal decongestant. *See* vasoconstrictor.

四氫萘唑啉 血管收縮藥，用作鼻腔減充血劑。

tetralogy of Fallot a form of congenital heart disease in which there is *pulmonary stenosis, enlargement of the right ventricle, a ventricular *septal defect, and in which the origin of the aorta lies over the septal defect. The affected child is blue (cyanosed) and frequently squats. The defect is corrected surgically.

法樂氏四聯徵 有肺動脉狹窄、右心室肥大、室間隔缺損，以及主動脉起端位於缺損間隔上方的一種先天性心臟病。患病兒童有紫紺，並常常蹲坐。手術可糾正這種缺損。

tetraplegia *n. see* quadriplegia.

四肢癱瘓

T-group *n.* a group of people who meet in order to increase their sensitivity and their skills in human relationships by discussing themselves and their relationships. Such groups are sometimes formed in the training of psychiatric staff (the *T* stands for *training*).

T人羣 聚集一起的一組人羣，通過討論他們自己及其相互關係，來增加他們在人際關係方面的感受和技能，在訓練精神病學工作人員時有時組織這樣的人羣(T意指"訓練")。

thalam- (thalamo-) *prefix denoting* the thalamus. Example: *thalamolenticular* (relating to the thalamus and lenticular nucleus of the brain).

〔前綴〕 **丘腦** 例如丘腦豆狀核的（有關丘腦和大腦豆狀核的）。

thalamencephalon *n.* the structures, collectively, at the anterior end of the brainstem, comprising the *epithalamus, *thalamus, *hypothalamus, and subthalamus, all of which are concerned with the reception and processing of information entering from sensory nerve pathways.

丘腦 集合在腦幹前端的一組結構，包括丘腦上部、丘腦、丘腦下部和丘腦底部，都與接受和處理來自感覺神經通路的信息有關。

thalamic syndrome a raised threshold to pain stimuli combined with a highly unpleasant burning quality to any pain that is experienced once the threshold is exceeded. It is caused by disease affecting the *thalamus at the upper end of the brainstem.

丘腦綜合徵 疼痛刺激的閾值提高，同時對任何疼痛有極不適的燒灼感，一旦超過此閾值時就有這種感受。是由於腦幹上端受損害所引起。

thalamotomy *n.* an operation on the brain in which a lesion is made in a precise part of the *thalamus. It has been used to control psychiatric symptoms of severe anxiety and distress, in which cases the lesion is made in the dorsomedial nucleus of the thalamus, which connects with the frontal lobe. *See also* psychosurgery.

丘腦切開術 一種腦部手術，即在丘腦的一定部位造成一種損傷。此法用於控制有嚴重焦慮和痛苦的精神症狀。在這些病例，是損傷與額葉相連的丘腦中線核。

thalamus *n.* (*pl.* **thalami**) one of two egg-shaped masses of grey matter that lie deep in the cerebral hemispheres in each side of the forebrain. The thalami are relay stations for all the sensory messages that enter the brain, before they are transmitted to the cortex. All sensory pathways, except that for the sense of smell, are linked to nuclei within the thalamus, and it is here that the conscious awareness of messages as sensations – temperature, pain, touch, etc. – probably begins.

丘腦 兩個卵圓形灰質團塊，位於大腦半球深部前腦的兩側。丘腦是所有感覺的信息在傳入大腦皮層之前的中繼站。除嗅覺外，所有感覺通路與丘腦內的核連接，就在此處可能開始對感覺的信息（如溫度、疼痛、觸覺等等）有有意識的辨認。

thalassaemia (Cooley's anaemia) *n.* a hereditary blood disease, widespread in the Mediterranean countries, Asia, and Africa, in which there is an abnormality in the protein part of the *hae-

地中海貧血（庫利氏貧血） 一種遺傳性疾病，廣泛分佈於地中海國家、亞洲和非洲。該病時血紅蛋白分子中的蛋白發生異

moglobin molecule. The affected red cells cannot function normally, leading to anaemia. Other symptoms include enlargement of the spleen and abnormalities of the bone marrow. Individuals inheriting the disease from both parents are severely affected (*thalassaemia major*), but those inheriting it from only one parent are usually symptom-free. Patients with the major disease are treated with repeated blood transfusions. The disease can be detected by prenatal diagnosis, including *amniocentesis.

常。病變的紅細胞不能正常地發揮作用而導至貧血。其它症狀有脾腫大和骨髓異常。從父母雙方遺傳患病者病變嚴重（重型地中海貧血），但僅從父母一方遺傳往往症狀不明顯。重症地中海貧血病人的治療是反覆輸血。通過產前診斷，如羊膜穿刺術，可以發現此病。

thalassotherapy *n.* treatment by remedial bathing in sea water.

海水療法 在海水中作治療性洗浴的療法。

thalidomide *n.* a drug that was formerly used as a sedative. If taken during the first three months of pregnancy, it was found to cause fetal abnormalities involving limb malformation; i.e. it has a teratogenic effect. For this reason thalidomide has now been withdrawn from clinical use.

反應停 過去用作鎮靜劑的一種藥物。若在妊娠開始三個月期間服用，可以引起胎兒發育異常，即致畸形作用。因此反應停在臨床應用中已被淘汰。

thallium *n.* a leadlike element that has several dangerously poisonous compounds. The poison is cumulative and causes liver and nerve damage and bone destruction. The victim's hair is likely to fall out and does not grow again. Treatment is by administration of *chelating agents. Symbol: Tl.

鉈 一種類似鉛的元素。它有幾種危險性毒性化合物。毒物蓄積，並引起肝和神經損害以及骨破壞，中毒者可能脫髮，並且不再生長。治療是採用絡合劑。符號：Tl

thanat- (thanato-) *prefix denoting* death.

〔前綴〕 **死**

theca *n.* a sheathlike surrounding tissue. For example, the *theca folliculi* is the outer wall of a *Graafian follicle.

膜 包圍組織的鞘狀膜，例如卵泡膜是格雷夫氏卵膜的外壁。

theine *n.* the active volatile principle found in tea (*see* caffeine).

咖啡因異構體 茶中發現的揮發性有效成分。

thenar *n.* **1.** the palm of the hand. **2.** the fleshy prominent part of the hand at the base of the thumb. *Compare* hypothenar. —**thenar** *adj.*

①**手掌** ②**魚際** 指手的拇指根部肉厚的隆起部分。

theobromine *n.* an alkaloid, occurring in cocoa, that has a weak diuretic action

可可鹼 可可內的一種鹼，有弱的利尿作用，並

and dilates coronary and other arteries. It was formerly widely used to treat angina.

能擴張冠狀動脈和其它動脈，過去曾廣泛用於治療心絞痛。

theomania *n.* a delusional belief that one is God.

神仙妄想 相信某人是神仙的一種妄想。

theophylline *n.* an alkaloid, occurring in the leaves of the tea plant, that has a diuretic effect and relaxes smooth muscles, especially of the bronchi. Theophylline preparations, particularly *aminophylline, are used mainly to control bronchial asthma.

茶鹼 茶葉中所含的生物鹼。具有利尿、鬆弛平滑肌，特別是支氣管平滑肌的作用。茶鹼製劑，尤其是氨茶鹼，主要用於控制支氣管哮喘。

theotherapy *n.* faith healing.

宗教療法 信仰療法。

therapeutics *n.* the branch of medicine that deals with different methods of treatment and healing (*therapy*), particularly the use of drugs in the cure of disease.

治療學 研究不同治療方法的醫學分支。尤指應用藥物治療疾病的方法。

therm *n.* a unit of heat equal to 100,000 British thermal units. 1 therm = 1.055 × 10^8 joules.

克卡 熱單位，相等於 100 000 英國的熱單位，1 克卡＝1.055×10^8 焦耳。

therm- (thermo-) *prefix denoting* **1.** heat. **2.** temperature.

〔前綴〕 ①**熱** ②**溫度**

thermoalgesia (thermalgesia) *n.* an abnormal sense of pain that is felt when part of the body is warmed. It is a type of *dysaesthesia and is a symptom of partial damage to a peripheral nerve or to the fibre tracts conducting temperature sensation to the brain.

熱性痛覺 身體某部分熱時所感到的異常疼痛感覺。這是感覺遲鈍的一種類型。是周圍神經或向大腦傳導溫覺的纖維束部分受損的症狀。

thermoanaesthesia *n.* absence of the ability to recognize the sensations of heat and coldness. When occurring as an isolated sensory symptom it indicates damage to the spinothalamic tract in the spinal cord, which conveys the impulses of temperature to the thalamus.

溫覺缺失 辨認熱和冷感覺的能力缺失。若作爲孤立的感覺症狀出現時，提示脊髓中向丘腦傳送溫度衝動的的脊髓丘腦束受損害。

thermocautery *n.* the destruction of unwanted tissues by heat (*see* cauterize).

熱烙術 用熱破壞無用的組織。

thermocoagulation *n.* the coagulation and destruction of tissues by cautery.

熱凝固術 用燒灼術將組織凝固或破壞。

thermography *n.* a technique for measuring and recording the heat produced by different parts of the body: by using photographic film sensitive to infrared radiation. The picture produced is called a *thermogram*. The heat radiated from the body varies in different parts according to the flow of blood through the vessels; thus areas of poor circulation produce less heat. On the other hand a tumour with an abnormally increased blood supply may be revealed on the thermogram as a 'hot spot'. The technique has been used in the diagnosis of tumours of the breast (*mammothermography*).

溫度記錄法 應用對紅外線輻射敏感的照相底片測定和記錄身體不同部位產熱的一種技術。所得的照片叫做溫度記錄圖。身體不同部位的熱輻射隨血管內的血流情況而不同，循環較差的部位產熱較少。相反，血液供應異常增加的腫瘤在溫度記錄圖上可顯示出"熱斑"區，此方法曾用於診斷乳房腫瘤（乳房溫度記錄法）。

thermolysis *n.* (in physiology) the dissipation of body heat by such processes as the evaporation of sweat from the skin surface.

熱放散 （生理學）通過汗液從皮膚表面蒸發的過程使身體散熱。

thermometer *n.* a device for registering temperature. A *clinical thermometer* consists of a sealed narrow-bore glass tube with a bulb at one end. It contains mercury, which expands when heated and rises up the tube. The tube is calibrated in degrees, and is designed to register temperatures between 35°C (95°F) and 43.5°C (110°F). An *oral thermometer* is placed in the mouth; a *rectal thermometer* is inserted into the rectum.

溫度計 記錄溫度的儀表。臨床用的體溫計是一個密封的細玻璃管，在其一端有一個小球，球中充有水銀。遇熱時水銀膨脹並上昇到玻管內，玻管上標記刻度，可記錄 35℃（95℉）和 43.5℃（110℉）之間的溫度。口溫度計是置於口腔內的。而肛門溫度計是將溫度計插入直腸。

thermophilic *adj.* describing organisms, especially bacteria, that grow best at temperatures of 48–85°C. *Compare* mesophilic, psychrophilic.

嗜熱的 形容在溫度 48～85℃時生長最好的微生物，特別是細菌。

thermophore *n.* any substance that retains heat for a long time, such as kaolin, which is often used in hot poultices.

保熱劑 能長時間保熱的一種物質，例如高嶺土，它常用於泥敷劑內。

thermoreceptor *n.* a sensory nerve ending that responds to heat or to cold. Such *receptors are scattered widely in the skin and in the mucous membrane of the mouth and throat.

溫度感受器 對熱或冷反應的感覺神經末梢。這種感受器廣泛分佈於皮膚以及口腔和咽部的黏膜裏。

thermotaxis *n.* the physiological process of regulating or adjusting body temperature.

體溫調節 調節和調整人體溫度的生理過程。

thermotherapy *n.* the use of heat to alleviate pain and stiffness in joints and muscles and to promote an increase in circulation. *Diathermy provides a means of generating heat within the tissues themselves.

溫熱療法 應用熱來減輕關節和肌肉的疼痛和僵硬，並使循環量增加，透熱療法是使肌肉內產熱的方法。

thiacetazone (thioparamizone) *n.* a drug used in the treatment of leprosy and (in combination with *isoniazid) tuberculosis. The drug is administered by mouth. Toxic effects, though infrequent, are severe and include anorexia, hepatitis, and exfoliative dermatitis.

氨硫脲 用於治療麻瘋和結核（與異烟肼聯合應用）的藥物。該藥用於口服。毒性反應雖然少見，但却嚴重，有食慾喪失、肝炎和剝脫性皮炎。

thiamin *n. see* vitamin B_1.

硫胺〔素〕

Thiersch's graft (split-skin graft) a type of skin graft in which thin partial thicknesses of skin are cut in narrow strips and placed onto the wound area to be healed.

提爾施氏移植片（分層皮移植片） 一種皮膚移植片，即將分層（不是全層）皮膚片切成窄條，置於傷口區上面，以使其癒合。

thioguanine *n.* a drug that prevents the growth of cancer cells and is used in the treatment of leukaemia. It is given by mouth and commonly reduces the numbers of white blood cells and platelets. Other side-effects include nausea, vomiting, loss of appetite, and jaundice. Trade name: **Lanvis**.

硫鳥嘌呤 防止腫瘤細胞生長的藥物，可治療白血病。用於口服，通常會使白細胞和血小板減少。副作用有噁心、嘔吐、食慾喪失和黃疸。

thioparamizone *n. see* thiacetazone.

氨硫脲

thiopentone *n.* a short-acting *barbiturate. It is given by intravenous injection to produce general *anaesthesia or as a premedication prior to surgery. Possible complications of thiopentone anaesthesia include respiratory depression, laryngeal spasm, and thrombophlebitis. The drug is not used when respiratory obstruction is present. Trade name: **Pentothal**.

硫噴妥鈉 短時作用的巴比妥酸鹽。用於靜脉注射以產生全身性麻醉，或作爲外科術前用藥。硫噴妥鈉麻醉可能發生的併發症有呼吸抑制、喉痙攣和血栓性靜脉炎。當有呼吸道阻塞時，此藥不宜應用。

thiophilic *adj.* growing best in the presence of sulphur or sulphur compounds. The term is usually applied to bacteria.

嗜硫的 在有硫或硫化物存在時生長最佳的。通常指細菌。

thiopropazate *n.* a major *tranquillizer similar to *chlorpromazine in its actions and effects. It is given by mouth to treat agitated psychotic patients with anxiety states and to control nausea and vomiting. Trade name: **Dartalan**.

奮乃靜醋酯 一種重要的鎮靜藥，其作用和療效與氯丙嗪相類似。此藥用於口服治療有焦慮狀態的精神病患者，亦用於控制噁心與嘔吐。

thioridazine *n.* a major *tranquillizer used in the treatment of a wide range of mental and emotional disturbances, including schizophrenia and senile dementia. The drug is given by mouth; side-effects include faintness, dizziness, dry mouth, and impairment of sexual function. Trade name: **Melleril**.

甲硫噠嗪 一種重要的鎮靜劑，廣泛用於治療精神和情緒紊亂，如精神分裂症和老年性痴呆。此藥用於口服，副作用有暈厥、頭暈、口乾以及性功能減退。

thiotepa *n.* a *cytotoxic drug. It is given by injection to treat cancer of the breast or ovary, lymphoma, and sarcoma. The most serious side-effects are on the blood-forming tissues, resulting in a reduction in white blood cells and platelets. Headache, nausea, and vomiting may also occur.

噻替哌 細胞毒性藥物。用於注射治療乳腺癌或卵巢癌、淋巴瘤和肉瘤。最嚴重的副作用是在造血組織，可引起白細胞和血小板減少，也可發生頭痛、噁心和嘔吐。

thiouracil *n.* a drug that is used in the treatment of overactivity of the thyroid gland (thyrotoxicosis). It is given by mouth; side-effects include fever, skin reactions, jaundice, and *agranulocytosis.

硫尿嘧啶 治療甲狀腺功能亢進（甲狀腺毒症）的藥物。口服。副作用有發熱、皮膚反應、黃疸和粒細胞缺乏。

thorac- (thoraco-) *prefix denoting* the thorax or chest.

〔前綴〕 **胸，胸廓**

thoracectomy *n.* an operation in which the chest cavity is opened (thoracotomy) and a rib or part of a rib is removed.

胸廓部分切除術 打開胸腔的一種手術（胸廓切開術），並將肋骨或肋骨的一部分切除。

thoracentesis *n. see* pleurocentesis.

胸腔穿刺術

thoracic cavity the chest cavity. *See* thorax.

胸腔

thoracic duct one of the two main trunks of the *lymphatic system. It receives lymph from both legs, the lower abdomen, left thorax, left side of the head, and left arm and drains into the left innominate vein.

胸導管 淋巴系統的兩個主幹之一。它接受來自雙下肢、下腹部、左胸、左側頭部和左臂的淋巴液，導入左側無名靜脈。

thoracic vertebrae the 12 bones of the *backbone to which the ribs are

胸椎 脊柱與肋骨相連接的 12 個脊柱骨，它們位

attached. They lie between the cervical (neck) and lumbar (lower back) vertebrae and are characterized by the presence of facets for articulation with the ribs. *See also* vertebra.

於頸椎和腰椎之間，與肋骨相接處有一小平面。

thoracocentesis *n. see* pleurocentesis.

胸腔穿刺術

thoracoplasty *n.* the surgical repair of abnormalities or defects of the thorax.

胸廓成形術 修復胸廓的異常和缺陷的手術。

thoracotomy *n.* surgical opening of the chest cavity to inspect or operate on the heart, lungs, or other structures within.

胸廓切開術 手術切開胸腔對心臟、肺或胸腔內其它結構進行探查或手術。

thorascope *n.* an instrument used to inspect the *pleural cavity.

胸腔鏡 探查胸腔的器械。

thorax *n.* the chest: the part of the body cavity between the neck and the diaphragm. The skeleton of the thorax is formed by the sternum, costal cartilages, ribs, and thoracic vertebrae of the backbone. It encloses the lungs, heart, oesophagus, and associated structures. *Compare* abdomen. —**thoracic** *adj.*

胸廓 頸和膈之間的體腔部分。胸廓是由胸骨、肋軟骨、肋骨和脊柱的胸椎構成的骨架。它將肺、心臟、食管和相關結構包圍在內。

thorium-X *n.* the radioactive isotope radium-224, which emits alpha radiation and has several applications in *radiotherapy. *See also* radium.

釷-X 放射性同位素 ^{224}鐳，它發射 α 射線，在放射治療方面有幾種不同的用途。

threadworm *n. see* pinworm.

線蟲

threonine *n.* an *essential amino acid. *See also* amino acid.

蘇氨酸（β-羥丁氨酸） 一種必需氨基酸。

threshold *n.* (in neurology) the point at which a stimulus begins to evoke a response, and therefore a measure of the sensitivity of a system under particular conditions. A *thermoreceptor that responds to an increase in temperature of only two degrees is said to have a much lower threshold than one that will only respond to a change in temperature of ten degrees or more. In this example the threshold can be measured directly in terms of degrees.

閾值 （神經病學）刺激開始引起反應的起始點，因而也是對特定情況下的一個系統的敏感性的測量。溫度僅升高 2 度時就起反應的溫度感受器的閾，比僅對溫度變化 10 度以上才起反應的溫度感受器閾值要低得多，在這個例子中閾值可直接以度數來測定。

thrill *n.* a vibration felt on placing the hand on the body. A heart murmur that

震顫 將手置於身體上感到的顫動。心臟雜音可在

is felt by placing the hand on the chest wall is said to be accompanied by a thrill.

胸壁上被手感覺到，稱之爲伴有震顫。

-thrix *suffix denoting* a hair or hairlike structure.

〔後綴〕 **毛** 指毛髮或類似毛髮的結構。

thromb- (thrombo-) *prefix denoting* **1.** a blood clot (thrombus). **2.** thrombosis. **3.** blood platelets.

〔前綴〕 ①**血凝塊（血栓）** ②**血栓形成** ③**血小板**

thrombasthenia *n.* a hereditary blood disease in which the function of the *platelets is defective although they are present in normal numbers. The manifestations are identical to those of thrombocytopenic *purpura.

血小板機能不全 一種遺傳性血液病，病時血小板數雖正常，但血小板功能有缺陷，臨床表現與血小板減少性紫癜相似。

thrombectomy *n.* a surgical procedure in which a blood clot (thrombus) is removed from an artery or vein (*see* endarterectomy, phlebothrombosis).

血栓切除術 一種外科手術，將血凝塊（血栓）從動脉或靜脉內切除。

thrombin *n.* a substance (*coagulation factor) that acts as an enzyme, converting the soluble protein fibrinogen to the insoluble protein fibrin in the final stage of *blood coagulation. Thrombin is not normally present in blood plasma, being derived from an inactive precursor, *prothrombin*.

凝血酶 在凝血過程的最後階段使可溶性纖維蛋白原轉變成不溶性纖維蛋白的起酶作用的物質（凝血因子）。正常血漿內不存在凝血酶，它是從非活動性的前體——凝血酶原衍生而來。

thromboangiitis obliterans *see* Buerger's disease.

閉塞性血栓性脉管炎

thrombocyte *n. see* platelet.

血小板

thrombocythaemia *n.* a disease in which there is an abnormal proliferation of the cells that produce blood *platelets (*megakaryocytes), leading to an increased number of platelets in the blood. This may result in an increased tendency to form clots within blood vessels (thrombosis); alternatively the function of the platelets may be abnormal, leading to an increased tendency to bleed. Treatment is by radiotherapy or by *cytotoxic drugs.

血小板增多症 生成血小板的細胞（巨核細胞）異常增生，導至血液中血小板增多的疾病。可使血管內形成血凝塊（血栓形成）的傾向增加。另一方面，血小板的功能可不正常，導至出血傾向增加。治療是用放射療法或用細胞毒藥物。

thrombocytopenia *n.* a reduction in the number of *platelets in the blood. This results in bleeding into the skin

血小板減少症 血液中血小板數減少。可引起皮膚出血（紫癜），自發性的

(*see* purpura), spontaneous bruising, and prolonged bleeding after injury. Thrombocytopenia may result from failure of platelet production or excessive destruction of platelets. —**thrombocytopenic** *adj.*

皮膚青腫和損傷後出血不止。血小板減少症可由於血小板生成不足或破壞過多造成。

thrombocytosis *n.* an increase in the number of *platelets in the blood. It may occur in a variety of diseases, including chronic infections, cancers, and certain blood diseases and is likely to cause an increased tendency to form blood clots within vessels (thrombosis).

血小板增多 血內血小板數的增多。可發生於不同疾病，如慢性感染、癌和某些血液病。使血管內形成血凝塊（血栓形成）的傾向增加。

thromboembolism *n.* the condition in which a blood clot (thrombus), formed at one point in the circulation, becomes detached and lodges at another point. It is most commonly applied to the association of phlebothrombosis and *pulmonary embolism (*pulmonary thromboembolic disease*).

血栓栓塞 在血循環內某處形成的血凝塊（血栓）脫落並停留在其它部位。這最常指的是靜脈血栓形成時併發的肺栓塞（肺血栓栓塞性疾病）。

thromboendarterectomy *n. see* endarterectomy.

血栓動脈內膜切除術

thromboendarteritis *n.* thrombosis complicating *endarteritis, seen in temporal *arteritis, *polyarteritis nodosa, and syphilis. It may cause death of part of the organ supplied by the affected artery.

血栓性動脈內膜炎 併有動脈內膜炎的血栓形成，見於顳動脈炎，結節性多動脈炎和梅毒，可引起被受損動脈供應的器官部分壞死。

thrombokinase *n. see* thromboplastin.

凝血激酶

thrombolysis *n.* the dissolution of a blood clot (thrombus) by the infusion of an enzyme, such as *streptokinase, into the blood. It may be used in the treatment of *phlebothrombosis or *pulmonary embolism.

血栓溶解 血內注入一種酶（例如鏈激酶），使血凝塊溶解。此法可用於治療靜脈血栓形成或肺栓塞。

thrombolytic *adj.* describing an agent that breaks up blood clots (thrombi). *See* anticoagulant.

溶解血栓的 描述能將血凝塊（血栓）分解的藥物。

thrombophlebitis *n.* a condition in which thrombosis is associated with inflammation of a vein wall (*see* phlebitis).

血栓性靜脈炎 靜脈壁炎症併發血栓形成的症狀。

thromboplastin (thrombokinase) *n.* a substance formed during the earlier

凝血激酶 在凝血早期形成的物質，起酶的作用，

stages of *blood coagulation. It acts as an enzyme, converting the inactive substance prothrombin to the enzyme *thrombin.

可使非活動性凝血酶原轉變成凝血酶。

thrombopoiesis *n.* the process of blood *platelet production. Platelets are formed as fragments of cytoplasm shed from giant cells (*megakaryocytes) in the bone marrow by a budding process.

血小板生成 巨核細胞在骨髓內發育過程中其胞漿脫落的碎片即形成血小板。

thrombosis *n.* a condition in which the blood changes from a liquid to a solid state and produces a blood clot (*thrombus*). Thrombosis may occur within a blood vessel in diseased states. Thrombosis in an artery obstructs the blood flow to the tissue it supplies: obstruction of an artery to the brain is one of the causes of a *stroke and thrombosis in an artery supplying the heart – *coronary thrombosis – results in a heart attack (*see* myocardial infarction). Thrombosis can also occur in a vein, and it may be associated with inflammation (*see* phlebitis, phlebothrombosis). The thrombus may become detached from its site of formation and carried in the blood to lodge in another part (*see* embolism).

血栓形成 血液由液體變成固體狀態並產生血凝塊（血栓）的情況。血栓形成可發生於病變的血管內。動脉血栓形成阻止血液流向它供應的組織。腦動脉阻塞是卒中的原因之一。供應心臟的動脉血栓形成，即冠狀動脉血栓形成，可引起心臟病發作（心肌梗死）。靜脉內也可發生血栓形成，它可併發於炎症。血栓可從其形成的部位脫落進入血液停留於其它部位。

thrombus *n.* a blood clot (*see* thrombosis).

血栓 血凝塊。

thrush *n. see* candidiasis.

鵝口瘡

thym- (thymo-) *prefix denoting* the thymus.

〔前綴〕 **胸腺**

thymectomy *n.* surgical removal of the thymus gland.

胸腺切除術 切除胸腺的手術。

-thymia *suffix denoting* a condition of the mind. Example: *cyclothymia* (marked alternation of mood).

〔後綴〕 **心境** 一種心理狀態。例如：循環情感性氣質（精神狀態的明顯交替變換）。

thymic aplasia failure of development of the *thymus gland. This was formerly thought to predispose to *hyper-

胸腺發育不全 胸腺發育不良，過去認爲這種情況易患過敏反應和感染，並

sensitivity reactions and to infection and so to death in childhood (*see* status lymphaticus), a concept no longer held.

在兒童期死亡，現已不再支持這種觀點。

thymidine *n.* a compound containing thymine and the sugar ribose. *See also* nucleoside.

胸腺嘧啶核苷 胸腺嘧啶與核糖的化合物。

thymine *n.* one of the nitrogen-containing bases (*see* pyrimidine) occurring in the nucleic acids DNA and RNA.

胸腺嘧啶 脫氧核糖核酸和核糖核酸中存在的一種含氮碱基。

thymitis *n.* inflammation of the thymus gland (the mass of lymphatic tissue behind the breastbone).

胸腺炎 胸腺（胸骨後淋巴組織）的炎症。

thymocyte *n.* a lymphocyte within the *thymus.

胸腺細胞 胸腺內的淋巴細胞。

thymoma *n.* a benign or malignant tumour of the *thymus gland. It is sometimes associated with *myasthenia gravis, a chronic disease in which muscles tire easily. Surgical removal of the tumour may result in improvement of the muscle condition, but the response is often slow.

胸腺瘤 胸腺的良性或惡性腫瘤。有時可伴有重症肌無力，是肌肉易疲勞的一種慢性病，手術切除腫瘤可改善肌肉狀況，但這種效果往往是緩慢的。

thymoxamine *n.* a drug that causes peripheral blood vessels to dilate (*see* vasodilator). It is administered by mouth in the treatment of Raynaud's disease and similar conditions. Side-effects include mild nausea, diarrhoea, headache, and flushing. The drug should be used with caution in patients with diabetes mellitus or heart disease. Trade name: **Opilon**.

百里胺（腎上腺素能阻斷藥） 使週圍血管擴張的藥物，用於口服，治療雷諾氏病和類似病變。副作用有輕度噁心、腹瀉、頭痛和面紅。糖尿病患者用此藥應謹慎。

thymus *n.* a bilobed organ in the root of the neck, above and in front of the heart. The thymus is enclosed in a capsule and divided internally by cross walls into many lobules, each full of lymphocytes (white blood cells associated with antibody production). In relation to body size the thymus is largest at birth. It doubles in size by puberty, after which it gradually shrinks, its functional tissue being replaced by fatty tissue. In infancy the

胸腺 在頸的根部心臟前上方的雙葉器官。胸腺由被膜包裹，其內部被結締組織分成許多小葉，每個小葉充滿淋巴細胞（與抗體產生有關的細胞）。與身體大小相比，胸腺在出生時最大。在青春期時增大一倍，以後就逐漸萎縮，它的有功能的組織被脂肪組織所代替。嬰兒期胸腺控制淋巴組織的發育

thymus controls the development of *lymphoid tissue and immune response to microbes and foreign proteins (accounting for allergic response, autoimmunity, and rejection of organ transplants). Its function in the adult is unclear. —**thymic** *adj.*

及對微生物和異體蛋白的免疫反應（為過敏反應、自身免疫，和對移植器官的排斥反應的原因）。成人期的功能不明。

thyro- *prefix denoting* the thyroid gland. Example: *thyroglossal* (relating to the thyroid gland and tongue).

〔前綴〕 **甲狀腺** 例如：甲狀舌的（與甲狀腺和舌有關的）。

thyrocalcitonin (calcitonin) *n.* a hormone, produced by certain cells in the thyroid gland, that lowers the levels of calcium and phosphate in the blood. Thyrocalcitonin is given by injection to treat hypercalcaemia and Paget's disease of the bone. *Compare* parathyroid hormone.

甲狀腺降鈣素（降鈣素） 甲狀腺的某種細胞分泌的激素。它降低血內鈣和磷的濃度。用於注射，可治療高鈣血症和變形性骨炎。

thyrocele *n.* a swelling of the thyroid gland. *See* goitre.

甲狀腺腫 甲狀腺腫脹。

thyroglobulin *n.* a protein in the thyroid gland from which the *thyroid hormones (thyroxine and triiodotyrosine) are synthesized.

甲狀腺球蛋白 甲狀腺的蛋白，它合成甲狀腺激素（甲狀腺素和三碘酪氨酸）。

thyrohyoid *adj.* relating to the thyroid cartilage and hyoid bone. The *thyrohyoid ligaments* form part of the *larynx; contraction of the *thyrohyoid muscle* raises the larynx.

甲狀舌骨的 與甲狀軟骨和舌骨有關的。甲狀舌骨韌帶組成喉的一部分。甲狀舌骨肌收縮時將喉向上移動。

thyroid cartilage the main cartilage of the *larynx, consisting of two broad plates that join at the front to form a V-shaped structure. The thyroid cartilage forms the *Adam's apple* in front of the larynx.

甲狀軟骨 喉部主要的軟骨。由兩個寬板組成，在前緣連結成一個V形結構。甲狀軟骨形成喉部前面的喉結。

thyroidectomy *n.* surgical removal of the thyroid gland. In *partial thyroidectomy*, only the diseased part of the gland is removed; in *subtotal thyroidectomy*, a method of treating *thyrotoxicosis, the surgeon removes 90% of the gland.

甲狀腺切除術 切除甲狀腺的手術。部分甲狀腺切除術時，僅切除腺體的病變部分，甲狀腺次全切除術是治療甲狀腺毒症的方法，外科切除腺體的90%。

thyroid gland a large *endocrine gland situated in the base of the neck

甲狀腺 位於頸根部的、大的內分泌腺（見圖）。

(see illustration). It consists of two lobes, one on either side of the trachea, that are joined by an *isthmus* (sometimes a third lobe extends upwards from the isthmus). The thyroid gland consists of a large number of closed follicles inside which is a jelly-like colloid, which contains the principle active substances that are secreted by the gland. The thyroid gland is concerned with regulation of the metabolic rate by the secretion of *thyroid hormone, which is stimulated by *thyroid-stimulating hormone from the pituitary gland and requires trace amounts of iodine. Thyroid extract is used in the treatment of thyroid deficiency diseases.

由兩葉組成，每葉在氣管的一側，由峽部相連（有時從峽部向上伸出第三葉）。甲狀腺由大量密閉的濾泡組成，其中是凍狀的膠體，它含有甲狀腺所分泌的主要活性物質。甲狀腺通過其分泌的甲狀腺素參與代謝率的調節。甲狀腺素的分泌是受垂體的促甲狀腺激素的刺激，並需要微量的碘。甲狀腺浸出物可以用於治療甲狀腺機能低下的疾病。

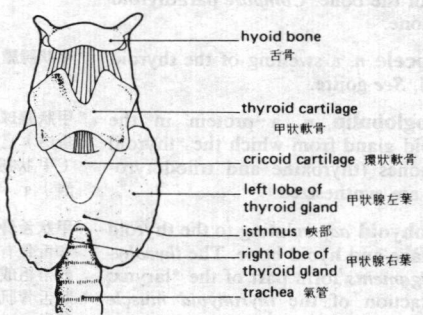

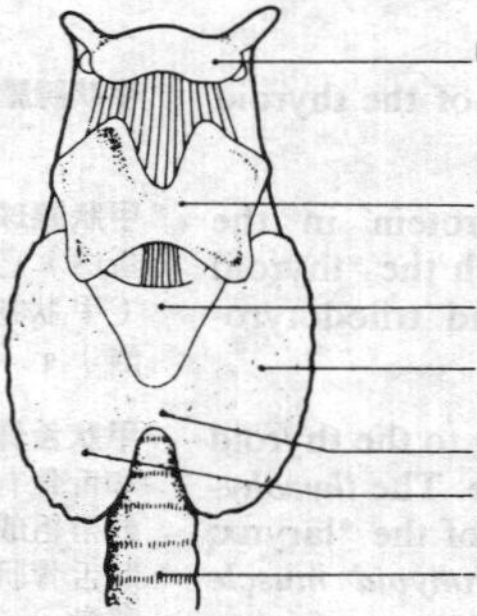

Position of the thyroid gland
甲狀腺的位置

thyroid hormone an iodine-containing substance, synthesized and secreted by the thyroid gland, that is essential for normal metabolic processes and mental and physical development. There are two thyroid hormones, *triiodothyronine* and *thyroxine*. Lack of these hormones gives rise to *cretinism in infants and *myxoedema in adults. Excessive production of thyroid hormones gives rise to *thyrotoxicosis.

甲狀腺激素 甲狀腺合成和分泌的含碘的物質。是正常代謝過程和精神與體格發育所必需的。有兩種甲狀腺激素，即三碘甲狀腺氨酸和甲狀腺素。嬰兒缺乏這些激素時引起獃小症，而成人引起黏液水腫。甲狀腺激素過度分泌會引起甲狀腺毒症。

thyroiditis *n.* inflammation of the thyroid gland. *Acute thyroiditis* is due to bacterial infection; *chronic thyroiditis* is

甲狀腺炎 甲狀腺發炎。急性甲狀腺炎是由於細菌感染；慢性甲狀腺炎通常

commonly caused by an abnormal immune response (*see* autoimmunity) in which lymphocytes invade the tissues of the gland. *See* Hashimoto's disease, struma.

是因異常免疫反應引起，此時淋巴細胞侵入到腺體組織。

thyroid-stimulating hormone (thyrotrophin, TSH) a hormone, synthesized and secreted by the anterior pituitary gland under the control of *thyrotrophin-releasing hormone, that stimulates activity of the thyroid gland. Defects in TSH production lead to over- or under-secretion of *thyroid hormones. TSH may be given by injection to test thyroid gland function.

促甲狀腺激素　垂體前葉在促甲狀腺激素釋放激素的調節下合成和分泌的激素。它刺激甲狀腺的活性。促甲狀腺激素分泌異常會導至甲狀腺激素分泌過多或過少。注射促甲狀腺激素可用於測定甲狀腺功能。

thyrotomy *n.* surgical incision of either the thyroid cartilage in the neck or of the thyroid gland itself.

甲狀〔腺〕切開術　手術切開頸部的甲狀軟骨或甲狀腺本身。

thyrotoxicosis *n.* the syndrome due to excessive amounts of thyroid hormones in the bloodstream, causing a rapid heart beat, sweating, tremor, anxiety, increased appetite, loss of weight, and intolerance of heat. Causes include simple overactivity of the gland, a hormone-secreting benign tumour or carcinoma of the thyroid, and *Graves's disease* (*exophthalmic goitre*), in which there are additional symptoms including swelling of the neck (*goitre*) due to enlargement of the gland and protrusion of the eyes (*exophthalmos*). Treatment may be by surgical removal of the thyroid gland, administration of radioactive iodine to destroy part of the gland, or by the use of drugs (such as *carbimazole or *propylthiouracil) that interfere with the production of thyroid hormones. —**thyrotoxic** *adj.*

甲狀腺毒症　由於血流中甲狀腺素量過多所致的綜合症。可引起心率快、出汗、震顫、焦慮、食慾亢進、體重下降和怕熱。原因有：單純的甲狀腺功能亢進；分泌激素的良性腫瘤或甲狀腺癌以及突眼性甲狀腺腫（格雷夫氏病），後者另有因甲狀腺腫大而頸部腫脹（甲狀腺腫）和眼睛突出（眼球突出）等症狀。治療採用手術切除甲狀腺、用放射性碘毀壞部分腺體、或服用阻礙甲狀腺激素合成的藥物（如甲亢平或甲基硫氧嘧啶）。

thyrotrophin *n. see* thyroid-stimulating hormone.

促甲狀腺激素

thyrotrophin-releasing hormone (TRH) a hormone-like substance from the hypothalamus (in the brain) that acts on the anterior pituitary gland to

促甲狀腺激素釋放激素　來自下丘腦（大腦內）的激素樣的物質。它作用於垂體前葉，刺激促甲狀腺

stimulate the release of *thyroid-stimulating hormone. TRH is given by intravenous injection to test thyroid gland function and to estimate reserves of thyroid-stimulating hormone in the pituitary.

激素釋放。靜脈注射促甲狀腺激素釋放激素可用來測定甲狀腺功能和判斷促甲狀腺激素在垂體內的儲備。

thyroxine *n.* one of the hormones synthesized and secreted by the thyroid gland (*see* thyroid hormone). Thyroxine can be administered by mouth to treat underactivity of the thyroid gland (*see* cretinism, myxoedema).

甲狀腺素 由甲狀腺合成和分泌的一種激素。甲狀腺素可口服治療甲狀腺功能低下。

tibia *n.* the shin bone: the inner and larger bone of the lower leg (see illustration). It articulates with the *femur above, with the *talus below, and with the *fibula to the side (at both ends); at the lower end is a projection, the medial *malleolus, forming part of the articulation with the talus.

脛骨 小腿內側的大骨（見圖），上面與股骨相關節，下與距骨相關節，在側面（兩端）與腓骨相關節。在其下端有一隆突，爲內踝，是與距骨形成關節的部分。

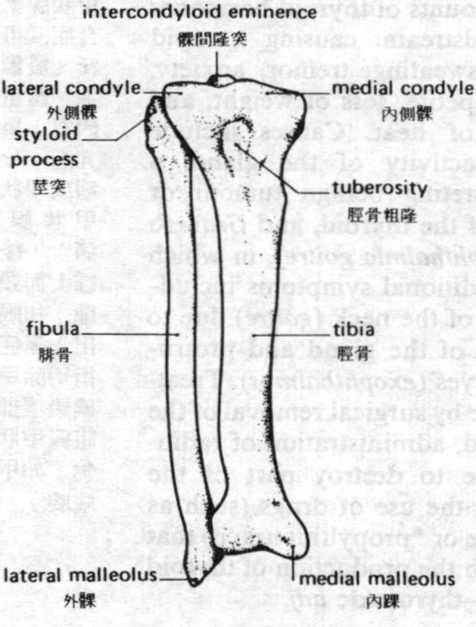

Right tibia and fibula
右側脛骨與腓骨

tibialis *n.* either of two muscles in the leg, extending from the tibia to the metatarsal bones of the foot. The *tibialis anterior* turns the foot inwards and

脛骨肌 從脛骨延伸至足部蹠骨的兩塊小腿肌肉之一。脛骨前肌使足向內翻，並使足趾向背屈曲。

flexes the toes backwards. Situated behind it, the *tibialis posterior* extends the toes and inverts the foot.

脛骨後肌在其後方，使足趾下伸，足內翻。

tibio- *prefix denoting* the tibia. Example: *tibiofibular* (relating to the tibia and fibula).

〔前綴〕 **脛，脛骨** 例如：脛腓的（有關脛骨和腓骨的）。

tic *n.* a repeated and largely involuntary movement varying in complexity from the twitch of a muscle to elaborate well-coordinated actions. Tics most often become prominent when the individual is exposed to emotional stress.

抽搐 反覆發生的、大都是不隨意的運動。其複雜程度有所不同：從一條肌肉的顫動，到精細協調的動作。當人的情緒激動時，抽搐常變得突出而明顯。

tic douloureux *see* neuralgia.

三叉神經痛

tick *n.* a bloodsucking parasite belonging to the order of arthropods (Acarina) that also includes the *mites. Tick bites can cause serious skin lesions and occasionally paralysis (*see* Ixodes, Amblyomma), and certain tick species transmit *typhus and *relapsing fever. Dimethyl phthalate is used as a tick repellent. There are two families: Argasidae (soft ticks), including *Ornithodoros*, with mouthparts invisible from above and no hard shield (*scutum*) on the dorsal surface; and Ixodidae (hard ticks), including *Dermacentor*, *Haemaphysalis*, and *Rhipicephalus*, with clearly visible mouthparts and a definite scutum.

蜱（壁蝨） 屬於節肢動物類（蟎目）的一種吸血的寄生蟲，也包括蟎。蜱叮咬引起嚴重的皮膚損害，偶可造成癱瘓。有的蜱類傳播斑疹傷寒和回歸熱。酞酸二甲酯（驅蚊酯）是蜱的驅除劑。蜱有兩種：隱喙蜱科（軟蜱），包括鈍喙蜱屬，從上面可看見它的口部，但在背部表面無硬盾（盾片）；硬蜱科（硬蜱），包括有革蜱屬、立蜱屬和扇頭蜱屬，有明顯可見的口部，並有一明確的盾片。

tick fever any infectious disease transmitted by ticks, especially *Rocky Mountain spotted fever.

蜱熱 由蜱傳播的各種傳染病，特別是落基山斑疹熱。

Tietze's syndrome (costochondritis) a painful swelling of a rib in the region of the chest, over the junction of bone and cartilage. The cause is unknown and the condition usually resolves without treatment, but in some cases local injections of corticosteroids are required.

提策氏綜合徵（肋骨軟骨炎） 胸部肋骨與軟骨連接處疼痛性腫脹。原因不明，病情往往不治自癒，但有時需局部注射皮質類固醇。

time sampling (in psychology) a way of recording behaviour in which the presence or absence of particular kinds

時間抽樣 （精神病學）一種記錄行爲的方法，是在預先安排的幾段固定時

of behaviour is noted during each of several fixed prearranged periods of time. *See also* event sampling.

間內記錄有無某種特殊的行爲。

tincture *n.* an alcoholic extract of a drug derived from a plant.

酊劑 從植物提取的酒精浸出藥物。

tinea *n. see* ringworm.

癬

tinnitus *n.* any noise (buzzing, ringing, etc.) in the ear. The many causes include wax (*cerumen) in the ear; damage to the eardrum; diseases of the inner ear, such as *otosclerosis and *Menière's disease; drugs such as aspirin and quinine, and abnormalities of the auditory nerve and its connections within the brain.

耳鳴 耳內有某種噪音（嗡嗡聲、鈴聲等等）鳴響。原因很多，如耳內耵聹（耳垢）；鼓膜損傷；內耳疾病：例如耳硬化症，美尼爾氏病；藥物中毒：例如阿司匹林和奎寧；聽神經及其在大腦內的傳導路發生異常。

tintometer *n.* an instrument for measuring the depth of colour in a liquid. The colour can then be compared with those on standard charts so that the concentration of a particular compound in solution can be estimated.

液體比色器 測量液體顏色深度的儀器。可將待測液體的顏色與標準比色表比較，以此測定溶液內某種特殊化合物的濃度。

tissue *n.* a collection of cells specialized to perform a particular function. The cells may be of the same type (e.g. in nervous tissue) or of different types (e.g. in connective tissue). Aggregations of tissues constitute organs.

組織 專門完成特定功能的細胞集團。這些細胞可以是同一類型的（例如神經組織），或是不同類型的（例如結締組織）。組織的聚集構成器官。

tissue culture the culture of living tissues, removed from the body, in a suitable medium supplied with nutrients and oxygen.

組織培養 在一個供給營養和氧氣的適宜培養基內培養從人體取出的活組織。

titre *n.* (in immunology) the extent to which a sample of blood serum containing antibody can be diluted before losing its ability to cause agglutination of the relevant antigen. It is used as a measure of the amount of antibody in the serum.

滴度 （免疫學）含有抗體的血清標本被稀釋至一定程度，即將失去與相關抗原起凝集作用的能力。用於測定血清中抗體的量。

titubation *n.* a rhythmical nodding movement of the head, sometimes involving the trunk. Occasionally the use of this term is extended to include a stumbling gait.

顫搖 有節律的點頭運動（有時包括軀幹）。有時詞義擴大包括蹣跚狀態。

tobacco *n.* the dried leaves of the plant *Nicotiana tabacum* or related species,

煙草 植物煙草或其近緣品種的乾葉，用於吸煙或

used in smoking and as snuff. Tobacco contains the stimulant but poisonous alkaloid *nicotine, which enters the bloodstream during smoking. The volatile tarry material also released during smoking contains chemicals known to produce cancer in animals.

作爲鼻煙。煙草含有興奮劑，但吸煙時有毒的生物鹼尼古丁（煙鹼）進入血流。吸煙時也釋放揮發性的柏油樣物質，已知其中所含的化學物質可引起動物癌症。

toco- *prefix denoting* childbirth or labour.

〔前綴〕 **分娩或生育**

tocopherol *n. see* vitamin E.

生育酚

Todd's paralysis (Todd's palsy) transient paralysis of a part of the body that has previously been involved in a focal epileptic fit (*see* epilepsy). It is thought to be due to the exhaustion of the cells of the motor cortex of the brain.

托德氏麻痹 在局灶性癲癇發作後身體某一部分發生的暫時麻痹。據認爲這是由於大腦皮層運動區細胞衰竭所致。

Tofranil *n. see* imipramine.

鹽酸丙咪嗪

tolazamide *n.* a drug administered by mouth in the treatment of maturity-onset diabetes. Side-effects include nausea, loss of appetite, diarrhoea, weakness, and lethargy. Trade name: **Tolanase**. *See also* sulphonylurea.

甲磺氮䓬脲 治療壯年期糖尿病的一種口服藥。副作用有噁心、食慾喪失、腹瀉、無力和嗜眠。

tolazoline *n.* a *vasodilator drug, given by mouth for the treatment of peripheral vascular disorders, such as *Raynaud's disease. Side-effects include flushing, nausea, vomiting, diarrhoea, and a fall in blood pressure on standing. The drug should not be given to patients with peptic ulcers or heart disease. Trade name: **Priscol**.

妥拉蘇林 血管擴張藥，用於口服治療周圍血管病變，例如雷諾氏病。副作用有面紅、噁心、嘔吐、腹瀉以及直立性低血壓。消化性潰瘍和心臟病患者不宜用此藥。

tolbutamide *n.* a drug given by mouth in the treatment of diabetes mellitus. It is believed to act directly on the pancreas to stimulate insulin production and is particularly effective in elderly patients with mild diabetes. Side-effects are similar to those of the *sulphonamides and include skin reactions and transient jaundice. Trade names: **Pramidex, Rastinon**.

甲磺丁脲 治療糖尿病的一種口服藥。據認爲它是直接作用於胰腺，刺激胰島素生成，尤其對老年輕型糖尿病患者有效。副作用與磺胺類藥物相似，並有皮膚反應和一過性黃疸。

tolerance *n.* the reduction or loss of the normal response to a drug or other substance that usually provokes a reac-

耐受性 藥物或通常能引起人體反應的物質的正常效應減低或喪失。藥物耐

tion in the body. *Drug tolerance* may develop after taking a particular drug over a long period of time. In such cases increased doses are necessary to produce the desired effect. Some drugs that cause tolerance also cause *dependence. *See also* glucose tolerance test, immunological tolerance, tachyphylaxis.

受性可發生於長時間服用一種特殊藥物之後。有耐藥性的病例，爲達到要求的效果，需要增加藥物劑量。有些引起耐藥性的藥物也引起賴藥性。

tolnaftate *n.* an antiseptic applied topically as a cream, powder, or solution in the treatment of various fungal infections of the skin, including ringworm. It is not effective in candidiasis. Trade names: **Tinactin, Tinaderm.**

髮癬退 作爲乳膏、粉劑或溶液應用於局部的一種抗菌劑，治療各種不同的皮膚黴菌感染，例如癬。對念珠菌無效。

toluidine blue a dye used in microscopy for staining *basophilic substances in tissue specimens.

甲苯胺藍 使顯微鏡檢查用的組織標本中嗜鹼物質染色的一種染料。

-tome *suffix denoting* a cutting instrument. Example: *microtome* (instrument for cutting microscopical sections).

〔後綴〕 **刀具** 如：切片機（製備顯微鏡切片的器械）。

tomo- *prefix denoting* **1.** section or sections. **2.** surgical operation.

〔前綴〕 ①**切面，節** ②**外科手術**

tomography *n.* the technique of using X-rays or ultrasound waves to produce an image of structures at a particular depth within the body, bringing them into sharp focus while deliberately blurring structures at other depths. The visual record of this technique is called a *tomogram* (*see also* orthopantomogram). *See* computerized axial tomography, positron emission tomography.

體層照像術 一種X線或超聲波檢查技術。調節焦距使身體的特定深度的結構產生清晰影像，而使其它深度的結構模糊不清。用這種方法所得的圖像叫做體層照像。

tomotocia *n.* the delivery of a baby by cutting open the mother's abdomen and womb (*see* Caesarean section).

剖腹產術 切開母親腹部和子宮而娩出嬰兒。

-tomy (-otomy) *suffix denoting* a surgical incision into an organ or part. Example: *gastrotomy* (into the stomach).

〔後綴〕 **切開術** 手術切開某器官或一部分，例如胃切開術。

tone *n. see* tonus.

音調

tongue *n.* a muscular organ attached to the floor of the mouth. It consists of a *body* and a *root*, which is attached by muscles to the hyoid bone below, the

舌 與口腔底部相連的一肌肉器官，由體和根組成。其肌肉附着在下面的舌骨上，並與後方的莖突

styloid process behind, and the palate above. It is covered by mucous membrane, which is continuous with that of the mouth and pharynx. On the undersurface of the tongue a fold of mucous membrane, the *frenulum linguae*, connects the midline of the tongue to the floor of the mouth. The surface of the tongue is covered with minute projections (*papillae*), which give it a furred appearance (see illustration). *Taste buds are arranged in grooves around the papillae, particularly the fungiform and circumvallate papillae. The tongue has three main functions. It helps in manipulating food during mastication and swallowing; it is the main organ of taste; and it plays an important role in the production of articulate speech. Anatomical name: **glossa**.

和上方的腭相連接。表面有黏膜，此黏膜和口腔和咽部黏膜相連接。在舌的下面有一黏膜皺襞，即舌繫帶將舌中線與口底部連接。舌表面密佈小的突起（乳頭），外表呈絨毛狀（見圖）。味蕾分佈於乳頭周圍的溝內，特別是菌狀乳頭和輪廓乳頭。舌有三個主要功能，在咀嚼和吞咽時它能協助攪拌食物；又是味覺的主要器官；並在構成清晰發音中起重要作用。

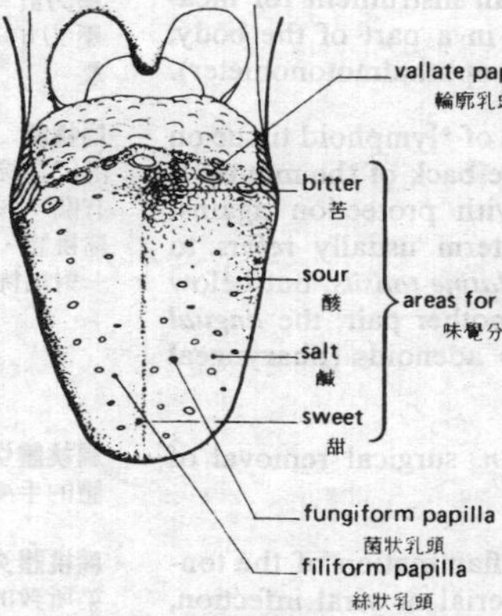

The upper surface of the tongue
舌的上表面

tonic 1. *adj.* **a.** relating to normal muscle tone. **b.** marked by continuous tension (contraction), e.g. a tonic muscle *spasm. **2.** *n.* a medicinal substance taken to increase vigour and liveliness and produce a feeling of well-being.

①**緊張的** a. 肌緊張正常的。b. 表現持續性緊張（收縮）的，例如，緊張性肌肉痙攣。②**强壯劑** 一種增加精力、活力和產生舒適感的藥劑。

tonicity *n.* **1.** the normal state of slight contraction, or readiness to contract, of

①**緊張性** 健康肌纖維收縮或準備收縮的正常狀

healthy muscle fibres. **2.** the effective osmotic pressure of a solution. *See* hypertonic, hypotonic, osmosis.

態。②**張力** 溶液的有效滲透壓。

tono- *prefix denoting* **1.** tone or tension. **2.** pressure.

〔前綴〕 ①**緊張或張力** ②**壓力**

tonofibril *n.* a tiny fibre occurring in bundles in the cytoplasm of cells that lie in contact, as in epithelial tissue. Tonofibrils are concerned with maintaining contact between adjacent cells. *See* desmosome.

張力原纖維 在細胞漿中互相接觸成束的細纖維，例如在上皮細胞內。張力原纖維與維持相鄰細胞之間的接觸有關。

tonography *n.* measurement of the pressure within the eyeball in such a way as to allow a record to be made on a chart of variations in pressure occurring over periods of several minutes at a time.

張力描記術 測量眼球內壓力的方法。這種方法可將每次幾分鐘的壓力變化描記在曲線圖上。

tonometer *n.* an instrument for measuring pressure in a part of the body, e.g. the eye (*see* ophthalmotonometer).

壓力計 測量身體某部位壓力的器械，例如測眼壓。

tonsil *n.* a mass of *lymphoid tissue on either side of the back of the mouth. It is concerned with protection against infection. The term usually refers to either of the *palatine tonsils*, but below the tongue is another pair, the *lingual tonsils*. *See also* adenoids (pharyngeal tonsils).

扁桃體 口腔後部兩側的淋巴組織。它與防禦感染有關。該名詞通常是指腭扁桃體，而在舌下面有另一對扁桃體。

tonsillectomy *n.* surgical removal of the tonsils.

扁桃體切除術 摘除扁桃體的手術。

tonsillitis *n.* inflammation of the tonsils due to bacterial or viral infection, causing a sore throat, fever, and difficulty in swallowing. If tonsillitis due to streptococcal infection is not treated (by antibiotics) it may lead to *rheumatic fever or *nephritis.

扁桃體炎 細菌或病毒感染所致的扁桃體發炎，可引起咽喉痛、發熱和吞咽困難。如果鏈球菌感染所致的扁桃體炎未經治療（用抗生素），可導至風濕病或腎炎。

tonsillotomy *n.* surgical incision of a tonsil or removal of part of a tonsil.

扁桃體切開術 切開扁桃體或切除部分扁桃體的手術。

tonus (tone) *n.* the normal state of partial contraction of a resting muscle, maintained by reflex activity.

緊張 靜止肌肉在正常情況下由反射活動保持的收縮狀態。

tooth *n.* (*pl.* **teeth**) one of the hard structures in the mouth used for cutting and chewing food. Each tooth is embedded in a socket in part of the jawbone (mandible or maxilla) known as the *alveolar bone* (or *alveolus*), to which it is attached by the *periodontal membrane. The exposed part of the tooth (*crown*) is covered with *enamel and the part within the bone (*root*) is coated with *cementum; the bulk of the tooth consists of *dentine enclosing the *pulp (see illustration). The group of embryological cells that gives rise to a tooth is known as the *tooth germ*. There are four different types of tooth (*see* canine, incisor, premolar, molar). *See also* dentition.

牙 口腔中用來切咬或咀嚼食物的堅硬結構。每顆牙嵌入牙槽骨（上頜骨或下頜骨的一部分）的窩臼中，以牙周膜相連接。牙暴露的部分（冠）被牙釉質覆蓋，埋在骨中的部分（牙根）由牙骨質覆蓋。牙體積的大部分是牙本質，其內部包裹牙髓（見圖）。使牙生長的一組胚胎期細胞稱爲牙胚。有四種不同型的牙。

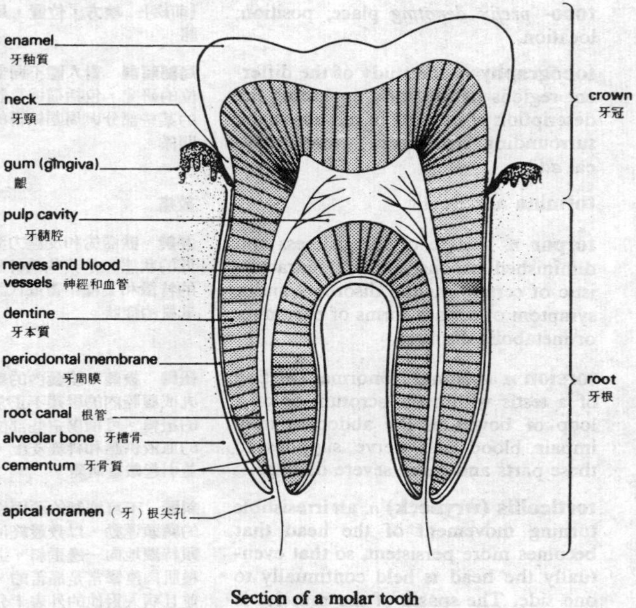

Section of a molar tooth
磨牙的切面

tooth extraction *see* extraction.

拔牙

topagnosis *n.* inability to identify a part of the body that has been touched.

位置（感）覺缺乏 不能確定身體被觸及的部位。

It is a symptom of disease in the parietal lobes of the brain. The normal ability to localize touch is called *topognosis*.

這是大腦頂葉病變的症狀。確定接觸部分的正常能力稱爲位置覺。

topectomy *n.* an obsolete operation for the control of psychiatric symptoms by excising selected areas of the cerebral cortex. *See also* psychosurgery.

額葉皮層局部切除術 爲控制精神症狀而切除大腦皮層選擇區的一種業已廢除的手術。

tophus *n.* (*pl.* **tophi**) a hard deposit of crystalline uric acid and its salts in the skin, cartilage (especially of the ears), or joints; a feature of *gout.

痛風石 在皮膚、軟骨（特別是耳）或關節處的尿酸結晶和其鹽的堅硬沉積物，是痛風的特徵。

topical *adj.* local: used for the route of administration of a drug that is applied directly to the part being treated (e.g. to the skin or eye).

局部的 指給藥途徑，將藥直接施用於被治療部位。

topo- *prefix denoting* place; position; location.

〔前綴〕 **地方，位置，局部**

topography *n.* the study of the different regions of the body, including the description of its parts in relation to the surrounding structures. —**topographical** *adj.*

局部解剖 對人體不同部位的研究，包括描述身體的某些部分與周圍結構的關係。

tormina *n. see* colic.

絞痛

torpor *n.* a state of sluggishness and diminished responsiveness: a characteristic of certain mental disorders and a symptom of certain forms of poisoning or metabolic disorder.

遲鈍 獃滯的和反應力減低的狀態。是某些精神病的特徵和某種中毒或代謝紊亂的症狀。

torsion *n.* twisting. Abnormal twisting of a testis within the scrotum or of a loop of bowel in the abdomen may impair blood and nerve supplies to these parts and cause severe damage.

扭轉 捩轉。陰囊內的睾丸或腹腔內的腸襻不正常的扭轉。可損傷這些部位的血液供應和神經支配，並引起嚴重病變。

torticollis (wryneck) *n.* an irresistible turning movement of the head that becomes more persistent, so that eventually the head is held continually to one side. The spasm of the muscles is often painful and the patient is sensitive about his appearance. It may be caused by a birth injury to the sternomastoid muscle (*see* sternomastoid tumour). Relief may be obtained by cutting the

斜頸 不可控制的頑固性的轉頭運動，以致最終使頭持續地向一邊歪斜。這種肌肉痙攣常是痛苦的，並且病人對他的外表十分敏感。可能是由於分娩時損傷胸鎖乳突肌造成。切斷頸部脊神經的運動神經根可使症狀緩解。

motor nerve roots of the spinal nerves in the neck region.

toruloma *n.* a tumour-like lesion in the lungs resulting from *cryptococcosis. **隱球菌結節** 隱球菌病引起的肺部腫瘤樣病變。

torulosis *n. see* cryptococcosis. **隱球菌病**

tourniquet *n.* a device to press upon an artery and prevent flow of blood through it, usually a cord, rubber tube, or tight bandage tightened around a limb. Tourniquets are no longer recommended as a first-aid measure to stop bleeding from a wound because of the danger of reducing the supply of oxygen to other tissues (direct pressure on the wound itself is considered less harmful). However, a temporary tourniquet to increase the distension of veins when a sample of blood is being taken does no harm. **止血帶** 壓迫動脉以阻止血液從動脉流出的器具。通常是圍繞肢體縛緊的一根帶子，橡皮管或緊的綳帶。止血帶已不再被推薦爲傷口止血的急救措施，因爲有減少對其它組織供氧的危險（直接壓迫傷口本身傷害較小）。但是在抽取血液標本時，爲使靜脉擴張，短時間用止血帶是無害的。

tow *n.* the teased-out short fibres of flax, hemp or jute, used in swabs for cleaning, in *packs or *stupes for the application of poultices, and for a variety of other purposes. **麻短纖維** 從亞麻、大麻或黃麻梳下來的短纖維，用作擦洗用的拭子，泥罨（敷）劑的包裹巾，或用於其他用途。

Towne's projection a *posteroanterior X-ray film to show the entire skull and mandible. **湯氏位（額枕位）投照** 爲顯示整個頭顱和下頜骨的前後位X線像片。

tox- (toxi-, toxo-, toxic(o)-) *prefix denoting* **1.** poisonous; toxic. **2.** toxins or poisoning. 〔前綴〕 **毒** ①有毒的，中毒的。②毒素或中毒。

toxaemia *n.* blood poisoning that is caused by toxins formed by bacteria growing in a local site of infection. It produces generalized symptoms, including fever, diarrhoea, and vomiting. *Compare* pyaemia, sapraemia, septicaemia. **毒血症** 細菌在局部感染處繁殖形成毒素所致血液中毒。它引起全身症狀，包括發熱、腹瀉和嘔吐。

toxaemia of pregnancy an illness of unknown cause affecting pregnant women. It includes the conditions of *pre-eclampsia and *eclampsia. **妊娠毒血症** 妊娠婦女所患的原因不明的疾病，包括子癎前期狀態和子癎。

toxic *adj.* having a poisonous effect; potentially lethal. **有毒的** 有毒性作用的；潛在致死性的。

toxicity *n.* the degree to which a substance is poisonous. *See also* LD_{50}. **毒性** 物質有毒的程度。

toxicology *n.* the study of poisonous materials and their effects upon living organisms. —**toxicologist** *n.*

毒理學 研究有毒物質和它對活機體的作用。

toxicosis *n.* the deleterious effects of a toxin; poisoning: includes any disease caused by the toxic effects of any substances.

中毒 毒素的有害作用；中毒，包括由任何物質的毒性作用所致的各種疾病。

toxin *n.* a poison produced by a living organism, especially by a bacterium (*see* endotoxin, exotoxin). In the body toxins act as *antigens, and special *antibodies (*antitoxins*) are formed to neutralize their effects.

毒素 活微生物，特別是細菌產生的毒物。在人體毒素起抗原作用，並形成特異性抗體（抗毒素），以中和其作用。

Toxocara *n.* a genus of large nematode worms that are intestinal parasites of vertebrates. *T. canis* and *T. cati*, the common roundworms of dogs and cats respectively, have life cycles similar to that of the human roundworm, **Ascaris lumbricoides*. *See* toxocariasis.

弓蛔蟲屬 脊椎動物腸道寄生的一種大型線蟲類：常見的犬弓蛔蟲與貓弓蛔蟲的生活週期與人的蛔蟲相似。

toxocariasis (visceral larva migrans) *n.* an infestation with the larvae of the dog and cat roundworms, *Toxocara canis* and *T. cati*. Man, who is not the normal host, becomes infected on swallowing eggs of *Toxocara* present on hands or in food and drink contaminated with the faeces of infected domestic pets. The larvae, which migrate around the body, cause destruction of various tissues; the liver becomes enlarged and the lungs inflamed (*see* pneumonitis). Symptoms may include fever, joint and muscle pains, vomiting, an irritating rash, and convulsions. Larvae can also lodge in the retina of the eye where they cause inflammation and *granuloma. The disease, widely distributed throughout the world, primarily affects children. There is no satisfactory treatment.

弓蛔蟲病（內臟遊走性幼蟲病） 犬弓蛔蟲和貓弓蛔蟲的幼蟲感染。正常時人並不是宿主，在咽下手上的蟲卵、或已感染的馴養家畜大便所污染的食物和飲料中的蟲卵時就引起感染。幼蟲在全身遊走，引起各組織的破壞，肝臟腫大，肺部發炎。症狀有發熱、關節和肌肉疼痛、嘔吐、刺激性皮疹和驚厥。幼蟲也可停留在眼睛視網膜上，並引起炎症和肉芽腫。該病廣泛分佈全世界，主要侵犯兒童，無有效的療法。

toxoid *n.* a preparation of the poisonous material (toxin) that is produced by dangerous infective organisms, such as those of tetanus and diphtheria, and has been rendered harmless by chemi-

類毒素 某些危險的致病微生物（如破傷風和白喉桿菌）產生的有毒物質（毒素）的製劑。可通過化學處理使它變成無毒

cal treatment while retaining its antigenic activity. Toxoids are used in *vaccines.

性，而保留它的抗原性。類毒素用於預防接種。

Toxoplasma *n.* a genus of crescent-shaped sporozoans that live as parasites within the cells of various tissues and organs of vertebrate animals, especially birds and mammals, and complete their life cycle in a single host. *T. gondii* infects sheep, cattle, dogs, and man, sometimes provoking an acute illness (*see* toxoplasmosis).

弓形體屬 半月形的孢子蟲類，寄生於脊椎動物、尤其是鳥和哺乳動物的不同組織和器官的細胞內，並在一個宿主身上完成它的生活周期。鼠弓形體感染羊、貓、狗和人，有時引起急性病。

toxoplasmosis *n.* a disease of mammals and birds due to the protozoan *Toxoplasma gondii*, which is transmitted to man via undercooked meat, contaminated soil, or by direct contact. Generally symptoms are mild but severe infection of lymph nodes can occur. *Congenital toxoplasmosis*, in which a woman infected during pregnancy transmits the organism to her fetus, can produce blindness or mental retardation in the newborn. Severe cases are treated with sulphonamides and pyrimethamine.

弓形體病 由鼠弓形體原蟲引起哺乳動物和鳥的疾病，通過未煮熟的肉、被污染的泥土或直接接觸傳播給人。全身症狀輕，但可發生淋巴結的嚴重感染。先天性弓形體病，是在妊娠期感染的婦女將微生物傳給胎兒，可引起新生兒的失明或精神發育遲緩，嚴重病例可用磺胺類加乙胺嘧啶治療。

trabecula *n.* (*pl.* **trabeculae**) **1.** any of the bands of tissue that pass from the outer part of an organ to its interior, dividing it into separate chambers. For example, trabeculae occur in the penis. **2.** any of the thin bars of bony tissue in spongy *bone. —**trabecular** *adj.*

小樑 ①把器官從外部到內部分成幾個分隔小腔的組織帶，例如陰莖的小樑。②鬆質骨的骨組織內纖細的樑柱。

trabeculectomy *n.* an operation for glaucoma, one part of which is the removal of a small segment of tissue from part of the wall of *Schlemm's canal. This area is known as the *trabecular meshwork*.

小樑切除術 治療青光眼的一種手術。手術的一部分是從施累姆氏管壁切除一小塊組織。該區域叫做小樑網。

tracer *n.* a substance that is introduced into the body and whose progress can subsequently be followed so that information is gained about metabolic processes. Radioactive tracers, giving off radiation that can be detected on a *scintigram or with a *gamma camera,

示踪劑 導入體內後可被追踪觀察，從而可得到關於代謝過程信息的一種物質。放射性示踪劑在放出射線時可在閃爍圖上或用γ照相機測知，它可用於各種目的，例如用於檢查

are used for a variety of purposes, such as the investigation of thyroid disease or possible brain tumours.

甲狀腺疾病或疑有腦腫瘤時。

trache- (tracheo-) *prefix denoting* the trachea.

〔前綴〕 **氣管**

trachea *n.* the windpipe: the part of the air passage between the *larynx and the main *bronchi, i.e. from just below the Adam's apple, passing behind the notch of the *sternum (breastbone) to behind the angle of the sternum. The upper part of the trachea lies just below the skin, except where the thyroid gland is wrapped around it. —**tracheal** *adj.*

氣管 在喉與支氣管間的一部分氣道，即從喉結下面經過胸骨切跡後面，到達胸骨角的後面。除了被甲狀腺環繞覆蓋部分外，上部氣管位於皮下。

tracheal tugging a sign that is indicative of an *aneurysm of the aortic arch: a downward tug is felt on the windpipe when the finger is placed in the midline at the root of the neck.

氣管牽引感 主動脉弓動脉瘤的體徵。將手指置於頸根部中線處，在氣管上可感到往下牽拉的感覺。

tracheitis *n.* inflammation of the *trachea, usually secondary to bacterial or viral infection in the nose or throat. Tracheitis causes soreness in the chest and a painful cough and is often associated with bronchitis. In babies it can cause asphyxia, particularly in *diphtheria. Treatment includes appropriate antibacterial drugs, humidification of the inhaled air or oxygen, and mild sedation to relieve exhaustion due to persistant coughing.

氣管炎 氣管發炎，通常繼發於鼻或咽喉部的細菌或病毒感染。氣管炎引起胸痛和疼痛性咳嗽，並經常伴有支氣管炎。在嬰兒，特別在百日咳時氣管炎可能會引起窒息。治療包括用恰當的抗菌藥物，空氣或氧氣濕化吸入，以及用緩和的鎮靜劑以減輕因持續咳嗽引起的疲憊。

tracheostomy (tracheotomy) *n.* a surgical operation in which a hole is made into the *trachea through the neck to relieve obstruction to breathing, as in diphtheria. A curved metal, plastic, or rubber tube is usually inserted through the hole and held in position by tapes tied round the neck. It may be possible for the patient to speak by occluding the opening with his fingers. The tube must be kept clean and unblocked. It often helps breathing if secretions are sucked out of the bronchial tree.

氣管造口術（氣管切開術） 爲減輕呼吸道阻塞在頸部"造口"通入氣管的外科手術，例如在白喉時。通常是通過造口插入一根彎曲的金屬的或塑料的或橡皮的管子，用帶子繞頸把它縛在恰當的位置。用手指堵住開口處病人就可以說話。管子必須保持清潔和通暢。若能吸出支氣管的分泌物，則常對呼吸有利。

tracheotomy *n. see* tracheostomy.

氣管切開術

trachoma *n.* a chronic contagious eye disease – a severe form of *conjunctivitis – caused by the virus-like organism *Chlamydia trachomatis*; it is common in tropical regions. The conjunctiva of the eyelids becomes inflamed, leading to discharge of pus. If untreated, the conjunctiva becomes scarred and shrinks, causing the eyelids to turn inwards so that the eyelashes scratch the cornea (*trichiasis); blindness usually follows. Treatment with tetracyclines is effective.

沙眼 類病毒微生物沙眼衣原體引起的慢性接觸傳染的眼病。本病是一種嚴重型結膜炎，常見於熱帶地區。瞼結膜發炎引起膿性分泌物，若不治療，結膜形成瘢痕收縮，使眼瞼向內翻，使睫毛摩擦角膜（倒睫），常引起失明。用四環素治療有效。

tract *n.* **1.** a group of nerve fibres passing from one part of the brain or spinal cord to another, forming a distinct pathway, e.g. the spinothalamic tract, pyramidal tract, and corticospinal tract. **2.** an organ or collection of organs providing for the passage of something, e.g. the digestive tract.

①**束** 從大腦或脊髓的某一部位通向另一部位形成獨特通路的一組神經纖維，如脊髓丘腦束、錐體束以及皮層脊髓束。 ②**管道** 可使某些東西通過的器官，例如消化道。

traction *n.* the application of a pulling force as a means of counteracting the natural tension in the tissues surrounding a broken bone. This tension makes correct alignment of the fragments difficult. Considerable force, exerted with weights, ropes, and pulleys, may be necessary to ensure that a broken femur is kept correctly positioned during the early stages of healing.

牽引 應用拉力抵抗骨折周圍組織的自然張力的方法，這種張力使斷骨的復位發生困難。爲保證在治療早期骨折的股骨保持正確的位置，則需要用重錘、繩索和滑輪產生適當的拉力。

tractotomy *n.* a neurosurgical operation for the relief of intractable pain. The nerve fibres that carry painful sensation to consciousness travel from the spinal cord through the brainstem in the spinothalamic tracts. This procedure is designed to sever the tracts within the medulla oblongata. *See also* cordotomy.

神經束切斷術 減輕難治性疼痛的神經外科手術。神經纖維是循脊髓丘腦束從脊髓通過腦幹將疼痛感覺傳達到意識的，這種手術方法旨在切斷延髓內的神經束。

tragus *n.* the projection of cartilage in the *pinna of the outer ear that extends back over the opening of the external auditory meatus.

耳屏 外耳耳廓上的軟骨性突起，向後延伸到外耳道開口的上方。

Training Opportunities Scheme *see* Employment Service Division.

就業培訓大綱

Training Services Division *see* Employment Service Division.

培訓服務處

trance *n.* a state in which reaction to the environment is diminished although awareness is not impaired. It can be caused by hypnosis, meditation, catatonia, hysteria, drugs (such as hallucinogens), and religious ecstasy.

恍惚 對周圍環境的反應減退而意識尚未損害的一種狀態。這可能由催眠、沉思、緊張症、癔症、藥物（例如引起幻覺的）和宗教的入迷等引起。

tranquillizer *n.* a drug that produces a calming effect, relieving anxiety and tension. *Major tranquillizers*, such as the phenothiazines (e.g. *chlorpromazine, and *trifluoperazine), and *haloperidol, are used to treat severe mental disorders (psychoses), including schizophrenia and mania. *Minor tranquillizers*, such as the benzodiazepines (e.g. *chordiazepoxide and *diazepam) and *meprobamate, are used to treat neuroses and to relieve anxiety and tension due to various causes. Some drowsiness and dizziness are side-effects of most tranquillizers, and abnormal muscle action and movements sometimes occur with major tranquillizers at high doses. Minor tranquillizers sometimes cause *dependence with prolonged use.

安定藥 減輕焦慮和緊張，起鎭靜作用的藥物。强安定藥，如吩噻嗪（即氯丙嗪和三氟拉嗪）和氟哌啶醇用於治療嚴重精神紊亂（精神病），包括精神分裂症和躁狂。弱安定藥，例如苯〔幷〕二氮草類（如利眠寧和安定）和眠爾通用於治療神經官能症和減輕不同原因的焦慮和緊張。多數安定藥的副作用是倦睡和頭暈。用大劑量强安定藥有時可出現異常的肌肉活動和運動，長期應用弱安定藥有時可產生賴藥性。

trans- *prefix denoting* through or across. Example: *transurethral* (through the urethra).

〔前綴〕 **經，透過** 例：經尿道的（通過尿道）。

transaminase *n.* an enzyme that catalyses the transfer of an amino group from an amino acid to an α-keto acid in the process of *transamination. Examples are *glutamic oxaloacetic transaminase (GOT), catalysing the transamination of glutamate and oxaloacetate to α-ketoglutarate and aspartate, and *glutamic pyruvic transaminase (GPT), converting glutamate and pyruvate to α-ketoglutarate and alanine.

轉氨酶 從一種氨基酸轉變爲 α -酮酸的過程中催化氨基轉移的酶。例如，穀氨酸草醯乙酸轉氨酶（GOT）催化穀氨酸和草醯乙酸轉移爲 α -酮戊二酸天門冬氨酸，穀氨酸丙酮酸轉氨酶（GPT）是將穀氨酸轉爲 α -酮戊二酸和丙氨酸。

transamination *n.* a process involved in the metabolism of amino acids in which amino groups ($-NH_2$) are transferred from amino acids to certain α-keto acids, with the production of a

氨基轉移〔作用〕 氨基酸的代謝過程。在此過程中氨基從氨基酸轉移到某種 α -酮酸和形成另一個酮酸和氨基酸。這種反應

second keto acid and amino acid. The reaction is catalysed by enzymes (*see* transaminase), which require pyridoxal phosphate as a coenzyme.

由酶催化，並需要磷酸吡哆醛作為輔酶。

transcription *n.* the process in which the information contained in the *genetic code is transferred from DNA to RNA: the first step in the manufacture of proteins in cells. *See* messenger RNA, translation.

轉錄〔作用〕 將有遺傳密碼的信息從脫氧核糖核酸轉移至核糖核酸的過程。這是細胞內蛋白製造的第一步。

transduction *n.* the transfer of DNA from one bacterium to another by means of a *bacteriophage (phage). Some bacterial DNA is incorporated into the phage. When the host bacterium is destroyed the phage infects another bacterium and introduces the DNA from its previous host, which may become incorporated into the new host's DNA.

轉導作用 通過噬菌體使脫氧核糖核酸從一種細菌轉移到另一種細菌的過程。一些細菌的脫氧核糖核酸併入噬菌體內，當受體細菌被破壞時，噬菌體就感染另外的細菌，並將脫氧核糖核酸從以前的受體誘導出來，併入新的受體的脫氧核糖核酸中去。

transection *n.* **1.** a cross section of a piece of tissue. **2.** cutting across the tissue of an organ (*see also* section).

橫切 ①一塊組織的橫斷面。 ②橫過組織或器官切開。

transferase *n.* an enzyme that catalyses the transfer of a group (other than hydrogen) between a pair of substrates.

轉移酶 催化兩種底物之間的基團（不是氫）轉移的酶。

transference *n.* (in psychoanalysis) the process by which a patient comes to feel and act towards the therapist as though he were somebody from the patient's past life, especially a powerful parent. The patient's transference feelings may be of love or of hatred, but they are inappropriate to the actual person of the therapist. *Countertransference* is the reaction of the therapist to the patient, which is similarly based on his own past relationships.

移情 （精神分析）病人逐漸將感情移向治療醫生，把他當作病人過去生活中的某個人，，特別是當作病人的有權威的父母來對待。病人的移情可能是愛，也可能是恨，但都與現實的這位醫生不符合。反移情作用是治療醫生對病人的反應，這同樣也是基於他自己過去的人際關係而形成的。

transferrin (siderophilin) *n.* a *glycoprotein, found in the blood plasma, that is capable of binding iron and thus acts as a carrier for iron in the bloodstream.

轉鐵蛋白 能在血中與鐵結合並攜帶鐵的一種血漿糖蛋白。

transfer RNA a type of RNA whose function is to attach the correct amino acid to the protein chain being synthe-

轉移核糖核酸 核糖核酸的一種，其功能是將相應的氨基酸結合到核糖體

sized at a *ribosome. *See also* translation.

（核蛋白體）正在合成中的多肽鏈上，以形成蛋白質。

transfusion *n.* **1.** the injection of a volume of blood obtained from a healthy person (the *donor*) into the circulation of a patient (the *recipient*) whose blood is deficient in quantity or quality, through accident or disease. Direct transfusion from one person to another is rarely performed; usually bottles of carefully stored blood of different *blood groups are kept in *blood banks for use as necessary. During transfusion the blood is allowed to drip, under gravity, through a needle inserted into one of the recipient's veins. Blood transfusion is routine during major surgical operations in which much blood is likely to be lost. **2.** the administration of any fluid, such as plasma or saline solution, into a patient's vein by means of a *drip.

①**輸血** 將從健康人（供血者）取得的血注入因意外或疾病造成血液量和質不足的病人（受血者）的血循環中。直接輸血很少施行。通常是把不同血型的血液妥善裝在瓶中，保存在血庫以供需要時應用。輸血時血液通過插入靜脈的針頭，依靠重力滴入。在失血可能多的大手術時輸血是常規。 ②**輸液** 各種液體，如血漿或鹽溶液用滴入法注入病人靜脉。

transillumination *n.* the technique of shining a bright light through part of the body to examine its structure. Transillumination of the sinuses of the skull is a means of detecting abnormalities.

透照法 用亮光照射身體某部以檢查其結構的方法。對顱骨各種竇的透照是檢查有無異常的一種方法。

translation *n.* (in cell biology) the manufacture of proteins in a cell, which takes place at the ribosomes. The information for determining the correct sequence of amino acids in the protein is carried to the ribosomes by *messenger RNA, and the amino acids are brought to their correct position in the protein by *transfer RNA.

轉譯 （細胞生物學）在細胞內核糖體製造蛋白質的過程。通過信使核糖核酸將確定蛋白質中氨基酸正確順序的信息傳遞給核糖體，而轉移核糖核酸則將氨基酸帶至其在蛋白質中的正確位置上。

translocation *n.* (in genetics) a type of chromosome mutation in which part of a chromosome is transferred to another part of the same chromosome or to a different chromosome. This changes the order of the genes on the chromosomes and can lead to serious genetic disorders, e.g. chronic myeloid leukaemia.

易位 （遺傳學）染色體突變的一種類型。染色體的一部分轉移至同一染色體的另一部分或不同的染色體中去，這改變了染色體上基因的排列，並可能導至嚴重的遺傳性病變，例如，慢性粒細胞性白血病。

transmethylation *n.* the process whereby an amino acid donates its terminal methyl ($-CH_3$) group for methylation of other compounds. Methionine is the principal methyl donor in the body and the donated methyl group may subsequently be involved in the synthesis of such compounds as choline or creatinine or in detoxification processes.

甲基轉移 氨基酸提供其甲基末端以使其它化合物甲基化的過程。蛋氨酸是體內重要的甲基供體，提供的甲基隨後可參與一些化合物的合成，如膽鹼或肌酐，或參與解毒過程。

transmigration *n.* the act of passing through or across, e.g. the passage of blood cells through the intact walls of capillaries and venules (*see* diapedesis).

移行（血細胞滲出） 通過或穿過某物的活動。例如血細胞通過完整的毛細血管壁或小靜脈壁而滲出。

transplantation *n.* the implantation of an organ or tissue (*see* graft) from one part of the body to another or from one person (the donor) to another (the recipient). Skin and bone grafting are examples of transplantation techniques in the same individual. A kidney transplant involves the grafting of a healthy kidney from a donor to replace the diseased kidney of the recipient. Heart transplants have also been carried out with limited success and a few liver transplants have also been attempted. Transplanting organs or tissues between individuals is a difficult procedure because of the natural rejection processes in the recipient of the graft. Special treatment (e.g. with *immunosuppresive drugs) is needed to prevent graft rejection.

移植術 將器官或組織從身體的一部分植入另一部分，或從一個人（供者）到另一個人（受者）。同體移植技術的例子是皮和骨的移植。腎臟移植技術是把供者的健康腎臟移植給受者以代替有病的腎。心臟移植術也有部分病例獲得成功，少數肝移植也有所探索。由於受體對移植物有自然排異作用，故在不同個體間移植器官或組織是困難的過程。需用特殊治療（例如免疫抑制藥）以防止移植物的排異反應。

transposition *n.* the abnormal positioning of a part of the body such that it is on the opposite side to its normal site in the body. For example, it may involve the heart (*see* dextrocardia).

錯位（反位） 身體某部分的位置異常，甚至其位置恰與正常部位相反。例如右位心。

transposition of the great vessels a congenital abnormality of the heart in which the aorta arises from the right ventricle and the pulmonary artery from the left ventricle. Life is impossible unless there is an additional abnormality, such as a septal defect, that permits the mixing of blood between

大血管錯位 一種先天性的心臟畸形，主動脈起始於右心室和肺動脈起始於左心室。除非有另外畸形，如中隔缺損，以使肺循環和體循環主動脈的血液混合，否則就不能存活。不治療的很少能活過

the pulmonary and systemic (aortic) circulations. Few of those untreated survive infancy and childhood, but the defect may be improved or corrected surgically.

嬰兒期或兒童期，可通過手術改善或矯正缺損。

transsexualism *n.* the condition of one who firmly believes that he (or she) belongs to the sex opposite to his (or her) biological gender. The roots of such a belief usually go back to childhood. Children with such beliefs are treated with encouragement to engage in the activities appropriate to their biological sex and to work through their difficulties in psychotherapy. Adults with such beliefs can seldom be persuaded to change them; surgical sex reassignment is sometimes justifiable, to make the externals of the body conform to the individual's view of himself (or herself). —**transsexual** *adj.*, *n.*

異性轉化心理變態 他（或她）堅定認爲自己的性別與其生理性別相反的一種病態。這種想法的根源常可追溯到兒童時期，對有這樣想法的兒童，可用鼓勵他參加適合其生理性別的活動來治療，並且以心理療法解決他們的困難。成人有這種想法時就很難以說服使他們改變，有時需做性徵再造手術，使身體外表符合他（或她）對自己的看法。

transudation *n.* the passage of a liquid through a membrane, especially of blood through the wall of a capillary vessel. The liquid is called the *transudate*.

漏出 液體通過膜的移動，特別是指血液通過毛細血管壁，此液體稱爲漏出液。

transurethral resection (TUR) *see* resection.

經尿道（前列腺）切除術

transverse *adj.* (in anatomy) situated at right angles to the long axis of the body of an organ.

橫的 （解剖學）與身體器官長軸成直角的。

transverse process the long projection from the base of the neural arch of a *vertebra.

橫突 脊椎神經弓基底部的長突。

transvestitism *n.* the condition in which sexual pleasure is obtained by dressing in the clothes of the opposite sex. It may occur in both heterosexual and homosexual people and may be directly related to masturbatory or other sexual behaviour. Treatment may be by behavioural techniques such as *aversion therapy, but is not always needed. *See also* perversion. —**transvestite** *n.*

易裝癖 由穿異性的衣服而得到性快感的情況。它可發生於異性和同性戀者，與手淫和其他性行爲直接相關。可通過用行爲療法，如厭惡療法進行治療，但並不經常需要。

tranylcypromine *n.* an antidepressant drug – one of the *MAO inhibitors – given by mouth for the treatment of severe mental depressive states. Common side-effects include restlessness, insomnia, giddiness, and a fall in blood pressure. Trade name: **Parnate**.

反苯環丙胺 一種抗抑鬱藥，爲單胺氧化酶抑制劑。口服用於治療嚴重的精神抑鬱狀態。常見的副作用有焦慮、失眠、眩暈和血壓降低。

trapezium *n.* a bone of the wrist (*see* carpus). It articulates with the scaphoid bone behind and with the first metacarpal in front.

大多角骨 腕部的一塊骨，與後面的舟骨、前面的第一掌骨相關節。

trapezius *n.* a flat triangular muscle covering the back of the neck and shoulder. It is important for movements of the scapula and it also draws the head backwards to either side.

斜方肌 覆蓋頸背部和肩膀的一塊扁平三角形肌肉。它對肩胛骨的運動有重要作用，並可使頭部向後仰，轉向任何一側。

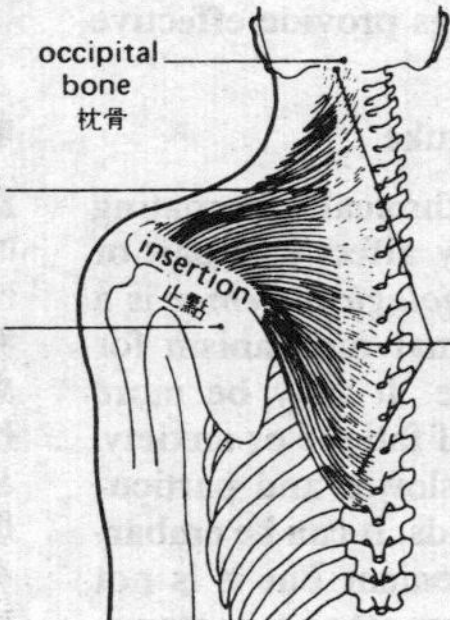

Left trapezius muscle
左斜方肌

trapezoid bone a bone of the wrist (*see* carpus). It articulates with the second metatarsal bone in front, with the scaphoid bone behind, and with the trapezium and capitate bones on either side.

小多角骨 腕部的一塊骨。與前面的第二掌骨、後面的舟骨、以及旁邊的大多角骨、頭狀骨相關節。

trauma *n.* **1.** a physical wound or injury, such as a fracture or blow. **2.** (in psychology) an emotionally painful and harmful event. Theorists have speculated that some events (such as birth) are always traumatic. Symptoms of neurosis may follow an overwhelm-

①**外傷** 軀體的傷害或損傷，如骨折或跌打。 ②**創傷** （心理學）感情上痛苦和受傷害的事件。理論家曾推測某些事件（如分娩）常是創傷性的。神經症狀可能在極爲緊張的

ingly stressful event, such as battle or serious injury. —**traumatic** *adj.*

事件後發生，如戰爭或嚴重外傷。

traumatic fever a fever resulting from a serious injury.

創傷性發熱 由於嚴重外傷而引起的發燒。

traumatology *n.* accident surgery: the branch of surgery that deals with wounds and disabilities arising from injuries.

創傷學 創傷外科。研究創傷和由外傷所致殘疾的外科學分支。

travel sickness (motion sickness) nausea, vomiting, and headache caused by motion during travel by sea, road, or air. The symptoms are due to overstimulation of the balance organs in the *inner ear by repeated small changes in the position of the body and are aggravated by movements of the horizon. *Antihistamine drugs provide effective treatment.

旅行病（暈動病） 由於乘船、汽車或飛機等旅行的運動而引起噁心、嘔吐和頭暈。這種症狀是由於體位反覆的輕微變化使內耳的平衡器官過度興奮，並由於水平運動而加重。抗組織胺藥物治療有效。

trematode *n. see* fluke.

吸蟲

tremor *n.* a rhythmical alternating movement that may affect any part of the body. The *physiological tremor* is a feature of the normal mechanism for maintaining posture. It may be more apparent in states of fatigue or anxiety. *Essential tremor* is slower and particularly affects the hands. It can be embarrassing and inconvenient but it is not accompanied by any other symptoms. A similar tremor may also occur in several members of one family or in elderly people. Tremor is a prominent symptom of *parkinsonism. An *intention tremor* occurs when a patient with disease of the cerebellum tries to touch an object. The closer the object is approached the wilder become the movements.

震顫 累及身體任何部分的節律性交替運動。生理性震顫是維持姿勢的正常機制的特徵。在疲勞或焦慮情況下更加明顯。特發性震顫是較慢的，特別是易發於兩手，這可能使人煩惱和不方便，但它不伴有其他症狀。同樣的震顫可發生於一個家庭中的幾個成員或老年人。震顫是帕金森氏病突出的症狀。意向性震顫發生於有小腦疾病的患者試圖去拿物體時，手愈接近物體，震顫運動愈甚。

trench foot (immersion foot) blackening of the toes and the skin of the foot due to death of the superficial tissues and caused by prolonged immersion in cold water.

浸泡足 由於淺表組織壞死和長時間浸泡在冷水中所引起的脚趾和足部皮膚發黑。

Trendelenburg position a special operating-table posture for patients undergoing surgery of the pelvis or for

特倫德倫伯格氏臥位 骨盆手術病人或休克病人在手術台上的特殊體位，骨

patients suffering from shock. The patient is laid on his back with the pelvis higher than the head, inclined at an angle of about 45°.

盆高於頭部，傾斜大約45°。

trephine *n.* a surgical instrument used to remove a circular area of tissue, usually from the cornea of the eye or from bone (the latter for microscopical examination). It consists of a hollow tube with a serrated cutting edge.

環鋸 用於切除一塊環狀組織的外科器械，常用在切除角膜或骨組織（後者爲顯微鏡檢查用）。它由一個帶有鋸齒切割邊緣的中空管組成。

Treponema *n.* a genus of anaerobic spirochaete bacteria. All species are parasitic and some cause disease in animals and man: *T. carateum* causes *pinta, *T. pallidum* *syphilis, and *T. pertenue* *yaws.

密螺旋體 一種厭氧的螺旋體。所有種屬都是寄生的，有些可使動物和人患病。品他病密螺旋體引起品他病，蒼白密螺旋體引起梅毒，細弱密螺旋體引起雅司疹。

treponematosis *n.* any infection caused by spirochaete bacteria of the genus *Treponema*. *See* pinta, syphilis, yaws.

密螺旋體病 由密螺旋體類引起的感染病。

triad *n.* (in medicine) a group of three united or closely associated structures or three symptoms or effects that occur together. A *portal triad* in a portal canal of the liver consists of a branch of the portal vein, a branch of the hepatic artery, and an interlobular bile tubule.

三聯〔徵〕 （醫學）三種成分聯合的或密切有關的一組結構，或共同發生的三種症狀或作用。肝門三聯就是由靜脈分支、肝動脈分支和葉間膽小管組成。

triamcinolone *n.* a synthetic corticosteroid hormone with uses similar to *cortisone; it reduces inflammation but does not cause salt and water retention. It is administered by mouth and common side-effects include dizziness, headache, somnolence, muscle weakness, and a fall in blood pressure, particularly on the sudden withdrawal of treatment. Trade names: **Adcortyl**, **Ledercort**.

氟羥潑尼松龍 作用與考的松相似的合成的皮質類固醇激素，它減輕炎症，但不引起水鈉瀦留。用於口服。常見的副作用有頭暈、頭痛、瞌睡、肌無力和血壓下降，尤其是在突然中止治療時。商品名：去炎松。

triamterene *n.* a *diuretic that is given by mouth and produces an effect within two hours. It causes the loss of sodium and chloride from the kidneys and is used in the treatment of various forms of fluid retention (oedema). Common side-effects include nausea, vomiting,

氨苯蝶啶 口服利尿劑，2小時內起效，可使腎臟排出鈉和氯，用於治療各種液體瀦留（水腫）。常見的副作用有噁心、嘔吐、無力、血壓降低和消化不良。

weakness, reduced blood pressure, and digestive disorders. Trade name: **Dytac**.

triangle *n.* (in anatomy) a three-sided structure or area; for example, the *femoral triangle.

三角 （解剖學）三邊的結構或部位，例如股三角。

triangular bandage a piece of material cut or folded into a triangular shape and used for making an arm sling or holding dressings in position.

三角帶 一塊被剪成或疊成三角形的材料，用來做手臂懸帶或將敷料固定在適當的位置。

Triatoma *n.* a genus of bloodsucking bugs (*see* reduviid). *T. infestans* is important in transmitting *Chagas' disease in Argentina, Uruguay, and Chile.

錐蝽屬 一類吸血的昆蟲。在阿根廷、烏拉圭和智利，騷擾錐蝽是傳播南美錐蟲病的重要的昆蟲。

triaziquone *n.* a drug used in the treatment of various forms of cancer and administered by mouth, injection, or directly into the tumour. It has toxic actions on normal tissues, particularly the bone marrow; other side-effects include nausea, vomiting, loss of hair, and skin reactions. Trade name: **Trenimon.**

三亞胺醌 治療各種癌瘤的藥物，可用於口服、注射或直接注入腫瘤。對正常組織有毒性，特別是對骨髓。其它副作用有噁心，嘔吐，脫髮和皮膚反應。

triceps *n.* a muscle with three heads of origin, particularly the *triceps brachii*, which is situated on the back of the upper arm and contracts to extend the forearm. It is the *antagonist of the *brachialis.

三頭肌 有三個起點的肌肉，特指肱三頭肌，位於上臂的後側，司前臂伸展作用。它是肱肌的拮抗肌。

trich- (tricho-) *prefix denoting* hair or hairlike structures.

〔前綴〕 毛髮或毛髮樣結構。

trichiasis *n.* a condition in which the eyelashes rub against the eyeball, producing discomfort and sometimes ulceration of the cornea. It may result from inflammation of the eyelids, which makes the lashes grow out in abnormal directions, or when scarring of the conjunctiva (lining membrane) turns the eyelid inwards. It accompanies all forms of *entropion.

倒睫 睫毛摩擦眼球引起不適，有時由角膜潰瘍形成。可能是由於眼瞼炎症使得睫毛向不正常方向生長，或結膜形成瘢痕，使眼瞼向內翻捲。各種形式的瞼內翻均伴有倒睫。

Trichinella *n.* a genus of minute parasitic nematode worms. The adults of *T. spiralis* live in the small intestine of man, where the females release large numbers of larvae. These bore through

毛線蟲屬 一種小的寄生性線蟲。旋毛線蟲的成蟲生活在人的小腸中，雌蟲在此生產大量的幼蟲。它們穿過腸壁可引起疾病。

the intestinal wall and can cause disease (*see* trichinosis). The parasite can also develop in pigs and rats.

這種寄生蟲也可在豬和鼠身上生長。

trichiniasis *n. see* trichinosis.

旋毛蟲病

trichinosis (trichiniasis) *n.* a disease of cold and temperate regions caused by larvae of the nematode worm **Trichinella spiralis*. Man contracts trichinosis after eating imperfectly cooked meat infected with the parasite's larval cysts. Larvae, released by females in the intestine, penetrate the intestinal wall and cause diarrhoea and nausea. They migrate around the body and may cause fever, vertigo, delirium, and pains in the limbs. The larvae eventually settle within cysts in the muscles, and this may result in pain and stiffness. Trichinosis, rarely a serious disease, is treated with thiabendazole.

旋毛蟲病 旋毛線蟲在寒帶和溫帶地區引起的疾病。人食入有幼蟲包囊寄生的未煮熟的肉而得旋毛蟲病。幼蟲在腸道釋出，穿過腸壁並引起腹瀉、嘔吐。它們在全身移行，可引起發燒、眩暈、譫妄和肢體疼痛。幼蟲最終留在肌肉中形成包囊，可能引起疼痛和僵硬。旋毛蟲病很少是嚴重疾病，可用噻苯咪唑治療。

trichloracetic acid an *astringent used in solution for a variety of skin conditions. It is also applied topically to produce sloughing, especially for the removal of warts.

三氯乙酸 一種收斂藥。製成溶液用於各種皮膚病。它也用於局部作爲腐蝕劑，特別是用於去除疣贅。

trichobezoar *n.* hairball; a mass of swallowed hair in the stomach. It may be the patient's own hair or animal hairs. *See* bezoar.

毛團 毛髮團。胃內一團被吞下的毛髮。可以是患者自己的毛髮或動物的毛髮。

Trichocephalus *n. see* whipworm.

鞭毛蟲

trichoglossia *n.* hairiness of the tongue, due to the growth of fungal organisms infecting its surface.

毛舌 由於眞菌感染舌表面引起的毛樣舌。

trichology *n.* the study of hair.

毛髮學 對毛髮的研究。

Trichomonas *n.* a genus of parasitic flagellate protozoans that move by means of a wavy membrane, bearing a single flagellum, projecting from the body surface. *T. vaginalis* often infects the vagina, where it may cause severe irritation and a foul-smelling discharge (*see* vaginitis), and sometimes also the male *urethra; it can be transmitted during sexual intercourse. *Metronidazole is used in treatment. *T. hominis* and *T. tenax*, which live in the large intes-

毛滴蟲屬 有鞭毛的一類寄生性原蟲。具有波動膜和一根鞭毛從體表伸出，借以使蟲體運動。陰道毛滴蟲常侵犯陰道，引起嚴重刺激和惡臭分泌物。有時也侵犯男性尿道，可能是通過性交傳播，可用滅滴靈治療。分別生活在大腸和口腔的人毛滴蟲被認爲是不致病的。

tine and mouth respectively, are not believed to cause disease.

trichomoniasis *n.* **1.** an infection of the digestive system by the protozoan *Trichomonas hominis*, causing dysentery. **2.** an infection of the vagina due to the protozoan *Trichomonas vaginalis*, causing inflammation of genital tissues with vaginal discharge. It can be transmitted to males in whom it causes urethral discharge. Treatment with *metronidazole is effective.

毛滴蟲病 ①由引起痢疾的人毛滴蟲所致的消化系統感染。 ②陰道毛滴蟲所致的陰道感染。可引起生殖器官炎症和陰道分泌物增多。它可以傳染給男性，引起尿道分泌物。用滅滴靈治療有效。

trichomycosis *n.* any hair disease caused by infection with a fungus.

毛髮菌病 眞菌感染引起的毛髮疾病。

Trichophyton *n.* a genus of fungi, parasitic to man, that frequently infect the skin, nails, and hair and cause *favus and *ringworm.

髮癬菌 寄生於人的眞菌屬，經常侵及皮膚、指甲和毛髮，引起黃癬病和白癬病。

trichorrhexis *n.* a condition in which the hairs break easily. It may be due to a hereditary condition or it may occur as a consequence of repeated physical or chemical injury. The latter condition may follow the use of heat or bleach on the hair or be caused by persistent rubbing.

脆髮病 頭髮易斷的一種病。由於遺傳因素或反覆的物理或化學性損傷所致。後者可於頭髮熱燙或漂白之後，或因持久摩擦引起。

trichosis *n.* any abnormal growth or disease of the hair.

毛髮病 毛髮的異常生長或疾病。

Trichosporon *n.* a genus of fungi, parasitic to man, that infect the scalp and beard (*see* piedra).

毛孢子菌屬 寄生於人、侵及頭皮和鬍鬚的一種眞菌。

trichotillomania *n.* loss of hair caused by a person persistently and neurotically rubbing or pulling it.

拔毛髮狂 病人頑固地和神經失常地摩擦和扯拽頭髮，致使頭髮脫失的一種病態。

trichromatic *adj.* describing or relating to the normal state of colour vision, in which a person is sensitive to all three of the primary colours (red, green, and blue) and can match any given colour by a mixture of these three. *Compare* dichromatic, monochromat.

三色視的 形容正常的色覺狀態。表明該人對三種基本顏色（紅、綠、藍）都敏感，而且能夠將此三種顏色適當混合，配出任何要配的顏色。

trichuriasis *n.* an infestation of the large intestine by the whipworm, *Trichuris trichiura*; it occurs principally in

鞭蟲病 毛首鞭蟲在人大腸寄生所致的疾病。主要發生在潮濕的熱帶地區。

humid tropical regions. Man acquires the infection by eating food contaminated with the worms' eggs. Symptoms, including bloody diarrhoea, anaemia, weakness, and abdominal pain, are evident only in heavy infestations. Trichuriasis can be treated with various anthelmintics, including thiabendazole and piperazine salts.

人由於食入被鞭蟲卵污染的食物而被感染，症狀有血性腹瀉、貧血、無力和腹痛，僅在嚴重感染時表現明顯。鞭蟲病可用不同的驅蟲藥治療，如噻苯咪唑和哌嗪鹽類。

Trichuris *n. see* whipworm.

鞭蟲屬

triclofos *n.* a *sedative and *hypnotic, given by mouth, usually as a syrup. It is used to induce sleep or as a daytime sedative, particularly in children. Prolonged administration may lead to *dependence. It is similar in its actions and effects to *chloral hydrate. Trade name: **Tricloryl.**

三氯乙磷酸 口服的鎮靜藥和催眠藥，常爲糖漿。用於引導睡眠或爲白天使用的鎮靜劑，特別是對兒童。長時間服用可導至賴藥性。其作用和效果與水合氯醛相似。

tricuspid valve the valve in the heart between the right atrium and right ventricle. It consists of three cusps that channel the flow of blood from the atrium to the ventricle and prevent any backflow.

三尖瓣 心臟右心房和右心室間的瓣膜，由三個尖瓣組成，它使血液由心房流到心室，而制止其返流。

tridactyly *n.* a congenital abnormality in which there are only three digits on a hand or foot.

三指（趾） 只有三個手指或三個脚趾的先天性畸形。

trifluoperazine *n.* a major *tranquillizer with uses and effects similar to those of *chlorpromazine. Common side-effects include drowsiness, dizziness, dryness of mouth, muscular spasm and tremor, and amenorrhoea. Trade names: **Stelazine, Terfluzine.**

三氟拉嗪 一種重要的安定藥。應用和效果與氯丙嗪相似。常見的副作用有瞌睡、頭暈、口乾、肌痙攣和震顫以及閉經。

trifocal lenses lenses in which there are three segments. The upper provides a clear image of distant objects; the lower is used for reading and close work; and the middle one for the intermediate distance. Musicians sometimes find the middle segment useful for reading the score during performance.

三焦距鏡片 分成三段的眼鏡鏡片，上面的一段獲得遠距清晰物像，下面一段用於讀書和精細工作，中間一段用於中距離視物。音樂家們發現中段可用於在演出時閱讀樂譜。

trigeminal nerve the fifth and largest *cranial nerve (V), which is split into three divisions: the ophthalmic, maxil-

三叉神經 第五對顱神經。是顱神經中最大的一對。它分出三支：眼神

lary, and mandibular nerves (see illustration). The motor fibres are responsible for controlling the muscles involved in chewing, while the sensory fibres relay information about temperature, pain, and touch from the whole front half of the head (including the mouth) and also from the meninges.

經、上頜神經和下頜神經（見圖）。運動纖維支配咀嚼肌，而感覺纖維傳遞整個頭的前半部（包括口部）和腦膜溫度、疼痛和觸覺的信息。

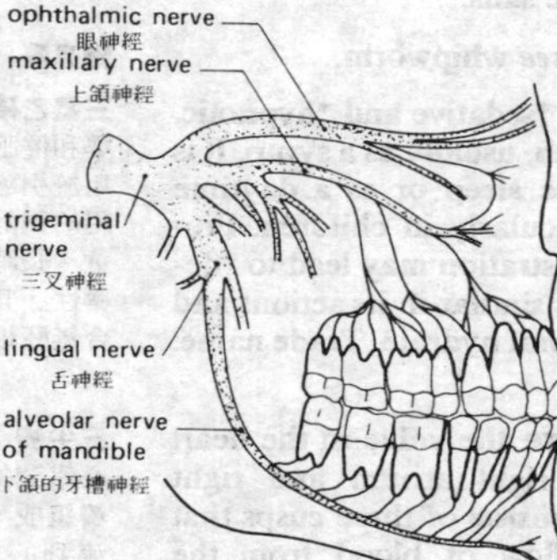

The trigeminal nerve
三叉神經

trigeminal neuralgia (tic douloureux) *see* neuralgia.

三叉神經痛

trigeminy *n.* a condition in which the heart beats can be subdivided into groups of three. The first beat is normal, but the second and third are premature beats (*see* ectopic beat).

三聯搏症 心臟搏動可被分成每三搏一組的異常情況。第一搏動是正常的；第二和第三是期前搏動。

trigger finger an impairment in the ability to extend a finger, resulting either from a nodular thickening in the flexor tendon or a narrowing of the flexor tendon sheath. On unclenching the fist, the affected finger (usually the third or fourth) at first remains bent and then, on overcoming the resistance, suddenly straightens ('triggers'). Treatment is by incision of the tendon sheath.

扳機狀指 由於屈肌肌腱結節狀增厚或其腱鞘狹窄而引起伸指能力的損害。在鬆開拳頭時，病指（常是第三或第四）先是保持彎曲狀，隨後克服阻礙突然伸直（扳機狀）。治療方法是切開腱鞘。

triglyceride *n.* a lipid or neutral *fat consisting of glycerol combined with

甘油三酸酯 由甘油和三個脂肪分子組成的脂類或

three fatty-acid molecules. Triglycerides are synthesized from the products of digestion of dietary fat: they are the form in which fat is stored in the body.

中性脂肪。甘油三酸酯是從飲食脂肪的消化產物合成，它是身體內脂肪貯存的形式。

trigone *n.* a triangular region or tissue, such as the triangular region of the wall of the bladder that lies between the openings of the two ureters and the urethra.

三角區 三角形的區域或組織，如膀胱壁的三角區，位於兩輸尿管開口和尿道口之間。

trigonitis *n.* inflammation of the trigone (base) of the urinary bladder. This can occur as part of a generalized *cystitis or it can be associated with inflammation in the urethra, prostate, or neck of the womb. The patient experiences an intense desire to pass urine frequently; treatment includes the clearing of any underlying infection by antibiotic administration.

膀胱三角炎 膀胱三角區的炎症。它可是整個膀胱炎的一部分，也可伴發於尿道炎、前列腺炎或子宮頸炎。患者有頻繁排尿的强烈慾望。可用抗生素淸除感染。

trigonocephaly *n.* a deformity of the skull in which the vault of the skull is sharply angled just in front of the ears, giving the skull a triangular shape. —**trigonocephalic** *adj.*

三角頭 頭顱畸形。顱骨穹窿在兩耳前方呈陡角，使顱骨成三角形。

trigravida *n. see* tertigravida.

孕$_3$

triiodothyronine *n.* one of the hormones synthesized and secreted by the thyroid gland. *See* thyroid hormone.

三碘甲狀腺氨酸 由甲狀腺合成和分泌的一種激素。

trimeprazine *n.* an *antihistamine drug (a *phenothiazine derivative) that also possesses sedative properties. Given by mouth, it is mainly used in the treatment of pruritus (itching) and as a preoperative medication, especially in children. Common side-effects include drowsiness, dizziness, dryness of mouth, muscular tremor and incoordination, and confusion. Trade name: **Vallergan**.

異丁嗪 一種抗組織胺藥，也具有鎭靜的特性（吩噻嗪的衍生物）。口服主要用於治療瘙癢，和作爲手術前用藥，特別是對兒童。常見副作用有瞌睡、頭暈、口乾、肌肉震顫和不協調，以及精神錯亂。

trimester *n.* (in obstetrics) any one of the three successive three-monthly periods (the *first*, *second*, and *third trimesters*) into which a pregnancy may be divided.

三月期 （產科學）按每三個月爲一期劃分的妊娠分期（第一、第二和第三個三月期）。

trimethoprim *n.* an antiseptic that is active against a range of microorganisms. It is used mainly in the treatment of chronic urinary-tract infections and malaria and is often administered, by mouth, in a combined preparation with sulphamethoxazole (*see* co-trimoxazole (Bactrim, Septrin)). Long-term treatment may cause depression of the bone marrow function.

甲氧苄氨嘧啶 對一系列微生物有效的抗菌藥。它主要用於治療慢性尿道炎和瘧疾，常與磺胺甲基異噁唑製劑聯合用於口服。長期治療可導至骨髓功能受抑制。

trimipramine *n.* a tricyclic *antidepressant drug that also possesses sedative properties. It is given by mouth or by injection for the treatment of acute or chronic mental depression. Common side-effects include drowsiness, dizziness, dry mouth, and a fall in blood pressure. Trade name: **Surmontil**.

三甲丙咪嗪 一種兼有鎮靜作用的三環結構的抗抑鬱藥，用於口服或注射治療急性或慢性精神抑鬱症。常見副作用爲瞌睡、頭暈、口乾和血壓下降。

trinitrophenol *n. see* picric acid.

三硝基酚

triose *n.* a carbohydrate with three carbon units: for example, glyceraldehyde.

丙糖 有三個碳單位的碳水化合物。如甘油醛。

tripara *n. see* tertipara.

產$_3$

triploid *adj.* describing cells, tissues, or individuals in which there are three complete chromosome sets. *Compare* haploid, diploid. —**triploid** *n.*

三倍體的 描述有三個完整染色體組的細胞、組織或個體。

triquetrum (triquetral bone) *n.* a bone of the wrist (*see* carpus). It articulates with the ulna behind and with the pisiform, hamate, and lunate bones in the carpus.

三角骨 腕部的一塊骨。它與後面的尺骨及腕部豌豆狀骨、鈎骨和月狀骨相關節。

trismus *n.* spasm of the jaw muscles, keeping the jaws tightly closed. This is the characteristic symptom of *tetanus but it also occurs less dramatically with overuse of the *phenothiazine drugs and in disorders of the *basal ganglia.

牙關緊閉 咬肌痙攣使上下頜緊閉。是破傷風的典型症狀，但在吩噻嗪類藥用量過多和基底神經節病變時，也可出現不甚顯著的這種症狀。

trisomy *n.* a condition in which there is one extra chromosome present in each cell in addition to the normal (diploid) chromosome set. A number of chromosome disorders are due to trisomy,

三倍體病 在每一個細胞內除了正常染色體組（二倍體）之外存在額外染色體的疾病。一些染色體病是由三倍體引起的，包括

including *Down's syndrome and *Klinefelter's syndrome. —**trisomic** *adj.*

先天愚型綜合徵和先天性睾丸發育不全綜合徵。

tritanopia *n.* a rare defect of colour vision in which affected persons are insensitive to blue light and confuse blues and greens. *Compare* deuteranopia, protanopia.

藍色盲 一種少見的視色障礙，患者對藍色不敏感，並且將藍色和綠色混淆。

tritium *n.* an isotope of hydrogen that emits beta particles (electrons) during its decay. It has been used as a *tracer in the investigation of diseases of the heart and the lungs. Symbol: T or ^{3}H.

氚 氫的同位素，在其衰變時放射出 β 粒子（電子），可作爲示踪劑檢查心臟和肺的疾病。符號：T 或 ^{3}H。

trocar *n.* an instrument used to draw off fluids from a body cavity (such as the peritoneal cavity). It comprises a metal tube containing a removable shaft with a sharp three-cornered point; the shaft is withdrawn after the trocar has been inserted into the cavity.

套針 用於從體腔（如腹腔）抽取液體的器械。它是一個金屬套管，內有一個可抽出的針芯，針尖銳利，將套針插入腔中後即將針芯拔出。

trochanter *n.* either of the two protuberances that occur below the neck of the *femur.

轉子 存在於股骨頸下的兩個隆凸之一。

troche *n.* a medicinal lozenge, taken by mouth, used to treat conditions of the mouth or throat and also of the alimentary canal.

錠劑 含藥糖錠，含化以治療口、咽喉和食道的病變。

trochlea *n.* an anatomical part having the structure or function of a pulley; for example the groove at the lower end of the *humerus or the fibrocartilaginous ring in the frontal bone (where it forms part of the orbit), through which the tendon of the superior oblique eye muscle passes. —**trochlear** *adj.*

滑車 有滑輪樣結構和功能的解剖部分，例如在肱骨下端的溝或眼上斜肌肌腱通過的額骨的纖維軟骨環（組成眼眶的一部分）。

trochlear nerve the fourth *cranial nerve (IV), which supplies the superior oblique muscle, one of the muscles responsible for movement of the eyeball in its socket. The action of the trochlear nerve is coordinated with that of the *oculomotor and *abducens nerves.

滑車神經 第四對顱神經，它支配上斜肌（負責眼球在眼窩中運動的肌肉之一）。滑車神經的作用是與動眼神經和展神經相配合的。

trochoid joint (pivot joint) a form of *diarthrosis (freely movable joint) in

車軸關節，旋轉關節 是動關節（移動自由的關

which a bone moves round a central axis, allowing rotational movement. An example is the joint between the atlas and axis vertebrae.

節）的一種類型。骨在關節中可圍繞中心軸作旋轉運動。例如在寰椎和樞椎間的關節。

Trombicula *n.* a genus of widely distributed mites – the harvest mites. The six-legged parasitic larvae (chiggers) are common in fields during the autumn and frequently attack man, remaining attached to the skin for several days while feeding on the lymph and digested skin tissues. Their bite causes intense irritation and a severe dermatitis. Various repellents, e.g. benzyl benzoate, can be applied to clothing. *Trombicula* larvae are responsible for transmitting scrub typhus in southeast Asia.

恙蟎屬 廣泛分佈的一類蟎，又稱沙蟎（或沙蝨）。六腿寄生幼蟲（恙蟲）在秋天田地中常見，且常襲擊人，在皮膚持續停留幾天，此時以淋巴液爲食，並消化皮膚組織。它們叮咬後引起劇烈的刺激和嚴重的皮炎。預防可用各種驅蟲劑，如用苯甲酸苄酯噴洒衣服。在東南亞恙蟲幼蟲是傳播恙蟲病的媒介。

trometamol *n.* a *diuretic that also reduces the acidity of body fluids. It is given by intravenous injection in conditions of acidosis to adjust the pH of the blood to normal levels. Trade name: **Tham-E**.

氨基丁三醇 一種利尿劑，尚可使體液酸度降低，酸中毒情況下靜脉注射可將血漿 pH 糾正到正常水平。

troph- (tropho-) *prefix denoting* nourishment or nutrition.

〔前綴〕 **營養**

trophoblast *n.* the tissue that forms the wall of the *blastocyst. At implantation it forms two layers, an inner cellular layer (*cytotrophoblast*) and an outer syncytial layer (*plasmidotrophoblast*), which forms the outermost layer of the placenta and attains direct contact with the maternal bloodstream.
Trophoblast sampling is a new screening technique for the prenatal diagnosis of congenital disorders, such as Down's syndrome and thalassaemia, as early as the ninth week of pregnancy. Still being developed, the technique involves the extraction of cells of the trophoblast, by suction through a flexible tube inserted through the cervix of the uterus, and their subsequent examination for genetic abnormalities.

滋養層 形成胚泡壁的組織。在植入時它形成兩層，內部細胞層（細胞滋養層）和外部合胞體層（合體滋養層），後者形成胎盤最外層，直接與母血接觸。
滋養層取樣檢驗是一種新的在胎兒期診斷先天性病變的技術，例如對早在妊娠第 9 週時的先天愚型綜合徵和地中海貧血。進一步發展，此項技術還可以通過一個插入子宮頸的可曲的管子抽吸滋養層的細胞，然後檢查有無遺傳性的異常。

trophozoite *n.* a stage in the life cycle of the malarial parasite (*Plasmodium*)

滋養體原蟲 瘧原蟲生活史中的一個期，在紅細胞

that develops from a merozoite in the red blood cells. The trophozoite, which has a ring-shaped body and a single nucleus, grows steadily at the expense of the blood cell; eventually its nucleus and cytoplasm undergo division to form a *schizont containing many merozoites.

內由裂殖子發育而來。滋養體有一環狀體和一單核，在膨脹的紅細胞內穩定地生長，最後核和胞漿分裂，形成含有許多裂殖子的裂殖體。

-trophy *suffix denoting* nourishment, development, or growth. Example: *dystrophy* (defective development).

〔後綴〕 **營養，發育，生長** 如：營養障礙（發育不全）。

-tropic *suffix denoting* **1.** turning towards. **2.** having an affinity for; influencing. Example: *inotropic* (muscle).

〔後綴〕 **①趨向……的 ②有親和力的，影響……的** 例如：影響收縮力的。

tropical medicine the study of diseases more commonly found in tropical regions than elsewhere, such as *malaria, *trypanosomiasis, *schistosomiasis, and *leishmaniasis.

熱帶醫學 研究在熱帶地區較其他地方常見的疾病的醫學分支。例如研究瘧疾、錐蟲病、血吸蟲病和利什曼病。

tropical ulcer (Naga sore) a skin disease prevalent in wet tropical regions. A large open sloughing sore usually develops at the site of a wound or abrasion. The ulcer, commonly located on the feet and legs, is often infected with spirochaetes and bacteria and may extend deeply and cause destruction of muscles and bones. Treatment involves the application of mild antiseptic dressings and intramuscular doses of *penicillin. Skin grafts may be necessary in more serious cases. The exact cause of the disease has not yet been determined.

熱帶潰瘍 流行於潮濕熱帶地區的一種皮膚病。通常是大塊的開放性爛瘡長在傷口或擦傷處。這種潰瘍常位於脚和腿，往往有螺旋體和細菌感染，可擴展到深處並引起肌肉和骨骼的損傷。治療可應用作用緩和的抗菌敷料和青黴素肌肉注射，在較重病例可能需做皮膚移植。該病的確切原因尚未能確定。

tropocollagen *n.* the molecular unit of *collagen. It consists of a helix of three collagen molecules: this arrangement confers on the fibres structural stability and resistance to stretching.

膠原單位 膠原蛋白的分子單位。它是由三個膠原分子組成的一個螺旋結構。這種排列使得纖維結構穩定和對牽拉有抗力。

troxidone *n.* an *anticonvulsant drug given by mouth, alone or in conjunction with other drugs, in the treatment of epilepsy. It is highly toxic and, in addition to producing nausea, vertigo,

三甲雙酮 一種抗驚厥藥，單獨口服或與其它藥合用治療癲癇。它是高毒性的，除了引起噁心、眩暈、視覺障礙和皮膚反應

visual disturbances, and skin reactions, it can affect the bone marrow and cause anaemia. Trade name: **Tridione**.

外，還可影響骨髓，引起貧血。

truncus *n.* a *trunk: a main vessel or other tubular organ from which subsidiary branches arise.

幹 主要血管或其它管道器官，由此分出從屬的分支。

truncus arteriosus the main arterial trunk arising from the fetal heart. It develops into the aorta and pulmonary artery.

動脉幹 從胎兒心臟發出來的主要動脉幹，它發育為主動脉和肺動脉。

trunk *n.* **1.** the main part of a blood vessel, lymph vessel, or nerve, from which branches arise. **2.** the body excluding the head and limbs.

①**主幹** 分出分支的主要血管和神經部分。 ②**軀幹** 不包括頭和肢體的身體。

truss *n.* a device for applying pressure to a hernia to prevent it from protruding. It usually consists of a pad attached to a belt with straps or spring strips and it is worn under the clothing.

疝帶 加壓力於疝以防止其突出的一種器件，通常是由一個連接搭扣帶的腰帶或彈性布條做成，它穿在衣服裏面。

trypanocide *n.* an agent that kills trypanosomes and is therefore used to treat infestations caused by these parasites (*see* trypanosomiasis). The main trypanocides are arsenic-containing compounds.

殺錐蟲劑 殺錐蟲的藥劑。可用於治療由這些寄生蟲引起的感染。主要的殺錐蟲劑是含砷的化合物。

Trypanosoma *n.* a genus of parasitic protozoans that move by means of a long trailing flagellum and a thin wavy membrane, which project from the body surface. Trypanosomes undergo part of their development in the blood of a vertebrate host. The remaining stages occur in invertebrate hosts, which then transmit the parasites back to the vertebrates. *T. rhodesiense* and *T. gambiense*, which are transmitted through the bite of *tsetse flies, cause *sleeping sickness in Africa. *T. cruzi*, carried by *reduviid bugs, causes Chagas' disease in South America.

錐蟲屬 一種寄生性的原蟲。具有長的鞭毛和薄的波動膜突出於體表之外，借以使蟲體運動。它在脊椎動物宿主的血中發育到一定階段，其餘各期在無脊椎動物身上進行，然後再傳播給脊椎動物。羅德西亞錐蟲和岡比亞錐蟲由彩彩蠅叮咬傳播，在非洲引起昏睡病。克斯錐蟲由獵椿象攜帶，在南美引起恰加斯氏病。

trypanosomiasis *n.* any disease caused by the presence of parasitic protozoans of the genus **Trypanosoma*. The two most important diseases are *Chagas' disease (South American

錐蟲病 由錐蟲類寄生性原蟲引起的疾病。最主要的兩種病是恰加斯氏病（南美錐蟲病）和昏睡病（非洲錐蟲病）。

trypanosomiasis) and *sleeping sickness (African trypanosomiasis).

tryparsamide *n.* a drug used in the treatment of trypanosomiasis (sleeping sickness). Usually given by injection, it penetrates the cerebrospinal fluid and is highly active against the infective organism (*Trypanosoma gambiense*). Trade name: **Tryparsam**.

錐蟲砷胺 治療錐蟲病（昏睡病）的藥物。通常用於注射，可透過腦脊液，對抗病原體（岡比亞錐蟲）的效力很强。

trypsin *n.* an enzyme that continues the digestion of proteins by breaking down peptones into smaller peptide chains (*see* peptidase). It is secreted by the pancreas in an inactive form, trypsinogen, which is converted in the duodenum to trypsin by the action of the enzyme enteropeptidase.

胰蛋白酶 通過將蛋白腖分解成小肽鏈使蛋白繼續消化的酶。胰腺分泌非活性的胰蛋白酶原，在十二指腸經腸肽酶的作用轉化爲胰蛋白酶。

trypsinogen *n. see* trypsin.

胰蛋白酶原

tryptophan *n.* an *essential amino acid. *See also* amino acid.

色氨酸 一種必需氨基酸。

tsetse *n.* a large bloodsucking fly of tropical Africa belonging to the genus *Glossina*. Tsetse flies, which have slender forwardly projecting biting mouthparts, feed during the day on man and other mammals. They transmit the blood parasites that cause *sleeping sickness. *G. palpalis* and *G. tachinoides*, which are found along river banks, transmit *Trypanosoma gambiense*; *G. morsitans*, *G. swynnertoni*, and *G. pallidipes*, which are found in savannah country, transmit *T. rhodesiense*.

彩彩蠅 熱帶非洲的一種大型吸血蠅，屬於舌蠅屬。彩彩蠅有一細長向前突出的能叮咬的嘴部，白天取食於人和其它哺乳動物。它們傳播可引起昏睡病的血液寄生蟲。鬚舌蠅等見於沿河岸地帶，傳播岡比亞錐蟲；淡足舌蠅等見於熱帶草原國家，傳播羅德西亞錐蟲。

TSH *see* thyroid-stimulating hormone.

甲狀腺刺激素

tsutsugamushi disease *see* scrub typhus.

恙蟲病

tubal pregnancy (oviducal pregnancy) *see* ectopic pregnancy.

輸卵管妊娠

tube *n.* (in anatomy) a long hollow cylindrical structure, e.g. a *Fallopian tube.

管 （解剖學）長而中空的結構。例如輸卵管。

tuber *n.* (in anatomy) a thickened or swollen part. The *tuber cinereum* is a

結節 （解剖學）厚的或腫脹的部位。灰結節是大

part of the brain situated at the base of the hypothalamus, connected to the stalk of the pituitary gland.

腦的一部分，位於下丘腦底部，與腺垂體蒂相接。

tubercle *n.* **1.** (in anatomy) a small rounded protuberance on a bone. For example, there are two tubercles at the upper end of the humerus. **2.** the specific nodular lesion of *tuberculosis.

小結節 ①（解剖學）在骨骼上的小圓形突起，例如在肱骨上端有兩個結節。②**結核結節**，結核病的特異性結節狀病變。

tubercular *adj.* having small rounded swellings or nodules, not necessarily caused by tuberculosis.

結節性的 具有小圓形腫脹或結節的，不一定是由結核病引起。

tuberculid *n.* a papular lesion in the skin, probably due to an allergic reaction to tuberculosis infection.

結核疹 皮膚的丘疹樣病變，可能是對結核菌感染的過敏反應。

tuberculin *n.* a protein extract from cultures of tubercle bacilli, used to test whether a person has suffered from or been in contact with tuberculosis. In the *Mantoux test* a quantity of tuberculin is injected beneath the skin and a patch of inflammation appearing in the next 18–24 hours is regarded as a positive reaction, meaning that a degree of immunity is present.

結核菌素 從結核菌中提取出來的一種蛋白浸液，用於檢查一個人是否患有結核病或與結核病有過接觸。芒圖氏反應是注射一定量的結核菌素於皮內，18～24 小時內出現炎症斑塊，則是陽性反應，表明存在一定程度的免疫。

tuberculoma *n.* a mass of cheeselike material resembling a tumour, seen in some cases of *tuberculosis. Tuberculomas are found in a variety of sites, including the lung or brain, and a single mass may be the only clinical evidence of disease. Treatment is by surgical excision, together with antituberculous drugs.

結核瘤 於某些結核病例見到的乾酪樣類似腫瘤的團塊物。結核瘤可見於不同部位，包括肺和腦，並且單獨一個腫塊可以是疾病的僅有的臨床證據。治療是行手術切除，同時用抗結核藥。

tuberculosis *n.* an infectious disease caused by the bacillus *Mycobacterium tuberculosis* (first identified by Koch in 1882) and characterized by the formation of nodular lesions (*tubercles*) in the tissues.

In *pulmonary tuberculosis* – formerly known as *consumption* and *phthisis* (wasting) – the bacillus is inhaled into the lungs where it sets up a primary tubercle and spreads to the nearest lymph nodes (the *primary complex*). Natural immune defences may heal it at this stage; alternatively the disease

結核病 結核分支桿菌（1882 年首次爲郭霍氏確定）引起的傳染病，其特徵是在組織內形成小結狀病變（結核結節）。

肺結核（以前稱爲癆病或肺癆）是結核菌吸入肺後，在肺內形成原發性結節，並且擴散到隣近的淋巴結（原發綜合徵）。在此期內自然免疫性防禦可使之痊癒。另一種情況是疾病可遷延數月或數年，並且隨着患者的抵抗力而

may smoulder for months or years and fluctuate with the patient's resistance. Many people become infected but show no symptoms. They can, however, act as carriers, transmitting the bacillus by coughing and sneezing. Symptoms of the active disease include fever, night sweats, weight loss, and the spitting of blood. In some cases the bacilli spread from the lungs to the bloodstream, setting up millions of tiny tubercles throughout the body (*miliary tuberculosis*), or migrate to the meninges to cause tuberculous *meningitis. Bacilli entering by the mouth, usually in infected cows' milk, set up a primary complex in abdominal lymph nodes, leading to *peritonitis, and sometimes spread to other organs, joints, and bones (*see* Pott's disease).

波動。許多人被感染但無症狀，他們可作爲帶菌者，通過咳嗽、打噴嚏傳播細菌。活動性結核病的症狀有發熱、夜汗、體重下降和咳血。在有些病例，細菌從肺部擴散入血，在全身引起數百萬個結節（粟粒型結核），或轉到腦膜引起腦膜炎。經口進入的結核菌，常是通過結核病牛的牛奶，在腹部淋巴結引起原發綜合徵，導至腹膜炎，有時可播散到其他器官、關節和骨。

Tuberculosis is curable by the antibiotics streptomycin, isoniazid (INH), and para-aminosalicylic acid (PAS). Preventive measures in the UK include the detection of carriers by X-ray screening of vulnerable populations and inoculation with *BCG vaccine of those with no immunity to the disease (the *tuberculin test identifies which people require vaccination).

結核病可以用鏈黴素、異煙肼和對氨基水楊酸治療。在英國，預防措施包括：對易感人羣進行X射線集體檢查以發現攜帶者，並且對無免疫力的人接種卡介苗（以結核菌素試驗確定誰需要接種）。

tuberose *see* tuberous.

結節狀的

tuberosity *n.* a large rounded protuberance on a bone. For example, there is a tuberosity at the upper end of the tibia.

粗隆 骨骼上的圓形突出，例如在脛骨上端有一粗隆。

tuberous (tuberose) *adj.* knobbed; having nodules or rounded swellings.

結節狀的（有結節的） 球狀突出的；有結節或圓形腫脹的。

tuberous sclerosis (epiloia) a congenital disorder in which the brain, skin, and other organs are studded with small plaques or tumours. Symptoms include epilepsy and mental retardation.

結節性硬化（結節性腦硬化） 腦、皮膚或其它器官散佈有小斑塊或腫物的先天性病變。症狀有癲癇和精神發育遲滯。

tubo- *prefix denoting* a tube, especially a Fallopian tube or auditory tube (meatus).

〔前綴〕**管** 尤指輸卵管或咽鼓管。

tuboabdominal *adj.* relating to or occurring in a fallopian tube and the abdomen.

輸卵管腹腔的 有關於或發生於輸卵管和腹腔的。

tubocurarine *n.* a drug given by intravenous injection to produce relaxation of voluntary muscles before surgery and in such conditions as tetanus, encephalitis, and poliomyelitis (*see* muscle relaxant). Toxic side-effects are usually only seen with overdosage, when respiratory failure due to paralysis of respiratory muscles may occur. Trade name: **Tubarine**.

筒箭毒鹼 靜脉注射以使隨意肌鬆弛的藥物。用於手術前以及破傷風、腦炎和脊髓灰質炎等病。毒性副作用通常僅見於過量時，此時因呼吸肌麻痺可能發生呼吸衰竭。

tubo-ovarian *adj.* relating to or occurring in a Fallopian tube and an ovary.

輸卵管卵巢的 關於或發生於輸卵管和卵巢的。

tubotympanal *adj.* relating to the tympanic cavity and the *Eustachian tube.

咽鼓管鼓室的 有關於鼓室和歐氏管的。

tubule *n.* (in anatomy) a small cylindrical hollow structure. *See also* renal tubule, seminiferous tubule.

小管 （解剖學）小而長的空心結構。

tularaemia (rabbit fever) *n.* a disease of rodents and rabbits, caused by the bacterium *Pasteurella tularense*, that is transmitted to man by deer flies (*see* Chrysops), by direct contact with infected animals, by contamination of wounds, or by drinking contaminated water. Symptoms include an ulcer at the site of infection, enlarged lymph nodes, headache, aching pains, loss of weight, and a fever lasting several weeks. Treatment with chloramphenicol, streptomycin, or tetracycline is effective.

兔熱病 由土拉桿菌引起的嚙齒動物和兔類的一種疾病。細菌是通過斑虻、直接與被感染的動物接觸、傷口汚染、或飲用被汚染的水而傳播給人的。症狀表現在感染部位有一潰瘍，淋巴結腫大，頭痛，全身疼痛，體重下降和持續數週的發熱。用氯黴素、鏈黴素或四環素治療有效。

tulle gras a soft dressing consisting of open-woven silk (or other material) impregnated with a waterproof soft paraffin wax.

潤膚薄紗 一種軟的敷料，用紗織成的稀疏的絲織品（或其他材料）浸漬不透水的軟石蠟組成。

tumbu fly a large non-bloodsucking fly, *Cordylobia anthropophaga*, widely distributed in tropical Africa. The female fly lays her eggs on ground contaminated with urine or excreta or on clothing tainted with sweat or urine. The maggots are normally parasites of

嗜人瘤蠅 一種大型的非洲吸血蠅，廣泛分佈於熱帶非洲。雌蠅產卵於被糞尿汚染的土地上，或汗和尿沾汚的衣服上。其蛆常寄生於鼠類，但如果它與人接觸，就可穿過皮膚引

rats, but if they come into contact with man they penetrate the skin, producing boil-like swellings (*see also* myiasis). The maggots can be gently eased out by applying oil to the swellings.

起癤樣腫物，在腫脹處塗油可使蛆逐漸減少。

tumefaction *n.* the process in which a tissue becomes swollen and tense by accumulation within it of fluid under pressure.

腫脹 組織受壓液體積聚，使組織膨脹而緊張的過程。

tumescence *n.* a swelling, or the process of becoming swollen, usually because of an accumulation of blood or other fluid within the tissues.

腫 腫物或腫脹的過程。通常是由於組織內血液或其它液體積聚造成。

tumid *adj.* swollen.

腫脹的

tumor *n.* swelling: one of the classical signs of *inflammation in a tissue, the other three being *calor (heat), *rubor (redness), and *dolor (pain). The swelling of an inflamed area is due to the leakage from small blood vessels of clear protein-containing fluid, which accumulates between the cells.

腫脹 組織炎症的一個典型症狀。炎症的其它三個症狀是發熱、發紅和疼痛。炎症區的腫脹是由於清亮的含蛋白液體從小血管中滲出聚集於細胞間。

tumour *n.* any abnormal swelling in or on a part of the body. The term is usually applied to an abnormal growth of tissue, which may be *benign or *malignant. *Compare* cyst.

腫瘤 身體某部任何不正常的腫物。該詞常指組織的異常生長，可爲良性或惡性的。

Tunga *n.* a genus of sand fleas found in tropical America and Africa. The fertilized female of *T. penetrans*, the chigoe or jigger, burrows beneath the skin of the foot, where it becomes enclosed in a swelling of the surrounding tissues and causes intense itching and inflammation. Surgical removal of the fleas is recommended.

潛蚤屬 見於熱帶非洲和美洲的一種沙蚤類。受精的雌性穿皮潛蚤、沙蚤鑽藏在足部皮膚下面，被封閉於腫脹的周圍組織中，引起劇烈刺癢和皮炎症。建議用手術去除蚤。

tunica *n.* a covering or layer of an organ or part; for example, a layer of the wall of a blood vessel (*see* adventitia, intima, media). The *tunica albuginea* is a fibrous membrane comprising one of the covering tissues of the ovary, penis, and testis.

膜 器官或局部的一個層或被膜，例如血管壁的一層。白膜是一種纖維膜，包裹卵巢、陰莖和睾丸的組織之一。

tunnel *n.* (in anatomy) a canal or hollow groove. *See also* carpal tunnel.

隧道 （解剖學）管道或凹溝。

TUR (transurethral resection) *see* resection.

經尿道（前列腺）切除術

turbinate bone *see* nasal concha.

鼻甲

turbinectomy *n.* the surgical removal of one of the bones forming the nasal cavity (nasal conchae, or turbinate bones).

鼻甲切除術 手術切除形成鼻腔的一塊骨（鼻甲骨）。

turgescence *n.* a swelling, or the process by which a swelling arises in tissues, usually by the accumulation of blood or other fluid under pressure.

腫脹 腫物，或組織發生腫脹的過程，通常是由於組織受壓，以致血液或液體積聚。

turgor *n.* a state of being swollen or distended.

脹滿 一種腫脹或膨脹的狀態。

Turner's syndrome a genetic defect in women in which there is only one X chromosome instead of the usual two. Affected women are infertile: they have female external genitalia but no ovaries and therefore no menstrual periods (*see* amenorrhoea). Characteristically they are short, mentally retarded, and have a webbed neck; other developmental defects are common.

特納氏綜合徵 婦女的一種遺傳性缺陷，她不像一般婦女有兩個 X 染色體，而只有一個。患病的婦女是不育的，她們有女性外生殖器，但無卵巢，所以無月經週期。她們的特徵是體矮，精神發育遲滯和有蹼頸，並常有其它的發育缺陷。

turricephaly *n. see* oxycephaly.

尖頭

tussis *n.* the medical name for *coughing.

咳 咳嗽的醫學專用詞。

twilight state a condition of disturbed consciousness in which the individual can still carry out some normal activities but is impaired in his awareness and has no memory of what he has done. It is encountered after epileptic attacks, in alcoholism, and in organic states of confusion. It may be associated with other symptoms, such as physical and mental slowing, episodes of rage, and hallucinations. Twilight states last only for a short time. commonly a few hours.

朦朧狀態 一種意識混亂，人在這種狀態時可以進行某些正常的活動，但他的意識有障礙，並且記不得他所做的事。可發生於癲癇發作後，酒精中毒和器質性精神錯亂時。可伴有其他症狀，例如體力和腦力活動減慢，暴怒發作和幻覺。朦朧狀態僅持續短時間，通常爲幾小時。

twins *n.* two individuals who are born at the same time and of the same parents. *Fraternal* (or *dizygotic*) *twins* are the result of the simultaneous fertilization of two egg cells; they may be of different sexes and are no more alike

雙生（孿生） 由同父母同時出生的兩個人，雙卵性（或雙合子的）雙胎是兩個卵細胞同時受精的結果，他們的性別可不同，並不比一般兄弟姐妹長得

than ordinary siblings. *Identical* (or *monozygotic*) *twins* result from the fertilization of a single egg cell that subsequently divides to give two separate fetuses. They are of the same sex and otherwise genetically identical; any differences in their appearance are due to environmental influences. *See also* Siamese twins.

更相像。單卵性（單合子的）雙胎是由單個卵細胞受精，然後再分爲兩個胎兒。他們性別相同，且其他方面遺傳性也相同。他們在外表方面的任何不同都是由於環境的影響。

tylosis *n.* the development of a callus on the skin (*see* callosity).

胼胝形成 在皮膚上形成胼胝。

tympan- (tympano-) *prefix denoting* **1.** the eardrum. Example: *tympanectomy* (surgical excision of). **2.** the middle ear.

〔前綴〕①**鼓膜** 例如鼓膜切除術（手術切除）。②**中耳**

tympanic cavity *see* middle ear.

鼓室

tympanic membrane (eardrum) the membrane at the inner end of the external auditory meatus, separating the outer and middle ears. It is formed from the outer wall of the lining of the tympanic cavity and the skin that lines the external auditory meatus. When sound waves reach the ear the tympanum vibrates, transmitting these vibrations to the malleus – one of the auditory *ossicles in the middle ear – to which it is attached.

鼓膜 外耳道內端的膜，分隔外耳和中耳。由鼓室外壁的上皮和外耳道的皮膚形成。當聲波到達耳朶時，鼓膜振動，並將振動傳遞到中耳的一塊聽小骨——錘骨（鼓膜與錘骨是連在一起的）。

tympanites (meteorism) *n.* distension of the abdomen with air or gas: the abdomen is resonant (drumlike) on *percussion. Causes include intestinal obstruction, *irritable bowel syndrome, and *aerophagy.

鼓脹（腸脹氣） 腹內因有空氣和氣體而膨脹，在叩診時腹部有共鳴（鼓音）。原因有腸梗阻、腸激惹綜合徵和吞氣症。

tympanoplasty *n. see* myringoplasty.

鼓膜成形術

tympanotomy *n. see* myringotomy.

鼓膜切開術

tympanum *n.* the *middle ear (tympanic cavity) and/or the eardrum (*tympanic membrane).

鼓室 中耳（鼓室腔）和/或鼓膜。

typhlitis *n.* inflammation of the caecum: formerly a common diagnosis of the condition now recognised as appendicitis.

盲腸炎 盲腸的炎症。以前常下盲腸炎的診斷，現在認爲是闌尾炎。

typhlosis *n.* an obsolete term for *blindness.

視覺缺失 失明的舊稱，現已不用。

typho- *prefix denoting* **1.** typhoid fever. **2.** typhus.

〔前綴〕①**傷寒** ②**斑疹傷寒**

typhoid fever an infection of the digestive system by the bacterium *Salmonella typhi*, causing general weakness, high fever, a rash of red spots on the chest and abdomen, chills, sweating, and in serious cases inflammation of the spleen and bones, delirium, and erosion of the intestinal wall leading to haemorrhage. It is transmitted through food or drinking water contaminated by the faeces or urine of patients or carriers. In most cases recovery occurs naturally but treatment with ampicillin or chloramphenicol reduces the severity of symptoms. Vaccination with *TAB provides temporary immunity. *Compare* paratyphoid fever.

傷寒 傷寒沙門氏菌所致的消化系統傳染病。引起全身虛弱、高熱、胸部和腹部紅斑狀疹、寒顫和出汗，嚴重病例有脾和骨骼發炎、譫妄以及腸壁糜爛導至出血。通過被病人或帶菌者的糞便或尿污染的食物或飲水傳播。多數情況可不治而癒，但用氨苄青黴素或氯黴素治療可減輕症狀的嚴重性。接種傷寒菌苗可得到暫時性免疫。

typhus (spotted fever) *n.* any one of a group of infections caused by *rickettsiae and characterized by severe headache, a widespread rash, prolonged high fever, and delirium. They all respond to treatment with chloramphenicol or tetracyclines. *Epidemic typhus* (also known as *classical* or *louse-borne typhus*) is caused by infection with *Rickettsia prowazeki* transmitted by lice. It was formerly very prevalent in overcrowded insanitary conditions (as during wars and famines), with a mortality rate approaching 100%. *Endemic typhus* (*murine* or *flea-borne typhus*) is a disease of rats due to *Rickettsia mooseri*; it can be transmitted to man by rat fleas, causing a mild typhus fever. There are in addition several kinds of *tick typhus* (in which the rickettsiae are transmitted by ticks), including *Rocky Mountain spotted fever, and typhus transmitted by mites (*see* rickettsial pox, scrub typhus).

斑疹傷寒（斑疹熱） 立克次氏體引起的一組傳染病，其特徵是嚴重的頭痛，廣泛的皮疹，持續高熱和譫妄。用氯黴素和四環素治療均有效。流行性斑疹傷寒（也稱爲經典的或蝨傳的斑疹傷寒）是由蝨傳播普氏立克次氏體引起。過去在擁擠的不衛生的情況下（如戰爭和飢荒時）很易流行，死亡率近於 100%。地方性斑疹傷寒（鼠型斑疹傷寒或蚤傳斑疹傷寒）是由莫氏立克次氏體引起的鼠病；可由鼠蚤傳播給人，引起病情緩和的斑疹傷寒。另一些蜱熱類型（由蜱傳播立克次氏體）包括有落基山斑疹熱和由螨引起的斑疹傷寒。

tyramine *n.* an amine naturally occurring in cheese. It has a similar effect in the body to that of *adrenaline. This effect can be dangerous in patients taking *MAO inhibitors (antidepres-

酪胺 天然存在於奶酪中的一種胺。在身體內與腎上腺素有相似作用，這種作用對服用單胺氧化酶抑制劑的患者可能有危險

sants), in whom blood pressure may become very high. Cheese is therefore not advised when such drugs are prescribed.

性，其血壓可能明顯升高。所以給病人用這類藥時建議不吃奶酪。

Tyroglyphus *n. see* Acarus.

粉螨屬

tyrosine *n. see* amino acid.

酪氨酸

tyrosinosis *n.* an inborn defect of metabolism of the amino acid tyrosine causing excess excretion of parahydroxyphenylpyruvic acid in the urine, giving it abnormal reducing power.

酪氨酸代謝紊亂症　先天性的酪氨酸代謝障礙，尿中過多地排出羥苯丙酮酸，使尿具有異常的還原能力。

tyrothricin *n.* an *antibiotic derived from the bacterium *Bacillus brevis*. It is used, alone or in combination with other drugs, mainly in the treatment of infections of the mouth, throat, skin, wounds and burns; it is applied topically as it is very toxic if taken into the body. Trade name: **Hydrotricine**.

短桿菌素　從短桿菌中提取的抗生素。可單獨應用或與其它藥物聯合應用，主要治療口腔、咽喉、皮膚、創傷和燒傷的感染。由於此藥進入人體後毒性很大，故只用於局部。

U

U

ubiquinone *n.* a *coenzyme that acts as an electron transfer agent in the mitochondria of cells (*see* electron transport chain).

輔酶Q　在細胞線粒體內起電子轉移物作用的一種輔酶。

ulcer *n.* a break in the skin or in the mucous membrane lining the alimentary tract that fails to heal and is often accompanied by inflammation. Ulcers in the skin include *varicose ulcers* complicating *varicose veins, due to defective circulation; *bedsores (decubitus ulcers), due to pressure; and *rodent ulcers, due to malignant growth. For ulcers of the alimentary tract, *see* aphtha, duodenal ulcer, gastric ulcer, peptic ulcer.

潰瘍　不易癒合和常伴發炎症的皮膚或消化道黏膜的破潰。皮膚潰瘍包括因循環障礙所致的靜脈曲張性潰瘍，因壓迫所致的褥瘡（褥瘡性潰瘍）和由於惡性腫瘤所致的侵蝕性潰瘍。關於消化道潰瘍參閱阿弗他、十二指腸潰瘍、胃潰瘍和消化性潰瘍。

ulcerative colitis inflammation and ulceration of the colon and rectum. *See* colitis.

潰瘍性結腸炎　結腸和直腸的炎症和潰瘍形成。

ulcerative gingivitis acute painful gingivitis with ulceration, in which the

潰瘍性齦炎　急性疼痛性有潰瘍形成的齒齦炎症。

tissues of the gums are rapidly destroyed. Occurring mainly in debilitated patients, it is associated with anaerobic microorganisms (*see* Borrelia, Fusobacterium) and is accompanied by an unpleasant odour. Treatment is with *metronidazole and a careful and thorough regime of oral hygiene supplemented with oxidizing mouthwashes. In the past ulcerative gingivitis has been called *Vincent's angina*; in its severe form it is known as *noma.

齒齦組織很快被破壞，主要發生於衰弱患者，併發厭氧菌感染，伴有難聞的氣味。治療是應用滅滴靈，嚴格講究口腔衛生，輔之以使用有氧化作用的含漱劑。以往潰瘍性齦炎被稱爲奮森氏咽峽炎，其嚴重型稱爲走馬疳。

ule- (ulo-) *prefix denoting* **1.** scars; scar tissue. **2.** the gums.

〔前綴〕 **①疤痕，疤痕組織 ②牙齦**

ulna *n.* the inner and longer bone of the forearm (see illustration). It articulates with the humerus and radius above and with the radius and indirectly with the wrist bones below. At its upper end is the *olecranon process and *coronoid process; at the lower end is a cone-shaped *styloid process*. —**ulnar** *adj.*

尺骨 前臂內側的長骨（見圖）。上端與肱骨和橈骨相關節，下端與橈骨，並間接地與腕骨相關節。尺骨的上端有鷹嘴突和喙狀突，下端有圓錐形的莖狀突。

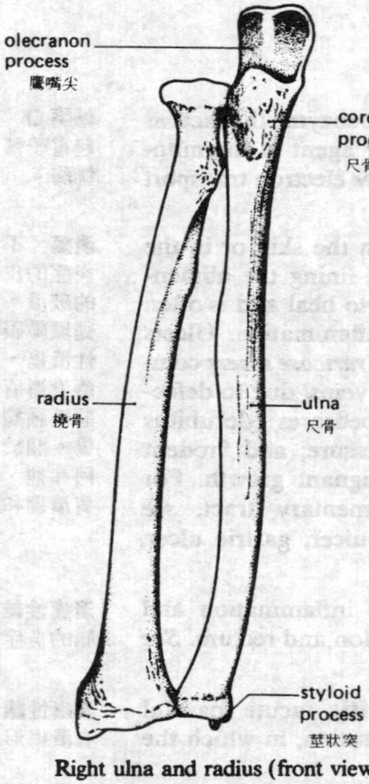

Right ulna and radius (front view)

右尺骨與橈骨（前面）

ulnar artery a branch of the brachial artery arising at the elbow and running deep within the muscles of the medial side of the forearm. It passes into the palm of the hand, where it unites with the arch of the radial artery and gives off branches to the hand and fingers.

尺動脉 肱動脉的分支，起自肘部，在前臂中間肌肉深處走行，穿入手掌與橈動脉弓吻合，分出動脉分支到手和手指。

ulnar nerve one of the major nerves of the arm. It originates in the neck, from spinal roots of the last cervical and first thoracic divisions, and runs down the inner side of the upper arm to behind the elbow. In the forearm it supplies the muscles with motor nerves; lower down it divides into several branches that supply the skin of the palm and fourth and fifth fingers.

尺神經 手臂主要的神經之一。起自頸部，從最後一個頸神經根和第一胸神經根分出，沿上臂的內側下行到肘的背部。在前臂它以運動神經支配肌肉；再向下尺神經分成若干分支，支配手掌皮膚、以及第四和第五手指。

ultra- *prefix denoting* **1.** beyond. **2.** an extreme degree (e.g. of large or small size).

〔前綴〕 ①**超，超出** ②**極端** （例如，極大或極小的）

ultracentrifuge *n.* a *centrifuge that works at extremely high speeds of rotation: used for separating large molecules, such as proteins.

超離心機 能作極高速旋轉的離心機，用來分離大分子，例如蛋白。

ultrafiltration *n.* filtration under pressure. In the kidney, blood is subjected to ultrafiltration to remove the unwanted water, urea, and other waste material that goes to make up urine.

超濾法 加壓下濾過。血液在腎臟受到超濾，以排出不需要的水分、尿素和其它廢物，這些物質組成了尿液。

ultramicroscope *n.* a microscope for examining particles suspended in a gas or liquid under intense illumination from one side. Light is scattered or reflected from the particles, which can be seen through the eyepiece as bright objects against a dark background.

超顯微鏡 在一側强光照明下檢查懸浮在氣體或液體中微粒的顯微鏡。通過接目鏡能看到微粒散射或反射的光線，呈現爲黑暗背景上發亮的物體。

ultramicrotome *n.* an instrument for cutting extremely thin sections of tissue (not more than 0.1 μm thick) for electron microscopy. *See also* microtome.

超微切片機 供電子顯微鏡檢查切割極薄層組織切片的器械（厚度不超過 0.1μm）。

ultrasonics *n.* the study of the uses and properties of sound waves of very high frequency (*see* ultrasound). **—ultrasonic** *adj.*

超聲學 研究超高頻聲波的特徵和應用的學科。

ultrasonography *n.* the use of *ultrasound to produce pictures of structures within the body.

超聲描記術 應用超聲產生身體內部結構圖象的技術。

ultrasonotomography (echotomography) *n.* the use of *ultrasound to examine the internal structure of the body by producing images of the reflections from different depths. A picture of the structures within a 'slice' of the body can be built up, much in the same way as X-rays can be employed to produce a tomogram (*see* tomography).

超聲體層攝影術（回聲體層攝影術） 通過應用超聲產生不同深層的反射影像來檢查身體內部結構的技術。與X線可應用來產生體層攝影圖像的方法一樣，可以產生身體某一層結構的圖像。

ultrasound (ultrasonic waves) *n.* sound waves of extremely high frequency (above 20,000 Hz), inaudible to the human ear. Ultrasound can be used to examine the structure of the inside of the body, in the same way that X-rays can be used to build up pictures but with the advantages that the patient is not submitted to potentially harmful radiation and that structures not opaque to X-rays can be seen. The vibratory effect of these sound waves can also be used in the treatment of various disorders of deep tissues, and even to break up stones in the kidney or elsewhere. *See also* echography.

超聲（超聲波） 人耳聽不到的超高頻率的聲波（20000 Hz以上）。超聲可用來檢查人體內部結構，與X線的方法相同能形成圖像，但它的優點是病人可免受可能有危害的照射，以及能看到可被X線穿透的結構。超聲波的振動作用也可用來治療各種深部組織的疾病，甚至可粉碎腎臟或其它部位的結石。

ultraviolet rays invisible short-wavelength radiation beyond the violet end of the visible spectrum. Sunlight contains ultraviolet rays, which are responsible for the production of both suntan and – on overexposure – sunburn. The dust and gases of the earth's atmosphere absorb most of the ultraviolet rays in sunlight (*see* ozone). If this did not happen, the intense ultraviolet radiation from the sun would be lethal to living organisms.

紫外線 可見紫光光譜以外的看不見的短波長的射線。太陽光含有紫外線，能使皮膚曬黑，過度照射可造成曬傷。地球大氣中的灰塵和氣體能吸收陽光中大部分紫外線。如果不是這樣，從太陽射來的强烈的紫外線照射就將殺傷活着的生物。

umbilical cord the strand of tissue connecting the fetus to the placenta. It contains two arteries that carry blood to the placenta and one vein that returns it to the fetus. It also contains remnants of the *allantois and *yolk sac and becomes ensheathed by the *amnion.

臍帶 將胎兒和胎盤連接起來的組織紐帶。它有兩條向胎盤輸送血液的動脉。臍帶也含有尿囊和卵黄囊的殘餘，並且不被羊膜覆蓋。

umbilicus (omphalus) *n.* the navel: a circular depression in the centre of the abdomen marking the site of attachment of the *umbilical cord in the fetus. —**umbilical** *adj.*

臍 肚臍：位於腹部中心的圓形凹窩。

umbo *n.* a projecting centre of a round surface, especially the projection of the inner surface of the eardrum to which the malleus is attached.

突 圓形表面突起的中心，特別是與錘骨相連接的鼓膜內面的突起。

unciform bone *see* hamate bone.

鈎形骨

uncinate fits a form of temporal lobe *epilepsy in which hallucinations of taste and smell and inappropriate chewing movements are prominent features.

鈎回發作 顳葉癲癇的一種類型，其突出的特徵是有味和嗅的幻覺，以及不合適的咀嚼運動。

unconscious *adj.* **1.** in a state of unconsciousness. **2.** describing mental processes of which a person is not aware. **3.** (in psychoanalysis) denoting the part of the mind that includes memories, motives and intentions that are not accessible to awareness and cannot be made conscious without overcoming resistances. *Compare* subconscious.

①**神志不清的** 處於不省人事的狀態。 ②**無意識的** 描述一種人沒有意識到的心理過程。 ③**潛意識的** （精神分析）包括記憶、動機和意向等心理活動的一部分，沒有達到意識的水平，若不克服阻力，就不能變成有意識狀態。

unconsciousness *n.* a condition of being unaware of one's surroundings, as in sleep, or of being unresponsive to stimulation. An unnatural state of unconsciousness may be caused by factors that produce reduced brain activity, such as lack of oxygen, a blow on the head, poisoning, blood loss, and many diseases, or it may be brought about deliberately during general *anaesthesia. *See also* coma.

意識喪失 對周圍事物失去知覺的狀態，例如在睡眠時，或對刺激無反應狀態。非自然的意識喪失狀態可能由導至腦活動減低的某些因素造成的，例如缺氧、打擊頭部、中毒、失血和很多疾病，或在全身麻醉過程中故意造成的。

uncus *n.* any hook-shaped structure, especially a projection of the lower surface of the cerebral hemisphere that is composed of cortex belonging to the temporal lobe.

鈎 任何鈎形結構，特別是大腦半球下部顳葉皮層表面的突起。

undecenoic acid an antifungal agent, applied to the skin in the form of powder, ointment, lotion, or aerosol spray for the treatment of such infec-

十一酸 抗眞菌藥物，以粉劑、軟膏、洗劑或氣霧的形式用於皮膚病治療，如脚癬。

tions as athlete's foot. Trade name: **Mycota**.

undine *n.* a small rounded container, usually made of glass, for solutions used to wash out the eye. It has a small neck for filling and a long tapering spout with a narrow outlet to deliver a fine stream of fluid to the eye.

洗眼壺 盛洗眼溶液的小的圓形容器。通常由玻璃製成，有一個裝水用的短頸和一個細長的流出管，傾注細流冲洗眼睛。

undulant fever *see* brucellosis.

波狀熱

ungual *adj.* relating to the fingernails or toenails (ungues).

指(趾)甲的 和手指甲或足趾甲有關的。

unguentum (in pharmacy) *n.* an ointment.

軟膏 (藥劑學)一種油膏。

unguis *n.* a fingernail or toenail. *See* nail.

指(趾)甲 手指甲或足趾甲。

uni- *prefix denoting* one.

〔前綴〕 **單一**

unicellular *adj.* describing organisms or tissues that consist of a single cell. Unicellular organisms include the Protozoa, most bacteria, and some fungi.

單細胞的 指由單一細胞組成的微生物或組織。單細胞的微生物包括原蟲、多數細菌和某些眞菌。

unigravida *n. see* primigravida.

初孕婦

unilateral *adj.* (in anatomy) relating to or affecting one side of the body or one side of an organ or other part.

單側的 (解剖學)與身體、器官或某部位的一側有關的。

union *n.* (in a fractured bone) the successful result of healing of a fracture, in which the previously separated bone ends have become firmly united by newly formed bone. Failure of union (*non-union*) may result if the bone ends are not immobilized or from infection or bone diseases. *Compare* malunion.

癒合 骨折(指折斷的骨骼)治療成功的結果。此時，原先分開的骨端因新骨形成而牢固地癒合。骨端沒有固定，或因感染和骨骼疾病可以造成骨端聯接的失敗(不癒合)。

unipara *n. see* primipara.

初產婦

unipolar *adj.* (in neurology) describing a neurone that has one main process extending from the cell body. *Compare* bipolar.

單極的 (神經病學)形容從細胞體伸出一個主突的神經元。

urachus *n.* the remains of the cavity of the *allantois, which usually disappears during embryonic development. In the adult it normally exists in the form of a solid fibrous cord connecting the blad-

臍尿管 尿囊腔的殘餘，通常在胚胎發育期間消失。成人正常存在的形式是連接膀胱與臍的堅韌的纖維帶，但也可以異常地

der with the umbilicus, but it may persist abnormally as a patent duct. —**urachal** *adj.*

存留下形似未閉的管道。

uracil *n.* one of the nitrogen-containing bases (*see* pyrimidine) occurring in the nucleic acid RNA.

尿嘧啶 存在於核糖核酸內的一種含氮鹼基。

uraemia *n.* the presence of excessive amounts of urea and other nitrogenous waste compounds in the blood. These waste products are normally excreted by the kidneys in urine; their accumulation in the blood occurs in kidney failure and results in nausea, vomiting, lethargy, drowsiness, and eventually (if untreated) death. Treatment may require *haemodialysis on a kidney machine. —**uraemic** *adj.*

尿毒症 血內存在過多的尿素和其它含氮的廢物。正常時這些廢物是通過腎臟由尿排出。腎功能衰竭時它們在血內蓄積。引起噁心、嘔吐、嗜睡和最終死亡（若不治療）。治療：需用人工腎機器進行血液透析。

uramustine *n.* a *cytotoxic drug used in the treatment of various forms of cancer, particularly chronic lymphatic leukaemia. It is administered by intravenous injection and is highly toxic; common side-effects are nausea, vomiting and diarrhoea, and depression of bone marrow function. Trade name: **Uracil Mustard**.

尿嘧啶氮芥 治療各種癌症，尤其是慢性淋巴細胞性白血病的細胞毒藥物。用作靜脉注射，毒性大，常見的副作用有噁心、嘔吐和腹瀉，以及骨髓抑制。

uran- (urano-) *prefix denoting* the palate.

〔前綴〕 腭

uraniscorrhaphy *n. see* staphylorrhaphy.

腭裂縫合術

uranism *n.* lead poisoning. *See* lead[1].

鉛中毒

urataemia *n.* the presence in the blood of sodium urate and other urates, formed by the reaction of uric acid with bases. In *gout, urataemia leads to deposition of urates in various parts of the body.

尿酸鹽血症 由於尿酸和鹼的反應形成的尿酸鈉和其它尿酸鹽在血內蓄積。痛風時尿酸鹽血症可導至尿酸鹽沉積於身體各部分。

uraturia *n.* the presence in the urine of urates (salts of uric acid). Abnormally high concentrations of urates in urine occur in *gout.

尿酸鹽尿 尿內存在尿酸鹽。痛風時尿內尿酸鹽濃度異常升高。

urea *n.* the main breakdown product of protein metabolism. It is the chemical form in which unrequired nitrogen is

尿素 蛋白代謝的主要分解產物。身體以這種化合物的形式把不需要的氮由

excreted by the body in the urine. Urea is formed in the liver from ammonia and carbon dioxide in a series of enzyme-mediated reactions (the *urea cycle*). Accumulation of urea in the bloodstream together with other nitrogenous compounds is due to kidney failure and gives rise to *uraemia.

尿排出體外。尿素是在一系列酶的誘導反應下在肝內由氨形成的。由於腎功能不全時血流內尿素與其它含氮化合物的積蓄，引起尿毒症。

urease *n.* an enzyme that catalyses the hydrolysis of urea to ammonia and carbon dioxide.

尿素酶 催化尿素水解成氨和二氧化碳的酶。

urecchysis *n.* the escape of uric acid from the blood into spaces in the connective tissue.

尿浸潤 尿酸從血液漏到結締組織的空隙中。

ureter *n.* either of a pair of tubes, 25–30 cm long, that conduct urine from the pelvis of kidneys to the bladder. The walls of the ureters contain thick layers of smooth muscle, which contract to force urine into the bladder, between an outer fibrous coat and an inner mucous layer. —**ureteral, ureteric** *adj.*

輸尿管 將尿從腎盂導入膀胱的一對長 25～30 cm 的管道。輸尿管壁有厚的平滑肌層，其外面爲纖維膜，其內面爲黏膜層，收縮時促使尿進入膀胱。

ureter- (uretero-) *prefix denoting* the ureter(s). Example: *ureterovaginal* (relating to the ureters and vagina).

〔前綴〕 **輸尿管** 例如：輸尿管陰道的（與輸尿管和陰道有關的）。

ureterectomy *n.* surgical removal of a ureter. This usually includes removal of the associated kidney as well (*see* nephroureterectomy). If previous nephrectomy has been performed to remove a kidney destroyed by *vesicoureteric reflux or because of a tumour of the renal pelvis, subsequent ureterectomy may be necessary to cure reflux into the stump of the ureter or tumour in the ureter, respectively.

輸尿管切除術 切除輸尿管的手術。常同時切除有關的腎臟。如果以前曾因膀胱輸尿管逆流損傷了腎臟或因腎盂腫瘤而做了腎切除術，則隨後可能需要做輸尿管切除術，消除輸尿管殘段的尿液返流或輸尿管中的腫瘤。

ureteritis *n.* inflammation of the ureter. This usually occurs in association with inflammation of the bladder (*see* cystitis), particularly if caused by *vesicoureteric reflux. Tuberculosis of the urinary tract can also cause ureteritis, which progresses to *stricture formation.

輸尿管炎 輸尿管的炎症。其發生經常和膀胱炎有關，尤其是當它由膀胱輸尿管逆流引起時。尿路結核也可以引起輸尿管炎，可發展形成狹窄。

ureterocele *n.* a cystic swelling of the wall of the ureter at the point where it passes into the bladder. It is associated with stenosis of the opening of the ureter and it may cause impaired drainage of the kidney with dilatation of the ureter and *hydronephrosis. If urinary obstruction is present, the ureterocele should be dealt with surgically.

輸尿管疝 輸尿管通入膀胱處輸尿管壁的囊性腫脹，它與輸尿管開口狹窄有關，可引起伴有輸尿管擴張和腎盂積水的腎臟排尿障礙。如果存在尿路阻塞，輸尿管疝需做手術處理。

ureteroenterostomy *n.* an artificial communication, surgically created, between the ureter and the bowel. In this form of urinary diversion, which bypasses the bladder, the ureters are attached to the sigmoid colon (*see* ureterosigmoidostomy).

輸尿管吻合術 人爲地建立輸尿管與腸腔之間的交通手術。這種尿路的改道是繞過膀胱將輸尿管連接到乙狀結腸。

ureterolithotomy *n.* the surgical removal of a stone from the ureter (*see* calculus). The operative approach depends upon the position of the stone within the ureter. If the stone occupies the lower portion of the ureter, it may be extracted by *cystoscopy, thus avoiding open surgery.

輸尿管石切除術 去除輸尿管結石的手術。手術方法取決於輸尿管結石的位置。如果結石位於輸尿管的下部，可以通過膀胱鏡取出，而避免做切開手術。

ureteroneocystostomy *n.* the surgical reimplantation of a ureter into the bladder. This is most commonly performed to cure *vesicoureteric reflux. The ureter is reimplanted obliquely through the bladder wall to act as a valve and prevent subsequent reflux. The operation is usually referred to as an *antireflux procedure* or simply *reimplantation of ureter*.

輸尿管膀胱吻合術 將輸尿管再植入膀胱的手術。最常用於治療膀胱輸尿管返流。將輸尿管呈 45° 角再植入膀胱壁，起活瓣的作用以防止以後的返流。手術通常稱爲抗逆流術或單純輸尿管再植入術。

ureteronephrectomy *n. see* nephroureterectomy.

輸尿管腎切除術

ureteroplasty *n.* surgical reconstruction of the ureter using a segment of bowel or a tube of bladder (*Boari flap*). This is necessary if a segment of ureter is damaged by disease or injury.

輸尿管成形術 用一段腸管或膀胱管重建輸尿管的手術。如果由於疾病或外傷損害了輸尿管，就必須做輸尿管成形術。

ureteropyelonephritis *n.* inflammation involving both the ureter and the renal pelvis (*see* ureteritis, pyelitis).

輸尿管腎盂腎炎 既侵犯輸尿管也累及腎盂的炎症。

ureterosigmoidostomy *n.* the operation of implanting the ureters into the

輸尿管乙狀結腸吻合術 將輸尿管植入乙狀結腸的

sigmoid colon (*see* ureterenterostomy). This method of permanent urinary diversion may be used after *cystectomy or to bypass a diseased or damaged bladder. The urine is passed together with the faeces, and continence depends upon a normal anal sphincter. The main advantage of this form of diversion is the avoidance of an external opening and appliance to collect the urine; the disadvantages include possible kidney infection and acidosis.

手術。這個暫時性尿路改道的方法，可用於膀胱切除術後，或爲了繞過有病或受損的膀胱。尿同糞便同時排出，並且依賴正常的肛門括約肌控制。這種類型的改道主要優點是避免額外的開口和應用器械收集尿液，缺點是可能發生腎臟感染和酸中毒。

ureterostomy *n.* the surgical creation of an external opening into the ureter. This usually involves bringing the ureter to the skin surface so that the urine can drain into a suitable appliance (*cutaneous ureterostomy*). The divided dilated ureter can be brought through the skin to form a spout, but ureters of a normal size need to be implanted into a segment of bowel used for this purpose (*see* ileal conduit) to avoid narrowing and obstruction.

輸尿管造口術　建立一個額外的輸尿管開口的手術。通常是將輸尿管通到皮膚表面，以使尿液排在適合的容器內（皮膚輸尿管造口術）。分離的擴張的輸尿管可以直接在皮膚上做一出口，但是正常大小的輸尿管則需植入一段腸道內再造口，目的是防止其狹窄和阻塞。

ureterotomy *n.* surgical incision into the ureter. The commonest reason for performing this is to allow removal of a stone (*see* ureterolithotomy).

輸尿管切除術　手術切除輸尿管。做此手術最經常的原因是摘除結石。

urethr- (urethro-) *prefix denoting* the urethra.

〔前綴〕 **尿道**

urethra *n.* the tube that conducts urine from the bladder to the exterior. The female urethra is quite short (about 3.5 cm) and opens just within the *vulva, between the clitoris and vagina. The male urethra is longer (about 20 cm) and runs through the penis. As well as urine, it receives the secretions of the male accessory sex glands (prostate and Cowper's glands and seminal vesicles) and spermatozoa from the *vas deferens; thus it also serves as the ejaculatory duct.

尿道　將尿從膀胱排向體外的管道。女性尿道短（大約 3.5 cm），開口在外陰內，在陰蒂和陰道之間。男性尿道長些（大約 20 cm），通過陰莖。除尿外，它也接受男性附屬的性腺（前列腺、庫珀氏腺和精囊）分泌物和從輸精管來的精子。因而也起到射精管的作用。

urethritis *n.* inflammation of the urethra. This may be due to gonorrhoea (*specific urethritis*), a nonspecific venereal infection (*nonspecific urethritis*), or

尿道炎　尿道的炎症。可由淋病（特異性尿道炎）、非特異性的性病感染（非特異性尿道炎），

to the presence of a catheter in the urethra. The symptoms are those of urethral discharge with painful or difficult urination (*dysuria). Treatment of urethritis due to infection is by administration of appropriate antibiotics after the causative organisms have been isolated from the discharge. Untreated or severe urethritis results in a urethral *stricture.

或尿道中放置導管引起。症狀爲排尿疼痛和排尿困難。感染引起的尿道炎的治療是在從尿中分離出致病菌後，再使用相應的抗生素。未治療的或嚴重的尿道炎可引起尿道狹窄。

urethrocele *n.* **1.** a pouch formed from a weakened portion of the wall of the *urethra that encroaches on the vaginal canal. It may result from infection or from the pressure of the fetal head in prolonged labour. **2.** downward displacement (prolapse) of the female urethra through its external opening.

①**尿道憩室**　於尿道壁薄弱部位形成的一個凹陷，且侵犯到陰道。它可由於感染或分娩延長時胎兒頭壓迫所致。　②**尿道突出**　女性尿道通過尿道口向下移位（脫垂）。

urethrography *n.* X-ray examination of the urethra, after introduction of a *radio-opaque fluid, so that its outline and any narrowing or other abnormalities may be observed in X-ray photographs (*urethrograms*). In *ascending urethrography* a radio-opaque jelly is injected up the urethra using a special syringe and penile clamp. In *descending urethrography* (*micturating cystourethrography*, *MCUG*), X-rays of the urethra can be taken during the passing of water-soluble contrast material previously inserted into the bladder.

尿道X線造影術　在導入不透X線的液體後，進行尿道X線檢查。在X線照像上可觀察到尿道外形、尿道的狹窄或其他的異常（尿道像片）。在上行尿道X線造影時，用特殊注射器和陰莖夾把造影劑射入尿道。在下行尿道X線造影（排泄性膀胱尿道造影術）時，可在預先注入膀胱的水溶性造影劑通過尿道時進行X線照像。

urethroplasty *n.* surgical repair of a urethral *stricture. The operation entails the insertion of a flap or patch of skin from the scrotum or perineum into the urethra at the site of the stricture, which is laid widely open. The operation can be performed in one stage, although two stages are usual in the reconstruction of a posterior urethral stricture (*see* urethrostomy).

尿道成形術　尿道狹窄的修復手術。手術的任務是把從陰囊或會陰皮膚取出的皮瓣和皮片植入尿道狹窄處，使其開口增大。手術可以一步完成。但通常後尿道狹窄的重建術則分兩步完成。

urethrorrhaphy *n.* surgical restoration of the continuity of the urethra. This may be required following laceration of the urethra.

尿道縫合術　手術修復尿道。可用於尿道撕裂後。

urethrorrhoea *n.* a discharge from the urethra. This is a symptom of *urethritis.

尿道液溢 從尿道不斷流出滲液，這是尿道炎症狀之一。

urethroscope *n.* an *endoscope, consisting of a fine tube fitted with a light and lenses, for examination of the interior of the male urethra, including the prostate region. —**urethroscopy** *n.*

尿道鏡 檢查男性尿道內部（包括前列腺區）的內窺鏡，由裝有光束和透鏡的細管組成。

urethrostenosis *n.* a *stricture of the urethra.

尿道狹窄 尿道的狹窄。

urethrostomy *n.* the operation of creating an opening of the urethra in the perineum in men. This can be permanent, to bypass a severe *stricture of the urethra in the penis, or it can form the first stage of an operation to cure a stricture of the posterior section of the urethra (*urethroplasty).

尿道造口術 在男性會陰部建立一個尿道開口的手術。可以是永久性的，目的是繞過陰莖內嚴重狹窄的尿道，或作爲治療尿道後部狹窄手術的第一步。

urethrotomy *n.* the operation of cutting a *stricture in the urethra. It is usually performed with a *urethrotome*. This instrument, a type of *endoscope, consists of a sheath down which is passed a fine knife, which is operated by the surgeon viewing the stricture down an illuminated telescope.

尿道切開術 切開狹窄尿道的手術。常用尿道刀來完成。這種器械是由一個有小刀通過的鞘組成的內窺鏡，由外科醫生通過照明鏡觀察而作手術。

-uria *suffix denoting* **1.** a condition of urine or urination. Example: ***polyuria*** (passage of excess urine). **2.** the presence of a specified substance in the urine. Example: ***haematuria*** (blood in).

〔後綴〕 **尿** ①尿或排尿的情況。如多尿（排尿過多） ②尿中出現的特殊物質。如血尿（血在尿內）。

uric acid a nitrogen-containing organic acid that is the end-product of nucleic acid metabolism and is a component of the urine. Crystals of uric acid are deposited in the joints of people suffering from *gout.

尿酸 含氮的有機酸，是核酸代謝的終末產物，也是尿液的一部分。尿酸結晶沉積於痛風患者的關節內。

uricosuric drug a drug, such as *probenecid or *sulphinpyrazone, that increases the amount of *uric acid excreted in the urine. Uricosuric drugs are used to treat gout and other conditions in which the levels of uric acid in the blood are increased, as during treat-

促尿酸尿藥物 促使尿酸從尿排出量增加的藥物，如丙磺舒和苯磺唑酮，用於治療痛風和血中尿酸增加，例如在用某些利尿劑治療期間。促尿酸尿藥物有時與某種抗生素（如青

ment with some *diuretics. Uricosuric drugs are sometimes administered with certain antibiotics (such as penicillin) to maintain high blood levels since they inhibit their excretion.

黴素）合用，以維持其高血藥水平，因爲促尿酸尿藥物抑制抗生素的排泄。

uridine *n.* a compound containing uracil and the sugar ribose. *See also* nucleoside.

尿核苷 含尿嘧啶和核糖的複合物。

uridrosis *n.* the presence of excessive amounts of urea in the sweat; when the sweat dries, a white flaky deposit of urea may remain on the skin. The phenomenon occurs in *uraemia.

尿汗症 汗中出現過多的尿素，當汗乾後，尿素的白色絮片狀沉積物留於皮膚上，這種現象見於尿毒症。

urin- (urino-, uro-) *prefix denoting* urine or the urinary system.

〔前綴〕 **尿，泌尿系統**

urinalysis *n.* the analysis of *urine, using physical, chemical and microscopical tests, to determine the proportions of its normal constituents and to detect alcohol, drugs, sugar, or other abnormal constituents.

尿分析 用物理，化學或顯微鏡方法檢查尿以判斷其正常成分的比例，和檢測尿中的酒精、藥物、糖或其它異常成分。

urinary bladder *see* bladder.

膀胱

urinary tract the entire system of ducts and channels that conduct urine from the kidneys to the exterior. It includes the ureters, the bladder, and the urethra.

尿路 將尿從腎向體外排出的整個管道系統。包括輸尿管、膀胱和尿道。

urination (micturition) *n.* the periodic discharge of urine from the bladder through the urethra. It is initiated by voluntary relaxation of the sphincter muscle below the bladder and maintained by reflex contraction of the muscles of the bladder wall.

排尿 定期從膀胱經尿道排出尿液。排尿的開始是通過膀胱下的括約肌隨意的鬆弛，而由膀胱壁肌肉收縮反射維持尿液排出。

urine *n.* the fluid excreted by the kidneys, which contains many of the body's waste products. It is the major route by which the end-products of nitrogen metabolism – *urea, *uric acid, and *creatinine – are excreted. The other major constituent is sodium chloride. Over 100 other substances are usually present, but only in trace amounts. Biochemical analysis of urine

尿 從腎臟排出的含有身體許多廢物的液體。它是含氮代謝終末產物尿素、尿酸和肌酐排出的主要途徑。另外的主要成分是氯化鈉。通常尿中有100多種其它物質，但僅是微量的。尿液生化分析常用於診斷疾病（如糖尿病時尿糖水平增高，酮尿症時酮

is commonly used in the diagnosis of diseases (for example, there are high levels of urinary glucose in diabetes and of ketone bodies in ketonuria) and in *pregnancy tests.

體水平增高）和作姙娠試驗。

uriniferous tubule *see* renal tubule.

腎小管

urinogenital (urogenital) *adj.* of or relating to the organs and tissues concerned with excretion and reproduction, which are anatomically closely associated.

泌尿生殖的　解剖上密切相關的泌尿和生殖器官組織。

urinogenital sinus the duct in the embryo that receives the ureter and mesonephric and paramesonephric ducts and opens to the exterior. The innermost portion forms most of the bladder and the remainder forms the urethra with its associated glands. Part of it may also contribute towards the vagina.

泌尿生殖竇　胚胎期接受輸尿管、中腎管、副中腎管、開口於體外的管道。其最裏面部分形成膀胱的大部分，其餘部分形成尿道及其有關的腺體，部分也可形成陰道。

urinometer *n.* a hydrometer for measuring the specific gravity of urine.

尿比重計　測量尿液比重的儀器。

urobilinogen *n.* a colourless product of the reduction of the *bile pigment bilirubin. Urobilinogen is formed from bilirubin in the intestine by bacterial action. Part of it is reabsorbed and returned to the liver; part of it is excreted in the faeces (a trace may also appear in the urine). When exposed to air, urobilinogen is oxidized to a brown pigment, *urobilin*.

尿膽素原　一種膽汁色素（膽紅素）的無色還原產物。尿膽素原是膽紅素在腸道內受細菌作用形成。部分被重吸收並回到肝臟，部分從糞中排出（尿內也可有微量）。當尿膽素原暴露於空氣中時，被氧化形成褐色色素——尿膽素。

urocele *n.* a cystic swelling in the scrotum, containing urine that has escaped from the urethra. This may arise following urethral injury. Immediate treatment is to divert the urine by suprapubic *cystotomy, local drainage of the swelling, and antibiotic administration.

陰囊積液　陰囊的囊性腫脹，含有從尿道溢出的尿液。這可發生在尿道損傷後。即時的治療是作恥骨弓上膀胱切開術以排出尿液，腫脹局部引流和應用抗生素。

urochesia *n.* the passage of urine through the rectum. This may follow a penetrating injury involving both the lower urinary tract and the bowel.

肛門排尿　尿通過直腸排出。它可發生在下部尿路和腸道的穿透性損傷後。

urogenital *adj. see* urinogenital.

泌尿生殖的

urography *n. see* pyelography.
尿道照影術

urolith *n.* a stone in the urinary tract. *See* calculus.
尿石 尿路的結石。

urology *n.* the branch of medicine concerned with the study and treatment of diseases of the urinary tract. —**urological** *adj.* —**urologist** *n.*
泌尿科學 研究和治療尿路疾病的醫學分支。

uroporphyrin *n.* a porphyrin that plays an intermediate role in the synthesis of *protoporphyrin IX. It is excreted in significant amounts in the urine in porphyria.
尿卟啉 合成原卟啉 IX 中起中介作用的卟啉，在卟啉症時大量的尿卟啉從尿中排出。

urticaria (hives, nettle rash) *n.* an acute or chronic allergic reaction in which red round wheals develop on the skin, ranging in size from small spots to several inches across. These itch intensely and may last for hours or days; the cause is sensitivity to certain foods, such as shellfish or strawberries. Sometimes urticaria may affect areas other than the skin, causing swelling on the tongue and lips: this serious variety, *angioneurotic oedema*, needs urgent medical attention.
蕁麻疹 急性的或慢性的過敏反應，皮膚出現大小不等的紅色圓形風團，小至點狀，大到幾英寸。有劇烈刺癢，可持續幾小時或幾天，其原因是對某些食物過敏，例如水生貝殼類動物或草莓。有時蕁麻疹除了累及皮膚外，可引起舌和唇的腫脹，這種嚴重情況稱爲血管神經性水腫，需要緊急的治療。

uter- (utero-) *prefix denoting* the womb (uterus). Examples: *uterocervical* (relating to the cervix (neck) of the womb); *uterovaginal* (relating to the womb and vagina); *uterovesical* (relating to the womb and bladder).
〔前綴〕 **子宮** 例如子宮頸的，子宮陰道的，子宮膀胱的。

uterine *adj.* of or relating to the womb (uterus).
子宮的 與子宮有關的。

uterocele *n. see* hysterocele.
子宮突出

uterogestation *n.* the development of a fetus in the womb, i.e. a normal pregnancy. *Compare* ectopic pregnancy.
子宮姙娠 胎兒在子宮內生長，即正常的姙娠。

uterography *n.* *radiography of the womb.
子宮造影術 子宮的放射線照像術。

utero-ovarian *adj.* relating to or occurring in the womb and an ovary.
子宮卵巢的 關於或發生於子宮和卵巢的。

uterosalpingography (hysterosalpingography) *n.* *radiography of the
子宮輸卵管造影術 注入不透射線的液體後，子宮

interior of the womb and the Fallopian tubes following injection of a *radio-opaque fluid.
和輸卵管的放射線顯影技術。

uterus (womb) *n.* the part of the female reproductive tract that is specialized to allow the embryo to become implanted in its inner wall and to nourish the growing fetus from the maternal blood. The nonpregnant uterus is a pear-shaped organ, about 7.5 cm long. It is suspended in the pelvic cavity by means of peritoneal folds (ligaments) and fibrous bands. The upper part is connected to the two *Fallopian tubes and the lower part joins the vagina at the cervix. The uterus has an inner mucous lining (*endometrium) and a thick wall of smooth muscle (*myometrium). During childbirth the myometrium undergoes strong contractions to expel the fetus through the cervix and vagina. In the absence of pregnancy the endometrium undergoes periodic development and degeneration (*see* menstrual cycle). —**uterine** *adj.*
子宮 女性生殖器的一部分，專爲胚胎植入其內壁和從母血中給生長着的胎兒以營養。未妊娠的子宮是一梨形器官，大約 7.5 cm 長。藉腹膜韌帶和纖維性帶懸於盆腔內。上部與兩個輸卵管相連接，下部以子宮頸與陰道相連接。子宮有內黏膜層（子宮內膜）和厚的平滑肌壁（子宮肌層）。在分娩時子宮肌層進行强有力的收縮，將胎兒通過子宮頸和陰道娩出。未妊娠的子宮，其內膜周期性增生和退化。

utricle (utriculus) *n.* **1.** the larger of the two membranous sacs within the vestibule of the ear: it forms part of the membranous *labyrinth. It is filled with fluid (endolymph) and contains a *macula. This responds to gravity and relays information to the brain about the position of the head. **2.** a small sac (the *prostatic utricle*) extending out of the urethra of the male into the substance of the prostate gland.
①**橢圓囊** 內耳前庭部的兩個膜性囊中較大的一個。它形成膜迷路的一部分。充滿液體（內淋巴）和含有聽斑。它把重力和有關頭部位置的信息傳遞到大腦。 ②**小囊（前列腺囊）** 從男性尿道伸到前列腺實質中的小囊。

uvea (uveal tract) *n.* the vascular pigmented layer of the eye, which lies beneath the outer layer (sclera). It consists of the *choroid, *ciliary body, and *iris. —**uveal** *adj.*
眼色素層 眼球外層（鞏膜）底下的血管色素層。它由脉絡膜、睫狀體和虹膜組成。

uveal tract *see* uvea.
葡萄膜 即眼色素層。

uveitis *n.* inflammation of any part of the uveal tract of the eye, either the iris (*iritis*), ciliary body (*cyclitis*), or choroid (*choroiditis*). Inflammation confined to
眼色素層炎（葡萄膜炎） 眼色素層任何一部分的炎症：虹膜（虹膜炎）、睫狀體（睫狀體炎）以及脉

the iris and ciliary body, which are commonly inflamed together, is called *anterior uveitis*; that confined to the choroid is termed *posterior uveitis*. In general, the causes of anterior and posterior uveitis are different; anterior uveitis (unlike choroiditis) is usually painful. All types may lead to visual impairment, and uveitis is an important cause of blindness. In most cases the disease appears to originate in the uveal tract itself, but it may occur secondarily to disease of other parts of the eye, particularly of the cornea and sclera. Treatment consists of the use of drugs that suppress the inflammation, combined with measures to relieve the discomfort and more specific drug treatment if a specific cause of the uveitis is found. The drugs may be given as drops, injections, or tablets, often in combination.

絡膜（脈絡膜炎）。限於虹膜和睫狀體的炎症常常是同時發生，稱爲前眼色素層炎。限於脉絡膜的炎症稱爲後眼色素層炎。通常，引起前眼色素層炎和後眼色素層炎的原因是不同的，前眼色素層炎（不同於脉絡膜炎）常常是很痛的。所有類型都引起視力損傷，並且眼色素層炎是失明的重要原因之一。多數情況下此病原發於眼色素層本身，但也可繼發於眼其他部分的疾病，特別是角膜和鞏膜。治療包括用藥控制炎症，同時採用減輕不適的措施。如果找到眼色素層炎的特殊原因，可用特異性藥物治療。藥物可用滴劑、注射劑或片劑，經常是聯合應用。

uveoparotitis (uveoparotid fever) *n.* inflammation of the iris, ciliary body, and choroid regions of the eye (the uvea) and swelling of the parotid salivary gland: one of the more common varieties of the chronic disease *sarcoidosis.

眼色素層腮腺炎 眼內虹膜、睫狀體和脉絡膜（眼色素層）的炎症和腮腺腫脹同時發生，這是慢性結節病中較常見的一種。

uvula *n.* a small soft extension of the soft palate that hangs from the roof of the mouth above the root of the tongue. It is composed of muscle, connective tissue, and mucous membrane.

懸壅垂 位於舌根上方，懸於口腔底部軟腭上的一小塊軟的延伸物。它由肌肉、結締組織和黏膜組成。

uvulectomy *n.* surgical removal of the uvula.

懸壅垂切除術 切除懸壅垂的手術。

uvulitis *n.* inflammation of the uvula.

懸壅垂炎 懸壅垂發炎。

V

V

vaccination *n.* a means of producing immunity to a disease by using a *vaccine, or a special preparation of antigenic material, to stimulate the

接種 一種用疫苗或抗原物質的特殊製劑刺激機體形成相應的抗體，以產生對疾病免疫力的方法。這

formation of appropriate antibodies. The name was applied originally only to treatment with vaccinia (cowpox) virus, which gives protection not only against cowpox itself but also against the related smallpox. However, it is now used synonymously with *inoculation* as a method of *immunization against any disease. Vaccination is often carried out in two or three stages, as separate doses are less likely to cause unpleasant side-effects. A vaccine is usually given by injection but may be introduced into the skin through light scratches; for some diseases, oral vaccines are available.

名詞原來僅用在使用牛痘病毒疫苗上，這種病毒疫苗不僅可預防牛痘，並且可抗天花。然而現在它被用來作爲任何疾病進行免疫接種的同義詞。接種常採用兩或三步進行，因每次使用較小劑量可減少副作用。接種常採用注射法，但也可通過輕輕劃紋而導入皮膚，對某些疾病可用口服疫苗。

vaccine *n.* a special preparation of antigenic material that can be used to stimulate the development of antibodies and thus confer active *immunity against a specific disease or number of diseases. Many vaccines are produced by culturing bacteria or viruses under conditions that lead to a loss of their virulence but not of their antigenic nature. Other vaccines consist of specially treated toxins (*toxoids) or of dead bacteria that are still antigenic. Examples of live but attenuated (weakened) organisms in vaccines are those against tuberculosis, rabies, and smallpox. Dead organisms are used against cholera and typhoid; precipitated toxoids are used against diphtheria and tetanus. *See* immunization.

疫苗　一種特異的抗原製劑，用於刺激機體產生抗體，從而對某特殊疾病或一組疾病產生自動免疫。許多疫苗的製成是通過細菌和病毒的培養使之喪失毒力，但保持它的抗原性，有些疫苗是經過特殊處理的仍有抗原性的毒素（類毒素）或死菌製成。例如毒力減弱的活菌疫苗有抗結核病、狂犬病和天花等疫苗。抗霍亂和梅毒的是死菌疫苗；類毒素沉澱劑用於抗白喉和破傷風。

vaccinia *n. see* cowpox.

牛痘

vaccinoid *adj.* resembling a local infection with vaccinia (cowpox) virus. A vaccinoid reaction is one of the possible results of vaccination against smallpox in individuals who already have partial immunity. The swelling, reddening, and blistering are considerably less than the so-called primary reaction that occurs after the inoculation of a person with no immunity against smallpox.

假牛痘　類似於牛痘病毒的局部感染。假牛痘反應是對天花已有部分免疫者種痘時可能引起的結果。腫脹、發紅和水疱比無天花免疫者在種痘後發生的所謂的初發反應明顯地輕。

vacuole *n.* a space within the cytoplasm of a cell, formed by infolding of

空泡　由細胞膜內折形成的細胞漿內的空間，其中

the cell membrane, that contains material taken in by the cell. White blood cells form vacuoles when they surround and digest bacteria and other foreign material.

含有被細胞攝入的物質。當白細胞包圍和消化細菌與其他異物時形成空泡。

vacuum extractor a suction cup that can be attached to the head of a fetus in order to aid delivery.

真空吸取器 爲了幫助分娩而放在胎兒頭部的吸杯。

vagin- (vagino-) *prefix denoting* the vagina.

〔前綴〕 **陰道**

vagina *n.* the lower part of the female reproductive tract: a muscular tube, lined with mucous membrane, connecting the cervix of the uterus (womb) to the exterior. It receives the erect penis during coitus: semen is ejaculated into the upper part of the vagina and from there the sperms must pass through the cervix and womb in order to fertilize an ovum in the Fallopian tube. The wall of the vagina is sufficiently elastic to allow the passage of the newborn child. —**vaginal** *adj.*

陰道 女性生殖道的最低部分，是襯有黏膜的肌肉管道，將子宮頸和外部相連接。性交時接受勃起的陰莖，精液射入陰道上部，然後精子必須通過子宮頸和子宮腔，才能在輸卵管使卵受精。陰道壁有充足的彈性可允許新生兒通過。

vaginismus *n.* sudden and painful contraction of the muscles surrounding the vagina, usually in response to the *vulva or vagina being touched. Sexual intercourse may be impeded, and the condition may be associated with fear of or aversion to coitus. Other causative factors include vaginal injury or ulceration, dryness or shrinkage of the lining membrane of the vagina, and inflammation of the vagina or bladder. *See also* dyspareunia.

陰道痙攣 常因接觸外陰和陰道而引起陰道周圍肌肉突然的和疼痛的收縮反應。可能妨礙性交。這種情況常與對性交害怕和反感有關，其他原因可有陰道損傷或潰瘍、陰道黏膜乾燥或皺縮以及陰道或膀胱的炎症。

vaginitis *n.* inflammation of the vagina, which may be caused by infection (commonly with **Trichomonas vaginalis*), ill-fitting contraceptive devices, dietary deficiency, or poor hygiene. There is often irritation, increased vaginal discharge, and pain on passing urine. Vaginitis may indicate the presence of venereal disease. *Postmenopausal vaginitis* is caused by a deficiency of female sex hormones.

陰道炎 陰道的炎症。可能由感染（常爲陰道滴蟲）和不恰當的避孕措施，飲食不足或衛生不佳引起。經常有刺激感，陰道分泌物增加和排尿時疼痛。陰道炎可能提示有性病，月經後陰道炎是由於缺乏女性激素引起的。

vaginoplasty (colpoplasty) *n.* a tissue-grafting operation on the vagina.

陰道成形術 陰道的組織移植手術。

vaginoscope *n. see* colposcope.

陰道鏡

vago- *prefix denoting* the vagus nerve.

〔前綴〕 **迷走神經**

vagotomy *n.* the surgical cutting of any of the branches of the vagus nerve. This is usually performed to reduce secretion of acid and pepsin by the stomach in order to cure a peptic ulcer. *Truncal vagotomy* is the cutting of the main trunks of the vagus nerve; in *selective vagotomy* the branches of the nerve to the gall bladder and pancreas are left intact. *Highly selective* or *proximal vagotomy* is the cutting of the branches of the vagus nerve to the body of the stomach, leaving the branches to the outlet (pylorus) intact: this makes additional surgery to permit emptying of the stomach contents unnecessary.

迷走神經切斷術 切斷迷走神經任何分支的手術。常用於治療消化性潰瘍，可減少胃酸和蛋白酶的分泌。迷走神經幹切斷術是切斷迷走神經的主幹；選擇性迷走神經切斷術時，支配膽囊和胰腺的神經分支保留完整。高度選擇性或近端迷走神經切斷術是切斷支配胃體部的迷走神經，留下支配幽門的分支完整無損，這就不需要做使胃內容物排空的附加手術。

vagus nerve the tenth *cranial nerve (X), which supplies motor nerve fibres to the muscles of swallowing and parasympathetic fibres to the heart and organs of the chest cavity and abdomen. Sensory branches of the vagus carry impulses from the viscera and the sensation of taste from the mouth.

迷走神經 第十對顱神經。以運動神經纖維支配吞嚥活動的肌肉和以副交感神經纖維支配心臟和胸腔、腹腔的臟器。迷走神經的感覺分支接受來自內臟的衝動和來自口腔的味覺。

valgus *adj.* describing any deformity that displaces the hand or foot away from the midline. *See* club-foot (talipes valgus), knock knee (genu valgum).

外翻的 指手或足離開中線錯位的畸形。

validity *n.* an indication of the extent to which a clinical sign or test is a true indicator of disease. Reduced validity can arise if the tests produce different results when conducted several times on the same person under identical conditions (i.e. *reduced reproducibility*, *reliability*, or *repeatability*). This may be because the same observer gets different results on successive occasions (*intraobserver error*) or because a series of different observers fail to obtain the same result (*interobserver error*). Such errors may arise because of a true

準確性 指一個臨床徵象或試驗結果作爲疾病指標的準確程度。若在相同條件下，對同一個人實施幾次試驗所得的結果不同時，可能使準確性降低（即再現性、可靠性和重複性減少）。這可能是因同一個觀察者對逐次的情況得出不同的結果（觀察者的誤差），或者是不同觀察者們不能得到同樣的結果（觀察者之間的誤差）。這類誤差之發生可

difference in observation and/or interpretation or because of a preconceived notion (often unconscious) by the observer, which influences either his judgment or the tone and manner with which he questions the patient. *Compare* intervention study.

能是由於在觀察方面和/或解釋方面的眞正差異，或由於觀察者有先入之見（往往是不自覺的），這會影響他的判斷，或影響他在問病人時說話的音調和方式。

valine *n.* an *essential amino acid. *See also* amino acid.

纈氨酸 一種必需氨其酸。

Valium *n. see* diazepam.

安定

vallecula *n.* a furrow or depression in an organ or other part. On the undersurface of the cerebellum a vallecula separates the two hemispheres.

谷 器官或其他部分的溝或凹陷。在小腦下部表面的谷將小腦分爲兩個半球。

valve *n.* a structure found in some tubular organs or parts that restricts the flow of fluid within them to one direction only. Valves are important structures in the heart, veins, and lymphatic vessels. Such a valve consists of two or three *cusps fastened like pockets to the walls of the vessel. Blood flowing in the right direction flattens the cusps to the walls, but when flow is reversed the cusps become filled with blood or lymph and dilate to block the opening (see illustration). *See also* mitral valve, tricuspid valve, semilunar valve.

瓣 一種在管道器官或其他部位的結構，以限制其中的溶液只向一個方向流動。瓣膜是心臟、靜脈和淋巴管的重要結構。一個瓣膜包括兩個或三個瓣尖，呈袋狀與管壁連接。正方向的血液使瓣尖倒向管壁，但當逆流時，由於瓣尖充滿血液或淋巴液而膨大，以致阻塞其開口（見圖）。

valvotomy (valvulotomy) *n.* surgical cutting through a valve. The term is usually used to describe the operation to relieve obstruction caused by stenosed valves in the heart.

瓣膜切開術 切開瓣膜的手術。此名詞常用在描述爲減輕心臟瓣膜狹窄引起阻塞的手術。

valvula *n.* (*pl.* **valvulae**) a small valve. The *valvulae conniventes* are circular folds of mucous membrane in the small intestine.

瓣（襞） 小的瓣膜。環狀襞是小腸黏膜的環形皺襞。

valvulitis *n.* inflammation of one or more valves, particularly the heart valves. This may be acute or chronic and is most often due to rheumatic fever (*see* endocarditis).

瓣膜炎 一個或多個瓣膜的炎症，特別是在心臟瓣膜。可以是急性或是慢性的，最常見是由於風濕熱引起。

vancomycin *n.* an *antibiotic, derived from the bacterium *Streptomyces orien-*

萬古黴素 從東方鏈球菌屬中得到的抗生素。對多

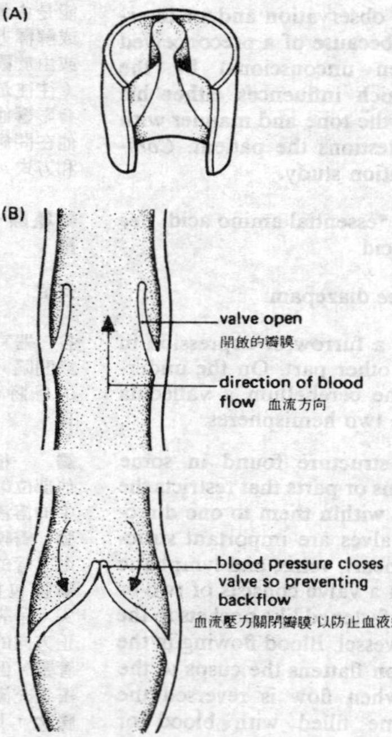

(A) cut vein showing the two cusps of a valve; (B) action of a venous valve

(A)切斷的靜脈顯示一個瓣膜的兩個瓣尖

(B)靜脈瓣的功用

talis, that is effective against most Gram-positive organisms (e.g. streptococci and staphylococci). It is given by intravenous infusion for infections due to strains that are resistant to other antibiotics. It usually has a low toxicity but may cause deafness or thrombophlebitis. Trade name: **Vancocin**.

數的革蘭氏陽性菌有效（例如：葡萄球菌和鏈球菌）。靜脈輸注用於對其他抗生素耐藥的菌株感染時。其毒性較低，但也可引起耳聾或血栓性靜脈炎。

van den Bergh's test a test to determine whether jaundice in a patient is due to *haemolysis or to disease of the liver or bile duct. A sample of serum is mixed with sulphanilic acid, hydrochloric acid, and sodium nitrite. The immediate appearance of a violet col-

范登伯格氏試驗 一種測定病人的黃疸是由於溶血或肝病或膽道疾病的試驗。血清標本與對氨基苯磺酸、鹽酸和亞硝酸鈉混合，立刻顯示出紫色叫做直接反應，表示由於肝損

our is called a *direct reaction* and indicates that the jaundice is due to liver damage or obstruction of the bile duct. If the colour appears only when alcohol is added, this is an *indirect reaction* and points to haemolytic jaundice.

傷或膽道梗阻造成的黃疸。如果僅在加入酒精後才顯示此色，則是間接反應，提示爲溶血性黃疸。

vaporizer *n.* a piece of equipment for producing an extremely fine mist of liquid droplets by forcing a jet of liquid through a narrow nozzle with a jet of air. Vaporizers are used to produce aerosols of various medications for use in inhalation therapy.

霧化器 借空氣的射流，使液體通過狹窄的嘴管噴射出來，產生極細小的液滴薄霧的一種器具。噴霧器用來使不同藥物產生氣溶膠（氣霧劑）而用於吸入療法。

Vaquez-Osler disease *see* polycythaemia vera.

瓦凱-奧斯勒氏病

variable *n.* (in biostatistics) a characteristic (e.g. morbidity, life style, or habit) relating to a single individual or group. *Qualitative variables* are descriptive characteristics, such as sex, race, or occupation; *quantitative variables* relate to a numerical scale and are subdivided into *discrete variables*, found only at fixed points (e.g. number of children), and *continuous variables*, found at any point on a scale (e.g. weight).

變量 （生物統計）與個人或一組人羣有關的特徵（如發病率、生活方式、或習慣）。質的變量是描述如性別、種族、職業等特徵；量的變量是關於數的大小，可以再分爲只存在於固定點的離散型變量（如兒童的數量）和在座標上任何點的連續型變量（如重量）。

variance *n. see* standard deviation.

方差

varicectomy *n. see* phlebectomy.

曲張靜脈切除術

varicella *n. see* chickenpox.

水痘

varices *pl. n. see* varix.

靜脈曲張

varicocele *n.* a collection of dilated veins in the spermatic cord, more commonly affecting the left side of the scrotum than the right. It usually produces no symptoms apart from occasional aching discomfort. In some cases varicocele is associated with a poor sperm count (*see* oligospermia) sufficient to cause infertility. Surgical correction of the varicocele in such patients (*varicocelectomy*) usually results in a considerable improvement in the quality and motility of the sperm.

精索靜脈曲張 擴張的靜脈聚集在精索，往往左側陰囊受累多於右側。除偶有疼痛不適外常無症狀。在某些病例精索靜脈曲張件有引起不育症的精子缺乏。這種病人在手術治療精索靜脈曲張後，精子的數量和運動能力都可得到明顯的改善。

varicose veins veins that are distended, lengthened, and tortuous. The superficial veins (saphenous veins) of the legs are most commonly affected; other sites include the rectum (*haemorrhoids) and testes (*varicocele). There is an inherited tendency to varicose veins but obstruction to blood flow is responsible in some cases. Complications including thrombosis, *phlebitis, and haemorrhage may occur. Treatment includes elastic support and *sclerotherapy, but *avulsion (stripping) or excision (*phlebectomy) is required in some cases.

靜脉曲張 靜脉擴張、拉長和彎曲。腿部的表淺靜脉（隱靜脉）最常受侵犯。另外也包括直腸（痔）和睾丸（精索靜脉曲張）。靜脉曲張有一定的遺傳傾向，但在某些病例是由於血流阻塞。併發症可能有血栓形成、靜脉炎，且可併發出血。治療有彈性支持法和硬化療法。但有些病例需做撕脫術（剝脫）或切除術（靜脉切除術）。

varicotomy *n.* incision into a varicose vein (*see* phlebectomy).

曲張靜脉切開術 切開曲張的靜脉。

variola *n. see* smallpox.

天花

varioloid **1.** *n.* a mild form of smallpox in people who have previously had smallpox or have been vaccinated against it. **2.** *adj.* resembling smallpox.

①**輕天花** 以前患過天花或已種痘者得的一種輕型天花。 ②**天花樣的**

varix *n.* (*pl.* **varices**) a single varicose vein.

靜脉曲張

varus *adj.* describing any deformity that displaces the hand or foot towards the midline. *See* bowleg (genu varum), club-foot (talipes varus).

內翻的 指手或脚向中線錯位的畸形。

vas *n.* (*pl.* **vasa**) a vessel or duct.

脉管或管道

vas- (vaso-) *prefix denoting* **1.** vessels, especially blood vessels. **2.** the vas deferens.

〔前綴〕 ①**脉管** 特別指血管。 ②**輸精管**

vasa efferentia (*sing.* **vas efferens**) the many small tubes that conduct spermatozoa from the testis to the epididymis. They are derived from some of the excretory tubules of the embryonic *mesonephros.

輸出管 將精子從睾丸傳送入附睾的許多小管，來自於胚胎的中腎管的一些排泄管。

vasa vasorum *pl. n.* the tiny arteries and veins that supply the walls of blood vessels.

血管滋養管 指營養血管壁的細小動脉和靜脉。

vascular *adj.* relating to or supplied with blood vessels.

血管的 與血管有關的或由血管供應的。

vascularization *n.* the development of blood vessels (usually capillaries) within a tissue.

血管化 組織中血管形成（常爲毛細血管）。

vascular system *see* cardiovascular system.

血管系統

vasculitis *n. see* angiitis.

血管炎

vas deferens (*pl.* **vasa deferentia**) either of a pair of ducts that conduct spermatozoa from the *epididymis to the *urethra on ejaculation. It has a thick muscular wall the contraction of which assists in ejaculation.

輸精管 射精時把精子從附睾中送入尿道的一對管。它有厚的肌層，在收縮時可幫助射精。

vasectomy *n.* the surgical operation of cutting the duct (vas deferens) connecting the testis to the seminal vesicle and urethra. Vasectomy of both ducts causes sterility and is an increasingly popular means of birth control. Vasectomy does not affect sexual desire or potency.

輸精管切除術 手術切除連接睾丸與精囊和尿道的輸精管，兩側輸精管的切除術引起不育，是一種日益普及的絕育方法。輸精管切除術不影響性慾或性交能力。

vaso- *prefix. see* vas-.

〔前綴〕 **血管**

vasoactive *adj.* affecting the diameter of blood vessels, especially arteries. Examples of vasoactive agents are emotion, pressure, carbon dioxide, and temperature. Some exert their effect directly, others via the *vasomotor centre in the brain.

血管活性的 影響血管尤其是動脉直徑的。例如：血管活性的因素有情緒、血壓、二氧化碳和體溫。有些是直接施加作用，另一些是通過大腦的血管運動中樞。

vasoconstriction *n.* a decrease in the diameter of blood vessels, especially arteries. This results from activation of the *vasomotor centre in the brain, which brings about contraction of muscular walls of the arteries and hence an increase in blood pressure.

血管收縮 血管口徑的縮小，特別是指動脉。這是由於腦部血管運動中樞的活動引起動脉肌層的收縮，因此導至血壓升高。

vasoconstrictor *n.* an agent that causes narrowing of the blood vessels and therefore a decrease in blood flow. Examples are *cyclopentamine, *methoxamine, and *phenylephrine. Vasoconstrictors are used to raise the blood pressure in disorders of the circulation, shock, or severe bleeding and to maintain blood pressure during surgery. Some vasoconstrictors (e.g. *xylometa-

血管收縮藥 引起血管狹窄致使血流減少的藥。如環戊丙甲胺、甲氧胺、苯福林。血管收縮藥用於循環障礙、休克和嚴重出血時以升高血壓，以及手術中維持血壓。一些收縮劑（如丁苄唑啉）用於黏膜時有速效，可用於減輕鼻充血。如果血壓升高太

zoline) have a rapid effect when applied to mucous membranes and may be used to relieve nasal congestion. If the blood pressure rises too quickly headache and vomiting may occur. A vasoconstrictor is often added to local anaesthetic solutions used in dentistry to prolong their effectiveness.

快，可發生頭痛和嘔吐。血管收縮藥常加入局麻溶液，用於牙科以延長局麻作用。

vasodilatation *n.* an increase in the diameter of blood vessels, especially arteries. This results from activation of the *vasomotor centre in the brain, which brings about relaxation of the arterial walls and a consequent lowering of blood pressure.

血管舒張 血管特別是動脉直徑的擴大。由於大腦血管運動中樞的活動引起動脉壁鬆弛，然後導至血壓下降。

vasodilator *n.* a drug that causes widening of the blood vessels and therefore an increase in blood flow. Vasodilators are used to lower blood pressure in cases of hypertension. *Coronary vasodilators*, such as *glyceryl trinitrate and *pentaerithrytol, increase the blood flow through the heart and are used to relieve and prevent angina. Large doses of coronary vasodilators cause such side-effects as flushing of the face, severe headache, and fainting. *Peripheral vasodilators*, such as *cyclandelate, *phenoxybenzamine, and *tolazoline, affect the blood vessels of the limbs and are used to treat conditions of poor circulation such as acrocyanosis, chilblains, and Raynaud's disease.

血管舒張藥 引起血管直徑擴大使血流增加的藥。血管舒張藥用於某些高血壓時降低血壓。冠狀血管擴張劑，如硝酸甘油和季戊四醇用來增加通過心臟的血流，以減輕和防止心絞痛。大量舒血管藥能引起面部潮紅，嚴重頭痛和暈厥等副作用。外用舒血管藥，如環扁桃酯，酚芐明和芐唑啉作用於肢體血管，用於治療循環不佳的病變，如手足發紺、凍瘡和雷諾氏病。

vaso-epididymostomy *n.* the operation of joining the vas deferens to the epididymis in a side-to-side manner in order to bypass an obstruction to the passage of sperm from the testis. The obstruction, which may be congenital or acquired, is usually present in the mid-portion or tail of the epididymis. Vaso-epididymostomy is therefore usually performed by anastomosing the head of the epididymis to a longitudinal incision in the lumen of the adjacent vas.

輸精管附睪吻合術 爲精子從睪丸出來的通道堵塞建立旁路而作輸精管和附睪側吻合使之相通的手術。阻塞可以是先天的或後天的，常常位於附睪的中部或尾部。輸精管附睪吻合術常使附睪頭部與鄰近的輸精管縱切口吻合。

vasoligation *n.* the surgical tying of the vas deferens (the duct conveying

輸精管結扎術 把輸精管（精子輸出睪丸的管道）

sperm from the testis). This is performed to prevent infection spreading from the urinary tract causing recurrent *epididymitis. It is sometimes performed at the time of *prostatectomy to prevent the complication of epididymitis in the postoperative period.

綁紮起來的手術。故這種手術是爲防止來自尿道的感染傳播引起復發性附睾炎。有時也用於前列腺切除術時防止術後合併附睾炎。

vasomotion *n.* an increase or decrease in the diameter of blood vessels, particularly the arteries. *See* vasoconstriction, vasodilatation.

血管舒縮 血管口徑的增加或縮小，特別是動脉。

vasomotor *adj.* controlling the muscular walls of blood vessels, especially arteries, and therefore their diameter.

血管舒縮的 控制血管的肌層，特別是動脉，從而控制它們的直徑。

vasomotor centre a collection of nerve cells in the medulla oblongata that receives information from sensory receptors in the circulatory system (*see* baroreceptor) and brings about reflex changes in the rate of the heart beat and in the diameter of blood vessels, so that the blood pressure can be adjusted. The vasomotor centre also receives impulses from elsewhere in the brain, so that emotion (such as fear) may also influence the heart rate and blood pressure. The centre works through *vasomotor nerves of the sympathetic and parasympathetic systems.

血管運動中樞 位於延髓的一個神經細胞集合體，它從循環系統的感受器接受信息，引起心率及血管口徑的反射性變化，以調整血壓。血管運動中樞也接受來自腦的刺激，所以情緒（特別是恐懼）也影響心率和血壓。中樞是通過交感和副交感系統的血管運動神經進行調節的。

vasomotor nerve any nerve, usually belonging to the autonomic nervous system, that controls the circulation of blood through blood vessels by its action on the muscle fibres within their walls or its action on the heart beat. The *vagus nerve slows the heart and reduces its output, but sympathetic nerves increase the rate and output of the heart and increase blood pressure by causing the constriction of small blood vessels at the same time.

血管運動神經 通常屬於自主神經系統的神經，通過作用於血管壁的肌纖維和作用於心臟跳動而控制血液循環。迷走神經減慢心臟活動，減少心輸出量，而交感神經則加快心率和增加心輸出量，並同時引起小血管收縮而升高血壓。

vasopressin (antidiuretic hormone, ADH) *n.* a hormone, released by the pituitary gland, that increases the reabsorption of water by the kidney, thus preventing excessive loss of water from

加壓素（抗利尿激素） 垂體釋放的激素，增加腎臟對水的重吸收以防止身體過多的失水，加壓素也可收縮血管，可通過鼻吸

the body. Vasopressin also causes constriction of blood vessels. It is administered either nasally or by injection to treat *diabetes insipidus.

入法或注射方法治療尿崩症。

vasopressor *adj.* stimulating the contraction of blood vessels and therefore bringing about an increase in blood pressure.

血管加壓的 刺激血管收縮以導至血壓的升高。

vasospasm *n. see* Raynaud's disease.

血管痙攣

vasotomy *n.* a surgical incision into the vas deferens (the duct conveying sperm from the testis). This is usually undertaken to allow catheterization of the vas and the injection of radio-opaque contrast material for X-ray examination (*vasography*), to test for patency of the duct in patients with *azoospermia.

輸精管造口術 手術切開輸精管（從睾丸輸出精子的管道）。此手術常用於檢查精子缺乏症患者管道開放情況時作導管插入術，和作X線檢查時注入不透X線的對比劑。

vasovagal *adj.* relating to the action of impulses in the *vagus nerve on the circulation. The vagus reduces the rate at which the heart beats, and so lowers its output.

血管迷走神經的 有關迷走神經衝動對循環的作用。迷走神經減慢心率，因此減少心輸出量。

vasovagal attack excessive activity of the vagus nerve, causing slowing of the heart and a fall in blood pressure, which leads to fainting. *See* syncope.

血管迷走神經發作 迷走神經過度興奮導至心跳減慢和血壓下降，從而引起暈厥。

vasovasostomy *n.* the surgical operation of reanastomosing the vas deferens after previous vasectomy: the reversal of vasectomy, undertaken to restore fertility.

輸精管吻合術 在做過輸精管切除後重新將輸精管吻合的外科手術，以恢復生育力。

vasovesiculitis *n.* inflammation of the *seminal vesicles and *vas deferens. This usually occurs in association with *prostatitis and causes pain in the perineum, groin, and scrotum and a high temperature. On examination the vasa and seminal vesicles are thickened and tender. Treatment includes administration of antibiotics.

輸精管精囊炎 精囊和輸精管的炎症。常伴發於前列腺炎，引起會陰、腹股溝、陰囊的疼痛和高燒。檢查輸精管和精囊有增厚並有觸痛。治療可應用抗生素。

vastus *n.* any of three muscles (*vastus intermedius*, *vastus lateralis*, and *vastus medialis*) that form part of the *quadriceps muscle of the thigh.

股肌 組成大腿股四頭肌的三塊肌肉（股中間肌、股外肌和股內肌）。

vectis *n.* a curved instrument used to assist the delivery of an infant.

助產杠桿 用來幫助分娩嬰兒的一種彎曲器具。

vector *n.* an animal, usually an insect or a tick, that transmits parasitic micro-organisms – and therefore the diseases they cause – from person to person or from infected animals to human beings. Mosquitoes, for example, are vectors of malaria, filariasis, and yellow fever.

媒介物 一種動物，常爲昆蟲或蜱，可以傳播寄生性微生物，並引起疾病，使之從人傳播給人或從已感染的動物傳播給人。例如：蚊子是瘧疾、絲蟲病和黃熱病的媒介物。

vectorcardiography *n. see* electrocardiography.

心向量描記法

vegetation *n.* (in pathology) an abnormal outgrowth from a membrane, fancied to resemble a vegetable growth. In ulcerative endocarditis, such outgrowths, consisting of *fibrin with enmeshed blood cells, are found on the membrane lining the heart valves.

贅生物 （病理學）一種膜上的不正常的贅疣。設想與植物的生長相似。在潰瘍性心內膜炎，這樣的贅疣由纖維及網絡中的血細胞組成，可於心瓣表面的膜上見到。

vegetative *adj.* **1.** relating to growth and nutrition rather than to reproduction. **2.** functioning unconsciously; autonomic.

①**生長的** 與生長和營養有關，而與生殖無關的。②**植物性的** 無意識地發生作用的，自主的。

vehicle *n.* (in pharmacy) any substance that acts as the medium in which a drug is administered. Examples are sterile water, isotonic sodium chloride, and dextrose solutions.

載劑 （藥學）投藥時運載藥物的物質。例如：蒸餾水、等張氯化鈉溶液和葡萄糖溶液。

vein *n.* a blood vessel conveying blood towards the heart. All veins except the *pulmonary vein carry deoxygenated blood from the tissues, via the capillaries, to the vena cava. The walls of veins consist of three tissue layers, but these are much thinner and less elastic than those of arteries (see illustration). Veins contain *valves that assist the flow of blood back to the heart. Anatomical name: **vena**. —**venous** *adj.*

靜脉 向心臟運送血液的血管。除肺靜脉外，所有靜脉從組織携帶脫氧的血經過毛細血管進入腔靜脉。靜脉壁由三層組織構成，但是它較薄且較動脉的彈性小（見圖）。靜脉有瓣膜，可協助血流回心臟。

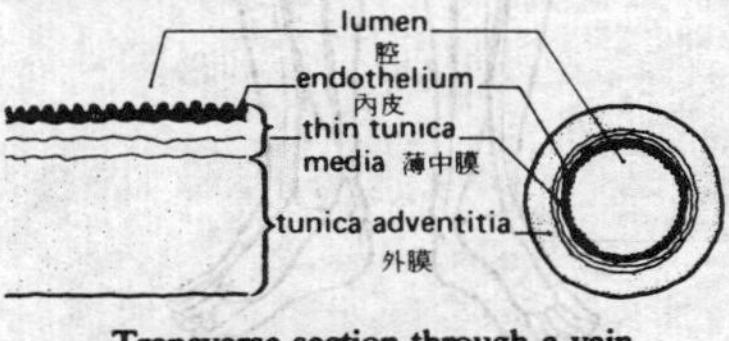

Transverse section through a vein
靜脉橫切面

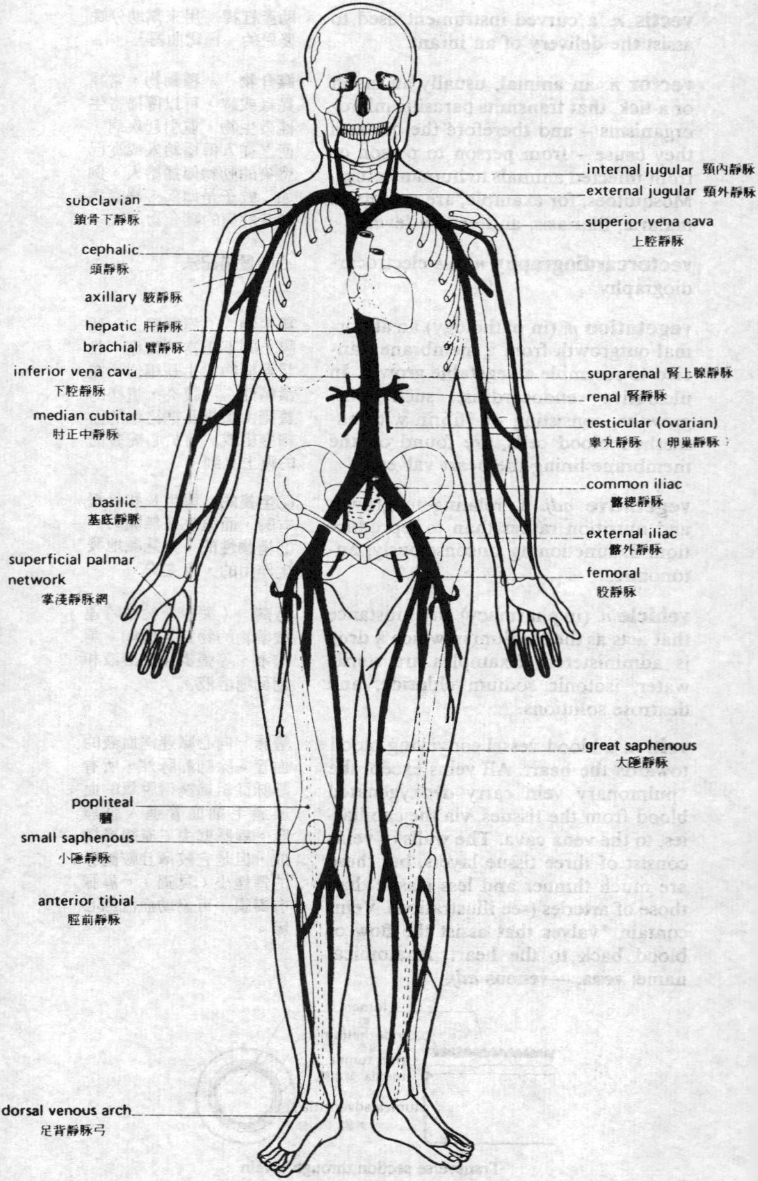
internal jugular 頸內靜脈
external jugular 頸外靜脈
superior vena cava 上腔靜脈
suprarenal 腎上腺靜脈
renal 腎靜脈
testicular (ovarian) 睪丸靜脈 (卵巢靜脈)
common iliac 髂總靜脈
external iliac 髂外靜脈
femoral 股靜脈
great saphenous 大隱靜脈
subclavian 鎖骨下靜脈
cephalic 頭靜脈
axillary 腋靜脈
hepatic 肝靜脈
brachial 臂靜脈
inferior vena cava 下腔靜脈
median cubital 肘正中靜脈
basilic 基底靜脈
superficial palmar network 掌淺靜脈網
popliteal 膕
small saphenous 小隱靜脈
anterior tibial 脛前靜脈
dorsal venous arch 足背靜脈弓

The principal veins of the body
人體主要靜脈

velamen (velamentum) *n.* a covering membrane.

膜 覆蓋的膜。

vellus *n.* the fine hair that occurs on the body before puberty is reached.

毫毛 青春期以前身體長出的細毛。

velum *n.* (in anatomy) a veil-like covering. The *medullary velum* is either of two thin layers of tissue that form part of the roof of the fourth ventricle of the brain.

帆 （解剖學）帆樣的覆蓋物。髓帆是構成第四腦室頂部的兩片薄層組織。

vena *n.* (*pl.* **venae**) *see* vein.

靜脉

vena cava either of the two main veins, conveying blood from the other veins to the right atrium of the heart. The *inferior vena cava*, formed by the union of the right and left common iliac veins, receives blood from parts of the body below the diaphragm. The *superior vena cava*, originating at the junction of the two innominate veins, drains blood from the head, neck, thorax, and arms.

腔靜脉 從靜脉將血液送到右心房的兩條主要靜脉。下腔靜脉是由左、右髂總靜脉連接而成，接受來自膈以下身體部位的血液。上腔靜脉起於兩無名靜脉連接處，收集來自頭、頸、胸和上肢的血液。

vene- (veno-) *prefix denoting* veins.

〔前綴〕 **靜脉**

venene *n.* a mixture of two or more *venoms: used to produce antiserum against venoms (*antivenene*).

蛇毒 一種或多種毒液的混合液。用來製成抗毒液（抗蛇毒）的抗血清。

venepuncture (venipuncture) *n.* the puncture of a vein for any therapeutic purpose; for example, to extract blood for laboratory tests. *See also* phlebotomy.

靜脉穿刺 爲了各種治療目的向靜脉中作穿刺術。例如取血作實驗室檢查。

venereal disease (VD) an infectious disease transmitted by sexual intercourse. The most important are *soft sore (chancroid), *gonorrhoea, and *syphilis.

性病 通過性交而傳遞的傳染病。最重要的有軟下疳、淋病和梅毒。

venereology *n.* the study of venereal diseases, including syphilis and gonorrhoea.

性病學 對性病的研究，包括梅毒和淋病。

venesection *n. see* phlebotomy.

靜脉切開術

veno- *prefix. see* vene-.

〔前綴〕 **靜脉**

venoclysis *n.* the continuous infusion into a vein of saline or other solution.

靜脉輸注 連續向靜脉內輸入鹽水或其他溶液。

venography (phlebography) *n.* X-ray examination to show up the course of veins in a particular region of the body. A *radio-opaque contrast medium is injected slowly into a vein and X-ray photographs (*venograms*) taken as the compound is carried towards the heart. Damage, obstruction, or abnormal communication with other vessels will be seen where the medium does not fill the vein properly or apparently leaks from it. *See also* angiography.

靜脉造影術 顯示身體某一區域靜脉的X線檢查法。不透射線的對比劑被緩慢地注入靜脉，當這化合物流向心臟時進行X線照像（靜脉照像），在對比劑不能使靜脉完全充盈或從靜脉明顯漏出時，就會發現靜脉的損傷、阻塞或與其他脉管有不正常的交通。

venom *n.* the poisonous material produced by snakes, scorpions, spiders, and other animals for injecting into their prey or enemies. Some venoms produce no more than local pain and swelling; others produce more general effects and can prove lethal.

毒液 蛇、蠍、蜘蛛和其他動物在刺咬被它們捕食的動物或敵人時產生的有毒物質。有些毒液只引起局部疼痛和腫脹，有些引起全身性反應並可致死。

venosclerosis *n. see* phlebosclerosis.

靜脉硬化

ventilation *n.* the passage of air into and out of the respiratory tract. The air that reaches only as far as the conducting airways cannot take part in gas exchange and is known as *dead space ventilation* – this may be reduced by performing a *tracheostomy. In the air sacs of the lungs (alveoli) gas exchange is most efficient when matched by adequate blood flow (*perfusion). Ventilation/perfusion imbalance (ventilation of under-perfused alveoli or perfusion of under-ventilated alveoli) is an important cause of *anoxia and *cyanosis.

通氣 空氣出入呼吸道的流通過程。空氣只能到達導氣管而不能參加氣體交換的稱爲死腔樣通氣，這種情況可進行氣管造口術使之減少。當有充分的血流相配時，肺泡的氣體交換（瀰散）是最有效的。通氣血流比例失衡（肺泡低瀰散性通氣或肺泡低通氣性瀰散）是缺氧和紫紺的主要原因。

ventilator *n.* **1.** a device to ensure a supply of fresh air. **2.** equipment that is manually or mechanically operated to maintain a flow of air into and out of the lungs of a patient who is unable to breathe normally. *See also* respirator.

①**通風機** 保證供給新鮮空氣的機器。 ②**呼吸機** 維持不能正常呼吸的病人氣流進出肺部的手工的或機械操作的裝置。

ventouse *n.* a cupping glass: a bell-shaped glass vessel from which the air can be removed, used for drawing blood to the surface of the skin. *See* cupping.

吸（瘀）杯 可吸出其中空氣的鐘形玻璃杯，用於將血吸到皮膚表面。

ventral *adj.* relating to or situated at or close to the front of the body or to the anterior part of an organ.

腹的，腹側的 位於或接近身體前部的，或與一器官的前部有關的。

ventricle *n.* **1.** either of the two lower chambers of the *heart, which have thick muscular walls. The left ventricle, which is thicker than the right, receives blood from the pulmonary vein via the left atrium and pumps it into the aorta. The right ventricle pumps blood received from the venae cavae (via the right atrium) into the pulmonary artery. **2.** one of the four fluid-filled cavities within the brain (see illustration). The paired first and second ventricles (*lateral ventricles*), one in each cerebral hemisphere, communicate with the third ventricle in the midline between them. This in turn leads through a narrow channel, the *cerebral aqueduct*, to the fourth ventricle in the hindbrain, which is continuous with the spinal canal in the centre of the spinal cord. *Cerebrospinal fluid circulates through all the cavities. —**ventricular** *adj.*

室 ①心臟的兩個下腔，有厚肌層，左室厚於右室，接受通過左心房來自肺靜脉的血，並將血泵入主動脉。右室將來自腔靜脉的血（通過右心房）泵入肺動脉。 ②大腦內四個充滿腦脊液的腔（見圖）。成對的第一和第二腦室（側腦室）各位於一側大腦半球，與中線上的第三腦室相通，經過狹窄的大腦導水管通到後腦的第四腦室，第四腦室與脊髓中央管相連續。腦脊液循環通過所有這些腦室。

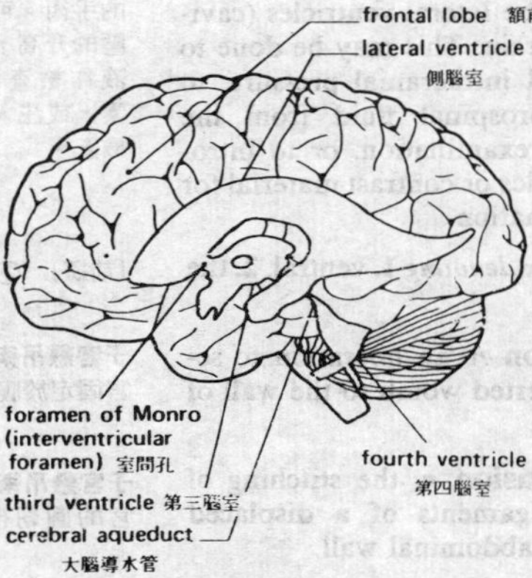

Ventricles of the brain (side view)

腦室（側面）

ventricul- (ventriculo-) *prefix denoting* a ventricle (of the brain or heart).

〔前綴〕 **室** （腦室或心室）

ventricular folds *see* vocal cords.

室襞

ventriculitis *n.* inflammation in the ventricles of the brain, usually caused by infection. It may result from the rupture of a cerebral abscess into the cavity of the ventricle or from the spread of a severe form of *meningitis from the subarachnoid space.

腦室炎 常由感染引起的腦室炎症。是由腦膿腫破潰進入腦室腔，或由來源於蛛網膜下腔的嚴重腦膜炎擴散而來。

ventriculoatriostomy *n.* an operation for the relief of raised pressure due to the build-up of cerebrospinal fluid that occurs in *hydrocephalus. Using a system of catheters, the fluid is drained into the jugular vein in the neck.

腦室心房造口〔引流〕術 減輕因腦積水腦脊液聚集壓力升高的一種手術。用導管系統將腦脊液導入頸部的頸靜脈。

ventriculography *n.* X-ray examination of the ventricles of the brain after the introduction of a contrast medium, such as air or radio-opaque material.

腦室造影術 在導入對比劑如空氣和不透射線的物質後作腦室的X線檢查。

ventriculoscopy *n.* observation of the ventricles of the brain through a fibre-optic instrument. *See* endoscope, fibre optics.

腦室鏡 檢查腦室的一種光學纖維儀器。

ventriculostomy *n.* an operation to introduce a hollow needle (cannula) into one of the lateral ventricles (cavities) of the brain. This may be done to relieve raised intracranial pressure, to obtain cerebrospinal fluid from the ventricle for examination, or to introduce antibiotics or contrast material for X-ray examination.

腦室造口引流術 將空針（套管）引入大腦側腦室的手術。可用於減輕顱內壓的升高，從腦室取腦脊液作檢查，或注入抗生素，或注入對比劑作X線檢查。

ventro- *prefix denoting* **1.** ventral. **2.** the abdomen.

〔前綴〕 **①前側的** **②腹**

ventrofixation *n.* an operation to secure a retroverted womb to the wall of the abdomen.

子宮懸吊術 將後傾的子宮固定於腹壁的手術。

ventrosuspension *n.* the stitching of the round ligaments of a displaced womb to the abdominal wall.

子宮懸吊術 將錯位的子宮的圓韌帶縫合到腹壁上。

venule *n.* a minute vessel that drains blood from the capillaries. Many venules unite to form a vein.

小靜脈 收集毛細血管血液的小血管。許多小靜脈滙合成靜脈。

verbigeration *n.* repetitive utterances of the same words over and over again.

言語重複 多次重複說出同樣的詞，這是一種影響

This is a kind of *stereotypy affecting speech and is most common in institutionalized schizophrenics.

言語的刻板症，常見於住院的精神分裂症患者。

vermicide *n.* a chemical agent used to destroy parasitic worms living in the intestine. *Compare* vermifuge.

殺蟲劑 一種用於除滅腸道寄生蟲的化學製劑。

vermiform appendix *see* appendix.

闌尾

vermifuge *n.* any drug or chemical agent used to expel worms from the intestine. *See also* anthelmintic.

驅蟲劑 用於驅除腸道蠕蟲的藥物或化學製劑。

vermis *n.* the central portion of the *cerebellum, lying between its two lateral hemispheres and immediately behind the pons and the medulla oblongata of the hindbrain.

蚓部 小腦的中間部分，位於兩側小腦半球中間，直接在後腦的橋腦和延髓的背部。

vermix *n.* the vermiform *appendix.

闌尾

vernier *n.* a device for obtaining accurate measurements of length, to 1/10th, 1/100th or smaller fractions of a unit. It consists of a fixed graduated main scale against which a shorter vernier scale slides. The vernier scale is graduated into divisions equal to nine-tenths of the smallest unit marked on the main scale. The vernier scale is often adjusted by means of a screw thread. A reading is taken by observing which of the markings on the scales coincide.

游標尺 一種精確的測量某單位長度的1/10、1/100或更小分數的儀器。它是在一個固定的有刻度的主標尺上滑動的小游標尺。游標尺的刻度等於主標尺上的最小單位的十分之九。游標刻度常用螺紋調整。觀察到與標尺的刻度重合之處，即爲讀數。

vernix caseosa the layer of greasy material that covers the skin of a fetus or newborn baby. It is produced by the oil-secreting glands of the skin and contains skin scales and fine hairs.

胎兒皮脂 一層蓋於胎兒和新生兒皮膚的油脂層，由皮脂腺產生，包括皮鱗屑和細毛。

verruca *n.* *see* wart.

疣

verrucous carcinoma an *indolent pre-invasive wartlike carcinoma of the oral cavity, which is associated with chewing tobacco.

疣狀癌 一種與嚼煙草有關的口腔侵襲前期無痛性疣狀癌。

version *n.* the changing of the position of a fetus in the womb. This may be done to facilitate delivery by applying manual pressure to the outside of the abdomen, by inserting the hand into

胎位倒轉術 改變子宮內胎兒位置，可用腹部外人工加壓、把手置入子宮內、或同時用兩種手法以促進胎兒分娩。在自發性

the womb, or by combining both methods (*see* cephalic version, podalic version). In *spontaneous version* the position of the fetus alters because of the natural contractions of the womb muscles.

倒轉時，胎兒位置變化是子宮肌肉自然收縮的緣故。

vertebra *n.* (*pl.* **vertebrae**) one of the 33 bones of which the *backbone is composed. Each vertebra typically consists of a *body*, or *centrum*, from the back of which arises an arch of bone (the *neural arch*) enclosing a cavity (the *vertebral canal*, or *foramen*) through which the spinal cord passes. The neural arch bears one *spinous process* and two *transverse processes*, providing anchorage for muscles, and four *articular processes*, with which adjacent vertebrae articulate (see illustration). Individual vertebrae are bound together by ligaments and *intervertebral discs. —**vertebral** *adj.*

椎骨 組成脊柱的三十三塊骨之一。每一個椎骨的特徵是有一個椎體，其背面形成一骨弓（神經弓），圍成一個腔（椎管或椎孔），脊髓從其中通過。神經弓具有一個棘突和供肌肉附着的兩個橫突，以及四個與鄰近椎骨相關節的關節突（見圖）。單個的椎骨被韌帶和椎間盤連接在一起。

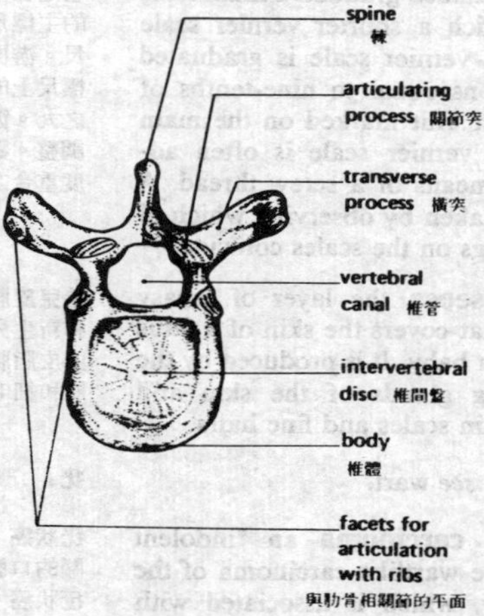

A typical thoracic vertebra (from above)
典型胸椎（上面觀）

vertebral column *see* backbone.

脊柱

vertigo *n.* a disabling sensation in which the affected individual feels that

眩暈 一種失去能力的感覺，患者覺得他或他周圍

either he himself or his surroundings are in a state of constant movement. It is most often a spinning sensation but there may be a feeling that the ground is tilting. It is a symptom of disease either in the *labyrinth of the inner ear or in the *vestibular nerve or its nuclei in the brainstem, which are involved in the sense of balance.

的環境處於不斷的運動狀態，經常是旋轉的感覺，但也可能有地傾斜的感覺。這是與平衡感覺有關的內耳迷路、腦幹前庭神經、或其核的病變的症狀。

vesical *adj.* relating to or affecting a bladder, especially the urinary bladder.

囊泡的 與囊泡有關或侵及囊泡的。特別是指膀胱。

vesicant (epispastic) *n.* an agent that causes blistering of the skin.

起疱劑 引起皮膚起疱的藥劑。

vesicle *n.* **1.** a very small blister in the skin, often no bigger than a pinpoint, that contains a clear fluid (serum). Vesicles occur in a variety of skin disorders, including eczema and herpes. **2.** (in anatomy) any small bladder, especially one filled with fluid. —**vesicular** *adj.*

①**小疱** 位於皮膚很小的疱，含清亮的物體（血清），常有釘頭大小。疱可出現於各種皮膚病時，如濕疹、疱疹。 ②（解剖學）**小囊** 特別是充滿液體的。

vesico- *prefix denoting* the urinary bladder. Example: *vesicovaginal* (relating to the bladder and vagina).

〔前綴〕 **膀胱** 如膀胱陰道的（與膀胱和陰道有關的）。

vesicofixation *n. see* cystopexy.

膀胱固定術

vesicoureteric reflux the backflow of urine from the bladder into the ureters. This is due to defective valves (which normally prevent reflux). Infection is conveyed to the kidneys, causing recurrent attacks of acute *pyelonephritis and scarring of the kidneys in childhood. Children with urinary infection must be investigated for reflux by *cystoscopy; if the condition does not settle with antibiotic therapy corrective surgery must be performed.

膀胱輸尿管回流 尿液從膀胱回流入輸尿管。這是由於瓣膜缺損（正常時瓣膜是防止回流的）。感染傳到腎臟引起急性腎盂腎炎的反覆發作和童年期的腎瘢痕形成。泌尿系感染的兒童必須用膀胱鏡檢查有否回流。如果抗生素治療不能奏效，則需做矯正手術。

vesicular breathing *see* breath sounds.

肺泡性呼吸

vesiculectomy *n.* surgical removal of a *seminal vesicle. This operation, which is rarely undertaken, may be performed for a tumour of the seminal vesicles.

精囊切除術 手術切除精囊。這種手術很少做，可用於治療精囊腫瘤。

vesiculitis *n.* inflammation of the seminal vesicles. *See* vasovesiculitis.

精囊炎 精囊的炎症。

vesiculography *n.* X-ray examination of the seminal vesicles. This is usually performed by injecting radio-opaque contrast material into the exposed vasa deferentia. It can also be undertaken by inserting a catheter into the ejaculatory duct (which discharges semen from the vesicle into the vas deferens) via an *endoscope. This examination is rarely undertaken for the specific purpose of outlining the seminal vesicles; it is more commonly performed to test for the patency of the vas deferens in patients with *azoospermia.

精囊造影術 精囊的X線檢查。這種檢查通常通過向暴露的輸精管注射不透射線的對比劑來進行，也可通過由窺鏡向射精管（把精子從精囊送至輸精管）內插一導管而實施，本檢查偶爾用於了解精囊輪廓，較常用於檢查精子缺乏症患者輸精管的開放情況。

vesiculopapular *adj.* describing a skin condition typified by having both vesicles (blisters) and papules (raised spots).

水疱丘疹的 描述皮膚病變，其特徵是同時有疱（水疱）和丘疹（凸起的斑疹）。

vesiculopustular *adj.* describing a skin condition that has both vesicles (blisters) and pustules (pus-filled blisters).

水疱膿疱的 描述皮膚病變。其特徵是同時有疱（水疱）和膿疱（充滿膿的疱）。

vessel *n.* a tube conveying a body fluid, especially a blood vessel or a lymphatic vessel.

管 指運輸體液的管道，特別是血管和淋巴管。

vestibular glands the two pairs of glands that open at the junction of the vagina and vulva. The more posterior of the two are the *greater vestibular glands* (*Bartholin's glands*); the other pair are the *lesser vestibular glands*. Their function is to lubricate the entrance to the vagina during coitus.

前庭腺 開口於陰道和外陰連接處的兩對腺體，其中較後面的一對是前庭大腺（巴多林氏腺），另一對是前庭小腺。它們的功能是在性交時使陰道入口處滑潤。

vestibular nerve the division of the *vestibulocochlear nerve that carries impulses from the semicircular canals, utricle, and saccule of the inner ear to the brain, conveying information about the body's posture and movements in space and allowing coordination and balance.

前庭神經 前庭耳蝸神經的一部分，從內耳的半規管、橢圓囊和球囊傳導衝動到大腦，傳遞體位和空間運動的信息，主管協調和平衡。

vestibule *n.* (in anatomy) a cavity situated at the entrance to a hollow part. The vestibule of the ear is the cavity of the bony *labyrinth that contains the *saccule and *utricle – the organs of equilibrium.

前庭 （解剖學）位於一凹陷部入口處的腔。耳前庭是骨迷路的空腔，它包括平衡器——球囊和橢圓囊。

vestibulocochlear nerve (acoustic nerve, auditory nerve) the eighth cranial nerve (VIII), responsible for carrying sensory impulses from the inner ear to the brain. It has two branches, the *vestibular nerve* and the *cochlear nerve*. The cochlear nerve carries impulses from the spiral *cochlea and is therefore the nerve of hearing, while the vestibular nerve serves equilibrium, carrying impulses from the semicircular canals, utricles, and saccules with information about posture, movement, and balance.

前庭耳蝸神經（聽神經） 第八對腦神經，傳遞內耳的感覺衝動到大腦。它有兩支，前庭神經和耳蝸神經。耳蝸神經從螺旋管傳出衝動，所以是聽神經。前庭神經則是起平衡作用，從半規管、球囊和橢圓囊傳出有關位置、運動和平衡信息的衝動。

vestigial *adj.* existing only in a rudimentary form. The term is applied to organs whose structure and function have diminished during the course of evolution until only a rudimentary structure exists.

退化的 只以痕跡形式存在的。該詞常用於在進化過程中器官的結構和功能減退至只存留殘餘結構的情況。

viable *adj.* capable of surviving. The term is applied to a fetus from about the 28th week of gestation at which stage it can survive.

能存活的 能生存的。該詞常應用於姙娠 28 周左右能存活的胎兒。

Vibramycin *n. see* doxycycline.

强力黴素

vibrator *n.* a machine used to generate vibrations of different frequencies, which have a stimulating effect when applied to different parts of the body. A vibrator may also be used to loosen thick mucus in the sinuses or air passages.

振動器 用於產生不同頻率的震動的機器。當應用於身體不同部位時可產生刺激效應。振動器也可用於使鼻竇或氣道內的濃稠黏液排出。

Vibrio *n.* a genus of Gram-negative motile comma-shaped bacteria widely distributed in soil and water. Most species are saprophytic but some are parasites, including *V. cholerae*, which causes *cholera.

弧菌 一類革蘭氏陰性的能運動的弧形細菌，廣泛分佈於泥土和水中，多數是腐生細菌類，也有一些是寄生的。例如引起霍亂的霍亂弧菌。

vibrissa *n.* (*pl.* **vibrissae**) a stiff coarse hair, especially one of the stiff hairs that lie just inside the nostrils.

鼻毛 粗硬的毛，特別指鼻孔內粗硬的毛。

vicarious *adj.* describing an action or function performed by an organ not normally involved in the function. For example, *vicarious menstruation* is a

異位的 指一個器官產生在正常情況下所沒有的功能和作用。例如：替代月經，是一種少見的病變，

rare disorder in which monthly bleeding occurs from places other than the vagina, such as the sweat glands, breasts, nose, or eyes.

此時從陰道以外的部位如汗腺、乳房、鼻或眼每月按時出血。

villus *n.* (*pl.* **villi**) one of many short finger-like processes that project from some membranous surfaces. Numerous *intestinal villi* line the small *intestine. Each contains a network of blood capillaries and a *lacteal. Their function is to absorb the products of digestion and they greatly increase the surface area over which this can take place. *Chorionic villi* are folds of the chorion (the outer membrane surrounding a fetus). They are particularly numerous in the *placenta, where they provide an extensive area for the exchange of oxygen, carbon dioxide, food, and waste products between maternal and fetal blood. *See also* arachnoid villus.

絨毛 從一些膜狀表面伸出的許多短指狀突起，大量小腸絨毛位於小腸表面，每個絨毛含有毛細血管網和乳糜管。它們的功能是吸收消化產物，並大大地增加了吸收的面積。絨毛膜（胎兒周圍的外膜）的絨毛是絨毛膜的皺褶，在胎盤中其數量特別多，爲母親和胎兒血液交換氧、二氧化碳、食物以及廢物等提供了廣大區域。

vinblastine *n.* a *cytotoxic drug that is given by intravascular injection mainly in the treatment of cancers of the lymphatic system, such as Hodgkin's disease. It is highly toxic, since it also acts on normal tissues; common side-effects include nausea, vomiting, diarrhoea, and depression of bone marrow function. Trade names: **Velban, Velbe**.

長春花鹼 靜脉注射用的細胞毒藥物，主要用於治療淋巴系統腫瘤。它是高毒性的，因爲它也作用於正常組織。常見的副作用有噁心、嘔吐、腹瀉和骨髓功能的抑制。

Vincent's angina an obsolete term for *ulcerative gingivitis.

奮森氏咽峽炎 潰瘍性齦炎的廢用詞。

vincristine *n.* a cytotoxic drug with uses and side-effects similar to those of vinblastine. Trade name: **Oncovin**.

長春新鹼 一種細胞毒藥物。用途和不良反應與長春花鹼類似。

vinculum *n.* (*pl.* **vincula**) a connecting band of tissue. The *vincula tendinum* are threadlike bands of synovial membrane that connect the flexor tendons of the fingers and toes to their point of insertion on the phalanges.

紐 組織的連接帶。腱紐是滑膜的絲樣帶，將指或趾的屈肌肌腱連接到指（趾）骨的附着點。

vindesine *n.* a cytotoxic drug with similarities to *vinblastine and vincris-

長春鹼醯胺 一種與長春花鹼和長春新鹼類似的細

tine. Additional side-effects include alopecia and peripheral neuropathy. Trade name: **Eldisine.**

胞毒藥，另外的副作用有脫髮和周圍神經病變。

vinyl ether a general anaesthetic, used mainly for inducing anaesthesia and for minor surgery under short anaesthesia. Both induction and recovery are more rapid than with ether. It is not used alone for long operations because of the dangers of overdosage and liver damage, but it is sometimes given in combination with nitrous oxide or ether. Trade name: **Vinethene.**

乙烯醚 一種全身痲醉劑。主要用於誘導痲醉或爲小手術短時間痲醉。誘導痲醉和恢復都較乙醚快。因爲有過量的危險和肝損傷，所以不單獨用於長時間的手術，但有時與氧化亞氮或乙醚聯合應用。

viomycin *n.* an *antibiotic derived from bacteria of the genus *Streptomyces.* It is given by intramuscular injection in the treatment of tuberculosis, particularly against strains that are resistant to other antibiotics (such as *streptomycin and *isoniazid). Side-effects, including ear and kidney damage, may occur in some patients. Trade name: **Viocin.**

紫黴素 鏈黴菌類細菌中提取出來的抗生素，用於肌肉注射治療結核病，特別是對其他抗生素（如鏈黴素和異煙肼）耐藥的菌株。副作用是部分患者可以出現耳和腎的損害。

viprynium *n.* a drug administered by mouth for the treatment of threadworm infestation. It has low toxicity but may cause nausea and vomiting. It stains the stools a red colour. Trade name: **Vanquin.**

撲蟯靈 一種口服藥，用於治療蟯蟲感染。此藥毒性低，但可引起噁心、嘔吐。它可使大便染成紅色。

viraemia *n.* the presence in the blood of virus particles.

病毒血症 血液中有病毒顆粒。

virilism *n.* the development in a female of a combination of increased body hair, muscle bulk, and deepening of the voice (*masculinization) and male psychological characteristics.

男性化（女子） 女性體毛增多，肌肉發達，嗓音低沉，以及出現男性心理特徵。

virilization *n.* the induction in a female of increased body hair, muscle bulk, and deepening of the voice as a result of hormone imbalance or hormone therapy.

男性化（女子） 女性體毛增多，肌肉發達，嗓音低沉。是由於激素失衡或激素治療的結果。

virology *n.* the science of viruses. *See also* microbiology.

病毒學 有關病毒的科學。

virulence *n.* the disease-producing (pathogenic) ability of a microorganism. *See also* attenuation.

毒力 微生物致病的能力。

virus *n.* a minute particle that is capable of replication but only within living cells. Viruses are too small to be visible with a light microscope and too small to be trapped by filters. They infect animals, plants, and microorganisms (*see* bacteriophage). Each consists of a core of nucleic acid (DNA or RNA) surrounded by a protein shell. Some bear an outer lipid capsule. Viruses cause many diseases, including the common cold, influenza, measles, mumps, chickenpox, herpes, smallpox, polio, and rabies. Antibiotics are ineffective against them, but many viral diseases are controlled by means of vaccines. —**viral** *adj.*

病毒 只在活細胞內有複製能力的微小顆粒。病毒很小，以至於不能在光學顯微鏡下看見，也不能被濾過器阻留。它們可侵襲動物、植物和微生物。每個病毒由蛋白質殼包繞的核酸核心（DNA 或 RNA）組成，有的具有一個脂質的外囊。病毒能引起許多疾病，如普通感冒、流感、麻疹、流行性腮腺炎、水痘、疱疹、天花、脊髓灰質炎和狂犬病。抗生素對它無效，但用疫苗可以控制許多病毒性疾病。

viscera *pl. n.* (*sing.* **viscus**) the organs within the body cavities, especially the organs of the abdominal cavities (stomach, intestines, etc.). —**visceral** *adj.*

內臟 在體腔中的器官。尤指腹腔中的器官。

visceral arch *see* pharyngeal arch.

鰓弓

visceral cleft *see* pharyngeal cleft.

鰓裂

visceral pouch *see* pharyngeal pouch.

咽囊

viscero- *prefix denoting* the viscera.

〔前綴〕 **內臟的**

viscus *n. see* viscera.

內臟

visual acuity sharpness of vision. How well one sees things depends on how well they are illuminated and upon such factors as practice and motivation, but the essential requirements are a healthy retina and the ability of the eye to focus incoming light to form a sharp image on the retina. The commonest way of assessing visual acuity is the *Snellen chart, which measures the *resolving power* of the eye.

視敏度 視覺的敏銳性。一個人視物的清晰程度依賴於物體受照明的强弱以及他的習慣和動機等因素，但其基本的要求是要有健全的視網膜和眼睛集中光線於視網膜上形成清晰影像的能力。最常用的確定視敏度的方法是斯內倫氏視力表。它能衡量眼睛的分辨能力。

visual field the area in front of the eye in any part of which an object can be seen without moving the eye. With both

視野 不動眼可以看見眼前任一部位物體的區域。雖然眼眉和眼瞼會在一定

eyes open and looking straight forward it is possible to see well-illuminated objects placed anywhere in front of the eyes, although the eyebrows and eyelids reduce the extent of the field somewhat. This is the *binocular visual field*. With only one eye open the field is *uniocular* and is restricted inwards by the nose. If the object is small or poorly illuminated it will not be seen until it is moved closer to the point at which the eye is actually looking, i.e. nearer to the centre of the visual field. Similarly, coloured objects are not seen so far away from the centre as are white objects of the same size and brightness. This is because the retina is not uniformly sensitive to light of different colours or intensities (*see* rod, cone): retinal sensitivity increases towards its centre (the *macula). Thus, while there is an absolute visual field beyond which things cannot be seen, no matter how large or bright they are, a relative field exists for objects of different brightness, size, and colour. *See also* campimetry, perimeter.

程度上減少視野的範圍、但兩眼睜開直視前方時，可以看見眼前任何地方照明很好的物體，這是雙眼視野。若僅睜一隻眼，則是單眼視野，其內側受鼻的限制。如果物體小或照明差，只有將它移近眼睛直視之處，即接近視野中央才能看見。同樣，有色物體在遠離中央處是看不見的，而同樣大小和亮度的白色物體却可以看見。這是因爲視網膜對不同顏色和明暗度敏感性不一所致。視網膜近中央處（黃斑）敏感度增加。因此，有一個絕對視野，還有一個相對視野。前者，無論物體多麼大和亮，超出它就不能看見；後者因物體的顏色、大小和亮度不同而異。

visual purple *see* rhodopsin.

視紫質

vital capacity the maximum volume of air that a person can exhale afer maximum inhalation. It is usually measured on an instrument called a *spirometer*.

肺活量　當一個人在最大吸氣後呼出的最大氣體容積，通常用稱爲肺量計的儀器進行測量。

vital centre any of the collections of nerve cells in the brain that act as governing centres for different vital body functions – such as breathing, heart rate, blood pressure, temperature control etc. – making reflex adjustments according to the body's needs. Most lie in the hypothalamus and brainstem.

生命中樞　腦中的神經細胞集團，它們是控制身體不同生命活動的中樞，如呼吸、心率、血壓和體溫調節等，按照身體需要來調節反射。多數位於下丘腦和腦幹。

Vitallium *n. Trademark.* an alloy of chromium and cobalt that is used in instruments, prostheses, surgical appliances, and dentures.

活合金　（商品名）鉻和鈷的合金。用於儀器、修復體、外科器械和假牙。

vital staining (intravital staining) the process of staining a living tissue by injecting a stain into the organism. *Compare* supravital staining.

活體染色法 通過把染料注入機體以使活體組織染色的過程。

vital statistics *see* biostatistics.

生命統計學

vitamin *n.* any of a group of substances that are required, in very small amounts, for healthy growth and development: they cannot be synthesized in the body and are therefore essential constituents of the diet. Vitamins are divided into two groups, according to whether they are soluble in water or fat. The water-soluble group includes the vitamin B complex and vitamin C; the fat-soluble vitamins are vitamins A, D, E, and K. Lack of sufficient quantities of any of the vitamins in the diet results in specific vitamin deficiency diseases.

維生素 健康生長和發育所需要的一組極小量的物質，它們不能在身體內合成，所以是飲食的重要成分，維生素按其溶於水或脂肪可劃分爲兩類：水溶性類包括維生素 B 複合物和維生素 C，脂溶性類有維生素 A、D、E 和 K。飲食中任何一種維生素量的不足，將引起特異的維生素缺乏病。

vitamin A (retinol) a fat-soluble vitamin that occurs preformed in foods of animal origin (especially milk products, egg yolk, and liver) and is formed in the body from the pigment β-carotene, present in some vegetable foods (for example cabbage, lettuce, and carrots). Retinol is essential for growth, vision in dim light, and the maintenance of soft mucous tissue. A deficiency causes stunted growth, *night blindness, *xerophthalmia, *keratomalacia, and eventual blindness. The recommended daily intake is 750 μg retinol equivalents for an adult (1 μg retinol equivalent = 1 μg retinol or 6 μg β-carotene).

維生素 A（維生素 A 醇） 爲一種脂溶性維生素。自然存在於動物性食物，特別是奶製品、蛋黃、肝中。在體內可從 β 胡蘿蔔素形成，後者是一種色素，存在於一些蔬菜中（如捲心菜、萵苣和胡蘿蔔）。維生素 A 醇是生長、暗視覺和維持柔軟的的黏膜組織所必需的。維生素 A 缺乏可引起生長障礙、夜盲、乾眼病、角膜軟化。建議成人每日攝入 750 μg 維生素 A 醇當量（1 μg 維生素 A 醇當量＝1 μg 維生素 A 醇或 6 μg β 胡蘿蔔素）。

vitamin B any one of a group of water-soluble vitamins that, although not chemically related, are often found together in the same kinds of food (milk, liver, cereals, etc.) and all function as *coenzymes. *See* vitamins B_1, B_2, B_6, B_{12}, biotin, folic acid, nicotinic acid, pantothenic acid.

維生素 B 一組水溶性維生素。雖然無化學聯繫，却常發現共同存在於同一的食物中（牛奶、肝、穀物類等），其功用是起輔酶作用。

vitamin B_1 (thiamin, aneurin) a vitamin of the B complex that is active in the form of *thiamin pyrophosphate*, a

維生素 B_1（硫胺） 維生素 B 複合物中的一種。硫胺焦磷酸鹽型有活

coenzyme in decarboxylation reactions in carbohydrate metabolism. A deficiency of vitamin B_1 leads to *beriberi. Good sources of the vitamin are cereals, beans, meat, potatoes, and nuts. The recommended daily intake is 1 mg for an adult.

性，是糖代謝中脫羧反應的輔酶。維生素B_1缺乏可導至脚氣病。穀類、豆類、肉、土豆和堅果爲此維生素的重要來源。成人每日攝入量是 1 mg。

vitamin B_2 (riboflavin) a vitamin of the B complex that is a constituent of the coenzymes *FAD (flavine adenine dinucleotide) and *FMN (flavine mononucleotide). Riboflavin is therefore important in tissue respiration. A deficiency of riboflavin causes a condition known as *ariboflavinosis, which is not usually serious. Good sources of riboflavin are liver, milk, and eggs. The recommended daily intake for an adult is 1.7 mg.

維生素B_2（核黃素） 維生素 B 複合物中的一種。爲輔酶 FAD（黃素腺嘌呤二核苷酸）和 FMN（黃素嘌呤單核苷酸）的一個成分。所以核黃素對組織呼吸是重要的，核黃素缺乏時引起核黃素缺乏症，通常是不嚴重的。肝、牛奶和蛋類是核黃素豐富的來源。成人每日攝入量是 1.7 mg。

vitamin B_6 (pyridoxine) a vitamin of the B complex from which the coenzyme *pyridoxal phosphate, involved in the transamination of amino acids, is formed. The vitamin is found in most foods and a deficiency is therefore rare.

維生素B_6（吡哆醇） 維生素 B 複合物中的一種。它形成磷酸吡哆醛，後者參與氨基酸的轉氨基反應，這種維生素存在於多種食物中，故缺乏症少見。

vitamin B_{12} (cyanocobalamin) a vitamin of the B complex. The form of vitamin B_{12} with coenzyme activity is *5-deoxyadenosyl cobalamin*, which is necessary for the synthesis of nucleic acids, the maintenance of *myelin in the nervous system, and the proper functioning of *folic acid, another B vitamin. The vitamin can be absorbed only in the presence of *intrinsic factor*, a protein secreted in the stomach. A deficiency of vitamin B_{12} affects nearly all the body tissues, particularly those containing rapidly dividing cells. The most serious effects of a deficiency are *pernicious anaemia and degeneration of the nervous system. Vitamin B_{12} is manufactured only by certain microorganisms and is contained only in foods of animal origin. Good sources are liver, fish, and eggs. The daily recommended adult intake is 3–4 μg.

維生素B_{12} B 族維生素中的一種。有輔酶活性的維生素B_{12}是 5-脫氧腺苷鈷胺素，後者是合成核酸和維持神經系統中的髓鞘所必需的，也是使葉酸和其他維生素 B 起正常作用所必需的。維生素B_{12}只有在胃分泌的一種蛋白——內因子存在情況下才能被吸收，維生素B_{12}缺乏影響到幾乎全身組織，特別是那些快速分裂細胞的組織。維生素B_{12}缺乏最嚴重的後果是惡性貧血和神經系統的變性。維生素B_{12}只由某些微生物產生，只在動物源性食物中含有，肝、魚類、蛋類都是重要的來源。成人每日攝入量爲 3～4μg。

vitamin C (ascorbic acid) a water-soluble vitamin that is essential in maintaining healthy connective tissues and the integrity of cell walls. It is necessary for the synthesis of collagen. A deficiency of vitamin C leads to *scurvy. The recommended daily intake is 30 mg for an adult; rich sources are citrus fruits and vegetables.

維生素 C（抗壞血酸） 一種水溶性維生素。主要是維持健全的結締組織和細胞壁（膜）的完整性，是合成膠原所必需的。維生素 C 缺乏導至壞血病。成人每日攝入量需 30 mg。其豐富來源是柑橘類水果和蔬菜。

vitamin D a fat-soluble vitamin that enhances the absorption of calcium and phosphorus from the intestine and promotes their deposition in the bone. It occurs in two forms: *ergocalciferol* (*vitamin D_2, calciferol*), which is manufactured by plants when the sterol ergosterol is exposed to ultraviolet light, and *cholecalciferol* (*vitamin D_3*), which is produced by the action of sunlight on 7-dehydrocholesterol, a sterol widely distributed in the skin. A deficiency of vitamin D, either from a poor diet or lack of sunlight, leads to decalcified bones and the development of *rickets and *osteomalacia. Good sources of vitamin D are liver and fish oils. The recommended daily intake is 10 μg for a child up to five years and 2.5 μg thereafter. Vitamin D is toxic and large doses must therefore be avoided.

維生素 D 一種脂溶性維生素。可加强鈣和磷在腸道內吸收和促進它們在骨中沉積。它以兩種形式出現：麥角鈣化醇（維生素 D_2）是植物中麥角固醇暴露於紫外線而生成的，膽鈣化醇（維生素 D_3）是由廣泛分佈於皮膚中的膽固醇類——7-脫氫膽固醇在陽光作用下生成。無論是因飲食中不足或缺乏陽光造成的維生素 D 缺乏，均可導至骨骼脫鈣，發生佝僂病和軟骨病。肝和魚肝油爲維生素 D 豐富的來源。五歲前兒童每日建議攝入量爲 10 μg，以後每天 2.5 μg。維生素 D 是有毒性的，故應避免大劑量應用。

vitamin E any of a group of chemically related compounds (*tocopherols* and *tocotrienols*) that have antioxidant properties and are thought to stabilize cell membranes by preventing oxidation of their unsaturated fatty acid components. The most potent of these is *α-tocopherol*. Good sources of the vitamin are vegetable oils, eggs, butter, and wholemeal cereals. It is fairly widely distributed in the diet and a deficiency is therefore unlikely.

維生素 E 一組化學上相關的有抗氧化劑特性的複合物（生育酚和生育三烯酚類）。人們認爲它能防止不飽和脂肪酸氧化而使細胞膜穩定。最常見的成分是 α-生育酚。植物油、蛋類、黃油和粗面粉穀類是這種維生素的豐富的來源。它於食物中廣泛存在，所以不大可能發生缺乏。

vitamin K a fat-soluble vitamin occurring in two main forms: *phytomenadione* (of plant origin) and *menaquinone* (of animal origin). It is necessary for the formation of *prothrombin in the liver,

維生素 K 以兩種形式存在的脂溶性維生素，維生素 K_1（植物源性）和維生素 K_2（動物源性）。它是肝臟合成凝血酶原所

which is essential for blood clotting, and it also regulates the synthesis of other clotting factors. A dietary deficiency does not often occur as the vitamin is synthesized by bacteria in the large intestine and is widely distributed in green leafy vegetables and meat.

必需的。而凝血酶原在凝血中必不可少。它也與其它凝血因子的合成有關。因爲維生素K可由大腸內細菌合成，並廣泛存在於綠色蔬菜和肉類中，故很少因飲食中含量不足而缺乏。

vitellus *n.* the yolk of an ovum.

vitiligo (leucoderma) *n.* a condition in which areas of skin lose their pigment and become white. There are no other changes, but the white patches, which appear anywhere, grow in size until much of the body is affected. The cause is unknown and treatment is unsatisfactory in Europeans.

白斑（白斑病） 皮膚某部位失去色素和變白。雖無其它病變，但白斑可出現在任何部位，並且會擴大，直至全身許多部位受累。在歐洲人中發病原因尚不清楚，治療也不滿意。

vitrectomy *n.* the removal of the whole or part of the vitreous humour of the eye.

玻璃體摘除術 摘除全部或部分眼內玻璃體。

vitreous humour (vitreous body) the transparent jelly-like material that fills the chamber behind the lens of the eye.

玻璃體 充滿眼晶狀體後腔的透明膠樣物質。

viviparous *adj.* describing animal groups (including most mammals) in which the embryos develop within the body of the mother so that the young are born alive rather than hatch from an egg. —**viviparity** *n.*

胎生的 描寫一類動物（主要指哺乳動物），其胚胎在母體內生長發育，出生時爲活的幼小動物，而不是從卵孵化的動物。

vivisection *n.* a surgical operation on a living animal for experimental purposes.

活體解剖 爲實驗目的而在活的動物身上進行的外科手術。

vocal cords (vocal folds) the two folds of tissue which protrude from the sides of the *larynx to form a narrow

聲帶 從咽部兩側凸出的兩條組織皺襞（見圖），在呼吸道中形成一條狹縫

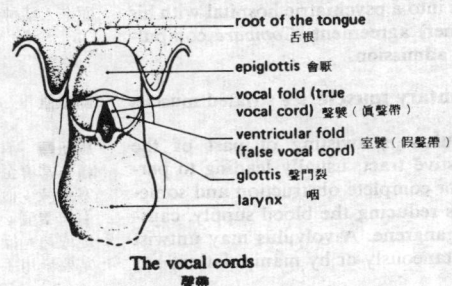

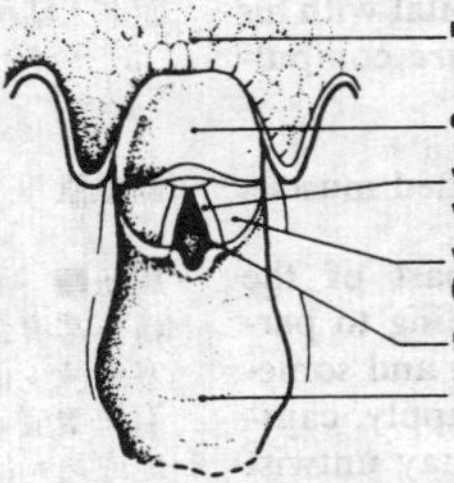

The vocal cords
聲帶

slit (glottis) across the air passage (see illustration). Their controlled interference with the expiratory air flow produces audible vibrations that make up speech, song, and all other vocal noises. Alterations in the vocal cords themselves or in their nerve supply by disease interferes with phonation.

（聲門）。它們對呼出的氣流能控制調節，產生聽得見的振動，這就是說話唱歌的聲音和其他的噪聲，由於疾病使聲帶本身或其神經支配發生變化，可影響發音。

vocal fremitus *see* fremitus.

語音震顫

vocal resonance the sounds heard through the stethoscope when the patient speaks ("ninety nine"). These are normally just audible but become much louder (*bronchophony*) if the lung under the stethoscope is consolidated, when they resemble the sounds heard over the trachea and main bronchi. Vocal resonance is lost over pleural fluid except at its upper surface, when it has a bleating quality and is called *aegophony*. *See also* pectoriloquy.

語音 當患者說話（"九十九"）時通過聽診器聽到的聲音。這些聲音在正常情況下剛可聽到，若聽診器下的肺實變時，聲音就會顯著增響（支氣管語音）。與在氣管和支氣管上聽到的聲音相似，在胸腔積液部位語音消失，但在積液以上的表面則不同，此時聽到的音類似羊鳴，稱爲"羊音"。

volar *adj.* relating to the palm of the hand or the sole of the foot (the *vola*).

掌的（蹠的） 指手掌和脚底（蹠）。

volsella (vulsella) *n.* surgical forceps with clawlike hooks at the ends of both blades.

雙爪鉗 末端有爪樣鈎的外科用鉗。

volt *n.* the *SI unit of electric potential, equal to the potential difference between two points on a conducting wire through which a constant current of 1 ampere flows when the power dissipated between these points is 1 watt. Symbol: V.

伏〔特〕 電位的國際標準單位。等於一安培恒定電流通過導線上消耗電功率爲 1 瓦〔特〕時的兩點間的電位差。符號：V。

voluntary admission entry of a patient into a psychiatric hospital with his (or her) agreement. *Compare* compulsory admission.

自願入院 通過病人同意而進入精神病院。

voluntary muscle *see* striated muscle.

隨意肌

volvulus *n.* twisting of part of the digestive tract, usually leading to partial or complete obstruction and sometimes reducing the blood supply, causing gangrene. A volvulus may untwist spontaneously or by manipulation, but

腸扭轉 消化道的部分扭轉，常導至部分或全部阻塞或減少血液供應，以致引起壞疽。腸扭轉可自發地或通過操作而鬆解，但常要施用手術探查。胃扭

surgical exploration is usually performed. *Gastric volvulus* is a twist of the stomach, usually in a hiatus *hernia. *Small-intestinal volvulus* is twisting of part of the bowel around an *adhesion. *Sigmoid volvulus* is a twist of the sigmoid colon, usually when this loop is particularly long.

轉常發生於食管裂孔疝。小腸扭轉是在黏連周圍的部分腸扭轉。乙狀結腸扭轉常因該段腸襻特別長而發生。

vomer *n.* a thin plate of bone that forms part of the nasal septum (*see* nasal cavity). *See also* skull.

犁骨 構成鼻中隔部分的薄板狀骨。

vomica *n.* **1.** an abnormal cavity in an organ, usually a lung, sometimes containing pus. **2.** the abrupt expulsion from the mouth of a large quantity of pus or decaying matter originating in the throat or lungs.

①**空洞** 某器官不正常的空腔。常在肺內，有時含有膿液。 ②**咳膿痰** 從口腔突然排出來自喉部或肺部的大量膿液或腐爛物。

vomit 1. *vb.* to eject the contents of the stomach through the mouth (*see* vomiting). **2.** *n.* the contents of the stomach ejected during vomiting. Medical name: **vomitus.**

①**嘔吐** 從口中排出胃內容物。 ②**嘔吐物** 嘔吐時排出的胃內容物。

vomiting *n.* the reflex action of ejecting the contents of the stomach through the mouth. Vomiting is controlled by a special centre in the brain that may be stimulated by drugs (e.g. *apomorphine) acting directly on it; or by impulses transmitted through nervous pathways either from the stomach (e.g. after ingesting irritating substances, in gastritis and other stomach diseases), the intestine (e.g. in intestinal obstruction), or from the inner ear (in travel sickness). The stimulated vomiting centre sets off a chain of nerve impulses producing coordinated contractions of the diaphragm and abdominal muscles, relaxation of the muscle at the entrance to the stomach, etc., causing the stomach contents to be expelled. Medical name: **emesis.**

嘔吐 經口排出胃內容物的反射活動。嘔吐是由大腦特殊中樞控制，可被藥物直接作用而興奮（例如：阿朴嗎啡），也可由神經通路傳遞來的衝動所興奮，包括胃的衝動（例如：在食入刺激性食物後，胃炎和其他胃病時），腸的衝動（例如：腸梗阻）或內耳的衝動（暈車時）等。嘔吐中樞興奮時引起一系列神經衝動，產生膈肌和腹部肌肉協調的收縮，胃入口處肌肉鬆弛等，使胃內容物排出。

von Hippel-Lindau disease a syndrome in which *haemangioblastomas, particularly in the cerebellum, are associated with renal and pancreatic cysts, *angiomas in the retina, cancer of the kidney cells, and red birthmarks.

希-林二氏病 一種成血管細胞瘤的綜合徵，特別是在小腦，它伴有腎和胰腺囊腫、視網膜血管瘤、腎細胞癌和紅色胎痣。

von Recklinghausen's disease 1. a syndrome due to excessive secretion of *parathyroid hormone (hyperparathyroidism), characterized by loss of mineral from bones, which become weakened and fracture easily, and formation of kidney stones. Medical name: **osteitis fibrosa**. **2.** *see* neurofibromatosis.

雷克林霍會氏病 ①由於甲狀旁腺激素分泌過多（甲狀旁腺機能亢進）引起的綜合徵。其特徵是骨丟失礦物質而變得脆弱和易骨折，以及腎結石形成。醫學名稱纖維性骨炎。 ②神經纖維瘤病。

voyeurism *n.* the condition of obtaining sexual pleasure by watching other people undressing or enjoying sexual relations. *See also* perversion. —**voyeur** *n.*

觀淫癖 通過看其他人裸體或性交而得到性快樂的一種病態。

vulsella *n. see* volsella.

雙爪鉗

vulv- (vulvo-) *prefix denoting* the vulva.

〔前綴〕 **外陰**

vulva *n.* the female external genitalia. Two pairs of fleshy folds – the *labia majora* and *labia minora* – surround the openings of the vagina and urethra and extend forward to the clitoris (see illustration). *See also* vestibular glands.

外陰 女性外生殖器。兩對多肉的皺襞（大陰唇和小陰唇）圍繞於陰道和尿道的開口，向前伸展至陰蒂（見圖）。

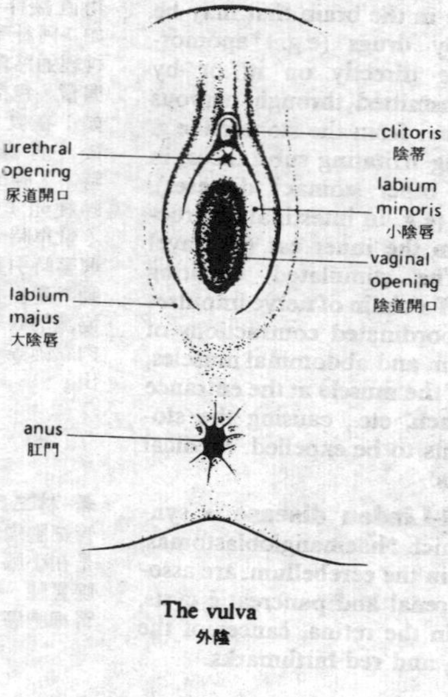

The vulva
外陰

vulvectomy *n.* surgical removal of the external genitals (vulva) of a woman.

外陰切除術 切除婦女外生殖器的手術。

vulvitis *n.* inflammation of the vulva, which is often accompanied by intense itching and burning pain. It may be caused by infection with the fungus *Candida albicans* or the bacterium *Neisseria gonococcus* or by ill-fitting underwear (which causes the lips of the vulva to rub together).

外陰炎 外陰的炎症，伴劇烈的瘙癢和灼痛。可由眞菌"白色念珠菌"或細菌"淋病雙球菌"感染引起，或由穿着不合體的襯褲引起（使陰唇相互摩擦）。

vulvovaginitis *n.* **1.** inflammation of the vulva and vagina (*see* vaginitis, vulvitis). **2.** *see* bartholinitis.

外陰陰道炎 ①外陰和陰道的炎症。②見前庭大腺炎。

W

W

wafer *n.* a thin sheet made from moistened flour, formerly used to enclose a powdered medicine that is taken by mouth.

糯米紙囊劑 由糯米粉加水製成的薄紙，過去常用於包裹口服的藥粉。

waiting list a list of the names of patients who are awaiting admission to hospital after having been assessed either as an out-patient or on a domiciliary consultation involving a specialist. In general the patients are offered places in the order in which their names were placed on the list, but in certain circumstances (e.g. if the condition is potentially dangerous or painful) the consultant may recommend urgent or even immediate admission. One of the facts recorded in relation to hospital admissions is the length of time between the name being placed on the list and the patient being admitted (*waiting time*). General practitioners may also request *direct admission* (immediate) for urgent cases who have not been seen by the consultant; such admission may be arranged by phone with the consultant or his deputy or channelled through the accident and emergency department of the hospital.

入院候診單 等候入院的病人的名單。他們或者是在門診上確定要入院的病人，或者是在地段上通過專家會診確定要入院的病人。通常，病人入院順序是按照名單上的順序，但在某些情況下（例如，如果病情有潛在危險性或疼痛劇烈），經治醫師可建議緊急或甚至立即接收入院。入院登記的目的之一就是確定從在名單上登記的時間到得以入院的時間的長短（等候時間）。全科醫師也可安排一些未經經治醫師診斷的緊急病人直接入院，他們可以通過電話與經治醫師或他的代理人聯繫，或者是通過醫院急診室安排病人入院。

Walcher's position a position in which the patient lies on the back with the legs hanging down: sometimes adopted to aid childbirth.

瓦爾歇氏臥位 病人仰臥掛腿的體位。有時用來幫助分娩。

Waldeyer's ring the ring of lymphoid tissue formed by the tonsils.

瓦爾代爾氏扁桃體環 扁桃體構成的淋巴組織環。

warfarin *n.* an *anticoagulant used mainly in the treatment of coronary or venous thrombosis to reduce the risk of embolism. It is given by mouth or injection. The principal toxic effect is local bleeding, usually from the gums and other mucous membranes. Warfarin has also been used as a rat poison. Trade names: **Coumadin, Marevan**.

苄丙酮香豆素（華法令） 一種主要用來治療冠狀動脉或靜脉血栓形成以減少栓塞危險性的抗凝藥。口服或注射。主要的毒性反應是局部出血，通常發生在牙齦部和其他黏膜。華法令也可用作滅鼠藥。

wart *n.* a small (often hard) benign growth in the skin. Caused by a virus, warts are commoner in young people, usually occurring on the face, fingers, hands, elbows, and knees. There are several types. *Juvenile warts* occur profusely on the hands and face of children; *common warts* are larger, with a rougher surface, and occur on the hands. *Plantar warts* occur on the sole of the foot; they are subject to pressure and are therefore painful and may be covered by a thick callus. They spread rapidly in communities, such as schools. *Venereal warts* are found on the genitals or around the anus in both sexes. Warts usually disappear spontaneously but there is a wide range of treatments, including local application of chemicals, removal with a *curette, and *electrocautery. Medical name: **verruca**.

疣 一種小的（常是硬的）皮膚良性新生物。由病毒引起，常見於青年人，多出現在面部、手指、手、肘和膝部。有幾種類型，青年疣多見於兒童的手和面部；尋常疣稍大，表面粗糙，並見於手上；足蹠疣見於足底，易受壓而疼痛，可被一厚胼胝覆蓋。它們在公共場所如學校傳播很快。性病濕疣見於兩性生殖器或肛門周圍。疣常自發消失，但也有很多治療方法，包括局部用藥、用刮術和電烙術去除。

Wassermann reaction the most commonly used test for the diagnosis of *syphilis. A sample of the patient's blood is examined, using a *complement-fixation reaction, for the presence of antibodies to the organism *Treponema pallidum*. A positive reaction (WR+) indicates the presence of antibodies and therefore infection with syphilis.

乏色曼氏反應 最常用的診斷梅毒的試驗。用補體結合反應來檢查病人的血標本中梅毒螺旋體的抗體。陽性反應（WR+）說明有抗體存在，因此有梅毒感染。

water bed a bed with a flexible water-containing mattress. The surface of the bed adapts itself to the patient's posture, which leads to greater comfort and fewer bedsores.

充水床墊 一種有柔軟可變形的含水床墊。床的表面可隨病人的姿勢而變化，以使病人舒適和少患褥瘡。

waterbrash *n.* a sudden filling of the mouth with dilute saliva. This often accompanies dyspepsia, particularly if there is nausea.

泛酸 口腔內突然充滿稀薄唾液。經常伴有消化不良，特別是噁心。

Waters' projection a *posteroanterior X-ray film to show the maxillae, maxillary sinuses, and zygomatic bones.

瓦特氏投影 顯示上頜骨，上頜竇和顴骨的前後位X線相片。

watt *n.* the *SI unit of power, equal to 1 joule per second. In electrical terms it is the energy expended per second when a current of 1 ampere flows between two points on a conductor between which there is a potential difference of 1 volt. 1 watt = 10^7 ergs per second. Symbol: W.

瓦特 功率的標準國際單位。相等於 1焦耳/秒。在電學上指 1 安培/秒的電流通過導體中電壓差爲 1 伏的兩點所耗的電能。1 瓦特 = 10^7爾格/秒，符號：W。

weal *n. see* wheal.

風塊

weber *n.* the *SI unit of magnetic flux, equal to the flux linking a circuit of one turn that produces an e.m.f. of 1 volt when reduced uniformly to zero in 1 second. Symbol: Wb.

韋伯 磁通量的標準國際制單位。相當於電路中一個線圈中 1 伏電動勢均勻地減到零時產生的電磁通量。符號：Wb。

Weber-Christian disease *see* panniculitis.

韋-克二氏病 結節性非化膿性脂膜炎。

Weber's test a hearing test in which a vibrating tuning fork is placed at the midpoint of the forehead. A normal individual hears it equally in both ears, but if one ear is affected by conductive *deafness the sound appears louder in the affected ear.

韋伯氏試驗 一種聽力試驗，把顫動的音叉放在額部中點，正常人兩耳聽到的聲響是相同的，若一個耳朵患有傳導性耳聾，該耳聽到的聲響顯得較響。

Wegener's granuloma a disease predominantly affecting the nasal passages, lungs, and kidneys, characterized by *granuloma formation in addition to arteritis. It is usually fatal but can be controlled (sometimes for years) with steroids and/or cyclophosphamide.

韋格內氏肉芽腫 一種主要侵犯鼻道、肺和腎的疾病。其特徵除動脈炎外爲肉芽腫形成。該病常常是致命的，但可以用固醇類或環磷醯胺控制（有時達幾年）。

Weil-Felix reaction a diagnostic test for typhus. A sample of the patient's serum is tested for the presence of antibodies against the organism *Proteus vulgaris*. Although this relatively harmless organism is not the cause of typhus, it possesses certain antigens in common with the causative agent of the disease and can therefore be used instead of it in laboratory tests. Typhus is suspected if antibodies are found to be present.

外斐氏反應 診斷斑疹傷寒的試驗，檢測病人血清標本中是否存在普通變形桿菌的抗體。雖然這種相對無害的細菌不是引起傷寒的病原體，但是它與致病菌有某種相同的抗原成分，所以在實驗室試驗中可用之代替。如果發現抗體則可疑有斑疹傷寒。

Weil's disease *see* leptospirosis.

外爾氏病

Welch's bacillus *see* Clostridium.

魏爾希氏桿菌

wen *n. see* sebaceous cyst.

皮脂囊腫

Wernicke's encephalopathy mental confusion or delirium occurring in combination with paralysis of the eye muscles, *nystagmus, and an unsteady gait. It is caused by a deficiency of vitamin B_1 (thiamin) and is most commonly seen in alcoholics and in patients with persistent vomiting. Treatment with thiamin relieves the symptoms.

韋尼克氏腦病 精神錯亂或譫妄伴有眼肌麻痹、眼球震顫和步態不穩。由維生素 B_1（硫胺）缺乏引起，常見於酒精中毒者和持久性嘔吐病人。用硫胺可以緩解症狀。

Wertheim's hysterectomy an operation performed for cancer of the womb or ovary, in which the womb, Fallopian tubes, ovaries, upper vagina, broad ligaments, and regional lymph nodes are removed.

韋太姆氏子宮切除術 子宮或卵巢惡性腫瘤的手術。手術切除子宮、輸卵管、卵巢、上陰道、闊韌帶和局部淋巴結。

Wharton's duct the secretory duct of the submandibular *salivary gland.

下頜腺管 下頜下唾液腺的分泌管。

Wharton's jelly the mesoderm tissue of the umbilical cord, which becomes converted to a loose jelly-like *mesenchyme surrounding the umbilical blood vessels.

華頓氏膠 臍帶中胚層組織，轉變爲圍繞着臍血管的疏鬆膠樣間質。

wheal (weal) *n.* a temporary red or pale raised area of the skin, often accompanied by severe itching. Wheals may be caused by scratching or rubbing the skin and are sometimes the sign of a local or general allergy (*see* urticaria). *See also* dermographia.

風塊 皮膚暫時隆起的發紅或蒼白的區域，常伴有嚴重瘙癢。風塊也可由搔抓或摩擦皮膚引起，常是局部或全身過敏的現象。

wheeze *n.* low-pitched breathing sounds associated with *bronchospasm, such as occurs in asthma and byssinosis. *Compare* stridor.

喘鳴 低調的伴有支氣管痙攣的呼吸音。例如發生於哮喘或棉屑沉着病時。

whiplash injury damage to the ligaments, vertebrae, spinal cord, or nerve roots in the neck region, caused by sudden jerking back of the head and neck. At its most severe death or permanent paralysis (*quadriplegia or *paraplegia) may result. Sudden deceleration in a motor accident is the commonest cause. Immobilization using a special collar is the principal treatment.

頭部衝擊傷 由於頭和頸部被突然猛烈向後推引起的韌帶、脊柱、脊髓和神經根的損傷。嚴重者可致死或永久性麻痹（四肢癱瘓和截癱）。最常見的原因是摩托車事故中突然減速。用特殊硬領固定是主要治療方法。

Whipple's disease a rare disease, occurring only in males, in which absorption of digested food in the intestine is reduced. As well as symptoms and signs of *malabsorption there is usually skin pigmentation and arthritis. Diagnosis is made by *jejunal biopsy; microorganisms have been found in the mucosa, and the disease usually responds to prolonged antibiotic treatment.

惠普爾氏病 一種罕見的疾病，只發生於男性，表現爲腸道內消化的食物吸收減退。除營養不良的症狀和體徵外，通常尚有皮膚色素沉着和關節炎。診斷有賴於空腸活組織檢查，可發現黏膜中有微生物存在。長期抗生素治療往往對該病有效。

Whipple's operation *see* pancreatectomy.

惠普可氏手術 胰腺切除術。

whipworm *n.* a small parasitic whiplike nematode worm, *Trichuris trichiura* (*Trichocephalus dispar*), that lives in the large intestine. Eggs are passed out of the body with the faeces and human infection (*see* trichuriasis) results from the consumption of water or food contaminated with faecal material. The eggs hatch in the small intestine but mature worms migrate to the large intestine.

鞭蟲 一種小的寄生性鞭毛樣線蟲。毛首鞭毛蟲生活在大腸中，蟲卵通過糞便排出體外。人通過食用有糞便污染的水和食物而感染。卵在小腸孵化，而成蟲移行至大腸。

white blood cell *see* leucocyte.

白細胞

white leg (milk leg) a condition that may affect women after childbirth in which there is clotting and inflammation in a vein in the leg. The leg becomes pale, swollen, and tense and is painful; the condition resolves only

股白腫 腿部靜脉中有血凝塊和炎症的一種疾病。可侵犯分娩後的婦女。腿變得蒼白，腫脹和緊張，並有疼痛，症狀消除緩慢。

slowly. Medical name: **phlegmasia alba dolens.**

white matter nerve tissue of the central nervous system that is paler in colour than the associated *grey matter because it contains more nerve fibres and thus larger amounts of the insulating material *myelin. In the brain the white matter lies within the grey layer of cerebral cortex; in the spinal cord it is between the arms of the X-shaped central core of grey matter.

白質 中樞神經系統的神經組織。因爲它含有較多的神經纖維和較大量的隔離物質髓鞘，顏色比相隣的灰質白些。在腦中白質位於大腦皮層的灰質層內部；在脊髓它位於X形的中央灰質的各柱之間。

whites *n. see* leucorrhoea.

白帶

whitlow (felon) *n.* an abscess affecting the pulp of the fingertip. *See also* paronychia.

瘭疽（指頭膿炎） 侵及指頭肉墊的膿腫。

whoop *n.* a noisy convulsive drawing in of the breath following the spasmodic coughing attack characteristic of *whooping cough.

哮吼 百日咳典型的痙攣性咳嗽發作後發生的痙攣性吸氣聲。

whooping cough an acute contagious disease, primarily affecting children, due to infection of the mucous membranes lining the air passages by the bacterium *Haemophilus pertussis*. After an incubation period of 1–2 weeks catarrh, mild fever, coughing, and loss of appetite gradually develop and persist for 1–2 weeks. The cough becomes paroxysmal: series of short coughs are followed by involuntary drawing in of the breath, which produces the whooping sound. Bleeding from the nose and mouth and vomiting often occur after a paroxysm. This stage lasts about two weeks and the child is infectious throughout. Over the following 2–3 weeks symptoms slowly decline but the cough may persist for many weeks. Whooping cough is seldom serious but the child is susceptible to pneumonia and tuberculosis. Immunization reduces the incidence and severity of the disease: the vaccine is usually given in a combined form (*see* DPT vaccine). An attack usually also confers immunity. Medical name: **pertussis**.

百日咳 一種主要侵犯兒童的急性傳染病。由於呼吸道內黏膜受到百日咳嗜血桿菌感染。在1～2周潛伏期後逐漸發生卡地、低熱、咳嗽和食慾喪失，持續1～2周，然後咳嗽變爲發作性：在一陣短促的咳嗽後，發生伴有哮吼聲的不自主吸氣。陣咳發作後常發生鼻腔和口腔出血和嘔吐。該期持續2～3周，此期內患兒都有傳染性。2～3周後症狀漸漸減輕，但咳嗽可持續許多周。百日咳很少是嚴重的，但患兒易患肺炎和結核病。免疫接種可降低疾病的發病率和嚴重性。通常用聯合疫苗接種。一次患病往往可以獲得免疫。

Widal reaction an *agglutination test for the presence of antibodies against the *Salmonella* organisms that cause typhoid fever. It is thus a method of diagnosing the presence of the disease in a patient and also a means of identifying the organisms in infected material.

肥達氏反應 一種檢驗抗傷寒沙門氏菌抗體的凝集試驗。它是診斷傷寒病人與鑑定被污染物質細菌種類的方法。

Wilms' tumour *see* nephroblastoma.

維爾姆斯氏瘤 腎胚細胞瘤。

Wilson's disease an inborn defect of copper metabolism in which there is a deficiency of *caeruloplasmin (which normally forms a nontoxic complex with copper). The free copper may be deposited in the liver, causing jaundice and cirrhosis, or in the brain, causing mental retardation and symptoms resembling *parkinsonism. There is a characteristic brown ring in the cornea (the *Kayser-Fleischer ring*). If the excess copper is removed from the body by regular treatment with *penicillamine both mental and physical development may be normal. Medical name: **hepatolenticular degeneration**.

威爾遜氏病 先天性的銅代謝障碍。本病銅藍蛋白（正常時與銅形成無毒性結合物）缺乏，游離的銅可以沉積在肝臟，引起黃疸和肝硬化；或沉積在腦，引起精神發育遲緩和酷似帕金森氏病的症狀。在角膜有一特徵性的褐色環（凱-弗二氏環）。若用青黴胺正規治療能使過多的銅排出體外，則智力和體力的發育都可正常。醫學名稱：肝豆狀核變性。

windigo *n.* a delusion of having been transformed into a *windigo*, a mythical monster that eats human flesh. It is often quoted as an example of a syndrome confined to one culture (that of some North American Indian tribes, such as the Cree).

溫第高妄想 一種變成神話中的吃人肉的怪物溫第高的妄想。常用以描述僅出現於某種民族（北美印第安部落，如克瑞族）的人的綜合徵。

windpipe *n. see* trachea.

氣管

wisdom tooth the third *molar tooth on each side of either jaw, which erupts normally around the age of 20.

智齒 兩側上下頜的第三個磨牙。正常在 20 歲左右萌出。

witch hazel (hamamelis) a preparation made from the leaves and bark of the tree *Hamamelis virginiana*, used as an *astringent, especially for the treatment of sprains and bruises.

北美金縷梅 用北美金縷梅的葉和樹皮做成的收斂劑。多用於治療扭傷和青腫。

withdrawal *n.* 1. (in psychology) the removal of one's interest from one's surroundings. *Thought withdrawal* is the

①**退縮** 心理學用語。某人對環境失去興趣。思想退縮（被奪）是指某人感

experience of one's thoughts being removed from one's head, which is characteristic of *schizophrenia. **2.** *see* coitus interruptus.

到思想從其頭腦中被去除掉的體驗，是精神分裂症的一個特徵。 ②**中斷性交**

withdrawal symptoms *see* dependence.

戒斷綜合徵

Wohlfahrtia *n.* a genus on non-blood-sucking flies. The females of *W. magnifica* and *W. vigil* deposit their parasitic maggots in wounds and the openings of the body. This causes *myiasis, particularly in children.

汚蠅屬　一種非吸血的蠅類。雌性壯麗汚蠅和邁氏汚蠅把它們產生的蛆堆積於傷口和人體孔口處，引起蠅蛆病。多見於兒童。

Wolffian body *see* mesonephros.

舞非氏體

Wolffian duct the mesonephric duct (*see* mesonephros).

舞非氏管　中腎管。

womb *n. see* uterus.

子宮

wood point *see* tooth pick.

牙簽

word blindness *see* alexia.

文字盲

worm *n.* any member of several groups of soft-bodied legless animals, including flatworms, nematode worms, earthworms, and leeches, that were formerly thought to be closely related and classified as a single group – Vermes.

蠕蟲　不同種類的無腿軟體動物。包括扁蟲、線蟲、蚯蚓和水蛭。它們以前被認爲是密切相關的，並被歸類在一個組——蠕蟲類中。

wormian bone one of a number of small bones that occur in the cranial sutures.

縫間骨　位於顱骨骨縫處的一些小骨。

wound *n.* a break in the structure of an organ or tissue caused by an external agent. Bruises, grazes, tears, cuts, punctures, and burns are all examples of wounds.

創傷　由於外界因素引起某一器官或組織結構的破壞。挫傷、擦傷、撕裂傷、刀割傷、刺傷、燒傷都是創傷的例子。

wrist *n.* **1.** the joint between the forearm and hand. It consists of the proximal bones of the *carpus, which articulate with the radius and ulna. **2.** the whole region of the wrist joint, including the carpus and lower parts of the radius and ulna.

①**腕關節**　前臂和手之間的關節。由橈骨、尺骨與近端腕骨組成。 ②**腕部**　腕關節的全部，包括腕和橈骨，尺骨的下部。

wrist drop paralysis of the muscles that raise the wrist, which is caused by

腕下垂　由於橈神經損傷導至的抬腕肌肉的麻痹。

damage to the *radial nerve. This may result from compression of the nerve against the humerus in the upper arm or from selective damage to the nerve, which is a feature of *lead poisoning.

可由於壓迫上臂肱骨處的神經或是選擇性神經損傷所致。後者是鉛中毒時的特徵。

wryneck *n. see* torticollis.

斜頸

Wuchereria *n.* a genus of white threadlike parasitic worms (*see* filaria) that live in the lymphatic vessels. *W. bancrofti* is a tropical and subtropical species that causes *elephantiasis, lymphangitis, and chyluria. The immature forms concentrate in the lungs during the day. At night they become more numerous in the blood vessels of the skin, from which they are taken up by blood-sucking mosquitoes, acting as carriers of the diseases they cause.

吳策線蟲屬 一屬生活在淋巴管內的白色線樣寄生蟲。班氏吳策絲蟲是一熱帶或亞熱帶種，引起象皮病、淋巴管炎與乳糜尿。白天微絲蚴集中於肺臟，夜間它們大量出現於皮膚血管中，被吸血蚊子吸走，後者起傳播絲蟲病的作用。

X

X

xanthaemia (carotenaemia) *n.* the presence in the blood of the yellow pigment *carotene, from excessive intake of carrots, tomatoes, or other vegetables containing the pigment.

胡蘿蔔素症 由於過多攝入胡蘿蔔、西紅柿和其他含有胡蘿蔔素的蔬菜，血中出現黃色的色素——胡蘿蔔素。

xanthelasma *n.* one or more yellow deposits of fatty material in the skin around the eyes. In elderly people it is quite common and of no more than cosmetic importance, but severe cases may be seen in certain disorders of fat metabolism.

黃斑瘤 眼周皮膚一處或多處黃色脂肪沉積。於老年人常見，這僅是容貌的問題，但嚴重病例可能出現於某種脂肪代謝障礙。

xanthine *n.* a nitrogenous breakdown product of the purines adenosine and guanine. Xanthine is an intermediate product of the breakdown of nucleic acids to uric acid.

黃嘌呤 腺嘌呤和鳥嘌呤的含氮分解產物。黃嘌呤是核酸分解成尿酸的中間產物。

xanthinuria *n.* excess of the purine derivative *xanthine in the urine, usually the result of an inborn defect of metabolism. It is both rare and symptomless.

黃嘌呤尿 尿內有過多的由嘌呤衍生的黃嘌呤。通常爲先天性代謝障礙的結果，本病既少見也無症狀。

xantho- *prefix denoting* yellow colour.
〔前綴〕 **黃色**

xanthochromia *n.* yellow discoloration, such as may affect the skin (for example, in jaundice) or the cerebrospinal fluid (when it contains the breakdown products of haemoglobin from red blood cells that have entered it).
黃變 變成黃色。可發生於皮膚（例如黃疸時）或腦脊液（當腦脊液中有紅細胞的血紅蛋白分解產物時）。

xanthoma *n.* (*pl.* **xanthomata**) a yellowish swelling, nodule, or plaque in the skin resulting from deposits of fat. The presence of xanthomata is usually accompanied by a raised blood *cholesterol level. There are several types; for example, *xanthomata palpebrarum*, in which the plaques appear on the eyelids in the elderly (*see* xanthelasma). *See also* xanthomatosis.
黃瘤 由於脂肪沉積於皮膚而引起的帶黃色的腫脹結節、斑塊。黃瘤常伴有血中膽固醇水平的增高。它有幾種類型，例如：黃斑瘤是出現於老年人眼瞼的斑塊。

xanthomatosis *n.* the presence of multiple small fatty tumours in the skin, the eyes, and the internal organs due to an excess of fats in the blood (hyperlipidaemia). *See* xanthoma.
黃瘤病 由於血中脂肪過多（高脂血症）引起皮膚、眼和內臟器官的多發的小脂肪瘤。

xanthophyll *n.* a yellow pigment found in green leaves. An example of a xanthophyll is *lutein*.
胡蘿蔔醇 一種存在於綠色葉中的黃色素。例如葉黃素。

xanthopsia *n.* yellow vision: the condition in which all objects appear to have a yellowish tinge. It is sometimes experienced in digitalis poisoning.
黃視症 視任何物體都顯示帶黃色色調，有時出現於洋地黃中毒時。

X chromosome the sex chromosome present in both sexes. Women have two X chromosomes and men one. Genes for some important genetic disorders, including *haemophilia, are carried on the X chromosomes; these genes are described as *sex-linked. *Compare* Y chromosome.
X染色體 兩性都具有的性染色體。女性有兩條X染色體，男性有一條。某些重要遺傳病變的基因位於X染色體上，如血友病，這些基因稱爲性連鎖基因。

xeno- *prefix denoting* different; foreign; alien.
〔前綴〕 **不同，外來的，相異的**

xenodiagnosis *n.* a procedure for diagnosing infections transmitted by insect carriers. Uninfected insects of the species known to carry the disease in question are allowed to suck the blood of a patient suspected of having the
動物接種診斷 診斷由病媒昆蟲傳播的傳染病的方法。用已知能傳播該病但未感染的昆蟲去刺吸疑有此病的病人的血，若該病的寄生蟲在昆蟲體內出

disease. A positive diagnosis is made if the disease parasites appear in the insects. This method has proved invaluable for diagnosing Chagas' disease, using reduviid bugs (the carriers), since the parasites are not always easily detected in blood smears.

現，則爲陽性診斷。用獵椿科昆蟲病媒在診斷恰加斯氏病時這種方法十分有用，因爲寄生蟲很難在血塗片上找到。

xenograft *n. see* heterograft.

異種移植物

xenophobia *n.* excessive fear of strangers and foreigners. *See* phobia.

生客恐怖 對陌生人和外國人過分害怕。

Xenopsylla *n.* a genus of tropical and subtropical fleas, with some 40 species. The rat flea, *X. cheopis*, occasionally attacks man and can transmit plague from an infected rat population; it also transmits murine typhus and two tapeworms, **Hymenolepis nana* and *H. diminuta*.

客蚤屬 一種熱帶、亞熱帶蚤屬。約有 40 種。鼠蚤（印鼠客蚤）偶然侵襲人類，並可從感染的鼠羣中將鼠疫傳染給人，它也可以傳播鼠型斑疹傷寒和兩種絛蟲：短膜殼絛蟲和長膜殼絛蟲。

xero- *prefix denoting* a dry condition.

〔前綴〕 **乾燥**

xeroderma *n.* a mild form of the hereditary disorder *ichthyosis, in which the skin develops slight dryness and forms branlike scales.

乾皮病 輕型的遺傳性鱗癬病變：皮膚輕度乾燥和形成糠皮樣鱗屑。

xerophthalmia *n.* a progressive disease of the eye due to deficiency of vitamin A. The cornea and conjunctiva become dry, thickened, and wrinkled. This may progress to *keratomalacia and eventual blindness.

乾眼病 由於維生素A缺乏的進行性眼病。角膜和結膜變乾燥，厚和有皺紋，可發展成角膜軟化和最後失明。

xerosis *n.* abnormal dryness of the conjunctiva, the skin, or the mucous membranes. Xerosis affecting the conjunctiva is due not to decreased production of tears but to changes in the membrane itself, which becomes thickened and grey in the area exposed when the eyelids are open.

乾燥病 眼結膜、皮膚或黏膜異常的乾燥。乾燥病侵及眼結膜不是由於眼淚分泌過少，而是由於結膜本身的改變，在眼瞼睁開時的暴露區結膜變厚變灰。

xerostomia *n.* dryness of the mouth resulting from diminished secretion of saliva. The phenomenon may be caused by drugs or poisons or be associated with disease. *Compare* ptyalism.

口腔乾燥 由於唾液分泌過少引起的口乾。這種現象可因藥物或毒物引起或在某種疾病中發生。

xiphi- (xipho-) *prefix denoting* the xiphoid process of the sternum. Example: *xiphocostal* (relating to the xiphoid process and ribs).

〔前綴〕 **劍** 指胸骨的劍突，如劍突肋骨的（與劍突和肋骨有關的）。

xiphisternum *see* xiphoid process.

劍突

xiphoid process (xiphoid cartilage) the lowermost section of the breastbone (*see* sternum): a flat pointed cartilage that gradually ossifies until it is completely replaced by bone, a process not completed until after middle age. It does not articulate with any ribs. Also called: **ensiform process** *or* **cartilage, xiphisternum**.

劍突（劍突軟骨） 胸骨最下端處的一塊扁平的尖形軟骨。此軟骨逐漸骨化直到完全被骨代替。這一過程直到中年後纔完成。它不連接任何肋骨，也稱爲劍形軟骨或軟骨劍突。

X-rays *n.* electromagnetic radiation of extremely short wavelength (beyond the ultraviolet), with great penetrating powers in matter opaque to light. X-rays are produced when high-energy beams of electrons strike matter. They are used in diagnosis in the techniques of *radiography and also in certain forms of *radiotherapy. Great care is needed to avoid unnecessary exposure, because the radiation is harmful in large quantities to all living things. *See* radiation sickness.

X射線 波長特別短的（超過紫外線）電磁波射線，有穿過不透光物體的强穿透力。當高能電子束撞擊物質時發出X射線，用於放射診斷及某種類型的放射治療。由於大劑量照射對所有活體都是有害的，所以需注意避免不必要的照射。

xylene (dimethylbenzene) *n.* a liquid used for increasing the transparency of tissues prepared for microscopic examination after they have been dehydrated. *See* clearing.

二甲苯 在製備顯微鏡檢查組織標本時脫水後用以增加透明度的液體。

xylometazoline *n.* a drug that constricts blood vessels (*see* vasoconstrictor). It is rapidly acting and long lasting and is applied topically as a nasal decongestant in the relief of the common cold and sinusitis. Toxic effects are rare. Trade name: **Otrivine**.

丁苄唑啉 一種血管收縮藥。作用快且持續時間長，作爲鼻的減充血劑用於局部以減輕感冒和鼻竇炎症狀。毒性反應少見。

xylose *n.* a pentose sugar (i.e. one with five carbon atoms) that is involved in carbohydrate interconversions within cells.

木糖 一種戊糖（有五個碳原子）。它參與細胞內碳水化合物的互變。

Y

Y

yawning *n.* a reflex action in which the mouth is opened wide and air is drawn into the lungs then slowly released. It is a result of drowsiness, fatigue, or boredom.

呵欠 把嘴張大讓空氣吸入肺然後再慢慢呼出的一種反射活動，是瞌睡、疲勞、厭煩的結果。

yaws (pian, framboesia) *n.* a tropical infectious disease caused by the presence of the spirochaete *Treponema pertenue* in the skin and its underlying tissues. Yaws occurs chiefly in conditions of poor hygiene. It is transmitted by direct contact with infected persons and their clothing and possibly also by flies of the genus *Hippelates*. The spirochaetes enter through abrasions on the skin. Initial symptoms include fever, pains, and itching, followed by the appearance of small tumours, each covered by a yellow crust of dried serum, on the hands, face, legs, and feet. These tumours may deteriorate into deep ulcers. The final stage of yaws, which may appear after an interval of several years, involves destructive and deforming lesions of the skin, bones, and periosteum (*see also* gangosa, goundou). Yaws, which commonly affects children, is prevalent in hot humid lowlands of equatorial Africa, tropical America, the Far East, and the West Indies. It responds well to treatment with *penicillin and other antibiotics.

雅司病 由於皮膚及皮下組織存在着雅司螺旋體而引起的一種熱帶傳染病。雅司病發生主要是因爲衛生條件差，它可以通過直接接觸患者和他們的衣服而感染，也可以通過潛蠅屬的蒼蠅傳播，雅司螺旋體通過皮膚破損處進入身體。開始的症狀是發燒、疼痛和瘙癢，繼而是在手、臉、腿和脚出現小腫塊，每個腫塊被乾血清的黃痂覆蓋。這些腫塊可惡化變成深的潰瘍。雅司病的最後階段可以間隔幾年後纔出現，有皮膚、骨、骨膜的破壞和變形病變。雅司病常侵及兒童，流行於赤道非洲國家、美洲熱帶地區、遠東和印度羣島潮濕炎熱的低地。用青黴素和其他抗生素治療效果良好。

Y chromosome a sex chromosome that is present in men but not in women; it is believed to carry the genes for maleness. *Compare* X chromosome.

Y染色體 存在於男性而不存在於女性的染色體。人們認爲它是攜帶男性基因的。

yeast *n.* any unicellular fungus of the genus *Saccharomyces*. Yeasts reproduce asexually by budding and sexually by the formation of spores. They ferment carbohydrates, producing alcohol and carbon dioxide, and are important in brewing and breadmaking. Yeasts

酵母 任何酵母屬的單細胞眞菌。酵母菌是以無性芽生和有性孢子形成的方式進行繁殖。它們使碳水化合物發酵，產生酒和二氧化碳，在釀造飲料和製作麵包上很重要。酵母菌

are a commercial source of proteins and of vitamins of the B complex.

是商品生產蛋白質和維生素B複合物的原料。

yellow fever an infectious disease, caused by an *arbovirus, occurring in tropical Africa and the northern regions of South America. It is transmitted by mosquitoes, principally *Aëdes aegypti*. The virus causes degeneration of the tissues of the liver and kidneys. Symptoms, depending on severity of infection, include chill, headache, pains in the back and limbs, fever, vomiting, constipation, a reduced flow of urine (which contains high levels of albumin), and *jaundice. Yellow fever often proves fatal, but recovery from a first attack confers subsequent immunity. The disease can be prevented by vaccination.

黃熱病 由蟲媒病毒引起的傳染病，發生於熱帶非洲和南美北部地區。它由蚊子傳播，尤其是埃及伊蚊。病毒引起肝和腎組織的變性。症狀決定於感染的嚴重程度，有寒顫、頭痛、背部和肢體疼痛、發燒、嘔吐、便秘、尿量減少（含有較多白蛋白）和黃疸。本病常是致命的，但第一次得病恢復後可獲得免疫。此病可用接種預防。

yellow spot *see* macula (lutea).

黃斑

yolk (deutoplasm) *n.* a substance, rich in protein and fat, that is laid down within the egg cell as nourishment for the embryo. It is absent (or nearly so) from the eggs of mammals (including man) whose embryos absorb nutrients from their mother.

卵黃（滋養質） 一種富有蛋白和脂肪的物質。作爲胚胎的營養物質而存在於卵細胞中。哺乳動物的胚胎是從他們的母體吸收營養的。

yolk sac (vitelline sac) the membranous sac, composed of mesoderm lined with endoderm, that lies ventral to the embryo. Its initially wide communication with the future gut is later reduced to a narrow duct passing through the *umbilicus. It probably assists in transporting nutrients to the early embryo and is one of the first sites where blood cells are formed.

卵黃囊 位於胚盤腹側的膜狀囊。由中胚層組成，內面襯以內胚層。它早期與原腸廣泛相通，以後變成一狹窄的通過臍的管道，它可能有助於向早期胚胎運輸營養，也是最早生成血細胞的部位。

yttrium-90 *n.* an artificial radioactive isotope of the element yttrium, used in *radiotherapy. Yttrium-90, which emits beta rays, can be used in the form of 1 mm spheres scattered around a tumour or injected directly into a tumour in the form of a solution.

^{90}釔 釔元素的人工放射性同位素。用於放射療法。^{90}釔發射出β射線，可採用直徑 1 mm 的球圍繞腫瘤散射的形式，或以溶液形式直接注入腫瘤。

Z

Z

zein *n.* a protein found in maize.

玉米蛋白 玉米中含有的蛋白。

zinc chloride a *caustic substance having strong *astringent properties. It is used as a solution for cleansing wounds and ulcers and also as a mouth wash and deodorant; in paste form it is the main component of zinc dental cement. Toxic effects are essentially due to poisoning by ingestion.

氯化鋅 有强大收斂特性的苛性物質。其溶液用於清潔傷口和潰瘍，也用作漱口和除臭劑；其糊劑是牙科鋅黏固粉的主要成分。毒性反應主要是攝入引起的。

zinc oxide a mild *astringent used in various skin conditions, usually mixed with other substances. It is applied as a cream, ointment, dusting powder, or as a paste, sometimes in the form of an impregnated bandage.

氧化鋅 溫和的收斂劑。用於各種皮膚病。往往和其他物質合用，可製成乳膏、軟膏、撒粉劑或糊劑使用。有時也用於加固繃帶。

zinc sulphate an *astringent applied in a lotion for the treatment of ulcers of the skin and mouth and to assist wound healing. It is also used in eye drops and, occasionally, as an emetic.

硫酸鋅 一種收斂劑。以其洗劑治療皮膚和口腔潰瘍，促進傷口癒合，也可用於滴眼，偶可用作爲催吐藥。

zinc undecenoate (zinc undecylenate) an antifungal agent with uses similar to those of *undecenoic acid.

十一烯酸鋅 一種抗眞菌藥。與十一碳烯酸作用相似。

Zollinger-Ellison syndrome a rare disorder in which there is excessive secretion of gastric juice due to high levels of circulating *gastrin, which is produced by a pancreatic tumour (benign or malignant) or an enlarged pancreas. The high levels of stomach acid cause peptic ulcers, which may be multiple, in unusual sites (e.g. jejunum), or which quickly recur after *vagotomy or partial *gastrectomy. Treatment with a histamine-blocking drug, by removal of the tumour (if benign), or by total gastrectomy is usually effective.

卓-艾二氏綜合症 由於胰腺腫瘤（良性或惡性）或胰腺增生向血循環內分泌大量胃泌素而造成胃液分泌過多的一種少見的疾病。高胃酸可以引起消化性潰瘍，可多發，並發生在罕發的部位（如空腸），在迷走神經切斷或部分胃切除術很快復發。用組織胺阻滯劑，切除腫瘤（如果是良性的）或全胃切除等治療往往有效。

zona pellucida the thick membrane that develops around the mammalian oocyte within the ovarian follicle. It is penetrated by at least one spermato-

透明帶 在哺乳動物卵泡中圍繞着卵細胞生長的一層厚膜。受精時至少可被一個精子穿透，在受精卵

zoon at fertilization and persists around the *blastocyst until it reaches the womb. *See* ovum.

到達子宮之前一直存在於胚泡周圍。

zonula *n. see* zonule.

小帶

zonule (zonula) *n.* (in anatomy) a small band or zone; for example the *zonule of Zinn* (*zonula ciliaris*) is the suspensory ligament of the eye. **—zonular** *adj.*

小帶　解剖學用語。小帶狀物或條狀物。如睫狀小帶是眼球的懸韌帶。

zonulolysis *n.* dissolution of the suspensory ligament of the lens of the eye (the *zonule of Zinn*), which facilitates removal of the lens in cases of cataract. A small quantity of a solution of an enzyme that dissolves the zonule without damaging other parts of the eye is injected behind the iris a minute or two before the lens is removed.

睫狀小帶鬆解法　鬆解眼晶狀體的懸韌帶（秦氏小帶）以便在白內障時有利於晶狀體的切除。在晶狀體切除之前 1～2 分鐘，在虹膜後注入少量某種酶溶液，可只溶解小帶而不損傷眼睛其他部位。

zoo- *prefix denoting* animals.

〔前綴〕 **動物**

zoonosis *n.* an infectious disease of animals that can be transmitted to man. *See* anthrax, brucellosis, cat-scratch fever, cowpox, glanders, Q fever, Rift Valley fever, rabies, rat-bite fever, toxoplasmosis, tularaemia, typhus.

動物傳染病　可傳染給人的動物傳染病。

zoophilism *n.* sexual attraction to animals, which may be manifest in stroking and fondling or in sexual intercourse (*bestiality*). **—zoophilic** *adj.*

嗜獸癖　對動物發生的性戀。可以表現爲撫愛動物或與之性交（獸姦）。

zoophobia *n.* excessively strong fear of animals. *See* phobia.

動物恐怖　對動物特別强烈的懼怕。

zoopsia *n.* visual hallucinations of animals. These can occur in any condition causing hallucinations but are most typical of *delirium tremens.

動物幻視　幻視中出現動物。可發生在任何幻覺時，但主要見於震顫性譫妄。

zwitterion *n.* an ion that bears a positive and a negative charge. Amino acids can yield zwitterions.

兩性離子　一個有正電荷和負電荷的離子。氨基酸可產生兩性離子。

zygoma *n. see* zygomatic arch, zygomatic bone.

顴　顴弓或顴骨。

zygomatic arch (zygoma) the horizontal arch of bone on either side of the

顴弓　位於兩邊面頰的眼睛下方水平位的骨弓，由

face, just below the eyes, formed by connected processes of the zygomatic and temporal bones. *See* skull.

顴骨和顳骨的突起連接而成。

zygomatic bone (zygoma, malar bone) either of a pair of bones that form the prominent part of the cheeks and contribute to the orbits. *See* skull.

顴骨 構成面頰突出部分的一對骨骼。也是眼眶的一部分。

zygote *n.* the fertilized ovum before *cleavage begins. It contains both male and female pronuclei.

合子 在卵裂開始前的受精卵。包括男性和女性的原核。

zygotene *n.* the second stage of the first prophase of *meiosis, in which the homologous chromosomes form pairs (bivalents).

偶線 減數分裂的第一前期的第二階段，此時同源染色體配對（二價體）。

zym- (zymo-) *prefix denoting* **1.** an enzyme. **2.** fermentation.

〔前綴〕 ①**酶** ②**發酵**

zymogen *n. see* proenzyme.

酶原

zymology *n.* the science of the study of yeasts and fermentation.

酶學 研究酵母和發酵的科學。

zymolysis *n.* the process of *fermentation or digestion by an enzyme.

酶解作用 發酵的過程或酶促消化的過程。

zymosis *n.* **1.** the process of *fermentation, brought about by yeast organisms. **2.** the changes in the body that occur in certain infectious diseases, once thought to be the result of a process similar to fermentation. —**zymotic** *adj.*

①**發酵** 由酵母菌引起的發酵過程。 ②**發酵病** 過去認爲在患某種傳染病時體內發生的一種類似於發酵過程的變化。

zymotic disease an old name for a contagious disease, which was formerly thought to develop within the body following infection in a process similar to the fermentation and growth of yeast.

發酵病 一種傳染病的舊名。以前認爲傳染病是在感染後於體內類似發酵和酵母生長過程中發生的。